U0267491

中西医结合心血管病
基础与临床

主　编　陈可冀

副主编　史大卓　徐　浩　殷惠军

编　者　（按姓氏拼音顺序排序）

冯新庆　李立志　马晓昌

缪　宇　薛　梅　杨　琳

张京春

北京大学医学出版社

ZHONGXIYI JIEHE XINXUEGUAN BING JICHU YU LINCHUANG

图书在版编目（CIP）数据

中西医结合心血管病基础与临床 / 陈可冀主编. —北京：
北京大学医学出版社，2014.6
ISBN 978-7-5659-0832-3

Ⅰ. ①中… Ⅱ. ①陈… Ⅲ. ①心脏血管疾病-中西医
结合-诊疗 Ⅳ. ①R54

中国版本图书馆CIP数据核字（2014）第070273号

中西医结合心血管病基础与临床

主　　编：陈可冀
出版发行：北京大学医学出版社（电话：010-82802230）
地　　址：（100191）北京市海淀区学院路38号　北京大学医学部院内
网　　址：http://www.pumpress.com.cn
E - m a i l：booksale@bjmu.edu.cn
印　　刷：北京佳信达欣艺术印刷有限公司
经　　销：新华书店
责任编辑：刘　燕　　责任校对：金彤文　　责任印制：张京生
开　　本：889mm×1194mm　1/16　　印张：50　　字数：1504千字
版　　次：2014年6月第1版　2014年6月第1次印刷
书　　号：ISBN 978-7-5659-0832-3
定　　价：320.00元

主编、副主编简介

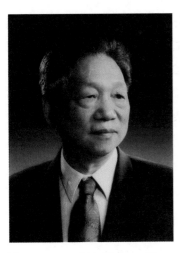

陈可冀，1991 年当选中国科学院院士 (学部委员)，长期从事心血管病与老年医学临床研究。现为中国中医科学院首席研究员及终身研究员，香港浸会大学及澳门科技大学荣誉博士；中国科协荣誉委员，中华医学会及中国医师协会常务理事，中国药典委员会执委，中国中西医结合学会名誉会长，中国老年学学会名誉会长，中国医师协会中西医结合医师分会会长，北京大学医学部兼职教授，首都医科大学中西医结合学系学术委员会主任，世界中医药学会联合会高级专家顾问委员会主席。《Chinese Medical Journal》(中华医学杂志英文版)、《中华心血管病杂志》及《中华老年医学杂志》顾问；《中国中西医结合杂志》及《Chinese Journal of Integrative Medicine》杂志主编，eCAM《Evidence-Based Complementary and Alternative Medicine》杂志心血管专栏特邀主编(2010 —)，曾任中国科学院生物学部副主任（1993 — 2001），中国科学院学部主席团成员（2004 — 2008），世界卫生组织传统医学顾问（1979 — 2009）。曾获首届立夫中医药学术奖（1994），国家科技进步奖一等奖（"血瘀证与活血化瘀研究"，2003）和二等奖（"证效动力学研究"，2001），首届世界中医药联合会首届中医药国际贡献奖（2007），中国非物质文化遗产传统医药项目代表性传承人（2007），吴阶平医学奖（2009）。主编《清宫医案集成》获国家新闻出版总署颁发的中国出版政府奖（2011）等奖项。

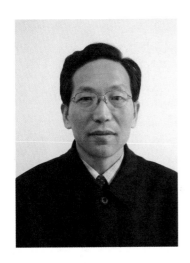

史大卓，中国中医科学院首席研究员，心血管病研究所所长，西苑医院副院长，国家中医心血管病重点专科主任，全国政协委员，九三学社中央委员，国家药典委员会委员，中国中西医结合活血化瘀专业委员会候任主任委员，世界中医联合会心血管病专业委员会常务副会长，北京市中西医结合心血管专业委员会主任委员。

从事心血管病临床和科研工作 25 年，相继负责国家"973"项目、国家科技攻关、国家自然基金重点项目等国家课题 15 项；获国家科技成果奖 1 项、省部级奖 13 项；主持研发新药 4 项，获发明专利 6 项。在国内外发表学术论文 230 余篇，主编医学专著 13 本。

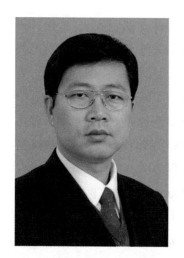

徐浩，医学博士，主任医师，博士生导师，科技部中青年科技创新领军人才。现为中国中医科学院心血管病研究所副所长、西苑医院心血管病中心常务副主任，兼任中华医学会老年医学分会秘书长，世界中医药学联合会心血管病专业委员会副秘书长，中国中西医结合学会循证医学专业委员会常委，《中国结合医学杂志英文版》(SCI收录) 副主编等职务。作为课题负责人承担国家及省部级课题10项，获成果奖11项，发表论文104篇（SCI收录30篇）。

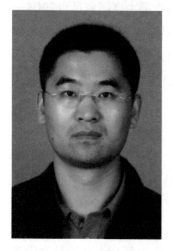

殷惠军，医学博士，生物学博士后，博士生导师，研究员。任中华医学会心血管病学专科分会委员，中华全国青年联合会十一届委员等多项社会及学术职务。主持国家863、国家自然科学基金等课题8项，作为骨干参加国家"973""十一五"攻关、国家自然基金重大研究计划及重点项目等10余项，获国家及省部级多项奖励，国家专利2项，获北京市科技新星，中华中医药科技之星。发表学术论文100余篇，其中SCI收录17篇，主编著作11部。

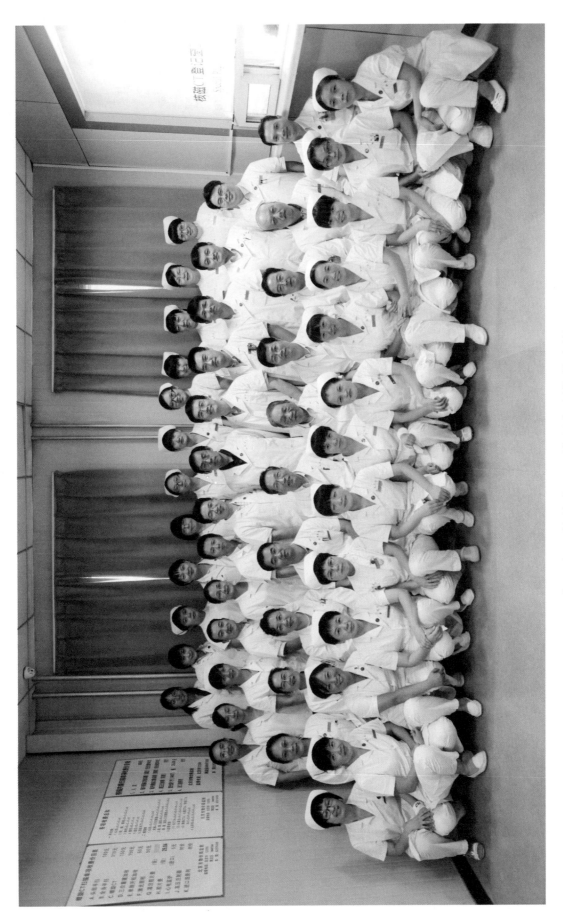

中国中医科学院心血管研究所集体合影

前　言

心血管病现在已是全球性的流行病，根据我国心血管病年度报告指出的调查和分析，我国总人群心血管病（包括心脏病和卒中）患病人数估计已达 2.3 亿人左右，大约每 10 秒钟就有 1 人死于本病。2013 年，美国《Circulation》杂志发布了一批心血管病专家合作调查的结果，也表明美国约有 8360 万成人患有心血管病，大约每 40 秒钟有 1 人因此病而死亡。心血管病向全球包括中国和美国心血管科医生都发出了严峻的挑战，不可轻视。

在"中国心脏大会 2013"即将在国家会议中心召开的时刻，首届"中西医结合论坛"也在此大会召开时作为一个新开辟的分会场应时召开，并将在每年上述大会召开的同时，召开一次同样的论坛盛会。中国中医科学院心血管病研究所今年也将同时宣告成立，并与全国及海内外同道一起加强交流防治的经验和研究成果，共襄进步。

作为中国中医科学院心血管病研究所前身的中国科学院西苑医院心血管病中心，曾经在 2009 年 8 月收集了以往 50 年间在防治心血管病中的种种临床经验和成果，正式公开出版了 130 多万字的《心血管病与活血化瘀》一书，除了重点总结了我们在传承、应用、发展和创新传统活血化瘀理论、研究血瘀证现代科学机理，以及应用活血化瘀治法和方药治疗心血管病的进展及其机理研究方面的进步之外，也总结了其他防治心血管病方面的经验和进展。在之后的这五年时间里，全体医护人员及临床与实验研究工作者，大家锐意进取，实事求是，以积硅步而至千里的勤勉精神，努力工作，在既往获得国家科技进步奖一等奖的起点上，谱写华丽的新篇章，取得了新的临床和基础研究的进展。

本书《中西医结合心血管病基础与临床》就是生动地凝结着同志们经年累月奋斗的历程和经历的足迹，大家执着追求，励志创新，研究内涵丰富，其中涵盖了心血管病血瘀证证治研究，心血管病瘀毒病机研究，防治心绞痛研究，防治心肌梗死及介入后再狭窄干预研究、防治心力衰竭及休克研究、防治高血压及动脉粥样硬化研究、有关心肌缺血损伤和心室重构的实验研究、防治血栓形成及抗血小板以及有关血管新生的实验研究，等等。反映了我们这个集体愿为中医药和中西医结合防治心血管病作出新的业绩的崇高理想和志向，自信而不畏艰难。

我们和全国中医药、中西医结合朋友们，和全球心血管病医学界的同道们，在同一条战线上。我们一定能在中医药学术传承、发展、创新及研发方面，做出新的业绩。在防治心血管病领域方面，做出新的成果，为人类健康谱写出新的篇章。

中国科学院资深院士　陈可冀

2013 年 8 月，北京

目　　录

第三章　中西医结合防治心血管病的临床研究

第四章　中医药防治心血管疾病的药理研究

第五章　糖、脂代谢异常的相关研究及其他

第六章　名老中医经验继承

第七章　综述与系统评价

第 一 章

冠心病血瘀证病证结合研究

第一章

冠心病血瘀证诊断标准研究 *

付长庚　高铸烨　王培利　王承龙　徐　浩　史大卓　陈可冀

20 世纪 80 年代以来，随着血瘀证诊断标准的提出，血瘀证和活血化瘀研究取得了显著进展，活血化瘀治法在临床上得到了广泛应用。血瘀证的诊断标准在不同疾病中具有普适性，但也存在范畴较为宽泛的缺点。有研究证实，不同疾病的血瘀证患者在中医证候特点、实验室检查指标等方面存在差异，现行的诊断标准难以准确衡量某一特定疾病的血瘀证证候。因此，建立病证结合的血瘀证诊断标准，成为当前血瘀证研究的一个发展趋势。

冠状动脉粥样硬化性心脏病（简称冠心病）血瘀证是血瘀证研究中最为活跃的领域。近三十年来，中医对冠心病病因病机的认识逐渐趋于统一，认为本病病机属"本虚标实，标实中血瘀贯穿发病过程始终"，由此带来了以"活血化瘀"为主的冠心病治疗方法学的改变，并在此基础上衍化出理气活血、益气活血、化浊活血、温阳活血等治法，显著提高了临床疗效。但是，冠心病血瘀证有哪些独特的临床表征？冠心病患者血瘀程度的轻重如何判断？血瘀的程度对心血管事件的发生有着怎样的预测价值？这些成为现代中医和中西医结合冠心病防治领域亟待探讨研究的问题。

近年来，冠状动脉造影、血管内超声等已成为冠心病诊断的金标准[1-3]，越来越多的理化指标被发现可以在不同程度上反映冠心病患者的血瘀程度，这为冠心病血瘀证病证结合诊断标准的建立奠定了基础。因此，笔者综合文献研究、专家咨询和临床流行病学调查的结果，结合现代信息生物学分析，从宏观临床表征和微观理化指标变化两方面，在既往血瘀证诊断标准的基础上结合临床所见，建立了冠心病血瘀证病证结合的诊断标准。

1. 冠心病血瘀证诊断标准的构建（表 1）

采用系统评价的标准化步骤整理古今文献，通过检索中文古籍数据库发现中医古籍中与冠心病血瘀证相关的临床表现主要包括胸满、胸痛、胸闷、心痛、怔忡、舌青、脉涩等 22 项；检索中国期刊全文数据库 CNKI（1999—2009）、中国生物医学文献数据库 CBM（1999—2009）、中文科技期刊全文数据库 VIP（1999—2009）、中国重要会议论文全文数据库（1999 年至今）、美国国立医学图书馆 PubMed（1989—2009），共检出与冠心病血瘀证相关的研究 1825 项，经反复筛选后有"冠心病血瘀证与高敏 C 反应蛋白（high-sensitive C-reactive protein，hs-CRP）相关性研究"等 74 项诊断性试验最终纳入分析。Meta 分析显示共有 hs-CRP、同型半胱氨酸（homocysteine，Hcy）、D- 二聚体等 122 项指标与冠心病血瘀证明显相关。根据文献研究结果设计专家咨询问卷，在全国范围内选择 80 位在冠心病中西医结合研究领域有代表性的专家，采用德尔菲法进行专家咨询，对相关指标进行筛选。在此基础上制订 CRF，采用横断面研究设计，对全国 15 家分中心 2007 年 10 月—2008 年 8 月期间经冠状动脉造影确诊至少有 1 支冠状动脉血管狭窄 ≥ 50% 或既往有陈旧性心肌梗死病史的冠心病患者进行流行病学调查，共 4274 例被纳入研究，其中无症状者 816 例，稳定劳累性心绞痛患者 992 例，急性冠状动脉综合征（acute coronary syndrome，ACS）超过 1 个月病情稳定者 2034 例，不稳定型心绞痛 432 例，既往有心肌梗死病史者 1911 例。按照 1986 年第二届全国活血化瘀研究学术会议制订的《血瘀证诊断标准》[4] 进行辨证，血瘀证 3257 例，非血瘀证 1017 例。通过单因素分析、Logistic 回归分析和逐步判别分析反复筛选，结合临床所见，根据病史、症状、体征、舌象、脉象、理化指标等不同变量的 OR 值判定其权重，制订了冠心病血瘀证诊断标准（草案）。

2. 冠心病血瘀证诊断标准敏感度、特异度检验（表 2）

采用病例对照研究设计，将 6 名有临床经验的心内科副主任医师分成相互独立的 A、B 两组，每组 3 人。A 组以 1986 年的《血瘀证诊断标准》[4]

* 原载于《中国中西医结合杂志》，2012，32（9）：1285-1286

第一章

表1　冠心病血瘀证诊断标准（草案）

	赋分	宏观指标	理化指标
主要指标	3分/项	1. 胸痛位置固定	4. 冠状动脉CT血管造影或冠状动脉造影显示任何一支血管有明显的狭窄（≥75%）
		2. 舌质色紫或暗	5. 超声显示心脏或血管内有附壁血栓
		3. 舌有瘀斑、瘀点	
次要指标	2分/项	1. 胸痛夜间加重	5. 造影或血管超声显示其他血管狭窄（≥50%）
		2. 口唇或齿龈色暗	6. 活化部分凝血活酶时间或凝血酶原时间缩短
		3. 舌下脉络粗胀或曲张，或色青紫、紫红、绛紫、紫黑	7. 纤维蛋白原升高
			8. D-二聚体升高
		4. 脉涩	
辅助指标	1分/项	1. 肌肤甲错	4. 冠状动脉CTA显示血管明显钙化或弥漫性病变
		2. 面色黧黑	5. 全血黏度、血浆黏度升高
		3. 四肢末端发绀	

注：符合2条主要指标，或3条次要指标，或1条主要指标加2条次要指标即可诊断血瘀证；辅助指标主要用于血瘀证的量化诊断，不作为血瘀证诊断的必须指标；冠心病血瘀证诊断必须包含主要指标、次要指标中至少1项宏观指标，单纯理化指标不能诊断；各项指标的计分用于评价冠心病血瘀证的程度

表2　冠心病血瘀证诊断标准检验

诊断标准	参考标准		合计
	阳性	阴性	
阳性	318	12	330
阴性	19	101	120
合计	337	113	450

为诊断依据，B组以新建诊断标准草案为诊断依据，分别在两个诊室，根据病例记录情况，相互独立对450例冠心病患者进行辨证，辨证结果有争议时，以人数较多的结果为准。结果显示与1986年的《血瘀证诊断标准》比较，新建冠心病血瘀证诊断标准敏感度为94.36%，特异度为89.38%，准确度为93.11%，阳性似然比为8.89，证明本标准有较好的可靠性和临床实用性。

3. 讨论

本研究采用病证结合研究模式，通过系统评价方法总结古今文献，采用德尔菲法完成专家咨询，按照横断面研究设计进行临床观察，最终制订出包含症状、体征、实验室指标综合评定的冠心病血瘀证病证结合的诊断标准，并通过病例对照研究检验其诊断效能，在方法学上比较可靠。

与既往标准相比，本标准具有以下特点：（1）重视宏观指标在诊断中的作用。本标准规定，冠心病血瘀证的诊断必须包含主要指标、次要指标中至少1项宏观指标，单纯理化指标不能诊断，这是因为在传统血瘀证的诊断中完全依靠患者的症状、体征确诊，我们现在所进行的证候客观化研究必须以符合传统血瘀证的定义为前提，单纯依靠理化指标无法保证诊断结果与传统的辨证结果相一致。（2）重视影像及理化指标在诊断中的意义。本标准中首次明确提出了8项对冠心病血瘀证有诊断意义的理化指标，其中影像指标4项，血液指标4项。影像指标反映了血管有明确的狭窄或堵塞，或有血栓形成的确切证据，血液指标反映了血液处于高凝状态。（3）对指标的诊断价值进行了分层和评分。研究证据多、专家认可度高的指标在诊断中的分值较高，反之则较低，通过总的积分情况来反映冠心病血瘀证的严重程度。（4）重视诊断指标的实用性。所选的各项指标都是临床上常用的检查指标，各级各类医院都可以根据自身条件选择适合的指标对冠心病血瘀证进行诊断和评价。

参考文献

[1] Onat A, Can G, Hergenc G, et al. Coronary disease risk prediction algorithm warranting incorporation of C-reactive protein in Turkish adults, manifesting sex difference. Nutr Metab Cardiovasc Dis, 2011, 2(9): 21-31.

[2] Bhatti S, Hakeem A, Yousuf MA, et al. Diagnostic

performance of computed tomography angiography for differentiating ischemic *vs* non-ischemic cardiomyopathy. J Nucl Cardiol, 2011, 2(17): 22.

[3] Garcìa-Garcìa HM, Gogas BD, Serruys PW, et al. IVUS-based imaging modalities for tissue characterization: similarities and differences. Int J Cardiovasc Imaging, 2011, 2(17): 213-229.

[4] 中国中西医结合学会活血化瘀研究专业委员会. 血瘀证诊断标准. 中西医结合杂志, 1987, 7 (3): 129.

冠心病血瘀证血小板差异功能蛋白
筛选、鉴定及功能分析 *

李雪峰　蒋跃绒　高铸烨　殷惠军　陈可冀

动脉粥样硬化（atherosclerosis，AS）易损斑块的破裂和急性血栓形成是急性冠脉综合征发病的主要病理因素[1]。相关研究证实，血小板的活化程度与冠心病患者的远期预后及不良事件发生率明显相关[2,3]。中医学"血瘀"与血小板高聚集状态密切相关，许多学者以血小板为切入点探索了中医学"血瘀"理论和活血化瘀治法的作用机制。我们对冠心病血瘀证差异基因表达谱的构建及目标基因的功能进行了研究，结果从核酸水平揭示了炎症免疫反应与冠心病血瘀证的相关性[4,5]。基于冠心病、血瘀证、血小板活化的关联性，我们进一步提出了研究假说：血小板功能蛋白的异常表达可能在冠心病血瘀证事件发生、发展中起关键作用。为此，本研究采用荧光差异显示二维凝胶电泳（two-dimensional fluorescence difference gel electro-phoresis，2-D DIGE）技术对冠心病血瘀证患者进行了血小板差异功能蛋白筛选，用基质辅助激光解析/电离-飞行时间质谱（matrix-assisted laser desorption/ ionization-time of flight time of flight mass spectrometry，MALDI-TOF-TOF）技术[6]对目标蛋白进行了鉴定，并对目标功能蛋白在冠心病血瘀证发生、发展中的作用进行了分析。

1. 资料与方法

1.1 诊断标准

参照：（1）1999 年美国心脏病学会（American College of Cardiology，ACC）/美国心脏协会（American Heart Association，AHA）/美国医师学会及美国内科学会（American College of Physicians-American Society of Internal Medicine，ACP-ASIM）联合协定关于《慢性稳定型心绞痛诊疗指南》[7]、2002 年 ACC/AHA《不稳定型心绞痛、无 ST 段抬高心肌梗死诊疗指南》[8]。（2）经冠状动脉造影证实 1 支或 1 支以上冠状动脉主支直径狭窄≥ 50%。

1.2 中医辨证分型标准

参考中国中西医结合学会活血化瘀专业委员会制订的血瘀证诊断标准[9]。

1.3 纳入及排除标准

纳入标准：符合诊断标准和血瘀证诊断标准；签署知情同意书。排除标准：（1）年龄＜ 35 岁或＞ 75 岁。（2）急性心肌梗死患者。（3）合并 1 型糖尿病、Ⅲ级高血压病、高血压急症、心功能 3 级等患者。（4）过敏体质及对多种药物过敏者。

1.4 临床资料

22 例为 2008 年 5—11 月北京安贞医院、西苑医院心血管内科住院的冠心病患者（冠心病血瘀证组），其中男 19 例，女 3 例，年龄 46 ~ 74 岁，平均（62.64±7.60）岁。所有患者符合纳入标准，均行冠脉造影。同期选择西苑医院体检中心健康志愿者 24 名（正常对照组），其中男 11 名，女 13 名，年龄 23 ~ 61 岁，平均（33.54±11.24）岁。

1.5 分组

每组分 4 个小组，即两组各有 4 次重复。正常对照组 24 名，分 4 个小组（A1、A2、A3、A4）。冠心病血瘀证组 22 例，分 4 个小组（B1、B2、

* 原载于《中国中西医结合杂志》，2010，30 (5)：467-476

B3、B4）。将每一小组的各血小板蛋白样本等体积混合（以消除个体间差异），然后定量。取等量各小组分析样本混合作为内标用 Cy2 标记。即正常对照组和冠心病血瘀证组各有 4 次重复，见表 1。

表 1　DIGE 上样设计

样本	Cy2	Cy3	Cy5
Gel1	内标	A1	B1
Gel2	内标	B2	A2
Gel3	内标	A3	B3
Gel4	内标	B4	A4

1.6　样本采集及制备

冠心病患者入院后，准备进行冠脉造影前，按以下方法采集、制备样本：（1）早晨空腹，用 BD 枸橼酸钠抗凝真空采血管采集 12mL 空腹全血。（2）将前 2mL 弃用。（3）余 10mL 轻轻平置采血管混匀，加入 0.7mL ACD（枸橼酸钠 22.0g、枸橼酸 8.0g、葡萄糖 24.5g，加水至 1000mL），轻轻混匀，900r/min 离心 10min，取上层富含血小板血浆（Platelet-rich plasmal，PRP）；在 PRP 中加入前列环素 2（Prostacycline2，PGI$_2$），轻轻混匀[10,11]，3000r/min，离心 10min，去上清，得 PLT 沉淀。（4）洗涤 PLT。在 PLT 沉淀中加入 Hepes-Tyrode buffer[12] 0.3mL，加入 PGI$_2$，轻轻重悬 PLT，3000r/min，离心 10min，去上清，重复 2 次。（5）洗涤 PLT 沉淀中加入 Hepes-Tyrode buffer，轻轻重悬 PLT，调 PLT 数至 $8 \times 10^8 \sim 1 \times 10^9$/ml，室温下孵育 20min；上样 12000r/min 离心 5min，立即加入罗氏蛋白酶抑制剂（complete protease inhibitor）20μL，并投入液氮中冻存，备用。

1.7　样品的蛋白提取

将细胞溶于 lysis buffer 中（7mmol/L 尿素，2mmol/L 硫脲，4%CHAPS，30mmol/L Tris-HCl，pH 8.6），提取后定量。

1.8　DIGE

差异凝胶分析：（1）将 Cy2、Cy3、Cy5（GE healthcare 公司）用 DMF 溶解成 1nmol/μL 的母液，分装，–20℃保存。（2）将荧光染料母液稀释成 400pmol/μL。（3）测样品蛋白溶液的 pH，用 30mmol/L Tris-HCl，或 50mmol/L NaOH 调 pH，使其 pH 为 8.0 ～ 9.0。（4）每一小组样本各 50μg 蛋白分别采用 400 pmol Cy3 和 Cy5 标记，各小组分析样本等量混合作为内标用 Cy2 标记，标记量同上，混匀，标记反应需避光，冰上放置 30min，然后用 1μL 10mmol/L 赖氨酸终止反应，混匀，冰上放置 10min。（5）将每块胶需上样的小组（表 1）蛋白样品，分别标记后混合，加入等体积的 2×sample buffer（7mol/L 尿素，2mol/L 硫脲，4% CHAPS，2% IPG buffer，2% DTT），再加入水化液（7mol/L 尿素，2mol/L 硫脲，4% CHAPS，1% IPG buffer，0.5%DTT）补足体积至 450μL。（6）等电聚焦及 SDS PAGE 电泳（均避光）。等电聚焦程序略。SDS PAGE 参数：12% SDS-PAGE 凝胶，电泳参数 3W/gel，时间 13h。（7）图像扫描及差异分析。用 Typhoon 9410 扫描仪在 488、532、633nm 波长分别对 Cy2、Cy3、Cy5 荧光染料标记的 DIGE 图像进行扫描。获取的各胶图（图 1）导入 DeCyder 2D version 6.5 software，对 Ettan DIGE 系统凝胶图像进行蛋白点检测、定量、匹配以及分析。胶内差异分析——同一张胶的一组图像上的蛋白点识别和定量。生物学差异分析——不同胶的多张图像进行匹配，提供不同组之间的差异蛋白表达水平的统计分析数据（单因素方差分析）。取 t 检测值 $P < 0.01$，差异倍数大于 2.0 倍的结果，进行差异分析。

1.9　制备胶

按 1mg 蛋白 / 凝胶，上样，进行 2-DIGE，并用考马斯亮蓝染色，得制备胶。扫描后胶图与 DeCyder 2D version 6.5 software 分析得到的 DIGE 差异点图（图 2）进行匹配，确定制备胶上对应的蛋白差异点位置，切胶。

1.10　质谱分析

1.10.1　胶内酶解　将切割蛋白差异点对应胶粒置于 Eppendorf 管中，将切取的胶粒冻干，加入测序级胰蛋白酶溶液（Sigma 公司，浓度：0.1mg/mL），于 37℃水浴酶解 16h，以 TFA 水溶液提取酶解肽段，提取液 0.5μL 点于质谱仪的靶上，基质：α-氰基 -4- 羟基 - 肉桂酸（Sigma 公司）溶液，溶于 0.1% TFA + 50% ACN 水中，浓度：5mg/mL。

1.10.2　质谱分析　质谱仪：美国 ABI-4800 型反射式基质辅助激光解析 / 电离飞行时间串联质谱（MALDI-TOF-TOF）；扫描方式：反射式；扫描范围：700 ～ 4000 Da；激光能量：MS 4800，MSMS 5600。

1.11 数据库检索

GPS 软件将鉴定蛋白点质谱数据（MS/MSMS）在 IPI-human 数据库中进行匹配，获得鉴定蛋白质的相关信息。检索参数：GPS 软件检索；误差 MS 0.3 Da；MSMS 0.2Da。数据库：人的数据库 IPI Human 3.23；数据取舍标准：蛋白质打分 > 64 分，置信水平 > 95%。

2. 结果

2.1 DIGE 差异凝胶分析（图1、2）

将所得的 DIGE 胶图导入 DeCyder 2D version 6.5 software，进行差异分析，获得正常对照组和冠心病血瘀证组间血小板差异蛋白点 13 个。

2.2 差异蛋白的验证（图3-6）

采用 Western-Blotting 方法验证 7 个差异蛋白点中的 isoform 2 of integrinalpha-Ⅱb（CD41，

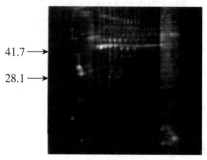

分子量pI ⟶ 3 ~ 10

41.7 →
28.1 →

图 1　冠心病血瘀证组与正常对照组的 DIGE 胶图

注：该图为 Cy2（代表内标）、Cy3（代表某一小组蛋白）、Cy5（代表另一组蛋白）3 张图叠加而成，因组成每一点的来自内标和其他两小组的蛋白表达量不同，形成不同颜色。pI（等电点）从左至右为 3 ~ 10；蛋白点分子量从上到下依次变小

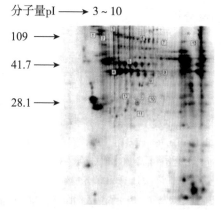

分子量pI ⟶ 3 ~ 10

109 →
41.7 →
28.1 →

图 2　冠心病血瘀证和正常对照组间血小板差异表达蛋白点胶图

注：该图根据 DIGE 分析结果，将初步筛选出的冠心病血瘀证和正常对照组间血小板差异蛋白点在胶图中位置手工标示（与表 2 中差异点编号对应）

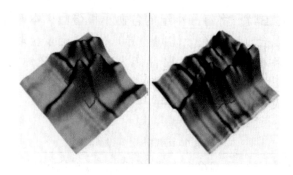

图 3　DeCyder 2D version 6.5 生成的 IPI00218628 对应差异蛋白点胶上三维图

注：左侧为正常对照组，右侧为冠心病血瘀证组，红色线内为差异点体积计算范围。冠心病血瘀证组是正常对照组的 2 倍

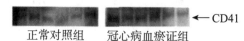

← CD41

正常对照组　　　冠心病血瘀证组

图 4　血小板 CD41 正常对照组和冠心病血瘀证组表达比较

注：左侧 6 例为正常对照组，右侧 6 例为冠心病血瘀证组

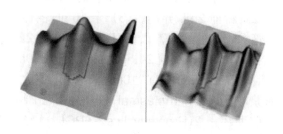

图 5　DeCyder 2D version 6.5 生成的 IPI00021440 对应差异蛋白点胶上三维图

注：左侧为正常对照组，右侧冠心病为血瘀证组。红色线内为差异点体积计算范围，冠心病血瘀证组是正常对照组的 2.13 倍

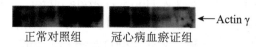

← Actin γ

正常对照组　　　冠心病血瘀证组

图 6　血小板 Actin γ 在对照组和冠心病血瘀证组表达比较

注：左侧 4 例为正常对照组，右侧 4 例为冠心病血瘀证组

Abcam 一抗）和 actin-cytop lasmic 2（Actin γ，Millipore 一抗）。CD41、Actin γ 在冠心病血瘀证组表达量分别是正常对照组的 2.00、2.13 倍。

2.3 差异蛋白点质谱鉴定（表 2，图2、7、8）

质谱通过测定蛋白质的一级结构（包括分子量、肽链氨基酸序列、多肽或二硫键数目和位置等），在认识蛋白质分子研究中发挥关键作用。特别是 MALDI-TOF-TOF 所具有的高通量、高灵敏度、高特异性、准确度高等优点，使其成为蛋白质研究的重要设备。在本研究中，筛选出 13 个差异

表 2 冠心病血瘀证组和正常对照组血小板差异蛋白搜库鉴定结果

蛋白编号	蛋白名称	蛋白分子量	蛋白等电点	蛋白打分	蛋白打分置信区间	离子打分	离子打分置信区间	差异蛋白点编号
IPI00218628	Gene_Symbol=ITGA 2B Isoform 2 of Integrin alpha-Ⅱb	109518.5	5.17	662	100	547	100	1
IPI00295976	Gene_Symbol=ITGA 2B Isoform 1 of Integrin alpha-Ⅱb	113319.5	5.21	330	100	220	100	2
IPI00218628	Gene_Symbol= ITGA 2B Isoform 2 of Integrin alpha-Ⅱb	109518.5	5.17	751	100	651	100	3
IPI00021440	Gene_Symbol=ACTG1 Actin，cytop lasmic 2	41765.8	5.31	505	100	405	100	4
IPI00894365	Gene_Symbol=ACTB cDNA FLJ52842，highly similar to Actin，cytop lasmic 1	39200.5	5.4	480	100	410	100	5
IPI00922240	Gene_Symbol=-cDNA FLJ55253，highly similar to Actin，cytop lasmic 1	38608.2	5.19	153	100	112	100	6
IPI00021439	Gene_Symbol=ACTB Actin，cytop lasmic 1	41709.7	5.29	379	100	245	100	8
IPI00794523	Gene_Symbol=ACTG1 cDNA FLJ43573fis，clone RECTM 2001691，highly similar to Actin，cytop	28193	5.2	289	100	252	100	11
<u>IPI00794523</u>	Gene_Symbol=ACTG1 cDNA FLJ43573fis，clone RECTM 2001691，highly similar to Actin，cytop	28193	5.2	145	100	94	100	12
IPI00873150	Gene_Symbol=-Putative cytochrome	33483	6.4	54	67.676	—	—	7
IPI00219713	Gene_Symbol= FGG Isoform Gamma-A of	49465	5.7	43	0	13	0	9
IPI00873150	Gene_Symbol=-Putative cytochrome	33483	6.4	78	99.883	—	—	10
IPI00009865	Gene_Symbol=KRT10 Keratin，type I cytoskeletal 10	59474.9	5.13	85	99.977	27	15.6	13

注：其中编号有下划线的是冗余；斜体为搜库未鉴定成功血小板差异蛋白点

蛋白点，质谱成功鉴定 9 个。去除两个冗余，找到 7 个有可靠数据支撑的血小板差异表达蛋白点。图 3、4 是用 Western-blotting 验证的 isoform 2 of CD41 和 Actin 的质谱图。

3. 讨论

蛋白质组学可整体上反映疾病各阶段蛋白表达的演变过程，研究蛋白在不同证型及正常状态下的表达情况，能够在分子水平揭示证的实质。鉴于冠心病、血小板功能状态、血瘀证三者之间存在密切的内在联系。我们以血小板为切入点，探索冠心病血瘀证血小板蛋白表达变化。

血小板蛋白的研究，从初步分离鉴定 25 个蛋白点，到用 2-D 银染技术获得约 2300 个血小板蛋

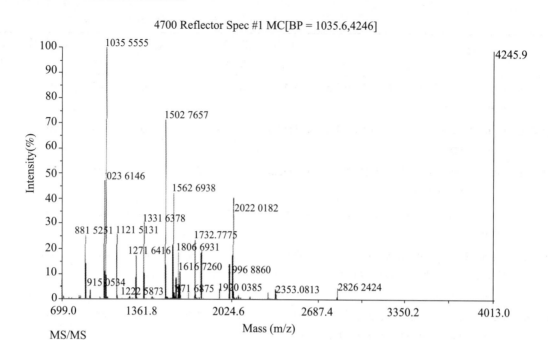

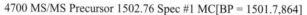

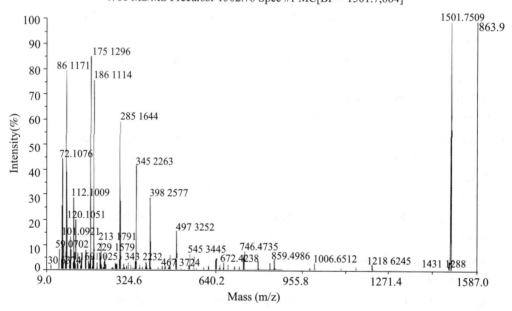

图 7　IPI00218628 Integrin alpha-Ⅱb 质谱图

注：此为冠心病血瘀证组与正常对照组间血小板差异蛋白点 3，质谱鉴定该蛋白为 IPI00218628 integrin alpha-Ⅱb

白点图，再到活化前后蛋白磷酸化修饰的研究和新的蛋白分子信号（Dok-2）的发现等[13-16]，均用健康人血小板，未见对健康人和患者之间血小板蛋白表达差异的研究。

本研究应用 2D-DIGE，筛选健康人群和冠心病血瘀证患者之间血小板差异蛋白，初步找到 7 个血小板差异表达蛋白点，对其中 2 个已有较深入研究的蛋白点，进行了 Western-blotting 验证。CD41 和 integrin Ⅲa（β_3）以复合体形式组成血小板最重要的膜受体 α Ⅱb-Ⅲa。在诱导剂等的刺激下，α Ⅱb-Ⅲa 发生构象改变，与 Fibrinogen 结合，借此与其他血小板聚集，并向胞内传递信号，引发血小板内的信号传递。血小板骨架蛋白接到传入信号后的重组装，控制 OCS 的功能、α 颗粒分泌，决定血小板活化进程、血栓形成和血栓形成速度。CD41 在冠心病血瘀证患者较之健康人的高表达，说明冠心病血瘀证患者血小板有异常增高的活化敏感性和血栓形成能力。这也反证了血瘀证在冠心病

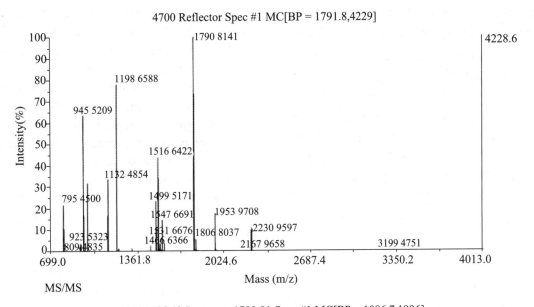

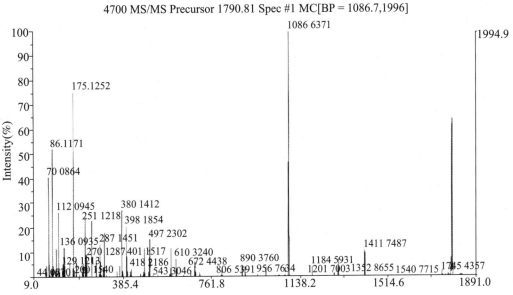

图 1-8　IPI00021440 Actin γ 质谱图

注：此为冠心病血瘀证组与正常对照组间血小板差异蛋白点 4，质谱鉴定该蛋白为 IPI00021440 Actin γ

患者群中的高比例和高事件发生率。

　　Actin γ 是血小板骨架蛋白的组成部分。如前述，骨架蛋白在血小板的活化进程中和 Locomotion 中发挥作用。如 α 颗粒释放和致密体分泌，释放血小板活化级联放大效应物质；骨架蛋白重构，与膜 α Ⅱ b-Ⅲ a 牢固连接，随之继发血小板变形、相互黏附、与纤维蛋白交接，形成血栓。有研究发现，通过转基因技术用 -cytoactin 在小鼠骨骼肌中替代 α-actin 达 40%，尽管骨骼肌细胞的超微结构基本与野生型一致，但并不能替代 α-actin 的功能 [17]。本研究发现 Actin γ 在冠心病血瘀证组表达量明显升高，推测在冠心病血瘀证患者，各种诱

导血小板活化的因素刺激血小板，使血小板内活化与抗活化进入新的平衡状态，在血小板完全活化前，骨架蛋白构形发生早期变化，Actin γ 表达量增加，为后续血小板分泌、变形、移动做准备。据此推测，Actin γ 可能是冠心病血瘀证发生发展中的重要蛋白。

　　其他尚待进一步验证的冠心病血瘀证血小板差异功能蛋白，isoform 1 of integrin alpha-Ⅱ b 是 CD41 的亚型 1，可能与 CD41 一起在冠心病血瘀证形成和事件中扮演重要角色，有待进一步研究。cDNA FLJ52842（highly similar to actin，cytop-lasmic 1）、cDNA FLJ55253（highly similar to actin-cytop lasmic 1）、actin-cytop lasmic1、cDNA FLJ43573 fis，clone RECTM 2001691（highly similar to actin，cytop））均可能是Actin γ的亚型，或修饰产物，或前蛋白。它们的高表达说明这些血小板骨架蛋白在冠心病血瘀证血小板活化与血栓形成中发挥作用，其确切机制有待深入探索。

综上所述，血小板CD41、Actin γ是冠心病血瘀证的标志蛋白，在冠心病血瘀证的发生、发展和事件发生中可能起重要作用。血小板其他异常表达功能蛋白可能在冠心病血瘀证形成中发挥作用。随着对这些血小板差异表达功能蛋白功能的认识和研究的深入，会有助于冠心病血瘀证及其事件发生分子机制的阐明。

参考文献

［1］ Fuster V, O'Rourke RA, Walsh RA, et al. editors Hurst's the heart. 12th ed. New York: The McGraw-Hill Companies, 2008: 1311-1316.

［2］ Gurbel PA, Bliden KP. The stratification of platelet reactivity and activation in patients with stable coronary artery disease on aspirin therapy. Thromb Res, 2003, 112(1-2): 9-12.

［3］ 陈可冀，薛梅，殷惠军. 血小板活化与冠状动脉粥样硬化性心脏病和血瘀证的关系. 首都医科大学学报，2008, 29(3): 266-269.

［4］ Yin HJ, Ma XJ, Chen KJ, et al. Investigation of gene expression profiles in coronary heart disease and functional analysis of target gene. China Sci Bull, 2009, 54(5): 759-765.

［5］ Ma XJ, Yin HJ, Chen KJ. Differential gene expression profiles in coronary heart disease patients of blood stasis syndrome in traditional Chinese medicine and clinical role of target gene. Chin J Integr Med, 2009, 15(2): 101-106.

［6］ Richard JS, editor. Proteins and proteomics: a laboratory manual. New York: Cold Spring Harbor Laboratory Press, 2003: 3-17.

［7］ Gibbons RJ, Chatterjee K, Daley J, et al. ACC/AHA/ACP-ASIM guidelines for the management of patients with chronic stable angina: a report of the American College of Cardiology/American Heart Association task force on practice guidelines (Committee on management of patients with chronic stable angina).

Jam Coll Cardiol, 1999, 33(7): 2092-2197.

［8］ Braunwald E, Antman EM, Kupersmith JW, et al. ACC/ AHA 2002 guideline update for the management of patients with unstable angina and non-ST-segment elevation myocardial infarction——summary article: a report of the American College of Cardiology/American Heart Association task force on practice guidelines (committee on the management of patients with unstable angina). J Am Coll Cardiol, 2002, 40(7): 1366-1374.

［9］ 中国中西医结合学会活血化瘀专业委员会. 血瘀证诊断标准. 中西医结合杂志，1987, 7（3）: 129.

［10］ Jarman DA, Du Boulay GH, Kendall B, et al. Responses of baboon cerebral and extracerebral arteries to prostacyclin and prostaglandin endoperoxide *in vitro* and *in vivo*. J Neurol Neurosurg Psychiatry, 1979, 42(8): 677-686.

［11］ Higgs EA, Higgs GA, Moncada S, et al. Prostacyclin (PG I_2) inhibits the formation of platelet thrombi in arterioles and venules of the hamster cheŵ pouch. Br J Pharmacol, 1978, 63(3): 535-539.

［12］ Garcia A, Prabhakar S, Brock CJ, et al. Extensive analysis of the human platelet proteome by two-dimensional gel electrophoresis and mass spectrometry. Proteomics, 2004, 4(3): 656-668.

［13］ Gravel P, Sanchez JC, Walzer C, et al. Human blood platelet protein map established by two-dimentional polyacrylamide gel electrophoresis. Electrophoresis, 1995, 16(7): 1152-1159.

［14］ O'Neill EE, Brock CJ, von Kriegsheim AF, et al. Towards complete analysis of the platelet proteome. Proteomics, 2002, 2(3): 288-305.

［15］ Maguire PB, Wynne KJ, Harney DF, et al. Identification of the phosphotyrosine proteome from thrombin activated platelets. Proteomics, 2002, 2(6): 642-648.

［16］ Garcia A, Prabhakar S, Hughan S, et al. Differential proteome analysis of TRAP-activated platelets: involvement of DOK-2 and phosphorrylation of RGS proteins. Blood, 2004, 103(6): 2088-2095.

［17］ Jaeger MA, Sonnemann KJ, Fitzsimons DP, et al. Context-dependent functional substitution of α-skeletal actin by γ-cytoplasmic actin. FASEB J, 2009, 23(7): 2205-2214.

冠心病稳定期血瘀证与冠状动脉病变特点的相关性 *

杜健鹏　史大卓　李田昌　徐浩　陈浩

第一章

冠心病（coronary heart disease，CHD）是在冠状动脉粥样斑块的基础上形成血管狭窄、痉挛或血栓，导致心肌供血不足，临床出现一系列心肌缺血症状的一类疾病，属于中医学胸痹心痛、真心痛的范畴。中医学认为心脉瘀阻为冠心病的一个主要病机，血瘀证为 CHD 最常见的一个证型。本研究采用 Gensini 评分方法，分析患者冠状动脉造影结果、中医血瘀证及其兼证与 Gensini 评分的关系，以期为临床辨证治疗 CHD 提供影像学依据。

1. 资料与方法

1.1 临床资料

1.1.1 研究对象 选取 2007 年 1 月至 2008 年 6 月于北京同仁医院经冠状动脉造影确诊的 CHD 患者，在其冠心病症状稳定期统一进行临床信息采集。

1.1.2 诊断标准 (1) CHD 诊断标准：参照世界卫生组织临床命名标准化联合专题组报告的《缺血性心脏病的命名及诊断》标准[1]，并且选择性冠状动脉造影左主干狭窄 ≥ 30%，或其他血管狭窄 ≥ 50% 者。(2) 中医辨证标准：CHD 辨证分型标准参照中国中西医结合学会心血管病专业委员会 1990 年 10 月修订的《冠心病中医辨证标准》[2]。(3) 血瘀证诊断、计分标准参照中国中西医结合学会活血化瘀专业委员会制定的《血瘀证诊断标准》[3]，血瘀证计分方法参照《活血化瘀研究与临床》[4] 进行评分。

1.1.3 纳入标准 (1) 所有入选病例均为符合诊断标准，经冠状动脉造影确诊的 CHD 患者。(2) 冠心病稳定期患者（临床冠心病稳定定义为稳定劳累性心绞痛 4 周以上无心绞痛发作，急性冠状动脉综合征治疗后病情稳定 4 周以上，无心绞痛发作）。(3) 年龄 ≤ 75 岁；(4) 签署知情同意书。

1.1.4 排除标准 (1) 合并严重充血性心力衰竭、重度心律失常、重度肺功能不全等急性疾病者。(2) 合并肝、肾、造血系统等严重原发性疾病者。(3) 恶性肿瘤患者。(4) 未控制的高血压（1 周内静息偶测血压 ≥ 140/90mmHg）。⑤糖尿病血糖控制不良者。

1.2 研究方法

1.2.1 冠状动脉造影特点 采用 Access 数据库详细记录患者冠状动脉造影情况，对患者冠状动脉狭窄血管和部位、狭窄程度及病变长度以及支架置入情况进行详细记录。根据文献方法采用 Gensini 评分对患者冠状动脉狭窄严重程度进行计分。Gensini 评分法：首先将冠状动脉分成 14 段，左主干 5 分，前降支及回旋支近段 2.5 分，前降支中段 1.5 分，前降支远段，回旋支中、远段 1 分，右冠状动脉 1 分，其余分支血管 1 分，根据病变血管的不同节段制定不同的权重系数。其次，根据冠状动脉管腔狭窄程度分别给予不同的权重系数：狭窄 1% ～ 25% 的权重系数为 1，26% ～ 50% 的权重系数为 2，51% ～ 75% 的权重系数为 4，76% ～ 90% 的权重系数为 8，91% ～ 99% 的权重系数为 16，100% 的权重系数为 32; 评分方法：每处病变的积分为狭窄程度评分乘以病变部位评分，每例患者的积分为所有病变积分的总和。

1.2.2 中医证候记录及血瘀证计分 在病历报告表中详细记录入选患者的病史、症状、舌象、脉象和辨证分型。中医辨证为本虚标实证，包括痰浊（偏热、偏寒）、血瘀、气滞、寒凝、气虚（心气虚、脾气虚、肾气虚）、阳虚（心阳虚、肾阳虚）、阴虚（心阴虚、肝肾阴虚）和阳脱等证候类型。根据患者症状、舌质、口唇及牙龈、舌下络脉和脉象情况，详细记录患者稳定期血瘀证计分，并根据血瘀证计分进行分级，计分 ≤ 9 为第一级，计分 > 9 为第二级。

1.3 统计学方法

使用 Access 建立数据库，数据导入 SPSS 13.0 软件进行统计分析，计量资料采用 $\bar{x} \pm s$ 表示，符合正态分布时采用 t 检验，方差不齐时采用校正 t 检验，不符合正态分布时采用秩和检验。相关性分析采用双变量相关分析，资料服从正态分布选择 Pearson 相关系数。

* 原载于《中国中西医结合杂志》，2010，8（9）：848-852

2. 结果

2.1 患者一般情况

共入选患者131例，其中男性87例（66.4%），女性44例（33.6%），平均年龄为（61.34±10.16）岁。根据既往诊断，有高血压病史92例（70.2%），糖尿病病史58例（44.3%），高脂血症病史67例（51.1%）。

2.2 中医辨证分型

131例经冠状动脉造影证实的CHD患者中，根据中医证型特点的分类如下：痰浊83例（63.4%），寒痰29例（22.1%），热痰54例（41.2%），血瘀85例（64.9%），寒凝3例（2.3%），气滞19例（14.5%），气虚85例（64.9%），阴虚27例（20.6%），阳虚27例（20.6%），阳脱0例。根据有无血瘀征象分类，血瘀证85例（64.9%），非血瘀证46例（35.1%）；对于血瘀证患者，根据血瘀证相兼证的不同又分为血瘀兼痰浊证56例（42.7%），气虚血瘀证55例（42.0%），阴虚血瘀证18例（13.7%），阳虚血瘀证17例（13.0%）。

2.3 血瘀证各兼证与非血瘀证冠状动脉病变长度、最重狭窄以及Gensini评分

血瘀、痰浊血瘀、热痰血瘀患者的冠状动脉病变长度、最重狭窄及Gensini评分的数值均高于非血瘀证，差异均有统计学意义（$P < 0.05$）；气虚血瘀、寒痰血瘀患者的冠状动脉病变长度和最重狭窄的数值高于非血瘀证，差异有统计学意义（$P < 0.05$）；阳虚血瘀患者的最重狭窄程度较非血瘀证严重，差异有统计学意义（$P < 0.05$）。见表1。

2.4 各证型冠状动脉病变长度、最重狭窄以及Gensini评分

根据患者是否为某种证候类型分为血瘀和非血瘀、痰浊和非痰浊、气滞和非气滞、寒凝和非寒凝、气虚和非气虚、阳虚和非阳虚、阴虚和非阴虚。血瘀证患者冠状动脉病变长度、最重狭窄和Gensini评分均高于非血瘀患者（$P < 0.05$，$P < 0.01$），痰浊患者的最重狭窄较非痰浊患者严重（$P < 0.05$），其余各证型比较，差异均无统计学意义。见表2。

2.5 血瘀证计分与Gensini评分

将血瘀证一级和二级患者的Gensini评分、冠状动脉病变长度、支架长度以及最重狭窄进行比较。血瘀证计分≤9分患者的冠状动脉病变长度、支架长度、最重狭窄和Gensini评分分别为（52.04±33.48）mm、（27.00±25.03）mm、（79.40±27.42）%和37.13±34.60，计分>9分患者分别为（67.87±39.06）mm、（46.53±30.60）mm、（85.27±25.03）%和44.87±30.32。与血瘀证计分≤9分的患者相比，计分>9分的患者冠状动脉病变长度更长，差异有统计学意义（$P < 0.05$）；二者支架长度、最重狭窄程度和Gensini评分比较，差异均无统计学意义（$P > 0.05$）。

2.6 血瘀证计分与Gensini评分的相关性

血瘀证计分与Gensini评分双变量相关分析显示，冠心病稳定期患者血瘀证计分与Gensini评分无明显相关性（Pearson相关系数为0.104，$P = 0.241$）。

表1　血瘀证各兼证与非血瘀证冠状动脉病变长度、支架长度、最重狭窄以及Gensini评分（$\bar{x} \pm s$）

Syndrome type	n	Lesion length（mm）	Stent length（mm）	Serious narrowness（%）	Gensini score
Non-blood stasis	46	47.02±33.56	27.00±25.03	73.54±32.24	34.08±35.90
Blood stasis	85	69.04±37.53*	46.53±30.60	87.95±20.54*	46.11±29.71*
Blood stasis accompanied by turbid phlegm	56	75.75±35.98*	44.00±25.52	91.16±15.83*	49.58±29.80*
Blood stasis accompanied by qi deficiency	55	71.29±39.66*	43.71±33.71	85.47±23.34*	42.67±28.32
Blood stasis accompanied by yin deficiency	18	53.89±44.76	30.00±27.50	75.17±31.93	38.33±34.31
Blood stasis accompanied by yang deficiency	17	64.47±40.14	68.50±29.00	86.35±16.37*	40.85±28.89
Blood stasis accompanied by cold phlegm	20	71.50±39.51*	43.00±44.58	88.65±22.71*	47.78±34.05
Blood stasis accompanied by heat phlegm	36	78.11±34.21*	44.60±12.03	92.56±10.40*	50.58±27.64*

*$P < 0.05$，vs non-blood stasis syndrome

表 2　各证型冠状动脉病变长度、最重狭窄以及 Gensini 评分（$\bar{x} \pm s$）

Syndrome type	n	Lesion length（mm）	Serious narrowness（%）	Gensini score
Blood stasis	85	69.04±37.53**	87.95±20.54**	46.11±29.71*
Non-blood stasis	46	47.02±33.56	73.54±32.24	34.08±35.90
Turbid phlegm	83	66.12±37.85	86.78±22.61△	45.84±32.74
Non-turbid phlegm	48	53.11±35.99	76.17±30.28	34.65±30.32
Qi stagnation	19	62.56±37.40	78.68±30.18	35.26±23.65
Non-qi stagnation	112	61.23±37.77	83.61±25.41	42.84±33.41
Cold stagnation	3	57.67±9.07	83.33±5.77	22.67±11.02
Non-cold stagnation	128	61.50±38.00	82.88±26.38	42.19±32.43
Qi defficiency	85	62.40±39.93	81.53±27.08	39.01±30.50
Non-qi defficiency	46	59.56±33.02	85.41±24.22	46.79±34.95
Yang deficiency	27	58.37±34.20	80.67±27.64	41.98±34.85
Non-yang deficiency	104	62.21±38.53	83.47±25.77	41.68±31.67
Yin deficiency	27	49.41±41.56	68.26±34.04	32.74±37.13
Non-yin deficiency	104	64.56±36.02	86.69±22.26	44.08±30.58

*$P < 0.05$, **$P < 0.01$, vs non-blood stasis syndrome；△$P < 0.05$, vs non-turbid phlegm syndrome

3. 讨论

冠状动脉造影一直被人们视为诊断 CHD 的金标准，可直观地显示出冠状动脉粥样硬化斑块所致的血管腔狭窄程度、狭窄的部位以及病变累及的冠状动脉长度。为了更好地评价冠状动脉病变严重程度，需要既考虑到冠状动脉病变的范围，又要考虑到冠状动脉病变的狭窄程度。目前冠状动脉评分的方法有多种，通过冠状动脉评分可以得到计量指标，便于比较。本研究采用的冠状动脉造影 Gensini 评分是一种非常有意义的冠状动脉严重程度评估方法，并广泛应用于临床[5-7]。Gensini 评分法评价冠状动脉病变的严重程度更精确、更敏感。冠状动脉病变越严重，Gensini 评分越高，心脏事件发生率也更高[8]。

近年来，CHD 患者中医证型与冠状动脉造影特点相关性研究有较多的报道。刘红旭等[9]对 113 例 CHD 患者中医证候与冠状动脉造影特点进行研究，发现 3 支病变患者中血瘀证占 95.65%，2 支病变患者中血瘀证占 63.64%，单支病变患者中血瘀证占 34.78%。鞠镐等[10]对经过冠状动脉造影检查确诊的 89 例 CHD 心绞痛患者进行中医证候分析，结果发现 88 例患者均有不同程度的血瘀证表现。徐浩等[11]从冠状动脉病变类型、累及血管数目和狭窄程度角度，分析冠状动脉造影与冠

心病患者发作时血瘀证及血瘀证计分的相关性，发现血瘀证与冠状动脉病变最终狭窄程度、病变计分、病变支数及有无 B2 和 C 型病变均明显相关，血瘀证计分越高，病变复杂程度及严重程度越明显，血瘀轻重可作为反映冠状动脉病变轻重程度的参考指标之一。既往研究多将重点放在冠状动脉狭窄程度、病变支数与中医证候之间的相关性，在分析冠状动脉病变严重性方面存在局限性。本研究引入 Gensini 评分，对 CHD 患者冠状动脉病变部位、范围、狭窄程度综合考虑，能较全面反映出冠状动脉病变的严重程度。以此为依据进行与中医证候相关性分析，可增加分析结果的客观性。

CHD 心绞痛的病机多属本虚标实，以心的阴阳气血不足为核心，属本；血瘀、痰湿、气滞、寒凝则是诱发因素，属标。本研究中 CHD 稳定期患者的证型以血瘀证、痰浊证和气虚证最为常见，并相互兼夹为患，与我们既往的研究相似[12]。本研究的 CHD 患者中，血瘀证患者的冠状动脉病变长度、最重狭窄与 Gensini 评分数值均显著高于非血瘀证患者；在血瘀证各兼证中，血瘀证兼痰浊患者的冠状动脉病变长度、最重狭窄及 Gensini 评分数值均高于非血瘀证患者，且痰浊患者的狭窄程度较非痰浊患者严重，提示瘀血、痰浊阻滞脉络是 CHD 的主要病机。由于本研究选取了 CHD 稳定

期患者，没有胸闷、胸痛的情况，因此血瘀证计分明显低于急性期患者。血瘀证计分＞9分的患者，其冠状动脉病变长度大于积分小的患者，但狭窄程度和 Gensini 评分没有统计学差异。相关性分析显示，CHD 稳定期的患者血瘀证计分与其发病时冠状动脉病变 Gensini 评分没有明显相关性，可能由于 Gensini 评分较高的患者多为经过介入治疗或者冠状动脉旁路移植术治疗后病情稳定的患者，冠状动脉病变的狭窄程度已经减轻或者消失，影响了患者血瘀证的严重程度，降低了血瘀证计分，有待以后扩大样本量继续研究证实。以往研究表明，血瘀证计分高的患者再狭窄发生率也相应增加[11]，进行长期随访事件发生率统计，可望得出更客观的评价。

参考文献

[1] 陈灏珠. 实用内科学. 第12版. 北京：人民卫生出版社，2005：1472-1473.

[2] 中国中西医结合学会心血管病专业委员会. 冠心病中医辨证标准. 中西医结合杂志，1991，11（5）：257-258.

[3] 中国中西医结合学会活血化瘀专业委员会. 血瘀证诊断标准. 中西医结合杂志，1987，7（3）：129-131.

[4] 陈可冀. 活血化瘀研究与临床. 北京：北京医科大学、中国协和医科大学联合出版社，1993，7-10.

[5] Jia EZ, Yang ZJ, Yuan B, et al. Relationship between high-sensitivity C-reactive protein level and angiographical characteristics of coronary atherosclerosis. Chin Med J (Engl)，2006, 119 (4): 319-323.

[6] Peppes V, Rammos G, Manios E, et al. Correlation between myocardial enzyme serum levels and markers of inflammation with severity of coronary artery disease and Gensini score: a hospital-based, prospective study in Greek patients. Clin Interv Aging, 2008, 3 (4): 699-710.

[7] Liu YX, Li XP, Peng DQ, et al. Usefulness of serum cathepsin L as an independent biomarker in patients with coronary heart disease. Am J Cardiol, 2009, 103 (4): 476-481.

[8] Dai DF, Lin JW, Kao JH, et al. The effects of metabolic syndrome versus infectious burden on inflammation, severity of coronary atherosclerosis, and major adverse cardiovascular events. J Clin Endocrinol Metab, 2007, 92 (7) :2532-2537.

[9] 刘红旭，王振裕，彭伟，等. 113 例冠状动脉造影病人中医证候与造影特点分析. 中日友好医院学报，2006，20（1）：35-37.

[10] 鞠镐，程文立，柯元南，等. 冠心病心绞痛病人冠状动脉造影与中医辨证分型关系的研究. 中西医结合心脑血管病杂志，2005，3（7）：569-571.

[11] 徐浩，鹿小燕，陈可冀，等. 血瘀证及其兼证与冠状动脉造影所示病变及介入治疗后再狭窄的相关性研究. 中国中西医结合杂志，2007，27（1）：8-13.

[12] 郑峰，曲丹，徐浩，等. 冠心病稳定期患者中医辨证与超敏 C 反应蛋白相关性研究. 中国中西医结合杂志，2009，29（6）：485-488.

冠心病差异基因表达谱的构建及目标基因的功能分析 *

殷惠军　马晓娟　蒋跃绒　史大卓　陈可冀

冠心病的发生涉及脂质代谢障碍、血管内皮细胞损伤、单核细胞迁移并分化为巨噬细胞、平滑肌细胞从中膜迁移至内膜并增殖、泡沫细胞的形成、细胞坏死和脂质沉积等许多过程。大量研究表明，炎症反应与冠心病的发生，尤其是不稳定斑块的形成与发展及血栓的形成关系密切[1]，而炎症介导冠心病的分子靶标及其作用的病理环节尚有待研究。

随着人类基因图谱的日益完善和后基因组研究的进展，世界正进入一个以生物信息为重要内容的生命科学时代，疾病基因组学逐渐成为国际医学界的重要研究方向。遗传流行病学研究表明，遗传因素在冠心病的发生、发展中起着至关重要的作用[2]，故从分子生物学角度研究冠心病病因，可为冠心病的预防和治疗提供新的途径。

* 原载于《科学通报》，2009，54（3）：354-359

本研究以基因芯片技术为主要研究手段，构建冠心病相关差异基因表达谱，并运用实时荧光定量逆转录聚合酶链式反应（reverse transcription polymerase chain reaction，RT-PCR）对目标基因进行鉴定，并进一步通过临床血清学实验验证所筛选的目标基因与疾病的相关性，并对目标基因进行功能分析，以探讨其作用机制。

1. 材料与方法

1.1 芯片实验

本研究选用 Affymetrix 公司的 Human Genome U133 Plus 2.0 芯片，该芯片一共有 54 614 个探针组，分析 47 000 个转录本和变异体，其中包括了可能的 38 500 个已知基因。在正式基因芯片杂交实验前选用 affymetrix 芯片系列中的质控芯片 Test-3 进行样本检测。

1.2 临床资料

病例来源于北京西苑医院门诊及住院患者，冠心病组入选标准参照世界卫生组织临床命名标准化联合专题组报告《缺血性心脏病的命名及诊断》：经选择性冠状动脉造影术证实至少有 1 处狭窄 > 50% 以上者[3]，16 例。正常对照组均为本研究室人员及本院职工查体者，经病史调查以及体检、血常规、肝功能、X 线胸部透视、心电图等检查，排除精神及重大躯体疾病、本人及家庭无精神病史者 8 例。以上入选对象均为无血缘关系汉族人，年龄在 35 ～ 75 岁，告知实验内容及目的并签署知情同意书。该研究符合赫尔辛基宣言，不违背医学伦理道德。

1.3 探针制备及芯片杂交

每例受试者采血 2mL，用淋巴细胞分离液法分离白细胞，按 Trizol（Trizol Reagent，Invitrogen Life Technologies，P/N 15596-018）一步法抽提总 RNA，采用 Nucleo-Spin®RNA Clean-up（MN，740.948.10）试剂盒进行过柱纯化，GeneChip IVT Labeling Kit 进行生物素标记，凝胶电泳和紫外分光光度计进行定性和定量检测，并进一步将探针片段化。处理后的探针先与质控芯片 Test-3 进行杂交，确认探针质量可靠后再与 U133 Plus 2.0 芯片进行杂交，在杂交炉（Affymetrix Hybridization Oven 640）中 45℃杂交 16h，然后于 Affymetrix Fluidics Station 450 工作站中洗脱、染色，再用 Affymetrix GeneChip Scanner 3000 进行探针阵列扫描。

1.4 数据处理和生物信息学分析

芯片扫描后，用 Affymetrix GeneChip operating software version 1.4 进行信号值提取、归一化处理及芯片间比较分析，根据 Ratio 值筛选冠心病相关差异基因。通过 http://www.gosurfer.org 网站进行基因本体论（gene ontology，GO）分析[4]，找到每一个差异基因的分子功能、生物学途径和细胞组件，结合疾病病理生理过程和相关研究，筛选冠心病相关的目标基因。通过 http://www.biorag.org 网站找到差异基因所在通路，并利用超几何分布统计学方法[5,6]分析通路结果，通过 P 值（$P < 0.05$）来判断显著性，筛选有意义的目标通路。

1.5 实时荧光定量 RT-PCR 鉴定

基于芯片结果，结合疾病病理生理过程及相关研究，进一步回归临床，筛选冠心病相关的 6 个目标基因，并用实时荧光定量逆转录聚合酶链式反应对目标基因进行验证，以排除基因芯片实验的假阳性。

1.6 临床验证

筛选冠心病患者 30 例和健康对照者（诊断标准同前）40 例为研究对象，采用双抗体夹心 ABC-ELISA 法检测目标基因 IL-8 的血清浓度，以验证目标基因与疾病的相关性。

1.7 目标基因 IL-8 功能分析

立足于基因芯片筛选和临床验证结果，选择与冠心病密切相关的目标基因 IL-8 作为诱导因素，研究炎症因子对血小板活化的影响，并对其作用机制进行初步探讨。以 12 例健康自愿者为研究对象，采取静脉全血 10mL，制备富血小板血浆（PRP）。将 PRP 分装到 12 个 1.5mL 离心管中。（1）血小板聚集率（platelet aggregation percentage，PAP）测定：1 ～ 4 号分别用低（50ng/mL）、中（100ng/mL）、高（150ng/mL）3 个浓度的 IL-8（美国 Peprotech）和生理盐水（normal saline，NS）温浴（IADPS 组、IADPM 组、IADPH 组、NADP 组）后加 ADP 测 PAP；5 ～ 8 号用 IL-8，ADP（美国 Chronolog），IL-8+ADP，NS 直接作诱导剂（ADP 组、IL-8 组、ADP+IL-8 组、NS 组）测 PAP。PAP 用比浊法测定。（2）血小板活性测定：9 ～ 12 号用 3 个浓度（同上）的 IL-8 和 NS 温浴后（IL-8AS 组、IL-8AM 组、IL-8AH 组、NSA 组），流式细胞术测其血小板 CD62p 表达（美国 Becton Dickinson 试剂盒）。（3）显微镜观察血小板聚集情况：对各组测完聚集率的样品（1 ～ 8 号）和 PRP 使用细胞离心机进行制片，在光学显微镜下观察不同处理情况下血小板的聚集情况。

1.8 统计学分析

采用 SPSS 分析软件进行统计分析，计数资料用卡方检验，计量资料用 t 检验，$P < 0.05$ 被认为具有统计学意义。

2. 结果

2.1 芯片实验

2.1.1 一般临床资料　入选对象中，年龄、性别、吸烟及饮酒情况经统计学分析，各组之间无显著性差异，具有可比性（$P > 0.05$）（表1）。

表1　各组临床资料比较

特性	冠心病组	正常对照组	P 值
例数	16	8	-
年龄	57.38±7.22	52.25±11.16	0.19
性别（男/女）	16/2	7/1	1.00
吸烟（%）	31.25	25.00	1.00
饮酒（%）	43.75	37.50	1.00

2.1.2 芯片质控及扫描结果　RNA 样品电泳条带清晰，28S 比 18S rRNA 条带亮度接近 2：1，紫外分光光度计检测 RNA 在波长 260 和 280nm 处的吸光度（absorbance，A），$A_{260}/A_{280} = 1.8 \sim 2.1$，质量符合表达谱芯片实验要求（图1）。Test-3 芯片与探针杂交扫描结果显示，芯片正中"+"清晰可见，外围连线清楚，明暗交替规律，进一步通过信号分析发现管家基因均表达，说明 RNA 样品质量可靠。U133 Plus 2.0 芯片与探针杂交扫描结果显示，芯片中上部清晰呈现阵列的名称"GeneChip HG-U133 Plus2"，平均背景值与噪音值均在正常范围，管家基因 β-actin 和 GAPDH（磷酸甘油醛

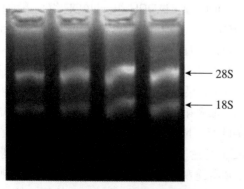

28S
18S

图1　冠心病组 RNA 电泳结果

脱氢酶）3' 端与 5' 端信号比值符合标准，芯片质控良好。

2.1.3 芯片结果分析　通过差异基因筛选，与冠心病相关的差异基因共有 107 个，其中上调 48 个，下调 59 个。冠心病相关差异基因涉及炎症免疫、细胞周期、信号转导、凋亡、细胞黏附、细胞活动、细胞结构、发育、应激反应、转录调控、转运、代谢等多个方面，通过 GO 和通路分析发现炎症免疫相关基因具有比例和显著性优势。冠心病相关的 107 个差异基因中分子功能和生物学途径涉及炎症免疫反应的有 14 个，占 13.1%（表2）。通路显著性分析发现，冠心病相关有意义通路共 15 个，其中有 4 个涉及炎症和免疫反应（表3）。

2.2 目标基因鉴定

基于芯片结果，结合疾病病理生理过程以及前人的研究，进一步回归临床，筛选冠心病相关的目标基因，共有 6 个目标基因：PRKCB1（蛋白激酶 C，β1）、IL-8（白介素 8）、HLA-DQB1（主要组织相容性复合体 Ⅱ β1）、FCGR3A（免疫球蛋白 IgG 结晶片段受体 Ⅲ a）、FOLR3（叶酸受体 γ3）

表2　冠心病相关涉及炎症免疫的差异基因

基因号	基因名称	fold change*
AF043337	白介素 8	2.46
NM_000570	免疫球蛋白 IgG 结晶片段受体 Ⅲ a	3.64
BC020691	前 B 细胞克隆增强因子 1	2.44
X00452	主要组织相容性复合体 Ⅱ α₁	3
AA994334	B 细胞慢性淋巴细胞性白血病 10	2.35
AF400602	C 型凝集素结构域家族 7A	2.29
NM_012445	脊椎蛋白 2，细胞外基质蛋白	−2.13
AW007751	T 细胞受体 α	−2.08
NM_000647	趋化因子受体 2	−2.34
BF110792	肿瘤蛋白 D52	−2.03
AI092511	二肽基肽酶 4	−2.37
AU145682	前 B 细胞因子	−2.54
NM_002261	杀伤细胞凝集素样受体亚家族 C3	−2.5
AF211977	白细胞受体簇 10	−2.62

* fold change 值为实验样品与对照样品的基因转录产物表达比值

表 3　冠心病相关涉及炎症免疫的有意义通路

通路	基因芯片识别基因数 / 个	差异基因数 / 个	P 值
B 细胞受体信号	63	12	< 0.001
自然杀伤细胞介导的细胞毒作用	131	18	< 0.001
T 细胞受体信号通路	93	13	< 0.05
免疫球蛋白 IgG 结晶片段高亲和受体信号	75	10	< 0.05

和 PTGDS（前列腺素 D_2 合成酶）。对目标基因进行 RT-PCR 鉴定，结果显示，6 个目标基因的差异倍数与基因芯片检测结果不完全相同，但变化方向均一致（图 2），表明基因芯片结果准确可靠。

2.3　临床验证

入选对象中，年龄、性别经统计学分析，冠心病组和健康对照组无显著性差异（$P > 0.05$），具有可比性（表 4）；而冠心病组血清 IL-8 水平显著高于健康对照组（$P < 0.05$），说明了炎症因子 IL-8 与冠心病的临床相关性（图 3）。

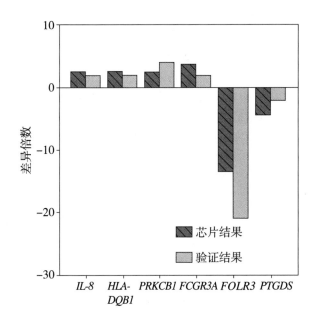

图 2　基因芯片检测结果与实时荧光定量 RT-PCR 验证结果的比较

表 4　两组临床资料比较

冠心病组	健康对照组	P 值
例数 / 个	30	40	-
年龄	58.50±8.16	54.73±10.64	0.11
男性人数（%）	17（56.7%）	14（35.0%）	0.71

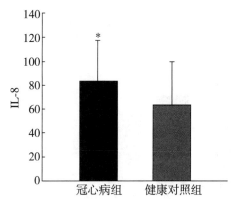

图 3　冠心病组与健康对照组 IL-8 水平比较
冠心病组 IL-8 浓度为（83.21±34.33）pg/mL，健康对照组 IL-8 浓度为（63.34±36.36）pg/mL*，$P < 0.05$，与健康对照组比较

2.4　目标基因 IL-8 对血小板活化的作用

2.4.1　血小板聚集率　IADPS 组、IADPM 组和 IADPH 组分别用 3 个不同剂量 IL-8 温浴后，PAP 显著高于 NS 温浴 NADP 组（$P < 0.05$），而 3 组 PAP 之间无显著性差异（$P > 0.05$）（图 4）。

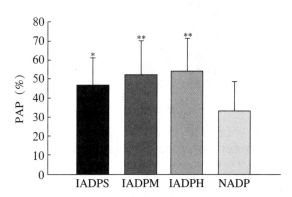

图 4　温浴处理后各组 PAP
IADPS 组 PAP 为（46.92±16.78）%，IADPM 组 PAP 为（52.27±17.74）%，IADPH 组 PAP 为（54.30±18.18）%，NADP 组 PAP 为（33.30±15.19）%。与 NADP 组比较，* 示 $P < 0.05$，** 示 $P < 0.01$

分别用 ADP 和 IL-8 做诱导剂，两组 PAP 之间无显著性差异（$P > 0.05$），但两组 PAP 均显著高于 NS 组（$P < 0.01$），而以 ADP+IL-8 作为诱导剂组 PAP 则明显高于 ADP，IL-8 和 NS 组（$P < 0.01$）（图 5）。

2.4.2　血小板 CD62p 表达　低量 IL-8 温浴 IL-8 AS 组 CD62p 平均荧光强度（mean fluorescen-tintensity，MFI）显著高于 NS 温浴 NSA 组及中量 IL-8 温浴 IL-8 AM 组和高量 IL-8 温浴 IL-8 AH 组（$P < 0.01$），IL-8 AM 组和 IL-8 AH 组 CD62p MFI 有高于 NSA 组的趋势，但是差异无统计学意义（$P > 0.05$）（图 6）。

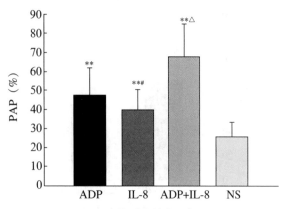

图 5　直接诱导的各组 PAP

ADP 组 PAP 为（47.61±14.42）%，IL-8 组 PAP 为（40.49±10.55）%，ADP+IL-8 组 PAP 为（67.68±17.55）%，NS 组 PAP 为（25.91±8.05）%。**，$P < 0.01$，与 NS 组比较；#示 $P > 0.05$，△示 $P < 0.01$，与 ADP 组比较

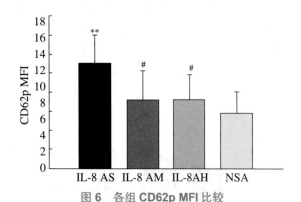

图 6　各组 CD62p MFI 比较

CD62p MFI 值 IL-8 AS 组 为 13.09±3.45，IL-8 AM 组 为 8.57±3.55，IL-8 AH 组为 8.61±3.07，NSA 组为 6.95±2.57 与 NSA 组比较，#示 $P > 0.05$，**示 $P < 0.01$

2.4.3　显微镜观察血小板聚集情况　瑞氏染色血片观察不同处理组血小板聚集情况（图 7）。未处理 PRP 组血小板呈点状散在分布；单纯 NS 处理组血小板较 PRP 组密集，多数血小板还呈散在分布状态；单纯 IL-8 处理组血小板有轻度聚集现象，可见血小板聚集体，但聚集体较小，散在分布血小板明显减少；所有 ADP 处理组均可见明显聚集现象，血小板聚集体均匀、紧密且体积较大。

　　结果表明，IL-8 对血小板聚集率有一定影响，存在增强 ADP 诱导作用的趋势，但其作用不随剂量增加而增加；小量 IL-8 与阴性对照相比较而言明显增加血小板活化标志物 CD62p 活性。显微镜下形态学观察，IL-8 可使血小板聚集，但聚集程度没有 ADP 处理组明显。

3. 讨论

　　本研究以全基因组芯片为主要研究手段，筛查冠心病患者和健康对照者的差异表达基因，通过对冠心病相关差异基因的功能和通路分析，发现冠心病在分子水平与炎症免疫反应具有密切相关性。传统观点认为，冠心病的主要病理机制为冠状动脉粥样硬化和冠脉痉挛，但是近年来，在冠心病尤其是在急性冠脉综合征的发病过程中，炎症作为一种促进因素越来越得到重视[7]。炎症反应不仅促进了动脉粥样硬化的发生，而且参与了不稳定性斑块形成、斑块破裂、继发冠状动脉痉挛及血栓形成等病理过程，激活的炎性细胞在冠心病的发生、发展中起着重要作用[8]。调查显示，仅有 14% 急性冠脉事件存在 70% 以上的冠状动脉狭窄，而越来越多的研究表明，冠状动脉粥样硬化斑块内的炎症反应促使冠状动脉内不稳定斑块的形成和破裂，并在此基础上发生细胞成分的活化且介导血栓的形成，是大多数急性冠状动脉综合征发生的主要原因[9]。作为炎症启动因素的免疫反应，其在动脉粥样硬化发生和冠心病进展中发挥着不可忽视的作用[10]。本研究发现，B 细胞受体信号通路和 T 细胞受体信号通路均与冠心病显著相关，说明体液免疫和细胞免疫介导了冠心病的发病。

　　IL-8 主要由单核 - 巨噬细胞、中性粒细胞和血管内皮细胞合成，是一种具有内源性白细胞趋化性和活化性作用的碱基 - 肝素结合性蛋白质[11]。本研究通过临床实验证明了目标基因 IL-8 血清水平与冠心病的相关性。研究表明[12]，IL-8 不仅具有中性粒细胞的活化和趋化作用，而且介导了 T 淋巴细胞的定向迁移，而中性粒细胞和 T 淋巴细胞在炎症和动脉粥样硬化形成过程中都发挥着重要的作用。在动脉粥样硬化过程中，IL-8 除了具有血管新生活性外，还可能具有内皮细胞和平滑肌细胞的趋化和促有丝分裂的作用，与冠状动脉粥样硬化的形成具有一定相关性[13]。正常血小板活化是体内生理性止血的必需步骤，而病理性血小板活化则与血栓性疾病密切相关。动脉血栓形成的基础病变是动脉粥样硬化，血小板在受损血管内膜下的黏附和聚集是血栓形成的重要启动因素之一[14]，而血小板在破溃斑块上的黏附聚集作用在动脉血栓形成中发挥了"扳机"作用，同时血小板作为炎症介质的来源，炎症触发的血小板活化也是动脉血栓形成的关键步骤[15]。动脉粥样硬化斑块破裂处炎症反应与血小板的激活及其相互介导是导致急性冠脉综合征等心脑血管事件的重要病理基础[16]。近年来炎症因子激活血小板的机制研究也有了初步进

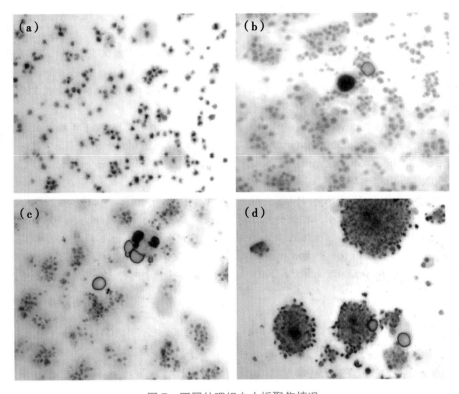

图 7　不同处理组血小板聚集情况

（a）PRP 组；（b）单纯 NS 处理组；（c）单纯 IL-8 处理组；（d）ADP 处理组。瑞氏染色，在光
学显微镜下观察各组血小板聚集情况。原始放大倍数：×400

展，如对肿瘤坏死因子（tumor necrosis factor-α，TNF-α）的研究显示[17,18]：TNF-α 可放大血小板对胶原的反应，是血小板通过花生四烯酸通路活化的触动因子，这一效应可以被 TNF-α 受体拮抗剂所抑制；TNF-α 超家族成员 CD40 与可溶性 CD40L 结合可使血小板表面 CD62P 表达增加，同时使血小板形态发生典型的活化改变，在血小板活化、血栓形成和炎症反应中起重要作用。

本研究的血小板聚集率、CD62p 活性、血小板聚集形态学研究结果均表明，IL-8 具有激活血小板的作用，对血小板的黏附、聚集、释放功能均有一定程度的影响，提示 IL-8 可能通过影响血小板活化程度而介导了冠心病的发病过程，而 IL-8 的作用机制及通路尚有待进一步研究。

参考文献

[1] Malpartida F, Vivancos R, Urbano C, et al. Inflammation and plaque instability. Arch Cardiol Mex, 2007, 77 (14): 16-22.

[2] Candore G, Balistreri CR, Caruso M, et al. Pharmacogenomics: a tool to prevent and cure coronary heart disease. Curr Pharm Des, 2007, 13 (36): 3726-3734.

[3] 徐浩，鹿小燕，陈可冀，等. 血瘀证及其兼证与冠脉造影所示病变及介入治疗后再狭窄的相关性研究. 中国中西医结合杂志，2007，27 (1)：8-13.

[4] Zhong S, Storch KF, Lipan O, et al. GoSurfer: a graphical interactive tool for comparative analysis of large gene sets in Gene Ontologyspace. Appl Bioinformatics, 2004, 3 (4): 261-264.

[5] Wu J, Mao X, Cai T, et al. KOBAS server: webbased platform for automated annotation and pathway identification. Nucleic Acids Res, 2006, 34 (1): 720-724.

[6] Mao X, Cai T, Olyarchuk JG, et al. Automated genome annotation and pathway identification using the KEGG Orthology (KO) as a controlled vocabulary. Bioinformatics, 2005, 21 (15): 3787-3793.

[7] Brunetti ND, Correale M, Pellegrino PL, et al. Acute phase proteins in patients with acute coronary syndrome: correlations with diagnosis, clinical features, and angiographic findings. Eur J Intern Med, 2007, 18 (2): 109-117.

[8] Napoleão P, Santos MC, Selas M, et al. Variations in inflammatory markers in acute myocardial infarction: A longitudinal study. Rev Port Cardiol, 2007, 26 (12):

第一章

1357-1363.

[9] Davies MJ. The pathophysiology of acute coronary syndromes. Heart, 2000, 83 (3): 361-366.

[10] Wick G, Knoflach M, Xu Q. Autoimmune and inflammatory mechanisms in atherosclerosis. Annu Rev Immunol, 2004, 22: 361-403.

[11] Qi X, Li J, Gu J, et al. Plasma levels of IL-8 predict early complications in patients with coronary heart disease after percutaneous coronary intervention. Jpn Heart J, 2003, 44 (4): 451-461.

[12] Poddar R, Sivasubramanian N, DiBello P M, et al. Homocysteine induces expression and secretion of monocyte chemoattractant protein-1 and interleukin-8 in human aortic endothelial cells implications for vascular disease. Circulation, 2001, 103 (22): 2717-2723.

[13] Simonini A, Moscucci M, Muller D W, et al. IL-8 is an angiogenic factor in human coronary atherectomy tissue. Circulation, 2000, 101 (13): 1519-1526.

[14] Jackson SP, Schoenwaelder SM. Antiplatelet therapy: in search of the "magic bullet". Nat Rev Drug Discov, 2003, 2 (10): 775-789.

[15] Davì G, Patrono C. Platelet activation and athero-thrombosis. N Engl J Med, 2007, 357 (24): 2482-2494.

[16] Michael RF, David FM. Unstable angina and non-ST elevation MI: IIb or not IIb？The evidence points to a better long-term outcome. J Crit Illness, 2002, 17 (2): 52-65.

[17] Pignatelli P, De Biase L, Lenti L, et al. Tumor necrosis factor-alpha as trigger of platelet activation in patients with heart failure. Blood, 2005, 106 (6): 1992-1994.

[18] Inwald DP, McDowall A, Peters MJ, et al. CD40 is constitutively expressed on platelets and provides a novel mechanism for platelet activation. Circ Res, 2003, 92 (9): 1041-1048.

汉族人血小板膜糖蛋白Ⅲa PLA 基因多态性与冠心病血瘀证的相关性[*]

薛　梅　陈可冀　殷惠军

血小板活化在冠心病等血栓性疾病的发生发展过程中起重要作用。血瘀证是冠心病最常见的证候之一，血瘀证患者多存在血小板活化现象，血小板膜糖蛋白在血小板黏附、聚集和释放反应中起关键作用，是血小板活化的特异性分子标志物[1]。多项研究[2-5]证实某些血小板膜糖蛋白Ⅰb（glycoprotein Ⅰb，GPb）、GP Ⅱb-Ⅲa 和 GP Ⅰa-Ⅱa 的基因多态性增加了冠状动脉血栓形成和冠状动脉事件发生的危险性。但冠心病血瘀证是否与上述基因多态性有关尚未见报道。GP Ⅱb-Ⅲa 在血小板聚集和血栓增长中起关键作用[6]，本研究正是以 GP Ⅲa 多态性为研究切入点，观察 PLA1/PLA2 基因多态性在汉族人中的分布状况，分析该多态性与冠心病和冠心病血瘀证易感性的相关性。

1. 资料与方法

1.1 临床资料

1.1.1 研究对象的选择　所收集病例为北京、河北地区无血缘关系汉族人，全部来源于 2005 年 3 月至 2007 年 5 月就诊于北京西苑医院和安贞医院者。据入选标准将所收集病例分为冠心病血瘀证组和冠心病非血瘀证组，并设健康对照，健康人群为来自西苑医院体检中心的本院职工或其他查体者，均经病史调查、体格检查，以及血常规、肝功能、X 线胸部透视、心电图等检查，排除精神及重大躯体疾病，本人及家庭无精神病史，告知检查内容并自愿参加。所有入选者皆签署知情同意书。

1.1.2 诊断标准　冠心病的诊断均符合 1979 年世界卫生组织临床命名标准化联合专题组报告《缺血

* 原载于《中西医结合学报》，2009，7（4）：325-329

性心脏病的命名及诊断》[7] 标准，选择有心绞痛症状和（或）心肌缺血的客观证据，且冠状动脉造影证实冠状动脉有显著狭窄（＞50%）者。中医辨证标准参照中国中西医结合学会冠心病中医辨证标准[8]。

1.1.3　纳入标准　缺血性心脏病，中医辨证分型不限；患者有心绞痛症状和（或）心肌缺血的客观证据；近期冠状动脉造影证实冠状动脉有显著狭窄（＞50%）；年龄在35～75岁。凡同时具备以上4条者，均纳入试验范围。

1.1.4　排除标准　严重感染；严重心功能不全（射血分数＜35%）；未控制的Ⅲ级高血压；严重瓣膜性心脏病；1型糖尿病；合并严重肝、肾、造血系统、神经系统等原发性疾病及精神病、恶性肿瘤；患者拒绝签署知情同意书，或估计依从性较差；参加其他临床试验的患者；妊娠期或哺乳期妇女。

1.2　观察指标及方法

1.2.1　基因多态性主要检测仪器及试剂　高速冷冻离心机（Sigma 3k-30、SORVALL RT7）；美国生物科学公司 ABI 9700 型聚合酶链反应（polymerase chain reaction，PCR）仪；ABI 7700 HT 型荧光定量 PCR 仪；DNA 提取试剂盒 Wizard Genomic DNA Purification Kit（Promega）；普通 PCR 试剂 Ex Taq DNA 聚合酶（P/N：DRR100B；Lot：CKA 1801A；大连宝生物工程有限公司）；荧光定量试剂为 ABI TaqMan 2×PCR master mix（P/N: 432 6614；Lot：G15502）。

1.2.2　基因多态性检测位点确认　GP Ⅲa 存在多个基因位点的变异，从美国国家生物技术信息中心（National Center for Biotechnology Information，NCBI）网站可以确认 GP Ⅲa PLA1/PLA2 多态位点位于 GP Ⅲa 的第3外显子。见表1。

1.2.3　基因多态性检测方法和步骤　按 Wizard Genomic DNA Purification Kit 试剂盒说明提取全基因组 DNA[9]，−20℃存放备检。

GP Ⅲa PLA1/PLA2 多态位点探针和引物采用 ABI Primer Express 2.0 软件设计：XM-rs5918-FAM（t），

FAM-CCCTGCCTCT GGGCT CACCT C-TAMRA，Tm ＝ 66.3，GC% ＝ 71.4，Length ＝ 21; XM-rs5918-VIC（c），VIC-CCT GCCTCCGGGCTCA CCTTAMRA，Tm ＝ 65.6，GC% ＝ 73.7，Length ＝ 19; XM-rs5918-FP，CAGGAGGTAGAGA GT CGCCAT AG，Tm ＝ 58.2，GC% ＝ 56.5，Length ＝ 23; XM-rs5918-RP，TAT CCT T CAGCAGA TT CTCCT TCA，Tm ＝ 58.2，GC% ＝ 41.7，Length ＝ 24; Amplicon: Tm ＝ 82，GC% ＝ 55，Length ＝ 118。

GP Ⅲa 的多态性检测采用 TaqMan 探针技术。TaqMan 探针技术包括普通 TaqMan、TaqMan MGB 和 TaqMan LNA，虽然后两者灵敏度和特异性较前者要高，但由于所检测的序列 GC 含量较高，所以采用更为适合的普通 TaqMan 探针。按文献方法[9] 检测 PCR 产物荧光强度变化，用 ABI 7700 HT 型荧光定量 PCR 仪，按 7700 用户手册操作。

1.3　统计学方法

统计分析采用 SPSS 11.5 统计软件，α ＝ 0.05 为检验水准。计数资料用卡方检验，计量资料用 t 检验或方差分析。

2.　结果

2.1　一般资料

入选对象中，冠心病血瘀证组110例，男性79例，女性31例，平均年龄（61.0±9.0）岁，体重指数（25.7±2.8）kg/m^2，心肌梗死11例，非心肌梗死99例，有心肌梗死病史者22例，有高血压病史者49例，有高脂血症病史者29例，有糖尿病病史者24例，有吸烟史者40例；冠心病非血瘀证组102例，男性75例，女性27例，平均年龄（60.0±9.4）岁，体重指数（25.7±2.7）kg/m^2，心肌梗死11例，非心肌梗死91例，有心肌梗死病史者23例，有高血压病史者46例，有高脂血症病史者21例，有糖尿病病史者27例，有吸烟史者37例。经统计学分析，两组间比较，差异无统计学意义（P ＞ 0.05）。健康对照组年龄、性别、体重指数与冠心病血瘀证组和冠心病非血瘀证

表 1　GP Ⅲa PLA1/PLA2 多态位点

Amino acid pos	HPA classification	Personal name classification	dbSNP allele	dbSNP rs# cluster ID
GP Ⅲa	HPA-1a	PLA1	T	rs5918
Leu 33 Pro	HPA-1b	PLA2	C	

HPA：human platelet antigen；dbSNP：single nucleotide polymorphism database

组比较，差异均无统计学意义，具有可比性（*P* > 0.05）。

2.2 PLA1/PLA2 多态位点分型

所有入选患者 TaqMan 探针检测图谱表明，rs5918 多态位点分型皆为纯合子 TT 型，即 PLA1/PLA1 型（图 1）。

2.3 PLA1/PLA2 多态位点基因型分析

冠心病血瘀证组、冠心病非血瘀证组和健康对照组 GP Ⅲ a 基因多态性均呈 PLA1/ PLA1（TT）型，而 PLA1/PLA2（TC）型和 PLA 2/ PLA2（CC）型缺如，未再进一步作统计学分析。

3. 讨论

GP Ⅱb - Ⅲa 的基因编码定位于第 17 号 q$^{21~22}$ 带一个约 260kb 大小的片段内，GP Ⅱb 基因长约 17kb，含有 30 个外显子，GP Ⅲa 基因长约 60kb，含有 14 个外显子。二者不能单独表现于细胞膜表面，需先在内质网形成复合物再表达于胞浆膜上，形成完整的功能单位。GP Ⅱb - Ⅲa 有多个多态位点，本研究选取发现最早的 PLA1/PLA2 基因多态位点为研究对象。

既往研究显示美国和英国人群中 PLA2/PLA2（CC）型等位基因约占 15%，芬兰和澳大利亚各占 11% 和 14%[10]。对于该基因多态性是否与冠心病的易感性和严重程度有关，各相关研究[11,12]得到了不同结论。本研究所有入选病例（冠心病血瘀证组 110 例、冠心病非血瘀证组 102 例和健康对照组 39 例）GP Ⅲa 基因多态性均呈 PLA1/PLA1（TT）型，PLA1/PLA2（TC）型和 PLA2/PLA2（CC）型缺如，该基因多态位点不是汉族人冠心病和冠心病血瘀证的危险因素，与国内外近年研究报道[13-15]结果一致。可见 GP Ⅲa 的 PLA1/PLA2 多态表型因地域种族的不同而存在显著差异。

PLA1/PLA2 基因多态性与冠心病之间的关系尚有争议。本课题组分析认为，地域分布和种族差异是产生差别的客观原因，所以对不同地域、人群分别进行研究比较，对阐明多态性与冠心病之间的关系，实现临床患者的个体化诊疗具有重要意义。实验设计、诊断标准和样本含量等研究方法的不同是产生结果差异的另一重要原因，也是后续研究中需要尽量完善、改进的部分。

冠心病、血小板功能状态、血瘀证三者之间

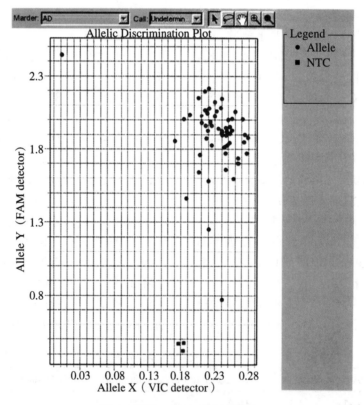

图 1 基因 rs5918 位点分型图

Abscissa：VIC signal intensity；Ordinate：FAM signal intensity；NTC：No template control. Round spot：Allele T homozygote

存在密切的内在联系。中医的证既与致病因素的性质、强弱有关，更与患者个体的体质因素有关，而正是基因的差异表达决定了个体的差异，推测冠心病血瘀证与某些相关基因的多态性之间存在内在联系[9]。本研究选择在血小板聚集和血栓增长中起关键作用的 GP Ⅱb - Ⅲa 作为切入点，结果显示 PLA1/PLA2 多态位点在我国人群中突变率极低，与冠心病血瘀证并无相关性。由于 GP Ⅱb - Ⅲa 具有数个多态位点，与血瘀证具有相关性的位点也可能存在于其他位点，或是多个位点的共同作用。在进一步研究中，扩大样本量并对多个目标基因的不同多态位点进行分析，对阐释冠心病血瘀证的部分发病机制具有积极作用。

参考文献

［1］ 陈可冀，薛梅，殷惠军. 血小板活化与冠状动脉粥样硬化性心脏病和血瘀证的关系. 首都医科大学学报，2008，29（3）：266-269.

［2］ Melus V, Pullmann R, Hybenova J, et al. Is PLA1/ PLA2 gene polymorphism of platelet membrane glycoprotein Ⅲa a risk factor for myocardial infarct？ Bratisl Lŵ Listy, 1999, 100 (11): 593-597.

［3］ Mikkelsson J, Perola M, Penttil A, et al. Platelet glycoprotein Ⅰb alpha HPA-2 Met/VNTR B haplotype as a genetic predictor of myocardial infarction and sudden cardiac death. Circulation, 2001, 104 (8): 876-880.

［4］ Beer JH, Pederiva S, Pontiggia L. Genetics of platelet receptor single-nucleotide polymorphisms: clinical implications in thrombosis. Ann Med, 2000, 32（Suppl 1）: 10-14.

［5］ Bray PF, Howard TD, Vittinghoff E, et al. Effect of genetic variations in platelet glycoproteins Ⅰb alpha and Ⅵ on the risk for coronary heart disease events in postmenopausal women taking hormone therapy. Blood, 2007, 109 (5): 1862-1869.

［6］ Jackson SP, Schoenwaelder SM. Antiplatelet therapy: in search of the "magic bullet". Nat Rev Drug Discov, 2003, 2 (10): 775-789.

［7］ 陈灏珠. 实用内科学. 第 12 版. 北京：人民卫生出版社，2005，1472-1473.

［8］ 中国中西医结合学会心血管专业委员会. 冠心病中医辨证标准. 中国中西医结合杂志，1991，11（5）：257.

［9］ 薛梅，陈可冀，马晓娟，等. 血府逐瘀口服液对冠心病血瘀证患者血液流变学的影响及其与人类血小板抗原 3 基因多态性的相关性. 中西医结合学报，2008，6（11）：1129-1135.

［10］ Di Castelnuovo A, de Gaetano G, Benedetta Donati M, et al. Platelet glycoprotein GP Ⅱb- Ⅲa polymorphism and coronary artery disease: implications for clinical practice. Am J Pharmacogenomics, 2005, 5 (2): 93-99.

［11］ Lagercrantz J, Bergman M, Lundman P, et al. No evidence that the PLA1/PLA2 polymorphism of platelet glycoprotein Ⅲa is implicated in angiographically characterized coronary athero-sclerosis and premature myocardial infarction. Blood Coagul Fibrinolysis, 2003, 14 (8): 749-753.

［12］ Abu-Amero KK, Wyngaard CA, Dzimiri N. Association of the platelet glycoprotein receptor Ⅲa (PLA1/ PLA1) genotype with coronary artery disease in Arabs. Blood Coagul Fibrinolysis, 2004, 15 (1): 77-79.

［13］ Pegoraro RJ, Ranjith N. Plasminogen activator inhibito rtype 1 (PAI-1) and platelet glycoprotein Ⅲa (PG Ⅲa) polymorphisms in young Asian Indians with acute myocardial infarction. Cardiovasc J S Afr, 2005, 16 (5): 266-270.

［14］ 油红文，高东升，王佩显. 血小板糖蛋白 Ⅱb - Ⅲa 的 PLA 基因多态性与心肌梗死关系的研究. 济宁医学院学报，2004，27（4）：25-26.

［15］ 杨胜利，何秉贤，何作云，等. 乌鲁木齐地区维汉两民族中糖蛋白 Ⅲa 基因多态性与冠心病危险性的关系. 中国微循环，2003，7（3）：136-139.

汉族人血小板 GP Ⅱb HPA-3 基因多态性与冠心病的相关性研究 *

薛　梅　陈可冀　殷惠军

随着人类基因组计划的迅速发展，冠心病相关基因的定位与识别已成为研究的热点。有证据表明血小板膜糖蛋白Ⅰb（glycoprotein Ⅰb，GP Ⅰb）、血小板膜糖蛋白Ⅱb、Ⅲa（glycoprotein Ⅱb-Ⅲa，GP Ⅱb-Ⅲa）、血小板膜糖蛋白Ⅰa-Ⅱa（glycoprotein Ⅰa-Ⅱa，GP Ⅰa-Ⅱa）的基因多态性增加了冠状动脉血栓形成和冠状动脉事件发生的危险性[1-4]。在冠心病形成过程中，GP Ⅱb-Ⅲa 在血小板聚集和血栓增长中起关键作用[5]，而关于 GP Ⅱb 人类血小板抗原-3（human platelet antigen-3，HPA-3）基因多态位点与冠心病相关性研究，目前国内尚未见报道。我们以此为研究的切入点，观察其 HPA-3（Bak^a/Bak^b）基因多态性在汉族人中的分布状况，分析该多态性与冠心病易感性的相关性。

1. 材料和方法

1.1 对象

所收集病例为北京、河北地区无血缘关系汉族人，全部来源于 2005 年 3 月至 2007 年 5 月就诊于西苑医院和安贞医院者，据入选标准分为冠心病组、健康对照组。健康对照组来自西苑医院体检中心查体者及本院职工查体者，为经病史调查、体检、血常规、肝功能、X 线胸部透视、心电图等检查，排除精神及重大躯体疾病，本人及家庭无精神病史，告知检查内容并自愿参加者。冠心病的诊断均符合 1979 年世界卫生组织临床命名标准化联合专题组报告《缺血性心脏病的命名及诊断》标准[6]，选择有心绞痛症状和 / 或心肌缺血的客观证据，且冠状动脉造影证实冠状动脉有显著狭窄（＞50%）者。纳入病例标准：缺血性心脏病，患者有心绞痛症状和 / 或心肌缺血的客观证据；近期冠状动脉造影证实冠状动脉有显著狭窄（＞50%）；年龄在 35 ～ 75 岁。凡同时具备以上 3 条者，均纳入试验范围。排除标准：严重感染；严重心功能不全（EF ＜ 35%）；未控制的Ⅲ级高血压患者；严

重瓣膜性心脏病；1 型糖尿病；合并严重肝、肾、造血系统、神经系统等原发性疾病及精神病、恶性肿瘤患者；患者拒绝签署知情同意书，或估计依从性较差；参加其他临床试验的患者；妊娠期或哺乳期妇女。所有入选对象中，冠心病组 212 例，男 154 例，女 58 例，平均年龄（60.4±9.2）岁；健康对照组 106 例，男 48 例，女 58 例，平均年龄（52.5±8.8）岁，均签署知情同意书。

1.2 方法

1.2.1 主要实验仪器及试剂
高速冷冻离心机（Sigma 3k-30、SORVALL^R RT7）；ABI 9700 型 PCR 仪；ABI 7700HT 型荧光定量 PCR 仪；DNA 提取试剂盒 Wizard genomic DNA purification kit（Promega）；普通 PCR 试剂：Ex Taq DNA 聚合酶，P/N：DRR 100B；Lot：CKA 1801A（大连宝生物工程有限公司）；荧光定量试剂：ABI TaqMan 2×PCR Master mix，P/N：4326614；Lot：G 15502 等。

1.2.2 基因组 DNA 提取
入选病例皆空腹抽取静脉血 2mL，EDTA 抗凝。将 300μL 血样加入含 900μL cell lysis solution 的离心管中，室温放置 10min，（13000 ～ 16000）×g 离心 20s，移弃大部分上清液，剩余 10 ～ 20μL。振荡离心管 10 ～ 15s 后，加入 nucleilysis solution 300μL，并吹吸 5 ～ 6 次后，加入 RNase solution 1.5μL，37℃水浴 15min，冰上冷却 5min。加入 protein precipitation solution 100μL 振荡 10 ～ 20s，（13000 ～ 16000）×g 离心 3min。取上清液加入含 300μL 异丙醇的离心管中，摇动直至出现大量白色 DNA 沉淀，离心 1min，弃上清液，加入 75% 乙醇翻转冲刷管壁，离心 1min，吸去上清液，室温干燥 10 ～ 15min，加入 DNA rⓌydration solution 100μL 4℃过夜，–20℃存放。

1.2.3 基因多态性检测
GP Ⅱb 存在多个基因位点的变异，关于 HPA-3（Bak^a/Bak^b）基因多态位点描述如下。

---

* 原载于《中国病理生理杂志》，2009，25（10）：1898-1902

表 1 GP Ⅱb HPA-3（Bakᵃ/Bakᵇ）多态位点

Amino acid pos	HPA classification	Personal name classification	db SNP allele	dbSNP rs# cluster id
GP Ⅱ b	HPA-3a	Bakᵃ	A	Rs5911
lle 843 Ser	HPA-3b	Bakᵇ	C	

SNP：single nucleotide polymorphism.

GP Ⅱb 的多态性检测采用 TaqMan 探针技术。TaqMan 探针技术包括普通 TaqMan、TaqMan MGB、TaqMan LNA，虽然后两者灵敏度和特异性较前者要高，但由于我们所检测的序列 GC 含量较高，所以采用更为适合的普通 TaqMan 探针。

GP Ⅱb HPA-3（Bakᵃ/Bakᵇ）多态位点探针和引物采用 ABI Primer Express 2.0 软件设计：XM-rs5911-FAM（t）：FAM-TGCCCAtCCCCAGCCCC-TAMRA，Tm=66，GC%=76.5，Length=17；XM-rs5911-VIC（g）：VIC-CTGCCCAgCCCCAGCCC-TAMRA，Tm=65.9，GC%=82.9，Length=17；XM-rs5911-FP：GGCCTGACCACTCCTTTGC，Tm=59.2，GC%=63.2，Length=19；XM-rs5911-RP：TCACTA CGAGAACTGGATCCTGAA，Tm=58.9，GC%=45.8，Length=24；amplicon：Tm=87，GC%=66，Length=157。

将所有样本 DNA 浓度（5～15μg/100μL）调整到 20～50mg/L。引物和探针检测 PCR 反应体系分别见表 2、表 3。GP Ⅱb 引物检测 PCR 循环条件：预变性 94℃ 5min，94℃ 30s，58℃ 30s，72℃ 30s，40 个循环，72℃ 延伸 10min，4℃ 保存。GP Ⅱb 探针检测 PCR 循环条件：预变性 95℃ 10min，95℃ 5s，60℃ 30s，60℃ 30s，40 个循环。引物和探针检测通过后，即按照上述反应条件进行正式实验，检测 PCR 产物荧光强度变化，用 ABI 7700 HT 型荧光定量 PCR 仪，按 7700 用户手册操作。

1.3 统计学处理

统计分析采用 SPSS 11.5 统计分析软件。计数资料用卡方检验，两组计量资料采用 t 检验，多组均数间的显著性检验采用方差分析。对冠心病与基因多态性相关性进行非条件 Logistic 回归分析。

2. 结果

2.1 HPA-3（Rs5911）多态位点分型图

HPA-3（Rs5911）基因多态位点分型图如图 1 所示。3 种基因型都有表达，其中纯合子 AA 型

表 2 GP Ⅱb 引物检测 PCR 反应体系

Reaction component	Concentration	Volume（μL）
10×PCR buffer	10×	2.5
dNTP	2.5μg/L	2
Forward primer	20μg/L	0.5
Reverse primer	20μg/L	0.5
Ex-Taq		0.125
H₂O		18.375
Template		1
Total		25

表 3 GP Ⅱb 探针检测 PCR 反应体系

Reaction component	Concentration	Volume （μL）
2×TaqMan Master Mix	2×	5.0
Forward primer	10μg/L	0.45
Reverse primer	10μg/L	0.45
TaqMan Fam probe	10μg/L	0.25
TaqMan Tet probe	10μg/L	0.25
Template DNA	10μg/L	2.0
ddH₂O		1.6
Total		10

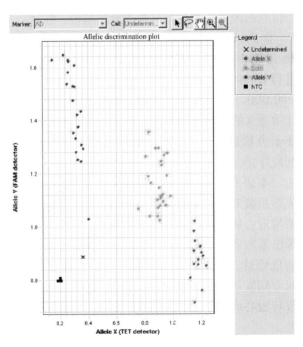

图 1 Rs5911 位点分型图

NTC：no template control，undetermined；red spot：allele Chomozygote；blue spot：allele A homozygote；green spot：heterozygote

即为 HPA-3a/3a，纯合子 CC 型即为 HPA-3b/3b，杂合子 AC 即为 HPA-3a/3b。

2.2 HPA-3（Rs5911）多态位点基因型分布比较

318 例受检者中，AA 型 98 例，AC 型 158 例，CC 型 62 例，A 等位基因频率 55.66%，C 等位基因频率 44.34%，经卡方检验，HPA-3 基因型分布频率观测值与预计值无显著差异（$P > 0.05$），符合 Hardy Weinberg 平衡。说明样本来自一个较大的、处于随机婚配平衡状态的群体，具有一定代表性。冠心病组和健康对照组比较基因型构成无显著差异（$P > 0.05$），见表 4。

2.3 冠状动脉病变支数与基因型分布比较

冠心病患者不同病变支数，基因型构成无显著差异（$P > 0.05$），见表 5。

2.4 根据年龄分层年龄 > 45 岁者基因型比较

至少含有 1 个 HPA-3b 等位基因者较 HPA-3a/3a 原生型纯合子，冠心病患者（72.4%/27.6%）多于健康人（57.1%/42.9%）。在年龄 > 45 岁的人群中，基因型在冠心病组和健康对照组两组间的分布具有显著差异（$P < 0.05$），见表 6。

2.5 校正年龄、性别、体重指数的冠心病 Logistic 回归分析

以是否患冠心病为因变量（赋值：健康 1，冠心病 2），以年龄、性别、体重指数、Rs5911 多态位点基因型为自变量（计数资料赋值：性别：男 1，女 2；GP Ⅱb 等位基因：含有至少 1 个 HPA-3b 为 1，不含有 HPA-3b 为 2）建立回归模型，进行 Binary Logistic 回归分析。似然比卡方检验 $P=0.000$，说明自变量中至少有 1 个的作用是有统计学意义的，模型有意义。对回归方程模型适配度作卡方检验，$P < 0.05$，有显著意义，模型适配度良好。

本研究结果显示（表 7），校正年龄、性别、体重指数对冠心病影响后，Rs5911 多态位点基因型与冠心病发病密切相关，含有至少 1 个 HPA-3b 等位基因者较 HPA-3a/HPA-3a 纯合型发生冠心病的危险性是 2.105 倍。年龄、性别、体重指数与冠心病发病密切相关（$P < 0.01$），年龄、体重指数与冠心病呈正相关，性别（男 1，女 2）呈负相关。

3. 讨论

冠心病是由遗传和环境因素共同作用所致的一种多基因疾病[7]，冠心病的发生、发展过程中，

动脉粥样硬化与血栓形成是两个重要的病理因素。血小板在动脉血栓形成过程中起着十分重要的作用，它的黏附、聚集和活化反应是通过血小板膜糖蛋白的功能实现的。其中重要的血小板膜糖蛋白有 GP Ⅰb-Ⅸ、GP Ⅰa-Ⅱa、GP Ⅰc-Ⅱa、GP Ⅱb-Ⅲa、GP Ⅳ 等。GP Ⅱb-Ⅲa 的基因编码定位于第 17 号上 q21-22 带 1 个约 260kb 大小的片段内，GP Ⅱb 基因长约 17kb，含有 30 个外显子，GP Ⅲa 基因长约 60kb，含有 14 个外显子。二者不能单独表现于细胞膜表面，需先在内质网形成复合物再表达于胞浆膜上，形成完整的功能单位。GP Ⅱb-Ⅲa 有多个多态位点，我们选取发现最早、研究最广泛的基因多态位点之一 -HPA-3 为研究对象。

关于 GP Ⅱ bHPA-3 基因多态位点与冠心病相关性研究，目前国内尚未见报道，多集中于人群分布情况的研究，国际人类基因组单体型图计划检测结果显示，45 位无血缘关系中国北京汉族人，3 种表型 HPA-3a/3a、HPA-3a/3b、HPA-3b/3b 分别占 33.1%、40.0%、26.7%，而近期的另一项研究结果显示[8]，在入选的 1000 例无血缘关系汉族人中，HPA-3a 和 HPA-3b 分别占 59.35% 和 40.65%。在本研究中冠心病组 3 种表型分别占 27.4%、52.3%、20.3%，健康对照组分别是 37.8%、44.3% 和 17.9%，组间比较无显著差异（$P > 0.05$）。冠心病患者不同病变支数基因型构成比较无显著差异（$P > 0.05$）。

国外该位点与冠心病相关性的研究多兼顾了冠心病的其他危险因素进行分析。来自于韩国的研究显示[9]，在小于 56 岁的人群中 HPA-3（GP Ⅱb）多态性与急性心肌梗死有关；另一关于 GP Ⅱb 的研究显示[10]，Ser843 多态性可能增加伴有其他冠心病危险因素的年轻女性患心肌梗死的危险性。在本研究按年龄进行分层比较时，我们发现大于 45 岁的人群中，至少含有 1 个 HPA-3b 等位基因者较 HPA-3a/3a 原生型纯合子，冠心病患者（72.4%/27.6%）多于健康人（57.1%/42.9%），此时不同基因型在冠心病组和健康对照组两组间的分布具有显著差异（$P < 0.05$）。可见年龄 > 45 岁含有 HPA-3b 等位基因者较携带 HPA-3a/3a 等位基因者发生冠心病的人数更多，HPA-3 多态性与年龄 > 45 岁的人群发生冠心病具有相关性，是冠心病发生的危险因素之一。以是否患冠心病为因变量的二分类 Binary Logistic 回归分析，校正年龄、性别、体重指数对冠心病的影响后，结果

表 4　HPA-3 多态位点基因型构成比较

Group	n	Genotypes n（%）			P
		HPA-3a/3a	HPA-3a/3b	HPA-3b/3b	
CHD patients	212	58（27.4）	111（52.3）	43（20.3）	0.166
Healthy subjects	106	40（37.8）	47（44.3）	19（17.9）	

表 5　冠状动脉病变支数与基因型分布比较

Different numbers of occlusive coronary artery	n	Genotypes n（%）			P
		HPA-3a/3a	HPA-3a/3b	HPA-3b/3b	
Single branch lesion	80	22（27.5）	38（47.5）	20（25.0）	
Two branch lesions	78	21（26.9）	43（55.2）	14（17.9）	0.731
Three branch lesions	54	15（27.8）	30（55.6）	9（16.6）	

表 6　年龄＞45 岁者基因型比较

Group	n	Geno types n（%）		P
		HPA-3a/3a	HPA-3a/3b+HPA-3b /3b	
CHD patients	203	56（27.6）	147（72.4）	0.012
Healthy subjects	84	36（42.9）	48（57.1）	

表 7　校正年龄、性别、体重指数的冠心病 Logistic 回归分析

Variables	B	S.E	P	Exp（B）
Age	0.116	0.017	0.000	1.123
Sex	−1.344	0.294	0.000	0.261
Body mass index	0.242	0.053	0.000	1.273
Genotype with at least one HPA-3b	0.744	0.301	0.013	2.105

显示 Rs5911 多态位点基因型与冠心病发病密切相关，含有至少 1 个 HPA-3b 等位基因者较 HPA-3a/HPA-3a 纯合型发生冠心病的危险性是 2.105 倍，Rs5911 多态位点基因型是冠心病发病的危险因素。本模型其他入选因素中，年龄、性别、体重指数与冠心病发病密切相关（$P < 0.01$），男性、年龄增长、体重指数增加都会增加发生冠心病的危险性。

综上所述，HPA-3 多态位点是北京地区汉族人冠心病发病的危险因素，在年龄＞45 岁的人群中表现明显。《难经·七十七难》提出了"上工治未病"的思想，对含有 HPA-3b 基因型的人群自年轻时即强化进行冠心病一级预防，这将为冠心病的预防提供一个全新的方向，并为实现个体化诊治提供初步的依据。

参考文献

[1] Melus V, Pullmann R, Hybenova J, et al. Is PLA1/PLA2 gene polymerphism of platelet membrane glycoprotein Ⅲa a risk factor for myocardial infarct？Bratisl Lŵ Listy, 1999, 100(11): 593-597.

[2] Mikkelsson J, Perola M, Penttila A, et al. Platelet glycoprotein Ⅰb alpha HPA-2 Met/VNTR B haplotype as a genetic predictor of myocardial infarction and sudden cardiac death. Circulation, 2001, 104(8): 876-880.

[3] Beer JH, Pederiva S, Pontiggia L. Genetics of platelet receptor single-nucleotide polymorphisms: clinical implications in thrombosis. Ann Med, 2000, 32(Suppl1):10-14.

[4] Bray PF, Howard TD, Vittinghoff E, et al. Effect of genetic variations in platelet glycoproteins Ib alpha and VI on the risk for coronary heart disease events in postmenopausal women taking hormone therapy. Blood, 2007, 109 (5): 1862-1869.

[5] Jackson SP, Schoenwaelder SM. Antiplatelet therapy: in search of the "magic bullet". Nat Rev Drug Discov, 2003, 2 (10): 775-789.

[6] 陈灏珠. 实用内科学. 12 版. 北京：人民卫生出版社，2005.1472-1473.

[7] 张玉玲，周淑娴，赵晓燕，等. 心肌梗死患者血管紧张素转换酶基因多态性与 ACE、PAI-1 活性的相关性. 中国病理生理杂志，2006，22 (12)：2336-2339.

[8] Huang H, Feng ML, Shen T, et al. Polymorphism of the human platelet alloantigens HPA-3 and HPA-9w in the Chinese Han population. Zhonghua Yi Xue Yi Chuan Xue Za Zhi, 2007, 24(5): 586-588.

[9] Park S, Park HY, Park C, et al. Association of the gene polymorphisms of platelet glycoprotein Ia and IIb-IIIa with myocardial infarction and extent of coronary artery disease in the Korean population. Yonsei Med J, 2004, 45(3): 428-434.

[10] Reiner AP, Schwartz SM, Kumar PN, et al. Platelet glycoprotein IIb polymorphism, traditional risk factors and non-fatal myocardial infarction in young women. Br J Haematol, 2001, 112(3): 632-636.

Correlation between Platelet Gelsolin Levels and Different Types of Coronary Heart Disease[*]

LIU Yue　YIN Hui-jun　JIANG Yue-rong　XUE Mei　CHEN Ke-ji

Coronary heart disease (CHD) remains a major global public health problem. Platelets play an important role in hemostasis but are also responsible for the formation of pathogenic thrombi underlying acute clinical manifestations of vascular atherothrombotic disease. Multiple pathways, including adenosine diphosphate (ADP), thromboxane A_2 (TXA_2), and thrombin are capable of activating platelets. Deregulated platelet activation can lead to the formation of platelet-rich thrombi that occlude the arterial lumen and are capable of causing ischemia and cardiovascular events. Oral antiplatelet drugs are a milestone in the therapy of cardiovascular atherothrombotic diseases. The efficacy of antiplatelet drugs, such as aspirin and clopidogrel, in decreasing the risk of adverse events in CHD patients has been well studied in the past 20 years. Despite oral antiplatelet therapy, a number of adverse CHD events continue to occur. In recent years, many reports have shown a possible relationship between residual platelet activity, as measured by a variety of laboratory tests, and clinical outcomes; raising the possibility that "resistance" to oral antiplatelet drugs may underlie many such adverse events[1]. These phenomena suggest that other pathways capable of stimulating platelet activation may exist. It is therefore meaningful to identify new therapeutic targets for anti-platelet therapy for CHD.

Using differential proteomics in platelets, our previous studies [2] found that gelsolin protein levels show the highest difference between the platelets of CHD patients and healthy controls. This suggests that the platelet cytoskeleton may play an important role in CHD development.

* 原载于 Chinese Science Bulletin，2012，57 (6)：631-638

Based on previous results, this paper further studied the distribution of gelsolin in human platelets and plasma, and studied any potential correlation with different types of CHD to verify the role of platelet gelsolin in CHD development.

1. Methods

1.1　Diagnostic Criteria

Patient diagnosis meet the standards established under the ACC/AHA/ACP-ASIM Guidelines (1999)[3]for the management of patients with chronic stable angina, and the ACC/AHA Guidelines (2002)[4] for the management of patients with unstable angina and non-ST-segment elevation myocardial infarction. We selected those patients having symptoms of angina and/or objective evidence of myocardial ischemia and those with at least one marked coronary stenosis (> 50%) shown by coronary arteriography examination.

1.2　Inclusion and Exclusion Criteria

The inclusion standard required that patients must meet all the following criteria, namely, (1) falls under one of the various classifications of ischemic heart diseases；(2) suffering from angina pectoris symptoms and/or showing signs of myocardial ischemia；(3) latest coronary arteriography examination showing significant stenosis (> 50%)；(4) age between 35 to 75 years.

Patients who met any one of the following conditions were excluded: severe valvuloplasty, diabetes mellitus type I, presence of severe primary diseases of the liver, kidney, hemopoietic system, presence of malignant tumors, calcium channel blockers (CCB) administration in the last two weeks, inability to obtain informed consent or deemed poor compliance case, participation in other clinical trials, and pregnant or lactating women.

Subjects enrolled in the healthy control group (31 cases) were identified as healthy by history and physical examination. Tests included routine blood count, liver function, chest X-ray, and electrocardiograph (ECG) , no history of prior administration of drugs affecting atherosclerotic or thrombotic processes in the last two weŵs, no history of significant mental or physical diseases nor history of familiar or self-psychiatric illnesses. This study is in accordance with the Helsinki Declaration [5], with no contravention to medical ethics.

1.3　Blood Preparation

Fresh blood (12mL) was drawn from an antecubital vein and collected into vacutainer tubes containing acid-citrate-dextrose (ACD) 9% v/v (trisodium citrate 22.0g/L, citric acid 8.0g/L, dextrose 24.5g/L) as anticoagulant, and the initial 2 mL of blood discarded to avoid spontaneous platelet activation. We collected the blood of patients before antithrombotic therapy and angiography examination. The blood was centrifuged for 10min at $150 \times g$ at room temperature to obtain platelet-rich plasma (PRP) and the remaining blood centrifuged for 20min at $800 \times g$ to obtain platelet poor plasma (PPP) 。

1.4　Determination of CD62p Expression in Platelets

We determined the level of platelet activation, as represented by the fluorescent intensity of platelet glycoprotein CD62p, by flow cytometry (EPICS Elite, Beckman Coulter Inc., Fullerton, CA, USA). We mixed the blood evenly and completed the following procedures within 4 h. Control and test tubes containing 50μL of blood had 20μL of homotype control CD61-FITC/CD62p-PE (CD61-FITC, Anti-GPIIIa, Cat: 348093；CD62p-PE, Anti-GMP-140, Cat: 348107；Becton Dickinson Co., Franklin Lakes, NJ, USA) added. Samples were mixed evenly by light shaking, and incubated in darkness at room temperature for 20 min. One milliliter of cold (2-8℃) fixative liquid was added into each tube, mixed well and incubated again in darkness at 2-8 ℃ for 30 min. Samples were then analyzed by flow cytometry to measure the mean fluorescence intensity (MFI) of CD62p. We used multi-parameter and multi-fluorescent flow cytometry with standard fluorescent micro-balloon adopted to correct the beam path and stream. Test data was obtained by Forward Scatter (FSC) *vs*. Side Scattering (SSC) gate, flow cytometry special software (Expo32, Beckman Coulter Inc.) .

1.5 Determination of Platelet Aggregation Rate (PAR)

We determined the PAR among different patients groups using turbidimetry (Platelet Aggregation Instrument, LBY-NJ2, Beijing Lipusheng Co., China). The inducer of platelet aggregation is arachidonic acid (AA, Helena Biosciences Co., Sunderland, Tyne and Wear, UK) .

1.6 Determination of $[Ca^{2+}]_i$ in Platelets

Platelet-rich plasma was prepared and incubated with 4μmol/L Fluo-3-AM (Sigma, Saint Louis, MO, USA) at 37 ℃ for 40 min. The Ca^{2+} concentration of platelets was determined using flow cytometry to measure their MFI, as previously described [6]. The platelet Ca^{2+} concentration (nmol/L) is calculated as $[Ca^{2+}]_i = K_d \times (F\text{-}F_{min}) / (F_{max}\text{-}F)$ [7].

1.7 Determination of Gelsolin, F-actin and Gc-globulin

The plasma concentration (PRP and PPP) of gelsolin (Cat: E0372h, R&D Co., Minneapolis, MN, USA) , F-actin (Cat: E1876h, R&D Co.) and Gc-globulin (Cat: E1910h, R&D Co.) were determined by enzyme-linked immunoadsorbent assay (ELISA) , as per the manufacturer's instructions.

1.8 Statistical Analysis

Statistical analysis was conducted using SPSS 13.0 software package. Data are expressed as mean±standard deviation ($\bar{x}\pm s$) or counts (percentage) , unless otherwise specified. We used Chi-square or rank sum test to evaluate enumeration data. For measurement data, we used variance analysis or t-tests. We assessed correlations of platelet gelsolin with other variables by Spearman correlation coefficient and unitary linear regression. A P-value of < 0.05 was considered statistically significant.

2. Results

2.1 General Clinical Materials

All CHD patients enrolled were in-patients admitted from August 2010 to February 2011 in Beijing Anzhen Hospital of Capital Medical University and were diagnosed and assigned to the SAP (33 cases) , UAP (39 cases) and AMI (42 cases) groups accordingly.

There was no statistical difference among the three groups in age, sex and platelet count ($P > 0.05$). The risk factors (smoking, hypertension, dyslipidemia and diabetes history), location of affected coronary artery and medication history (statins and aspirin) was comparable among the three groups ($P > 0.05$) (Table 1) .

2.2 Comparison of Plasma Gelsolin Concentration of CHD Patients among Each Patient Group

Compared with the control group, the gelsolin concentration in the PRP of the UAP and AMI groups was significantly higher ($P < 0.01$) , while that in the PPP of the three patients groups decreased markedly ($P < 0.01$). Compared with the SAP group, the gelsolin concentration in the PRP of the UAP and AMI groups was significantly higher ($P < 0.01$) (Table 2) .

2.3 Comparison of CD62p and $[Ca^{2+}]_i$ of Platelets for CHD Patients among Each Patient Group

Compared with healthy controls, the CD62p and $[Ca^{2+}]_i$ of platelets was significantly higher ($P < 0.01$) among the three patient groups. Compared with the SAP group, the CD62p and $[Ca^{2+}]_i$ of platelets among the UAP and AMI groups was significantly higher ($P < 0.01$) again (Figures 1 and 2) .

2.4 Comparison of PAR for CHD Patients among Each Patient Group

Compared with healthy controls, the PAR of the three patient groups was markedly increased ($P<0.01$). Compared with the SAP group, the PAR of the UAP and AMI groups was significantly increased ($P<0.01$) again (Figure 3).

2.5 Comparison of F-actin and Gc-globulin Concentration for CHD Patients among Each Patient Group

Compared with healthy controls, the F-actin of the UAP and AMI groups was significantly increased ($P < 0.05$ and $P < 0.01$ respectively).

Table 1 Clinical Features of Each Study Groups

Parameter	CHD patients			Control group（31 cases）
	SAP group（33 cases）	UAP group（39 cases）	AMI group（42 cases）	
Age（years，$\bar{\chi} \pm s$）	54.0±6.5	52.5±5.5	51.5±7.5	50.5±8.0
Male/females（case）	26/7	30/9	35/7	23/8
Risk factor [case（%）]				
Hypertension	15（45.5）	17（43.6）	20（47.6）	0
Dyslipidemia	14（42.4）	17（43.6）	19（45.2）	0
Diabetes	4（12.1）	4（10.3）	5（11.9）	0
Current smokers	22（66.7）	25（64.1）	29（69.05）	0
Medication [case（%）]				
Aspirin	20（60.6）	24（61.5）	26（61.9）	0
Statins	13（39.4）	15（38.5）	17（40.5）	0
Single-vessel disease [case（%）]	12（36.4）	15（38.5）	16（38.1）	0
Multi-vessel disease [case（%）]	21（63.6）	24（61.5）	26（61.9）	0
Platelet count（$\times 10^3$/μL）	214±56.9	215±38.8	216±22.8	210.9±42.7

Table 2 Comparison of Plasma Gelsolin Concentration among Different Patient Groups（$\bar{\chi} \pm s$，μg/mL）[a]

Group	Case	PRP	PPP
SAP	33	105.13±15.27[**]	109.17±18.12[**]
UAP	39	128.23±17.55[**][++]	112.58±11.47[**]
AMI	42	162.16±21.07[**][++]	112.40±8.66[**]
Control	31	117.55±9.91	121.44±6.77

a）[**]，$P < 0.01$，compared with the control group；[++]，$P < 0.01$，compared with the SAP group

The Gc-globulin of the three CHD groups was also significantly higher（$P < 0.01$）. Compared with the SAP group, the F-actin of the AMI group was significantly increased（$P < 0.01$）. However, the Gc-globulin of the other two groups was not statistically different（$P > 0.05$）（Figure 4）.

2.6 Analyses of Correlations Between Platelet Gelsolin Concentration and CD62p or Plasma F-actin Levels among Each Patient Group

Next, we investigated any potential correlation between the platelet gelsolin concentration and CD62p or plasma F-actin levels that may exist between the SAP, UAP and AMI groups. Correlation analysis showed that platelet gelsolin concentrations were high positively correlated with

CD62p or plasma F-actin levels in each of the three patient groups（Figure 5）.

3. Discussion

CHD is a leading cause of death in many developed countries. It is increasingly clear that cardiovascular outcomes depend on an understanding of the biology of CHD, which may involve vascular inflammation, endothelial dysfunction, and plaque instability[8], among others. Activated platelets play a pivotal role in the formation of arterial thrombi[9]. CD62p (P-selection) is a 140 kD glycoprotein that is present in the granules of platelets and translocates rapidly to the cell surface after platelet activation, and is generally

第一章

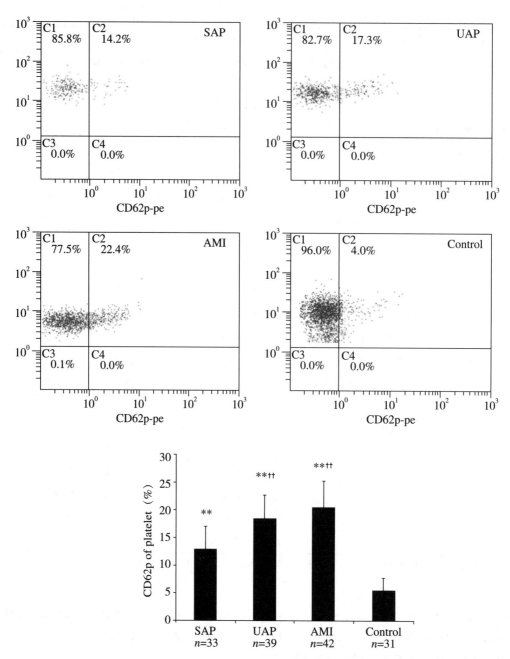

Figure 1　Comparison of CD62p of Platelet for CHD Patients among Different Groups(mean ± standard deviation). SAP group, 12.97% ± 4.01%; UAP group, 18.62% ± 4.05%; AMI group, 20.54% ± 6.75%; Control group, 5.55% ± 2.20%.**, $P < 0.01$, compared with the control group; ++, $P < 0.01$, compared with the SAP group

considered to be the gold marker of platelet activation[10,11]. There is evidence that patients with various types of CHD, including stable[12] and unstable[13] angina and acute myocardial infarction[14] have increased CD62p levels. Among all types of CHD, symptomatic stable angina is a clinical expression of myocardial ischemia associated with fixed atherosclerotic coronary stenosis；however,

patients with acute coronary syndrome (ACS) constitute the major proportion of persons who require admission to cardiac units for urgent care, including invasive treatment and aggregate anticoagulant and antiplaque drug therapy[15]. In this study, our results were consistent with these observations, indicating that varying degrees of platelet activation appear in all types of CHD and

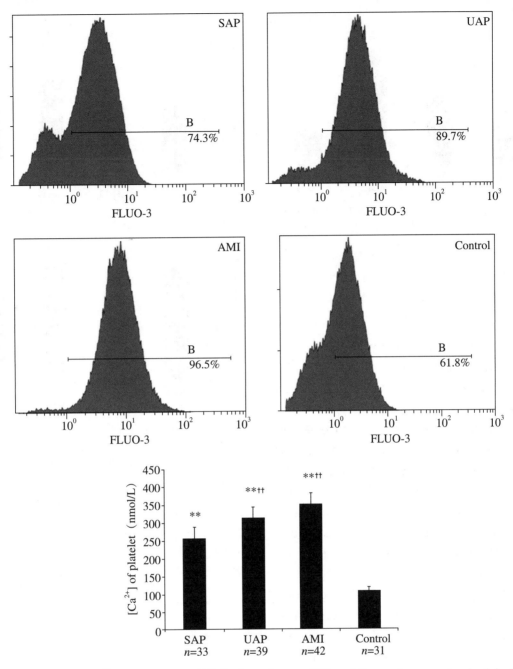

Figure 2　Comparison of $[Ca^{2+}]_i$ of Platelet for CHD Patients Among Different Groups(mean ± standard deviation). SAP group, 258.22 ± 30.19 nmol/L; UAP group, 315.98 ± 28.88 nmol/L; AMI group, 352.51 ± 32.51 nmol/L; Control group, 109.62 ± 9.84 nmol/L. **, $P < 0.01$, compared with the control group; ++, $P < 0.01$, compared with the SAP group

that ACS (including unstable angina and non-ST elevation MI) has a higher level of platelet activation and PAR compared with that of stable angina. These findings suggest an important role for CD62p in the arterial thrombosis of ACS.

Platelet activation not only causes membrane protein change, but also a series of morphological changes, from inviscid, discotic circulating platelets into a paste-like, protruding platelet jelly, that depends on the regulation of platelet cytoskeletal proteins.

Over the past ten years, laboratories have successfully applied proteomics technology to platelet research, contributing to the emerging field of platelet proteomics. Those studies led to the identification of a considerable number

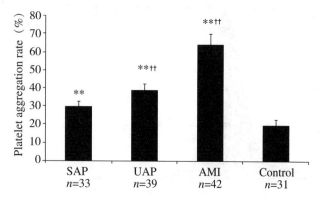

Figure 3　Comparison of Platelet Aggregation Rate(PAR) for CHD Patients among Different Groups (mean ± standard deviation). SAP group, 30.18% ± 2.6%; UAP group, 39.07% ± 3.41%; AMI group, 64.29% ± 5.67%; Control group, 20% ± 2.93%.**, $P < 0.01$, compared with the control group; ††, $P < 0.01$, compared with the SAP group

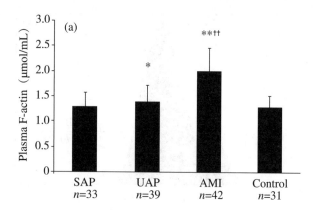

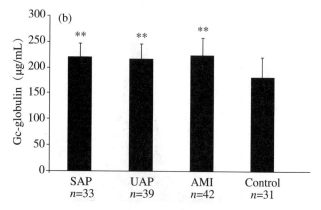

Figure 4　Comparison of F-actin and Gc-globulin Concentration for CHD Patients among Different Groups (mean ± standard deviation). (a)Plasma F-actin concentration for CHD patients among different groups. SAP group, 1.29 ± 0.29μmol/mL; UAP group, 1.41 ± 0.31μmol/mL; AMI group, 2.01 ± 0.46μmol/mL; Control group, 1.27 ± 0.25μmol/mL; (b)Plasma Gc-globulin concentration for CHD patients among different groups. SAP group, 220 ± 26.78μg/mL; UAP group, 218.27 ± 27.30μg/mL; AMI group, 224.49 ± 32.73μg/mL; Control group, 181.81 ± 37.67μg/mL. *, $P < 0.05$, **, $P < 0.01$, compared with control group; ††, $P < 0.01$, compared with SAP group

of novel platelet proteins, many of which have been studied further at a functional level[16]. Our previous study[2] had identified gelsolin as having the greatest difference in expression levels between the platelets of CHD patients and healthy subjects. However, the role of platelet gelsolin in the development of CHD is unclear.

Gelsolin is a calcium-activated F-actin severing and capping protein found in many cell types and that is expressed as both cytoplasmic and plasma isoforms, and is an important cytoskeletal protein [17]. Two regulatory mechanisms are thought to modulate gelsolin activity *in vivo*. Calcium activates gelsolin to allow capping and severing of F-actin, while phosphatidylinositol-4, 5-bisphosphate (PIP$_2$) at the cell membrane keeps gelsolin sequestered in an inactive state. Upon hydrolysis of PIP$_2$, gelsolin is released into the cytoplasm and Ca^{2+} dependent activation can occur [18]. Previous work on gelsolin has mainly focused on the calcium regulated remodeling of F-actin, while more recent data has begun to elucidate the importance of gelsolin-mediated function in pathological conditions, including cardiovascular disease [19].

During tissue injury and cell death, actin is released into the circulation where it can interact with components of the haemostatic and fibrinolytic systems, or polymerize and form F-actin. *In vitro* studies [20] have suggested that F-actin can lead to platelet aggregation directly, and the presence of F-actin in blood vessels, which can plug smaller vessels and decrease blood flow to promote the formation of blood clots, can be fatal. Infusion of high doses of G-actin in rabbits caused the rapid and fatal formation of massive actin filament-containing thrombi in arterioles and capillaries of pulmonary veins, as well as endothelial injury [21]. An actin scavenger system [22] is therefore likely to exist,

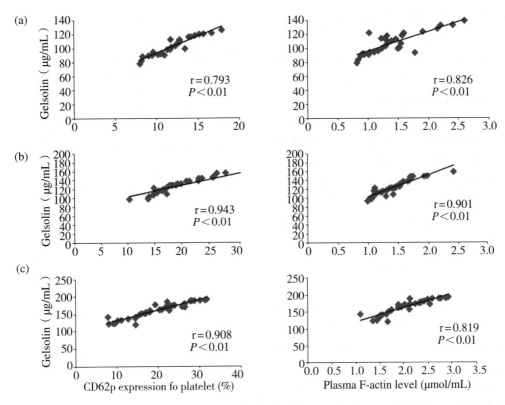

Figure 5 Analysis of Correlations Between Platelet Gelsolin Concentration and CD62p or Plasma F-actin Level among Different Groups, (a)SAP group(*n*=33); (b)UAP group(*n*=39); (c)AMI group (*n*=42)

plasma gelsolin, together with Gc-globulin, another extracellular actin-binding protein, were regarded as potentially important components of this system: capable of removing F-actin from the circulation and inhibiting F-actin elongation.

Our results were consistent with previous studies and showed that the gelsolin concentration of PPP decreased in SAP and ACS patients [23]. ACS is often associated with the rupture of vulnerable atherosclerotic plaques and coronary thrombus formation, leading to adverse outcomes. The results of this study clearly demonstrated that actin is released into the bloodstream, leading to accumulation of F-actin at the higher level of platelet activation of ACS, and that circulating actin concentrations in excess of plasma gelsolin or Gc-globulin have prothrombotic or cytotoxic activities resulting in the severe depletion of plasma gelsolin. Gc-globulin (vitamin D binding protein) is a multifunctional protein [24]; its main physiological importance is probably the binding of actin, or binding and transportation

of vitamin D analogous. Interestingly, in this study we observed that the plasma of CHD patients contains greater amounts of Gc-globulin compared with healthy subjects. Previous studies [25] demonstrated that three vitamin D binding protein isotypes were increased in asprin-resistant CHD patients and this could reduce the inhibitory effect of asprin on thromboxane A_2 production. Thus, this may suggest that the increased Gc-globulin level in this study may be associated with a large number of asprin-resistant patients included in our study or with increased reactively due to sudden severe depletion.

Another finding from our present study is the different levels of gelsolin in human platelet and plasma. Namely, an increase in platelet gelsolin levels, which was in agreement with our findings from a study of platelet proteomics [2], and a decrease in plasma gelsolin levels in ACS patients, compared to healthy subjects and stable angina patients. An analysis between platelet gelsolin concentrations and CD62p showed that platelet gelsolin levels have a high positive correlation with the level of platelet activation in ACS. Calcium ions not only promote gelsolin secretion but also play a vital role in the development of platelet activation. Studies have shown increased platelet $[Ca^{2+}]_i$ in patients with CHD [26], and that calcium chelators can reduce platelet $[Ca^{2+}]_i$ and inhibit platelet aggregation [27]. Our results showed an increased platelet $[Ca^{2+}]_i$ in ACS compared with healthy subjects and stable angina patients. The increased calcium influx in platelets could be one of the main mechanisms causing the abnormally increased platelet gelsolin levels observed in ACS.

Previous research has focused on gelsolin's possible role in cardiovascular diseases; several directions are currently being explored to test whether gelsolin itself can be used as a therapeutic molecule [28]. Our findings provide further insight into the important role of platelet gelsolin in the process of platelet activation in ACS. In this study, we have shown that platelet cytoskeletal proteins vary between different types of CHD, manifested mainly in gelsolin and F-actin. It is likely that plasma gelsolin clears away a great deal of F-actin released into circulation, and this is consistent with a role as an actin scavenger. At the onset of ACS, plasma gelsolin levels diminish significantly, while platelet gelsolin level increased abnormally, accompanied by an increased level of platelet activation and calcium influx. Platelet gelsolin levels are more highly correlated with ACS, compared to SAP. Therefore, does platelet gelsolin represent a novel therapeutic target of anti-platelet activation in ACS? We believe this is a significant area of further study, and it will be our research direction in the future.

References

[1] Gergely F, Andrea F, Gabriella P, et al. Clinical importance of aspirin and clopidogrel resistance. World J Cardiol, 2010, 2: 171-186.

[2] Li XF, Jiang YR, Wu CF, et al. Study on the correlation between platelet function proteins and symptom complex in coronary heart disease. Mol Cardiol China, 2009, 9: 326-331.

[3] Gibbons RJ, Chatterjee K, Daley J, et al. ACC/AHA/ACP-ASIM guidelines for the management of patients with chronic stable angina: a report of the American college of cardiology/American Heart Association task force on practice guidelines (committee on management of patients with chronic stable angina) . J Am Coll Cardio, 1999, 33: 2092-2197.

[4] Braunwald E, Antman EM, Kupersmith JW, et al. ACC/AHA 2002 guideline update for the management of patients with unstable angina and non-ST-segment elevation myocaridal infarction-summary article: a report of the American college of cardiology/American Heart Association task force on practice guidelines (committee on the management of patients with unstable angina) . J Am Coll Cardio, 2002, 40: 1266-1374.

[5] World Medical Association declaration of Helsinki. Recommendations guiding physicians in biomedical research involving human subjects. JAMA, 1997, 277: 925-926.

[6] Zhuang MM, Wen YX, Liu SL, et al. Determination of the level of cytopplasmic free calcium in human platelets with flow cytometry. J Xi'an Jiaotong Univ (Med Sci) , 2005, 26: 508-510.

[7] Grynkiewicz G, Poenie M, Tsien RY. A new generation of Ca^{2+} indicators with greatly improved fluorescence properties. J Biol Chem, 1985, 260: 3440-3450.

[8] Libby P. Inflammation and cardiovascular disease mechanisms. Am J Clin Nutr, 2006, 83: 456S-460S.

[9] Brydon L, Magid K, Steptoe A. Platelets, coronary heart disease, and stress. Brain BŴav Immun, 2006, 20: 113-119.

[10] Hsu-Lin S, Berman CL, Furie BC, et al. A platelet membrane protein expressed during platelet activation and secretion: studies using a monoclonal antibody specific for thrombin-activated platelets. J Biol Chem, 1984, 259: 9121-9126.

[11] Michelson AD, Furman MI. Laboratory markers of platelet activation and their clinical significance. Curr Opin Hematol, 1999, 6: 342-348.

[12] Furman MI, Benoit SE, Barnard MR, et al. Increased platelet reactivity and circulating monocyte-platelet aggregates in patients with stable coronary artery disease. J Am Coll Cardiol, 1998, 31: 352-358.

[13] Ikeda H, Takajo Y, Ichiki K, et al. Increased soluble

form of P-selectin in patients with unstable angina. Circulation, 1995, 92: 1693-1696.

[14] Shimomura H, Ogawa H, Arai H, et al. Serial changes in plasma levels of soluble P-selectin in patients with acute myocardial infarction. Am J Cardiol, 1998, 81: 397-400.

[15] Lichtman JH, Bigger JT Jr, Blumenthal JA, et al. Depression and coronary heart disease. Recommendations for screening, referral, and treatment: a science advisory from the American Heart Association Prevention Committee of the Council on Cardiovascular Nursing, Council on Clinical Cardiology, Council on Epidemiology and Prevention, and Interdisciplinary Council on Quality of Care and Outcomes Research. Endorsed by the American Psychiatric Association. Circulation, 2008, 118: 1768-1775.

[16] García A. Clinical proteomics in platelet research: challenges ahead. J Thromb Haemost, 2010, 8: 1784-1785.

[17] Kwiatkowski DJ, Stossel TP, Orkin SH, et al. Plasma and cytoplasmic gelsolins are encoded by a single gene and contain a duplicated actin-binding domain. Nature, 1986, 323: 455-458.

[18] Allen, PG. Actin filament uncapping localizes to ruffling lamellae and rocketing vesicles. Nat Cell Biol, 2003, 5: 972-979.

[19] Liu Y, Jiang YR, Yin HJ, et al. Gelsolin and cardiovascular diseases. Mol Cardiol China, 2011, 11: 50-53.

[20] Vasconcellos CA, Lind SE. Coordinated inhibition of actin-induced platelet aggregation by plasma gelsolin and vitamin D-binding protein. Blood, 1993, 82: 3648-3657.

[21] Haddad JG, Harper KD, Guoth M, et al. Angiopathic consequences of saturating the plasma scavenger system for actin. Proc Natl Acad Sci USA, 1990, 87: 1381-1385.

[22] Lee WM, Galbraith RM. The extracellular actin-scavenger system and actin toxicity. N Engl J Med, 1992, 326: 1335-1341.

[23] Suhler E, Lin W, Yin HL. Decreased plasma gelsolin concentrations in acute liver failure, myocardial infarction, septic shock and myonecrosis. Crit Care Med, 1997, 25: 594-598.

[24] White P, Cooke N. The multifunctional properties and characteristics of vitamin D-binding protein. Trends Endocrinol Metabol, 2000, 11: 320-327.

[25] López-Farré AJ, Mateos-Cáceres PJ, Sacristán D, et al. Relationship between vitamin D binding protein and aspirin resistance in coronary ischemic patients: a proteomic study. J Proteome Res, 2007, 6: 2481-2487.

[26] Kato M, Kambe M, Kajiyama G. Increased cytosolic free Mg^{2+} and Ca^{2+} in platelets of patients with vasospastic. Am J Physiol, 1998, 274: 548-554.

[27] Fujinishi A, Takahara K, Ohba C, et al. Effects of nisoldipine on cytosolic calcium, platelet aggregation, and coagulation/fibrinolysis in patients with coronary artery disease. Angiology, 1997, 48: 515-521.

[28] Li GH, Shi Y, Chen Y, et al. Gelsolin regulates cardiac remodeling after myocardial infarction through DNase I-mediated apoptosis. Circ Res, 2009, 104: 896-904.

Research on the Correlation between Platelet Gelsolin and Blood-Stasis Syndrome of Coronary Heart Disease[*]

LIU Yue   YIN Hui-jun   CHEN Ke-ji

Atherothrombosis, which directly threatens people's health and lives, is the main cause of morbidity and mortality all over the world. Atherogenesis and its underlying mechanisms has become the centre of intense research. Platelets play a key role in the development of acute coronary syndromes (ACS) and contribute to cardiovascular events. In addition, they participate in the process of forming and extending atherosclerotic plaques[1,2]. The activation of platelets may be the critical component of atherothrombosis which is the hot spot in basic and clinic research of cardiovascular diseases in recent years. Over the last decade, proteomics technology has been successfully applied to platelet research, contributing to the emerging field of platelet proteomics. Those studies led to the identification of a considerable amount of novel platelet proteins, many of which have been further studied at functional level[3]. During the last 3 years[4-6] a combination of two-dimensional gel electrophoresis and mass spectrometry-based proteomic approaches has been used to profile alterations in platelet proteins.

Our previous data demonstrate that coronary heart diseases (CHD), blood-stasis syndrome and platelet activation have close relationship[7,8]. We also study the correlation between blood stasis syndrome (BSS) /non-BSS and platelet function proteins in CHD by the differential proteomics of platelet, and find gelsolin is the main differential protein of platelet between them[9], which indicates the cytoskeleton of platelet may play a important role in the developing of BSS in CHD. Based on the previous results, this paper further studied the distribution of gelsolin in human platelet and plasma, and the correlation with BSS in CHD to verify the role of platelet gelsolin in the formation of BSS in CHD.

1. Methods

1.1 Diagnostic Criteria

Patients' diagnosis must fit the standard of the "Nomenclature and Diagnosis of Ischemic Heart Diseases" reported by the united special group for standardization of clinical nomenclature of the World Health Organization[10]. Of the patients selected were those having symptoms of angina or/and objective evidence of myocardial ischemia and those with at least one marked coronary stenosis (>50%) shown by coronary arteriongraphy examination. BSS typing was made based on the standard diagnostic criteria established by the Special Committee of Promoting Blood Circulation and Removing Blood Stasis, Chinese Association of Integrative Medicine[11]. Those enrolled must be diagnosed consistently by three Chinese medicine (CM) doctors by blind method.

1.2 Inclusion and Exclusion Criteria

The standard of inclusion required that patients must fit all the following criteria, i. e. suffering from ischemic heart diseases of any CM syndrome type; having symptoms of angina pectoris or/and objective evidence of myocardial ischemia; latest coronary arteriongraphy examination showing significant stenosis (>50%); age between 35 to 75 years.

The patient were excluded with any one of the following conditions: severe valvulopathy; type 1 diabetes mellitus; complicated with severe

* 原载于 Chinese Journal of integrative Medicine，2011，17（8）：587-592

primary diseases of the liver, kidney, hemopoietic system and malignant tumors; medication history of calcium channel blockers in the last 2 weeks; refusing to sign the informed consent or being estimated as with poor compliance; participating in other clinical trials; women in pregnancy or lactation stage.

1.3　General Clinical Materials

All CHD patients enrolled were the inpatients of Beijing Anzhen hospital, Capital Medical University, from August 2010 to December 2010, who were diagnosed and assigned to the BSS group (30 cases) and the non-BSS group (30 cases). The subjects recruited as the healthy control group (30 cases) were persons who had been identified as healthy by examination of history, physique, blood routine, live function, chest film, and ECG, etc., not taking drugs affecting atherosclerotic or thrombotic processes in the last 2 weeks, with those having mental or significant physical diseases as well as familial or self psychiatric history excluded. The study is in accord with the Helsinki Declaration, with no contravention to the medical ethics.

There was no statistic deference among the three groups in age, sex and platelet count ($P >$ 0.05). The risk factors (smoking, hypertension, dyslipidemia and diabetes history), different branches of affected coronary artery and taking medicine history (statins and aspirin) were comparable between BSS of CHD group and non-BSS of CHD group ($P > 0.05$, Table1).

1.4　Blood Preparation

Fresh blood (12mL) was drawn from an antecubital vein and collected into vacutainer tubes containing acid-citrate-dextrose (ACD) 9% v/v as anticoagulant, and the initial 2 mL of blood was discarded to avoid spontaneous platelet activation. The blood of the patients collected before the antithrombotic therapy and angiography examination. The blood was centrifuged for 10 minutes at 900 rpm ($150 \times g$) at room temperature to obtain platelet-rich plasma (PRP) and the rest of blood were centrifuged for 20 min at 3000 rpm ($800 \times g$) to obtain poor-platelet plasma (PPP).

1.5　Determination of CD62p Expression of Platelet

The level of the platelet activation repre-

Table 1　Clinical Features of the Studied Groups

Parameter	CHD patients		Healthy Control group (30 cases)
	BSS group (30 cases)	Non-BSS group (30 cases)	
Age (Years, $\bar{x} \pm s$)	53.0±7.5	52.0±8.5	49.5±9.0
Male/Females (Case)	21/9	23/7	22/8
Risk Factor [Case (%)]			
Hypertension	18 (60)	17 (56.7)	0
Dyslipidemia	17 (56.7)	15 (50)	0
Diabetes	6 (20)	7 (23.3)	0
Current smokers	19 (63.3)	20 (66.7)	0
Medication [Case (%)]			
Aspirin	23 (76.7)	25 (83.3)	0
Statins	8 (26.7)	10 (33.3)	0
Single-vessel disease [Case (%)]	11 (36.7)	12 (40)	0
Multi-vessel disease [Case (%)]	19 (63.3)	18 (60)	0
Platelet count ($\times 10^3/\mu L$)	210±45.8	207±47.3	208.9±39.1

sented by the fluorescent intensity of platelet glycoprotein CD62p was determined by flow cytometry. The blood was mixed evenly and the following procedures were finished with 4 hours. The control and test tubes contain 50μL of blood sample, then had homotype control CD61-FITC/CD62p-PE (CD61-FITC, Anti-GP Ⅲa, Cat: 348093, Lot: 49817, Becton Dickinson Co.; CD62P-PE, Anti-GMP-140, Cat: 348107, Lot: 60928, Becton Dickinson Co.) added into them respectively, 20μL in each tube. Then the samples were mixed evenly by light shaking, and incubated in darkness at room temperature for 20 min. One milliliter of cold (2-8℃) fixative liquid was added into each tube, mixed well and incubated again in darkness under 2-8℃ for 30 min; then the samples were put into the analyzer to measure the mean fluorescence intensity (MFI) of CD62p with muti-parameter and muti-color flurescent flow cytometry (EPICS Elite, Beckman Coulter Co., USA) used and standard flurescent micro-balloon adopted to correct the beam path and stream. The test data were obtained by FS vs. SS gate, Expo32 special software.

1.6　Determination of $[Ca^{2+}]_i$ of Platelet

Platelet-rich plasma was prepared and incubated with 4 μmol Fluo-3-AM (Sigma, USA) at 37℃ for 40 min, the mean fluorescence intensity (F) of Ca^{2+} of platelet was determined using flow cytometry as previously described[12], and the Ca^{2+} level of platelet (μmol/L) is calculated as follow: $[Ca^{2+}]_i = K_d \times (F-F_{min}) / (F_{max}-F)$ [13].

1.7　Determination of Gelsolin, F-actin and Gc-globulin

The plasma concentration (PRP and PPP) of gelsolin (Cat: E0372h, R&D Co., USA), F-actin (Cat: E1876h, R&D Co., USA) and Gc-globulin (Cat: E1910h, R&D Co., USA) were determined by double-antibody sandwich avidin-biotin peroxidase complex enzyme-linked immunosorbent assay (ABC-ELISA), following the instruction of Elisa-kit respectively.

1.8　Statistical Analysis

Statistical analysis was performed by SPSS 13.0 software. Chi-square or rank sum test was used to evaluate enumeration data. For measurement data, t-test or variance analysis was used. A P-value of < 0.05 was considered statistically significant.

2. Results

2.1　Comparison of Plasma Gelsolin Concentration of CHD Patients among Different Groups

Compared with the control group, the gelsolin concentration in PRP of BSS group increased significantly ($P < 0.01$), while that in PPP of BSS and non-BSS group decreased markedly ($P < 0.05$), Compared with the non-BSS group, the gelsolin concentration in PRP of BSS group increased significantly ($P < 0.01$, Table 2),

Table 2　Comparison of Plasma Gelsolin Concentration among Different Groups ($\bar{x} \pm s$, μg/mL)

Group	Case	PRP	PPP
BSS	30	$155.47 \pm 25.46^{**\triangle}$	$116.04 \pm 9.80^{*}$
Non-BSS	30	118.75 ± 26.48	$115.50 \pm 14.71^{*}$
Control	30	117.48 ± 10.08	121.45 ± 6.89

Note: $^{*}P < 0.05$, $^{**}P < 0.01$, compared with the control group; $^{\triangle}P < 0.01$, compared with the non-BSS group

2.2　Comparison of CD62p and $[Ca^{2+}]_i$ of Platelet for CHD Patients Among Different Groups

Compared with the control group, the CD62p and $[Ca^{2+}]_i$ of platelet of BSS group and non-BSS group increased significantly ($P < 0.01$). Compared with non-BSS group, $[Ca^{2+}]_i$ of platelet of BSS group increased markedly ($P < 0.01$, Table 3 and Figure 1).

2.3　Comparison of F-actin and Gc-globulin Concentration for CHD Patients among Different Groups

Compared with the control group, the F-actin and Gc-globulin of BSS and non-BSS groups increased significantly ($P < 0.01$). Compared with non-BSS of CHD group, F-actin and Gc-globulin

Table 3　Comparison of CD62p and $[Ca^{2+}]_i$ of Platelet for CHD Patients among Different Groups ($\bar{x} \pm s$)

Group	Case	CD62p（%）	$[Ca^{2+}]_i$ of platelet(nmol/L)
BSS	30	19±68±8.61*	366±87±23.34*△
Non-BSS	30	17±68±7.54*	286±49±41.99*
Control	30	5±56±2.24	109±39±9.92

Note：*$P < 0.01$，compared with the control group；△$P < 0.01$，compared with non-BSS group

Table 4　Comparison of F-actin and Gc-globulin Concentration for CHD Patients among Different Groups ($\bar{x} \pm s$)

Group	Case	F-actin (μmol/mL)	Gc-globulin (μg/mL)
BSS	30	1.74±0.52*	227.87±37.97*
Non-BSS	30	1.63±0.55*	224.20±30.39*
Control	30	1.27±0.26	181.33±38.22

Note：*$P < 0.01$，compared with the control group

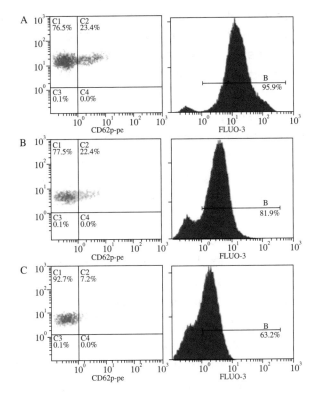

Figure 1　Flow Cytometry Analysis of CD62p-PE and $[Ca^{2+}]_i$ of Platelet

Notes：A：a CHD patient with BSS，B：a CHD patient with non-BSS，C：a healthy control subject

of BSS group have no statistic deference ($P >$ 0.05, Table 4),

3. Discussion

　　CHD is the leading cause of death throughout the world, and its development is associated with many pathogenic factors. A common feature of CHD is coronary artery occlusion, whether permanent or intermittent, as a result of the rupture of vulnerable plaque and resultant thrombosis. Activated platelets play a pivotal role in the formation of arterial thrombi[14]. BSS is the most

common CM syndrome typing, which is closely related to platelet activation and thrombosis. The combination research between disease and syndrome of BSS involves about pathology and clinical diagnostics of western medicine and traditional medicine, which makes us to know the disease deeply, and provides effective therapeutic target.

　　Platelets are anuclear cells derived from mega-karyocytes. They are produced in the bone marrow, released in the blood flow and circulate for 7 to 10 days. Under normal conditions platelets are in loose contact to the vascular wall, without adhering to the endothelium. Platelet activation leads to the release of numerous molecules stored in their granules, e.g., adenosine diphosphate (ADP), thromboxane A_2 (TXA_2), platelet-activating factor (PAF) [15]. CD62p is one of the human platelet membrane glycoprotein and only released on the activated platelet membrane, which is identified as the most specific biomarker of platelet activation now. Our results show that the expression of CD62p of BSS of CHD increased significantly compare with healthy group ($P < 0.01$), that indicate CHD has the status of platelet activation, which be consistent with previous research results[8].

　　Platelet activation can not only cause the membrane protein change, also a series of morphological changes, from inviscid, discotic circulating platelets into a paste, protruding platelet jelly, that depends on the regulation of platelet cytoskeletal protein.

　　Our previous study[9]demonstrates that gelsolin is the main differential protein of platelet between BSS of CHD and non-BSS of CHD patients. Gelsolin, discovered in 1979 by Yin and Stossel[16]based on its ability to activate the gel-sol transformation of actin filaments (F-actin) in a calcium-dependent manner, it was also one of the actin binding proteins (ABPs) that can sever or cap F-actin and as a secreted form in the plasma of vertebrates. The actin cytoskeleton plays a central role in many fundamental cellular processes involving the generation of force and facilitation of movement, which are enabled by the assembly of actin monomers (G-actin) into F-actin and cooperation with a wide variety of ABPs[17].

Some research suggests[18]that F-actin can lead to platelet aggregation directly, and the presence of filaments of actin in blood vessels can be fatal, which can plug smaller vessels and decrease blood flow to promote the formation of blood clot. Gelsolin, together with Gc-globulin, another extracellular actin-binding protein, functions as an "extracellular actin scavenger system" (EASS) responsible for the clearing of much more actin released by tissue injury[19]and hold back the lengthen of F-actin. By severing F-actin, gelsolin reduces blood viscosity by promoting polymer disassembly. Our results show that F-actin of BSS in CHD increased markedly ($P < 0.01$) while gelsolin in PPP decreased compare with healthy group ($P < 0.05$), which have coincides with the results of previous study[20]and indicates that F-actin released into the circulation at the status of platelet activation of BSS of CHD, results in the depletion of plasma gelsolin severely. Meanwhile, the plasma Gc-globulin of BSS group increased compare with the healthy group ($P < 0.01$), which may be association with elevation of irritability because of severe depletion.

Calcium ion plays a vital role in the development of platelet activation. The transformation, aggregation and release reaction of platelet are triggered by the increase of free calcium ion concentration of platelet ($[Ca^{2+}]_i$), which is the essential mechanism of thrombosis. Studies have found the increase of $[Ca^{2+}]_i$ in patient with CHD[21], meanwhile calcium antagonist can reduce $[Ca^{2+}]_i$ of platelet accompanied by inhibiting platelet aggregation[22]. Our results show that $[Ca^{2+}]_i$ and gelsolin concentration in PRP of BSS increased significantly compared with the non-BSS and control group ($P < 0.01$), which was agreement with our former study of platelet proteomic. Based on the change of $[Ca^{2+}]_i$ is the promoter of gelsolin secretion, we presume that platelet gelsolin may be as a new potential biomarker and/or therapeutic target of BSS of CHD, and the increased calcium influx of platelet could be one of the main mechanism.

The study shows that platelet cytoskeleton protein dynamic changes during the development of BSS of CHD, which focus on the gelsolin and F-actin. Plasma gelsolin clears a great deal of F-actin from circulation, and that results in depletion of plasma gelsolin severely, moreover the increased calcium influx of platelet, which may together lead to the gelsolin expression on platelet increased abnormally during the process of BSS of CHD. But could the excessive F-actin released by tissue injury at the status of platelet activation stimulate the platelet directly to secrete gelsolin increased abnormally? And are the platelet gelsolin the therapeutic target of anti-platelet activation of Chinese herbs for promoting blood circulation and removing blood stasis? These issues are well worth further investigation.

References

[1] Davi G, Patrono C. Platelet activation and athero-thrombosis. N Engl J Med, 2007, 357 (24): 2482-2494.

[2] Moliterno DJ. Advances in antiplatelet therapy for ACS and PCI. J Interv Cardiol, 2008, 21 (S11): S18-S24.

[3] Garcia A. Clinical proteomics in platelet research: challenges ahead. J Thromb Haemost, 2010, 8: 1784-1785.

[4] Thiele T, Steil L, Gebhard S, et al. Profiling of alterations in platelet proteins during storage of platelet concentrates. Transfusion, 2007, 47: 1221-

1233;

[5] Banfi C, Brioschi M, Marenzi G, et al. Proteome of platelets in patients with coronary artery disease. Experimental Hematology, 2010, 38: 341-350.

[6] Senzel L, Gnatenko DV, Bahou WF. The platelet proteome. Curr Opin Hematol, 2009, 16: 329-333.

[7] Chen KJ, Xue M, Yin HJ. The relationship between platelet activation and coronary heart disease and blood-stasis syndrome. Journal of Capital Medical University, 2008, 29 (3): 266-269.

[8] Xue M, Chen KJ, Yin HJ. Relationship between platelet activation related factors and polymorphism of related genes in patients with coronary heart disease of blood-stasis syndrome. Chin J Integr Med, 2008, 14 (4): 267-273.

[9] Li XF, Jiang YR, Wu C, et al. Study on the correlation between platelet function proteins and symptom complex in coronary heart disease. Molecular Cardiology of China, 2009, 9 (6): 326-331.

[10] Chen HZ, ed. Practical internal medicine. 12th ed. Beijing: People's Medical Publishing House, 2005, 1472-1473.

[11] Society of Cardiology, Chinese Association of the Integration of Traditional and Western Medicine. The diagnostic criteria of TCM in coronary heart disease. Chin J Integr Tradit West Med, 1991, 11 (5): 257.

[12] Zhuang MM, Wen YX, Liu SL, et al. Determination of the level of cytoplasmic free calcium in human platelets with flow cytometry. Journal of Xi'an Jiaotong University (Medical Science), 2005, 26 (5): 508-510.

[13] Grynkiewicz G, Poenie M, Tsien RY. A new generation of Ca^{2+} indicators with greatly improved fluorescence properties. J Biol Chem, 1985, 260 (6): 3440-3450.

[14] Brydon L, Magid K, Steptoe A. Platelets, coronary heart disease, and stress. Brain, Behavior, and Immunity, 2006, 20 (2): 113-119.

[15] Antoniades C, Bakogiannis C, Tousoulis D, et al. Platelet activation in atherogenesis associated with low-grade inflammation. Inflamm Allergy Drug Targets , 2010, 12, 9 (5): 334-345.

[16] Yin HL, Stossel TP. Control of cytop lasmic actin gelsol transformation by gelsolin, a calcium dependent regulatory protein. Nature, 1979, 281: 583-586.

[17] Spinardi L, Witke W. Gelsolin and diseases. Subcell Biochem, 2007, 45: 55-69.

[18] Vasconcellos CA, Lind SE. Coordinated inhibition of actin-induced platelet aggregation by plasma gelsolin and vitamin D-binding protein. Blood, 1993, 82 (12): 3648-3657.

[19] Lee WM, Galbraith RM. The extracellular actin scavenger systern and actin toxicity. N Engl J Med, 1992, 326 (20): 1335-1341.

[20] Suhler E, Lin W, Yin HL. Decreased plasma gelsolin concentrations in acute liver failure, myocardial infarction, septic shock and myonecrosis. Crit Care Med, 1997, 25: 594-598.

[21] Kato M, Kambe M, Kajiyama G. Increased cytosolic free Mg^{2+} and Ca^{2+} in platelets of patients with vasospastic. Am J Physiol, 1998, 274: 548-554.

[22] Fujinishi A, Takahara K, Ohba C, et al. Effects of nisoldipine on cytosolic calcium, platelet aggregation, and coagulation/fibrinolysis in patients with coronary artery disease. Angiology, 1997, 48: 515-521.

第
一
章

Aberrant Expression of FcγR ⅢA (CD16) Contributes to the Development of Atherosclerosis*

HUANG Ye   YIN Hui-jun   WANG Jing-shang   LIU Qian   WU Cai-feng   CHEN Ke-ji

1. Introduction

Despite considerable therapeutic advances over the past 50 years, atherosclerotic cardio-vascular disease is the leading cause of death worldwide[1]. Atherosclerosis, a chronic inflammatory state, is chiefly responsible for the development of coronary heart disease (CHD). The underlying mechanisms of CHD have not yet been elucidated. Additionally, there is little in the way of CHD-specific prevention and treatment.

The genetics of CHD has received great interest with the recent advancements in high-throughput genomics and genome-wide association studies[2]. We investigated the differential gene expression profiles of peripheral leukocytes from CHD patients with the oligonucleotide microarray technique[3]. We found that a few differentially expressed genes presumably played a crucial role in the initiation and development of CHD through the network topology analysis. Of them, Fc receptor ⅢA of immunoglobulin G (FcγR ⅢA, also called CD16) was identified to be involved in the development of CHD. We demonstrated that there was a significant increase of FcγR ⅢA at the mRNA level in leukocytes[3] and at the protein level for both soluble CD16 (sCD16) in sera and membrane CD16 on monocytes from CHD patients compared to the healthy control (data not shown). However, the mechanism of deregulated FcγR ⅢA expression implicated in the development of CHD has not yet been elucidated.

In the current study, we therefore investigated FcγR ⅢA-induced molecular events that might be responsible for the formation and development of CHD using human peripheral monocyte-umbilical vein endothelial cells (HUVECs) in vitro. We also used an aortic atherosclerosis mouse model of ApoE$^{-/-}$ mice, which has been confirmed as a model of human atherosclerotic disease. Our data together suggest that inhibition of FcγR ⅢA or its signaling may represent a promising strategy for prevention and treatment of CHD.

2. Materials and Methods

2.1　Cell Experiments

2.1.1　Purification of Monocyte and Human Umbilical Vein Endothelial Cells

Fresh whole blood was collected with informed consent from healthy donors into vacutainer tubes containing heparin. Monocytes were isolated by adherence after Ficoll-Hypaque purification of peripheral blood mononuclear cells and were cultured as described previously[4]. HUVEC isolations were carried out using the collagenase procedure developed by Jaffe[5]. Cells were cultured on gelatin and grown to subconfluence in DMEM culture medium (GIBCO, USA) containing 10% fetal calf serum supplemented with 40U/mL heparin, 10ng/mL EGF, 2mmol/L glutamine, 50U/mL penicillin, 50μg/mL streptomycin and 1 mmol/L sodium pyruvate at 37℃ under 5% CO_2. HUVECs were used for experiments at the post three passages.

2.1.2　Adhesion Assay

To investigate the role of FcγR ⅢA in regulating the adherence of monocytes to HUVECs, we

* 原载于Gene，2012，498（1）：91-95

increased the FcγR ⅢA level on monocytes stimulated by recombinant human M-CSF (Peprotech, USA) for 18 h and reduced its level by IVIG pretreatment for 1 h followed by 18-h M-CSF stimulation. The protein level of membrane CD16 on monocytes (the level of FcγR ⅢA protein) was assessed by FACS analysis. The adhesive efficiency of monocytes with HUVECs was measured by the Bradford method as described previously [6].

2.2　Animal Experimentation

2.2.1　Identification of Atherosclerosis Model

Eight-week-old male ApoE$^{-/-}$ mice and wt C57BL/6J mice with the same genetic background were obtained from Beijing University Laboratory Animal Center. Mice were housed in the facility at Xiyuan hospital, China Academy of Chinese Medical Sciences according to the guidelines for laboratory animals approved by Beijing Experimental Animal Management Center. After 1 weŵ of adaption, the ApoE$^{-/-}$ mice were switched from normal diet to high-fat diet[7] which contained 21% fat from lard with 0.15% (wt/wt) cholesterol purchased from the Experimental Animal Center of the Academy of Military Medical Sciences. Mice were maintained on this high-fat diet for 10 weeks. Twenty wt C57BL/6J mice were chosen as the control group, and 60 ApoE$^{-/-}$ mice were randomly divided into three groups, ApoE$^{-/-}$ group, ApoE$^{-/-}$ +IVIG group, ApoE$^{-/-}$ +simvastatin (Sm) group, with 20 mice in each group. Mice in the ApoE$^{-/-}$ +IVIG group received an intraperitoneal (I.P.) injection of IVIG (Chengdu Rongsheng Pharmaceutical Co., Ltd., China: 1 mg/g) daily over a 5-day period prior to the exposure to high-fat diet. Mice in the ApoE$^{-/-}$ +Sm group received Sm (Hangzhou Moshadong Pharmaceutical Co., Ltd., China: 0.026 g/kg) per gavage for 10 weŵs. Mice in C57 group and ApoE$^{-/-}$ group received PBS.

The establishment of the atherosclerosis model in ApoE$^{-/-}$ mice was evaluated by analyzing blood lipid levels and morphology of aortic roots with H&E staining as previously described[8].

2.2.2　ELISA Assay, Immunofluorescent Staining and Western Blot Analysis

Serum TNF-α, IL-1 and soluble E-selectin (sE-selectin) levels from mice were measured by ELISA according to the instructions from R&D Systems (USA). Immunofluorescent staining was performed according to the standard procedures described previously[9]. The protein level of MMP-9 in aorta was determined by Western blot analysis according to the standard procedure as previously described[10]. GAPDH was used as a loading control.

2.2.3　RT-PCR Assay

Total RNA samples were extracted from aorta using Trizol reagent (Invitrogen, USA). And then RT-PCR analysis was carried out. GAPDH was used as an internal control. The primer sequences for PCR analysis were shown below, MMP-9：forward, 5'-GCGTGTCTGGAGATTCGAC-3', reverse, 5'-CCATGGCAGAAATAGGCTTT-3': GAPDH：forward, 5'-GGGTGTGAACCATGAGAAGT-3', reverse, 5'-GGCATGGACTGT GGTCATGA-3'.

2.3　Statistical Analysis

The SPSS Statistics 13.0 package was utilized to analyze the data. Differences among groups were analyzed using the one-way analysis of variance (ANOVA), followed by multiple comparisons by LSD test. The $P < 0.05$ was considered statistically significant.

3. Results

To determine the role of FcγR ⅢA in vitro, we investigated the effect of elevation or inhibition of FcγR ⅢA level on the interaction between monocytes and HUVECs. Monocytes and HUVECs were purified first. Monocytes were characterized by their morphologies through microscopy with the Wright-Gimsa staining. The purity of monocytes was about 90% as determined by FACS analysis (Figure 1A). More than 99% HUVECs were identified to be endothelial cells by their characteristic cobblestone morphology under an inverted microscope (Leica DMIRB, Germany) and characterized by brown granules in cytoplasm using immunocytochemical staining of factor Ⅷ (Figure 1B). The CD16 level on monocytes were elevated with the stimulation of recombinant human M-CSF for 18 h. Increased protein level of membrane CD16 on monocytes was confirmed by flow cytometry. As shown in Figure 1C and D, the percentage of CD14+ CD16+ monocytes was largely increased by 59% compared to the control ($P < 0.01$; Figure 1C), and the average protein level of CD16 reflected by its fluorescent intensity was also increased by 82% ($P < 0.01$; Figure 1D). Then, we inhibited the CD16 level on monocytes by IVIG pretreatment for 1 h. The FACS analysis indicated that the portion of CD14+ CD16+ and the CD16 protein level reflected by fluorescent intensity were reduced compared to the M-CSF induction group ($P < 0.05$; Figure 1C), which is in agreement with a previous observation[11]. To assess the effect of FcγR ⅢA level changes on adherence of monocytes to HUVECs, we examined the adhesive efficiency of monocytes with elevation or inhibition of CD16 level to HUVECs. The adhesive efficiency of monocytes upon M-CSF stimulation to HUVECs was increased (> 8 fold, $P < 0.01$; Figure 1E) compared to the blank control. Correspondingly, the adhesive efficiency of monocytes with IVIG pretreatment to HUVECs was decreased by 42% compared to that of monocytes with M-CSF ($P < 0.01$; Figure 1E).

To further evaluate the role of FcγR ⅢA, we looked into its regulation on aortic atherosclerotic plaque destabilization using a mouse model of atherosclerosis in ApoE−/− mice. Aortic atherosclerotic plaque formation was induced in ApoE−/− mice after feeding on high-fat diet for 10 weeks which was confirmed by assessment of blood lipid levels and histological examination of aortic roots. As shown in Figure 2A, the levels of

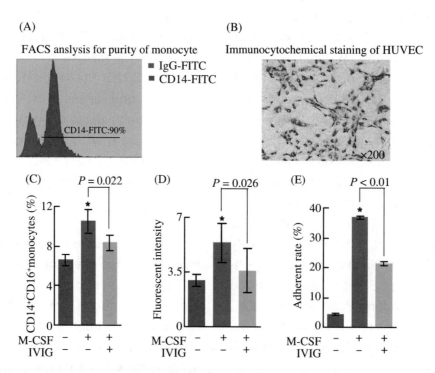

Figure 1　FcγR ⅢA Increases the Adherence of Monocytes to HUVECs. (A)FACS analysis for purity of monocyte. (B)Immunocytochemical staining of HUVEC. (C) The percentage of CD14+ CD16+ monocytes upon M-CSF stimulation for 18 h with or without 1-h IVIG pretreatment. (D) The CD16 protein level was quantified by its fluorescent intensity on the membrane of monocytes. (E) The adherent efficacy of monocytes to HUVECs. Results were presented as mean ± SD (n=6), *P < 0.01, compared to the control

TC, TG and LDL-C were increased, and HDL-C level was decreased in ApoE$^{-/-}$ mice on high-fat diet, compared to the C57 mice fed with normal rodent diet ($P < 0.01$). Correspondingly, thickened aortic intimal, massive foam cells accumulation, and atherosclerosis plaque formation were observed in ApoE$^{-/-}$ mice fed with high-fat diet evidenced by hematoxylin eosin staining (Figure 2B). Thereafter, to test whether there were FcγR ⅢA expression changes in mice with atherosclerotic plaque, we assayed the protein level of membrane CD16 on monocytes. As presented in Figure 3A and B, there was a significant increase of the protein level of membrane CD16 on monocytes reflected by the percentage of CD16-positive cells and CD16-PE fluorescent intensity in ApoE$^{-/-}$ mice compared to the control (> 3 fold, $P < 0.01$; Figure 3A), and the average protein level of CD16 reflected by fluorescent intensity was also increased by 47% ($P < 0.01$; Figure 3B). Additionally, we observed that the protein level

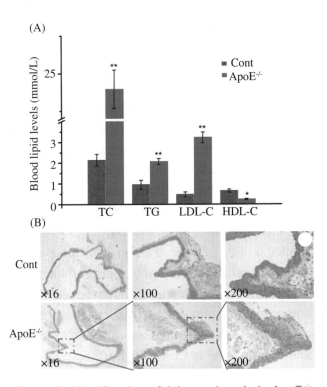

Figure 2　Identification of Atherosclerosis in ApoE$^{-/-}$ Mice. The ApoE$^{-/-}$ Mice Was Used to Be An Aortic Atherosclerosis Mouse Model. (A) TC, TG, LDL-C and HDL-C. Results were presented as mean ± SD (n=8) . $^{*}P < 0.05$, $^{**}P < 0.01$, compared with the control mice. (B) Representative images of histological examination of aortic atherosclerotic plaques in ApoE$^{-/-}$ mice through H&E staining. Dash box, which represents plaque formation, indicates the area which was magnified to 100 × image or 200 × image

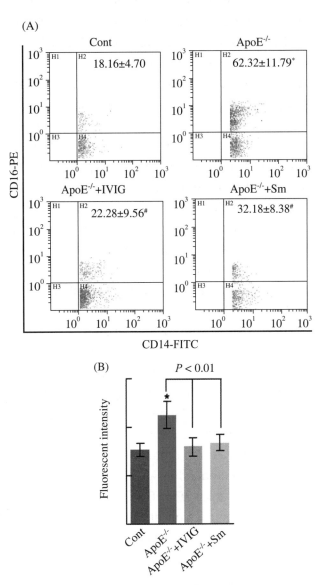

Figure 3　FcγR ⅢA Level in ApoE$^{-/-}$ Mice Fed with High-Fat Diet for 10 Weeks. (A) Representative data of FACS analysis of CD14^{+} CD16^{+} monocytes. Whole peripheral blood samples from ApoE$^{-/-}$ mice were stained with FITC- conjugated anti-CD14 antibody and PE-conjugated anti-CD16/32 antibody, followed by FACS. $^{*}P < 0.01$, compared with the control mice. $^{#}P < 0.01$, compared with the ApoE$^{-/-}$ mice. (B) The FcγR ⅢA level was reflected by its fluorescent intensity. Results were presented as mean ± SD (n=8). $^{*}P < 0.01$, compared with the control mice

of membrane CD16 on monocytes in IVIG pretreatment mice was decreased by 64% (P < 0.01; Figure 3A) compared to the ApoE$^{-/-}$mice, consistent with the *in vitro* observations (Figure 1C).

To further verify the potential role of FcγR ⅢA in atherosclerotic plaque destabilization and inflammatory response, we looked into the mRNA expression and protein level of MMP-9 in aorta and TNF-α, IL-1 and sE-selectin contents in sera, respectively. Previous studies suggested that statins (such as Simvastatin) exert a wide spectrum of pleiotropic effects on atherosclerosis in a few ways, including endothelial function improvement, nitric oxide bioavailability, inflammatory cell migration, plaque thrombogenicity, and ultimately enhancement of plaque stability, in addition to their effects on lowering LDL-C[12]. Thus, we used Simvastatin as a positive control to assess the effect of FcγR ⅢA on the atherosclerotic plaque destabilization and inflammation. Matrix-metalloproteinases (MMPs) are involved in several steps in plaque progression driving plaques into vulnerable rupture-prone states[13]. Of them, MMP-9 cleaves different bioactive molecules, implicated in plaque destabilization and inflammatory modulation in atherosclerosis[14]. As shown in Figure 4A and B, both the mRNA and protein levels of MMP-9 of aorta were increased in ApoE$^{-/-}$ mice compared to the control mice (P < 0.01). In contrast, both the mRNA expression and its protein level of MMP-9 in aorta were reduced by 36% and 15%, respectively, in IVIG pretreatment mice, compared with the ApoE$^{-/-}$ mice (Figure 4A and B). The role of FcγR ⅢA inhibition by IVIG in atherosclerotic plaque destabilization in ApoE$^{-/-}$ mice was Similar to that with Simvastatin treatment. To examine the impact of FcγR ⅢA on inflammation, we assessed TNF-α, IL-1 and sE-selectin content in sera via ELISA. We observed increased serum levels of TNF-α, IL-1 and sE-selectin in ApoE$^{-/-}$ mice, compared to the C57 mice: whilst the

serum levels of TNF-α, IL-1 and sE-selectin in ApoE$^{-/-}$ mice with inhibition of FcγR ⅢA were decreased compared to the ApoE$^{-/-}$ mice (Figure 4C). The effect of FcγR ⅢA inhibition by IVIG on inflammation was similar to the ApoE$^{-/-}$ mice treated with Simvastatin (Figure 4C).

4. Discussion

Cardiovascular disease is the leading cause of death worldwide, accounting for almost 16.7million deaths each year, with CHD as its major manifestation[15]. Little is known regarding the mechanism of CHD. However, inflammation, one of the main mechanisms, is implicated in several stages of CHD development including atherosclerosis, plaque destabilization and plaque rupture[16]. Fc receptors (FcRs), a group of membrane glycoproteins that belong to the immunoglobulin superfamily, are the specific receptors for the Fc regions of immunoglobulins expressed in most leukocytes. FcRs are defined by their specificity for immunoglobulin isotypes [17]. Fcγ receptor (FcγR) plays an essential role in the process of immunoinflammatory responses, which is used as an important trigger molecule for inflammation, allergy, and cytophagy[18]. Of them, FcγR ⅢA (CD16) is a transmembrane subtype and mainly expressed on monocytes[19]. Previous studies on FcγR ⅢA have extensively focused on the relationship between gene polymorphisms or gene expression differences and diseases[20-22]. In agreement with previous studies, our recent study also suggested that increased mRNA expression and protein level of FcγR ⅢA were correlated to CHD development, and FcγR ⅢA was mainly expressed on monocytes (data not shown).

The recruitment of monocytes to the vessel wall is an early step in the formation of atherosclerotic lesions[23]. Adhesion is a complex process characterized by rolling and tethering monocytes to the endothelial surface[24]. The majority of monocytes located in the luminal endothelium, differentiate into macrophages,

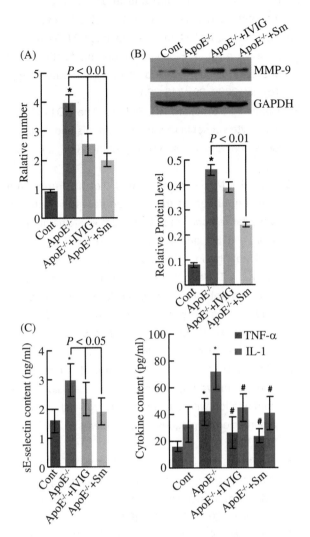

Figure 4　The Changes of MMP-9 and Inflammatory Cytokines in ApoE$^{-/-}$ Mice. (A)Relative expression level of MMP-9 in aorta evaluated by qRT-PCR. $^*P <$ 0.01, compared with the control mice. (B)Western blot analysis of MMP-9 in aorta. The band intensity was normalized to GAPDH, and the average band intensity after normalization was presented in the bar graph. $^*P <$ 0.01, compared with the control mice. (C) The levels of TNF-α, IL-1 and sE-selectin in sera. $^*P <$ 0.01, compared with the control mice. $^\#P <$ 0.01, compared with the ApoE$^{-/-}$ mice. Results were presented as mean ± SD (n=8)

which play an important role in engulfing normal or modified LDL, forming lesion and ultimately disrupting plaques[25]. Therefore, the monocyte-endothelial cell interaction is crucial for the development of atherosclerosis. We thus assumed that FcγR ⅢA might play a key role in

the adherence of monocytes to endothelial cells. In the current study, we demonstrated that the protein level of membrane CD16 on monocytes could be enhanced by recombinant human M-CSF *in vitro*, consistent with a previous observation [26], and IVIG could suppress the membrane CD16 level on monocytes. Furthermore, the elevated level of FcγR ⅢA on monocytes closely correlated to the adhesive efficiency of monocytes to HUVECs.

Some studies confirmed the validity of ApoE$^{-/-}$ mice as a model of human atherosclerotic disease[27]. Therefore, we further investigated the mechanisms underlying FcγR ⅢA induced events in the aortic atherosclerotic formation *in vivo* using the ApoE$^{-/-}$ mouse model. We showed that the protein level of membrane CD16 on monocytes was significantly increased in ApoE$^{-/-}$ mice exposed to high-fat diet and decreased in ApoE$^{-/-}$ mice with administration of IVIG. One previous study showed that FcγR ⅢA was able to stimulate proinflammatory cytokines, such as TNF-α and IL-1[28], which could provoke cell proliferation and migration of smooth muscle cells and macrophages in the atherosclerotic plaque and decrease the plaque stability[29]. We observed in our study that the levels of TNF-α and IL-1 were increased in ApoE$^{-/-}$ mice and decreased in response to IVIG pretreatment. E-selectin is critical for the firm arrest and transmigration of leukocytes out of blood vessels and into tissues[30]. E-selectin is constitutively present on endothelial cells, and its expression is increased by the stimulation of proinflammatory cytokines. sE-selectin was recognized as a marker to characterize endothelial damage[31]. In the current study, increased level of sE-selectin in ApoE$^{-/-}$ mice suggested that FcγR ⅢA enhancement was correlated to endothelial activation, and this also indicated our observations *in vitro*. Importantly, we demonstrated that mRNA expression and protein level of MMP-9 in aorta were increased in mice coupled with FcγR ⅢA elevation.

These data together suggest that FcγR ⅢA enhancement correlated to atherosclerotic plaque destabilization by promoting proinflammtory cytokine release and causing artery endothelium injury, and the inhibitory effect of IVIG on plaque destabilization was similar to Simvastatin.

5. Conclusion

Overall, the present work describes the crucial role of FcγR ⅢA in the development of atherosclerosis. The results together indicate that FcγR ⅢA contributes to the atherosclerotic formation by enhancing the adhesive efficiency of monocytes to HUVECs, stimulating expression of inflammatory cytokines and triggering the atherosclerotic plaque destabilization. Thus, inhibition of FcγR ⅢA or its signaling may represent a promising approach for the prevention and treatment of CHD.

References

[1] Sanz J, Fayad ZA. Imaging of atherosclerotic cardiovascular disease. Nature, 2008, 451: 953-957.

[2] van der Net JB, Janssens AC, Sijbrands EJ, et al. Value of genetic profiling for the prediction of coronary heart disease. Am Heart J, 2009, 158: 105-110.

[3] Yin HJ, Ma XJ, Jiang YR, et al. Investigation of gene expression profiles in coronary heart disease and functional analysis of target gene. Chin Sci Bull, 2009, 54: 1-7.

[4] Bennett S, Breit SN. Variables in the isolation and culture of human monocytes that are of particular relevance to studies of HIV. J Leukoc Biol, 1994, 56: 236-240.

[5] Jaffe EA. Culture of human endothelial cells derived from umbilical veins. Identification by morphologic and immunologic criteria. J Clin Invest, 1973, 52: 2745-2754.

[6] Zhu L, Wang S, Qn Y, et al. Effects of Huoxue injection on the adherence of human monocytes to endothelial cells and expression of vascular cell adhesion molecules. CJITWM, 2009, 29, 238-241.

[7] Johnson J, et al. Plaque rupture after short periods of fat feeding in the apolipoprotein E-knockout mouse: model characterization and effects of pravastatin treatment. Circulation, 2005, 111: 1422-1430.

[8] Soto-Rodriguezl, Campillo-Velazquez PJ, Alexander-Aguilera A, et al. Biochemical and histopathological effects of dietary oxidized cholesterol in rats. J Appl Toxicol, 2009, 29: 715-723.

[9] Cairns AP, Crockard AD, Bell AL. The CD14+CD16+ monocyte subset in rheumatoid arthritis and systemic lupus erythematosus. Rheumatol Int, 2002, 21: 189-192.

[10] Steed MM, Tyagi N, Sen U, et al. Functional consequences of the collagen/elastin switch in vascular remodeling in hyperhomocysteinemic wild-type, eNOS-/-, and iNOS-/- mice. Am J Physiol Lung Cell Mol Physiol, 2010, 299: L301-L311.

[11] Ichiyama T, Ueno Y, Hasegawa M, et al. Intravenous immunoglobulin inhibits NF-kappa B activation and affects Fc gamma receptor expression in monocytes/macrophages. Naunyn Schmiedebergs Arch Pharmacol, 2004, 369, 428-433.

[12] Chatzizisis YS, et al. Attenuation of inflammation and expansive remodeling by Valsartan alone or in combination with Simvastatin in high-risk coronary atherosclerotic plaques. Atherosclerosis, 2009, 203, 387-394.

[13] Schafers M, Schober O, HermannS. Matrix-metalloproteinases as imaging targets for inflammatory activity in atherosclerotic plaques. J Nucl Med, 2010, 51: 663-666.

[14] Back M, Ketelhuth DF, Agewall S. Matrix metalloproteinases in atherothrombosis. Prog Cardiovasc Dis, 2010, 52, 410-428.

[15] Dahlof B. Cardiovascular disease risk factors: epidemiology and risk assessment. Am J Cardiol, 2010, 105, 3A-9A.

[16] Hansson GK. Inflammation, atherosclerosis, and coronary artery disease. N Engl J Med, 2005, 352, 1685-1695.

[17] Nimmerjahn F, Ravetch JV. Fc gamma receptors: old friends and new family members. Immunity, 2006, 24: 19-28.

[18] Deo, YM, Graziano RF, Repp R, et al. Clinical significance of IgG Fc receptors and Fc gamma R-directed immunotherapies. Immunol Today, 1997, 18, 127-135.

[19] Masuda A, et al. Role of Fc receptors as a thera-peutic target. Inflamm Allergy Drug Targets, 2009, 8: 80-86.

[20] Abe J, Jibiki T, Noma S, et al. Gene expression profiling of the effect of high-dose intravenous Ig in patients with Kawasaki disease. J Immunol, 2005, 174, 5837-5845.

[21] Ivan E, Colovai AI. Human Fc receptors: critical targets in the treatment of autoimmune diseases and transplant rejections. Hum Immunol , 2006, 67, 479-491.

[22] Kawanaka N, Nagake Y, Yamamura M, et al. Expression of Fc gamma receptor III (CD16) on monocytes during hemodialysis in patients with chronic renal failure. Nephron, 2002, 90, 64-71.

[23] Mestas J, Ley K. Monocyte-endothelial cell interactions in the development of atherosclerosis. Trends Cardiovasc Med, 2008, 18: 228-232.

[24] Shantsila E, Lip GY. Monocytes in acute coronary syndromes. Arterioscler Thromb Vasc Biol, 2009, 29: 1433-1438.

[25] Bobryshev YV. Monocyte recruitment and foam cell formation in atherosclerosis. Micron , 2006, 37, 208-222.

[26] Munn DH, Garnick MB, Cheung NK. Effects of parenteral recombinant human macrophage colony-stimulating factor on monocyte number, phenotype, and antitumor cytotoxicity in nonhuman primates. Blood, 1990, 75: 2042-2048.

[27] Jawien J, Nastalek P, Korbut R. Mouse models of experimental atherosclerosis. J Physiol Pharmacol, 2004, 55, 503-517.

[28] Frankenberger M, Sternsdorf T, Pechumer H, et al. Differential cytokine expression in human blood monocyte subpopulations: a polymerase chain reaction analysis. Blood, 1996, 87, 373-377.

[29] de Bont N, et al. LPS-induced release of IL-1 beta, IL-1 Ra, IL-6, and TNF-alpha in whole blood from patients with familial hypercholesterolemia: no effect of cholesterol-lowering treatment. J Interferon Cytokine Res, 2006, 26, 101-107.

[30] Stefanadi E, Tousoulis D, Papageorgiou N, et al. Inflammatory biomarkers predicting events in atherosclerosis. Curr Med Chem, 2010, 17: 1690-1707.

[31] Samuelsson A, Towers TL, Ravetch JV. Anti-inflammatory activity of IVIG mediated through the inhibitory Fc receptor. Science , 2001 , 291, 484-486.

Investigation of Gene Expression Profiles in Coronary Heart Disease and Functional Analysis of Target Gene[*]

YIN Hui-jun　MA Xiao-juan　JIANG Yue-rong　SHI Da-zhuo　CHEN Ke-ji

The occurrence of coronary heart disease (CHD) is related to many pathogenetic processes, including lipid metabolic disorder, vascular endothelial injury, monocyte migration and its differentiation to macrophage, transportation of smooth muscle cells from tunica media to tunica intima, foam cell formation, cell necrosis, lipids deposition, etc. Increasing evidence indicates that there is a close relationship between inflammation and occurrence of CHD, especially with the formation and development of unstable plaque and thrombosis[1]. Whilst, the molecular target of inflammation inducing CHD and its acting pathological pivot are waiting for further studying.

Along with the unceasing improvement of the human gene map and the advancement of postgenome research, the world is entering an era of life sciences with bio-information as an important subject. Meanwhile, the noso-genomelogy is becoming gradually a vital orientation of researches

* 原载于 Chinese Science Bulletin，2009，50（5）：759-765

第
一
章

in the international medical field. The genetic epidemiological study showed that the hereditary factor plays the up-most action in the occurrence and development of CHD[2]. Hence, we use molecular biological methods to investigate the pathogenesis of CHD, which would offer a new pathway for prevention and treatment of the illness.

In the present study, we used high-density oligonu-cleotide microarrays to identify the genes associated with CHD. Herein, we further examined the possible pathogenic role of target gene IL-8 by several approaches, including both clinical and experimental studies.

1. Materials and Methods

1.1 Genechip Experiment

The Human Genome U133 plus 2.0 genechip produced by Affymetrix Co. was used in this study, which had 54,614 probe groups for analyzing 47,000 transcripts and variants, including the 38,500 eventual known genes. And the quality control of samples was disposed in advance by the chip Test-3.

1.2 Patients and Controls

The 16 CHD patients enrolled were the in-patients or out-patients in Beijing Xiyuan Hospital. The diagnosis of CHD was made referring to the standard in the "Nomenclature and diagnosis of ischemic heart disease" reported by the joint special group of WHO. Only those with at least one branch of coronary artery constricted over 50%, shown by coronary arteriography, were selected. Controls in the study were 8 healthy individuals. For ethical reasons, no angiography was performed in the control group. All the subjects enrolled, both patients and healthy persons, were of Han nationality, without any kindred relation among them, aged between 35 and 75 years. Informed consent for participation in the study was obtained from all individuals. The study is in accord with the Helsinki Declaration, with no contravention to the medical ethics.

1.3 Probe Preparation and Chip Hybridization

The blood sample was drawn from each testee to separate leucocytes by lymphocyte separating liquid, then total RNA was isolated with Trizol Reagent (Invitrogen Life Technologies, P/N 15596-018). The isolated RNA was purified with NucleoSpin® RNA Clean-up (MN, 740.948.10), and the quality and quantity of RNA were assessed with gel electrophoresis and an ultraviolet spectrophotometer. The probes were labeled with GeneChip IVT Labeling Kit and fragmentized in succession. Firstly, the reliability of probes was confirmed by hybridizing with the quality control chip Test-3. Then they were hybridized with U133 Plus 2.0 chip at 45℃ for 16h (Affymetrix Hybridization Oven 640). The elution and staining were carried out in Affymetrix Fluidics Station 450. Finally, the hybridized arrays were scanned by Affymetrix GeneChip Scanner 3000.

1.4 Microarray-data Analysis

The extraction of signal data and normalization were processed with Affymetrix genechip operating software version 1.4. Microarray-data of the two groups were compared and analyzed to screen out differential genes associated with CHD by the ratio figure. Gene ontological analysis[4] was performed through a network station (http://www.gosurfer.org) to find the molecular function, biological pathway and cell component of each differential gene. The pathways of differential genes were achieved through http://www.biorag.org, and analyzed by means of hypergeometric distribution statistical technique[5-6]. Meaningful target pathways were screened out, depending on P value (P<0.05). Based on above information of differential genes, target genes were screened out combining with the pathophysiologic process and literature review.

1.5 Real-time RT-PCR Identification

The 6 target genes, screened out from differential genes, were identified by real-time fluorescent quantitative RT-PCR, which could eliminate the false positive of the Genechip experiment to some extent.

1.6 Clinical Verification

Thirty CHD patients and 40 healthy volunteers

were selected depending on the same criteria as before. Their serum concentration of interleukin-8 (IL-8) was determined by double-antibody sandwich ABC-ELISA method for verifying the correlation between the target gene and CHD.

1.7　Functional Analysis of the Target Gene IL-8

IL-8, the CHD closely associated target gene, was taken as an inducing factor for studying the impact of the inflammatory factor on platelet activation, and the action mechanism was preliminarily explored as well. Platelet rich plasma (PRP) was prepared from 12 healthy volunteers, and divided into 13 centrifugal tubes of 1.5 mL, No.1 to 12 for experiment, No.13 as controls.

1.7.1　Platelet Aggregation Percentage (PAP). IL-8 (Peprotech Co.USA) at three different concentrations (50,100 and 150 ng/mL) was added to tube Nos. 1-3 respectively as the IADPS, IADPM and IADPH group, and to No. 4, an equal volume of normal saline (NS) was added instead as the NADP group. Then, Nos. 1-4 were warm-bathed for 3 m. Before PAP was detected by turbidimetry, ADP (Chrono-log Co.USA), an inducer, was added to every tube. For tube Nos. 5-8, PAP was detected directly after adding IL-8, ADP, IL-8+ADP and NS respectively as inducer (ADP, IL-8, ADP+IL-8 and NS group) .

1.7.2　Platelet CD62p Expression. IL-8 and NS, with the same volume and concentration used for tube Nos. 1-4, were added respectively into tube Nos. 9-12 as the IL-8AS, IL-8AM, IL-8AH and NSA group, and platelet CD62p expression was determined after warm-bathing by flow cytometry with the test kit produced by Becton Dickinson Co. USA.

1.7.3　Microscopic Observation of Platelet Aggregation Condition. The control PRP and Nos. 1-8 samples after PAP detection were prepared into slides using a cell centrifugal machine. Conditions of platelet aggregation after different treatments were observed under a light microscope.

1.8　Statistical Analysis

Statistical analysis was performed by SPSS software. Chisquare test was used to evaluate enumeration data, while for measurement data, t-test was used. $P < 0.05$ was considered to be statistically significant.

2. Results

2.1　Chip Experiment

2.1.1　Clinical materials. Subjects enrolled in the 2 groups (the CHD patient group and the normal control group) showed insignificantly statistical difference in aspects of age, sex, smoking, alcohol drinking ($P > 0.05$) (Table 1) .

Table 1　Comparison of Clinical Materials Between Groups

Item	CHD	Control	P value
Cases	16	8	–
Age	57.38±7.22	52.25±11.16	0.19
Sex (M/F)	16/2	7/1	1.00
Smoking (%)	31.25	25.00	1.00
Alcohol drinking (%)	43.75	37.50	1.00

2.1.2　Results of Chip Quality Control and Scanning. The electrophoretic band of RNA was clear, with the 28S/18S rRNA band luminance ratio approaching 2:1. Ultraviolet spectrophotometric examination showed that the ratio of absorbance at 260 and 280 nm was equal to 1.8-2.1, fitted to the requirements of the Genechip experiment (Figure 1) . The scanning result of Test-3 chip showed that the "+" symbol

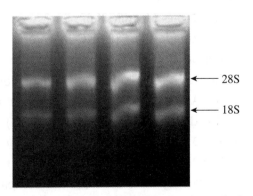

Figure 1　The Result of RNA Electrophoresis in the CHD Patient Group

at the chip center could be clearly seen, with distinct boundary lines and regular dark-bright alternation, and the expression of housekeeping gene was normal, indicating that the quality of RNA samples was reliable. Scanning of U133 plus 2.0 chip showed that the array designation "GeneChip HG-U133 Plus 2" presented clearly at the median-superior part of the chip, with mean background and the noise figure in the normal range, and the ratio of 3′ and 5′ end signal of house keeping gene β-actin and glyceraldehyde phosphate dehydrogenase (GAPDH) was up to the standard, indicating good-quality controlling.

2.1.3 Analysis of Chip Results. By differential gene screening, totally 107 differential genes were found associated with CHD. Among them, 48 were up-regulated and 59 down-regulated. They were related to many aspects like inflammation, immune, signal transduction, apoptosis, cell adhesion, cell activity, cell structure, development, stress response, transcription adjustment and control, transportation, metabolism, etc. The preponderance of inflammatory and immune related genes in proportion and significance could be found out in gene ontology and pathway analysis. The molecular function and biological pathway of 14 genes out of the 107 CHD associated differential genes were related with inflammation and immune reactions, accounting for 13.1% (Table 2). The analysis of pathway significance showed that there were 15 significant pathways associated with CHD, 4 of which involved inflammation and immune reactions (Table 3).

2.2 Target Genes Identification

Proteinkinase C-β1 (PRKC-β), interleukin-8 (IL-8), major histocompatibility complex Ⅱβ1 (HLA-DQB1), Fc-receptor ⅢA of immunoglobulin G (FCGR3A), folic acid receptor γ3 (FOLR3), prostaglandin D2 synthetase (PTGDS) and β-actin cDNAs were amplified by real-time RT-PCR. The differential scales of target genes showed by RT-PCR were not completely identical with the chip, but the orientation of changing in the two was identical (Figure 2) .

Hence, the reliability of chip outcomes could be ensured.

2.3 Clinical Verification

To elucidate the potential clinical relevance of this *in vitro* finding, we examined plasma levels of IL-8 in CHD patients and sex- and age-matched healthy controls (Table 4). As shown in Figure 3, patients with CHD (*n*=30) had significantly increased plasma levels of IL-8 compared with healthy controls (*n*=40) .

2.4 Effect of Target Gene IL-8 on Platelet Activation

2.4.1 Platelet Aggregation Percentage (PAP). PAP of the three groups treated with IL-8 was (46.92±16.78)% in the IADPS, (52.27±17.74)% in the IADPM and (54.30±18.18)% in the IADPH group, all were significantly higher than that of the NADP group treated with NS ((33.30±15.19)%, $P < 0.05$) . The difference between the three IL-8 treated groups showed statistical insignificance (*P* > 0.05) (Figure 4) .

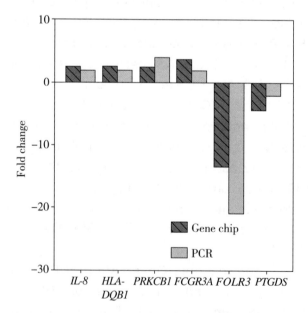

Figure 2　Comparison between Gene Chip Results and RT-PCR Identification

As shown in Figure 5, there were no significant differences in PAP between the ADP and IL-8 group ((47.61±14.42)% *vs* (40.49±10.55)%, *P* > 0.05). Both the ADP and

Table 2　Differential Genes of CHD Related to Inflammation and Immune Response

Gene ID	Gene title	Fold change[a]
AF043337	Interleukin 8	2.46
NM_000570	Fc fragment of IgG，low affinity ⅢA，receptor（CD16a）	3.64
BC020691	Pre-B-cell colony enhancing factor 1	2.44
X00452	Major histocompatibility complex，class Ⅱ，DQ alpha 1	3
AA994334	B-cell CLL/lymphoma 10	2.35
AF400602	C-type lectin domain family 7，member A	2.29
NM_012445	Spondin 2，extracellular matrix protein	−2.13
AW007751	T cell receptor alpha locus	−2.08
NM_000647	Chemokine（C-C motif）receptor 2	−2.34
BF110792	Tumor protein D52	−2.03
AI092511	Dipeptidyl-peptidase 4	−2.37
AU145682	Early B-cell factor	−2.54
NM_002261	Killer cell lectin-like receptor subfamily C，member 3	−2.5
AF211977	Leukocyte receptor cluster member 10	−2.62

a）Fold change is the expression ratio of gene transcription between the experimental sample and the control

Table 3　Significant Pathways Related to Inflammation and Immune Response

Pathway name	Identified genes	Differential expressed genes	P value
B cell receptor signaling	63	12	< 0.001
Natural killer cell mediated cytotoxicity	131	18	< 0.001
T cell receptor signaling	93	13	< 0.05
Fc epsilon RI signaling	75	10	< 0.05

Table 4　Clinical Materials of the Two Groups

	CHD Group	Control Group	P value
Cases	30	40	–
Age (y)	58.50 ± 8.16	54.73 ± 10.64	0.11
Male (%)	17 (56.7%)	14 (35.0%)	0.71

IL-8 group had increased PAP compared with the NS group ((25.91 ± 8.05)%, P < 0.01) . PAP of the ADP+IL-8 group was (67.68 ± 17.55) %, which was significantly higher than that of the other three groups (P < 0.01) .

2.4.2　Platelet CD62p Expression. Mean fluorescent intensity (MFI) of CD62p in the IL-8AS group was significantly higher than in the IL-

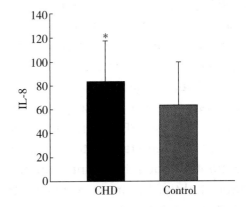

Figure 3　Comparison of IL-8 Levels between Groups. The Serum Level of IL-8 in CHD (83.21 ± 34.33 pg/ml) Was Significantly Higher than in the Control Group (63.34 ± 36.36 pg/mL) *, P < 0.05

55

第一章

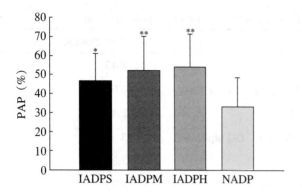

Figure 4   PAP in Different Groups after Warm-bathing. *
#shows P < 0.05 and " shows P < 0.01 vs the NADP group

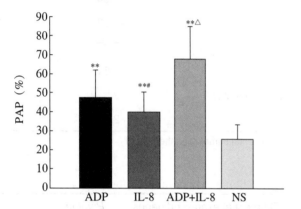

Figure 5   PAP in the Directly Induced Groups. "shows P < 0.01 vs the NS group; #shows P > 0.05 and △ shows P < 0.01 vs the ADP group

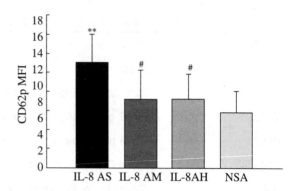

Figure 6   MFI of Platelet CD62p in Different Groups. # shows P > 0.05 and "shows P < 0.01 vs the NSA group

dispersed platelet markedly decreased. Obvious aggregation presented in all ADP treated groups, with homogenous, dense, and large platelet glomeration.

These results suggested that IL-8 has certain effect on platelet aggregation, and enhancing ADP induction, but the action is not dose-dependent. In comparison with the negative control, a small dose of IL-8 could apparently enhance the expression of CD62p, which is a major marker of platelet activation. Microscopic morphological observation showed that IL-8 could induce platelet aggregation, but the effect was not so obvious as ADP did.

3. Discussion

The differential genes associated with CHD were screened out by gene chip in this study, and it was found, through analyzing the function and pathway of these genes, that CHD is closely correlated with inflammation and immune reaction at the molecular level. Coronary atherosclerosis (AS) and spasm were recognized previously as the main pathogenetic mechanism of CHD. While in recent years, the promoting effect of inflammation in the pathogenetic process of CHD, particularly acute coronary syndrome has accepted increasing attention[7]. It has been known that inflammation not only could accelerate the occurring of AS, but also takes part in the pathological processes as formation of unstable

8AM, IL-8AH, and NSA group (13.09 ± 3.45) vs. (8.57 ± 3.55), (8.61 ± 3.07) and (6.95 ± 2.57), P < 0.01). CD62p expression of the IL-8AM and IL-8AH group was insignificantly different from that of the NSA group (P > 0.05), though a trend of ascending could be seen (Figure 6).

2.4.3   Microscopic Observation of Platelet Aggregation Condition. The platelet aggregation condition of various groups was observed by Wright's staining under microscope (Figure 7). Platelets in the raw PRP were distributed in a scattered spotted state. After treatment, in the NS treated group the distribution became compact slightly, but most of the platelets remained dispersed. In the group treated with IL-8, mild platelet aggregation could be seen, with some small platelet glomeration, and the

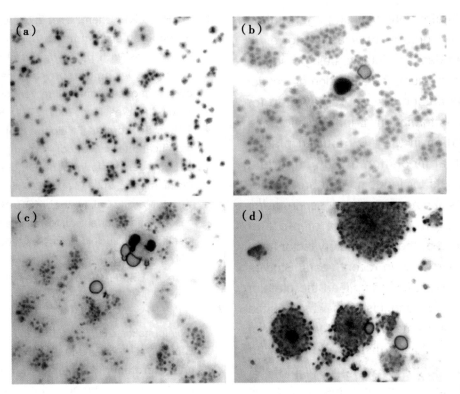

Figure 7　Condition of Platelet Aggregation in Various Groups. Wright's staining. (a) Untreated PRP；(b) NS treated group; (c)IL-8 treated group; (d)ADP treated group. ×400

plaque, rupture of plaque, secondary coronary spasm and thrombosis. Activated inflammatory cells play an important role in the development of CHD[8]. Investigations showed that coronary constriction over 70% presented in only 14% of acute coronary events. Inflammation in AS plaque could speed up the formation and rupture of unstable plaque, from which the activation of cell components arose together with thrombosis is the dominant cause for happening of acute coronary syndrome in most patients[9]. As an initiating factor of inflammation, the effect of immune reaction on the occurrence of AS and developing of CHD should not be neglected[10]. In this study, the B- and T-cell receptor signal pathways were found to be significantly associated with CHD, indicating that both humoral and cellular immune play a part in the occurrence of CHD.

IL-8, which is synthesized mainly by mononuclear phagocyte, neutrophil and vascular endothelial cells, is a basi-heparin conjugated protein possessing endogenous leucocyte chemotactic and activating action[11]. The correlation between CHD and plasma concentration of the target gene IL-8 has been proved in this study through clinical verification. IL-8[12] not only possessed the chemotactic and activating actions on neutrophilic granulocyte, but also could mediate the directional migration of T-lymphocyte, and both neutrophilic granulocyte and T-lymphocyte exerted important effect in the processes of inflammation and AS formation. IL-8, a CXC chemokine that induces the migration and proliferation of endothelial cells and smooth muscle cells, is a potent angiogenic factor that may play a certain role in AS[13].

Normal activation of platelets is a necessary procedure for physiological hemostasis, while pathological platelet activation is closely related with thrombotic diseases. Arterial thrombus is formed on the basis of AS, and one of its important initiating factors is the adhesion and aggregation of platelets in impaired endangium[14].

Meanwhile, platelet adhesion and aggregation on the ruptured plaque play as a trigger in thrombosis. Besides, as platelets being a source of inflammation medium, the activation of platelet set-off by inflammation is also a key step for arterial thrombus formation[15]. Inflammation and platelet activation in the AS ruptured plaque and their mutual mediation are an important pathological basis for inducing cerebro-cardio-vascular events like acute coronary syndrome[16]. Researches of the mechanism of platelet activating induced by the inflammatory factor have progressed preliminarily in recent years. Studies demonstrated that TNF-α amplified the platelet response to collagen, and this effect was inhibited by TNF-α receptor antagonist and inhibitors of arachidonic acid metabolism, which showed that TNF-α behaves as a trigger of platelet activation through stimulation of the arachidonic acid pathway[17]. CD40 combining with soluble CD40L could enhance the expression of platelet CD62p, and cause typical activated change of platelet shape, which plays an important role in platelet activation, thrombus formation and inflammation[18].

All the results in this study regarding PAP, CD62p activity and morphology of platelet aggregation showed that IL-8 has platelet activating action, which could impact the adhesion, aggregation and release of platelet to some extent. Our findings in the present study suggest IL-8 might mediate the development of CHD by way of influencing platelet activation. But its exact action mechanism and pathway are still waiting for further study.

References

[1] Malpartida F, Vivancos R, Urbano C, et al. Inflammation and plaque instability. Arch Cardiol Mex, 2007, 77 (14): 16-22.

[2] Candore G, Balistreri CR, Caruso M, et al. Pharmacogenomics: a tool to prevent and cure coronary heart disease. Curr Pharm Des, 2007, 13 (36): 3726-3734.

[3] Xu H, Lu XY, Chen KJ, et al. Study on correlation of blood-stasis syndrome and its accompanied syndromes with pathological changes showed in coronary angiography and restenosis after percutaneous coronary intervention. Chin J Integr Tradit Chin West Med, 2007, 27 (1): 8-13.

[4] Zhong S, Storch K F, Lipan O, et al. GoSurfer: a graphical interactive tool for comparative analysis of large gene sets in Gene Ontology space. Appl Bioinformatics, 2004, 3 (4) : 261-264.

[5] Wu J, Mao X, Cai T, et al. KOBAS server: a web-based platform for automated annotation and pathway identification. Nucleic Acids Res, 2006, 34 (1) : 720-724.

[6] Mao X, Cai T, Olyarchuk JG, et al. Automated genome annotation and pathway identification using the KEGG Orthology (KO) as a controlled vocabulary. Bioinformatics, 2005, 21 (15): 3787-3793.

[7] Brunetti ND, Correale M, Pellegrino PL, et al. Acute phase proteins in patients with acute coronary syndrome: correlations with diagnosis, clinical features, and angiographic findings. Eur J Intern Med, 2007, 18 (2): 109-117.

[8] Napoleão P, Santos MC, Selas M, et al. Variations in inflammatory markers in acute myocardial infarction: a longitudinal study. Rev Port Cardiol, 2007, 26 (12): 1357-1363.

[9] Davies MJ. The pathophysiology of acute coronary syndromes. Heart, 2000, 83 (3): 361-366.

[10] Wick G, Knoflach M, Xu Q. Autoimmune and inflammatory mechanisms in atherosclerosis. Annu Rev Immunol, 2004, 22: 361-403.

[11] Qi X, Li J, Gu J, et al. Plasma levels of IL-8 predict early complications in patients with coronary heart disease after percutaneous coronary intervention. Japan Heart J, 2003, 44 (4): 451-461.

[12] Poddar R, Sivasubramanian N, DiBello PM, et al. Homocysteine induces expression and secretion of monocyte chemoattractant protein-1 and interleukin-8 in human aortic endothelial cells implications for vascular disease. Circulation, 2001, 103 (22): 2717-2723.

[13] Simonini A, Moscucci M, Muller DW, et al. IL-8 is an angiogenic factor in human coronary atherectomy tissue. Circulation, 2000, 101 (13): 1519-1526.

[14] Jackson SP, Schoenwaelder SM. Antiplatelet therapy: in search of the "magic bullet". Nat Rev Drug Discov, 2003, 2 (10): 775-789.

[15] Davì G, Patrono C. Platelet activation and atherothrom-bosis. N Engl J Med, 2007, 357 (24): 2482-2494.

[16] Michael RF, David FM. Unstable angina and non-ST elevation MI: IIb or not IIb？ The evidence points to a better long-term outcome. J Crit IILness, 2002, 17 (2) : 52-65.

[17] Pignatelli P, De Biase L, Lenti L, et al. Tumor necrosis factor-alpha as trigger of platelet activation in patients with heart failure. Blood, 2005, 106 (6): 1992-1994.

[18] Inwald DP, McDowall A, Peters MJ, et al. CD40 is constitutively expressed on platelets and provides a novel mechanism for platelet activation. Circ Res, 2003, 92 (9): 1041-1048.

Differential Gene Expression Profiles in Coronary Heart Disease Patients of Blood Stasis Syndrome in Traditional Chinese Medicine and Clinical Role of Target Gene[*]

MA Xiao-juan　YIN Hui-jun　CHEN Ke-ji

Coronary heart disease (CHD) is a complex disease jointly influenced by heredity and environmental factors, the study on its polymorphism and differential gene expression profiles has become a hot topic for disease genomics research in recent years. Blood stasis syndrome (BSS), a major syndrome type of CHD, could happen in various diseases for its comprWensive pathological state and common pathological characteristics, but its development mechanism and progression are complex and different. Recently, BSS is a focus in the field of traditional Chinese medicine (TCM) and integrative medicine. Numerous researches on the combination of modern disease and TCM syndrome have demonstrated that BSS is closely related with the development of diseases in hemorheology, platelet function, vascular endothelium injury, microcirculation disturbance, inflammation, immunological regulation, etc[1]. Now, morbid genomics is an important direction for the diagnosis and treatment of diseases, and the gene chip technique is the production of accommodation. This research screened the differential gene expression profiles related with CHD patients of BSS by the gene chip technique, and target genes were confirmed with real-time reverse transcription polymerase chain reaction (RT-PCR). The pathological mechanism of occurrence and development of CHD with BBS was investigated by studying the correlation of target gene interleukin-8 (IL-8) with the disease.

1. Methods

1.1　Patients and Controls

All patients enrolled were the inpatients or out-patients from the Xiyuan Hospital, China Academy of Chinese Medical Sciences from March 2006 to April 2007, who were diagnosed and assigned to CHD patients with BSS group, CHD patients without BSS group, BSS patients without CHD group, with 8 in each group. Based on the diagnostic standard of CHD referring to the

* 原载于 Chinese Journal of Integrative Medicine，2009，15（2）：101-106

"Nomenclature and Diagnosis of Ischemic Heart Disease" reported by the jointed special group for standardization of clinical nomenclature of WHO, those with at least one coronary artery branch constricted over 50%[2], as shown by coronary arteriography, were selected. BSS were based on the diagnostic criteria established by the Special Committee of Promoting Blood Circulation and Removing Blood Stasis, Chinese Association of Integrative Medicine[3]. Those enrolled must be diagnosed consistently by 3 TCM doctors by blind method. In the normal control group, the 8 volunteers were selected from checkup clinic the hospital or the Cardiovascular Diseases Research Room. All the subjects enrolled were of Han nationality without any kindred relationships between them and aged between 35 to 75 years. They were informed on the contents and aim of the experiment, and had signed the written informed consent. The study is in accord with the Helsinki Declaration, with no contravention to the medical ethics.

1.2　Genechip Experiment

The Human Genome U133 Plus 2.0 genechip, produced by the Affymetrix Co., USA. was used in this study, which had 54,614 probe groups for analyzing 47,000 transcripts and variants, including the 3,800 currently known genes. The quality control chip Test 3 of the affymetrix chip series was selected and determined before the gene chip was hybridized.

The blood sample was drawn from each tester to separate leucocytes by a lymphocyte separating liquid. Then, total RNA was isolated with the Trizol Reagent (Invitrogen Life Technologies, PIN 15596-018), The isolated RNA was purified with NucleoSpin® RNA Clean-up (MN, 740.948.10), and the quality and quantity of RNA were assessed with gel electrophoresis and an ultraviolet spectrophotometer. The probes were labeled with the GeneChip IVT Labeling Kit and fragmentized in succession. Firstly, the reliability of probes was confirmed by hybridizing with the quality control chip Test-3. Then, they

were hybridized with the U133 Plus 2.0 chip at 45℃ for 16h (Affymetrix Hybridization Oven 640). The elution and staining were carried out in the Affymetrix Fluidics Station 450. Finally, the hybridized arrays were scanned by the Affymetrix GeneChip Scanner 3000.

1.3　Microarray-Data Analysis

The extraction of signal data and normalization were processed by the Affymetrix genechip operating software version 1.4. Microarray-data of the two groups were compared and analyzed to screen out differential genes associated with CHD and BSS according to the ratio figure. Gene ontological analysis[4] was performed through a network station (http: //www.gosurfer. org) to find the molecular function, biological pathway and cell component of each differential gene. The pathways of differential genes were achieved through http: //www.biorag.org, and the significance of target pathways screened out by means of hypergeometric distribution statistical technique[5,6]. Based on the above information of differential genes, target genes were screened out combining with the pathophysiologic process and literature review.

1.4　Real-time RT-PCR

Six target genes related with CHD with BBS were screened out based on the gene chip results, combined with pathophysiologic process and clinic progress. The target genes were identified and proofed by real-time RT-PCR, which could eliminate the false positives of the gene chip experiment.

1.5　Clinical Verification

Based on the above criteria, 30 CHD patients with BSS and 40 healthy persons were selected from Xiyuan Hospital. They were excluded inflammatory diseases including upper respiratory tract infection, urinary infection and digestive infection. The serum concentration of the target gene, IL-8, was determined by double-antibody sandwich avidin-biotin peroxidase complex enzyme-linked immunosorbent assay (ABC-ELISA) for verifying the correlation between the target gene and the disease.

1.6　Statistical Analysis

Statistical analysis was performed by SPSS 13.0 software. Chi-square or rank sum test was used to evaluate enumeration data. For measurement data, t-test or variance analysis was used. $P < 0.05$ was considered to be statistically significant.

2. Results

2.1　General Clinical Materials

There was no statistic deference among the four groups in age, sex and family history ($P > 0.05$). There was no significant difference between CHD with BSS group and BSS without CHD group in the blood stasis integral ($P > 0.05$), The hypertension, hyperlipidemia and diabetes history were comparable among the three disease groups ($P > 0.05$, Table 1),

2.2　Analysis of Differential Genes

The electrophoretic band of sample RNA was clear, the ratio of 28S to18S rRNA band luminance approaching 2：1. Ultraviolet spectrophotometric examination shows that the ratios of absorbance at 260 nm and 280 nm were equal to 1.8 to 2.1, fitting to the demand of the gene chip experiment. The scanning result of Test 3 chip shows that the "+" symbol at the chip center could be clearly seen, with distinct boundary lines and regular dark-bright alternation. Further signal expression of the housweeping gene was normal, indicating that the quality of RNA samples was reliable.

Scanning of U133 Plus 2.0 chip showed that the array designation "Gene Chip HG-U133 Plus 2" presented clearly at the median-superior part of the chip, with mean background and the noise figure in the normal range, and the ratio of 3' and 5' end signal of housekeeping gene β-actin and glyceraldehyde phosphate dehydrogenase (GAPDH) was up to the standard, indicating good-quality control.

A total of 107 different genes were screened out and found associated with CHD, including 48 up-regulated genes and 59 down-regulated genes. Among these 107 different genes, 14 genes (13.1%) were found to be related to the inflammatory reaction and immune response through Gene Ontoolgy (Go) analysis. In the pathway analysis, 4 of 15 conspicuous pathways were referred to the inflammation and immune response. Forty-eight different genes were associated with BSS, including 26 up-regulated genes and 22 down-regulated genes. Five of the 48 genes (10.4%) and 5 of 10 significant pathways were involved in inflammation and immune response (Tables 2-5).

2.3　Target Genes Identification

Six target genes related with CHD with BBS were screened based on the gene chip results combined with pathophysiologic process and literature study, then further identified and regressed to clinic. The six target genes were protein kinase C-β1 (PRKC-β), IL-8, major histocompatibility complex Ⅱ β1 (HLA-DQB1),

Table 1　Comparison of Clinical Materials

Group	Case	Age (Yr, $\bar{\chi} \pm s$）	Sex (Case, M/F)	Family history (%)	Blood stasis integral($\bar{\chi} \pm s$）	Hypertension history (%)	Hyperlipidemia history (%)	Diabetes history (%)
CHD with BSS	8	55.75±7.29	7/1	75.00	26.63±5.24	62.50	37.50	12.50
BSS with CHD	8	59.00±7.25	7/1	37.50	22.88±6.58	75.00	50.00	12.50
CHD without BSS	8	59.00±9.35	7/1	50.00	–	37.50	50.00	25.00
Control	8	52.25±11.16	7/1	37.50	–	–	–	–
P value		0.40	1.00	0.41	0.23	0.32	0.85	0.75

Table 2　Differential Genes of CHD Related to Inflammation and Immune Response

Gene ID	Gene title	Fold change 1	Fold change 2
AF043337	Interleukin-8	6.25	2.46
NM_000570	Fc fragment of IgG, low affinity ⅢA, receptor（CD16a）	2.35	3.64
BC020691	Pre-B-cell colony enhancing factor 1	3.3	2.44
X00452	Major histocompatibility complex, class Ⅱ, DO alpha 1	4.34	3.00
AA994334	B-cell CLL/lymphoma 10	2.46	2.35
AF400602	C-type lectin domain family 7, member A	2.46	2.29
NM_012445	Spondin 2, extracellular matrix protein	−4.24	−2.13
AW007751	T cell receptor alpha locus	−3.27	−2.08
NM_000647	Chemokine (C-C motif) receptor 2	−2.15	−2.34
BF110792	Tumor protein D52	−2.27	−2.03
AI092511	Dipeptidyl-peptidase 4	−2.52	−2.37
AU145682	Early B-cell factor	−2.32	−2.54
NM_002261	Killer cell lectin-like receptor subfamily C，member 3	−4.04	−2.5
AF211977	Leukocyte receptor cluster member 10	−2.74	−2.62

Notes：Fold change is the expression ratio of gene transcription between experimental sample and the control

Table 3　Differential Genes of BSS Related to Inflammation and Immune Response

Gene ID	Gene title	Fold change 1	Fold change 2
M16276	Major histocompatibility complex，class Ⅱ	2.5	2.19
AF043337	Interleukin-8	2.46	2.52
AW007751	T cell receptor alpha locus	−2.08	−2.67
NM_002261	Killer cell lectin-like receptor subfamily C	−2.5	−2.60
W68403	Integrin beta 2	−2.55	−2.29

Table 4　Significant Pathways of CHD Related to Inflammation and Immune Response

Pathway name	Identified gene	Differential expressed gene	P value
B cell receptor signaling	63	12	$P < 0.001$
Natural killer cell mediated cytotoxicity	131	18	$P < 0.001$
T cell receptor signaling	93	13	$P < 0.05$
Fc epsilon RI signaling	75	10	$P < 0.05$

Table 5　Significant Pathways of BSS Related to Inflammation and Immune Response

Pathway name	Identified gene	Differential expressed gene	P value
Natural killer cell mediated cytotoxicity	131	12	$P < 0.001$
B cell receptor signaling	63	8	$P < 0.001$
Antigen processing and presentation	87	9	$P < 0.001$
T cell receptor signaling	93	7	$P < 0.05$
Cell adhesion molecules	131	8	$P < 0.05$

Fc receptor ⅢA of immunoglobulin G (FCGR3A), folic acid receptor γ3 (FOLR3), prostaglandin D2 synthetase (PTGDS) and β-actin cDNAs, and they were amplified by real-time RT-PCR. The different scales of target genes showed with RT-PCR and the chip were not completely identical, but the orientations of changing in the two were identical (Figure 1). Hence, the reliability of chip outcomes could be ensured.

Table 6　Clinical Materials of the Two Groups

Group	Case	Age (Year, $\bar{\chi} \pm s$)	Male [Case (%)]
CHD with BSS	30	58.50±8.16	17 (56.7%)
Control	40	54.73±10.64	14 (35.0%)
P value		0.11	0.71

Table 7　Comparison of IL-8 Level between Groups

Group	Case	II-8 (ng/L, $\bar{x} \pm s$)	P value Normality test	t-test
CHD with BSS	30	83.21±34.33	0.78	0.04
Control	40	63.34±36.36	0.65	

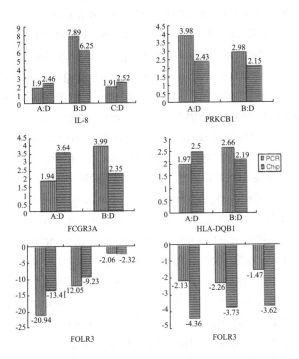

Figure 1　Comparison between Gene Chip Results and RT-PCR Identification

Notes: A: CHD patients with BSS group; B: CHD patients without BSS group; C: BSS patients without CHD group; D: healthy control group

2.4　Clinical Verification

There was no statistic difference in the age and sex between CHD patients with BBS group and the healthy control group ($P > 0.05$, Table 6). As shown in Table 7, the serum level of IL-8 in CHD patients with BSS was higher significantly than that in the healthy controls. It shows potential clinical correlation of inflammatory factor IL-8 with CHD patients with BSS.

3. Discussion

CHD, the main cause for cardiac disability and mortality, is a hot spot in the field of international cardiovascular disease researches in recent years. The morbidity of CHD shows an increase yearly. Coronary atherosclerosis (AS) and coronary spasm are recognized as the main pathogenetic mechanisms of CHD. While in recent years, the promoting effect of inflammation in the pathogenetic process of CHD, particularly in acute coronary syndrome has been paid more attention to. The degree of coronary artery stenosis in a few of patients with acute coronary syndrome is just mild or moderate. The serious clinical events are due to the inactive status of pathological changes plaques transferring to the active state, and inflammation plays a key role in the activation of pathological plaque[7].

It has been known that inflammation could not only accelerate the occurrence of AS, but also take part in the pathological processes as the formation of unstable plaque, rupture of plaque, secondary coronary spasm and thrombosis. Activated inflammatory cells play an important role in the development of CHD[8]. Investigations show that only 14% of acute coronary events presented above 70% stenosis of the coronary. Inflammation in AS plaque could speed up the formation and rupture of unstable plaque, which could further lead to the activation of cell components, and also cause the thrombosis formation. That is the dominant cause for the occurrence of acute coronary syndrome in most patients[9]. The course of CHD mainly relates to the biological characteristics of coronary plaque, rather than the extent of coronary artery stenosis. While, the continuous progress of plaque lesions is closely correlated with inflammation[10,11].

Stagnated blood is recorded as "bad blood", "stayed blood" "hemagglutination" in "Yellow Emperor's Internal Classic (黄帝内经)". Modern studies suggest that the stagnated blood can be divided into blood of stasis, blood away from meridian and vessels and contaminated blood. And contaminated blood can be divided into exogenous, endogenous and complexity types. The exogenous is induced by pathogenic biological and physical-chemical factors. While the endogenous is the result of metabolite accumulation caused by important organ failure. The compounded stagnation includes exogenous and endogenous[12]. BSS, as a comprehensive pathological state, could happen in many diseases, which must have common pathological features. Studies show that BSS has a similar change trend in a certain degree in different diseases, which implies its common material basis. Blood stasis is a major etiological factor and pathological product in various diseases. Inflammatory response is the important link in multiple systemic diseases of modern medicine. A lot of studies have shown that inflammatory responses and BBS must have a close relationship in the pathology, pathogenesis and treatment. In the process of different diseases, inflammatory factors are involved in the development of blood stasis to some extent, and the method of promoting blood circulation and removing stasis plays an important role in the treatment of inflammatory diseases. The animal model of BSS induced by inflammatory factors reflects the close relationship between blood stasis and inflammation from different aspects[12].

IL-8 is synthesized mainly by the mononuclear phagocytes, neutrophils vascular endothelial cells and is a heparin-conjugated protein possessing endogenous leucocyte chemotactic and activating action. Its receptor is composed of seven transmembrane units and IL-8 binds with its receptor and bird nucleotide-binding protein to develop the complex for conveying information. IL-8 belongs to the CXC subfamily and has the function of chemotaxis on neutrophils and basophils, which can induce neutrophil degranulation and the release of lysosomal enzyme, and basophils release histamine, participate in the immune reaction, metabolic and inflammatory response in the acute phase[13].

IL-8 could not only possess the activation factors on neutrophilic granulocytes, but also mediate the directional migration of T-lymphocyte[14]. Both neutrophilic granulocytes and T-lymphocytes play important roles on inflammation and the development of AS. IL-8 induces the migration and proliferation of endothelial cells and smooth muxcle cells, which is a potent angiogenic factor that may play a role in AS[15]. The acute diffuse inflammation of the endodermis stimulates thrombosis and activates the secretion of protein autolysis enzyme, which accelerates the rupture of plaque fibrous cap. IL-8 could promote the activation of the immune system and the formation of thrombus through the control of macrophages and metalloproteinases, which is involved in the pathogenesis of CHD, increasing the instability of atherosclerotic plaque[16].

In the present study, high-density oligonucleotide microarrays were used to identify the different gene profiles of CHD with BSS, which laid the foundation of the genetic diagnosis for BSS. Herein, we further analyzed the molecular function and biologic pathway of the different related genes screened with gene chips through data mining, and revealed the relevance between the development of CHD with BSS and inflammatory-immune reaction at the level of the nucleic acid, which may be a beneficial exploration for the syndrome study on BBS of TCM. In order to provide complete molecular biology evidence for syndrome study, the proteomic features of BSS still need to be further studied based on the summary of genomics characteristics.

References

[1] Ma M, Zhang G J. The progress of investigation on the objectification of blood stasis syndrome. J Shandong Univ Tradit Chin Med, 2002, 2: 155-158.

[2] Xu H, Lu XY, Chen KJ, et al. Study on correlation of blood-stasis syndrome and its accompanied syndromes with pathological changes showed in coronary angiography and restenosis after percutaneous coronary intervention. Chin J Integr Tradit West Med, 2007, 27: 8-13.

[3] Special Committee of Promoting Blood Circulation and Removing Blood Stasis, Chinese Association of Integrative Medicine. The diagnostic criteria of blood stasis syndrome. Chin J Integr Tradit West Med, 1987, 7: 129.

[4] Zhong S, Storch KF, Lipan O, et al. GoSurfer: a graphical interactive tool for comparative analysis of large gene sets in Gene Ontology space. Appl Bioinformat, 2004, 3: 261-264.

[5] Shi YH, Zhu SW, Mao XZ, et al. Transcriptome profiling, molecular biological, and physiological studies reveal a major role for ethylene in cotton fiber cell elongation. Plant Cell, 2006, 18: 651-664.

[6] Mao X, Cai T, Olyarchuk JG, et al. Automated genome annotation and pathway identification using the KEGG Orthology (KO) as a controlled vocabulary. Bioinformatics, 2005, 21: 3787-3793.

[7] Brunetti ND, Correale M, Pellegrino PL, et al. Acute phase proteins in patients with acute coronary syndrome: correlations with diagnosis, clinical features, and angiographic findings. Eur J Intern Med, 2007, 18: 109-117.

[8] Napoleão P, Santos MC, Selas M, et al. Variations in inflammatory markers in acute myocardial infarction: a longitudinal study. Rev Port Cart Cardiol, 2007, 26: 1357-1363.

[9] Davies M J. The pathophysiology of acute coronary syndromes. Heart, 2000, 83: 361-366.

[10] Wick G, Knoflach M, Xu Q. Autoimmune and inflammatory mechanisms in atherosclerosis. Annu Rev Immuno, 2004, 22: 361-403.

[11] Chen KJ, Shi ZX. Practical workbook of blood-stasis syndrome. Beijing: People's Medical Publishing House, 1999, 5-8.

[12] Ma XJ, Yin HJ, Chen KJ. Research progress of correlation between blood-stasis syndrome and inflammation. Chin J Integr Tradit West Med, 2007, 27: 669-672.

[13] Oi X, Li J, Gu J, et al. Plasma levels of IL-8 predict early complications in patients with coronary heart disease after percutaneous coronary intervention. Jpn Heart J, 2003, 44: 451-461.

[14] Poddar R, Sivasubramanian N, Dibello PM, et al. Homocysteine induces expression and secretion of monocyte chemoattractant protein-1 and interleukin-8 in human aortic endothelial cells implications for vascular disease. Circulation, 2001, 103: 2717-2723.

[15] Simonini A, Moscucci M, Muller DW, et al. IL-8 is an angiogenic factor in human coronary atherectomy tissue. Circulation, 2000, 101: 1519-1526.

[16] Guo M. Role of IL-8 in tumor angiogenesis. Chin J Gastroenterol Hepatol, 2003, 12: 409-411.

第 二 章

心血管瘀毒病因学研究

冠心病稳定期因毒致病的辨证诊断量化标准 *

陈可冀　史大卓　徐　浩　殷惠军　张京春

第二章

20 世纪 60 年代以后，基于冠心病"本虚标实，标实中血瘀贯穿发病过程始终"的病因病机认识，带来了临床以"宣痹通阳"为主转为以"活血化瘀"为主的冠心病治疗方法学的改变，且在此基础上衍化出理气活血、益气活血、化浊活血、温阳活血等治法，显著提高了临床疗效。但是，同样是"血瘀"为其主要病因病机，为什么有的患者长期病情稳定，有的却发生急性事件，甚至猝死？以"血瘀为主"能否概括冠心病的中医学病因病机？成为现代中医 / 中西医结合病因病机学上亟待探讨研究的问题。

动脉粥样硬化（AS）易损斑块的破裂和急性血栓形成是冠心病心血管事件发生的主要病理因素 [1]。大量研究证明，AS 基础上的血栓形成与炎症密切相关，两者相互促进，互为因果：一方面，炎症因子可以诱发血小板黏附聚集和血栓形成；另一方面，血栓形成也是炎症激活的主要因素。冠心病发病过程中的血小板活化、黏附聚集和血栓形成，中医学多将其病因病机归于"血脉瘀阻"的范畴；但组织坏死、过氧化应激损伤、炎症反应等病理改变，似尚难以用单一"血瘀"所能概括。结合传统中医学有关因毒致病特点的认识和冠心病的中医临床特点，应考虑存在因"毒"致病或"瘀"、"毒"互结致病的病因病机问题。

冠心病的病理改变，其中包括 AS 斑块破裂、血栓闭塞引发的组织损伤坏死、炎症瀑布反应、氧化脂质沉积、细胞凋亡等，与传统中医学因毒邪致病起病急骤、传变迅速、直中脏腑、腐肌伤肉的特点多有相似之处。在以往血瘀的基础上，结合对毒的认识，可望更全面诠释急性冠状动脉综合征（ACS）的中医临床发病点和病因病机。有小样本临床观察表明，清热解毒方药在防治不稳定性心绞痛（UA）方面具有较为可靠的临床疗效 [2]；有研究采用不同活血化瘀中药干预 ApoE 基因缺陷小鼠 AS 不稳定斑块，证明活血解毒中药消减和稳定 AS 斑块的作用优于单纯的活血化瘀中药 [3]。这也证明 AS 在血瘀的基础上，应考虑存在毒邪致病的病因病机。

血瘀作为中医学的一个病因病机，在致病特点、判别标准和微观病理改变研究方面取得了显著的进展。尽管毒和"瘀"、"毒"互结致病在心脑血管病发病中的作用古今皆多有相关的论述，但有关其致病特点、整体和微观病理改变认识尚不够统一，辨证辨病认识也不够规范，限制了中医药、中西医结合临床防治冠心病研究的深入和临床疗效的提高。因此，笔者综合文献研究、实验研究、小样本临床随机对照研究和前瞻性大样本队列研究结果，结合现代信息生物学分析，从宏观临床表征和微观理化指标变化两方面，在冠心病血瘀辨证诊断的基础上结合临床所见，建立了冠心病稳定期患者因毒致病的辨证诊断的量化标准。

文献研究系统总结了古今文献中有关"瘀"、"毒"病因的致病特点、临床表征和理化指标，发现"瘀"和毒皆有所不同；实验研究模拟临床瘀、毒作为病因致病的病理过程，建立了系列动物和细胞模型。通过活血（川芎、赤芍有效部位组成的芎芍胶囊）及活血解毒中药（芎芍胶囊 + 黄连胶囊）干预前后血栓形成、炎症反应和组织损伤相关指标的变化，以效测因，证明清热解毒中药作用的相关理化指标如炎症反应因子高敏 C 反应蛋白（hs-CRP）和胶原代谢相关因子基质金属蛋白酶 -9（MMP-9）等均有改善；小样本临床随机对照研究，入选 60 例 UA 患者，比较活血中药和活血解毒中药干预上述理化指标的变化，以效测因，证实活血解毒干预后 hs-CRP 水平较单纯活血组明显降低。包括 1503 例冠心病稳定期患者的前瞻性队列研究，以证求因，综合分析，进一步归纳了冠心病稳定期患者"毒"的临床表征和理化指标。在此基础上，对"毒"致病组（发生血栓性终点事件组）和非"毒"致病组（未发生血栓性终点事件组）的临床表征特点和理化指标进行生物信息学指标的比较和分析，然后采用 Logistic 逐步回归方法，结合中医学关于因毒致病的认识，根据病史、症状、体征、舌象、脉象、理化指标等不同变量的风险比值

* 原载于《中国中西医结合杂志》，2011，31（3）：313-314

（OR）判定其权重，制订了冠心病稳定期患者因毒致病诊断及量化标准，包括主要指标6项，次要指标6项。见表1。

表1 冠心病稳定期因毒致病辨证诊断及量化标准

指标类型		诊断指标	分值
主要指标	症状	1. 中、重度心绞痛	3
		2. 重度口苦	4
	舌象	3. 老舌	3
		4. 舌青或青紫	3
		5. 剥苔（不含类剥苔）	5
		6. 舌下络脉紫红或绛紫	3
次要指标	生化指标	1. hs-CRP > 3mg/L	1
		2. 纤维蛋白原短期内显著升高	1
		3. P-选择素短期内显著升高	1
	既往病史	4. 高胆固醇病史	1
		5. 高血压史2～3级	1
		6. 糖尿病病史，FBG ≥ 7.0mmol/L	2

注：符合1个主要指标，或2个次要指标（至少含1项生化指标）即可诊断

为了反证表1标准的可靠性，将1503例冠心病稳定期患者按照此标准分为符合以"毒"病因致病组（符合组）和不符合以"毒"为病因致病组（不符合组），分别计算其心血管血栓性事件发生的危险度、相对危险度及归因危险度。结果表明符合组786例患者发生事件63例，发生危险度8.02%；不符合组717例患者发生事件9例，发生危险度1.26%。符合组事件发生危险度明显高于不符合组（P < 0.001）。相对危险度（RR）= 6.39，即符合组事件发生的危险性是不符合组的6.39倍。归因危险度（AR）= 6.76%，即符合组心血管血栓性事件发生率为6.76%。血栓性事件发生率为归因危险度百分比（ARP）=（6.39–1）/6.39×100% = 84.35%，即符合组中发生的心血管事件84.35%归因于"毒"邪病因致病。OR= 6.85（95% CI 3.38 ～ 13.89），即符合组事件发生率是非不符合组6.85倍。说明此标准可用于冠心病稳定期高危患者的辨识和因毒致病的诊断。

在传统中医学的发展历程中，病因认识上的每一次发展和创新都会带来治疗方法学的进步和相应疾病临床疗效的提高，如温病学、疫病论及现代血瘀理论的认识等。在以往冠心病血瘀病因认识的基础上，在中医药学以毒病因认识和理论思维的指导下，笔者建立了冠心病稳定期因毒致病的辨证诊断和量化标准，对于进一步发挥传统中医药在冠心病防治领域"既病防变"相关治疗方药的优势，以提高临床疗效，具有重要的意义。

参考文献

[1] Ueda Y，Ogasawara N，Mastsuo K，et al. Acute coronary syndrome. Circulation，2010，74 (3)：411-417.

[2] 卢笑辉. 黄连解毒胶囊治疗不稳定型心绞痛临床疗效及作用机制研究. 山东中医药大学学报，2005，29（6）：457-460.

[3] 文川，徐浩，黄启福，等. 16种活血中药及芎芍胶囊对ApoE基因缺陷小鼠动脉粥样硬化斑块胶原沉积及其代谢的影响. 中国病理生理杂志，2005，21（8）：1640.

冠心病稳定期"瘀毒"临床表征的研究[*]

徐 浩 曲 丹 郑 峰 史大卓 陈可冀

20世纪90年代以来，随着对动脉粥样硬化（AS）危险因素的深入了解和积极控制，冠心病的一级预防取得了令人鼓舞的进展。然而，急性心血管病事件的一级预防仍缺乏确切有效的措施，全球每年约1900万人突发急性心血管事件。这不得不迫使我们在现有认识的基础上，对心血管病的中西医结合病因病机进行更为深入的分析和思考。以导师陈可冀院士为首的课题组[1-4]在既往研究基础上明确提出"瘀毒致变"引发急性心血管事件的假说，对于冠心病急性心血管事件的中医防治研究具

* 原载于《中国中西医结合杂志》，2010，30（2）：125-129

有重要的理论指导意义。本研究即采用前瞻性研究方法，结合临床心血管事件随访，探索稳定期冠心病患者"瘀毒"临床表征，以期早期识别和干预冠心病高危患者，这对于我国国情下的冠心病二级预防及进一步降低急性心血管事件的发生率具有重要意义。

1. 资料与方法

1.1 诊断标准

冠心病诊断标准：参照国际心脏病学会及世界卫生组织（WHO）临床命名标准化联合专题组报告《缺血性心脏病的命名及诊断》制定标准[5]。冠心病辨证分型标准参照中国中西医结合学会心血管专业委员会 1990 年 10 月修订的"冠心病中医辨证标准"[6]。

1.2 纳入标准

符合 WHO 缺血性心脏病诊断标准，并且选择性冠状动脉造影至少有 1 支冠脉血管狭窄≥50%者；临床表现为无症状、稳定劳累性心绞痛或急性冠状动脉综合征（ACS）超过 1 个月病情稳定者；年龄≤75 岁；签署知情同意书。

1.3 排除标准

近 1 个月内感染、发热、创伤、烧伤、手术史；活动性结核病或风湿免疫疾病患者；严重心力衰竭患者，EF＜35%；合并严重瓣膜疾病或心肌病；合并严重慢阻肺、肺心病或呼吸衰竭患者；已知的肾功能不全，血清肌酐（Cr）男性＞221μmol/L，女性＞177μmol/L；已知的肝功能不全，谷丙转氨酶（ALT）＞正常值的 3 倍或合并肝硬化；严重造血系统疾病；严重精神病患者；恶性肿瘤患者；脏器移植患者；患者的预期寿命小于 3 年。

1.4 临床资料

2007 年 9 月至 2008 年 3 月期间，入选中日友好医院全国中西医结合心血管病中心经冠状动脉造影检查确诊的冠心病稳定期患者 254 例，男 184 例，女 70 例，年龄 32 ～ 75 岁，平均（61.9±9.9）岁；病程 1.5 个月至 20 年，平均 4.5 年。有高血压病史 156 例（61.4%）；糖尿病病史 92 例（36.2%）；高脂血症病史 188 例（74.0%）；心肌梗死病史 115 例（45.3%）。冠状动脉造影单支病变 75 例（29.5%），双支病变 71 例（28.0%），3 支病变 108 例（42.5%）。

1.5 研究方法及观察指标

对入选的患者在病历报告表（CRF）中详细记录体质特点、个人史、既往史、家族史、目前症状、体征、舌象、脉象和辨证分型情况，并取血检测。信息采集、录入人员均为心血管科专科医师并接受过统一培训考核，所有录入信息由课题组主要研究人员进行核查确认后，方为有效。数据录入采用双人录入，以确保资料的准确可靠。中医的辨证分型由两名副高以上中西医结合心血管医师确认。血常规采用仪器法测定，总胆固醇（TC）采用氧化酶法测定，三酰甘油（TG）采用酶法测定，高密度脂蛋白 - 胆固醇（HDL-C）采用直接法测定，低密度脂蛋白 - 胆固醇（LDL-C）采用酶法测定，载脂蛋白 A（ApoA）、载脂蛋白 B（ApoB）和脂蛋白 a [LP（a）] 采用免疫透视比浊法测定，纤维蛋白原（Fib）采用定量法测定，空腹血糖（FBG）采用葡萄糖氧化酶法测定，丙氨酸氨基转移酶（ALT）采用 IFCC 推荐法测定，Cr 采用苦味酸法测定，hs-CRP 采用免疫比浊度法测定。患者均于清晨空腹静脉采血，由中日友好医院化验室统一检测以上各项指标。所有患者均随访 1 年，记录心血管事件发生情况。随访心血管事件定义为：（1）心源性死亡；（2）复苏成功的心搏骤停；（3）非致命性心肌梗死；（4）需行介入治疗（PCI）或冠状动脉旁路移植术（CABG）；（5）因不稳定性心绞痛住院。

1.6 统计学方法

计数资料的假设性检验使用 χ^2 检验。计量资料用均数 ± 标准差（$\bar{\chi}±s$）表示，两样本均数的比较采用 t 检验，方差不齐者用 t 检验。资料不服从正态分布采用 Mann-Whitney 检验。对随访心血管事件发生的相关因素首先进行单因素分析，对差异有统计学意义的变量进一步采用 Logistic 回归分析，变量进入回归模型的检验水准为 0.05，剔除水准为 0.10。

2. 结果

2.1 随访心血管事件情况

254 例患者中有 246 例患者到医院复查，8 例患者进行电话随访，失访 2 例（0.8%）。随访期间无死亡及急性心肌梗死患者，3 例（1.2%）行 PCI 治疗；25 例（9.8%）因不稳定性心绞痛住院。

2.2 冠心病稳定期患者心血管事件的单因素分析

2.2.1 基本临床资料与心血管事件单因素分析 28 例有心血管事件的患者年龄平均为（61.93±9.88）岁，无事件患者年龄平均为（60.19±9.72）岁，两组比较差异无统计学意义（$P > 0.05$）；184 例男性患者中 19 例（10.3%）出现心血管事件；70 例女性患者中 9 例（12.9%）有心血管事件发生，两组比较差异无统计学意义（$P > 0.05$）；体重指数、腰围（cm）有心血管事件患者平均分别为 25.61±3.46 和 90.89±9.02，无事件患者分别为 25.47±3.05 和 91.34±8.15，两组比较差异均无统计学意义（$P > 0.05$）。

2.2.2 个人史资料与心血管事件的单因素分析 对 254 例患者，就个人史信息[有无吸烟、饮酒、性格急躁、A 型性格、职业特点、工作劳累、紧张、平素饮食习惯（嗜辛辣、嗜油腻、嗜咸食、嗜甜食）、家庭是否和睦、平素是否锻炼身体]在发生心血管事件患者与未发生心血管事件患者间进行比较，结果发现，两组差异均无统计学意义（$P > 0.05$）。

2.2.3 合并病与心血管事件的单因素分析 本研究比较了发生心血管事件与无心血管事件患者在合并病，如心肌梗死、高血压、糖尿病、高脂血症、脑血管病和周围血管病方面的差异，两组均无统计学意义（均 $P > 0.05$）。

2.2.4 心绞痛发作的诱因与心血管事件的单因素分析 本研究比较了患者发生心绞痛诱因在出现心血管事件的患者与无心血管事件患者中的差异，结果发现，劳累、情绪、饱餐、平卧、吸烟和受寒在两组中差异均无统计学意义（$P > 0.05$）。

2.2.5 心绞痛发作的部位与心血管事件的单因素分析 有 52 例患者心绞痛部位在胸骨后，其中有 11 例（21.2%）出现心血管事件，202 例无胸骨后疼痛患者中，有 17 例（8.4%）有心血管事件，两组比较，差异有统计学意义（$P = 0.009$）；心绞痛部位在心前区、剑突下、左胸、背部及其他部位者在有心血管事件和无事件两组中比较，差异均无统计学意义（$P > 0.05$）。

2.2.6 心绞痛性质与心血管事件的单因素分析 254 例患者心绞痛的性质有多种，最多的是闷痛，后依次是绞痛、压迫痛和隐痛，胀痛和烧灼痛较少，仅有 1 例心绞痛发作表现为牙痛。本研究比较了多种心绞痛发作的性质在心血管事件发生与未发生患者之间的差异，结果发现，差异均无统计学意义（$P > 0.05$）。

2.2.7 血液指标与心血管事件的单因素分析 本研究将患者血常规、FBG、血脂、Fib、hs-CRP、ALT、Cr 与心血管事件发生进行了比较。有心血管事件患者 TG 为（1.21±0.60）mmol/L，无事件患者为（1.66±1.15）mmol/L，两组比较差异有统计学意义（$P = 0.009$）；有心血管事件患者 TC/HDL-C 为 3.48±0.99，无事件患者为 4.04±1.49，两组比较差异有统计学意义（$P = 0.025$）；FBG 在有心血管事件的患者中为（6.36±1.59）g/L，无事件患者为（5.97±1.83）g/L，两组比较差异有统计学意义（$P = 0.024$）；hs-CRP 在有心血管事件患者为（2.55±2.03）mg/L，无事件患者为（2.20±2.19）mg/L，两组比较差异无统计学意义（$P = 0.249$）；但将 hs-CRP 分为 ≥3mg/L 和 <3mg/L 两类比较，没有发生事件的 226 例患者中，hs-CRP ≥3mg/L 者 50 例，占 22.1%，随访发生事件的 28 例患者中，hs-CRP ≥3mg/L 者 11 例，占 3913%，两组比较差异有统计学意义（$P = 0.045$）。其他指标比较，两组差异无统计学意义（均 $P > 0.05$）。

2.2.8 冠状动脉病变部位、范围与心血管事件的单因素分析 对冠状动脉病变部位分析结果显示，左主干、左前降支、左回旋支、右冠状动脉病变在随访有无心血管事件组间差异均无统计学意义（均 $P > 0.05$）。对病变范围的分析结果发现，单支病变、双支病变和 3 支病变对心血管事件的发生均无明显影响（$P > 0.05$）。

2.2.9 中医兼症与心血管事件的单因素分析 254 例患者以眼花、头晕、口干欲饮、耳鸣、腰酸和肢麻症状多见。有头痛症状患者 52 例，其中 11 例（21.2%）有心血管事件发生；无头痛者有 202 例，17 例（8.4%）有事件发生，两组比较差异有统计学意义（$P = 0.009$）；有耳鸣症状者 99 例，17 例（17.2%）有心血管事件；155 例无耳鸣者 11 例（7.1%）有心血管事件，两组比较差异有统计学意义（$P = 0.012$）；平素经常咽痛者 45 例，其中 10 例（22.2%）有心血管事件，209 例平素无咽痛者 18 例（8.6%）有心血管事件，两组比较差异有统计学意义（$P = 0.015$）；其他兼症（发热、手足心热、自汗、面红、头晕、眼花、口干欲饮、口苦、口黏、口疮、胃痛、水肿、咳嗽、咳痰、畏寒、盗汗、头胀、口臭、脘痞、肢麻、腰酸、气喘）有心血管事件和无事件患者比较，差异均无统计学意义（$P > 0.05$）。

2.2.10 中医辨证分型与心血管事件的单因素分析 254 例患者中医辨证以血瘀证最多（245 例），1 年内出现心血管事件者 27 例（11.0%），9 例无血瘀证患者 1 例（11.1%）出现，两组比较差异无统计学意义（$P > 0.05$）；其余证型（气虚、痰浊、气滞、寒凝、阴虚、阳虚）有心血管事件和无事件患者比较，差异均无统计学意义（$P > 0.05$）。

2.2.11 脉象与心血管事件的单因素分析 患者脉象总体分布以弦脉、沉脉和滑脉为多，结脉、缓脉和涩脉为少。7 例有涩脉或结代脉患者中有 4 例（57.1%）出现心血管事件，247 例无涩脉或结代脉患者 24 例（9.7%）有心血管事件，两组比较差异有统计学意义（$P = 0.003$）；其他脉象有心血管事件和无事件患者比较差异均无统计学意义（$P > 0.05$）。

2.3 冠心病稳定期患者心血管事件相关危险因素的多元回归分析（表 1）

选择单因素分析有显著性差异的因素，采用 Logistic 多元逐步回归方法分析随访心血管事件影响因素，结果表明：可升高心血管事件发生率的影响因素有（以危险度从高到低排序）：脉涩或结代、胸骨后疼痛、平素经常咽痛、头痛（$P < 0.05$）。尽管 Logistic 多元逐步回归分析提示 hs-CRP 对心血管事件的影响未达到统计学差异（$P = 0.094$），但已显示明显趋势（hs-CRP $\geq$ 3mg/L 较 < 3mg/L 者更易发生心血管事件）。

3. 讨论

冠心病病因病机的认识目前逐渐趋于统一，认为本病属于本虚标实之证，本虚为气、血、阴、阳亏虚，病位在心，涉及肺、脾、肾；标实为气滞、血瘀、痰浊、寒凝，而尤以血瘀被公认为最重要的病因病机之一。随着炎症致 AS 学说的兴起，认为炎症反应在 AS 发生、发展及造成斑块不稳定

引发急性心血管事件中扮演了重要的角色。而炎症反应与中医"毒"的认识不谋而合。在此基础上，以陈可冀院士为首的课题组[1-4]明确提出"瘀毒致变"引发急性心血管事件的假说，对于深化冠心病发生发展过程的演变规律和病因病机的认识，进一步提高急性心血管事件中医药防治水平无疑具有重要意义，而探索冠心病稳定期"瘀毒"临床表征显尤为关键。

本研究从冠心病稳定期患者个人史、体质特点、既往史、家族史、症状、体征、证候、理化检查指标等多方面，分析随访心血管事件发生的相关影响因素，以期探索随访发生心血管事件的这部分患者的临床特点，而这可能正是在"瘀毒致变"理论指导下冠心病稳定期患者的"瘀毒"临床表征。结果显示，胸骨后疼痛、平素经常咽痛、头痛和脉涩或结代是稳定期冠心病患者随访发生心血管事件的独立危险因素。hs-CRP 作为炎症反应标记物，是不稳定斑块的一个敏感的预测指标[7]，并可独立预测冠心病患者临床不良心血管事件的发生[8]。2003 年 1 月，美国心脏协会和疾病控制中心发表声明，推荐 hs-CRP 作为临床检测指标在一级预防人群中用于对心血管疾病，以及在稳定性冠状动脉疾病或急性冠状动脉综合征患者复发心血管事件的危险评价（Ⅱa，证据强度 B）[9]。本研究结果显示 hs-CRP $\geq$ 3mg/L 随访心血管事件发生率明显升高，尽管没有达到差异有统计学意义，但鉴于 hs-CRP 目前公认的预测急性心血管事件的价值，hs-CRP $\geq$ 3mg/L 无疑可作为"瘀毒"微观表征之一。

冠心病"瘀毒"病机既有冠心病"瘀"的共性，也具有起病急骤、传变迅速、病变复杂、病势

表 1 心血管事件相关危险因素的 Logistic 多元逐步回归分析

影响因素	B	SE	Wald	Sig	Exp（B）	95%CIforExp（B）
胸骨后疼痛	1.118	0.491	5.180	0.023	3.058	1.168-8.007
头痛	0.994	0.501	3.942	0.047	2.702	1.013-7.207
耳鸣	0.635	0.469	1.831	0.176	1.886	0.752-4.729
平素咽痛	1.033	0.520	3.939	0.047	2.808	1.013-7.785
脉涩或结代	3.096	0.966	10.283	0.001	22.119	3.333-146.792
hs-CRP	0.846	0.505	2.809	0.094	2.331	0.866-6.272
TG	-0.712	0.481	2.192	0.139	0.490	0.191-1.260
TC/HDL-C	-0.386	0.254	2.300	0.129	0.680	0.413-1.119
FBG	0.163	0.119	1.864	0.172	1.177	0.931-1.488

酷烈等"毒"的特点,这在 ACS 患者中表现较为突出和典型。但基于"瘀毒致变"假说所立活血解毒治疗大法,其干预靶人群的重点绝不是已发生急性心血管事件的患者,而是在冠心病稳定期的"瘀毒内蕴"高危患者,这也是中医"未病先防""既病防变"的优势所在,因此,如何辨识冠心病稳定期的"瘀毒"临床表征显然具有更重要的临床意义。从临床实际来看,在"瘀毒致变"引发急性心血管事件之前的量变过程中,传统"毒"的临床表征如高热神昏、疮疡红肿热痛、舌质红绛、苔焦或起芒刺等,在冠心病稳定期患者中并不多见。在本研究显示的心血管事件重要影响因素中,胸骨后疼痛、头痛、脉涩或结代为血瘀征象,而平素经常咽痛和 hs-CRP 增高提示机体有慢性炎症反应,是"毒"的表征之一,这些症状、体征和实验室指标无疑可以考虑作为稳定期冠心病患者"瘀毒"的临床表征,为早期辨治高危患者提供依据。除临床事件随访外,本研究在入选后 6 个月、1 年两个时间点均进行了临床随访,内容包括主症、兼症及生化检查,与入选时一致,但由于本研究为阶段性结果,仅对入选时相关指标进行了随访心血管事件相关因素的多元 Logistic 逐步回归分析,因此所发现的"瘀毒"表征还只是初步的。随着样本数的扩大,结合是否发生心血管事件而进行不同时间点的对比分析,无疑将更有助于把握其动态变化规律,冠心病稳定期患者"瘀毒"临床表征会进一步完善,其敏感性和特异性也会进一步增加。在此基础上,对这部分冠心病高危患者及早给予活血解毒中药干预,可望进一步降低心血管事件发生,值得深入研究。

参考文献

[1] 徐浩. 活血解毒中药抗炎及稳定易损斑块的探索与思考. 中国中西医结合杂志, 2008, 28 (5): 393-394.

[2] 周明学, 徐浩, 陈可冀, 等. 活血解毒中药有效部位对 ApoE 基因敲除小鼠血脂和动脉粥样硬化斑块炎症反应的影响. 中国中西医结合杂志, 2008, 28 (2): 126-130.

[3] 徐浩, 史大卓, 殷惠军, 等. "瘀毒致变"与急性心血管事件: 假说的提出与临床意义. 中国中西医结合杂志, 2008, 28 (10): 934-938.

[4] 史大卓, 徐浩, 殷惠军, 等. "瘀"、"毒"从化——心脑血管血栓性疾病病因病机. 中西医结合学报, 2008, 6 (11): 1105-1108.

[5] 陈灏珠主编. 实用内科学. 12 版. 北京: 人民卫生出版社, 2005: 1472-1473.

[6] 中国中西医结合学会心血管专业委员会. 冠心病中医辨证标准. 中西医结合杂志, 1991, 11 (5): 257-258.

[7] Virmani R, Burke AP, Farb A, et al. Pathology of the vulnerable plaque. J Am Coll Cardiol, 2006, 47 (8 Suppl): C13-18.

[8] Goldstein JA, Chandra HR, O cNeill WW. Relation of number of complex coronary lesions to serum C-reactive prote in levels and major adverse cardiovascular events at one year. Am J Cardiol, 2005, 96 (1): 56-60.

[9] Pearson TA, Mensah GA, Alexander RW, et al. Markers of inflammation and cardiovascular disease: application to clinical and public health practice: a statement for healthcare professionals from the Centers for Disease Control and Prevention and the American Heart Association. Circulation, 2003, 107 (3): 499-511.

活血解毒中药配伍干预介入后不稳定型心绞痛的临床研究 *

陈 浩 高铸烨 徐 浩 史大卓 陈可冀 吕树铮 李田昌

不稳定型心绞痛(unstable angina, UA)是介于稳定型心绞痛和急性心肌梗死(AMI)之间的一组临床心绞痛综合征。近年来,在国家重大基础研究项目的资助下,本课题组根据现代医学研究进展,结合中医学有关"瘀毒"致病的病因病机学说,提出冠心病"瘀毒"致病理论,并进行基础研

* 原载于《中西医结合心脑血管杂志》, 2009, 7 (10): 1135-1137

究。研究证实活血解毒中药具有稳定易损斑块、抑制炎症、调节血脂等功效。那么临床上它是否能改善心绞痛症状，抑制炎症指标、改善 UA 患者的预后？本研究针对这一问题，进行小样本的临床随机对照研究。

1. 资料与方法

1.1 诊断标准

西医诊断标准：参考 WHO《缺血性心脏病的命名及诊断标准》[1]，2007 年中华医学会心血管病学分会、中华心血管病杂志编辑委员会公布的《不稳定型心绞痛诊断与治疗指南》[2]。中医证候诊断标准：参照 1990 年中西医结合心血管学会修订的《冠心病中医辨证标准》[3]。血瘀证计分标准：参照中国中西医结合学会活血化瘀专业委员会制定的血瘀证诊断标准[4]，并结合冠心病患者的发病特点，按文献[5]方法进行评分。

1.2 纳入标准

年龄 40～75 岁；符合不稳定型心绞痛诊断；在胸痛发作后 48h 内接受冠状动脉造影并行介入治疗成功的患者；中医辨证属血瘀型（包括气滞血瘀、气虚血瘀等复合证型）；具有"骤发性、酷烈性及顽固性"等毒邪致病特点；签署知情同意书者。

1.3 排除标准

稳定型心绞痛或急性心肌梗死患者；近 1 个月内感染、发热、创伤、烧伤、手术史和炎症；活动性结核病或风湿免疫疾病患者；已知的肾功能不全，已知的肝功能不全，基础肝酶检测＞正常值的 3 倍；严重心力衰竭患者，射血分数（ejection fraction，EF）＜35%；合并造血系统等严重原发性疾病、精神病患者；恶性肿瘤患者；脏器移植患

者；参加其他临床试验者；妊娠期或哺乳期妇女。

1.4 剔除标准

受试者依从性差，未按规定用药，无法判定疗效或资料不全等影响疗效或安全性判定者；观察中自然脱离、失访者，包括治疗过程中有效，但不能取得联系获得有效临床资料；发生严重不良反应或并发症，不宜继续接受研究而被迫中止研究者。

1.5 一般资料

选择 2008 年 3 月至 2008 年 9 月首都医科大学附属安贞医院和首都医科大学附属同仁医院心内科行冠状动脉内支架植入术成功的不稳定型心绞痛患者 61 例。采用随机、对照方法分为活血组（31 例）与活血解毒组（30 例）。两组一般资料、既往病史、病情分级、造影结果、支架长度及类型、中医主症计分、血瘀证计分、心绞痛计分基本相似，具有可比性（$P > 0.05$）。详见表 1。

1.6 治疗方法

1.6.1 PTCA 及冠脉支架植入术　采用股动脉或桡动脉径路按常规标准方法进行。

1.6.2 药物治疗　两组均给予西医标准化药物治疗，包括抗缺血治疗、抗血小板治疗 [阿司匹林和（或）氯吡格雷]、抗凝治疗及他汀类药物，并根据合并症给予对症处理。活血解毒组在常规西药治疗的同时加口服芎芍胶囊（由川芎、赤芍的有效部位组成，为北京市药监局批准的院内制剂，京药制字：Z20053499）2 粒，3 次 / 日；黄连胶囊（由湖北香连药业有限责任公司生产，国药准字：Z19983042）2 粒，3 次 / 日，用药 2 周。活血组在常规西药治疗的同时加口服芎芍胶囊 2 粒，3 次 / 日，用药 2 周。

1.7 随访

用药 2 周后复查心电图、血小板计数（ALT）、

表 1　两组病例临床资料比较

组别	n	年龄岁	性别（例）		既往病史（例）					病情分级（例）		
			男	女	高血压病	糖尿病	高脂血症	脑卒中	陈旧性心肌梗死	低危	中危	高危
活血组	31	61.84±8.41	22	9	18	7	11	2	4	0	26	5
活血解毒组	30	61.24±9.86	25	5	16	9	12	4	1	0	24	6

组别	病变范围（例）			病变类型（例）		中医主症计分	血瘀证计分	心绞痛计分
	单支	双支	三支	新病变	再狭窄			
活血组	8	12	11	28	3	17.97±6.74	10.89±4.62	14.42±4.86
活血解毒组	12	7	11	26	4	18.94±5.64	10.59±3.38	14.89±4.63

注：两组各项比较，$P > 0.05$

血肌酐（Cr）、高敏C反应蛋白（hs-CRP）、血脂，填写中医主症计分（包括胸痛、胸闷、气短、乏力、心悸症状）、心绞痛计分（包括心绞痛发作次数、持续时间、疼痛程度、硝酸甘油用量、体力活动大小）、血瘀证计分及中医兼症、舌脉情况。以后每3个月门诊或电话随访1次，随访6个月，重点观察生存质量、终点指标发生的情况。

1.8　观察指标

主要终点指标：心血管死亡、心肌梗死、脑卒中、需要行血运重建术（包括冠状动脉旁路移植术）、因不稳定型心绞痛再住院。治疗前后心绞痛计分、中医主症计分、血瘀证计分及心电图变化。实验性指标观测：全部研究对象分别于治疗前及治疗结束后清晨无菌抽取空腹静脉血检测 hs-CRP、Cr、ALT、总胆固醇（TC）、三酰甘油（TG）、低密度脂蛋白（LDL）、高密度脂蛋白（HDL）。

1.9　疗效判定标准

心绞痛症状疗效评定标准参照《胸痹心痛（冠心病心绞痛）诊疗规范》《中药新药治疗胸痹（冠心病心绞痛）的临床研究指导原则》[6] 及1979 年中西医结合治疗冠心病心绞痛及心律失常座谈会《冠心病心绞痛及心电图疗效评定标准》。

1.10　统计学处理

采用 SPSS 15.0 软件包进行统计学处理。计量资料以均数 ± 标准差（$\bar{x} \pm s$）表示。定性资料采用卡方检验、Fisher 精确概率法、Wilcoxon 秩和检验。定量资料符合正态分布用 t 检验（组间进行方差分析检验，方差不齐时选用校正的 t 检验），不符合正态分布用 Wilcoxon 秩和检验和 Wilcoxon 符号秩和检验。$P < 0.05$ 为有统计学意义。

2.　结果

2.1　两组治疗前后心绞痛计分、中医主症计分、血瘀证计分比较

两组治疗前后心绞痛计分、中医主症计分、血瘀证计分比较均有统计学意义（$P < 0.01$），但组间治疗后比较无统计学意义（$P > 0.05$）。详见表2。

表2　两组心绞痛、中医主症、血瘀证计分比较（$\bar{x} \pm s$）分

组别		心绞痛	中医主症	血瘀证
活血组	治疗前	14.42±4.86	17.97±6.74	10.89±4.62
	治疗后	4.84±7.32[1)	4.03±6.61[1)	8.03±4.79[1)
活血解毒组	治疗前	14.89±4.63	18.94±5.64	10.59±3.38
	治疗后	1.47±3.64[1)	3.83±6.13[1)	8.00±4.68[1)

与同组治疗前比较，1) $P < 0.01$

2.2　两组实验室指标比较

活血组治疗前后 hs-CRP 水平降低，但未达到统计学意义（$P > 0.05$）；活血解毒组治疗前后 hs-CRP 水平显著降低（$P < 0.05$）；两组 TC、LDL 水平治疗前后均显著降低（$P < 0.05$），但组间比较无统计学意义（$P > 0.05$）；两组 HDL 水平治疗前后未达到统计学意义（$P > 0.05$）。详见表3。

2.3　两组心绞痛、心电图、总体疗效比较（见表4）

两组病例在心绞痛、心电图和总体疗效方面，均无统计学意义（$P > 0.05$），二者疗效相当。

2.4　不良反应、随访3个月主要终点事件比较

治疗过程中，活血组2周随访时出现1例肝功能轻度异常，追问病史，考虑为服用他汀类药物所致，通过调整他汀类药物及保肝治疗后肝功能恢复正常。活血解毒组有4例患者服药期间出现腹泻，但不超过3次／日，调整药量为1粒／次，每日两次后症状缓解，完成2周疗程；随访3个月时，活血组有1例出现支架内再狭窄，需行血运重建术（冠状动脉旁路移植术）。两组均未发生严重出血事件、死亡和急性心肌梗死。因发生临床终点事件病例数较少，未进行统计分析。本研究服药2周，目前随访观察6个月，推测若延长用药时间，观察其远期疗效，则有可能得到阳性结果。

3.　讨论

冠心病不稳定型心绞痛属中医"胸痹心痛"

表3　两组实验室指标比较（$\bar{x} \pm s$）

	组别	hs-CRP（mg/L）	TC（mmol/L）	TG（mmol/L）	LDL（mmol/L）	HDL（mmol/L）
活血组	治疗前	4.18±7.84	4.97±1.52	1.93±0.84	3.18±1.91	0.94±0.28
	治疗后	3.10±3.83	3.96±0.72[1)	1.69±0.74	2.45±0.54[1)	0.99±0.26
活血解毒组	治疗前	5.75±8.54	4.32±1.04	1.66±0.79	2.81±0.99	1.05±0.28
	治疗后	2.62±2.66[1)	3.66±0.82[1)	1.45±0.77	2.28±0.87[1)	0.98±0.29

注：与同组治疗前比较，1) $P < 0.05$

表4 两组心绞痛、心电图、总体疗效比较

项目	组别	n	显效例	有效例	无效例	总有效率 %
心绞痛	活血组	31	1	30	0	100.0
	活血解毒组	30	1	28	1	96.7
心电图	活血组	31	8	23	0	100.0
	活血解毒组	30	7	23	0	100.0
总体	活血组	31	0	31	0	100.0
	活血解毒组	30	0	29	1	96.7

之范围，其发病多与饮食不当、情志失调、寒邪内侵、久病年迈等有关，病机有虚实之分。张仲景在《金匮要略》中将其病机概括为"阳微阴弦"，即上焦阳气不足，下焦阴寒气盛。阳微指胸阳不振，即气虚、阳虚，临床有时可兼阴虚，表现为气阴两虚或阴阳两虚；阴弦指瘀血、痰浊、寒凝为患；且诸多因素中瘀血尤为突出。

近年来，由于人们生活水平的提高，生活方式及饮食结构的改变，大气环境污染、疾病模式及疾病谱的变化，使现代人的体质乃至病理生理特点都与以前有了很大不同，这些变化显著地影响到冠心病的发生、发展。血瘀是贯穿于不稳定型心绞痛发展过程的中心环节，若瘀久化热、酿生毒邪，或从化为毒，可致瘀毒内蕴，如迁延日久、失治误治，则正消邪长，一旦外因引动、蕴毒骤发，则毒瘀搏结、痹阻心脉，"瘀毒致变"而导致不稳定型心绞痛的发生、发展。

动脉粥样硬化"炎症"学说得到了普遍的认可。易损斑块破裂、血栓形成导致急性冠状动脉综合征发病理论对冠心病的诊治产生了很大影响，同时也促进了中西医结合防治冠心病理论实践的发展。以往的研究发现活血解毒中药有效部位虎杖提取物、大黄醇提取物均可通过改善斑块内部成分来稳定易损斑块，较单纯活血药物或解毒药物效果更为显著[7]。

hs-CRP 是临床常用的炎症指标，目前已经有大量研究支持 hs-CRP 可用于心血管疾病危险的评估。Hartford 等[8]观察了 CRP 对 ACS 发生心血管事件的预测价值，结果发现，随着入院时 CRP 水平升高，病死率和充血性心力衰竭的发生率均明显增加。在多因素分析中，入院时 CRP 的水平是判断 ACS 预后最强的独立预测因子。JUPITER 研究[9]（Justification for the use of Statinsin Primary Prevention: An Intervention Trial Evaluating Rosuvastin）对 LDL-C 水平正常但 hs-CRP 水平升高（≥ 2mg/L）的健康人群，随机服用瑞舒伐他汀（rosuvastatin）20mg/d 或安慰剂组。随访1.9年，与安慰剂相比，瑞舒伐他汀 20mg 使心肌梗死、非致死性卒中、不稳定型心绞痛住院、血运重建和心血管死亡主要复合终点发生率显著降低44%。JUPITER 研究将一级预防的干预从 LDL-C 拓展至 LDL-C 和炎症双靶点，提供了针对 hs-CRP 水平升高治疗可有效减少心血管事件的证据。

本临床研究初步结果表明，在西医常规治疗基础上加用活血解毒中药在降低炎症指标、改善心绞痛症状方面有一定疗效，较加用单纯活血药效果明显，也反证了"瘀毒"在冠心病发生发展中有内在的关联性，为"瘀毒"致病理论提供了依据，值得进一步深入研究。

参考文献

[1] 国际心脏病学会和协会及世界卫生组织临床命名标准化联合专题组报告. 缺血性心脏病的命名及诊断标准. 中华内科杂志, 1981, 20 (4): 254.

[2] 中华医学会心血管病学分会. 不稳定性心绞痛和非 ST 段抬高心肌梗死诊断与治疗指南. 中华心血管病杂志, 2007, 35 (4): 295-304.

[3] 中国中西医结合学会心血管分会. 冠心病中医辨证标准. 中国中西医结合杂志, 1991, 11 (5): 257.

[4] 中国中西医结合学会活血化瘀专业委员会. 血瘀证诊断标准. 中西医结合杂志, 1987, 7 (3): 129.

[5] 王阶. 血瘀证诊断标准的研究. 北京: 北京医科大学、中国协和医科大学联合出版社, 1993: 7.

[6] 郑筱萸. 中药新药临床研究指导原则（试行）. 北京: 中国医药科技出版社, 2002: 57-61.

[7] 周明学, 徐浩, 陈可冀, 等. 活血解毒中药有效部位对 ApoE 基因敲除小鼠血脂和动脉粥样硬化斑块炎症反应的影响. 中国中西医结合杂志, 2008, 28 (2): 126-130.

[8] Goldstein JA, Chandra HR, O'NeillWW. Relation of number of complex coronary lesions to serum C-reactive protein levels and major adverse cardiovascular events at one year. Am J Cardiol, 2005, 96 (1): 56-60.

[9] Pearson TA, Mensah GA, Alexander RW, et al. Markers of inlammation and cardiovascular disease: application to clinical and public health practice: a statement for healthcare professionals from the Centers for Disease Control and Prevention and the American Heart Association. Circulation, 2003, 107 (3): 499-511.

活血解毒中药对稳定期冠心病患者血清
炎症标记物及血脂的影响*

郑 峰 周明学 徐 浩 陈可冀

研究表明，超敏 C 反应蛋白（hs-CRP）作为目前最可靠的动脉粥样硬化（AS）炎症标志物，与斑块的进展密切相关，现已被视为急性冠状动脉综合征（ACS）发病的独立危险因子，并用于判定其预后[1]。笔者既往实验研究表明，活血解毒中药酒大黄及其有效作用部位大黄醇提物具有明显的稳定斑块作用，其机制与抑制炎症反应有关[2-3]。但目前关于活血解毒中药对临床稳定期冠心病患者血清炎症标志物及血脂影响的相关研究甚少。为此，笔者以新清宁片（熟大黄）为活血解毒中药的代表药物、以丹七片为活血对照药，观察其对常规他汀类药物治疗的冠心病稳定期患者血清炎症标志物及血脂的影响。

1. 资料与方法

1.1 一般资料

选择 2007 年 10 月—2008 年 1 月在中日友好医院经冠状动脉造影检查确诊的冠心病稳定期患者 30 例，按随机数字表法分为 3 组：他汀对照组、活血中药组和活血解毒中药组，每组 10 例。他汀对照组 10 例，男 7 例，女 3 例，平均年龄（61.2±11.5）岁，单支病变 4 例，双支病变 3 例，三支病变 3 例；活血中药组 10 例，男 6 例，女 4 例，平均年龄（63.1±9.5）岁，单支病变 4 例，双支病变 4 例，三支病变 2 例；活血解毒中药组 10 例，男 7 例，女 3 例，平均年龄（60.1±12.4）岁，单支病变 4 例，双支病变 3 例，三支病变 3 例。3 组冠心病患者之间的性别、年龄及病变情况比较均无显著差异（$P > 0.05$）。

1.2 诊断标准

冠心病诊断标准：符合 1979 年 WHO 诊断标准，并且选择冠状动脉造影左主干狭窄 ≥ 30%，或其他血管狭窄 ≥ 50% 者。血瘀证诊断标准参照中国中西医结合学会活血化瘀专业委员会制订的血

瘀证诊断标准[4]，并结合冠心病患者的发病特点，按文献[5]方法进行血瘀证计分。

1.3 纳入标准

经冠状动脉造影确诊的冠心病患者；中医辨证为血瘀证（可兼有气虚、痰浊等其他证候要素）；临床表现为无症状、稳定劳累性心绞痛、其他类型心绞痛或急性冠状动脉综合征病程超过 1 个月病情稳定者；年龄 30 ~ 75 岁；血清学检测 hs-CRP > 3ng/mL；规律服用他汀类药物治疗 ≥ 2 个月的患者；签署知情同意书。

1.4 排除标准

近 1 个月内感染、发热、创伤、烧伤、手术史；未规律服用他汀类药物治疗；平素有脾虚腹泻症状的患者；有出血倾向的患者；活动性结核病或风湿免疫疾病患者；严重心力衰竭患者，EF < 35%；合并严重瓣膜疾病或心肌病；合并严重慢阻肺、肺心病或呼吸衰竭患者；已知的肾功能不全，男性血清肌酐 > 2.5mg/dl（221μmol/L），女性 > 2.0mg/dl（177μmol/L）；已知的肝功能不全，基础肝酶检测 > 正常值的 3 倍或合并肝硬化；严重造血系统疾病；严重精神病患者；恶性肿瘤患者；脏器移植患者。

1.5 剔除标准

入选后患者未能坚持按规律服药的；服药 1 个月后患者因故未能按时复查的；复查时发现患有感冒、发热、腹泻等急性感染性疾病。

1.6 试验分组与治疗方法

他汀对照组：按照 2007 中国成人血脂异常防治指南[6]给予他汀类药物（辛伐他汀、阿托伐他汀等）治疗；活血中药组：在常规他汀类药物治疗的基础上加用丹七片，每次 3 片（每片 0.3g），每天 3 次，主要成分为丹参和三七，由北京同仁堂科技发展股份有限公司制药厂提供，批号为 20070912；活血解毒中药组：在常规他汀类

*原载于《中华中医药杂志》，2009，24（19）：1153-1157

药物治疗基础上加用新清宁片，每次 3 片（每片 0.3g），每天 3 次，主要成分为熟大黄，由中国中医科学院实验药厂提供，批号为 20070509。疗程均为 1 个月。本试验经中日友好医院伦理委员会批准，编号：2007-60。

1.7 检测指标及方法

患者均于清晨空腹静脉采血，采用酶联免疫吸附试验（ELISA）检测服药前后血清 hs-CRP、肿瘤坏死因子 -α（tumor necrosis foctor α，TNF-α）浓度，试剂盒由 R&B 公司提供，严格按照说明书进行操作；血脂指标包括总胆固醇（TC）、甘油三酯（TG）、高密度脂蛋白胆固醇（HDL-C）、低密度脂蛋白胆固醇（LDL-C）、脂蛋白（a）[LP（a）]、载脂蛋白 A（ApoA）、载脂蛋白 B（ApoB），肝肾功能检测包括谷丙转氨酶（ALT）、肌酐（Cr），均由中日友好医院化验室统一检测。非 HDL-C（non-HDL-C）= TC - HDL-C，动脉粥样硬化指数（atherogenic index，AI）=（TC-HDL-C）/HDL-C。

1.8 统计学方法

所用数据用 SPSS 11.5 软件进行统计分析，计量资料用 $\bar{x} \pm s$ 表示，组间比较用单向方差分析（One-way ANOVA），方差齐性用 LSD 法，方差不齐时用 Tambane's T^2 法，同组治疗前后比较采用配对资料的 t 检验，以 $P < 0.05$ 为差异有统计学意义。

2. 结果

2.1 临床试验完成情况

实际完成病例 27 例，每组 9 例。1 例患者因心房颤动住院而未能按时复查，1 例患者因感冒发热未按时复查，1 例患者服药后大便次数增加而停药。

2.2 各组治疗前后血清 hs-CRP 浓度的变化

服药 1 个月后，与治疗前比较，活血解毒中药组和活血中药组患者血清 hs-CRP 浓度显著降低（$P < 0.05$，$P < 0.01$）。他汀对照组患者血清 hs-CRP 浓度有所降低，但无统计学意义（$P > 0.05$）。活血解毒中药组治疗前后血清 hs-CRP 浓度差值与他汀对照组比较有显著差异（$P < 0.05$），与活血中药组比较有非常显著差异（$P < 0.01$）。见表 1。

2.3 各组治疗前后血清 TNF-α 浓度的变化

服药 1 个月后，与治疗前比较，各组患者血清 TNF-α 浓度虽有程度不同的降低，但均无统计

表 1 各组治疗前后血清 hs-CRP 比较（$\bar{x} \pm s$）

组别	例数	hs-CRP(mg/L)		
		治疗前	治疗后	差值
他汀对照组	9	4.63±1.64	2.73±2.39	1.90±2.15
活血中药组	9	5.44±2.03	3.96±2.27*	1.49±1.48
活血解毒中药组	9	10.57±4.54	3.74±3.51**	6.83±4.99△▲

注：与本组治疗前比较，*$P < 0.05$，**$P < 0.01$；与他汀对照组比较，△$P < 0.05$，与活血中药组比较，▲$P < 0.01$

学意义（$P > 0.05$）；各组治疗前后 TNF-α 浓度差值比较亦无显著差异（$P > 0.05$）。见表 2。

表 2 各组治疗前后血清 TNF-α 比较（$\bar{x} \pm s$）

组别	例数	TNF-α(mg/L)		
		治疗前	治疗后	差值
他汀对照组	9	3.90±3.09	2.47±1.31	1.43±2.64
活血中药组	9	4.55±4.11	3.67±2.64	0.88±3.06
活血解毒中药组	9	3.51±1.44	2.52±0.54	0.99±1.70

2.4 各组治疗前后血脂水平的变化

服药治疗 1 个月后，与治疗前比较，活血解毒中药组可明显降低患者血清 TC 浓度和非 HDL-C 浓度，并可升高血清 HDL-C 浓度，同时还可降低血清 ApoB/A 比值以及 AI（$P < 0.05$，$P < 0.01$）。而活血中药组患者各项血脂指标除血清 ApoB/A 比值与治疗前比较明显降低外，其他虽有所改善，但无统计学差异（$P > 0.05$）。见表 3。

2.5 各组治疗前后血瘀证计分的变化

治疗 1 个月后，与治疗前比较，活血解毒中药组血瘀证计分明显降低（$P < 0.05$）；他汀对照组和活血中药组血瘀证计分虽有降低，但与治疗前比较无显著差异（$P > 0.05$）。3 组间治疗前后血瘀证计分差值比较无显著差异（$P > 0.05$）。见表 4。

2.6 安全性观察

研究过程中，各组患者治疗前后肝、肾功能均在正常范围，活血解毒中药组有 1 例患者自诉服药后大便次数明显增多，停药后症状仍存在，后患者自行停药，退出试验。其余患者未有药物不良反应报告。

表 3　各组患者治疗前后血脂指标比较（$\bar{x}\pm s$）

组别	例数	时间	TC	TG-C	LDL-C	HDL-C	LP (a)	non-HDL-C	ApoB/A	AI
他汀对照组	9	治疗前	5.59±1.49	2.03±1.43	1.64±0.63	1.12±0.30	0.26±0.13	4.46±1.41	0.90±0.15	4.11±1.56
		治疗后	4.09±0.76*	1.59±1.03	1.18±0.36	1.12±0.25	0.22±0.06	2.98±0.89*	0.71±0.21	2.96±1.81*
活血中药组	9	治疗前	4.32±1.31	1.54±0.97	2.09±0.89	1.14±0.42	0.20±0.07	3.19±1.24	0.90±0.27	2.99±1.21
		治疗后	4.39±1.21	1.44±0.91	2.55±1.05	1.25±0.47	0.18±0.09	3.14±1.13	0.63±0.17*	2.78±1.23
活血解毒中药组	9	治疗前	4.82±0.47	1.64±0.63	2.79±0.39	1.08±0.09	0.24±0.12	3.74±0.43	1.07±0.31	2.99±1.21
		治疗后	4.10±0.64*	1.18±0.36	2.45±0.57	1.21±0.15**	0.21±0.11	2.89±0.64**	0.64±0.07**	2.78±1.23

注：与治疗前比较，*$P < 0.05$，**$P < 0.01$。下表同

表 4　各组治疗前后血瘀证计分的比较（$\bar{x}\pm s$）

组别	例数	血瘀证计分		
		治疗前	治疗后	差值
他汀对照组	9	13.43±9.13	11.57±6.60	1.86±6.41
活血中药组	9	13.57±4.54	12.57±4.12	1.00±4.79
活血解毒中药组	9	17.14±3.63	11.86±4.53*	5.29±5.15

注：与治疗前比较，*$P < 0.05$

3. 讨论

越来越多的研究表明，AS 斑块由原来的稳定状态进入一种不稳定状态，在这种不稳定斑块（易损斑块）破裂的基础上合并血栓形成是造成急性心血管事件最重要的病理基础，炎症反应是影响冠状动脉 AS 斑块稳定性的重要因素，病变内外的炎症均加速或触发急性事件的发生[7]。笔者既往实验研究表明，活血解毒中药酒大黄及其有效作用部位大黄醇提物具有明显的稳定斑块作用，其机制与抑制炎症反应有关，效果优于活血中药[2-3]。然而，关于活血解毒中药对稳定期冠心病患者血清炎症标志物影响的相关研究甚少。新清宁片的主要成分是熟大黄，是大黄经酒蒸或酒炖而成，泻下成分大黄酸减少，而活血化瘀力量增强，可作为活血解毒中药的代表药物。本研究即在他汀降脂药常规治疗基础上加用新清宁片，并与加用活血中药丹七片以及单纯他汀类降脂药治疗作比较，观察其对冠心病稳定期患者血清炎症标志物及血脂的影响。

hs-CRP 作为炎症标记物之一，不仅标志着血管事件危险的增高，还可能参与疾病机制，有助于判断预后、危险分层，并可能会成为预防和治疗 AS 及其并发症的潜在靶点[8]。2003 年 1 月，美国心脏协会和疾病控制中心发表声明，推荐 hs-CRP 作为临床检测指标在一级预防人群中用于对心血管疾病，以及在稳定性冠状动脉疾病或急性冠状动脉综合征患者复发心血管事件的危险评价（Ⅱa，证据强度 B）[9]，表明炎性反应在血栓性疾病尤其是心脑血管疾病的发病中具有重要地位。本研究结果显示，在他汀类降脂药基础上加用活血解毒中药新清宁片可明显降低冠心病稳定期患者升高的血清 hs-CRP 水平，优于单纯他汀类降脂药治疗和他汀加用活血中药丹七片治疗，这与笔者既往动物实验中"活血解毒中药在抑制炎症反应、稳定易损斑块方面优于单纯活血药"的研究结论相一致。由于样本数较小，各组治疗前 hs-CRP 的基线水平不一致，活血解毒中药组明显高于其他两组，但治疗前后的差值仍然显示出活血解毒中药的作用。血清 TNF-α 作为冠心病患者全身炎症反应的非特异性标记物之一，对于评价冠心病患者未来心血管事件发生也有一定的预测价值[10]。本研究中各组都有降低 TNF-α 的趋势，但未见统计学差异，考虑可能与样本数较小有关。

脂质代谢紊乱是导致 AS 的重要机制，也是影响斑块稳定性的重要因素，通过调脂治疗可使冠心病患者获得远期受益已成共识。笔者的研究结果表明，他汀药常规治疗加用新清宁可明显降低患者血清 TC 浓度和非 HDL-C 浓度，并可升高血清 HDL-C 浓度，同时还可显著降低血清 ApoB/A 比值及 AI，对患者血清 LDL-C 浓度亦有降低趋势，提示这种治疗方案对冠心病稳定期患者的血脂具有广泛的调节作用，尤其在规范他汀治疗基础上，活血解毒中药的这种辅助调脂作用无疑为我们提供了一个有效的联合调脂策略。另外，HDL-C 参与 TC 的逆向转运，具有抗血栓、抗炎、抗氧化及增加内皮细胞抗 LDL-C 的毒性作用等功能[11]。本研究在常规他汀药治疗基础上，加用新清宁片治疗可进一

第二章

步升高血清 HDL-C 浓度，进而改善 ApoB/A 比值及 AI 等指标，这在当前降脂治疗同样关注 HDL-C 的背景下，显然具有重要的临床意义，值得深入研究。

本研究还发现，活血解毒中药组治疗后血瘀证计分较治疗前亦明显降低，而他汀对照组与活血中药组治疗后血瘀证计分虽有下降趋势，但较治疗前无显著差异，考虑与样本数较小、且入选患者均为冠心病稳定期患者有关，但同时提示，对于 hs-CRP > 3ng/ml 的冠心病稳定期患者，活血解毒中药在改善血瘀状态方面较单纯活血中药显示有一定的优势。

本研究结果表明，在他汀类降脂药基础上加用活血解毒中药新清宁片能进一步降低冠心病稳定期患者血清 hs-CRP 水平，改善血瘀状态，纠正血脂代谢紊乱，体现了中西医结合治疗的优势，而且两药合用未见明显不良作用，适宜临床推广应用。同时，hs-CRP 作为炎症标记物，可视作中医"毒"微观指标之一，本研究也为冠心病发展过程中的"瘀毒致变"假说[12] 提供了初步的临床依据。当然，本研究仅是小样本的预试验，且 hs-CRP 为替代指标之一，本试验用药方案对冠心病稳定期患者能否预防再发急性心血管事件，尚需大样本、长期随访的临床试验加以证实。

参考文献

[1] Futterman LG, Lemberg L. High-sensitivity C-reactive protein is the most effective prognostic measurement of acute coronary events. Am J Crit Care, 2002, 11（5）：482-486.

[2] 文川，徐浩，黄启福，等. 活血中药对 ApoE 缺陷小鼠血脂及 AS 斑块炎症反应的影响. 中国中西医结合杂志，2005，25（4）：345-348.

[3] 周明学，徐浩，陈可冀，等. 活血解毒中药有效部位对 ApoE 基因敲除小鼠血脂和 AS 斑块炎症反应的影响. 中国中西医结合杂志，2008，28（2）：126-130.

[4] 中国中西医结合学会活血化瘀专业委员会. 血瘀证诊断标准. 中国中西医结合杂志，1987，7（3）：129-131.

[5] 王阶. 血瘀证诊断标准的研究. 活血化瘀研究与临床. 北京：北京医科大学、中国协和医科大学联合出版社，1993：7.

[6] 中国成人血脂异常防治指南制定联合委员会. 中国成人血脂异常防治指南. 中华心血管病杂志，2007，35（5）：390-413

[7] Shah PK. Pathophysiology of plaque rupture and the concept of plaque stabilization. Cardiol Clin, 2003, 21（3）：303-14.

[8] Wilson AM, Ryan MC, Boyle AJ. The novel role of C-reactive protein in cardiovascular disease：risk marker or pathogen. Int J Cardiol, 2006, 106（3）：291-7.

[9] Pearson TA, Mensah GA, Alexander RW, et al. Markers of inflammation and cardiovascular disease：application to clinical and public health practice：a statement for health care professionals from the Centers for Disease Control and Prevention and the American Heart Association. Circulation, 2003, 107（3）：499-511.

[10] Libby P, Aikawa M. Stabilization of atherosclerotic plaques：new mechanisms and clinical targets. Nat Med, 2002, 8：1257-1262.

[11] Mavab M, Anantharamaiah GM, Reddy ST, et al. Mechanisms of disease：proatherogenic HDL-an evolving field. Nar Clin Pract Endocrino Metab, 2006, 2（9）：504-511.

[12] 徐浩，史大卓，殷惠军，等. "瘀毒致变"与急性心血管事件：假说的提出与临床意义. 中国中西医结合杂志，2008，28（10）：934-938.

Study on the Tongue Manifestations for the Blood-Stasis and Toxin Syndrome in the Stable Patients of Coronary Heart Disease[*]

FENG Yan　XU Hao　QU Dan　ZHENG Feng　SHI Da-zhuo　CHEN Ke-ji

As documented in ancient literature of Chinese medicine (CM), tongue reflects sign of Xin (心), thus the investigation of tongue manifestations has great significance to analyze CM pathogenesis of coronary heart disease (CHD) and its treatment based on syndrome-differentiation. The tongue manifestations of blood stasis syndrome were extensively studied in the past years, and dark purple tongue, petechia or ecchymosis, varicose sublingual vessel were all served as the main contents of diagnostic criteria for blood stasis syndrome. However, the relationship between the follow-up acute cardiovascular events (ACEs) and tongue manifestations in the stable CHD patients has not been investigated so far. Under the leadership of academician Prof. CHEN Ke-ji, our team definitely proposed a CM pathogenesis hypothesis of "blood-stasis and toxin causing catastrophe" in stable CHD on the basis of the previous studies[1-8], which can be summarized as follows: blood stasis is the key link throughout the evolution of CHD, and it is also the basic pathogenetic condition of the stable CHD patients as well. Blood-stasis and toxin will accumulate inside by long-duration blood-stasis and subsequent incubated heat, or originate from other pathogenetic factors. If it lasts for a long time or is delayed-treated and mistreated, the pathogenetic factors increase gradually accompanied by decreased body resistance, which results in breakout of accumulated toxin once invoked by external causes. The toxin injures the flesh, further entangles with blood-stasis, and finally blocks Xin vessel and lead to transformation of disease by manifesting acute and severe condition such as unstable angina, acute myocardial infarction and cardiac sudden death. This is the pivotal pathogenesis for the stable CHD patients who are about to experience ACEs in the future. This hypothesis will undoubtedly play an important role in theoretically guiding studies on preventing ACEs with CM treatment in CHD patients. This research adopted the method of prospective study to explore tongue manifestations of "blood-stasis and toxin" in the stable CHD patients according to the follow-up ACEs based on this hypothesis.

1. Methods

1.1 Diagnostic Criteria

The diagnostic criteria for CHD was referred to the report of "Naming and Diagnosis of Ischemic Heart Disease" formulated by the Joint Workshop of International Society of Cardiology and the World Health Organization (WHO) for standardized clinical naming[9]. The criterion of CM syndrome-differentiation for CHD was referred to "The Criterion of CM Syndrome-differentiation for CHD" revised by Cardiovascular Branch of Chinese Association of Integrative Western and Chinese Medicine in October 1990[10].

1.2 Inclusion Criteria

As the followings: with the diagnostic criteria of ischemic heart disease formulated by WHO, at least one coronary stenosis $\geq 50\%$ demonstrated

* 原载于 Chinese Journal of Integrative Medicine, 2011, 17 (5): 333-338

by selective coronary angiography; clinically manifested as asymptomatic, stable effort angina, or acute coronary syndrome (ACS) for more than 1 month who were in stable condition; aged ≤ 75 year old; signed informed consent form.

1.3 Exclusion Criteria

Having infection, fever, trauma, burns, surgical history within one month; active tuberculosis or patients with rheumatic autoimmune diseases; severe heart failure, ejection fraction (EF) < 35%; with severe valvular disease or cardiomyopathy; with severe chronic obstructive pulmonary disease, pulmonary heart disease or respiratory failure; known renal insufficiency, serum creatinine (Cr) > 2.5mg/dL (221μmol/L) for male, and Cr > 2.0mg/dL (177μmol/L) for female; known liver dysfunction, alanine aminotransferase (ALT) over 3 times more than the normal value or accompanied by cirrhosis; serious blood disorders; serious mental illness; cancer patients; organ transplant patients; with life expectancy less than 3 years.

1.4 Clinical Data

From September 2007 to March 2008, a total of 254 CHD patients diagnosed by coronary angiography with stable condition in the National Integrative Medicine Center for Cardiovascular Diseases of China-Japan Friendship Hospital were enrolled. There were 184 male and 70 female cases. The youngest was 32 years old, while the oldest was 75, with the mean age 61.9 ± 9.9 years old; 156 cases got a history of hypertension, accounting for 61.4%; diabetes mellitus in 92 patients (36.2%); 188 patients had a history of hyperlipidemia (74.0%); 115 cases of myocardial infarction (45.3%). In light of coronary angiography, 75 patients was single vessel disease (29.5%), two-vessel disease in 71 cases (28.0%), three vessel disease in 108 cases (42.5%).

1.5 Research Method and Observation Indices

The tongue pictures of all selected patients were record on the tongue manifestations with Canon IXUS 860 digital camera, the

judgment of tongue manifestations and CM syndrome differentiation were confirmed by two cardiovascular physicians of integrative medicine with professional title of associate professors or higher. All patients were followed up for 1 year to record the occurrence of ACEs. ACEs were defined as: (1) cardiac death; (2) cardiac arrest of successful resuscitation; (3) non-fatal myocardial infarction; (4) necessity for percutaneous coronary intervention (PCI) or coronary artery bypass grafting (CABG); (5) hospitalized for unstable angina pectoris.

1.6 Patients Selection and Matching Methods

Twenty-nine patients with ACEs during one-year follow-up were selected (including three PCI patients, 25 cases hospitalized for UA, and one case of recommending hospitalization for UA but not hospitalized for economic reasons), and the patients without ACEs were matched in proportion of 2:1 according to gender, age (± 2.5years), diabetes mellitus history and previous ACS hospitalization history. A total of 83 cases were included for analysis, of whom 29 cases with follow-up events (ACEs group), 54 cases without events (non-ACEs group).

1.7 Statistical Analysis

SPSS 11.5 statistical software was applied, count data using Chi-square test, while risk estimation of follow-up ACEs expressing as odds ratio (OR).

2. Results

2.1 Overall Distribution of All Kinds of Tongue Manifestations

The numbers of reddish tongue were 17 and were 20.5% in the total. Red tongue was 24, 28.9%, only two cases were full-red tongue, the rest were tongue with red color on the margin or tip. Crimson tongue was found only in one patient, being red in the whole tongue with crimson tip. Dark red tongue was 14, accounting for 16.9%. Twenty-four patients with light dark red tongue, 28.9%. Dark purple tongue was found in three patients. Light purple tongue was seen in

17 patients, covering 20.5%. Bluish tongue was found in 15 patients (Figure 1A), accounting for 18.1%, most of which were bluish-grounding on basis of other tongue color, while bluish purple tongue was seen in three patients (Figure 1B). Petechia was found in five patients, all presented on the margins of tongue.

White coating tongue was seen in 68 patients, 81.9%. Yellow coating tongue seen in 29 patients, 34.9%. Thick coating was found in 22 patients, 26.5%, mostly presented on the middle and rear. Slippery coating tongue was seen in one patient. Dry or rough coating was found in four patients. Greasy coating tongue was seen in 60 patients, covering 72.3%, of which 48 cases were sticky greasy coating, two was dirty greasy coating (Figure 1C), and ten was dry sticky coating (Figure 1D). Curdy coating was only found in one patient. Peeled coating was seen in three patients, all were exfoliated tongue.

Stiff tongue was found in four patients. Tender tongue was seen in three patients. Enlarged tongue was found in 43 patients, 51.8%. Teeth-marked tongue was found in all patients, but at different degrees. No case was thin tongue. Prickly tongue was seen in 47 patients, 56.6%. Fissured tongue was found in 38 cases, 45.8%

and most of them were in the middle of enlarged or teeth-marked tongue, while few of them were tongue with deep fissures. Deviated tongue only was found in one case with the sequelae of stroke. One case had a bleeding spot on the tongue.

Most sublingual vessels of the patients were abnormal, only four were almost normal, showing gradual variation from thin to thick, with light-purple color and little tortuous. The remaining patients indicated swelling or varicose sublingual vessel, most of whom more than half of the sublingual vessels (even the whole vessel) were involved (Figure 1E), or sublingual vessels with bluish purple (Figure 1E), purple red (Figure 1F) or even purple black color.

2.2　Comparison of Tongue Manifestation in ACEs and Non-ACEs Groups

Among 17 patients of reddish tongue, six had ACEs, 20.7% of ACEs group, while 11 patients without ACEs for 20.4% of non-ACEs group, showing no significant difference between the two groups. In 24 patients of red tongue, ten had ACEs, for 34.5%, while 14 without events for 25.9%, showing no significant difference. For 14 patients of dark red tongue, ACEs occurred in five cases, 17.2%, while nine cases without ACEs for

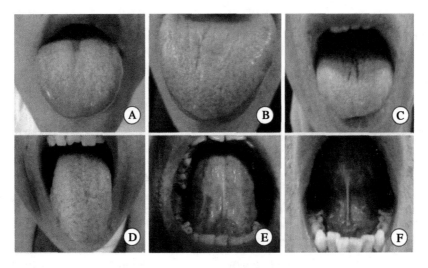

Figure 1　Different Tongue Manifestation

Notes: A. Bluish-grounding tongue；B. Bluish purple tongue；C. Dirty greasy coating
D. Dry greasy coating；E. Bluish purple sublingual vessels；F. Purple red sublingual vessels

16.7%, with no significant difference between the two groups; 24 patients had light dark red tongue, among which ACEs occurred in nine cases, for 31.0%, while 15 cases without ACEs for 27.8%, with no significant difference between the two groups. Seventeen cases was purple tongue, of which 3 cases got ACEs, 10.3%, while 14 patients without events, for 25.9%, with no significant difference between the two groups. Fifteen cases had bluish tongue, in which 11 cases occurred ACEs, for 37.9%, while four cases was non-

ACEs, covering 7.4%, with significant difference between the two groups (P= 0.002, Table 1) .

Among the 68 patients with white coating, 27 cases had ACEs, 93.1%, 41 had no events, covering 75.9%, which showed no significant difference between the two groups, but had a certain trend (P=0.052). In 29 patients with yellow coating, three had events, 10.3%, and 26 got no events, 48.1%, which showed significant difference between the two groups (P=0.001). For 22 patients with thick coating, 8 patients had

Table 1　Distribution Comparison of Tongue Manifestation between Two Groups [Cases (%)]

Tongue manifestation	Numbers (%)	Non-ACEs group (%)	ACEs group (%)	P
Tongue color				
Reddish	17 (20.5)	11 (20.4)	6 (20.7)	0.97
Red (mainly on tip and margin)	24 (28.9)	14 (25.9)	10 (34.5)	0.41
Dark red	14 (16.9)	9 (16.7)	5 (17.2)	1.00
Light dark red	24 (28.9)	15 (27.8)	9 (31.0)	0.75
Light-purple	17 (20.5)	14 (25.9)	3 (10.3)	0.09
Bluish	15 (18.1)	4 (7.4)	11 (37.9)	0.002**
Coating				
White coating	68 (81.9)	41 (75.9)	27 (93.1)	0.052
Yellow coating	29 (34.9)	26 (48.1)	3 (10.3)	0.001**
Thick coating	22 (26.5)	14 (25.9)	8 (27.6)	0.87
Greasy coating	60 (72.3)	41 (75.9)	19 (65.5)	0.31
Sticky greasy	48 (57.8)	36 (66.7)	12 (41.4)	0.026*
dry-greasy or dirty-greasy	12 (14.5)	5 (9.3)	7 (24.1)	0.10
Tongue shape				
Enlarged tongue	43 (51.8)	28 (51.9)	15 (51.7)	0.99
Prickly tongue	47 (56.6)	31 (57.4)	16 (55.2)	0.85
Fissured tongue	38 (45.8)	23 (42.6)	15 (51.7)	0.43
Sublingual vessel				
Swelling	33 (39.8)	23 (42.6)	10 (34.5)	0.47
Varicose	43 (51.8)	28 (51.9)	15 (51.7)	0.99
Swelling or varicose involving whole vessel	16 (19.3)	13 (24.1)	3 (10.3)	0.16
Bluish purple	49 (59.0)	36 (66.7)	13 (44.8)	0.054
Purple-red	23 (27.7)	11 (20.4)	12 (41.4)	0.041*

Notes: *P < 0.05, **P < 0.01, compared with the non-ACEs group

events, 27.6%, 14 patients didn't occur events, 25.9%, with no significant difference between the two groups. In 48 cases of sticky greasy coating, 12 patients had events, 36 patients got no events, 41.4% and 66.7% respectively, there were significant difference between the two groups (P=0.026). There were two cases of dirty greasy coating and ten of dry-greasy coating, of which 7 patients had ACEs, 24.1%, five cases without ACEs, 9.3%, which showed no significant difference between the two groups, but a certain trend.

Forty-three patients had enlarged tongue, of which 15 patients had ACEs, 51.7%, and 28 patients got no events, 51.9%, with no significant difference between the two groups. In 47 patients with prickly tongue, 16 patients had events, 55.2%, and 31 patients with no events, 57.4%, with no significant difference between the two groups. Among 38 cases of fissured tongue, 15 patients had ACEs, accounting for 51.7%, and 23 patients occurred no events, for 42.6%, which showed no significant difference between the two groups.

Among 33 patients with swelling sublingual vessels, ten patients had ACEs, 34.5%, and 23 patients got no events, 42.6%, which showed no significant difference between the two groups. Forty-three patients had varicose sublingual vessel, of which 15 cases got ACEs, 51.7%, and 28 patients without events, 51.9%, with no significant difference between the two groups. Sixteen cases had swelling or varicose involving the whole vessel, among which ACEs occurred in three patients, 10.3% and 13 patients occurred no events, 24.1%, with no significant difference between the two groups. In 49 cases of bluish purple sublingual vessel, 13 patients had ACEs, 44.8%, and 36 patients without events, 66.7%, with no significant difference between two groups (P=0.054). Purple-red sublingual vessel was found in 23 patients, of which 12 patients had ACES, 41.4%, and 11 patients without cardiovascular events, 20.4%, with significant

difference between the two groups (P=0.041).

2.3　Risk Estimation on Main Representation of Tongue Manifestation

The risk estimation of follow-up ACEs using OR on the bluish or bluish purple tongue, dry-greasy or dirty-greasy tongue, and purple-red sublingual vessel was performed to explore their values as clinical manifestations of "blood-stasis and toxin". The results showed that the OR of occurring ACEs during one-year follow-up in bluish or bluish purple tongue patients reached 11.67 ($P < 0.001$), and 95% confidence interval (CI) was 3.34 to 40.81, which meant 11.67 times risk of ACEs with such tongue more than whom without this tongue. The OR of experiencing follow-up ACEs in patients of purple-red sublingual vessel reached 2.76 ($P < 0.05$), and 95% CI was 1.02 to 7.44, which meant 2.76 times risk more than whom without such tongue. The OR of occurring ACEs during one-year follow-up in patients of dry-greasy or dirty-greasy coating attained 3.12 (P=0.066), and 95%CI was 0.89 to 10.92. It was just shy of significant difference between the patients with and without dry-greasy or dirty-greasy coating as for the risk of follow-up ACEs, considering to be related with inadequate sample size, which should be expanded for further demonstration.

3.　Discussion

Extensive studies were carried out on the tongue manifestations of blood stasis syndrome before, although the relationship between follow-up ACEs and tongue manifestation in stable CHD patients was not investigated. This study enrolled stable CHD patients, collected information on the tongue with unified type of digital camera and judged by two integrative cardiovascular physicians with deputy senior title to ensure its objectivity. The study selected 29 cases occurring ACEs, and the patients without ACEs were matched in proportion of 2 : 1 according to gender, age ($\pm$2.5 years), diabetes mellitus history and previous ACS hospitalization history, which reduced the impact of confounding factors to some extent.

The results showed that the most common tongues of the stable CHD patients were dark red, light dark red, light purple, dark purple or bluish purple; and sublingual vessels in almost all patients were abnormal, manifesting swelling or varicose in shape and bluish purple or purple red in color, which suggested that blood-stasis was the main pathogenesis of stable CHD. The majority of patients had greasy coating or fissures on the basis of swelling or teeth-marked tongue, reflecting pathogenesis features of qi and yang deficiency in fundamentality as well as exuberant phlegm-dampness in superficiality. Prickly tongues were not rare, but mostly limited to the tip, reflecting that some patients also had signs of exuberance heart fire. Pale, crimson or thin tongue, peeled coating, dry or rough coating were less common, suggesting that it was rare in CHD patients to have simple blood deficiency, yin deficiency and blood heat, or heat syndromes.

It was generally believed that turning into heat was one of the important ways of internal toxin production. However, according to this study, there was no significant difference in the patients with red and prickly tongues in light of with or without follow-up ACEs, and more patients with yellow tongue coating did not experience follow-up events. Further analysis showed that the patients with bluish or bluish purple tongue had more ACEs during the follow-up period, suggesting that the patients of obstruction in chest-yang were more prone to turn into toxin in addition to the common pathogenesis of stasis. On the other hand, the patients with sticky greasy and yellow coating were more stable, whereas those patients with dry-greasy or dirty-greasy tongue coating had an tendency of increasing ACEs, indicating that from white to yellow coating might not be the sign of transforming into heat and toxicity in stable CHD patients. Instead, the white coating rapidly transformed into dryness, turbidity and generated toxin before the transformation into yellow tongue coating, and changing from sticky greasy to dry greasy or dirty greasy coating might be an important clinical manifestation of transforming toxin.

The analysis on sublingual vessel showed that the patients with swelling or varicose involving whole vessel had no significant difference compared with the patients with and without follow-up ACEs, indicating that the severity of blood-stasis might not be a necessary condition of transforming toxin, which was consistent with our previous studies on the correlation between hs-CRP and blood-stasis syndrome score[11]. This result also suggested that clinical symptoms and blood stasis conditions of the stable CHD patients might be alleviated by activating blood circulation and removing blood-stasis, but only specific treatment targeting at key links in pathogenesis transformation could be expected to further reduce the occurrence of ACEs. The patients with purple-red sublingual vessel had a higher incidence of ACEs during one-year follow-up, suggesting the different tongue manifestations of coldness and heat in the pathogenesis of the stable CHD patients transforming into toxin, which is worthy of further study.

References

[1] Xu H. Exploration and consideration on anti-inflammatory of traditional Chinese herbs and stabilization of vulnerable plaque. Chin J Integr Tradit West Med, 2008, 28(5): 393-394.

[2] Zhou MX, Xu H, Chen KJ, et al. Effects of some active ingredients of Chinese drugs for activating blood circulation and detoxicating on blood lipids and atherosclerotic plaque inflammatory reaction in apoE-gene knockout mice. Chin J Integr Tradit West Med, 2008, 28(2): 126-130.

[3] Xu H, Shi DZ, Yin HJ, et al. Blood-stasis and toxin causing catastrophe hypothesis and acute cardiovascular events: proposal of the hypothesis and its clinical significance. Chin J Integr Tradit West Med, 2008, 28(10): 934-938.

[4] Shi DZ, Xu H, Yin HJ, et al. Combination and transformation of toxin and blood stasis in etiopathogenesis of thrombotic cerebrocardiovascular diseases. J Chin Integr Med, 2008, 6(11): 1105-1108.

[5] Zheng F, Zhou MX, Xu H, et al. Effects of herbs with function of activating blood circulation and detoxication on serum inflammatory markers and blood lipids in stable patients with coronary heart disease. China J Tradit Chin Med Pharm, 2009, 9(24): 1153-1157.

[6] Chen H, Gao ZY, Xu H, et al. Clinical study of unstable angina patients undergoing percutaneous coronary intervention treated with Chinese medicine for activating blood circulation and detoxicating. Chin J Integr Med Cardio-/Cerebrovasc Dis, 2009, 10(7): 1135-1137.

[7] Zhou MX, Xu H, Chen KJ, et al. Effects of several herbal extractives with the effect of promoting blood flow and detoxication on atherosclerotic plaque stability in aorta of ApoE-gene knockout mice. Chin J Pathophysiol, 2008, 24(11): 2097-2102.

[8] Xu H, Qu D, Zheng F, et al. Study on clinical manifestations for blood-stasis and toxin in stable coronary heart disease patients. Chin J Integr Tradit West Med, 2010, 30: 125-129.

[9] Chen HZ, ed. Practical internal medicine. 12 version. Beijing: People's Medical Publishing House, 2005: 1472-1473.

[10] Cardiovascular Institute of Traditional Chinese Medicine Professional Committee. The criterion of CM syndrome-differentiation for CHD. J Integr Tradit West Med, 1991, 11(5): 257-258.

[11] Zheng F, Qu D, Xu H, et al. Relationship between Chinese medicine syndrome and serum level of high-sensitivity C-reactive protein in patients with stable CHD. Chin J Integr Tradit and West Med, 2009, 29(6): 485-488.

ITIH4: A New Potential Biomarker of "Toxin Syndrome" in Coronary Heart Disease Patient Identified with Proteomic Method[*]

XU Hao   SHANG Qing-hua   CHEN Hao   DU Jian-peng   WEN Jian-yan   LI Geng
SHI Da-zhuo   CHEN Ke-ji

1. Introduction

Syndrome differentiation is a unique diagnostic method of traditional Chinese medicine (TCM)[1,2]. "Blood stasis syndrome" (BSS) is considered as a major and key syndrome in the process of coronary heart disease (CHD) in TCM [3,4], and activating blood circulation and dissolving stasis has been a mainstream treatment for CHD. However, some stable CHD patients develop acute cardiovascular events (ACEs), while others do not, why？ Based on this question, we proposed a hypothesis of "blood stasis and toxin" considering blood stasis was a constant pathogenesis in CHD, while "toxin" was the trigger in transforming to ACEs [5].

The original meaning of "toxin" is a kind of poisonous herb but it has been considered as a pathogenic factor in a narrow sense and pathogenesis, medicine, and syndrome in a broad sense. It is often seen in the fields of epidemic febrile diseases and surgical diseases (such as

* 原载于 Evidence-Based Complementary and Alternative Medicine，2013，Article ID 360149

carbuncle, abscess, hard furuncle, and sore). Zhang et al.[6] presented a theory of "artery carbuncle" according to previous studies that arteriosclerosis plaque has the characteristics such as redness, swelling, and being hot on the local scale, just like the traditional "toxin syndrome". Heat-clearing and detoxifying treatment has been widely used in CHD, especially acute coronary syndrome patients [7-9]. Previous studies showed that Rhizoma Coptidis, Cyrtomium Rhizome, compound simiaoyongan decoction, and Huanglian Jiedu decoction could improve clinical symptoms by multiple mechanisms such as anti-inflammatory action, lipid regulation, and AS plaque reduction[10-19]. Furthermore, a lot of researches indicated that drugs for activating blood circulation and detoxifying had a better effect on relieving angina than drugs for activating blood circulation only; it might be related to the effect of anti-inflammatory action [20-27].

Changes in macroscopic manifestation certainly have the corresponding microscopic biological basis. Inflammation has been proved to be a biomarker for CHD/ACS, and the proteome supported us with a new technology for studying it further. The proteome is a subject studying all the proteins in a cell, a kind of tissue, or an organism in specific conditions or at specific times and has been one of the most potential and effective approaches for decoding and revealing the biological foundation and essence of syndromes. Different syndromes consequentially have relevant differential protein expressions; meanwhile, one syndrome also has different protein expressions after treatment of different medicines. Therefore, the protein's characteristics of a specific syndrome can be reflected by the effectiveness of prescriptions corresponding to syndromes.

Berberine extracted from Rhizoma Coptidis, a representative herb of clearing heat and detoxifying, could inhibit the expressions of inflammatory factors such as thromboxane A_2 and prostaglandin I_2 after the injury of blood vessels [10]. Xiongshao capsule, consisting of active ingredients (Chuanxiongol and paeoniflorin), has shown beneficial effect in

atherosclerosis or CHD in clinical and experimental studies [28-34]. Therefore, it was served as a representative Chinese medicine for activating blood circulation.

The aim of this study was to look for the protein biomarker of "toxin syndrome" of CHD patients, which is anticipated to help early identification of high-risk CHD patients in stable period.

2. Design and Ethics Statement

There are two parts in this paper (Figure 1). The first one was a randomized controlled trial (RCT) with 2 study groups conducted at 2 cooperating hospitals (Anzhen Hospital and Tongren Hospital) to look for biomarkers for "toxin syndrome" of TCM. The other was a nested case-control study with a follow-up for ACEs conducted at 5 cooperating hospitals (China Academy of Chinese Medical Sciences Xiyuan Hospital,

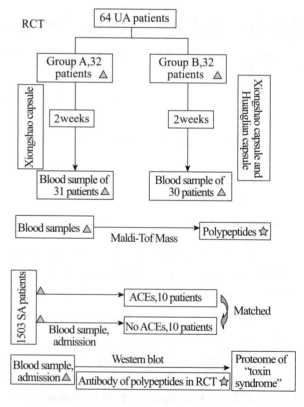

Figure 1 Flow Chart of the Study

Note: UA: unstable angina pectoris; SA: stable angina pectoris; RCT: randomized controlled trial; ACEs: acute cardiovascular disease

China-Japan friendship Hospital, Anzhen Hospital, Tongren Hospital, and Fujian Integrative Medicine Clinic) to verify the biomarker found in RCT. The trials were carried out according to the Declaration of Helsinki, and the protocols were approved by the institutional review boards and ethics committees at each center. All the patients provided written informed consent.

3. Materials and Methods

3.1 Randomized Controlled Trial

3.1.1 Patients Fasting serum samples were obtained from 64 patients with UA (ICD-10: I20.0/20.1/20.9) [35,36] aged between 40 and 75 years old. All of the patients who were admitted into the 2 cooperating hospitals were enrolled in the study. The inclusion criteria were successful PCI in 48 hours after the first severe angina and BSS of TCM (including Qi-stagnation-blood-stasis syndrome and Qi-deficiency-blood-stasis syndrome) [37-39]. Patients were excluded if they met any of the following criteria: presence of (1) stable angina or acute myocardial infarction; (2) inflammation, fever, trauma, bure, or surgery in one recent month; (3) active tuberculosis or rheumatic autoimmune disease; (4) known renal insufficiency and serum creatinine > 2.5 mg/dL in male and > 2.0 mg/dL in female; (5) known hepatic insufficiency and alanine transaminase (ALT) > three times value of the normal level; (6) severe heart failure (EF < 35%); (7) complication by severe primary disease such as hematologic systems and psychological abnormalities; (8) malignancies; (9) organ transplantation; (10) participants of other clinical trials; (11) taking other Chinese patent drugs; (12) pregnancy or breast-feeding. Patients were removed from analysis if they could not estimate the efficacy for they did not take any medicine or did not participate reexamination as proposal.

3.1.2 Groups and Drugs 64 eligible patients were randomly assigned in a 1:1 ratio to group of activating blood circulation (Xiongshao capsule, Z20053499, Hospital preparation approved by Beijing drug administration, group A) or group of activating blood circulation and detoxification (Huanglian capsule, Z19983042, Hubei Xianglian Pharmaceutical Co., Ltd and Xiongshao capsule, group B). Randomization table was performed centrally with the use of SAS software and reserved by a specific person who did not participate this clinic research. Randomized number was obtained by telephone if any patient was eligible.

In the group of activating blood circulation, Xiongshao capsule was taken as 500 mg (2 capsules) 3 times per day for 2 weeks. In the group of activating blood circulation and detoxification, Huanglian capsule was taken as 500 mg (2 capsules) 3 times per day, and Xiongshao capsule was taken as 500 mg (2 capsules) 3 times per day for 2 weŵs.

All patients received western standardized medication including antiplatelet drugs (aspirin and/or clopidogrel hydrogen sulfate), anticoagulant drugs (heparin or low molecular weight heparin), anti-ischemic drugs (nitrates, β-blocker, calcium channel blocker, and angiotensin converting enzyme inhibitors), and statins.

3.1.3 Data Collection At the beginning of the trial, all patients filled out a standardized questionnaire containing general information, past history, risk stratification of UA [40], angina score, primary symptom score of TCM [41], BSS score [42], medical treatment, and PCI surgery. In addition, to obtain the serum, at the beginning and the end of the trial, 2mL of blood from each patient with an empty stomach was drawn into common coagulation-promoting tubes, centrifuged at 3000 r for 10 min at room temperature to remove insoluble materials, cells, and debris, and supernatants were kept at −80℃ until use.

3.1.4 Reagents and Instruments The WCX magnetic bead kit (Bruker Daltonics Tech, Beijing, China), alpha-cyano-4-hydroxycinnamic acid

(HCCA), MALDI-TOF MS (type: microflex, Bruker Daltonics Biosciences, Bremen, Germany), 100% ethanol (chromatographic grade), and 100% acetone (chromatographic grade) were freshly prepared (sigma) .

3.1.5　WCX Fractionation and MALDI-TOF MS Analysis　The suspension in the WCX magnetic bead kit was mixed by shaking. After eluting and beating, the magnetic beads were separated from the protein, and the eluted peptide samples were transferred to a 0.5 mL clean sample tube for further MS analysis. Five microliters of HCCA substrate solution (0.4 g/L, dissolved in acetone and ethanol) and 0.8-1.2μL of elution were mixed. Then, 0.8-1.2μL of this mixture was applied to a metal target plate and dried at room temperature. Finally, the prepared sample was analyzed by MALDI-TOF MS. A range of 1000-10,000 Da peptide molecular weights was collected, and 400 shots of laser energy were used. Peptide mass fingerprints were obtained by accumulating 50 single MS signal scans.

3.1.6　Peptide Sequence　Experiment for 4280.13m/z peptide identification was performed using a nano-liquid chromatography-electrospray ionization-tandem mass spectrometry (nano-LC/ESI-mass spectrometry/mass spectrometry) system consisting of an Acquity UPLC system (Waters) and an LTQ Orbitrap XL mass spectrometer (Thermo Fisher) equipped with a nano-ESI source. The peptide solutions were loaded to a C18 trap column (nano-Acquity) (180μm × 20 mm × 5μm (symmetry)). The flow rate was 15μL/min. Then the desalted peptides were analyzed by C18 analytical column (nano-Acquity) (75μm × 150 mm × 3.5μm (symmetry)) at a flow rate of 400 nL/min. The mobile phases A (5% acetonitrile, 0.1% formic acid) and B (95% acetonitrile, 0.1% formic acid) were used for analytical columns. The gradient elution profile was as follows: 5%B-50%B-80%B-80%B-50%B-5%B in 100 min. The MS instrument was operated in a data-dependent model. The range of full scan was 400-2000m/z with a mass resolution

of 100, 000 (m/z400). The eight most intense monoisotope ions were the precursors for collision induced dissociation. Mass spectrometry was limited to two consecutive scans per precursor ion followed by 60 s of dynamic exclusion.

3.1.7　Statistical Analysis　ClinProTools (ClinProt software version 2.1, Bruker Daltonics) was used to subtract baseline, normalize spectra (using total ion current), and determine peak m/z values and intensities in the mass range of 1000 to 10,000 Da. The signal-to-noise (S/N) ratio should be higher than five. To align the spectra, a mass shift of no more than 0.1% was determined. The peak area was used as quantitative standardization. Student's t-test was used for analysis of normally distributed continuous data, while Wilcoxon test for nonnormally distributed continuous data. Chi-square test was used for categorical data analysis. A P value < 0.05 was considered significant.

3.2　Nested Case-Control Study

3.2.1　Patients　1503 patients with stable CHD (old myocardial infarction or at least one significant (> 50%) stenosis that was documented on a recent coronary angiogram and WHO [35]) younger than 80 years old were enrolled from 5 cooperating hospitals. Stable CHD was defined as no symptoms or stable exertional angina or patients in stable condition after ACS for at least 1 month. Patients were excluded if they met any of the following criteria: presence of (1) inflammation, fever, trauma, bure, or surgery in one recent month; (2) active tuberculosis or rheumatic autoimmune disease; (3) severe heart failure (EF < 35%); (4) complication by severe valvular heart disease, or myocardiopathy; (5) complication by severe chronic obstructive pulmonary disease (COPD), pulmonary heart disease or respiratory failure; (6) known renal insufficiency and serum creatinine > 2.5 mg/dL in male and > 2.0 mg/dL in female; (7) known hepatic insufficiency and alanine transaminase (ALT) > three times value of the normal level; (8) complication by severe primary disease such as hematologic systems; (9) severe psychological abnormalities; (10) malignancies; (11) viscera transplantation; (11) life expectancy less than 3 years. Patients were removed from analysis if a mistaken inclusion or lack of necessary record for analysis or failure to follow up for ACEs because of missing contact information took place.

3.2.2 Data Collection　In all patients, follow-up was scheduled at 0.5 and 1 year after inclusion of the trial. At every visit of the trial, information was obtained from each patient by use of a standardized questionnaire, the information regarding general information, past history, and the secondary cardiovascular events in follow-up. Physicians collecting information were unaware of the purpose of the study. Secondary cardiovascular events were defined as death from heart disease, nonfatal myocardial infarction (MI), or ischemic cerebrovascular events (stroke or transient ischemic attack) . All the cardiovascular events were estimated by consulting medical records. In addition, the serum also was collected at every visit, and the method of blood collection, centrifugation, and storage was the same as that of RCT.

　Twenty three patients were confirmed as ACEs during one-year follow-up, and 10 patients were selected for their well preserved serum sample. Another 10 patients with no follow-up ACEs were matched in a 1 : 1 ratio by sex, age (± 5 years), hypertension history, diabetes history, and myocardial infarction history. All the sera at the admission of these 20 patients were adopted for verifying the differential protein of "toxin syndrome" obtained from RCT by Western blot method.

3.2.3 Western Blot　To detect the inter-alpha-trypsin inhibitor heavy chain H4 (ITIH4) obtained from RCT (see results section), blood serum stored in $-80\ ℃$ refrigerator was assayed using Western blot as described before[43]. Additionally, ITIH4 antibody (1 : 2500, Sigma, USA) was used for detection of ITIH4. The horseradish peroxidase (HRP) conjugated anti-mouse IgG ($0.1 mL/cm^2$,

Santa Cruz Biotechnology, UAS) was used as the secondary antibody, and signals were visualized using the enhanced chemiluminescence system (ECL, Pierce, USA) .

3.3　Statistical Analysis

Statistical analysis was performed by a statistician in a blind fashion. Statistical analysis was performed with SPSS 15.0 software. All tests were two tailed, and a statistical probability of < 0.05 was considered significant. Normality test and homogeneity test of variances were conducted. Frequency table, percentage or constituent ratio for describing enumeration data; $\bar{x} \pm s$ for describing measurement data. χ^2 test or Fisher exact test if necessary was used for comparison of enumeration data, t-test was used for comparison of measurement data (corrected t-test was used if variant heterogeneity), and Wilcoxon tests were used for abnormal distribution.

4.　Results

4.1　Patients' Characteristics in RCT

64 participants with UA were enrolled in 5 centers and were randomized into two groups: 32 to receive Xiongshao capsule (group A) and 32 to receive Xiongshao capsule and Huanglian capsule (group B). During the course of the study, one patient was excluded in group A due to incomplete follow-up, while two patients were excluded in group B with 1 incomplete follow-up, and 1 noncompliance with medications. They were removed from statistics as the stated protocol. Thus finally, the population in analysis consisted of 61 patients, with 31 patients in group A and 30 patients in group B. The baseline characteristics of the UA patients were summarized in Table 1. The two groups were well matched with regard to baseline clinical and angiographic characteristics ($P > 0.05$) .

4.2　Sample Processing in RCT

During the course of the protein analysis, five blood samples were excluded from group A due to bad peptide mass spectrometry; thus,

第二章

the population in differential protein analysis consisted of 56 patients, with 26 patients in group A and 30 patients in group B. Acquisition mass range 500-10,000 Da (low-to-medium molecular mass range) would be studied in bioinformatics analysis.

4.3 MALDI-TOF Mass Spectrometry Analysis of Peptides in Serum of RCT

Statistical analysis of the data revealed that the expression of 24 spots was altered after treatment as compared with that at admission in group A (7 of them upregulated and 17 downregulated, Table 2, Figure 2). The expression of 15 spots was altered after treatment as compared with that at admission in group B (8 of them upregulated and 17 downregulated, Table 3, Figure 3), and 4 of the 15 spots were the same as group A. Twelve protein spots were found (Table 4) to be the differential protein for the significant differences between the difference of before-after treatment in group A and group B; 2 of them (3207.37 Da and 4279.95 Da) were considered to be unique to "toxin syndrome" for being differential proteins of group B but not group A. These 2 spots were identified by mass spectrometry (Figures 4 and 5) .

4.4 Identification of Protein Fragments by Proteome Analysis in RCT

Isoform 2 of inter-alpha-trypsin inhibitor heavy chain H4 (ITIH4) and Isoform 1 of Fibrinogen alpha chain precursor (FGA) were identified in different spots by proteome analysis which can be served as biomarkers of "toxin syndrome" in CHD patients (Table 5) .

4.5 Western Blot

A large multicenter nested case control study was conducted for verifying the unique protein biomarker to "toxin syndrome" of TCM obtained from RCT. The admission blood samples of 20 patients were collected for Western blot (10 patients, resp. in the ACEs group and the matched group). We assay the serum protein concentrations and based on the readings load the same amount of protein. In the posttranslational process, the protein ITIH4 was modified and cleaved by plasma kallikrein to yield 100 kDa and 35 kDa fragments. Statistics indicated that protein expression of ITIH4 in the ACEs group was significantly lower than that in the matched group (P = 0.027) (Table 6, Figure 6). Therefore, the results of nested case-control study further demonstrated the biomarker identified in the RCT, which indicated that the reduced ITIH4 might be a unique protein biomarker/ bioinformation of "toxin syndrome" in CHD patients.

5. Discussion

As the development of systems biology and the advancement of the human genome project increased, more and more attention has been paid on the importance of proteome. In this study, we identified 2 peptides (FGA and ITIH4) related to CHD "toxin syndrome" by "taking special drugs to ascertain syndromes" in RCT using MOLDI-TOF MS. Since fibrinogen has been proven to be a risk factor for ACEs in many previous studies[44-46], we only verified another differential protein, ITIH4, by Western blot in a subsequent nested case-control study. Finally, ITIH4 was ascertained to be a new biomarker for CHD "toxin syndrome", which can also be served as a new risk predictor for ACEs in stable CHD patients.

BSS is one of the basic syndromes in CHD, and "toxin syndrome" is the key in pathogenesis of disease progression. BSS and "toxin syndrome" can coexist or transform to each other, which make up the whole pathological process of CHD[5]. From the macroscopic point of view, Xu et al.[47,48] enrolled 254 stable CHD patients, collected the clinical information and ACEs in follow-up, and thus concluded a series of clinical manifestations for "toxin syndrome" in stable CHD patients including pain in substernal, headache, uneven or irregular pulse, frequent pharyngalgia, and increased high-sensitivity C-reactive protein (hs-CRP), Other scholars [49] collected clinical

Table 1　Baseline Information of Two Groups in RCT

Groups	Group A	Group B
Age		
Minimum value (years)	48	42
Maximum value (years)	74	75
Mean value (years)	61.94 ± 8.41	61.24 ± 9.86
Sex		
Male (proportion)	22 (71%)	25 (86.2%)
Female (proportion)	9 (29%)	5 (13.8%)
Angina score	14.42 ± 4.86	14.89 ± 4.63
Primary symptom score of TCM	17.97 ± 6.74	18.94 ± 5.64
BSS score	10.89 ± 4.62	10.59 ± 3.38
Past history		
Hypertension (N)	18	16
Diabetes (N)	7	9
Dislipidemia (N)	11	12
Stroke (N)	2	4
Peripheral vascular atherosclerosis (N)	5	3
Old myocardial infarction (N)	4	1
Western medicine		
Aspirin (N) 31	30	31
Clopidogrel hydrogen sulfate (N)	31	30
Nitrates (N)	21	16
β -blocker (N)	28	30
ACEI/ARB (N)	19	17
CCB (N)	3	9
Low molecular weight heparin (N)	16	19
Statins (N)	30	29
UA risk stratification		
Low risk (N)	0	0
Mediate risk (N)	26	24
High risk (N)	5	6
Number of stenosed coronary vessel		
1 vessel (N)	8	12
2 vessels (N)	12	7
3 vessels (N)	11	11
Lesions nature		
De novo (N)	28	26
Restenosis (N)	3	4
Stent type		
Sirolimus-eluting stent (N)	21	21
paclitaxel-eluting stent (N)	8	6
Mixed drug-eluting stents (N)	2	3
Total length of stents	22.94 ± 7.23	21.67 ± 9.69

Note: group A patients have taken the Xiongshao capsule; group B patients have taken the Xiongshao capsule and Huanglian capsule

93

Table 2　Comparison of before and after Treatment in Group A（$\bar{\chi}\pm s$）

Mass (Da)	Ave ± StdDev (A-Q)	Ave ± StdDev (A-H)	P
1076.12	3.77 ± 2.35	2.54 ± 1.24	0.016099
1136.37	7.25 ± 3.12	5.42 ± 2.08	0.008065
1205.62	9 ± 3.32	6.92 ± 4.43	0.018784
1329.42	14.44 ± 7.31	10.26 ± 4.92	0.000268
1348.81	10.41 ± 4.08	7.09 ± 2.89	0.000806
1464.89	24.93 ± 13.64	13.52 ± 6.44	0.000293
1519.06	18.49 ± 8.17	11.39 ± 5.92	0.000111
1544.61	30.66 ± 17.33	19.41 ± 16.3	0.011662
1616.74	33.35 ± 22.17	18.7 ± 9.09	0.002143
2209.31	37.24 ± 18.84	25.45 ± 17.84	0.01935
2279.51	50.15 ± 17.26	40.99 ± 14.08	0.018232
2644.01	30.08 ± 20.39	22.42 ± 14.8	0.000347
2660.01	288.15 ± 231.67	206.03 ± 161.86	0.003587
2862.02	77.55 ± 78.74	45.15 ± 29.33	0.00951
3261.70	125.1 ± 63.45	159.89 ± 62.44	0.043161
3277.49	45.57 ± 23.64	59.7 ± 29.1	0.015557
4053.87	71.26 ± 38.16	95.63 ± 53.55	0.047052
4710.25	15.53 ± 5.5	12.84 ± 4.04	0.028146
4936.10	17.25 ± 15.28	9.77 ± 2.99	0.015955
4964.02	147.4 ± 184.34	59.95 ± 34.25	0.019728
5807.76	52.08 ± 23.63	70.92 ± 24.68	0.010841
5822.51	22.33 ± 13.95	31.77 ± 10.34	0.007368
5904.69	881.7 ± 598.83	1266.04 ± 415.59	0.00471
6049.22	27.36 ± 10.77	32.41 ± 10.1	0.023583

Note: paired sample t test was used, 2-tailed, and $P < 0.05$ was considered significant; Ave: peak area/intensity average; StdDev: standard deviation of the peak area/intensity average; A-Q: before treatment in group A; A-H: after treatment in group A

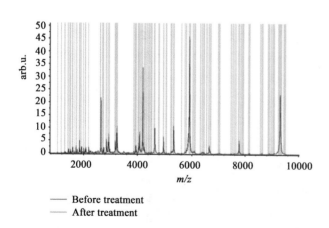

Figure 2　Peptide Mass Spectrometry Before and after Treatment in Group A

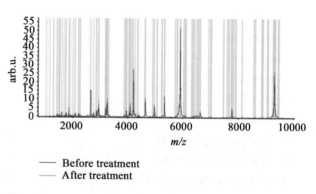

Figure 3　Peptide Mass Spectrometry before and after Treatment in Group B

Table 3　Comparison of before and after treatment in group B ($\bar{x} \pm s$)

Mass (Da)	Ave ± StdDev (B_Q)	Ave ± StdDev (B_H)	P
1616.74	32.83 ± 18.26	23.95 ± 12.74	0.033415
2209.31	29.04 ± 14.35	21.23 ± 10.27	0.022373
2881.04	49.8 ± 18.98	38.19 ± 10.15	0.010917
3207.37	56.15 ± 17.06	47.84 ± 12.01	0.023899
4053.87	60.23 ± 22.82	83.04 ± 42.14	0.010323
4266.31	35.94 ± 19.99	45.73 ± 19.4	0.020676
4279.95	18.9 ± 8.79	27.23 ± 23.79	0.025866
4817.85	20.34 ± 17.41	11.15 ± 7.93	0.012491
4936.10	21.91 ± 27.22	10.29 ± 3.94	0.02628
5066.25	25.87 ± 7.61	32.1 ± 11.2	0.019568
5248.63	21.01 ± 5.89	25.23 ± 8.04	0.025751
6378.01	47.98 ± 47.92	28.92 ± 10.34	0.045958
7833.86	10.85 ± 2.21	12.97 ± 4.82	0.040051
9064.40	30.36 ± 8.86	35.83 ± 10.12	0.012614
9290.26	907.98 ± 442.14	1126.48 ± 455.76	0.023601

Note: paired sample t-test was used, 2-tailed, and $P < 0.05$ was considered significant; Ave: peak area/intensity average; StdDev: standard deviation of the peak area/intensity average; B-Q: before treatment in group B; B-H: after treatment in group B; overstriking mass: unique to group B

Table 4　Comparison of Difference between before and after Treatment in the Two Groups

Mass (Da)	Ave ± StdDev (AH–AQ)	Ave ± StdDev (BH–BQ)	P
1329.42	−4.18 ± 5.02	0.4 ± 6.86	0.005918
1519.06	−7.1 ± 7.9	−2.47 ± 9.08	0.046435
2660.01	−82.12 ± 130.27	3.85 ± 184.48	0.047102
2881.04	4.86 ± 16.64	−11.62 ± 23.4	0.003442
3207.37	6.56 ± 21.34	−8.31 ± 19.09	0.008696
3277.49	14.13 ± 27.75	−9.87 ± 33.72	0.005087
3972.15	−8.69 ± 22.59	3.47 ± 15.5	0.02561
4279.95	−2.49 ± 14.27	8.32 ± 19.41	0.020196
5066.25	−0.43 ± 10.97	6.23 ± 13.8	0.049446
5807.76	18.84 ± 34.89	−2.2 ± 36.2	0.031283
5822.51	9.44 ± 16.49	−7.75 ± 32.03	0.013558
6088.68	8 ± 28.11	−8.21 ± 25.58	0.029233

Note: Paired sample t-test was used, 2-tailed, and $P < 0.05$ was considered significant; Ave: Peak area/intensity average；StdDev: standard deviation of the peak area/intensity average; "A_H-A_Q": subtraction between after and before treatment in group A; "B_H-B_Q": subtraction between after and before treatment in group B; overstriking mass: unique to "Toxin"

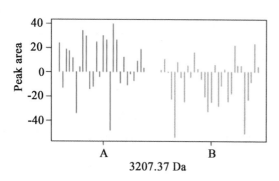

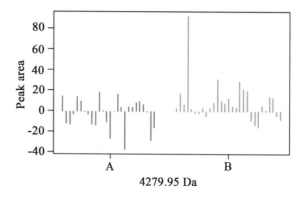

Figure 4　Difference of 3207 Da Protein Peak between Group A and Group B

Figure 5　Difference of 4279.95 Da Protein Peak between Group A and Group B

Table 5　Peptides Identification Unique to "Toxin"

Mass	IPI	GeneSymbol	Amino acid sequence
4280.13 Da	IPI00218192.3	ITIH4 Isoform 2 of inter-alpha-trypsin inhibitor heavy chain H4	R.NVHSAGAAGSRMNFRPGVLSSRQLGLPGPPDVPDHAAYHPF.R
3206.42 Da	IPI00021885.1	FGA Isoform 1 of Fibrinogen alpha chain precursor	K.SSSYSKQFTSSTSYNRGDSTFESKSYKM*.A

Table 6　ITIH4 Expression between ACEs Group and Matched Group

Groups	Patients	MOD	P
ACEs group	10	8.41 ± 4.04	0.027
Matched group	10	11.57 ± 5.34	

Note: paired sample t-test was used, 2-tailed, and $P < 0.05$ was considered significant; MOD: mean optical density

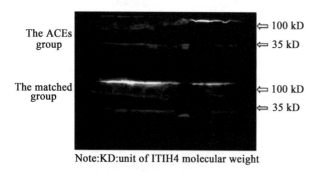

Note:KD:unit of ITIH4 molecular weight

Figure 6　ITIH4 Expression between the ACEs Group and the Matched Group

information and then summarized a differentiation standard for "toxin-stasis syndrome" of ACS in Chinese medicine. From the microcosmic point of view, "inflammatory reaction" is always a research focus for CHD "toxin syndrome." Wen et al. [23] investigated the effect on plaque

stabilization among herbs regulating blood circulation (Salvia Miltiorrhiza, Radix Paeoniae Rubra), activating blood circulation (Szechuan Lovage Rhizome, Panax Notoginseng), and breaking blood stasis (Peach Seed, Rhubarb Root Parched in Wine) from inflammation, pathomorphology, cellular composition, and so on; indicated Rhubarb root parched in wine was the best for its effect of breaking blood stasis and detoxification. Zhou et al. [26] proposed the hypothesis of "activating blood circulation and detoxification—inflammatory reaction inhibition—plaque stabilization", then compared the effect on plaque stabilization among herbs activating blood circulation (Panax Notoginsenosides), herbs for detoxification (Goldthread Rhizome extract) and herbs activating blood circulation and detoxification (Rhubarb alcohol extract and Polygonum Cuspidatum extract). The results indicated the superior effect of Rhubarb alcohol extract and Polygonum Cuspidatum extract on stabilizing vulnerable plaque, showing the "class effect" of herbs activating blood circulation and detoxification in inhibiting inflammatory reaction and stabilizing plaque.

The function of ITIH4 in European Molecular Biology Laboratory-The European Bioinformatics Institute (EMBLEBI) showed that ITIH4 is a type II acute-phase protein (APP) involved in inflammatory responses to trauma. And it may also play a role in liver development and regeneration [50]. Inter-alpha-trypsin inhibitor (ITI) family proteins are all composed by light chain (bikunin) and at least 6 heavy chains. Lots of researches have proved that bikunin could inhibit the activity of protease, but little studies have paid attention to heavy chains of ITI. In 2000, Japanese scholar Choi-Miura et al. found that inter-alpha-trypsin inhibitor family heavy chain-related protein (IHRP) could inhibit the aggregation and phagocytosis of actins in polymorphonuclear leukocyte, implying that IHRP might be a new APP involved in inflammatory responses [51]. In 2004, Fujita et al. showed that genetic locus mutation of ITIH4 might be one of possible factors for dyslipidemia [52]. Then, Piñeiro et al. proved that ITIH4 was a new APP isolated from cattle during experimental infection [53]. Recently, Kashyap et al. found that ITIH4 showed high expression in normal subjects but no expression or little expression in patients with acute ischemic stroke (AIS), and this protein could return to normal level in blood serum gradually as the patients were getting better. The scholars considered that ITIH4 was a novel biomarker in inflammatory responses for AIS due to its close relationship with S-100 β-β, neuron specific enolase (NSE), interleukin-2 (IL-2), and interleukin-10 (IL-10) expression [54].

Results in this study showed that the group of activating blood circulation and detoxification could significantly increase ITIH4 expression

and decrease FGA expression compared with the group of activating blood circulation and indicated that ITIH4 and FGA might be potential protein biomarkers for "toxin syndrome" of CHD. ITIH4 was further demonstrated in a nested case-control study, indicating its potential role as a new prewarning biomarker in stable CHD patients.

Before recommending the conclusion of this study to clinical practice, we have to consider the following weaknesses. We cannot ascertain whether the tendency of these two polypeptides is always the same in the process of "toxin syndrome" development. Therefore, a large prospective cohort study collecting information in more time points is necessary.

6. Conclusion

ITIH4 might be a new potential biomarker of CHD "toxin syndrome" in TCM, indicating the potential role as a prewarning biomarker in stable CHD patients.

References

[1] Ferreira AS, Lopes AJ. Chinese medicine pattern differentiation and its implications for clinical practice. Chinese Journal of Integrative Medicine, 2011, 17 (11) : 818-823.

[2] Mei MF. A systematic analysis of the theory and practice of syndrome differentiation. Chinese Journal of Integrative Medicine, 2011, 17 (11) : 803-810.

[3] Li O, Xu H. The occurrence of cardiovascular events of coronary heart disease inpatients and study on chinese medicine syndrome distribution laws. Chinese Journal of Integrated Traditional and Western Medicine, 2012, 32 (5) : 303-606.

[4] Gao ZY, Zhang JC, Xu H, et al. Analysis of relationships among syndrome, therapeutic treatment, and Chinese herbal medicine in patients with coronary artery disease based on complex networks. Chinese Journal of Integrated Traditional and Western Medicine, 2010, 8 (3) : 238-243.

[5] Xu H, Shi DZ, Yin HJ, et al. Blood-stasis and toxin causing catastrophe hypothesis and acute cardiovascular events: proposal of the hypothesis and its 10 Evidence-Based Complementary and Alternative Medicine clinical significance. Chinese

Journal of Integrated Traditional and Western Medicine, 2008, 28 (10) : 934-938.

[6] Zhang Z, Yang GL, Zhang HY, et al. A hypothesis of atherosclerosis plaque from the surgical carbuncle theory. Liaoning Journal of Traditional Chinese Medicine, 2008, 35 (2) : 201-202.

[7] Wang L, Wei LB, Liu XF, et al. Toxin theory and acute coronary syndrome. Chinese Journal of Integrative Medicine on Cardio-/Cerebrovascular Disease, 2005, 3 (12) : 1080-1081.

[8] Du WX, Liu CY, Zhang HX, et al. Acute myocardial infarction and TCM theory. Chinese Journal of Integrative Medicine on Cardio-/Cerebrovascular Disease, 2006, 4 (5) : 434-436.

[9] Wu W, Peng R. Progress of heat & toxin pathogenesis in coronary heart disease. Journal of New Chinese Medicine, 2007, 39 (6) : 3-4.

[10] Duan H, Zhang HK, Liu JJ, et al. Effect of berberine on IL-6 of carotid artery after ballon injury in rabbits. Journal of Medical Forum, 2006, 27 (10) : 6-9.

[11] Wu M, Wang J. Advance on study in anti-atherosclerosis mechanism of berberine. China Journal of Chinese Materia Medica, 2008, 33 (18) : 2013-2016.

[12] Lei ZQ, Chen SY, Gao XM. Traditional Chinese Pharmacology. Shanghai: Shanghai Science and Technology Press, 1995.

[13] He SW, Zhao RH, Wu HJ. Effect of wild purslane on atherosclerosis formation in rabbit. Chinese Journal of Preventive Medicine, 1997, 31 (2) : 91.

[14] Tan HB. Study of gynostemma pentaphylla on atherosclerosis in rabbit. Chinese Journal of Gerontology, 2007, 27 (6) : 519-521.

[15] Xie LD, Chen LX, Wu SX. Overview of clinical and basic research of Simiao Yong'an decoction in the treatment of coronary heart disease. Global Traditional Chinese Medicine, 2012, 5 (8) : 629-633.

[16] Zhu N, Cao XM, Cai YX. Effect of huanglian jiedu decoction on CRP and TNF-α in coronary heart disease. Journal of Emergency in Traditional Chinese Medicine, 2012, 21 (4) : 542-543.

[17] Li GQ, Huang P, Cheng HM, et al. Effect of huanglian jiedu decoction on T cell expression regulated by CD4$^+$ CD25$^+$ in rats with atherosclerosis. Guangdong Medical Journal, 2010, 31 (3) : 329-331.

[18] Guo ZY, Huang P, Li GQ. Effect of huanglian jiedu decoction on the expression of MCP-1/CCR2 mRNA in atherosclerosis rats. Traditional Chinese Drug Research and Clinical Pharmacology, 2010, 21 (6) : 583-586.

[19] Zheng F, Zhou MX, Xu H. Effects of herbs with function of activating blood circulation and detoxication on serum inflammatory markers and blood lipids in stable patients with coronary heart disease. China Journal of Traditional Chinese Medicine and Pharmacy, 2009, 24 (9) : 1153-11576.

[20] Lu XH, Ding SW. Clinical effect and mechanism on treating unstable angina pectoris by huanglian jiedu capsule. Journal of Shandong University of Traditional Chinese Medicine, 2005, 29 (6) : 457-460.

[21] Yu R, He SX, Ye XL, et al. The effect of therapeutic method of blood-activating and detoxifying of TCM on serumlevel of sCD40L in the patients with acute coronary syndrome. Journal of Emergency in Traditional Chinese Medicine, 2008, 17 (11) : 1500-1501.

[22] Yu R, Hu XS, He SX, et al. The effect of huoxuejiedu decoction on serum level of MMP-1, MMP-9, TIMP-1 in the patients with acute coronary syndrome. Journal of Emergency in Traditional Chinese Medicine, 2008, 17 (10) : 1337-1346.

[23] Wen C, Xu H, Chen QF, et al. Effects of herbs of activation blood on atherosclerotic plaque morphology in ApoE gene-deficient mice. Chinese Journal of Pathophysiology, 2005, 21 (5) : 864-867.

[24] Wen C, Xu H, Huang QF, et al. Effect of drugs for promoting blood circulation on blood lipids and inflammatory reaction of atherosclerotic plaques in ApoE gene deficiency mice. Chinese Journal of Integrated Traditional and Western Medicine, 2005, 25 (4) : 345-349.

[25] Zhou MX, Xu H, Chen KJ, et al. Effects of some active ingredients of Chinese drugs for activating blood circulation and detoxicating on blood lipids and atherosclerotic plaque inflammatory reaction in ApoE gene knockout mice. Chinese Journal of Integrated Traditional and Western Medicine, 2008, 28 (2) : 126-130.

[26] Zhou MX, Xu H, Chen KJ, et al. Effects of several herbal extractives with the effect of promoting blood flow and detoxication on atherosclerotic plaque stability in aorta of apoE-gene knockout mice. Chinese Journal of Pathophysiology, 2008, 24 (11) : 2097-2102.

[27] Zhang JC, Chen KJ, Zheng GJ, et al. Regulatory effect of Chinese herbal compound for detoxifying and activating blood circulation on expression of NF-kappaB and MMP-9 in aorta of apolipoprotein E gene knocked-out mice. Chinese Journal of Integrated Traditional and Western Medicine, 2007, 21 (1) : 40-44, 2007.

[28] Chen KJ, Shi DZ, Xu H, et al. XS0601 reduces the incidence of restenosis: a prospective study of 335 patients undergoing percutaneous coronary intervention in China. Chinese Medical Journal, 2006, 119 (1) : 6-13.

[29] Xu H, Chen KJ, Shi DZ, et al. Clinical study of Xiongshao capsule in preventing resterosisc after coronary interventional treatment. Chinese Journal of Integrative Medicine, 2002, 8 (3) : 162-166.

[30] Shang QH, Xu H, Lu XY, et al. A multi-center randomized double-blind placebo controlled trial of Xiongshao capsule in preventing restenosis after percutaneous coronary intervention: a subgroup analysis of senile patients. Chinese Journal of Integrative Medicine, 2011, 17 (9) : 669-674.

[31] Xu H, Shi DZ, Chen K, et al. Effect of Xiongshao capsule on vascular remodeling in porcine coronary balloon injury model. Chinese Journal of Integrative Medicine, 2000, 6 (4) : 278-282.

[32] Li LZ, Liu JZ, Ma LB, et al. Effect of Xiongshao capsule on lipid metabolism and platelet aggregation in experimental atherosclerosis rabbits. Chinese Journal of Integrated Traditional and Western Medicine, 2008, 28 (12) : 1100-1103.

[33] Zhang DW, Zhang L, Liu GZ. Effects of Xiongshao capsule combined with ischemic postconditioning on monocyte hemoattractant protein-1 and tumor necrosis factor-α in rat myocardium with ischemic reperfusion injury. Chinese Journal of Integrated Traditional and Western Medicine, 2010, 30 (12) : 279-1283.

[34] Xu FQ, Xu H, Liu JG, et al. Effects of Xiongshao capsule on the proliferation of vascular smooth muscle cells in rabbits with atherosclerosis. Chinese Journal of Integrated Traditional and Western Medicine, 2008, 28 (10) : 912-916.

[35] Report of the Joint International Society and Federation of Cardiology/World Health Organization Task Force on Standardization of Clinical Nomenclatures. Nomenclature and criteria for diagnosis of ischemic heart disease. Circulation, 1979, 59 (3): 607-609.

[36] Chinese Society of Cardiology. Guideline for diagnosis and treatment of patients with unstable angina and non-ST segment elevation myocardial infarction. Chinese Journal of Cardiology, 2007, 35 (4) : 295-304.

[37] Subcommittee of Cardiovascular Diseases of China Society of Integrated Traditional Chinese and Western Medicine. Criteria for TCM syndrome differentiation of patients with coronary heart disease. Chinese Journal of Integrated Traditional and Western Medicine, 1991, 11 (5) : 257-258.

[38] Professional Committee of Activating Blood Circulation in Chinese Association of the Integration of Traditional and Western Medicine. Criteria for diagnosis of blood stasis syndrome. Chinese Journal of Integrated Traditional and Western Medicine, 1987, 7 (3) : 129.

[39] Fu CG, Gao ZY, Wang PL, et al. Study on the diagnostic criteria for coronary heart disease patients of blood stasis syndrome. Chinese Journal of Integrated Traditional and Western Medicine, 2012, 32 (9) : 1285-1286.

[40] Chinese Society of Cardiology. Guildline on diagnosis and treatment of unstable angina pectoris and non-ST elecated myocardial infarcion. Chinese Journal of Cardiology, 2007, 35 (4) : 295-304.

[41] Zheng YY. Chinese Herbal Medicine Clinical Research Guilding Principles (for Trial Implementation), Chinese Medicine and Technology Publishing House, 2002.

[42] Chen KJ. Study on activating blood circulation and cllinical application. Beijing : Peking Union Medical College Press, 1993.

[43] Gong Y, Wang X, Liu J, et al. NSPc1, a mainly nuclear localized protein of novel PcG family members, has a transcription repression activity related to its PKC phosphorylation site at S183. FEBS Letters, 2005, 579 (1) : 115-121.

[44] Tataru MC, Schulte H, Von EA, et al. Plasma fibrinogen in relation to the severity of arterios-clerosis in patients with stable angina pectoris after myocardial infarction. Coronary Artery Disease, 2001, 12 (3) : 157-165.

[45] Naito M. Effects of fibrinogen, fibrin and their degradation products on the behavior of vascular smooth muscle cells. Nippon Ronenlgakkai Zasshi, 2000, 37 (6): 458-463.

[46] Ma HL, Lu X, Yang HJ, et al. Fibrinogen is the one of risk factors of coronary heart disease. Chinese Journal of Thrombosis and Hemostasis, 2008, 14 (1): 8-11.

[47] Xu H, Qu D, Zheng F, et al. Clinical manifestations of "Blood-stasis and Toxin" in patients with stable coronary heart disease. Chinese Journal of Integrated Traditional and Western Medicine, 2010, 30 (2) 125-129.

[48] Feng Y, Xu H, Qu D, et al. Study on the tongue manifestations for the blood-stasis and toxin syndrome in the stable patients of coronary heart disease. Chinese Journal of Integrative Medicine, 2011, 17 (5) : 333-338.

[49] Chen H. The clinical research on differentiation standard for toxin-stasis syndrome of ACS in Chinese medicine [Doctoral dissertation]. Beijing: China Academy of Chinese Medical Sciences, 2009.

[50] http://www.uniprot.org/uniprot/Q14624.

[51] Choi-Miura HN, Takahashi K, Yoda M, et al. The novel acute phase protein, IHRP, inhibits actin polymerization and phagocytosis of polymorphonuclear cells. Inflammation Research, 2000, 49 (6) : 305-310.

[52] Fujita Y, Ezura Y, Emi M, et al. Hypercholesterolemia associated with splice-junction variation of inter-α-trypsin inhibitor heavy chain 4 (ITIH4) gene. Journal of Human Genetics, 2004, 49 (1) : 24-28.

[53] Piñeiro M, Andrés M, Iturralde, et al. ITIH4 (inter-alphatrypsin inhibitor heavy chain 4) is a new acute-phase protein isolated from cattle during experimental infection. Infection and Immunity, 2004, 72 (7) : 3777-3782.

[54] Kashyap RS, Nayak AR, Deshpande PS, et al. Inter-α-trypsin inhibitor heavy chain 4 is a novel marker of acute ischemic stroke. Clinica Chimica Acta, 2009, 402 (1-2) : 160-163.

第 三 章

中西医结合防治心血管病的临床研究

第一节 中西医结合防治冠心病心绞痛

芎芍胶囊治疗冠心病心绞痛心血瘀阻证
112 例临床研究 *

彭 伟 史大卓 薛一涛 高洪春 张法荣

冠心病心绞痛是指冠状动脉硬化或痉挛致管腔狭窄，冠状动脉供血不足而导致的以心肌急剧的、暂时的缺血、缺氧为特征的临床综合征。其特点以阵发性的胸骨后压榨性疼痛为主。本病属于中医学"胸痹""心痛""厥心痛"等范畴。近年来，现代医学防治冠心病研究发展迅速，可概括为三个方面：(1) 增加冠状动脉血流量，改善缺血心肌血供。(2) 降低心肌耗氧量。(3) 增强心肌细胞本身耐缺血、缺氧的能力。已有研究证明，中药有扩张冠状动脉、抗血小板黏聚、防止血栓形成等作用[1]。芎芍胶囊是中国中医科学院西苑医院和北京国际生物制品研究所共同研制的治疗冠心病心绞痛的中药制剂（五类）。根据国家药品监督管理局2002ZL0215 号批文，经山东中医药大学附属医院伦理委员会批准，进行Ⅱ期临床研究。本研究采用芎芍胶囊治疗冠心病心绞痛心血瘀阻证112 例，收到了较好的治疗效果，现报道如下。

1. 资料与方法

1.1 诊断标准

1.1.1 西医诊断标准 入选病例均按国际心脏病学会和协会及世界卫生组织临床命名标准化联合专题组报告《缺血性心脏病的命名及诊断标准》[2] 诊断。

1.1.2 中医辨证分型标准 参照2002 年《中药

新药临床研究指导原则》[3] 制定。辨证属心血瘀阻证：主证：胸痛或胸闷；次证：疼痛部位固定不移，痛引肩背或臂内侧，心悸不宁，口唇紫暗；舌象：舌质紫暗或有瘀斑；脉象：脉涩。具有主证之一，次证具有2 项或2 项以上者，结合舌脉即可诊断。

1.2 纳入标准、排除标准及剔除标准

参照文献[3] 制订。纳入标准：(1) 符合冠心病心绞痛诊断标准及中医证候诊断标准，年龄在18 ~ 70 岁并签署知情同意书者。(2) 心绞痛发作时间持续3 分钟以上者。排除标准：(1) 冠心病急性心肌梗死、不稳定性心绞痛或有Ⅳ级劳累心绞痛以及其他心脏疾病、神经官能症、更年期症候群、甲状腺功能亢进症、颈椎病、胆心病、胃及食管反流等所致胸痛者。(2) 合并Ⅱ级以上高血压（血压＞ 160/100mmHg）控制不满意者、重度心肺功能不全、恶性心律失常（快速心房颤动、心房扑动、阵发性室性心动过速等）患者。(3) 有出血倾向患者。(4) 合并肝、肾、造血系统等严重原发性疾病，精神病患者。(5) 年龄在18 岁以下或70 岁以上患者，妊娠或哺乳期妇女，过敏体质者。(6) 正在参加其他临床试验的患者。剔除标准：符合入选标准，但因各种原因未接受治疗的患者。

1.3 心绞痛分级

参照1979 年9 月全国中西医结合防治冠心病

---

* 原载于《中国中西医结合杂志》，2011，31（2）：191-194

心绞痛、心律失常研究座谈会修订的标准[4]制定。（1）劳力型心绞痛分为Ⅰ级、Ⅱ级、Ⅲ级。（2）非劳力型心绞痛分为轻度、中度、重度。

1.4 一般资料

本研究采用多中心、随机、双盲、阳性药对照的试验方法。240 例病例分别来自山东中医药大学附属医院、天津中医学院附属第一医院、天津中医学院附属第二医院、陕西省中医药研究院附属医院、陕西中医学院附属医院 5 家研究中心的门诊及住院患者，按随机数字表法分为 2 组。试验组 120 例，男 66 例，女 54 例；年龄 43 ~ 68 岁，平均（58.39±5.71）岁；病程 4 个月至 24 年，平均（5.15±2.79）年；心绞痛程度轻度者 53 例，中度者 67 例；伴有高血压病 60 例，糖尿病 9 例，高脂血症 59 例，陈旧性心肌梗死 6 例。对照组 120 例，男 64 例，女 56 例；年龄 41 ~ 69 岁，平均（57.87±5.23）岁；病程 6 个月至 21 年，平均（5.19±2.82）年；心绞痛程度轻度者 51 例，中度者 69 例；伴有高血压病 62 例，糖尿病 8 例，高脂血症 57 例，陈旧性心肌梗死 6 例。治疗前两组在性别、年龄、婚姻状况、工作性质、病例来源、病程、一般体格检查、心绞痛及中医症状积分、血液流变学、血脂、心电图检查方面比较，差异无统计学意义（$P < 0.05$）。

1.5 治疗方法

试验组给予芎芍胶囊（药物组成：川芎、赤芍，生产厂家：北京国际生物制品研究所，批号：200410，规格：250mg/ 粒）加血府逐瘀胶囊安慰剂。对照组给予血府逐瘀胶囊（天津市第五中药厂，批号：C03014，规格：0.4g/ 粒）加芎芍胶囊安慰剂，均 2 粒 / 次，3 次 / 日，早、中、晚饭后 0.5 小时口服。疗程均为 4 周。服药前 7 天和服药期间停用抗血小板聚集和抗凝血药物、长效抗心绞痛药。特殊情况可临时加服速效抗心绞痛药物。芎芍胶囊安慰剂和血府逐瘀胶囊安慰剂均由北京国际生物制品研究所生产，二者分别与芎芍胶囊和血府逐瘀胶囊外观、色泽等相同，并进行统一包装。

1.6 观察指标

观察治疗前后心绞痛疗效、硝酸甘油服用量及其停减率、中医证候、心电图、血脂［总胆固醇（TC）、三酰甘油（TG）、高密度脂蛋白胆固醇（HDL-C）、低密度脂蛋白胆固醇（LDL-C）］、血液流变指标等变化。

1.7 疗效判定标准

1.7.1 冠心病心绞痛疗效标准 参考文献[3]标准。症状消失或基本消失为显效；疼痛发作次数、程度及持续时间明显减轻为有效；症状基本与治疗前相同为无效；疼痛发作次数、程度及持续时间有所加重为加重。

1.7.2 硝酸甘油停减率 硝酸甘油停减率（%）=［（治疗前每周用药片数 – 治疗后每周用药片数）/ 治疗前每周用药片数］×100%。

1.7.3 心电图改善标准 参考文献[4]标准。（1）显效：心电图恢复至"大致正常"或达到"正常心电图"。次极量分级运动试验由阳性转为阴性或较治疗前运动耐量上升二级以上者。（2）有效：S-T 段的降低，以治疗后同升 ≥ 0.05mV，但未达正常水平，在主要导联倒置 T 波改变变浅（≥ 25% 者），或 T 波由平坦变为直立者。次极量分级运动试验较治疗前运动耐量上升一级者。（3）无效：心电图基本与治疗前相同。（4）加重：治疗后 S-T 段降低 ≥ 0.05mV，主要导联倒置 T 波加深（≥ 25%），或直立 T 波变平坦，平坦 T 波变倒置，以及出现异位心律、房室或室内传导阻滞。次极量分级运动试验较治疗前运动耐量下降一级者。

1.7.4 中医证候疗效标准 参考文献[3]标准。根据积分法判定中医证候总疗效。疗效指数（n，%）=［（治疗前积分–治疗后积分）/ 治疗前积分]×100%。显效：n ≥ 70%；有效：30% ≤ n < 70%；无效：n < 30%。

1.7.5 中医单项症状疗效标准 参考文献[3]标准。（1）痊愈：症状消失。（2）显效：症状明显好转或减轻 2 级以上。（3）有效：症状好转或减轻 I 级以上。（4）无效：症状无改变或加重。

1.8 统计学方法

采用 DAS 1.0 软件进行数据分析。计量资料采用 t 检验，方差不齐时用 t' 检验，同组前后比较时采用配对 t 检验；计数资料采用校正 χ^2 检验、Fisher 精确检验等；等级资料采用 CMH 法；多中心分析时计数资料采用 CMH 法分析，计量资料采用方差分析；对用药后综合评价指标、主要疗效指标，同时进行 PP 分析和 ITT 分析。

2. 结果

2.1 脱落病例统计 试验共入组 240 例，其中试验组完成 112 例，脱落 8 例；对照组完成 115 例，脱落 2 例，剔除 3 例。脱落原因：试验组不良事件 1 例，受试者不合作 3 例，失访 3 例，缺乏疗效 1 例。对照组受试者不合作 1 例，出现其他并发症 1 例。两组脱落病例比较差异无统计学意义（$P > 0.05$）。

2.2 两组治疗后心绞痛疗效比较（表 1）

试验组治疗后心绞痛改善总有效率及显效率优于对照组，差异均有统计学意义（$P < 0.05$，$P < 0.01$）。

表 1 两组治疗后心绞痛疗效比较

组别	例数	显效（例）	有效（例）	无效（例）	加重（例）	显效率（%）	总有效率（%）
试验	112	48*	50	14	0	42.86	87.50**
对照	115	40	43	32	0	34.78	72.17

注：与对照组比较，*$P < 0.05$，**$P < 0.01$

2.3 两组治疗后硝酸甘油停减率比较

两组各有 43 例患者应用硝酸甘油。其中，治疗后试验组停药 32 例，减量 2 例，剂量不变 9 例，停减率 79.07%；对照组停药 30 例，减量 7 例，剂量不变 6 例，停减率 86.05%。两组硝酸甘油停减率比较差异无统计学意义（$P > 0.05$）。

2.4 两组治疗后心电图改善比较（表 2）

两组治疗后心电图改善总有效率及显效率比较差异均有统计学意义（$P < 0.05$，$P < 0.01$），试验组优于对照组。

表 2 两组治疗后心电图改善比较

组别	例数	显效（例）	有效（例）	无效（例）	加重（例）	显效率（%）	总有效率（%）
试验	112	41	41	30	0	36.61**	73.21*
对照	115	30	35	48	2	26.09	56.52

注：与对照组比较，*$P < 0.05$，**$P < 0.01$

2.5 两组治疗后中医证候疗效比较

试验组显效 34 例，有效 63 例，无效 15 例，显效率 30.36%，总有效率 86.61%；对照组显效 26 例，有效 73 例，无效 16 例，显效率 22.61%，总有效率 86.09%。两组治疗后中医证候总有效率及等级分析（显效、有效、无效）比较差异均无统计学意义（$P > 0.05$）。

2.6 两组治疗后中医单项症状疗效比较（表 3）

两组治疗后中医单项症状（胸痛、胸闷、心悸）愈显率（愈显率 = 痊愈率 + 显效率）及等级分析比较差异均无统计学意义（$P > 0.05$）。

2.7 两组治疗前后血液流变学及血脂各指标比较（表 4、5）

治疗后两组血液流变学及血脂各项指标与治疗前比较，差异均无统计学意义（$P > 0.05$）；治疗前后两组间比较差异均无统计学意义（$P > 0.05$）。

2.8 安全性评价

两组治疗后一般体格检查、大便常规未见异常。治疗后，两组受试者均部分出现肝肾功能、血尿常规异常，具体原因有待于进一步观察、研究。丙氨酸氨基转移酶在对照组有 1 例正常转异常（52U/L）；血清尿素氮测定在试验组有 1 例正常转异常（7.5mmol/L）。血常规检查有部分指标正常转异常：血红细胞在对照组有 1 例正常转异常（6.57×10^{12}/L）；中性粒细胞在试验组有 1 例正常转异常（47.5%）。另外，有 3 例出现不良反应，其中试验组 2 例，发生晨起空腹服药后胃痛或胃脘胀痛不适，改为饭后 30 分钟服药后胃部不适消失，不良反应发生率为 0.018%；对照组 1 例，发生月经过多，坚持治疗后上述反应消失，不良反应发生率为 0.009%。两组不良反应发生率比较差异无统计学意义（$P > 0.05$）。

表 3 两组治疗后中医单项症状疗效比较

组别	症状	例数	痊愈（例）	显效（例）	有效（例）	无效（例）	显效率（%）	痊愈率（%）	愈显率（%）
试验	胸痛	112	46	61	5	0	54.46	41.07	95.54
对照		115	39	70	6	0	60.87	33.91	94.78
试验	胸闷	112	46	1	29	36	0.89	41.07	41.96
对照		115	39	0	32	44	0.00	33.91	33.91
试验	心悸	110	36	0	45	29	0.00	32.73	32.73
对照		114	28	0	54	32	0.00	24.56	24.56

表4　两组治疗前后血液流变学各项指标比较（$\bar{\chi} \pm s$）

组别	例数	时间	全血黏度低切 （mPa.s）	全血黏度高切 （mPa.s）	血浆黏度 （mPa.s）	红细胞比容 （%）	纤维蛋白原 （g/L）
试验	112	治疗前	14.47±1.21	4.53±0.02	1.43±0.02	0.45±0.07	3.48±0.06
		治疗后	13.92±4.81	5.03±5.09	1.38±0.25	0.43±0.04	3.30±0.71
对照	115	治疗前	15.52±1.75	4.61±0.09	1.42±0.03	0.46±0.11	3.50±0.31
		治疗后	14.82±5.81	4.64±0.76	1.37±0.20	0.44±0.04	3.36±0.70

表5　两组治疗前后血脂各项指标比较（mmol/L，$\bar{\chi} \pm s$）

组别	例数	时间	TC	TG	HDL-C	LDL-C
试验	112	治疗前	5.56±0.07	2.01±0.20	1.36±0.01	3.36±0.05
		治疗后	5.50±1.04	1.90±1.30	1.42±0.39	3.25±0.84
对照	115	治疗前	5.46±0.06	1.98±0.19	1.36±0.03	3.24±0.14
		治疗后	5.26±0.95	1.98±1.12	1.33±0.37	3.12±0.97

3. 讨论

现代研究证实，本虚标实是冠心病心绞痛的基本病机。"本虚"主要指心脏的虚损，但有气虚、阳虚、阴虚、血虚之分；"标实"有气滞、血瘀、痰凝、热结之别，但其主要病机为瘀血内阻、心脉不通。心血瘀阻在冠心病心绞痛的病机演变中占有特殊重要的地位，故活血化瘀、通脉止痛是冠心病心绞痛的重要治疗方法。李学勇[5]运用传统活血化瘀、理气止痛方血府逐瘀汤治疗冠心病心绞痛心血瘀阻型患者124例，疗效显著。董卫民[6]研究表明血府逐瘀汤在治疗冠心病心绞痛发作次数、心电图及症状改善方面疗效确切。杜桂琴等[7]研究表明应用活血化瘀、通脉止痛方法治疗冠心病心绞痛心血瘀阻证安全、有效。

芎芍胶囊中川芎辛、温，归肝、胆、心包经，活血行气，祛风止痛；赤芍苦、微寒，归肝经，清热凉血，散瘀止痛。二药配合共奏活血化瘀、通脉止痛之效。药效学、毒理学研究也证明，川芎所含川芎嗪能扩张冠状动脉，抑制血管平滑肌的收缩，增加冠状动脉血流量[8]，降低心肌耗氧量，提高耐缺氧能力，保护缺血心肌，并且有抑制血栓烷素活性及血小板聚集[9]、抗血栓、降血脂以及降血压等作用；赤芍能抑制血小板聚集及红细胞聚集，抗凝和抗血栓，抗动脉粥样硬化，扩张冠状动脉血管，增加冠状动脉血流量，保护缺血心肌，提高心肌对缺氧的耐受性，并且能降低肺血管阻力，减轻后负荷，改善微循环，降低门脉高压。

本研究结果表明治疗后芎芍胶囊试验组在改善心绞痛、心电图方面优于血府逐瘀胶囊对照组，差异均有统计学意义（$P < 0.05$，$P < 0.01$）。应用芎芍胶囊治疗冠心病心绞痛心血瘀阻证对减轻心绞痛程度，减少心绞痛持续时间，改善心电图，以及改善胸痛、胸闷、心悸等临床症状疗效确切，不良反应率低，说明芎芍胶囊治疗冠心病心绞痛心血瘀阻证安全、有效，其深入的作用机制则有待于进一步探讨。

参考文献

[1] 史大卓.中医临床研究冠心病心绞痛的思路方法.中医杂志，2000，41（1）：51-52.

[2] Report of the Joint International Society and Federation of Cardiology/Word Health Organization Task Force and Standardization of Clinical Nomenclature. Nomenclature and criteria for diagnosis of ischemic heart disease. Circulation, 1979, 59：607-608

[3] 郑筱萸主编.中药新药临床研究指导原则.北京：中国医药科技出版社，2002：69-73.

[4] 全国中西医结合防治冠心病心绞痛、心律失常座谈会.冠心病心绞痛及心电图疗效评定标准.1979.

[5] 李学勇.血府逐瘀汤治疗冠心病心绞痛（心血瘀阻型）124例.河南中医学院学报，2006，21（3）：49-50.

[6] 董卫民.血府逐瘀汤治疗冠心病心绞痛40例.现代中医药，2010，1（1）：8-9.

第三章

[7] 杜桂琴，孙兰军.七龙脉通胶囊治疗冠心病心绞痛（心血瘀阻证）临床观察.天津中医药大学学报，2007，26（4）：185-187.

[8] 成丽.浅议川芎的药理学作用.中国现代药物应用，

2010，4（6）：137-138.

[9] 张国，赵江花.川芎嗪在心血管疾病中的药理作用研究进展.中国当代医药，2009，16（4）：142.

冠心病住院患者心血管事件的发生与中医证候分布规律研究 *

李鸥　徐浩

以冠心病为主的心血管病是目前首要的致死原因，即使随着药物支架及冠心病二级预防药物的临床广泛应用，每年仍有大约2千万人突发急性心血管事件。多年的研究显示，中医药在防治冠心病方面表现出一定效果和良好的前景，尤以辨证论治的个体化治疗为特色[1]。如何进一步减少急性心血管事件的发生是目前冠心病防治研究的热点。冠心病中医证候分布特点相关研究报道正逐渐增多[2]，而冠心病患者中医证候分布特点与随访发生急性心血管事件有何关系的报道较少。本研究选择京津地区9家中医及中西医结合医院1072例冠心病住院患者进行前瞻性研究，结合随访心血管事件对中医证候分布特点进行分析，以期为冠心病中医临床辨证论治及药物研发提供参考。

1. 资料与方法

1.1 诊断标准

冠心病诊断标准参照国际心脏病学会及WHO临床命名标准化联合专题组报告《缺血性心脏病的命名及诊断》制定的标准[3]。

1.2 中医辨证分型标准

冠心病辨证分型标准参考中国中西医结合学会心血管专业委员会1990年修订的冠心病中医辨证标准[4]及《中医内科学》统编教材关于"胸痹心痛"章节所述内容。

1.3 纳入及排除标准

纳入标准：（1）符合冠心病诊断标准的住院患者。（2）临床可表现为心绞痛、心肌梗死、心功能不全、心律失常。（3）既往有陈旧性心肌梗死病史或曾行冠状动脉造影至少有一支冠状动脉狭窄≥50%。排除标准：患者虽有冠心病病史，但因其他原因住院，入院后第一诊断不是冠心病或冠心病引起的心力衰竭、心律失常。

1.4 研究方法

利用北京市科委重大项目支持的冠心病中医临床个体化诊疗研究数据平台，通过临床信息采集系统，由经过培训考核合格的临床研究人员实时采集患者的中医四诊信息及中西医诊断，并输入高度结构化的冠心病临床数据库。中医辨证要求由2名具有副主任医师及以上职称的中西医结合心内科专业医师进行。为便于分析，在广泛咨询专家基础上，将中医复合证型拆分为寒凝、火热、气滞、痰浊、痰热、血瘀、气虚、血虚、阴虚、阳虚、水饮11个证候要素。

1.5 临床资料

收集2003年1月1日—2006年9月30日期间中国中医科学院西苑医院、中国中医科学院广安门医院、卫生部中日友好医院、北京中医药大学附属东方医院、北京中医药大学附属东直门医院、北京市中西医结合医院、北京中医医院、天津中医药大学第二附属医院和天津市中医医院心血管科的住院患者，共计符合纳入标准者1072例，失访67例，共1005例，年龄26～96岁，平均（68.90±10.73）岁；男性616例（61.3%），女性389例（38.7%）。

1.6 心血管事件的定义

包括心源性死亡（含脑血管死亡）、急性心肌梗死、再行血运重建术。

* 原载于《中国中西医结合杂志》，2012，32（5）：603-606

1.7 随访时间

患者出院后 1 年。

1.8 统计学方法

将患者的中西医诊断从 SQL server 数据库导入到 SPSS 数据库，采用 SPSS 13.0 软件进行统计分析。一般资料采用描述性统计分析，计量资料用 $\bar{x} \pm s$ 表示。采用主成分 Logistic 回归分析冠心病中医证候要素与心血管事件发生的关系。

2. 结果

2.1 冠心病住院患者中医证候要素分布（表1）

1005 例冠心病住院患者中，寒凝 8 例（0.8%），火热 87 例（8.6%），气滞 74 例（7.4%），痰浊 556 例（55.3%），痰热 73 例（7.3%），血瘀 817 例（81.3%），气虚 560 例（55.7%），血虚 39 例（3.9%），阴虚 278 例（27.7%），阳虚 83 例（8.2%），水饮 28 例（2.8%）。提示冠心病中医证候要素总体分布以血瘀为最多，其次为气虚、痰浊和阴虚。

表 1　发生心血管事件与未发生心血管事件患者中医证候要素分布比较

证候要素	发生心血管事件组（66 例）	未发生心血管事件组（939 例）
寒凝	1（1.5）	7（0.7）
火热	3（4.5）	84（8.9）
气滞	5（7.6）	69（7.3）
痰浊	36（54.5）	520（55.4）
痰热	2（3.0）	71（7.6）
血瘀	56（84.8）	761（81.0）
气虚	44（66.7）	516（55.0）
血虚	4（6.1）	35（3.7）
阴虚	24（36.4）	254（27.0）
阳虚	3（4.5）	80（8.5）
水饮	4（6.1）	24（2.6）

2.2 冠心病住院患者中医证候要素与临床心血管事件发生的关系

2.2.1 急性心血管事件的发生情况（表1） 随访 1 年，1005 例患者中发生急性心血管事件的患者有 66 例，包括心源性死亡（含脑血管死亡）48 例，急性心肌梗死 12 例，再行血运重建术 6 例。未发生急性心血管事件的患者有 939 例。发生心血管事件组与未发生心血管事件组各证候要素分布比较，差异均无统计学意义（$P > 0.05$）。

2.2.2 主成分 Logistic 回归分析

2.2.2.1 提取特征值及方差（表2） 将 11 个中医证候要素分别进行主成分分析，取特征值（即相应该主成分引起变异的方差）在 1 以上的 6 个主成分，其累计贡献度占 75% 以上。从表 2 可看出，第一主成分解释了总变异的 18.721%，其特征根为 2.059，其余主成分同此。

2.2.2.2 旋转后的成分矩阵（表3） 经方差最大化正交旋转法旋转，迭代 6 次所得结果，得出旋转后的公因子的因子负荷。根据此结果，6 个主成分（以 FAC 表示），分别是：（1）FAC1：痰热（96.9%），火热（96.6%），痰浊（24.3%）；（2）FAC2：气虚（81.9%），阴虚（78.2%）；（3）FAC3：阳虚（77.3%），水饮（73.2%）；（4）FAC4：气滞（82.3%）；（5）FAC5：血瘀（52.9%），痰浊（21.8%）；（6）FAC6：寒凝（92.7%）。

2.2.2.3 Logistic 回归（表4） 将急性心血管事件作为因变量，发生心血管事件赋值 1，未发生心血管事件赋值 0，以 FAC1、FAC2、FAC3、FAC4、FAC5、FAC6 作为自变量进行 Logistic 回归分析。结果示：FAC2 在 Logistic 回归中差异有统计学意义，$P = 0.036$，OR = 1.305（CI：1.018 ~ 1.672）。而气虚、阴虚主要由 FAC2 解释，提示气虚阴虚可能是冠心病发生心血管事件相关的证候要素。

3. 讨论

证候在中医辨证论治中起着承上启下的作用，它由结合病因病机而启，承引着诊断与治则。深入研究冠心病证候分布特点，对于提高冠心病的中医辨证论治水平具有重要意义。近些年来，在中医证候学研究中，Logistic 回归分析、聚类分析、主成分分析、因子分析等多元统计学方法已取得不少成果。Logistic 回归分析属于概率型非线性回归，常用来分析疾病与各危险因素之间的定量关系[5]。然而，Logistic 回归应用虽然较为普遍，但如果自变量之间存在共线性，则会影响自变量对结局变量的关系，从而影响模型的稳定性，而主成分分析能够消除 Logistic 回归自变量之间的共线性。由于冠心病患者中医证候比较复杂，常虚实兼有，相互兼夹，各证候要素之间往往具有一定的相关性，即有较强的共线性存在，若将各个证候要素直接代入 Logistic 回归则会影响模型的可靠性和稳定性。而对于冠心病中医证候临床研究也证实了这一点。如

第三章

表2　特征值及方差

成分	初始特征值			提取平方和载入			旋转平方和载入		
	合计	方差（%）	累积（%）	合计	方差（%）	累积（%）	合计	方差（%）	累积（%）
1	2.059	18.721	18.721	2.059	18.721	18.721	1.970	17.980	17.908
2	1.669	15.171	33.893	1.669	15.171	33.893	1.541	14.013	31.921
3	1.379	12.535	46.427	1.379	12.535	46.427	1.381	12.557	44.478
4	1.120	10.178	56.605	1.120	10.178	56.605	1.203	10.940	55.418
5	1.040	9.454	66.059	1.040	9.454	66.059	1.144	10.400	65.818
6	1.015	9.226	75.285	1.015	9.226	75.285	1.041	9.467	75.285
7	0.892	8.108	83.392						
8	0.757	6.877	90.270						
9	0.614	5.578	95.848						
10	0.372	3.379	99.226						
11	0.085	0.774	100.00						

表3　旋转后的成分矩阵

证候要素	成分					
	FAC1	FAC2	FAC3	FAC4	FAC5	FAC6
寒凝	−0.008	0.005	−0.070	0.020	0.029	0.927
气滞	0.047	−0.299	−0.074	0.823	0.159	−0.062
痰热	0.969	0.003	−0.018	−0.077	0.006	−0.038
血瘀	−0.141	−0.083	−0.376	0.038	0.529	−0.287
气虚	−0.069	0.819	−0.213	0.016	−0.140	−0.107
血虚	−0.065	−0.015	−0.153	0.017	−0.872	−0.135
阴虚	0.077	0.782	0.069	−0.071	0.089	0.100
阳虚	−0.033	−0.247	0.773	−0.029	−0.018	0.102
水饮	−0.019	0.094	0.732	0.064	0.051	−0.175
火热	0.966	0.012	−0.010	−0.039	−0.007	0.045
痰浊	0.243	−0.304	−0.153	−0.711	0.218	−0.108

表4　Logistic 回归

步骤 1[a]	B	S.E	Wals	df	Sig.	Exp（B）	EXP（B）的95%CI	
							下限	上限
FAC1	−0.227	0.177	1.653	1	0.199	0.797	0.563	1.127
FAC2	0.266	0.126	4.419	1	0.036	1.305	1.018	1.672
FAC3	−0.013	0.130	0.010	1	0.919	0.987	0.765	1.274
FAC4	0.042	0.136	0.094	1	0.759	1.042	0.799	1.360
FAC5	−0.003	0.126	0.001	1	0.979	0.997	0.778	1.277
FAC6	−0.019	0.136	0.019	1	0.890	0.981	0.751	1.281
常量	−2.706	0.134	408.137	1	0.000	0.067		

王阶等[6]对冠心病不稳定型心绞痛患者中医证候之间的相关性分析发现，气虚血瘀证与痰瘀互阻证密切相关。

主成分分析的出发点是用较少的互相独立的因子变量来代替原有变量的绝大部分信息。运用主成分分析方法，可以确定对发生事件贡献度较大的几个变量，也就是所谓的"主成分"[5]。它可以将较为复杂的变量信息简化为几个因子。本研究将冠心病患者的中医证候要素作为自变量，使用主成分分析，取特征值在1以上的6个主成分，其累计贡献度占75%以上；将二者再次进行Logistic回归分析，结果表明主要由气虚和阴虚组成的主成分，随访1年内发生急性心血管事件的风险明显增加，为中医药干预减少心血管事件的发生提供了理论基础。

目前对于冠心病的中医病机多数认为属本虚标实，以血瘀证为最常见，并且贯穿于发病的整个过程。但应该充分认识到，血瘀是关键的病理因素，但不是唯一的。现有多种不同观点，如张晓东[7]认为阳虚为冠心病的主要病机，治疗冠心病要以温阳方药为主；王瑞科等[8]认为冠心病多与痰瘀互结相关，治疗以活血化痰方药为主；刘耀乾等[9]认为冠心病主要病因病机是气虚血瘀，提出治疗要以益气活血方药为主；近来，陈可冀院士课题组[10]提出"瘀毒致变"假说，指出瘀为常、毒为变，对冠心病稳定期易发生心血管事件的"瘀毒内蕴"患者，应在活血治疗基础上加以"解毒"；随后的多中心队列研究进一步证实了这一假说[11, 12]，并初步构建了冠心病稳定期因毒致病的量化标准[13]。

本研究所收集的病例均为"金标准"诊断的冠心病患者，这确保了研究的客观性。结果表明，冠心病住院患者的主要中医证候要素为血瘀、气虚、痰浊、阴虚等，其中血瘀证发生率最高，发生心血管事件组与未发生心血管事件组血瘀证均达80%之多，两者比较差异无统计学意义。主成分Logistic回归分析结果显示，由气虚和阴虚组成的主成分与发生急性心血管事件的关系密切，提示本虚尤其是气虚阴虚在冠心病病机转变中具有重要作用。中医学有"因虚致瘀，气虚生痰"等说法，久病伤气，气虚不能推动血行，血脉瘀滞更甚，从而加大冠心病心血管事件的风险；痰瘀互阻，久病蕴热，灼伤真阴，或久病耗伤气血，内及真阴，皆可导致阴虚，而阴虚生内热，煎灼津液，炼液为痰，加重血脉瘀滞，从而也能增大发生心血管事件的风险。

本研究未涉及"毒"证及随访心血管事件的分析，但气虚、阴虚是否为"毒"产生的基础？或者为"瘀毒致变"的促发因素，尚有待进一步探讨。总之，对冠心病患者重视早期干预气虚和阴虚证候，可能有助于血瘀、痰浊及其他变证的防治，减少心血管事件的发生，为稳定斑块、干预冠心病高危患者的组方选药提供了依据，值得进一步研究。

参考文献

[1] Gao ZY, Xu H, Shi DZ, et al. Analysis on outcome of 5284 patients with coronary artery disease: the role of integrative medicine. J Ethnopharmacology, Available online 7 September 2011, doi: 10.1016/j.jep. 2011.08.071.

[2] 张琳，于鑫婷，徐浩. 冠心病中医证候特点的分析与思考. 中西医结合心脑血管病杂志，2009，7（5）：578-581.

[3] Nomenclature and criteria for diagnosis of ischemic heart disease. Report of the Joint International Society and Federation of Cardiology/World Health Organization task force on standardization of clinical nomenclature. Circulation, 1979, 59（3）：607-609.

[4] 中国中西医结合学会心血管专业委员会. 冠心病中医辨证标准. 中西医结合杂志，1991，11（5）：257.

[5] 王雪华，夏春明，颜建军，等. 中医证候分类中常用多元统计分析方法及应用评析. 世界科学技术—中医药现代化思路与方法，2008，10（2）：15-20.

[6] 王阶，何庆勇，李海霞，等. 815例不稳定型心绞痛中医证候的因子分析. 中西医结合学报，2008，8（6）：788-792.

[7] 张晓东. 温阳养阴法治疗不稳定性心绞痛的理论探讨及实验研究. 南京：南京中医药大学优秀硕士毕业论文集，2005.

[8] 王瑞科，杨继平，李红. 葛丹稳心汤对不稳定性心绞痛患者LPA影响的临床研究. 湖南中医杂志，2007，23（2）：5-7.

[9] 刘耀乾，李小苹. 丹参滴丸和川芎嗪配合西药联合治疗不稳定型心绞痛临床观察. 中国中西医结合杂志，2003，23（7）：544-545.

[10] 徐浩，史大卓，殷惠军，等. "瘀毒致变"与急性心血管事件：假说的提出与临床意义. 中国中西医结合杂志，2008，28（10）：934-938.

[11] 徐浩，曲丹，郑峰，等. 冠心病稳定期"瘀毒"临床表征的研究. 中国中西医结合杂志，2010，30（2）：125-129.

[12] Feng Y, Xu H, Qu D, et al. Study on the tongue manifestations for the blood-stasis and toxin syndrome in the stable patients of coronary heart disease. Chin J Integr Med, 2011, 17 (5): 333-338.

[13] 陈可冀, 史大卓, 徐浩, 等. 冠心病稳定期因毒致病的辨证诊断量化标准. 中国中西医结合杂志, 2011, 31 (3): 313-314.

冠心病稳定期患者中医辨证与超敏C反应蛋白相关性研究 *

郑 峰 曲 丹 徐 浩 陈可冀

研究表明，冠状动脉内不稳定斑块（易损斑块）破裂引起急性血栓形成是触发心血管事件的病理基础[1]。炎症反应在冠状动脉粥样斑块的形成和破裂的过程中扮演了重要的角色。超敏C反应蛋白（hs-CRP）作为炎症反应标记物，是不稳定斑块的一个敏感的预测指标[2]，并可独立预测冠心病患者临床不良心血管事件的发生[3]。冠心病中医辨证与hs-CRP的相关性研究已有报道[4-7]，但既往研究多为不稳定型心绞痛（unstable angina, UA）、急性心肌梗死（acute myocardial infapction, AMI）或冠心病住院患者，且样本数较少。本研究探讨了冠心病稳定期患者中医辨证与hs-CRP的相关性，现报告于下。

1. 资料和方法

1.1 诊断标准

冠心病诊断标准：参照国际心脏病学会及世界卫生组织临床命名标准化联合专题组报告《缺血性心脏病的命名及诊断》制定标准[8]，并且选择性冠状动脉造影左主干狭窄 ≥ 30%，或其他血管狭窄 ≥ 50% 者。中医辨证标准：冠心病辨证分型标准参照中国中西医结合学会心血管专业委员会1990年10月修订的"冠心病中医辨证标准"[9]。血瘀证诊断、计分标准参照中国中西医结合学会活血化瘀专业委员会制定的血瘀证诊断标准[10]，血瘀证计分方法参照《活血化瘀研究与临床》[11]进行评分。

1.2 纳入标准

经冠状动脉造影确诊的冠心病患者；临床表现为无症状、稳定劳累性心绞痛、其他类型心绞痛或急性冠脉综合征病程超过1个月病情稳定者；年龄 ≤ 75 岁；签署知情同意书。

1.3 排除标准

近1个月内有感染、发热、创伤、烧伤、手术史；活动性结核病或风湿免疫疾病患者；严重心力衰竭患者，射血分数 < 35%；合并严重瓣膜疾病或心肌病；合并严重慢性阻塞性肺疾病、肺心病或呼吸衰竭患者；已知的肾功能不全，男性血清肌酐 > 221μmol/L，女性 > 177μmol/L；已知的肝功能不全，基础肝酶检测 > 正常值的3倍或合并肝硬化；严重造血系统疾病；严重精神病患者；恶性肿瘤患者；脏器移植患者；患者的预期寿命 < 3年。

1.4 临床资料

2007年9月—2008年11月，选择在中日友好医院经冠状动脉造影检查确诊的冠心病患者346例，在其冠心病症状稳定期统一进行临床信息采集，并取血测定hs-CRP。346例稳定期冠心病患者中，男256例，女90例；年龄32～75岁，平均（60.9±9.6）岁；有高血压病史225例（占65.0%），高脂血症病史261例（占75.4%），糖尿病病史121例（占35.0%），脑卒中病史46例（占13.3%），吸烟史203例（占58.7%）；中医辨证为痰浊140例（占40.5%），血瘀324例（占

* 原载于《中国中西医结合杂志》, 2009, 29 (6): 485-488

93.6%）、气滞 24 例（占 6.9%）、寒凝 1 例（占 0.3%）、气虚 189 例（占 54.6%）、阴虚 67 例（占 19.4%）、阳虚 139 例（占 40.2%），无阳脱患者。

1.5　研究方法及观察指标

对入选的患者在病历报告表（case report form，CRF）中详细记录病史、症状、舌象、脉象和辨证分型。中医的辨证分标实证、本虚证，包括痰浊（偏热、偏寒）、血瘀、气滞、寒凝、气虚、阳虚、阴虚和阳脱等证候。舌象采用佳能 IXUS860 数码相机记录存档，中医的辨证分型由两名副主任医师以上级中西医结合心血管医师确认。hs-CRP 采用免疫比浊度法测定，患者均于清晨空腹静脉采血，由中日友好医院化验室统一检测。

1.6　统计学方法数据

采用 SPSS 13.0 软件进行统计分析，计量资料用均数 ± 标准差（$\bar{x} \pm s$）表示，两样本均数的比较采用 t 检验，方差不齐者用 t' 检验。多组间的比较用单向方差分析（One-way ANOVA），方差齐性用 LSD 法，方差不齐时用 Tambane's T2 法。相关性分析采用双变量相关分析（Bivariate），资料服从正态分布选择 person 相关系数。

2. 结果

2.1　患者性别、年龄及既往病史对 hs-CRP 水平影响的比较（表 1）

346 例冠心病稳定期患者中，女性 hs-CRP 水平略高于男性，但两组差异无统计学意义（$P > 0.05$）；年龄 ≥ 60 岁患者 hs-CRP 水平明显高于年龄 < 60 岁患者（$P < 0.05$）；合并高血压病史、高脂血症病史、糖尿病病史、脑卒中病史及是否有吸烟史对 hs-CRP 水平未见显著影响（$P > 0.05$）。

2.2　患者不同证候对 hs-CRP 水平影响的比较（表 2）

346 例患者中根据是否具有某证候分为痰浊和非痰浊、血瘀和非血瘀、气滞和非气滞、寒凝和非寒凝、气虚（含阳虚）和非气虚、阳虚和非阳虚、阴虚和非阴虚 7 组，各组内 hs-CRP 水平比较差异均无统计学意义（$P > 0.05$）。

2.3　不同复合证型间 hs-CRP 水平的比较（表 3）

本组最常见的复合证型依次为气虚血瘀、阳

虚血瘀、气虚血瘀痰浊、阳虚血瘀痰浊、气虚阴虚血瘀和血瘀痰浊，各复合证型间 hs-CRP 水平比较，差异无统计学意义（$P > 0.05$）。

表 1　患者性别、年龄及既往病史对 hs-CRP 水平影响的比较（$\bar{x} \pm s$）

项目		例数	hs-CRP（mg/L）	P 值
性别	男性	256	1.94 ± 1.94	0.086
	女性	90	2.36 ± 2.07	
年龄	< 60 岁	146	1.80 ± 1.86	0.049
	≥ 60 岁	200	2.23 ± 2.05	
高血压病史	有	225	2.16 ± 2.03	0.148
	无	121	1.84 ± 1.88	
高脂血症病史	有	261	2.06 ± 2.01	0.899
	无	85	2.03 ± 1.89	
糖尿病史	有	121	2.22 ± 2.06	0.251
	无	225	1.96 ± 1.94	
脑卒中病史	有	46	2.17 ± 1.91	0.660
	无	300	2.03 ± 2.00	
吸烟史	有	203	2.07 ± 1.99	0.860
	无	143	2.03 ± 1.97	

表 2　冠心病患者不同证候对 hs-CRP 水平影响的比较（$\bar{x} \pm s$）

证候	例数	hs-CRP（mg/L）	P 值
痰浊	140	2.08 ± 1.91	0.819
非痰浊	206	2.03 ± 2.03	
血瘀	324	2.07 ± 2.00	0.492
非血瘀	22	1.77 ± 1.79	
气滞	24	2.16 ± 2.09	0.781
非气滞	322	2.04 ± 1.98	
寒凝	1	2.60	
非寒凝	345	2.05 ± 1.98	
气虚	189	2.12 ± 1.97	0.443
非气虚	157	1.96 ± 2.00	
阳虚	139	2.05 ± 2.01	0.978
非阳虚	207	2.05 ± 1.97	
阴虚	67	2.25 ± 2.13	0.363
非阴虚	279	2.00 ± 1.94	

表 3　冠心病患者不同复合证型间 hs-CRP 的比较（$\bar{x} \pm s$）

中医分型	例数	hs-CRP（mg/L）
气虚血瘀	56	2.02±1.90
阳虚血瘀	49	1.89±2.25
气虚血瘀痰浊	36	1.94±2.24
阳虚血瘀痰浊	31	1.81±1.31
气虚阴虚血瘀	20	2.03±1.84
血瘀痰浊	18	1.70±1.27

2.4　痰热与非痰热之间 hs-CRP 水平的比较（表 4）

为探讨冠心病稳定期患者辨证有无热象对 hs-CRP 水平的影响，我们对辨证痰热、非痰热患者进行了分析（按照本研究中医辨证标准仅痰浊辨证中明确提及热证）。346 例患者中辨证为痰热（痰浊偏热）94 例，非痰热者 252 例，痰热组 hs-CRP 水平较非痰热组有升高趋势，但差异无统计学意义（$P > 0.05$）。将非痰热患者进一步细分为阴虚（虚热）38 例和其他 214 例，结果 3 组间差异无统计学意义（$P > 0.05$），但痰热者较阴虚者有升高趋势。进一步分析有痰浊证 140 例（137 例合并血瘀）患者，其中偏热 94 例，偏寒 46 例，痰浊偏热组 hs-CRP 水平 [(2.32±2.12) mg/L] 明显高于痰浊偏寒组 [(1.59±1.27) mg/L]，两组比较差异有统计学意义（$P < 0.05$）。

表 4　痰热与非痰热之间 hs-CRP 水平的比较（$\bar{x} \pm s$）

证候		例数	hs-CRP（mg/L）	P 值
痰热（痰浊偏热）		94	2.32±2.12	0.120
非痰热		252	1.95±1.92	
痰热		94	2.32±2.12	
非痰热	阴虚	38	1.83±2.00	0.285
	其他	214	1.97±1.91	
痰浊	偏热	94	2.32±2.12	0.013
	偏寒	46	1.59±1.27	

2.5　血瘀证计分与 hs-CRP 之间相关性

血瘀证计分与 hs-CRP 水平双变量相关分析显示，冠心病稳定期患者血瘀证计分与 hs-CRP 水平无明显相关性（person 相关系数为 0.069，$P = 0.203$）。

3. 讨论

辨证论治是中医学的精髓，冠心病证型客观化的研究对于进一步认识证的实质、寻找辨证的客观依据、指导中医诊断和治疗有着积极意义。随着现代医学对冠心病研究的不断深入和诊断技术不断提高，探索冠心病证候实质及病因病机学说成为冠心病中医基础理论研究的热点。hs-CRP 作为炎症标记物之一，已证实是冠心病心血管事件的独立预测因子 [2,3]，受到广泛关注。冠心病中医辨证与 hs-CRP 的相关性研究已有报道 [4-8]，但既往研究多为 UA、AMI 或冠心病住院患者，hs-CRP 水平相对较高，反映的是急性期的炎症反应，受诊断和治疗因素影响较大，而且这些研究观察样本数较少。本研究探讨冠心病稳定期患者中医辨证与 hs-CRP 水平的相关性，以期为冠心病稳定状态早期识别高危患者提供线索。

对 346 例冠心病稳定期患者的证候分析发现，证候以血瘀证、气虚证、痰浊证居多，其中血瘀证高达 93.6%，高于文献报道水平，但和我们既往研究一致 [12]，这可能与本研究冠心病患者均为冠状动脉造影证实、且绝大多数患者行介入或旁路移植手术治疗有关；复合证型以气虚血瘀证、阳虚血瘀证和气虚血瘀痰浊证多见，尤其是阳虚血瘀证较其他研究为多，我们体会气虚、阳虚可能是冠心病介入治疗后患者本虚的主要特点，值得进一步研究。hs-CRP 水平检测结果发现，老年患者 hs-CRP 明显高于非老年患者；女性 hs-CRP 有高于男性的趋势，但差异无统计学意义；而患者是否有高血压病、糖尿病、高脂血症、脑卒中和吸烟史对血清 hs-CRP 水平未见显著影响。

既往基于 UA、AMI 及冠心病住院患者的研究结果显示，中医辨证实证患者、热证患者 hs-CRP 水平较高 [4-8]。本研究结果显示，冠心病稳定期患者各证候之间、常见复合证型之间 hs-CRP 水平均未见显著差异。在此基础上，我们探讨了辨证有无热象对 hs-CRP 水平的影响，由于本研究中医辨证标准仅痰浊辨证中明确提及热证，因此我们对辨证痰热、非痰热患者进行了分析，结果 346 例患者中辨证为痰热（痰浊偏热）94 例的 hs-CRP 水平较无痰热者有升高趋势，但无显著差异。进一步将非痰热患者细分为阴虚（虚热）38 例和其他 214 例，结果 3 组间比较差异亦无统计学意义，但痰热者较阴虚者有升高趋势。而通过分析有痰浊证140例患者（偏热94例，偏寒46例）发现，偏热组 hs-CRP 水平明显高于偏寒组，提示辨证实热者 hs-CRP 水平增高。血瘀证计分与 hs-CRP 水平双变量相关分析显示，冠心病稳定期患者血瘀证计分与 hs-CRP 水平无明显相关性。

中医学认为，冠心病为本虚标实之证，本虚为心之气、血、阴、阳亏虚，标实为血瘀、痰浊、寒凝、气滞，尤以血瘀为最常见。我们结合既往研究结果，首先提出"瘀毒致变与急性心血管事件"假说[13-16]，认为血瘀是贯穿于冠心病发展过程的中心环节，也是稳定期患者的基础病理状态。若瘀久化热、酿生毒邪，或从化为毒，在此基础上蕴毒骤发是稳定期冠心病发生急性心血管事件的主要病因和关键病理机转。hs-CRP 作为炎症标记物，可作为中医"毒"微观指标之一，本研究结果提示，血瘀严重程度并非转化为毒的必要条件，是否蕴热（多为实热）才是化毒的关键，为冠心病患者"蕴热化毒"这一病机提供了客观依据。在此基础上，我们将结合 hs-CRP 及临床终点事件随访进一步探索冠心病稳定期高危患者的病史、症状、体征、客观检测指标及证候特点，以期构建冠心病稳定期患者"瘀毒"临床表征，这对于冠心病稳定状态高危患者的早期识别和及早干预，无疑具有重要的意义。

参考文献

[1] Conti CR. Updated pathophysiolgic concepts in unstable coronary artery disease. Am Heart J, 2001, 141 (2 Suppl): S12-14.

[2] Vimani R, Burke AP, Farb A, et al. Pathology of the vulnerable plaque. Jam Coll Cardiol, 2006, 47 (8 Suppl): C13-18.

[3] Goldstein JA, Chandra HR, O'Neill WW. Relation of number of complex coronary lesions to serum C-reactive protein levels and major adverse cardiovascular events at one year. Am J Cardiol, 2005, 96 (1): 56-60.

[4] 杨徐杭, 汶医宁, 魏敏慧, 等. 冠心病中医辨证与血清 C 反应蛋白的相关性研究. 中医药学刊, 2004, 22 (9): 1649-1650.

[5] 林超, 郭进建, 林青, 等. 高敏 C 反应蛋白与不稳定型心绞痛中医证型相关性研究. 中国中医急症, 2007, 16 (10): 1221-1223.

[6] 易自刚, 王强, 张双旗. 急性冠脉综合征中医证型与 L-18、hs-CRP 的相关性研究. 江苏中医药, 2007, 39 (12): 22-23.

[7] 商秀洋, 石洁. 冠心病中医辨证与血清高敏 C 反应蛋白的关系研究. 现代中西医结合杂志, 2008, 17 (6): 818-819.

[8] 陈灏珠主编. 实用内科学. 12 版. 北京: 人民卫生出版社, 2005: 1472-1473.

[9] 中国中西医结合学会心血管专业委员会. 冠心病中医辨证标准. 中国中西医结合杂志, 1991, 11 (5): 257-258.

[10] 中国中西医结合学会活血化瘀专业委员会. 血瘀证诊断标准. 中国中西医结合杂志, 1987, 7 (3): 129-131.

[11] 陈可冀主编. 活血化瘀研究与临床. 北京: 北京医科大学、中国协和医科大学联合出版社, 1993: 7-10.

[12] 徐浩, 鹿小燕, 陈可冀, 等. 血瘀证及其兼证与冠脉造影所示病变及介入治疗后再狭窄的相关性研究. 中国中西医结合杂志, 2007, 27 (1): 8-13.

[13] 周明学, 徐浩, 陈可冀, 等. 黄连提取物对 ApoE 基因敲除小鼠主动脉易损斑块 Perilipin 和 PPAR-γ 基因表达的影响. 中国中西医结合杂志, 2008, 28 (6): 532-536.

[14] 周明学, 徐浩, 陈可冀, 等. 活血解毒中药有效部位对 ApoE 基因敲除小鼠血脂和动脉粥样硬化斑块炎症反应的影响. 中国中西医结合杂志, 2008, 28 (2): 126-130.

[15] 徐浩. 活血解毒中药抗炎及稳定易损斑块的探索与思考. 中国中西医结合杂志, 2008, 28 (5): 393-394.

[16] 徐浩, 史大卓, 殷惠军, 等. "瘀毒致变"与急性心血管事件: 假说的提出与临床意义. 中国中西医结合杂志, 2008, 28 (10): 934-938.

第三章

用复杂网络挖掘分析冠心病证候 - 治法 - 中药的关系 *

高铸烨　张京春　徐　浩　史大卓　付长庚　曲　丹　周雪忠

中医临床诊疗过程是患者机体反应、医生思维决策和复杂干预手段的非线性互动过程，具有局部复杂相关性、涌现性[1]等特点，着重于用证效关系来判别辨证的正确性，也就是以药测证、药证相应[2]。复杂网络（Complex Network）[3]是以网络化建模形式研究复杂现象的一种分析方法，在医学研究领域如分子结构研究、新药开发研究等方面都有应用，是一种描述组成复杂系统各元素间关系的一种表达形式。为了解冠心病证候特征、治法特点及药物应用之间的关系，根据"药证相应"理论[4,5]，对北京、天津地区9家三级甲等中医或中西医结合医院3018例冠心病患者进行住院诊疗状况的调查，用复杂网络挖掘分析冠心病证候 - 治法 - 中药关系。

1. 资料和方法

1.1　入选标准

1.1.1　诊断标准参照美国心脏病学院（American College of Cardiology，ACC）/美国心脏学会（American Heart Association，AHA）等2002年联合修订的"慢性稳定性心绞痛诊疗指南"[6,7]，以及中华医学会心血管病学分会2000年制定的"不稳定性心绞痛诊断和治疗建议"[8]和2001年制定的"急性心肌梗死诊断和治疗指南"[9]制定。中医辨证标准参照中国中西医结合学会心血管学会制定的冠心病中医辨证标准[10]。

1.1.2　纳入标准　符合上述诊断标准，且于住院期间服用中药的患者，年龄、性别、发病时间、用药、合并疾病不限（即不干预临床诊疗）；剔除无中医辨证的患者。

1.2　临床资料

病例为2003年1月1日—2006年9月30日期间在中国中医科学院西苑医院、中国中医科学院广安门医院、中日友好医院、北京中医药大学附属东方医院、北京中医药大学附属东直门医院、北京市中西医结合医院、北京中医医院、天津中医药大学第二附属医院、天津市中医

医院心血管科的冠心病住院患者。入选冠心病患者3018例，其中男1369例，女1649例，年龄33～96岁，平均（68.48±10.24）岁；疾病亚型以心绞痛为最多（1882例，62.36%），其后依次为心功能不全（1805例，59.81%），心律失常（1121例，37.14%），陈旧性心肌梗死（482例，15.97%），急性心肌梗死（418例，13.85%）。合并病以高血压最多（2238例，74.16%），其后依次为糖尿病（859例，28.46%），脑血管病（685例，22.7%），肺部感染（602例，19.95%），高脂血症（463例，15.34%），支气管炎（401例，13.29%）。

1.3　方法

1.3.1　资料收集整理方法　采用统一设计的调查表，利用冠心病中医临床个体化诊疗研究数据平台，通过临床信息采集系统，由经过培训考核合格的临床研究人员采集患者的全部住院信息，并输入数据库，再由北京交通大学计算机学院专业人员对数据进行转换、提取、清洗、分析。中药功效按照新世纪全国高等中医药院校规划教材《中药学》[11]进行拆分整理，如将化痰、祛痰、清痰、除痰、祛浊、泄浊、泻浊、清浊、化浊等整理为化浊。

1.3.2　分析方法　利用SQL Server 2000工具对人口学资料、一般临床特点、证候、治法及方药数据进行转换、加载，利用SPSS 13.0软件进行统计分析。一般资料采用频数统计分析，证治规律利用北京市科委重大项目"中医药防治重大疾病临床个体诊疗评价体系研究"所构建的数据挖掘平台，由北京交通大学数据挖掘人员利用Oracle 10.0g工具进行复杂网络分析[12,13]。以证候、治法、中药及其功效作为网络结点建立复杂网络图，通过计算机分析和处理，将反复出现的证候 - 治法、证候 - 药物、证候 - 功效关系连成网络结构。

2. 结果

2.1　中医证候要素分布情况

3018例中以血瘀最多（2328例，77.14%），

* 原载于《中西医结合学报》，2010，29（6）：485-488

其后依次是气虚（1654 例，54.8%）、痰浊（1050例，34.79%）、阴虚（722 例，23.92%）、阳虚（330例，10.93%）、气滞（207 例，6.86%）、痰浊偏热（158 例，5.24%）、痰浊偏寒（129 例，4.27%）、血虚（95 例，3.15%）、热证（88 例，2.92%）、水饮（87 例，2.88%）、阳亢（53 例，1.76%）、寒凝（23例，0.76%）、肾虚（15 例，0.5%），其他（27 例，0.89%）。

2.2　治法特点

临床常用治法以活血最多（2210 例，73.23%），其后依次是补气（1659 例，54.97%）、化浊（1282例，42.48%）、养阴（951 例，31.51%）、清热（702例，23.26%）、理气（623 例，20.64%）、宣痹（535例，17.73%）、通络（458 例，15.18%）、补脾（433例，14.35%）、温阳（357 例，11.83%）、疏肝（310例，10.27%）、安神（302 例，10.01%）、利水（284例，9.41%）、和胃（200 例，6.63%）、宣肺（191例，6.33%）、止咳（151 例，5%）、补肾（145 例，4.8%）、止痛（144 例，4.77%）。

2.3　方药使用情况

常用方剂依次是自拟方、血府逐瘀汤、生脉散、栝蒌薤白半夏汤、桃红四物汤、二陈汤、温胆汤、栝蒌薤白白酒汤、补阳还五汤、炙甘草汤、天麻钩藤饮。常用单味中药依次是丹参、茯苓、川芎、赤芍、桃仁、红花、当归、甘草、半夏、枳壳、陈皮、栝蒌、麦冬、地黄、柴胡。

2.4　证治规律复杂网络分析

对证候要素、治法、中药功效进行证候 - 治法、证候 - 药物、证候 - 功效之间的复杂网络分析，结果如下。

2.4.1　证候 - 治法复杂网络图分析（图 1）　从治法和证候要素的节点分布特征可以看出，常用于治疗冠心病的治法是活血、清热、补气、化浊（痰）、养阴、温阳、宣痹。

2.4.2　证候 - 药物复杂网络图分析（图 2）　从药物和证候要素的节点分布特征可以看出，冠心病核心药物组成是黄芪、陈皮、地黄、川芎、白术、桃仁、茯苓、甘草、半夏、泽泻、赤芍、当归、丹参、枳壳、桂枝、麦冬（按关联度由高到低依次排序），从药物性味可以看出临床用药多寒温并使，以温性药为多用。

2.4.3　证候 - 功效复杂网络图分析（图 3）　从证候要素和中药功效的节点分布特征可以看出，与常见证候要素构成关联关系的药物功效主要是止痛、化浊（痰）、清热、活血、补气、凉血、利水、化瘀、解毒、补血（按关联度由高到低依次排序）。

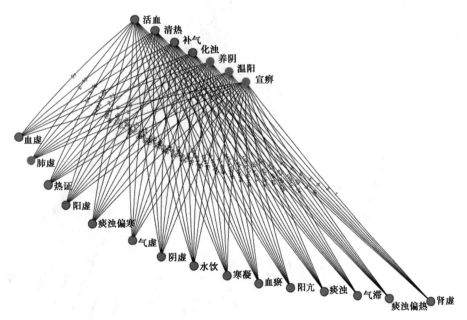

图 1　冠心病证候 - 治法复杂网络节点分布图

注：图中每条连线上的数字为两个节点之间关联的频数，如活血与血瘀共有 1648 次关联（下图同）

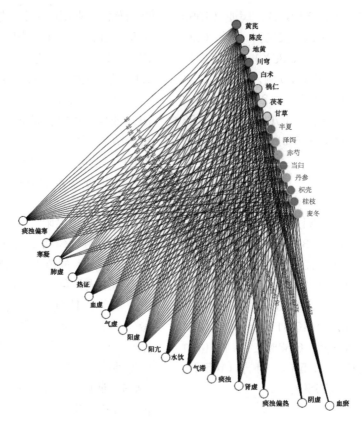

图 2　冠心病证候 - 药物复杂网络节点分布图
注：图中圆圈红色表示该药性温，黄色表示性平，绿色表示性寒

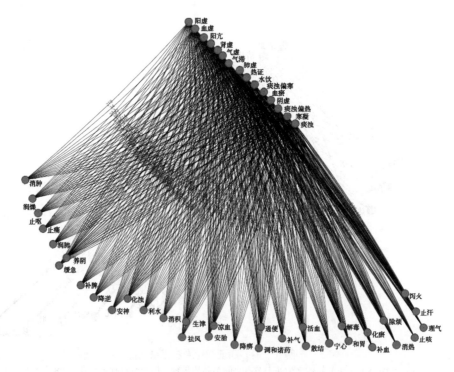

图 3　冠心病证候 - 功效复杂网络节点分布图

3. 讨论

复杂网络对于组成复杂系统的多个元素，其内在可以因某一种潜在关系而相互连接，并形成节点；大部分节点间只有少数几个连接，而某些节点却拥有与其他节点的大量连接。复杂系统是由少数集散节点所主控的网络系统，具有大量连接的集散节点所组成的功能团，可以反映其整体的、共性的部分或全部特征[12-15]。这与中医临床诊疗过程极其相似，辨证有主证、兼证、变证、夹杂证之分，治则有标本轻重缓急之别，治法有汗、和、下、补等之异，遣方用药有君、臣、佐、使等主次搭配关系。药证相应是中医辨证论治原则性的体现，在处方用药中存在君药对主证（症）、臣药和佐使药对兼证（症）的关系；主证、君药类似于网络的少数集散节点，治则治法则是这种复杂网络关系的抽象概括。复杂网络是数据挖掘的一种方法，即从大量数据中挖掘出隐含的、先前未知的、对决策有潜在价值的关系、模式和趋势[16]。很多情况下，数据挖掘的本质是很偶然地发现非预期但很有价值的信息[17]。

本研究应用北京市科委重大项目所构建的冠心病个体化诊疗信息数据挖掘平台，对 3018 例患者的分析结果提示冠心病核心证候要素主要是血瘀、气虚、痰浊、阴虚、阳虚、气滞，治法主要是活血、补气、化浊、养阴，所用药物功效主要是止痛、化浊（痰）、清热、活血、补气、凉血、利水、化瘀、解毒、补血，提示在胸痹临证时务以止痛为要，尽快解除患者的疼痛症状；另一方面清热、凉血、利水、解毒功效药物的应用可能与患者合并肺部感染、高血压等病症有关。从治法与证候的复杂网络分析结果看，清热治法应用较多，而在现有冠心病中医辨证标准[10]中并未单列"热证"，仅在"实证"——"痰浊"中分列"痰浊偏寒""痰浊偏热"两型，显然有一定局限性。由于工作紧张、饮食不节、情志刺激及空气污染等因素日益凸现，临床中冠心病患者热证比例逐渐增加，因此有必要在现有冠心病中医辨证分型"实证"中单列"火热"证，作为"血瘀"、"痰浊"、"寒凝"、"气滞"的补充，以更全面地体现冠心病证候的演变及特点。值得一提的是，解毒功效也与冠心病的基本证型不相一致，这种"毒"是否与热有关？还是冠心病患者病机转化中的潜在特点？就现有资料分析，这或许与患者合并不同疾病而用清热解毒类药

物有关，但更可能是一种"意外的"潜在规律被挖掘出来，这也与近年来所提出的"瘀毒致变"假说有殊途同归之妙[18-20]。但解毒是否应作为冠心病的治疗大法及如何选用解毒药物有待进一步研究。

参考文献

[1] 侯灿. 用系统方法探讨中医证的本质. 中国中西医结合杂志，2007，27（5）：461-465.

[2] 沈自尹. 以药测证对肾虚证基因网络和信号转导的研究. 中国中西医结合杂志，2005，25（12）：1125-1128.

[3] González MC, Barabási AL. Complex networks: from data to models. Nature Physics, 2007, 3（4）：224-225.

[4] 谢元华, 张京春, 陈可冀. 病证方药相应及其意义. 中西医结合心脑血管病杂志，2008，6（1）：1-2.

[5] 窦志芳, 郭蕾, 张俊龙, 张鑫. "方证对应"研究的思考. 中医杂志，2006，47（8）：563-564, 570.

[6] Gibbons RJ, Abrams J, Chatterjee K, et al. ACC/AHA 2002 guideline update for the management of patients with chronic stable angina--summary article: a report of the American College of Cardiology/American Heart Association Task Force on Practice Guidelines（Committee on the Management of Patients With Chronic Stable Angina）. Circulation, 2003, 107（1）：149-158.

[7] 廖晓星, 马虹. 慢性稳定型心绞痛诊疗指南（1999年）——美国心脏病学院（ACC）/美国心脏学会（AHA）/美国医师学院及美国内科学会 ACP-ASIM 联合议定. 岭南心血管病杂志，2000，6（3）：215-216.

[8] 中华医学会心血管病学分会, 中华心血管病杂志编辑委员会. 不稳定性心绞痛诊断和治疗建议. 中华心血管病杂志，2000，28（6）：409-412.

[9] 中华医学会心血管病学分会, 中华心血管病杂志编辑委员会, 中国循环杂志编辑委员会. 急性心肌梗死诊断和治疗指南. 中华心血管病杂志，2001，29（12）：710-725.

[10] 中国中西医结合学会心血管专业委员会. 冠心病中医辨证标准. 中西医结合杂志，1991，11（5）：257.

[11] 高学敏. 中药学. 北京：中国中医药出版社. 2004：8-592.

[12] 周雪忠, 刘保延, 王映辉等. 复方药物配伍的复杂网络方法研究. 中国中医药信息杂志，2008，15（11）：98-100.

[13] 倪青, 陈世波, 周雪忠, 等. 基于无尺度网络分析的2型糖尿病代谢综合征方-药-证关系. 中国中医药信息杂志，2006，13（11）：19-22.

[14] Ortega GJ，Sola RG，Pastor J. Complex network analysis of human ECoG data. Neurosci Lett，2008，447（2-3）：129-133.

[15] Boccaletti S，Latora V，Moreno Y，et al. Complex networks：structure and dynamics. Phys Rep，2006，424（4-5）：175-308.

[16] Feng Y，Wu Z，Zhou X，et al. Knowledge discovery in traditional Chinese medicine：state of the art and perspectives. Artif Intell Med，2006，38（3）：219-236.

[17] 高铸烨，徐浩，陈可冀，等．用随机行走模型评价生脉注射液治疗冠心病的临床疗效．中西医结合学报，2008，6（9）：902-906.

[18] 张京春，陈可冀．瘀毒病机与动脉粥样硬化易损斑块相关的理论思考．中国中西医结合杂志，2008，28（4）：366-368.

[19] 徐浩，史大卓，殷惠军，等．"瘀毒致变"与急性心血管事件：假说的提出与临床意义．中国中西医结合杂志，2008，28（10）：934-938.

[20] 史大卓，徐浩，殷惠军，等．"瘀"、"毒"从化——心脑血管血栓性疾病病因病机．中西医结合学报，2008，6（11）：1105-1108.

急性冠状动脉综合征中医证候要素分析 *

王承龙　张大武　王培利　史大卓

急性冠状动脉综合征（acute coronary syndrome，ACS）仍是目前人类健康的主要威胁。2006 年美国因 ACS 住院的患者有 1365 000 例，每 6 例死亡者中就有 1 例是冠心病患者，1 年内因冠状动脉事件死亡的患者占 34%，而其中 15% 死于心肌梗死 [1]。尽管现代医学采用冠状动脉介入治疗及抗心肌缺血、抗血小板、强化降脂等药物干预，但介入术后住院死亡率和再梗死率仍达 5% 左右 [2]。介入术后低或无复流、冠状动脉内血栓形成、支架内再狭窄等严重影响患者的预后及其生存质量。本研究通过总结 ACS 患者中医证候要素的分布规律，并结合全球急性冠状动脉事件注册研究（global registry of acute coronary event，GRACE）危险评分，探索中医证候要素与 ACS 危险分层的相关性，从而为中医药早期靶向干预 ACS 患者不良预后提供依据。

1. 临床资料

1.1　一般资料

于 2008 年 5 月至 2009 年 1 月纳入 241 例 ACS 患者，研究病例来自中国中医科学院西苑医院、卫生部中日友好医院、首都医科大学附属安贞医院、首都医科大学附属同仁医院、北京军区总医院、上海复旦大学附属中山医院。其中男 201 例，平均年龄（60.1±9.2）岁；女 40 例，平均年龄（65.5±6.9）岁。经冠状动脉造影证实单支病变者 47 例（19.5%），双支病变者 85 例（35.2%），三支病变者 109 例（45.3%）；合并高血压病 151 例（62.6%），糖尿病 68 例（28.2%），血脂异常 85 例（35.5%），脑卒中 13 例（5.4%），陈旧性心肌梗死 36 例（14.9%），有冠心病家族史 67 例（27.8%），吸烟史 151 例（62.6%）。

1.2　诊断及辨证标准

ACS 诊断标准参照《不稳定型心绞痛和非 ST 段抬高型心肌梗死诊断与治疗指南》[3] 和美国心脏病协会 / 心脏病学院 2007 年发布的 ST 段抬高型心肌梗死的治疗指南 [4]。

ACS 常多个证候要素相兼出现，故本研究采取证候分解的方法，将每位患者身上复杂的证候分解成若干个相对单纯的证候要素，便于分析。中医辨证标准参照《冠心病中医辨证标准》[5]。

1.3　纳入标准

符合 ACS 诊断标准及中医辨证标准者；年龄 40 ～ 75 岁；签署知情同意书。

1.4　排除标准

合并严重肝、肾、造血、神经系统等疾病及

* 原载于《中医杂志》，2011，52（19）：1654-1657

精神病、恶性肿瘤者；依从性较差者；妊娠期或哺乳期妇女；参加其他研究者。

2. 方法

2.1　研究方法

基于文献研究和专家咨询结果制定病例报告表，包括患者的基本资料（姓名、性别、年龄、文化程度、职业、病案号、联系方式）、病史相关内容、四诊资料（中医主症、兼症、舌象、脉象表现共 116 项）、生命体征、实验室检查资料以及经皮冠状动脉介入诊断和治疗相关情况。根据其病史、症状、体征和相关实验室检查进行全球急性冠状动脉事件注册（Global Registry of Acute Coronary Events，GRACE）危险评分，评分标准 [6-7] 包括患者年龄、慢性心力衰竭病史、心肌梗死病史、静息心率、收缩压、ST 段压低、血清肌酐水平、心肌损伤标志物、住院期间有无经皮冠状动脉介入治疗干预 9 个方面计算出 ACS 患者出院后 6 个月内可能发生全因死亡事件的百分比。根据相关文献报道 [8-9]，将 ≥ 120 分者设为高危组，< 120 分者设为中低危组。

按照中医诊断标准进行中医证候要素的分类，即气虚、阴虚、阳虚、血瘀、痰浊、气滞、寒凝。考虑中医证候要素之间存在较强的交互作用，Logistic 回归分析未能提取各变量间存在的交互作用项。故使用多因子降维法（multifactor dimensionality reduction，MDR）分析 [10]，提取复合中医证候要素。MDR 针对诸如疾病状态等分类变量，采用数据降维的思想，从而解决在有限样本量条件下，分析高维数据之间的交互作用。具体步骤如下：（1）将中医证候要素 7 个变量排成 7 列，设置变量 X1= 血瘀；X2= 痰浊偏寒；X3= 痰浊偏热；X4= 气虚；X5= 阴虚；X6= 阳虚；X7= 气滞，用 1 表示"有"，0 表示"无"进行赋值。（2）分类变量 class 用于区分高危和中低危患者。用 1 表示高危，0 表示中低危。（3）打开 MDR software 1.1.0 版本软件，载入已经清理好的数据，在程序默认的参数设置下运行。（4）多因子分类的集合中包含了 MDR 模型中各因子的组合，通过交叉验证和置换检验两个重要手段评估 MDR 模型是否有统计学意义。首先进行交叉验证一致性检验，即通过 10 次交叉验证，比较同一个因子组合被确定的次数，如果该因子组合有 1 次被确定，则交叉验证得分为最小值 1，如果该因子组合有 10 次

被确定，则交叉验证得分为最大值 10。通过十重交叉验证，在一定程度上可以避免因数据分组的偶然性而产生假阳性结果。其次看模型的假设检验，$P < 0.05$，认为该模型有统计学意义，假设检验使用置换检验结果分析。

2.2　统计学方法

采用 SPSS 16.0 软件包进行频数分析和 Logistic 回归等统计学分析，使用 MDR software 1.1.0 版本软件进行多因子降维方法分析。

3. 结果

3.1　中医证候要素分布情况

241 例 ACS 患者中血瘀证最为常见，为 213 例（88.4%），其次是气虚证 150 例（62.2%），阴虚证 79 例（32.8%），痰浊偏寒证 49 例（20.3%），痰浊偏热证 29 例（12.0%），阳虚证 21 例（8.7%），气滞证 2 例（0.8%）。标实证中以血瘀、痰浊为主；本虚证以气虚和阴虚为主。

3.2　GRACE 危险评分情况

241 例 ACS 患者经 GRACE 危险评分，其中高危组 21 例（8.7%），中低危组 220 例（91.3%）。表 1 示，高危组患者血瘀证最为常见 19 例（90.5%）；中低危组血瘀证 194 例（88.2%），两组患者中医证候要素分布无统计学差异（$P > 0.05$）。

表 1　241 例 ACS 患者不同 GRACE 危险分层的中医证候要素分布情况 ［例（%）］

证候要素	中低危组	高危组
血瘀	194（88.2）	19（90.5）
气虚	140（63.6）	10（47.6）
阴虚	73（33.2）	6（28.6）
痰浊偏寒	45（20.5）	4（19.0）
痰浊偏热	26（11.8）	3（14.3）
阳虚	17（7.7）	4（19.0）
气滞	2（0.9）	0

3.3　中医证候要素的多因子降维法分析

表 2 所示，血瘀 + 痰浊偏寒 + 阳虚的交叉验证一致性最好，10 次交叉验证均达到 100%，其次是血瘀 + 痰浊偏寒的交叉验证一致性较好，为 90%（9/10）；检验样本准确度方面以血瘀 + 痰浊偏寒 + 气虚 + 阳虚最高，为 0.6307，其中 4 个模型的置换检验均 $P < 0.05$，但血瘀 + 痰浊偏寒 + 痰浊偏热 +

气虚＋阳虚的交叉验证一致性差，故将其剔除。

表2　ACS中医证候要素的MDR模型

模型	检验样本准确度	P值	交叉验证一致性
X2	0.5758	0.095	9/10
X1X2	0.5859	0.027	9/10
X1X2X6	0.6092	0.024	10/10
X1X2X4X6	0.6307	0.003	8/10
X1X2X3X4X6	0.6023	0.002	4/10

将血瘀、痰浊偏寒、痰浊偏热、气虚、阳虚五因素的交互作用树状图进行交互作用效应和强度的分析，提示血瘀和痰浊偏寒显示有强的协同作用，但阳虚与血瘀、痰浊偏寒聚在一起时交互作用欠佳。

结合交互作用树状图，将血瘀、痰浊偏寒两因素交互作用体和血瘀、痰浊偏寒、阳虚3因素交互作用体与其他中医证候要素一起进行Logistic分析，结果见表3，进入回归方程的自变量是血瘀、痰浊偏寒、阳虚三因素交互作用体，卡方检验，$\chi^2=4.137$，$P<0.05$，故Logistic回归方程有统计学意义。Logistic回归方程为：logitP=－2.480+1.969（血瘀＋痰浊偏寒＋阳虚），结果表明同时表现为血瘀、痰浊偏寒和阳虚证候要素的与不出现这3证素的ACS患者相比，发生不良预后危险的比数比例为7.167，可以认为出现阳虚＋血瘀＋痰浊偏寒的ACS患者较不出现的患者6个月内发生全因死亡事件可能性的百分比要高。

4. 讨论

本研究以基于循证医学证据的GRACE危险评分结果作为评价标准，采用多因子降维法和Logistic回归分析评价241例ACS患者的中医证候要素分布，显示血瘀和气虚在ACS患者人群中占有较大比例，这与以往报道急性心肌梗死患者中医证候要素的分析结果一致[11-12]。

GRACE危险评分是GRACE研究中用于对ACS患者住院死亡率和出院后6个月死亡率的

预测评分系统[6]。ElbarouniB等[9]分析了12 242例加拿大ACS患者，平均GRACE危险评分是127分，第25%和75%的百分位数分别是103分和157分，从所有患者出现的全因死亡事件和GRACE危险评分的结果分析来看，GRACE危险评分是一个有效的和强有力的心血管事件预测模型。尽管有许多能够较准确地预测住院和30天死亡风险的因素[13-14]，但并不能增加GRACE危险评分对ACS患者住院和30天全因死亡事件预测的精确性。而且GRACE危险评分可以针对ACS的不同临床分型进行全因死亡的预测[8,15-16]。

MDR是一种分析交互作用的新方法，2001年由Ritchie等[17]研究散发性乳腺癌时首次提出。2004年，Coffey等[18]应用其分析心肌梗死基因-基因交互作用，他们将基因型组合区分为高、低风险后，以"低风险型"组合为参照，经Logistic回归拟合，分析发现"高风险型"罹患心肌梗死的危险度增高，差异有统计学意义（OR=1.44，95%CI：1.06～1.95）。本研究通过MDR模型筛选出影响ACS预后的具有交互作用的中医证候要素，并且经Logistic回归分析验证，结果表明同时表现为血瘀、痰浊偏寒和阳虚证候要素的患者与不出现这些复合中医证素的ACS患者相比，发生不良预后危险的比数比例为7.167（OR=7.167，95%CI：1.583～32.441），可以认为出现阳虚＋血瘀＋痰浊偏寒的ACS患者较不出现的患者6个月内发生全因死亡事件的可能性要高，这为中医药早期、合理干预ACS患者心血管事件的发生提供了依据。由于我们的样本量较少，阳虚＋血瘀＋痰浊偏寒复合中医证候要素在整个受试者人群中仅有8例，故分析和验证在出院后6个月发生的全因死亡率意义有限，需要扩大样本量进一步研究。

参考文献

[1] Writing group members, Lloyd-Jones D, Adams RJ, et al. Heart disease and stroke statistics—2010 update: a report from the American Heart Association. Circulation, 2010, 121 (7): e46-e215.

[2] Singh M, Rihal CS, Gersh BJ, et al. Twenty-five-

表3　241例ACS中医证候要素的Logistic回归分析

自变量	回归系数	标准误	Wald值	P值	OR值	95%置信区间
血瘀＋痰浊偏寒＋阳虚	1.969	0.770	6.535	0.011	7.167	1.583～32.441
常数项	-2.480	0.245	102.177	0.000	0.084	

year trends in in-hospital and long-term outcome after percutaneous coronary intervention: a single-institution experience. Circulation, 2007, 115 (22): 2835-2841.

[3] 中华医学会心血管病学分会. 不稳定型心绞痛和非 ST 段抬高心肌梗死诊断与治疗指南. 中华心血管病杂志, 2007, 35 (4): 295-304.

[4] Canadian Cardiovascular Society, American Academy of Family Physicians, American College of Cardiology, et al. 2007 focused update of the ACC/AH A 2004 guidelines for the management of patients with ST-elevation myocardial infaretion: a report of the American College of Cardiology/ American Heart Association Task Force on Practice Guidelines. J Am Coll Cardiol, 2008, 51 (2): 210-247.

[5] 中国中西医结合学会心血管病学会. 冠心病中医辨证标准. 中西医结合杂志, 1991, 11 (5): 257.

[6] Eagle KA, Lim MJ, Dabbous OH, et al. A validated prediction model for all forms of acute coronary syndrome: estimating the risk of 6-month postdischarge death in an international registry. JAMA, 2004, 291 (22): 2727-2733.

[7] Fox KA, Dabbous OH, Goldberg RJ, et al. Prediction of risk of death and myocardial infarction in the six months after presentation with acute coronary syndrome: prospective multinational observational study (GRACE). BMJ, 2006, 333 (7578): 1091.

[8] Ferreira-Gonzlez I, Permanyer-Miralda G, Heras M, et al. Patterns of use and effectiveness of early invasive strategy in non-ST-segment elevation acute coronary syndromes: an assessment by propensity score. Am Heart J, 2008, 156 (5): 946-953.

[8] Elbarouni B, Goodman SG, Yan RT, et al. Validation of the Global Registry of Acute Coronary Event (GRACE) risk score for in-hospital mortality in patients with acute coronary syndrome in Canada. Am Heart J, 2009, 158 (3): 392-399.

[10] 金明娟, 刘冰, 张爽爽, 等. 多因子降维法在人群散发性结直肠癌交互作用分析中的应用. 中华流行病学杂志, 2008, 29 (6): 535-539.

[11] 王玲, 刘红旭, 邹志东. 北京地区中医医院急性心肌梗死住院病人中医证候特征研究. 中西医结合心脑血管病杂志, 2008, 6 (4): 379-380.

[12] 毛静远, 牛子长, 张伯礼. 近 40 年冠心病中医证候特征研究文献分析. 中医杂志, 2011, 52 (11): 958-961.

[13] Timteo AT, Toste A, Ramos R, et al. Does admission NT-proBNP increase the prognostic accuracy of GRACE risk score in the prediction of short-term mortality after acute coronary syndromes？Acute Card Care, 2009, 11 (4): 236-242.

[14] Correia LC, Rocha MS, Bit tencourt AP, et al. Does acute hyperglycemia add prognostic value to the GRACE score in individuals with non-ST elevation acute coronary syndromes? Clin Chim Acta, 2009, 410 (1-2): 74-78.

[15] Jedrzkiewicz S, Goodman SG, Yan RT, et al. Temporal trends in the use of invasive cardiac procedures for non-ST segment elevation acute coronary syndromes according to initial risk stratification. Can J Cardiol, 2009, 25 (11): 370-376.

[16] Nallamothu B, Fox KA, Kennelly BM, et al. Relationship of treatment delays and mortality in patients undergoing fibrinolysis and primary percutaneous coronary intervention. The Global Registry of Acute Coronary Events. Heart, 2007, 93 (12): 1552-1555.

[17] Ritchie MD, Hahn LW, Roodi N, et a1. Multifactor-dimensionality reduction reveals high-order interactions among estrogen-metabolism genes in sporadic breast cancer. Am J Hum Genet, 2001, 69 (1): 138-147.

[18] Coffey CS, Hebert PR, Ritchie MD, et al. An application of conditional logistic regression and multifactor dimensionality reduction for detecting gene-gene interactions on risk of myocardial infarction: the importance of model validation. BMC Bioinformatics, 2004, 5: 49-58.

Analysis on Outcome of 5284 Patients with Coronary Artery Disease: The Role of Integrative Medicine[*]

Gao Zhu-ye   Xu Hao   Shi Da-zhuo   Wen Chuan   Liu Bao-yan

1. Introduction

In the beginning of 21st century, we are facing to serious challenges of coronary artery disease (CAD). Although it is becoming less lethal, CAD prevalence is incessantly increasing and it is still the most common cause of death. Extensive studies showed that risk factors such as hypertension, diabetes, dyslipidemia and smoking were positively correlated to CAD, and CAD incidence was significantly reduced with the reduction of risk factors (Helfand et al., 2009; Wilson, 2009; Morrow, 2010). European Society of Cardiology (ESC), American Heart Association (AHA), American College of Cardiology (ACC), Chinese Medical Association have published in succession clinical guidelines on stable angina pectoris (Gibbons et al., 2003; Fox et al., 2006), unstable angina pectoris (China Society of Cardiology, CSC, 2000; Braunwald et al., 2002; Anderson et al., 2007; CSC, 2007; Hoekstra and Cohen, 2009), acute myocardial infarction (CSC, 2001; Van de Werf et al. 2008; Kushner et al., 2009; Ferket et al., 2010), hypertension (The Drafting Committee of Chinese Guidelines for Hypertension Prevention and Treatment, 2000; Mancia et al., 2009) and dyslipidemia (Dyslipidemia Group of the Editorial Board of Chinese Journal of Cardiology, 1997; National Cholesterol Education Program NCEP, 2010; Joint Committee for Developing Chinese Guidelines on Prevention and Treatment of Dyslipidemia in Adults, 2007) in recent years, which have played an important role in improving secondary prevention of coronary heart disease.

Traditional Chinese Medicine (TCM) has a history of thousands of years and has made great contributions to the health and wellbeing of the people, and to the maintenance and growth of the population. Currently, more than 90% of the urban and rural Chinese population had ever sought for TCM in their lifetimes (Lu et al., 2008). Integrative medicine (IM) treatment has been the most representative characteristic for CAD patients in China, especially those in IM hospitals (Xu and Chen, 2008). However, the implementation of the above mentioned guidelines in clinical practice of IM hospitals in China and the potential benefit of IM therapy in improving CAD prognosis remain unclear. In this study, we performed a prospective research for CAD patients who were hospitalized in cardiovascular department in nine IM hospitals in Beijing and Tianjin between January 2003 and September 2006 for analyzing the secondary prevention status of CAD.

2. Materials and Methods

2.1 Patients

All patients were recruited from 9 IM hospitals (Xiyuan Hospital affiliated to China Academy of Chinese Medical Science, China-Japan Friendship Hospital, Guang'anmen Hospital affiliated to China Academy of Chinese Medical Science, Don fang Hospital affiliated to Beijing University of Chinese Medicine, Dongzhimen Hospital affiliated to Beijing University of Chinese Medicine, Beijing Hospital of Integrated Traditional Chinese with Western Medicine, Beijing Hospital of Traditional Chinese Medicine, Second affiliated hospital of Tianjin University of Traditional

[*] 原载于 Journal of Ethnopharmacology，2012，141（2）：578-583

Chinese Medicine, Tianjin Hospital of Traditional Chinese Medicine) in Beijing and Tianjin from January 2003 to September 2006. The research followed guidelines of the Declaration of Helsinki and Tokyo for humans, and was approved by the institutional human experimentation committee, and that informed consent was obtained.

5284 consecutive hospitalized CAD patients were enrolled into the study, which was approved by the local ethic committee. The average age in patients was 67.89 ± 10.97 years [range 26-98]. Patient's demographic and clinical characteristics are shown in Table 1. The primary diagnosis, comorbid diseases and TCM patterns are displayed in Table 2.

Table 1　Demographics and Clinical Characteristics

Variable	Number	Percentage of total
Age < 60	1190	22.52%
Age ≥ 60	4094	77.48%
Male	2717	51.40%
Female	2567	48.60%
Smoking	1460	27.60%
Drinking	602	11.40%

2.2　Inclusion and Diagnostic Criteria

All hospitalized patients in cardiovascular department in these hospitals who met any of the following diagnosis were enrolled in this study: (1) unstable angina pectoris, (2) acute myocardial infarction and (3) heart failure due to CAD.

Diagnostic criterion for CAD was referred to the report of "Nomenclature and criteria for diagnosis of ischemic heart disease" formulated by the Joint International Society and Federation of Cardiology/World Health Organization task force on standardization of clinical nomenclature (Nomenclature and Criteria for Diagnosis of Ischemic Heart Disease, 1979).

The criterion of TCM pattern diagnosis for CAD was referred to "The criterion of TCM pattern diagnosis for CAD" revised by Cardiovascular

Specialty Committee of Chinese Association of Integrative Western and Chinese Medicine in October 1990 (Specialty Committee of Cardiovascular Diseases, China Association of Integrative Western and Chinese Medicine, 1991).

Table 2　Primary Diagnosis, Comorbid Diseases and TCM Patterns

Type	Number	Percentage of total
Primary diagnosis		
Unstable angina pectoris	2992	62.07%
Heart failure	1036	19.61%
AMI	968	18.32%
Comorbid disease		
Hypertension	3796	71.8%
Diabetes mellitus	1503	28.4%
Cerebrovascular diseases	1024	19.4%
Dyslipidemia	973	18.4%
Renal insufficiency	542	10.3%
TCM patterns		
Blood stasis	2366	79.3%
Qi deficiency	1687	56.5%
Phlegm-turbidness	1080	41.1%
Yin deficiency	740	24.8%
Yang deficiency	337	11.3%
Qi stagnation	195	6.5%
Phlegm-heat	164	5.5%
Blood deficiency	101	3.4%
Excessive fluid	92	3.1%
Cold coagulation	25	0.8%

Note: AMI, acute myocardial infarction

2.3　Study Design and Treatment

The present registry study was designed as a prospective multi-center study. We developed a special questionnaire for interviewing the diagnostic and therapeutic status of hospitalized CAD patients. We collected data on demographic characteristics, medical history, diagnosis, treatment, endpoint events by means of a unified clinical and research information platform.

The information of treatment was recorded in detail, including but not limited to percutaneous coronary intervention (PCI), coronary artery bypass graft (CABG), Nitrates, anti-platelet agents, β-receptor blockers, angiotensin converting enzyme inhibitors (ACEI) and angiotensin receptor blockers (ARB), anticoagulants, statins, calcium channel blockers, diuretic agents, digitalis agents, phosphodiesterase inhibitors, etc. TCM therapies were administered to the enrolled patients according to corresponding pattern diagnosis, unless the patients declined TCM therapy or failed to take TCM due to other reasons. IM treatment was defined as prescribing TCM (in-hospital medication for seven days or more, and the post-discharge cumulative medication for three months or more), either Chinese medicine decoctions or Chinese patent drugs, in addition to routine conventional medicine. To ensure the compliance, patients were followed up monthly by telephone, clinical visits, or through calls to their primary care physician to determine the occurrence of major adverse cardiac events (MACEs) during one year after discharge from hospital.

2.4 Evaluation Methods

The diagnostic and therapeutic status of CAD patients was evaluated based on relevant clinical guidelines including Recommendations on the Diagnosis and Treatment of Unstable Angina Pectoris (CSC, 2000), Guidelines for Diagnosis and Treatment of Acute Myocardial Infarction (CSC, 2001), A draft of Chinese Guidelines for Hypertension Prevention and Treatment (The Drafting Committee of Chinese Guidelines for Hypertension Prevention and Treatment, 2000), Principles for the Prevention of Dyslipidemia (Dyslipidemia Group of the Editorial Board of Chinese Journal of Cardiology, 1997).

The primary endpoints consisted of in-hospital death and oneyear follow-up MACEs

including death due to any cause, acute myocardial infarction (AMI), PCI CABG. The outcome of patients was evaluated by an independent endpoint committee.

2.5 Management of Data

All of the data were validated by double entry methods. Using standardized data elements and definitions, this study managed systematic data with software Mysql 5.0, an onsite audit programme, and transmitted to a central data warehouse for additional review before analysis. Data of lost to follow-up were analyzed by last observation to carry forward.

2.6 Statistics

Statistical analysis of the experimental data was carried out using SPSS (version 11.0). Patients' demographic and clinical characteristics were analyzed with descriptive analytic method and the chi-square test for categorical variables. Continuous variables were presented as mean with standard deviation and categorical variables were expressed as frequencies with percentages. Logistic regression analysis using fractional polynomial modeling was conducted to determine the association between demographic and clinical information and mortality in MACEs. The criterion for statistical significance was at $P < 0.05$.

3. Results

3.1 The Standard-reaching Rate of Blood Lipid and Blood Pressure

Table 3 shows the standard-reaching rate of blood lipid and blood pressure. The standard-reaching rate of CAD patients with dyslipidemia was satisfied for total cholesterol (TC), while it was not optimistic for triglyceride, low-density lipoprotein cholesterol (LDL-C) and high-density lipoprotein cholesterol (HDL-C). As for those with hypertension, the standard-reaching rate of blood pressure was better than blood lipid, but there were still one third and one fifth patients who failed to control their systolic blood pressure (SBP) and diastolic blood pressure (DBP) respectively.

Table 3 Levels of Blood Lipid and Blood Pressure

Indices	Standard of evaluation	Standard-reaching rate（%）
TC （mmol/L）	＜ 4.68	85.6
LDL-C （mmol/L）	＜ 2.6	21.4
HDL-C （mmol/L）	≥ 1.0	52.5
Triglycerides （mmol/L）	＜ 1.7	31.2
SBP （mmHg）	＜ 140	61.9
DBP （mmHg）	＜ 90	80.9

Note：TC, total cholesterol；LDL-C, low-density lipoprotein cholesterol；HDL-C, highdensity lipoprotein cholesterol；SBP, systolic blood pressure；DBP, diastolic blood pressure

3.2 Status of Treatment

Displayed in Table 4 are the numbers and rates of each medications, coronary artery revascularization and Chinese herbal medicine which patients had received. A total of 4962 patients (93.9%) had received IM therapy including the Chinese patent medicine 85.7% and Chinese herbal formula 57.2% respectively. The injection usage of Chinese patent medicine was as follows: Danshen Injection (extractives from Salvia miltiorrhiza Bunge) 33.1%, Xuezhuantong injection (Panax Notoginseng Saponins) 32.0%, Shengmai injection (extractives from Ginseng, Radix Ophiopogonis and Schisandra Chinensis) 30.3%, Gegensu injection (puerarin) 29.8%, Dengzhanxixin injection (extractives from Erigeron breviscapus) 18.9%, Ciwujia injection (extractives from Radix Acanthopanacis Senticosi) 14.9%, Chuanxiongqin injection (Ligustrazine) 10.9% and Shenfu injection (extractives from Ginseng and Radix Aconiti Lateralis) 6.7%. Most TCM decoctions were self-formulated according to different TCM pattern diagnosis. The usage of classic Chinese herbal formula was as follows: Xuefuzhuyu decoction 4.9%, Shengmai san 4.6%, Gualouxiebaibanxia decoction 4.0%, Taohongsiwu decoction 3.3%, Erchen decoction 2.5%, Wendan decoction 2.0%, Gualouxiebaibaijiu decoction 1.9%, Buyanghuanwu decoction 1.8%, Zhigancao decoction 1.5%, Tianmagouteng yin 1.3%. The category and name of herbs most frequently administered have been

shown in Tables 5 and 6.

3.3 Prognostic Analysis

90 patients (1.7%) died in hospital, 162 patients died during one-year follow-up, 28 patients suffered AMI and 42 patients experienced coronary revascularization. There were 322 patients with MACEs, and the overall incidence of endpoints was 6.1% (322/5284). Table 7 displays the result of logistic stepwise regress analysis, in which AMI, heart failure, age ≥ 60 years, and medication of phosphodiesterase inhibitors were the independent negative prognostic factors for in-hospital mortality and follow-up MACEs, while statins and IM treatment were the independent protective factors.

4. Discussion

Nine IM hospitals of China were included in this study. The clinical data was collected by means of a unified clinical and research information platform and the results represented to some extent the general status of diagnostic

Table 4 Status of Medication and Therapy

Therapy	Number	Percentage of total
IM therapy	4962	93.9
PCI or CABG	757	14.3
Nitrates	4928	93.7
Anti-platelet agents	4454	84.7
β-receptor blockers	3442	65.5
ACEI and ARB	3265	62.1
Anticoagulants	2777	52.8
Statins	2732	51.9
Calcium channel blockers	2436	46.3
Diuretic agents	2150	40.9
Digitalis agents	1057	20.1
Phosphodiesterase inhibitors	752	14.2

Note: IM, integrative medicine: PCI, percutaneous coronary intervention; CABG, coronary artery bypass graft; ACEI, angiotensin converting enzyme inhibitors; ARB, angiotensin receptor blockers

Table 5　Top Ten Most Frequently Used Category of Herbs

Category	Number	Percentage of total
Qi-tonifying agents	2697	89.25%
Blood-activating agents	2600	86.04%
Qi-regulating agents	2345	77.60%
Heat-clearing agents	2040	67.50%
Dampness-draining agents	1993	65.95%
Phlegm-resolving agents	1943	64.30%
Stasis-removing agents	1892	62.61%
Blood-tonifying agents	1885	62.38%
Interior-warming agents	1590	52.61%
Yin-tonifying agents	1470	48.64%

Table 6　Top Ten Most Frequently Used Herbs

Herbs	Number	Percentage of total
Salvia miltiorrhiza Bunge	1907	63.10%
Poria	1813	59.99%
Raidx Astragali	1501	49.67%
Radix Paeoniae Rubra	1472	48.71%
Peach seed	1430	47.32%
Angelica	1415	46.82%
Radix Ligustici Chuanxiong	1401	46.36%
Safflower	1372	45.40%
Pinellia	1369	45.30%
Glycyrrhiza	1250	41.36%

and treatment for CAD patients objectively in Beijing and Tianjin. The analysis on the prognostic factors highlighted the potential role of IM in reducing MACEs and might have some implications for future clinical practice in second prevention of CAD.

Modern medical model is gradually moving

Table 7　Analysis of Prognostic Factors Using Multivariate Logistic Stepwise Regression

Variables	β	P	OR	95%CI
AMI	1.726	< 0.001	5.62	2.56 - 12.33
Heart failure	0.986	< 0.001	2.68	1.67 - 4.29
Age $\geqslant$ 60	0.696	0.006	2.01	1.22 - 3.30
Phosphodiesterase inhibitors	0.514	0.007	1.67	1.15 - 2.42
Statins	−1.456	0.036	0.23	0.06-0.91
IM treatment	−0.37	0.035	0.69	0.49-0.97

Note：AMI, acute myocardial infarction；IM, integrative medicine；OR, odds ratio；CI, confidence interval

from empirical medicine to evidence-based medicine (EBM). Aspirin, statins, ACEI/ARB, β-receptor blockers were all demonstrated their protective effect in second prevention of CAD. A variety of guidelines (angina, myocardial infarction, heart failure, hypertension, dyslipidemia, etc.) on the basis of EBM have been introduced one after another to clinical practice and played an important role in standardizing clinical management of cardiovascular diseases. However, the guideline implementation in real-world clinical settings seems not to be optimistic (Hobbs and Erhardt, 2002). This study showed the therapeutic patterns of CAD in these nine hospitals were basically consistent with relevant guidelines, but the application of ACEI/ARB, β-receptor blockers and statins agents is also needed to be intensified. The reasons we proposed in this study maybe related to following factors: less awareness of long-term benefit, only satisfied to the relieved clinical symptoms, overconcerning about drug adverse side-effects, etc.

In addition, the standardized treatment based on guidelines should also consider individual differences of the patients. The individualized treatment has been a trend of future development of medicine. In recent years, with the development of pharmacogenomics, it is possible to guide individual treatment by genetic differences of individual response to drug therapy.

However, it is obviously too early to put this idea into practice at this stage. Treatment based on pattern diagnosis is one of the basic principles and the characteristics of TCM. The patients were divided into different TCM patterns based on clinical data collected by four diagnostic methods (inspection, listening and smelling, interrogation, pulsefeeling and palpation) and further analysis on the cause, nature and location of disease. In this study, the patients were classified into several subgroups by TCM pattern diagnosis, and the corresponding TCM intervention by Chinese patent drugs and herbal medicines reflects the idea of individualized treatment. As shown in Tables 2 and 5, the patients were made pattern diagnosis and treated by administration of corresponding TCM. The top five TCM patterns in CAD patients were in turn blood stasis, Qi deficiency, phlegm-turbidness, Yin deficiency and Yang deficiency, indicating the most common sub-populations of CAD. Although it is hard to understand TCM pattern diagnosis for conventional clinicians, summarizing the symptom-signs characteristics of patients with different TCM patterns and analyzing pattern-treatment-outcome relationship might be helpful in searching for more specific target groups with better drug response and thus have valuable implications for future individualized medicine.

It is indisputable that the ultimate goal of any medicine is to improve health of mankind and enhance the therapeutic effect on preventing and treating diseases. Under this circumstance, the concept and practice of IM emerges as the times require (Rees and Weil, 2001; Eisenberg, 2011; Weil, 2011). However, most traditional medicines have not been successfully integrated into their national healthcare systems. For example, in Africa and Latin America, traditional medicines are completely separated from conventional medicine. There is no communication, no integration. In China, the integration of Chinese and Western medicine has been explored for more than a century. The experience has exemplified the tolerance, dependence, and assimilation of not only two medicines but also other science disciplines in IM (Xu and Chen, 2008), and provided a paradigm for worldwide IM (Dobos and Tao, 2011; Robinson, 2011). IM has shown potential benefit on alleviating clinical symptoms, reducing post-PCI restenosis, enhancing quality of life and improving post-PCI myocardial perfusion in CAD patients (Chen et al., 2006; Li et al., 2009; Qin and Huang, 2009; Zhang et al., 2009; Chu et al., 2010; He et al., 2010), while its role in second prevention of CAD and its effect on reducing MACEs remains unclear. In this prospective study, 5284 CAD patients were enrolled and logistic regression analysis showed that IM treatment and statins were the independent protective factors and could reduce the risk of MACEs by 31% and 77% respectively. The CAD patients with older age, more comorbid diseases and more complicated condition in IM hospitals also call for complicated intervention regimen. Although the influence of IM is less than a half of statins, the additional benefit on the basis of standardized conventional medicines can be anticipated to further improve second prevention of CAD in the future.

Although the advantages of TCM as a complementary medicine have been confirmed in management of CAD in this study, more investigations are still needed to be further determined how to integrate conventional medicine and TCM, the medication protocol, the time of intervention, drug dosage and the potential herb-drug interaction in clinical practice. On the whole, the key strategies of the secondary prevention of CAD are to intensify guideline implementation of CAD patients, to control their multiple risk factors and, maybe in the future, to highlight integrative complex intervention.

第三章

5. Conclusions

Results from this study showed that the implementation of relevant guideline in CAD management was not optimistic in IM hospitals in China. There was still certain gap between the usage of ACEI/ARB, β-receptor blockers, statins and clinical guideline. IM therapy, which integrates conventional medicine and TCM, has potential benefit for reducing MACEs in CAD patients. However, the schemes of intervention with IM therapy, the mechanism of action and the potential herb-drug interactions in clinical practice are still needed to be further determined.

References

［1］ Anderson, JL, Adams, CD, Antman, EM, et al. American College of Cardiology; American Heart Association Task Force on Practice Guidelines (Writing Committee to Revise the 2002 Guidelines for the Management of Patients With Unstable Angina/Non ST-Elevation Myocardial Infarction); American College of Emergency Physicians; Society for Cardiovascular Angiography and Interventions; Society of Thoracic Surgeons; American Association of Cardiovascular and Pulmonary Rehabilitation; Society for Academic Emergency Medicine, 2007. ACC/AHA 2007 guidelines for the management of patients with unstable angina/non-ST segment elevation myocardial infarction: a report of the American College of Cardiology/American Heart Association Task Force on Practice Guidelines (Writing committee to revise the 2002 guidelines for the management of patients with unstable angina/non-ST-elevation myocardial infarction) developed in collaboration with the American College of Emergency Physicians, the Society for Cardiovascular Angiography and Interventions, and the Society of Thoracic Surgeons endorsed by the American Association of Cardiovascular and Pulmonary Rehabilitation and the Society for Academic Emergency Medicine. Journal of the American College of Cardiology 50, e1-e157.

［2］ Braunwald E, Antman EM, Beasley JW, et al. American College of Cardiology; American Heart Association. Committee on the Management of Patients with Unstable Angina, 2002. ACC/AHA guideline update for the management of patients with unstable angina and non-ST-segment elevation myocardial infarction-2002: summary article: a report of the American College of Cardiology/American Heart Association Task Force on Practice Guidelines (Committee on the Management of Patients with Unstable Angina). Circulation 106, 1893-1900.

［3］ Chen KJ, Shi DZ, Xu H, et al. XS0601 reduces the incidence of restenosis: a prospective study of 335 patients undergoing percutaneous coronary intervention in China. Chinese Medical Journal, 2006, 119, 6-13.

［4］ Chinese Society of Cardiology of Chinese Medical Asso-ciation, Editorial Board of Chinese Journal of Cardiology, Guideline for diagnosis and treatment of patients with chronic stable angina. Chinese Journal of Cardiology, 2007, 35, 195-206.

［5］ Chinese Society of Cardiology of Chinese Medical Association, Editorial Board of Chinese Journal of Cardiology, Guideline for diagnosis and treatment of patients with unstable angina and non-ST-segment elevation myocardial infarction. Chinese Journal of Cardiology, 2007, 35, 295-304.

［6］ Chinese Society of Cardiology, Chinese Medical Association, Editorial Committee of Chinese Journal of Cardiology, Diagnosis and treatment recommendation of unstable angina pectoris. Chinese Journal of Cardiology, 2000, 28, 409-412.

［7］ Chinese Society of Cardiology, Chinese Medical Association, Guidelines for the diagnosis and treatment of patients with acute myocardial infarction. Chinese Journal of Cardiology, 2001, 29: 710-725.

［8］ Chu FY, Wang J, Yao K, et al. Effect of Xuefu Zhuyu Capsule on the symptoms and signs and health-related quality of life in the unstable angina patients with blood-stasis pattern after percutaneous coronary intervention: a randomized controlled trial. Chinese Journal of Integrative Medicine, 2010, 16, 301-304.

［9］ Dobos G, Tao I. The model of western integrative medicine: the role of Chinese medicine. Chinese Journal of Integrative Medicine, 2011, 17, 11-20.

［10］ Dyslipidemia Group of the Editorial Board of the Chinese Journal of Cardiology, Editor Committee of the Chinese Journal of Cardiology, Principles for the prevention of dyslipidemia. Chinese Journal of Cardiology, 1997, 25, 169-173.

［11］ Eisenberg D. Reflections on the past and future of integrative medicine from a lifelong student of the integration of Chinese and western medicine. Chinese Journal of Integrative Medicine, 2001, 17, 3-5.

[12] Ferket BS, Colkesen EB, Visser JJ, et al. Systematic review of guidelines on cardiovascular risk assessment: which recommendations should clinicians follow for a cardiovascular health check？ Archives of Internal Medicine, 2010, 170, 27-40.

[13] Fox K, Garcia MA, Ardissino D et al. Task Force on the Management of Stable Angina Pectoris of the European Society of Cardiology; ESC Committee for Practice Guidelines (CPG), Guidelines on the management of stable angina pectoris; executive summary; the Task Force on the Management of Stable Angina Pectoris of the European Society of Cardiology. European Heart Journal, 2006, 27, 1341-1381.

[14] Gibbons RJ, Abrams J, Chatterjee K, et al. American College of Cardiology; American Heart Association Task Force on Practice Guidelines; Committee on the Management of Patients with Chronic Stable Angina, 2003. ACC/AHA 2002 guideline update for the management of patients with chronic stable angina - summary article: a report of the American College of Cardiology/American Heart Association Task Force on Practice Guidelines (Committee on the Management of Patients with Chronic Stable Angina). Circulation, 107: 149-158.

[15] He QY, Wang J, Zhang YL, et al. Effect of Yiqi Yangyin Decoction on the quality of life of patients with unstable angina pectoris. Chinese Journal of Integrative Medicine, 2010, 16, 13-18.

[16] Helfand M, Buckley DI, Freeman M, et al. Emerging risk factors for coronary heart disease: a summary of systematic reviews conducted for the U. S. Preventive Services Task Force. Annals of Internal Medicine, 2009, 151, 496-507.

[17] Hobbs FD, Erhardt, L. Acceptance of guideline recommendations and perceived implementation of coronary heart disease prevention among primary care physicians in five European countries: the Reassessing European Attitudes about Cardiovascular Treatment (REACT) survey. Family Practice, 2002, 19, 596-604.

[18] Hoekstra J, Cohen M. Management of patients with unstable angina/non ST-elevation myocardial infarction: a critical review of the 2007 ACC/AHA guidelines. International Journal of Clinical Practice, 2009, 63, 642-655.

[19] Joint Committee for Developing Chinese Guidelines on Prevention and Treatment of Dyslipidemia in Adults, Chinese guidelines on prevention and treatment of dyslipidemia in adults. Chinese Journal of Cardiology, 2007, 35, 390-419.

[20] Kushner FG, Hand M, Smith Jr, SC, et al. Focused updates: ACC/AHA guidelines for the management of patients with ST-elevation myocardial infarction (updating the 2004 guideline and 2007 focused update) and ACC/AHA/SCAI guidelines on percutaneous coronary intervention (updating the 2005 guideline and 2007 focused update) a report of the American College of Cardiology Foundation/American Heart Association Task Force on Practice Guidelines. Journal of the American College of Cardiology, 2009, 54, 2205-2241.

[21] Li YQ, Jin M, Qiu SL, et al. Effect of Chinese drugs for supplementing Qi, nourishing Yin and activating blood circulation on myocardial perfusion in patients with acute myocardial infarction after revascularization. Chinese Journal of Integrative Medicine, 2009, 15, 19-25.

[22] Lu AP, Ding XR, Chen KJ, 2008. Current situation and progress in integrative medicine in China. Chinese Journal of Integrative Medicine, 2008, 14, 234-240.

[23] Mancia G, Laurent S, Agabiti-Rosei E, et al. Reappraisal of European guidelines on hypertension management: a European Society of Hypertension Task Force document. High Blood Pressure, 2009, 18, 308-347.

[24] Morrow DA. Cardiovascular risk prediction in patients with stable and unstable coronary heart disease. Circulation, 2010, 121, 2681-2691.

[25] National Cholesterol Education Program (NCEP) Expert Panel on Detection, Evaluation, and Treatment of High Blood Cholesterol in Adults (Adult Treatment Panel Ⅲ), Third report of the National Cholesterol Education Program (NCEP) expert panel on detection, evaluation, and treatment of high blood cholesterol in adults (adult treatment panel Ⅲ) final report. Circulation, 2002, 106, 3143-3421.

[26] Nomenclature and Criteria for Diagnosis of Ischemic Heart Disease. Report of the Joint International Society and Federation of Cardiology/World Health

Organization task force on standardization of clinical nomenclature. Circulation, 1979, 59: 607-609.

[27] Qin F, Huang X. Guanxin Ⅱ for the manage-ment of coronary heart disease. Chinese Journal of Integrative Medicine, 2009, 15, 472-476.

[28] Rees L, Weil A, Integrated medicine. British Medical Journal, 2001, 322, 119-120.

[29] Robinson N. Integrative medicine-traditional Chinese medicine, a model？ Chinese Journal of Integrative Medicine, 2011, 17: 21-25.

[30] Specialty Committee of Cardiovascular Diseases, China Association of Integrative Western and Chinese Medicine, Criterion of syndrome-differentiation in coronary heart disease. Chinese Journal of Integrated Traditional and Western Medicine, 1991, 11: 257.

[31] The Drafting Committee of Chinese Guidelines for Hypertension Prevention and Treatment. A draft of Chinese guidelines for prevention and treatment of hypertension. Chinese Journal of Hypertension, 2000, 8, 94-102.

[32] Van de Werf F, Bax J, Betriu A, et al. Management of acute myocardial infarction in patients presenting with persistent ST-segment elevation: the Task Force on the Management of ST-Segment Elevation Acute Myocardial Infarction of the European Society of Cardiology. European Heart Journal, 2008, 29: 2909-2945.

[33] Weil A. The state of the Integrative Medicine in the U. S. and western World. Chinese Journal of Integrative Medicine, 2011, 17: 6-10.

[34] Wilson, PW. Risk scores for prediction of coronary heart disease: an update. Endocrinology and Metabolism Clinics of North America, 2009, 38: 33-44.

[35] Xu H, Chen KJ. Integrative medicine: the experience from China. Journal of Alternative and Complementary Medicine, 2008, 14, 3-7.

[36] Zhang YC, Chen RM, Lu BJ, et al. Influence of shengmai capsule on recovery of living capacity in patients after myocardial infarction. Chinese Journal of Integrative Medicine, 2009, 15, 333-336.

The Significant Increase of FcγR ⅢA (CD16), A Sensitive Marker, in Patients with Coronary Heart Disease[*]

HUANG Ye   YIN Hui-jun   WANG Jing-shang   MA Xiao-juan   ZHANG Ying   CHEN Ke-ji

1. Introduction

Epidemiological and clinical studies have shown strong and consistent relationships between inflammatory markers and risk of future cardiovascular events, and measurement of inflammatory markers would contribute to identify individuals with a high risk of cardiovascular events who would benefit from treatment (Willerson and Ridker, 2004). In our previous study, we investigated the differential gene expression profiles of peripheral leukocytes from CHD patients with the oligonucleotide microarray technique (Yin et al., 2009). We confirmed the correlation between immune-inflammatory responses and the development of CHD using the pathway analysis tools, and demonstrated that a few differentially expressed genes related to inflammation presumably played a crucial role in the development of CHD through the network topology analyses. Of them, Fc receptor ⅢA of immunoglobulin G (FcγR ⅢA, also called CD16) was identified to be implicated in the development

* 原载于Gene，2012，504（2）：284-287

of CHD. Our recent data suggested an important role of FcγR ⅢA in the atherosclerotic formation by elevating the adhesive efficiency of monocytes to HUVECs *in vitro*, by increasing expression of inflammatory cytokines and also by kindling the atherosclerotic plaque destabilization in ApoE$^{-/-}$ mouse (Huang et al., 2012). However, whether or not deregulated Fcγ ⅢA expression is implicated in the pathogenesis of patients with CHD has not yet been elucidated.

In the current study, we therefore assessed the FcγR ⅢA mass at the mRNA level in leukocytes and at the protein level for soluble CD16 (sCD16) in sera and the membrane CD16 level on circulating monocytes from 100 patients with CHD and 40 healthy individuals. We also determined the level of a marker for activated monocytes, soluble CD14 (sCD14). Additionally, to clarify the correlation of the expression of CD16 molecule on monocytes to specific cytokines known to stimulate CD16 expression, serum macrophage colonystimulating factor (M-CSF) levels were assayed as well. Moreover, inflammatory cytokines related to CD16 such as intercellular adhesion molecule 1 (ICAM-1, CD54), TNF-α and IL-1 were also examined (Belge et al., 2002). Our data together suggest that FcγR ⅢA contributed to the development of CHD by triggering monocyte activation coupled to inflammatory cytokine stimulation. These findings stressed an important role of FcγR ⅢA in the development of CHD.

2. Materials and Methods

2.1 Patients and Control Individuals

The total patient population consisted of 100 diagnosed CHD patients based on the 1999 ACC/AHA/ACP-ASIM guidelines for the management of patients with chronic stable angina and the ACC/AHA 2002 guideline for the management of patients with unstable angina and non-ST-segment elevation myocardial infarction (Braunwald et al., 2002; Gibbons et al., 1999). A diameter stenosis of at least 50% was diagnosed by visible estimation in a major coronary artery from standard selective coronary angiography. There were 58 patients with stable angina pectoris and 42 patients with acute coronary syndrome from Beijing Anzhen Hospital. Patients with serious diseases, such as liver or kidney dysfunction, stroke or tumors were excluded. As a control group, we selected 40 age and sex-matched healthy volunteers without any history of chest pain or evidence of cardiac or systemic diseases, who were recruited from the physical examination center of Xiyuan Hospital. The healthy individuals were not on any medication. All the subjects for both patients and healthy individuals were Han nationality, with age between 35 and 75. Our study was in accordance with the Helsinki Declaration, with no contravention to the medical ethics. Ethical approval for the study was granted by the Ethics Committee at Xiyuan Hospital, China Academy of Chinese Medical Sciences. All participants were given informed consent prior to participation in the study, and the study protocol followed the guidelines of the Ethics Committee of Xiyuan Hospital, China Academy of Chinese Medical Sciences. The clinical characteristics of the patients are shown in Table 1.

2.2 CBC Counts and C-reactive Protein Level

Whole blood was collected from patients and healthy individuals. Blood was stored in EDTA precoated tubes (BD) followed by the CBC analysis with XS-800i (Sysmex, Japan). The level of C-reactive protein (CRP) was determined by a highly sensitive, latex particle enhanced immunoassay following the instruction provide by the manufacturer (Roche Diagnostics, Germany).

2.3 qRT-PCR Assay

Total RNA samples were extracted from leukocytes using Trizol reagent (Invitrogen, USA). And then qRT-PCR analysis was carried out. GAPDH was used as an internal control. The primer sequences for PCR analysis are shown below, FcγR ⅢA: forward, 5′-TGTT

Table 1 The Profiles of Patients and Healthy Control Individuals Enrolled in the Study

	Healthy control (n =40)	CHD group (n =100)	P value
Age (mean ± SD) [a]	48.10 ± 9.49	52.50 ± 6.35	0.072
Male (n, %) [b]	32 (80%)	82 (82%)	0.813
Body mass index, kg/m² (mean ± SD) [a,c]	23.40 ± 2.60	24.10 ± 3.50	0.04
Hypercholesterolemia (> 230 mg/dl)	–	15	–
Hypertension	–	62	–
Diabetes	–	34	–
Monocyte count (mmol/L) [c]	0.36 ± 0.16	0.38 ± 0.10	0.667

[a] Statistical comparison by the *t*-test for normal distributed continuous variables.

[b] By chi-square test for categorical variables.

[c] Data on monocyte count for 100 CHD patients and 40 healthy controls.

CAAGGAGGAAGACCCT-3′, reverse, 5′-GAA GTAGGAGCCGCTGTCTT-3′; GAPDH: forward, 5′- GGGTGTGAACCATGAGAAGT-3′, reverse, 5′- GGCATGGACTGTG GTCATGA-3′.

2.4 ELISA Assay, Immunofluorescent Staining and FACS Analysis

Serum sCD16, sCD14, TNF-α, IL-1 and M-CSF levels from CHD patients and healthy control were measured by ELISA according to the instructions from R&D Systems (USA). Immunofluorescent staining and FACS analysis were performed according to the standard procedures described previously (Cairns et al., 2002).

2.5 Statistical Analysis

The SPSS Statistics 13.0 package was utilized to analyze the data. Differences between two groups were analyzed using the Independent Simples *T* test. The $P < 0.05$ was considered statistically significant.

3. Results and Discussion

FcγR ⅢA (CD16) belongs to Fcγ receptor (FcγR) which plays an essential role in the process of immunoinflammatory responses

(Deo et al., 1997), and it is mainly expressed on monocytes (Masuda et al., 2009). FcγR ⅢA (CD16) is a transmembrane subtype and mainly expressed on monocytes (Masuda et al., 2009). Several studies have shown that FcγR ⅢA was implicated in various inflammatory conditions, such as sepsis (Fingerle et al., 1993), human immunodeficiency virus infection (Nockher et al., 1994), and hemodialysis (Nockher and Scherberich, 1998). To demonstrate the relevance of deregulated FcγR ⅢA expression to the development of CHD, we here assessed the expression of FcγR ⅢA in CHD patients and in healthy control at the mRNA level in leukocytes and at the protein level in sera. In agreement with previous studies, we observed that FcγR ⅢA at the mRNA level in leukocytes from CHD patients was largely increased by 57% compared to the healthy control ($P < 0.01$; Figure. 1A). Additionally, the protein level of FcγR ⅢA, i. e., serum sCD16 level, was also significantly increased in CHD patients, compared to the healthy control (> 2 fold, $P < 0.01$; Figure 1B). The C-reactive protein (CRP), a plasma protein synthesized by liver, is a sensitive and dynamic systemic marker of inflammation (Pepys and Hirschfield, 2003). Previous studies demonstrated that CRP is associated with the

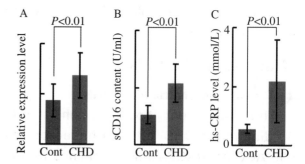

Fig 1 The Significance of FcγR ⅢA in Patients with CHD. (A) The relative expression level of FcγR ⅢA in leukocytes evaluated by qRT-PCR. (B) The level of sCD16 in sera analyzed by ELISA. (C) The level of hs-CRP in sera analyzed by a highly sensitive, latex particle enhanced immunoassay. Results were presented as mean ± SD (n =100 in the CHD group and n=40 in the healthy control group)

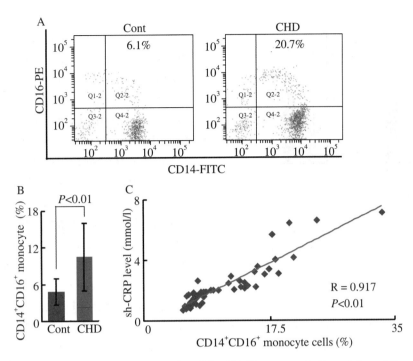

Figure2 The CD16⁺ Monocytes in Patients with CHD. (A) Representative data of the FACS analysis of CD14⁺CD16⁺ monocytes. Whole peripheral blood samples from patients with coronary heart disease (CHD) and healthy controls (cont)were stained with FITC-conjugated anti-CD14 antibody and PE-conjugated anti-CD16 antibody, followed by the FACS analysis. (B) The percentage of CD14⁺CD16⁺ monocytes in the whole CD14-positive cells. (C) The correlation between the percentage of CD14⁺CD16⁺ monocytes and the hs-CRP level

risk of CHD (Kaptoge et al., 2010) and predicts the incidence of CHD events (Buckley, et al., 2009). In agreement with previous studies, we observed a high level of CRP in CHD patients compared to that in the healthy control (~ 4 fold, $P < 0.01$; Figure1C). We further determined the protein level of membrane CD16 on monocytes, as characterized by 2-color immunofluorescent staining (Figure 2A). The FACS analysis indicated that the subpopulation of CD14⁺CD16⁺ monocytes in the whole CD14-positive cells was $10.5 \pm 5.5\%$ in patients with CHD and $4.8 \pm 2.2\%$ in healthy individuals (> 2.2 fold, $P < 0.01$; Figures 2A and B), without significant difference in the monocyte count based on the CBC results between the CHD patients and the healthy control. Moreover, we demonstrated that the percentage of CD14⁺CD16⁺ monocytes was positively correlated to the CRP level in patients with CHD ($P < 0.01$; Figure 2C), suggesting the contribution of the increase of CD16 to CHD development and its potential diagnostic value for CHD.

Monocytes play a crucial role in inflammatory diseases such as atherosclerosis (Randolph, 2009). Prior to their involvement in the pathogenesis of CHD, monocytes undergo phenotypic transformation, leading to their activation. Activated monocytes release sCD14 shedding its transmembrane form, which results in down-regulation of the cell surface CD14 (Bazil and Strominger, 1991). CD14, a monocyte endotoxin receptor, binds to lipopolysaccharides, together with tolllike receptors, to evoke monocyte activation (Shantsila and Lip, 2009). sCD14 may therefore be a marker for activation of monocytes/ macrophages (Krüger et al., 1991). In the current study, changes in the serum sCD14 level in CHD patients are shown in Figure 3A. We observed that sCD14 level in sera was increased by 78% in the CHD patients compared to the healthy control ($P < 0.01$; Figure 3A), suggesting the activation of monocytes in the CHD patients. M-CSF, a homodimeric

133

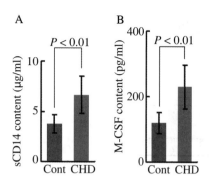

Figure3 The Levels of Inflammatory Cytokines Related to FcγR ⅢA in CHD. (A) The sCD14 level in sera determined by ELISA. (B) The M-CSF level in sera. Results were presented as mean ± SD (n =100 in the CHD group and n=40 in the healthy control group)

glycoprotein, specifically promotes the growth and differentiation of the monocyte/macrophage lineage (Devaraj et al., 2009), and plays a significant role in the process of atherosclerosis (Watanabe et al., 1995). M-CSF has been shown to induce CD16 expression on blood monocytes *in vivo* and *in vitro* (Johnson et al., 2005; Young et al., 1990). To shed light on the relationship between the expression of the CD16 on monocytes and the specific cytokines known to induce the CD16 molecule, M-CSF level in sera was measured by ELISA. The M-CSF level was largely increased by 90% in the CHD patients compared to the healthy control ($P < 0.01$; Figure 3B), similar to a previous observation (Munn et al., 1990). These findings together suggested that M-CSF might contribute to the CD14 and CD16 phenotypic differentiation on monocytes in CHD patients and during this phenotypic shift, CD14 on monocytes is shed from the surface which might then result in a high serum level of sCD14.

In a previous study, CD16[+] monocytes have been shown to possess several features of inflammatory tissue macrophages such as the expression of the intercellular adhesion molecule 1 (ICAM-1, CD54) (Thieblemont et al., 1995). ICAM-1 is a member of the immunoglobulin superfamily, and directly contributes to inflam-

matory responses within the blood vessel wall in the progression of CHD by increasing endothelial cell activation and augmenting atherosclerotic plaque formation (Lawson and Wolf, 2009). We thus looked into the expression of CD54 on CD16[+] monocytes from CHD patients and healthy control. As shown in Figure 4A, the mean fluorescent intensity (MFI) of CD54 was largely increased by 73% compared to the healthy control ($P < 0.01$). Previous studies indicated that circulation CD14[+]CD16[+] monocytes could spontaneously produce TNF and IL-1 (Frankenberger et al., 1996), which could provoke cell proliferation and migration of smooth muscle cells and macrophages in the atherosclerotic plaque (de Bont et al., 2006). Therefore, we also assessed TNF-α and IL-1 content in sera *via* ELISA. The significantly increased serum levels of TNF-α and IL-1 in the CHD patients were observed compared to the healthy control ($P < 0.01$; Figure 4B).

In the current study, we presumed that CD14[++] monocytes were induced by M-CSF and changed into CD14[+]CD16[+] monocytes. CD14 was shed off from monocytes and entered into blood circulation as soluble CD14, which indicated monocyte activation. CD14[+]CD16[+] monocytes were involved in the pathogenesis of CHD by stimulating CD54 on monocytes released as ICAM-1 and triggering a high level of proinflammatory cytokines such as TNF-α and IL-1 (Figure 5).

4. Conclusion

Overall, the present work confirmed the correlation between the increase of FcγR ⅢA at the mRNA and protein levels to CHD. FcγR ⅢA contributed to the development of CHD by triggering the monocyte activation and stimulating expression of inflammatory cytokines (Figure 5). Thus, the significant increase in CD14[+]CD16[+] monocytes and its downstream signaling in CHD patients indicated that the FcγR ⅢA level

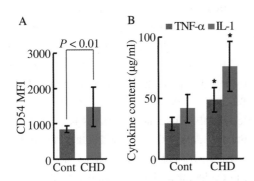

Figure4　The production of Inflammation in CHD Patients. **(A)** The CD54 level was quantified by its fluorescent intensity on CD14$^+$CD16$^+$ monocytes. Whole peripheral blood samples from patients with coronary heart disease (CHD) and healthy controls (cont) were stained with FITC-conjugated anti-CD14 antibody, PE-conjugated anti-CD16 antibody and CY5-conjugated anti-CD54 antibody, followed by the FACS analysis. **(B)** The levels of TNF-α and IL-1 in sera. *, $P < 0.01$, compared with the healthy control. Results were presented as mean ± SD (n =100 in the CHD group and n =40 in the healthy control group)

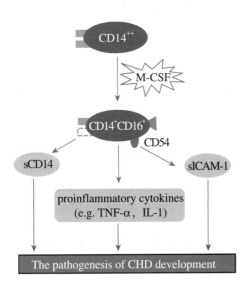

Figure 5　A Schematic Describing a Model Responsible for the Role of FcγR ⅢA in the Pathogenesis of CHD, M-CSF induces CD14^{++} monocytes to change into CD14$^+$CD16$^+$ monocytes. During this progress, CD14 on monocytes was shed off and entered into blood circulation as soluble CD14, which indicated monocyte activation. Additionally, FcγR ⅢA stimulated CD54 on monocytes to release in blood as soluble ICAM-1. Additionally, FcγR ⅢA also triggered a high level of proinflammatory cytokines such as TNF-α and IL-1. These together would enhance the pathogenesis of CHD development

might serve as a sensitive marker for the CHD diagnosis.

References

[1] Bazil V, Strominger JL. Shedding as a mechanism of down-modulation of CD14 on stimulated human monocytes. J Immunol, 1991, 147: 1567-1574.

[2] Belge KU, et al. The proinflammatory CD14$^+$ CD16$^+$DR^{++} monocytes area major source of TNF. J Immunol, 2002, 168: 3536-3542.

[3] Braunwald E, et al. ACC/AHA 2002 guideline update for the management of patients with unstable angina and non-ST-segment evation myocardial infarctionsummary article: a report of the American College of Cardiology/American Heart Association task force on practice guidelines (committee on the management of patients with unstable angina). J Am Coll Cardiol, 2002, 40: 1366-1374.

[4] Buckley DI, Fu R, Freeman M, et al. C-reactive protein as a risk factor for coronary heart disease: a systematic review and meta-analyses for the U.S. Preventive Services Task Force. Ann Intern Med, 2009, 151: 483-495.

[5] Cairns AP, Crockard AD, Bell AL. The CD14$^+$CD16$^+$ monocyte subset in rheumatoid arthritis and systemic lupus erythematosus. Rheumatol Int, 2002, 21: 189-192.

[6] de Bont N, et al. LPS-induced release of IL-1 beta, IL-1 Ra, IL-6, and TNF-alpha in whole blood from patients with familial hypercholesterolemia: no effect of cholesterol-lowering treatment. J Interferon Cytokine Res, 2006, 26: 101-107.

[7] Deo YM, Graziano RF, Repp R, et al. Clinical significance of IgG Fc receptors and Fc gamma R-directed immunotherapies. Immunol, 1997, 18: 127-135.

[8] Devaraj S, Yun JM, Duncan-Staley C, et al. C-reactive protein induces MCSF release and macrophage proliferation. J Leukoc Biol, 2009, 85: 262-267.

[9] Fingerle G, Pforte A, Passlick B, et al. The novel subset of CD14$^+$/CD16$^+$ blood monocytes is expanded in sepsis patients. Blood, 1993, 82: 3170-3176.

[10] Frankenberger, M, Sternsdorf T, Pechumer, H, et al. Differential cytokine expression in human blood monocyte subpopulations: a polymerase chain reaction analysis. Blood, 1996, 87: 373-377.

第三章

135

[11] Gibbons RJ, et al. ACC/AHA/ACP-ASIM guidelines for the management of patients with chronic stable angina: executive summary and recommendations. A report of the American College of Cardiology/ American Heart Association task force on practice guidelines (committee on management of patients with chronic stable angina). Circulation, 1999, 99: 2829-2848.

[12] Huang Y, Yin H, Wang J, et al. Aberrant expression of FcR IIIA (CD16) contributes to the development of atherosclerosis. Gene, 2012: 498, 91-95.

[13] Johnson J, et al. Plaque rupture after short periods of fat feeding in the apolipoprotein E-knockout mouse: model characterization and effects of pravastatin treatment. Circulation, 2005, 111: 1422-1430.

[14] Kaptoge S, et al. C-reactive protein concentration and risk of coronary heart disease, stroke, and mortality: an individual participant meta-analysis. Lancet, 2010, 375: 132-140.

[15] Krüger C, et al. Serum CD14 levels in polytraumatized and severely burned patients. Clin Exp Immunol, 1991, 85: 297-301.

[16] Lawson C, Wolf S. ICAM-1 signaling in endothelial cells. Pharmacol Rep, 2009, 61: 22-32.

[17] Masuda A, et al. Role of Fc receptors as a therapeutic target. Inflamm Allergy Drug Targets, 2009, 8: 80-86.

[18] Munn DH, Garnick MB, Cheung NK. Effects of parenteral recombinant human macrophage colony-stimulating factor on monocyte number, phenotype, and antitumor cytotoxicity in nonhuman primates. Blood, 1990, 75: 2042-2048.

[19] Nockher WA, Scherberich JE. Expanded CD14+CD16+ monocyte subpopulation in patients with acute and chronic infections undergoing hemodialysis. Infect Immun, 1998, 66: 2782-2790.

[20] Nockher WA, Bergmann L, Scherberich JE. Increased soluble CD14 serum levels and altered CD14 expression of peripheral blood monocytes in HIV infected patients. Clin Exp Immunol, 1994, 98: 369-374.

[21] Pepys MB, Hirschfield, GM. C-reactive protein: a critical update. J Clin Invest, 2003, 111 : 1805-1812.

[22] Randolph, GJ. The fate of monocytes in atherosclerosis. J Thromb Haemost, 2009, 7 (Suppl. 1): 28-30.

[23] Shantsila E, Lip GY. Monocytes in acute coronary syndromes. Arterioscler. Thromb Vasc Biol, 2009, 29: 1433-1438.

[24] Thieblemont N, Weiss L, Sadeghi HM, et al. CD14 low CD16 high: a cytokine-producing monocyte subset which expands during human immunodeficiency virus infection. Eur J Immunol, 1995, 25: 3418-3424.

[25] Watanabe Y, et al. Role of macrophage colony-stimulating factor in the initial process of atherosclerosis. Ann N Y Acad Sci, 1995, 748: 357-364.

[26] Willerson JT, Ridker PM. Inflammation as a cardiovascular risk factor. Circulation, 2004, 109 (Suppl.1): II2-II10.

[27] Yin HJ, Ma XJ, Jiang YR, et al. Investigation of gene expression profiles in coronary heart disease and functional analysis of target gene. Chin Sci Bull, 2009, 54: 1-7.

[28] Young DA, Lowe LD, Clark SC. Comparison of the effects of IL-3, granulocyte-macrophage colony-stimulating factor, and macrophage colony stimulating factor in supporting monocyte differentiation in culture: analysis of macrophage antibody-dependent cellular cytotoxicity. J Immunol, 1990, 145: 607-615.

第三章

The Expression of CD14$^+$CD16$^+$ Monocyte Subpopulation in Coronary Heart Disease Patients with Blood Stasis Syndrome[*]

HUANG Ye   WANG Jing-Shang   YIN Hui-jun   CHEN Ke-ji

1. Introduction

The way of disease-syndrome combination is an important style to diagnose and treat disease in traditional Chinese medicine (TCM) clinical practice today. Study on the blood stasis syndrome (BSS) is the most active field of integration of traditional and western medicine research in China[1]. To normalize and standardize the BSS, the way of disease-syndrome combination is used to explore the essence of BSS, which will be the inevitable tendency in the future. Study on CHD with BSS initiated by research team of Chen keji is the model of the way of disease syndrome combination. In our previous study, we found that Fc receptor IIIA of immunoglobulin G (FcγR IIIA, also called CD14$^+$CD16$^+$ monocyte subpopulation) is one of the differentially expressed genes related to coronary heart disease (CHD) patients using the oligonucleotide microarray technique [2], and high level of FcγR IIIA in CHD patients observed previously was verified by both mRNA level and its protein content [3]. Our recent study suggested an important role of FcγR IIIA in the atherosclerotic formation by elevating the adhesive efficiency of monocytes to HUVECs *in vitro*, by increasing expression of inflammatory cytokines and also by kindling the atherosclerotic plaque destabilization in ApoE$^{-/-}$ mouse [4]. Additionally, we also investigated that traditional Chinese medicine of activation of blood and dissolving stasis, effective components of Chuanxiong Rhizome and Red Peony Root, could stabilize the atherosclerotic plaque by suppressing inflammation, and its target was relative with FcγR IIIA[5]. However, whether or not the deregulation of the expression of CD14$^+$CD16$^+$ monocyte subpopulation is implicated in the pathogenesis of CHD patients with BSS has not yet been elucidated.

2. Methods

2.1 Patients and Healthy Control

All patients with coronary heart disease were the inpatients of Beijing Anzhen Hospital, from May 2010 to December 2010, diagnosed by a diameter stenosis of at least 50% from standard selective coronary angiography [6,7]. These CHD patients were selected into blood stasis syndrome (BSS) group and non-BSS group based on the standard diagnostic criteria established by the Special Committee of Promoting Blood Circulation and Removing Blood Stasis, Chinese Association of Integrative Medicine[8]. Patients with severe valvulopathy, serious primary diseases such as liver or kidney dysfunction, malignant tumors, medication history of antiplatelet therapy, and women in pregnancy or lactation stage were excluded from enrollment. Forty age- and sex-matched healthy individuals from the physical examination center of Xiyuan Hospital were selected as a control group. These individuals were without any history of chest pain or evidence of cardiac or other systemic disease verified by history examination, chest film, electrocardiogram, and blood routine examination, and none was taking any

* 原载于 Evidence-Based Complementary and Alternative Medicine，2013，Article id 416932

medication. Our study was in accordance with the Helsinki Declaration, with ethical approval granted by the Ethics Committee at Xiyuan Hospital, China Academy of Chinese Medical Sciences, and a written informed consent was obtained from all study participants. The clinical characteristics of the participants are shown in Table 1.

2.2 Blood Samples

Peripheral blood was collected from the CHD patients with BSS/non-BSS and healthy subjects under standardized conditions. Blood from CHD patients was drawn before coronary angiography was performed. For the analyses of cytometry or mRNA expression or flow cytometry, 2mL ethylenediaminetetraacetate- (EDTA-) anticoagulated blood was taken and immediately analyzed. For the detection of inflammatory cytokines by ELISA assay, blood was centrifuged at 3, 000 rpm for 20 min, and serum was frozen at −80℃ until analysis.

2.3 RT-PCR

FcγR ⅢA mRNA Expression was investigated by the quantitative real-time polymerase chain reaction (PCR) assay. Total RNA samples were extracted from leukocytes using Trizol reagent (Invitrogen, USA) according to the manufacturer's protocol. The purity and integrity of RNA were determined on a UV spectrophotometer (Eppendorf, Germany) by 260-280 nm absorbance ratio and agarose gel electrophoresis (1.5%) and ethidium bromide staining, respectively. cDNA preparations were performed at 42 ℃ for 1h, with reverse trans-criptase, 2μL RNase, 2μL of an oligo (dT) primer, and 10 mM of each dNTP in a total volume of 50μL of 1x first strand cDNA synthesis buffer, incubated at 70 ℃ for 10 min. PCR assays were carried out in a PCR (ABI 7500, USA). 1.5μL of cDNA mixture was subjected to amplification in a 20μL mixture. The following primer sequences with the predicted size were used for amplification: FcγR ⅢA: forward, 5'-TGTTCAAGGAGGAAGACCCT-3', reverse, 5'-GAAGTAGGAGCCGCTGTCTT-3'; GAPDH: forward, 5'-GGGTGTGAACCATGAG AAGT-3', reverse, 5'-GGCATGGACTGTGGTCATGA-3'. PCR conditions were as follows: initial denaturation at 94℃ for 15 min followed by 40 cycles of denaturation for 15s

Table 1　Characteristics of the CHD Patients with BSS/non-BSS and Healthy Individuals Participated in the Study

	CHD patients			
	BSS patients (*n*=50)	Non-BSS patients (*n*=50)	Healthy control (*n*=40)	*P* value
Age (year)	53.00 ± 6.43	52.92 ± 6.03	49.50 ± 8.71	0.507
Sex (male/female)	36/14	33/17	28/12	0.804
BMI (kg/m²)	25.50 ± 2.77	25.10 ± 2.57	24.29 ± 1.57	0.509
SAP (*n*)	12	13	—	—
ACS (*n*)	38	37	—	—
UAP (*n*)	31	31	—	—
AMI (*n*)	7	6	—	—
Hypercholesterolemia (> 230 mg/dL) (yes/no)	7/43	5/45	—	—
Hypertension (yes/no)	31/19	30/20	—	—
Diabetes (yes/no)	20/30	20/30	—	—
Monocyte count (mmol/L)	0.38 ± 0.11	0.37 ± 0.20	0.36 ± 0.11	0.891

BMI: body mass index; SAP: stable angina pectoris; ACS: acute coronary syndrome; UAP: unstable angina; AMI: acute myocardial infarction. Data are expressed as mean±SD

at 94℃ , annealing at 60℃ for 34 sec, extending at 72℃ for 15 sec, and a final extension at 72 ℃ for 10min. Glyceraldehydes-3-phosphate dehydrogenase (GAPDH) was used as an internal control in all PCR reactions. The PCR products were subjected to 2% agarose gel electrophoresis. The relative mRNA expression level of the target gene in each individual was calculated using the comparative cycle time (C_t) method[9].

2.4　Flow Cytometry

FcγR ⅢA protein level was assessed by flow cytometry. Ethyle-nediaminetetraacetic-Acid- (EDTA-) anticoagulated peripheral blood (PB) samples were collected from all patients and healthy controls for flow cytometric analysis performed previously described[10]. Briefly, PB samples were stained with saturating concentrations of fluorescein-isothiocyanate-(FITC-) conjugated anti-CD14 monoclonal antibody (mAb) (BD Biosciences, Lot: 74003) and phycoerythrin-(PE-) conjugated anti-CD16 mAb (BD Biosciences, Lot: 73903) or isotype-matched control mAb for 20 min at room temperature in the dark. After erythrocytes were lysed by incubation with lysing solution for 8 min, PB mononuclear cells were resuspended in PBS with 1% fetal calf serum. The surface expression of CD14 and CD16 on PB monocytes was performed by a fluorescence-activated cell sorter (FACS) cytometer (Becton Dickinson). The test data were obtained by FS versus SS gate and analyzed by Expo32 special software. Monocytes were identified by gating CD14$^+$ events, and all additional analyses were performed on this population. FcγR ⅢA protein content defined by the percentage of CD16 on the monocyte population (CD14$^+$/CD16$^+$%) was measured.

2.5　Enzyme-Linked Immunosorbent Assay (ELISA)

Concentrations of TNF-α (R&D, USA, Lot: 1007143), IL-1 (R&D, USA, Lot: 1007155), and soluble CD14 (sCD14) (R&D, USA, Lot: 1010179) in sera were determined by double-antibody sandwich avidin-biotin peroxidase complex enzyme-linked immunosorbent assay (ABC-ELISA), according to manufacturer's instructions.

2.6　Statistical Analysis

All data are expressed as mean±SD. The SPSS Statistics 15.0 package was utilized to analyze the data. Differences among groups were analyzed using the one-way analysis of variance (ANOVA), followed by multiple comparisons by LSD test. Difference was considered significant at $P < 0.05$.

3. Results and Discussion

BSS is a pathological state, which is the outward manifestation of some certain pathological stage of various diseases. Due to lack of objective diagnosis criteria, the essence of BSS is studied into the bottleneck stage. Recently, based on the way of disease-syndrome combination, much effective exploration of the essence of BSS was the foundation of BSS objective diagnosis criteria construction. During the past 50 years, we found a correlation between CHD with BSS and inflammatory, hemo-dynamics, platelet, and microcirculation [11].

Atherosclerosis, a chronic inflammatory immune state, is chiefly responsible for the development of CHD. Various leukocytes have been shown to influence atherogenesis. Monocytes and their descendant macrophages are central protagonists in the development of atherosclerosis [12]. Monocyte migration to the vessel wall is an initial event in the growth of atherosclerotic lesions [13]. Once monocytes are activated, adhesion to endothelial cells was induced by the transform of phenotype, which led to myocardium injury, inducing the proinflammatory cytokines such as TNF-α and IL-1 synthesis to initiate the inflammatory cascade reaction and oxidative stress injury, producing matrix metalloproteinase (MMP) and releasing many media to induce plaque instability and even fracture [14,15]. Therefore, monocytes played the key role in the chronic inflammationimmunoreaction of the arterial vessels. In our study, we investigated that there was no significant difference of monocyte count based on CBC count among CHD patients with BSS, non-BSS, and healthy control (Table 1). However, the level of sCD14 which is the indicator of activated monocyte [16] was obviously increased in CHD patients with BSS, compared to non-BSS and healthy control (Figure. 1). The increased level of sCD14 in sera in CHD patients with BSS indicated monocytes activation. To demonstrate the correlation between deregulated expression of $CD14^+CD16^+$ monocyte subpopulation and pathogenesis of CHD with BSS, its mRNA expression at the leukocyte level was assessed. As shown in Figure 2, relative expression level of $CD14^+CD16^+$ monocyte subpopulation in both CHD patients with BSS and non-BBS was largely increased by 99% and 77%, respectively, compared to the healthy control ($P < 0.01$). However, there was no significant difference of this relative expression level between CHD patients with. BSS and non-BSS (Figure. 2). The expression of biological traits was controlled by gene, and the biological traits were reflected by protein. To investigate whether or not the expression change of $CD14^+CD16^+$ monocyte subpopulation in both CHD patients with BSS and non-BSS at its protein level, therefore, we further analyzed the protein level of $CD14^+CD16^+$ on monocyte member using 2-color immunofluorescent staining (Figure 3a). The FACS results showed that the protein level of $CD14^+CD16^+$ on monocyte member was significantly increased in the CHD patients with BSS, when compared to the CHD patients with non-BSS and the healthy control ($P < 0.01$ or $P < 0.05$, Figure 3b).

TNF-α is one of the cytokines with various biological activation, and one previous study confirms that increased level of TNF-α was existed in the monocyte/macrophage, smooth muscle cells, and endothelial cells in the atherosclerotic

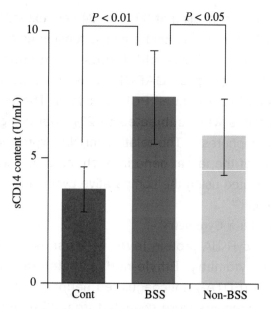

Figure 1 The Significant Level of Soluble CD14 in Sera in CHD Patients with BSS by ELSIA Assay. Results were presented as mean ± SD

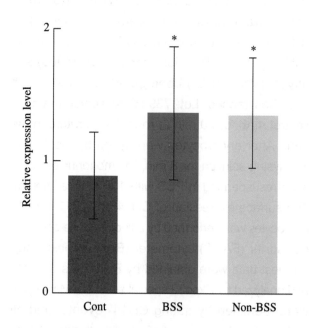

Figure 2 The mRNA Level of $CD14^+CD16^+$ Monocyte Subpopulation in Leukocytes in CHD Patients with BSS by qRT-PCR. *$P < 0.01$ compared to the control group. Results were presented as mean ± SD

plaque, and this high level was correlated to the severity of atherosclerosis [17]. IL-1 was released by active monocyte/macrophage, which induced the releasing of many cytokines and growth factors by monocyte/macrophage

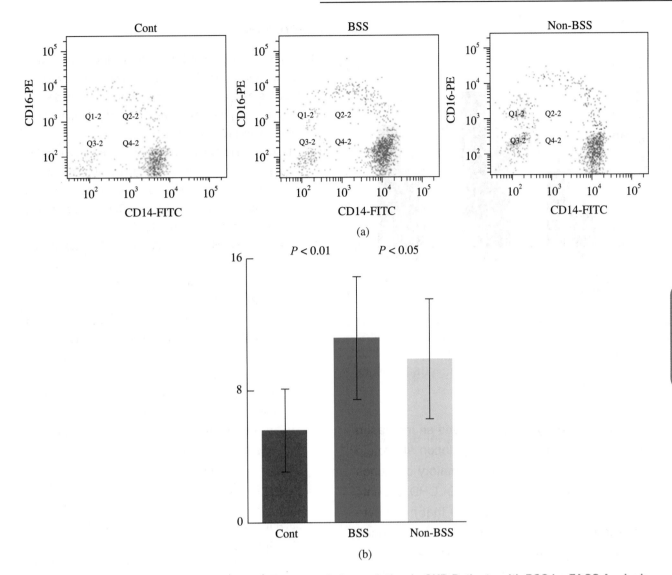

Figure 3　The Protein Level of CD14$^+$CD16$^+$ Monocyte Subpopulation in CHD Patients with BSS by FACS Analysis. (a) Representation data of FACS analysis of CD14$^+$CD16$^+$ monocyte subpopulation. Whole peripheral blood samples from patients and healthy individuals were stained with FITC-conjugated anti-CD14 antibody and PE-conjugated anti-CD16 antibody, followed by FACS. (b) The percentage of CD14$^+$CD16$^+$ monocoyte subpopulation in the whole CD14-positive cells. Results were presented as mean ± SD

and the expression of adhesion molecules such as ICAM-1. Additionally, IL-1 could stimulate vascular endothelium to produce many inflammatory factors such as TNF-α, aggravated local inflammatory reaction, and promote the development of atherosclerosis[18,19]. Additionally, previous studies indicated that the circulation of CD14$^+$CD16$^+$ monocytes could spontaneously produce TNF and IL-1[20], which could provoke cell proliferation and migration of smooth muscle cells and macrophages in the atherosclerotic plaque [21]. Therefore, protein level of TNF-α and IL-1 in sera was also assessed in our study by ELISA. The significant increased serum of TNF-α and IL-1 level was observed in CHD patients with BSS and non-BSS compared to the healthy control ($P < 0.01$, Figure 4), and the level of TNF-α and IL-1 in CHD patients with BSS was much higher than that in CHD patients with non-BSS ($P < 0.05$, Figure 4).

In the current study, we investigated that

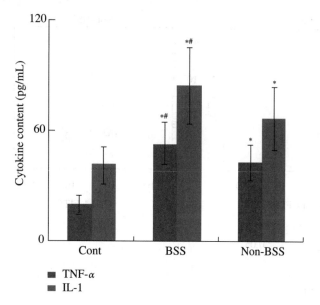

Figure 4 The Changes of Inflammatory Cytokines of TNF-α and IL-1 in Sera in CHD Patients with BSS. *P < 0.01 compared to the control group. #P < 0.05 compared to the CHD patients with non BSS. Results were presented as mean ± SD

第三章

there were monocyte activation and an increased CD14+CD16+ monocyte subpopulation at protein level and its downstream inflammatory cytokines such as TNF-α and IL-1 in sera in CHD patients with BSS. Herein, we presumed that monocyte activation in the CHD patient with BSS induced the phenotype of monocyte member transforming to CD14+CD16+ monocyte subpopulation which was involved in the pathogenesis of CHD with BSS.

4. Conclusion

Overall, the present work confirmed the correlation between increased CD14+CD16+ monocyte subpopulation at protein level and CHD patients with based on the way of disease syndrome combination. Thus, the increased CD14+CD16+ monocyte subpopulation and its downstream inflammatory cytokines in CHD patient with BSS indicated that CD14+CD16+ monocyte subpopulation was one of the sensitive markers in the pathogenesis of CHD with BSS.

References

[1] Liu Y, Yin HD, Shi DZ, et al. Chinese herb and formulas for promoting blood circulation and removing blood stasis and antiplatelet therapies. Evidence-Based Complementary and Alternative Medicine, 2012, Article ID 184503.

[2] Ma XJ, Yin HJ, Chen KJ. Differential gene expression profiles in coronary heart disease patients of blood stasis syndrome in traditional Chinese medicine and clinical role of target gene. Chinese Journal of Integrative Medicine, 2009, 15 (2): 101-106.

[3] Huang Y, Yin HJ, Wang JS, et al. The significant increase of FcγR ⅢA (CD16), a sensitive marker, in patients with coronary heart disease. Gene, 2012, 504 (2): 284-287.

[4] Huang Y, Yin HJ, Wang JS, et al. Aberrant expression of Fcγ R ⅢA (CD16) contributes to the development of atherosclerosis. Gene, 2012, 498 (1): 91-95.

[5] Huang H, Yin HJ, Ma XJ, et al. Correlation between FcγR ⅢA and aortic atherosclerotic plaque desta-bilization in ApoE knockout mice and intervention effects of effective components of Chuanxiong Rhizome and Red Peony Root. Chinese Journal of Integrative Medicine, 2011, 17 (5): 355-360.

[6] Braunwald E, Antman EM, Beasley JW, et al. ACC/AHA 2002 guideline update for the management of patients with unstable angina and non-ST-segment elevation myocardial infarction—summary article: a report of the American College of Cardiology/AmericanHeart Association Task Force on Practice Guidelines (committee on the management of patients with unstable angina). Journal of the American College of Cardiology, 2002, 40 (7): 1366-1374.

[7] Gibbons RJ, Chatterjee K, Daley J, et al. ACC/AHA/ACPASIM guidelines for the management of patients with chronic stable angina: executive summary and recommendations. A report of the American College of Cardiology/American Heart Association task force on practice guidelines (committee on management of patients with chronic stable angina). Circulation, 1999, 99 (21): 2829-2848.

[8] Society of Cardiology, Chinese Association of the Integrative Medicine. The diagnostic criteria of Chinese medicine in coronary heart disease. Chinese Journal of Integrated Traditional and Western Medicine, 1991, 11: 257.

[9] Meijerink JPP, Mandigers C, Van De Locht. A novel

method to compensate for different amplification efficiencies between patient DNA samples in quantitative real-time PCR. Journal of Molecular Diagnostics, 2001, 3 (2): 55-61.

［10］ Gremmel T, Kopp CW, Seidinger D, et al. The formation of monocyte-platelet aggregates is independent of on-treatment residual agonists' -inducible platelet reactivity. Atherosclerosis, 2009, 207 (2): 608-613.

［11］ Chen KJ. Exploration on the possibility of reducing cardiovascular risk by treatment with Chinese medicine recipes for promoting blood-circulation and relieving blood-stasis. Zhong Guo Zhong Xi Yi Jie He Za Zhi, 2008, 28 (5): 389.

［12］ Pittet MJ, Swirski FK. Monocytes link atherosclerosis and cancer. European Journal of Immunology, 2011, 41 (9): 2519-2522.

［13］ Woollard KJ, Geissmann F. Monocytes in atherosclerosis: subsets and functions. Nature Reviews Cardiology, 2010, 7 (2): 77-86.

［14］ Pamukcu B, Lip GYH, Devitt A. The role of monocytes in atherosclerotic coronary artery disease. Annals of Medicine, 2010, 42 (6): 394-403.

［15］ Saha P, Modarai B, Humphries J, et al. The monocyte/macrophage as a therapeutic target in atherosclerosis. Current Opinion in Pharmacology, 2009, 9 (2): 109-118.

［16］ Kruger C, Schutt C, Obertacke U, et al. Serum CD14 levels in polytraumatized and severely burned patients. Clinical and Experimental Immunology, 1991, 85 (2): 297-301.

［17］ Barath P, Fishbein MC, Cao J, et al. Detection and localization of tumor necrosis factor in human atheroma. American Journal of Cardiology, 1990, 65 (5): 297-302.

［18］ Merhi-Soussi F, Kwak BR, Magne D, et al. Interleukin-1 plays a major role in vascular inflammation and atherosclerosis in male apolipoprotein E-knockout mice. Cardiovascular Research, 2005, 66 (3): 583-593.

［19］ Isoda K, Sawada S, Ishigami N, et al. Lack of interleukin-1 receptor antagonist modulates plaque composition in apolipoprotein E-deficient mice. Arteriosclerosis, Thrombosis, and Vascular Biology, 2004, 24 (6): 1068-1073.

［20］ Frankenberger M, Sternsdorf T, Pechumer H. Differential cytokine expression in human blood monocyte subpopulations: a polymerase chain reaction analysis. Blood, 1996, 87 (1): 373-377.

［21］ de Bont N , Netea MG, Rovers C, et al. LPS-induced release of IL-1β, IL-1Ra, IL-6, and TNF-α in whole blood from patients with familial hyper cholesterolemia: no effect of cholesterol-lowering treatment. Journal of Interferon and Cytokine Research, 2006, 26 (2): 101-107.

第三章

Combination of Chinese Herbal Medicines and Conventional Treatment versus Conventional Treatment Alone in Patients with Acute Coronary Syndrome after Percutaneous Coronary Intervention (5C trial): An Open-Label Randomized Controlled, Multicenter Study[*]

WANG Shao-Li   WANG Cheng-long   WANG Pei-li   XU Hao   LIU Hong-ying   DU Jian-peng
ZHANG Da-wu   GAO Zhu-ye   ZHANG Lei   FU Chang-geng   LÜ Shu-zheng   YOU Shi-jie
GE Jun-bo   LI Tian-chang   WANG Xian   YANG Guan-lin   LIU Hong-xu   MAO Jing-yuan
LI Rui-jie   CHEN Li-dian   LU Shu   SHI Da-zhuo   CHEN Ke-ji

1. Intorduction

Acute coronary syndrome (ACS), encompassing unstable angina (UA) and acute myocardial infarction (AMI, non-ST elevation, and ST elevation), is one of the leading causes of morbidity and mortality. There has been a steady decline in mortality from coronary artery disease (CAD) in most developed countries over the last three decades [1], primarily due to dramatic advances in revascularization procedures such as percutaneous coronary intervention (PCI) and coronary artery bypass graft (CABG), as well as pharmacological treatments [2]. Approximately 10% of ACS survivors after PCI, however, will ultimately suffer a second AMI, stroke, or cardiovascular death [3,4] despite the availability of timely, appropriate treatments. Therefore, reducing the risk of recurrent cardiovascular events in patients with ACS after PCI remains a great challenge in the foreseeable future [5].

Chinese herbal medicines (CHMs) have been widely used in clinical practice for thousands of years. In the past few decades, CHMs have shown beneficial effects in improving clinical symptoms and clinical outcomes in CAD patients. Xinyue Capsule and Fufang Chuanxiong Capsule are commonly prescribed in mainland China, and both have been approved by the State Food and Drug Administration (SFDA) of China for clinical use in CAD patients. The major therapeutic effects of these drugs, as documented in previous trials, include relieving myocardial ischemia, decreasing symptoms, improving myocardial reperfusion after PCI, regulating blood lipids, and reducing recurrent angina [6-9]. However, no study has yet to focus on the efficacy of the two capsules in reducing recurrence of cardiovascular events in patients with ACS after PCI. Therefore, in this multicenter, open-label, randomized controlled trial (chictr. org number: ChiCTR-TRC-00000021), we evaluated the efficacy of Xinyue Capsule and Fufang Chuanxiong Capsule plus conventional treatment on cardiovascular events in patients with ACS after PCI.

2. Method

2.1 Design Overview

This study was conducted at thirteen hospitals in five provinces of mainland China. The participants were recruited from April 2008 to October 2009, and follow-up was completed by October 2010. The study protocol was approved by the ethics review board of Xiyuan Hospital.

* 原载于 Evidence-Based Complementary and Alternative Medicine, 2013, Article ID 741518

China Academy of Chinese Medical Sciences (CACMS), in accordance with the principles described in the Declaration of Helsinki [10], and all participants signed informed consent forms before enrollment.

2.2　Setting and Participants

Recruitment, intervention, and data collection were performed at the thirteen participating hospitals. Patients between 18 and 75 years of age were eligible for inclusion if they were hospitalized for ACS [11,12] involving either AMI (with or without ST segment elevation) or UA and also underwent successful PCI (defined as the target vessel with TIMI grade 3 flow). The exclusion criteria were as follows: (1) concomitant affliction with severe complications including hepatic, renal, and hematopoietic dysfunction, psychiatric disorders, or cancers; (2) absence of written informed consent, unwillingness to participate in follow-up, or refusal to receive treatment with study drugs; (3) pregnancy or breastfeeding; and (4) concurrent enrollment in other clinical studies.

2.3　Randomization and Intervention

An independent, offsite clinical trials statistician at CACMS used a computer-generated random allocation sequence to randomize the trial in blocks of four, stratified with each recruiting center. The details of the sequence remained unknown to any investigator or coordinator and were contained in sequentially numbered, opaque, sealed envelopes (SNOSE), bearing only the hospital name and a number on the outside. A pharmacist at each center who was independent of the clinical study kept the allocation sequence, took responsibility for the allocation, and prepared the treatment medication. After completing the baseline visit, participants who met the enrollment criteria were randomly assigned in a 1 : 1 ratio to receive either CHMs (Xinyue Capsule and Fufang Chuanxiong Capsule) plus conventional treatment or conventional treatment alone. Participants and investigators were masked to the treatment allocation until interventions were assigned. Data collectors and outcome adjudicators were masked until all data were entered into the database. Data management and statistical analyses were performed solely by data handlers and data analysts at Beijing Jiaotong University who were masked to the treatment assignments until the statistical report was completed. The study was open-label because the unique aroma and taste of Fufang Chuanxiong Capsule and Xinyue Capsule significantly challenged the successful blinding. In addition, even if we designed placebo capsules for the present study, the participants could easily distinguish between placebo and true capsules by the specific aftertaste left from oral intake of the true capsules.

All participants received conventional treatment in accordance with current guidelines [11,12], including aspirin (100 mg/day indefinitely), clopidogrel (75 mg/day for at least 12 months), and statins. All other medications were decided by physicians at each center who were not involved in the study. After participants were discharged, medication decisions and the option of revascularization were made by the responsible clinician without restriction. Angiographic follow-up was performed during the follow-up period, but it was not required in this study.

In addition to the conventional treatment, participants in the treatment group received Xinyue Capsule (two capsules orally, three times daily) and Fufang Chuanxiong Capsule (two capsules orally, three times daily) for six successive months. The Xinyue Capsule (SFDA Registry number: Z20030073; manufacturer: Jilin Jian Yisheng Pharmaceutical Co., Ltd., Jian City, Jilin Province, China) is an extract from leaves and stems of Panax quinquefolius L., containing 50 mg total ginsenosides. The Fufang Chuanxiong Capsule (SFDA Registry number: 0802205; manufacturer: Shandong Phoenix Pharmaceutical Co., Ltd., Dongying City, Shandong Province, China) is made from Chuanxiong and Ligusticum, with each capsule containing 3.20 mg/gm ligustrazine and 1.73 mg/gm ferulic acid. The quality of the two CHMs met the Chinese Medicine Standards of the SFDA. Capsules were distributed to the thirteen study sites with the same batch number. The companies that provided the two CHMs had no role in the design, analysis, or interpretation of the study.

From the baseline visit to the end of the study, the other CHMs used in the treatment of ACS after PCI, which might complicate the pharmacological effectiveness of Xinyue Capsule or Fufang Chuanxiong Capsule, were prohibited. A member of the executive committee in the study was responsible for monitoring quality control with respect to the management of all participants. The adherence of participants to study medication was assessed by independent nurses at each site.

2.4 Outcomes and Follow-up

At the baseline visit, investigators assessed the following characteristics which might have an impact on treatment: body mass index (BMI), heart rate, the number of diseased vessels, target vessels, smoking history, presence or absence of diabetes, hypertension, hyperlipidemia, CAD family history and medications, and so forth. The primary and secondary endpoints were adjudicated at 30 days, as well as at 3, 6, 9, and 12 months after the baseline visit.

The primary endpoint was the composite of cardiac death, nonfatal recurrent MI, or ischemia-driven revascularization. The secondary endpoint was the composite of readmission for ACS, stroke, or congestive HF. The safety endpoint concerned major bleeding events, defined as any intracranial bleeding, or any clinically relevant bleeding necessitated a blood transfusion judged by the investigators. All deaths were considered cardiac unless an unequivocal noncardiac cause was identified. Ischemia-driven revascularization was defined as repeat revascularization with either PCI or CABG because of recurrent myocardial ischemic events. Repeat PCI was defined as revascularization

of target lesions or target vessels. Stroke was defined as the development of disabling neurologic symptoms with objective findings lasting at least 24 hours. Recurrent MI was diagnosed based on reappearance of symptoms, and/or new electrocardiographic changes in association with a reelevation of creatine kinase-MB (CKMB) to levels greater than three times the upper limit of the reference level. Congestive HF was defined as a new diagnosis of congestive HF requiring hospitalization.

Subjects were followed up at each study center. The endpoint data were collected and recorded in a case report form (CRF) by the investigators at each visit (either a direct visit or telephone interview). For remote participants interviewed by telephone, local medical reports were collected by mail and a direct visit was performed at least once during the one year follow-up period. All clinical outcomes were adjudicated by independent outcome committees whose members were blinded to treatment assignment with review of original documentation.

2.5 Statistical Analysis

Sample size calculations were based on evidence from previous studies, which showed that the one-year composite incidence of cardiac death, nonfatal recurrent MI, or ischemia-driven revascularization in patients with ACS after PCI treated by conventional treatment was 8% to 18% [13,14]. Thus the incidence of the primary endpoint in this study during one-year in the control group was estimated at 13.5%, and treatment with additional CHMs reduced it to 7% [15]. For our study, a total of 676 participants would provide 80% power to test a difference in the primary endpoint at the 5%, two-sided level of significance. Allowing for a 20% dropout rate and adding power for analysis of the secondary endpoint, we recruited 808 total participants.

All participants were subject to baseline analysis as well as efficacy and safety evaluations. All data analysis was conducted according to a preestablished analysis plan. For categorical variables, the data were presented in a frequency table and expressed as percentages, and intergroup differences were compared by Chi-square or Fisher exact tests. For continuous variables, mean and standard deviation was used for normally distributed data, and median with interquartile range was calculated for not normally distributed data. A Student's t-test or Wilcoxon Rank-sum test was used, as appropriate, for the analyses of intergroup differences. The difference in cumulative incidence of the primary or secondary endpoints at one-year between groups was estimated by the Kaplan-Meier method with the logrank test. The treatment efficacy, as measured by the hazard ratio (HR) and its associated 95% confidence interval (CI), was estimated with the Cox proportional hazards regression. For the calculation of an adjusted HR with 95% CI for the primary or secondary endpoints, Cox proportional hazards regression was performed with 11 preidentified covariates of interest: age, gender, number of diseased vessels, target vessels, final diagnosis, smoking history, CAD family history, BMI, number of randomization centers, presence or absence of diabetes, hypertension, and hyperlipidemia. Participants who were lost to follow-up were censored at their last visit. The intention-to-treat method was applied in the analysis.

A two-sided P value less than 0.05 was considered to be statistically significant. The statistical analysis was performed with SPSS statistical software, Version 17.0 for Windows.

3. Results

3.1　Participant Characteristics

In this study, 808 participants with ACS after successful PCI from April 2008 to October 2010 were assigned to the control (404 participants) and treatment (404 participants) groups randomly. During follow-up, three participants died of cardiac events (two in the treatment group and one in the control group) and two participants in the control group died of cancer (both due to

lung cancer). Thirty eight participants (4.7%) were classified as dropout with no significant difference between the two groups [16 (4.0%) in the treatment group versus 22 (5.4%) in the control group, P = 0.319]. Among the dropouts, five declined to participate in the follow-up, two had noncardiac adverse events (cancer), twenty-eight were unreachable for data collection, and three in the control group received CHMs were excluded. A total of 765 participants completed the one-year follow-up (Figure 1). CHMs were administered to 378 (93.6%) participants in the treatment group for the six months. The baseline characteristics of the participants are shown in Table 1, and the two groups were well matched, except for the proportion of male participants.

3.2　Primary Endpoint

During the follow-up period, the cumulative incidence of the primary endpoint in the treatment group was significantly lower than that in the control group [11 (2.7%) versus 25 (6.2%); unadjusted HR 0.43, 95% CI 0.21–0.87, P=0.015]. After adjusting for the effects of covariates, the combination of CHMs with conventional treatment was associated with a significant reduction in the primary endpoint compared to conventional treatment alone (adjusted HR 0.44, 95% CI: 0.21-0.92, P=0.028) (Table 2 and Figure 2A). Among the components of the primary endpoint, cardiac death and recurrent MI did not differ significantly between the treatment and control groups (1.0% versus 2.0%, unadjusted HR 0.49, 95% CI: 0.15-1.64, adjusted HR 0.35, 95% CI: 0.09-1.33, P = 0.238) (Table 2 and Figure 2B). Ischemia-driven revascularization, however, was significantly reduced in the treatment group compared to the control group (2.0% versus 5.4%, unadjusted HR 0.35, 95% CI: 0.16-0.80, adjusted HR 0.36, 95% CI: 0.16-0.82, P =0.008) (Table 2 and Figure 2C).

3.3　Secondary Endpoint

The secondary endpoints occurred in 14 (3.5%) in the treatment group and 35 (8.7%) in the control group (unadjusted HR 0.39, 95% CI: 0.21-0.72, P =0.002). After adjusting for the

Table 1 Baseline Characteristics of Participants

Characteristic	Treatment group (n=404)	Control group (n=404)
Demographics		
Male, n (%)	322 (79.7)	281 (69.6)
Age, median (interquartile ranges)	60 (53, 67.75)	61 (53, 68)
Final diagnosis[§], n (%)		
NSTE-ACS	287 (71.0)	296 (73.3)
STE-ACS	117 (29.0)	108 (26.7)
Number of diseased vessels, n (%)		
One	104 (25.7)	110 (27.2)
Two	131 (32.4)	115 (28.5)
Three	169 (41.8)	179 (44.3)
Target vessels[&], n (%)		
LAD	322 (79.7)	319 (79.0)
LCX	226 (55.9)	209 (51.7)
RCA	231 (57.2)	234 (57.9)
LM	30 (7.4)	36 (8.9)
Risk factors, n (%)		
Hypertension	247 (61.1)	262 (64.9)
Diabetes mellitus	111 (27.5)	123 (30.4)
Hyperlipidemia	163 (40.3)	159 (39.4)
Smoking history	234 (57.9)	225 (55.7)
Family history of CAD	103 (25.5)	95 (23.5)
BMI[**] mean (SD)	25.31 (3.01)	25.60 (2.88)
Medication, n (%)		
Beta-blocker	157 (38.9)	160 (39.6)
ACEI	125 (30.9)	123 (30.4)
ARB	74 (18.3)	80 (19.8)
CCB	96 (23.8)	102 (25.2)
Statin	195 (48.3)	192 (47.5)

[§]NSTE-ACS: non-ST-segment elevation ACS; STE-ACS: ST-segment elevation ACS.

[&] LAD: left anterior descending artery; LCX: left circumflex artery; RCA: right coronary artery; LM: left main coronary artery.

[**]BMI: body mass index (kg/m^2).

effects of covariates, the addition of CHMs to conventional treatment was associated with a significant reduction in the secondary endpoint compared with conventional treatment alone (adjusted HR 0.37, 95% CI: 0.21-0.72, P = 0.002) (Table 2 and Figure 3A). Among the components of the endpoint, the cumulative incidence of readmission for ACS in the treatment group was lower than that in the control group (2.0% versus 5.9%, unadjusted HR 0.33, 95% CI: 0.15-0.72, adjusted HR 0.29, 95% CI: 0.13–0.65, P =0.004) (Table 2 and Figure 3B). However, the incidence of stroke (0.7% versus 1.5%, unadjusted HR 0.49, 95% CI: 0.12–0.97, adjusted HR 0.69, 95% CI: 0.16-3.02, P= 0.307) and congestive HF (0.7% versus 1.2%, unadjusted HR 0.59, 95% CI: 0.14 –2.48, adjusted HR 0.52, 95% CI: 0.12–2.36, P=0.469) did not differ between the two groups.

3.4　Safety

Major bleeding events were not observed in all participants. Aside from the cardiovascular events defined as primary and secondary endpoints in this study, four participants in the control group were afflicted with cancer. One dropped out due to esophageal cancer, one due to thyroid cancer, and two died of lung cancer. In the treatment group, no cancer-related events occurred, but slight stomach bloating was noted in two (0.5%) participants at one or three months after enrollment. The symptom of stomach bloating was relieved after extending the time interval between taking food and medicines.

4. Discussion

In this study, CHMs plus conventional treatment led to a more favorable outcome for patients with ACS after successful PCI compared to conventional treatment alone. The benefits included a reduction in the incidence of the primary endpoint and secondary endpoint, as well as incidence of ischemia-driven revascularization in components of primary endpoint and readmission for ACS in components of secondary endpoint. The safety of CHMs plus conventional treatment was also confirmed in the study.

We had searched the MEDLINE (1966 to 2012), OVID (1946 to 2012), and Cochrane

Table 2　Clinical Outcomes at 1 Year[††]

Endpoint	Treatment group (n = 404)[‡‡]	Control group (n = 404)[‡‡]	Unadjusted HR (95% CI)	Adjusted HR (95% CI)	P value[§§]
Primary endpoint	11 (2.7)	25 (6.2)	0.43 (0.21 to 0.87)	0.44 (0.21 to 0.92)	0.015
Death/MI	4 (1.0)	8 (2.0)	0.49 (0.15 to 1.64)	0.35 (0.09 to 1.33)	0.238
Revascularization	8 (2.0)	22 (5.4)	0.35 (0.16 to 0.80)	0.36 (0.16 to 0.82)	0.008
Secondary endpoint	14 (3.5)	35 (8.7)	0.39 (0.21 to 0.72)	0.37 (0.20 to 0.71)	0.002
Readmission for ACS	8 (2)	24 (5.9)	0.33 (0.15 to 0.72)	0.29 (0.13 to 0.65)	0.004
Stroke	3 (0.7)	6 (1.5)	0.49 (0.12 to 1.97)	0.69 (0.16 to 3.02)	0.307
Congestive HF	3 (0.7)	5 (1.2)	0.59 (0.14 to 2.48)	0.52 (0.12 to 2.36)	0.469

[††] Values are expressed as n (%).

[‡‡] Kaplan-Meier estimate.

[§§] P value derived from log-rank test.

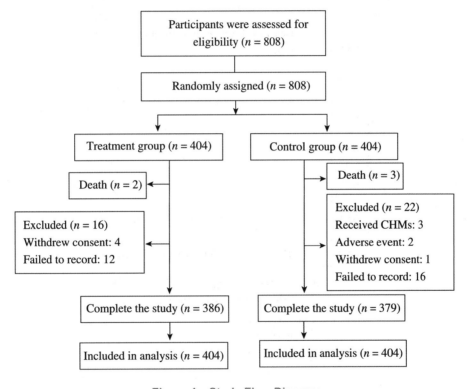

Figure 1　Study Flow Diagram

libraries (last search done on May 15, 2012) using the terms "Chinese herbal medicine", "percutaneous coronary intervention", and "coronary artery disease" to identify all randomized controlled clinical trials that had compared the efficacy of CHMs plus conventional treatment versus conventional treatment alone on cardiovascular events for CAD after PCI. Four trials met the selection criteria [15-18], but none of these addressed patients with a full spectrum of ACS after PCI. Thus, to our knowledge, our trial is the first randomized, controlled study in mainland China to assess the efficacy of CHMs plus conventional treatment versus conventional

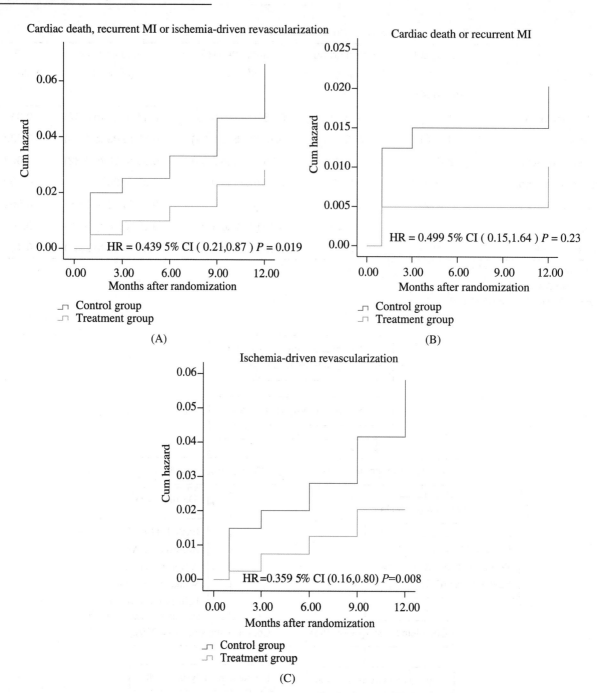

Figure 2   Kaplan-Meier Time to Event Curve for Primary Endpoint

treatment alone on ACS after PCI, as evaluated by cardiovascular events. Of the four trials that met selection criteria, three [15,17,18] demonstrated an association between CHMs pharmacologically similar in effect to Fufang Chuanxiong Capsule and reduction of restenosis in post-PCI patients. The benefits of CHMs in restenosis lend support to our finding of a reduction in ischemia-driven

revascularizations in the treatment group.

This study did not demonstrate a significant impact of CHMs on mortality or recurrent MI, a result that might be ascribed to the relatively small sample size of our trial. The reduction in the incidence of the composite primary endpoint in the treatment group was largely attributed to the benefits of CHMs plus conventional treatment in

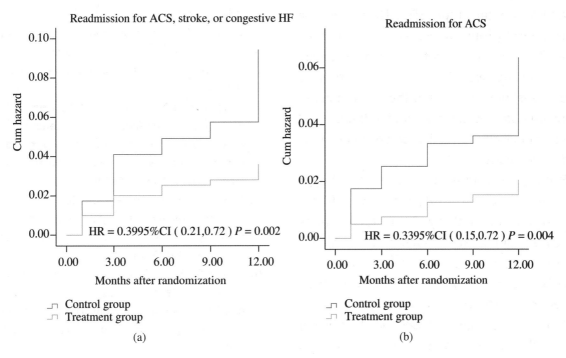

Figure 3　Kaplan-Meier Time to Event Curve for Secondary Endpoint

reducing ischemiadriven revascularization.

Our results also demonstrated a significant reduction in the secondary endpoint. The reduced incidence of the composite secondary endpoint was largely derived from a significant decrease in readmission for ACS in particular. However, we cannot exclude the possibility that CHMs might also provide benefits regarding stroke or congestive HF, because previous experimental studies have demonstrated that the active ingredients contained in Xinyue Capsule and Fufang Chuanxiong Capsule exert cardiovascular benefits in myocardial ischemia, myocardial hypertrophy, myocardial remodeling, HF, and thrombosis [19-21]. In recent randomized controlled trials, the benefits of CHMs on myocardial perfusion, infarcted area, and ventricular wall movement were demonstrated in patients with ST-segment elevation MI after PCI [22]. Given that no previous study has investigated the effects of CHMs on cardiovascular events in ACS patients after PCI, our trial provides the first evidence that Xinyue Capsule and Fufang Chuanxiong Capsule in combination with conventional treatment may

further improve clinical outcomes in ACS patients after PCI by reducing cardiovascular events.

In consideration of the potential pharmacological interplay between CHMs and antiplatelet agents, the major side effect of Xinyue Capsule and Fufang Chuanxiong Capsule in combination with conventional treatment in this study was predicted to be a possible increase in hemorrhagic events. Because no major bleeding events occurred in either of the two groups, our results suggest that CHMs plus conventional treatment with antiplatelet agents did not increase the risk of major bleeding events in patients with ACS after PCI.

Data from a previous meta-analysis [23] indicated a statistically increased risk of noncardiac mortality (cancer, stroke, or infectious diseases, etc.) in CAD patients treated with sirolimus-eluting stents (SES) versus bare metal stents, 40% of which was cancer-related death, implicating an association between the use of SES and an increase in cancer-related mortality. Our study found that four subjects were afflicted with cancer in the control group, and all had an implanted SES. No patients in the treatment group, however, suffered from cancer. The association between cancer-related events and the use of SES or CHMs require further investigation owing to the small number of cancer-related events observed in the present study and the lack of statistical evidence provided in previous reports.

Some limitations in this study should be noted. First, our study was not a blind, placebo-controlled study. To reduce biases from observation, data collection, and efficacy evaluation, all data collectors, outcome adjudicators, data handlers, and data analysts involved in this study were not knowledgeable of the study group assignment. Second, the number of enrolled participants was relatively small and the follow-up period was only one-year. As a result, the study may not have sufficient power to detect a statistically significant difference in each endpoint between the two groups. Finally, our trial was only conducted in mainland China and all participants were Chinese; thus, our findings may not be applicable to patients from different races or other countries.

However, our findings shed light on the benefits and safety of CHMs plus conventional treatment for ACS patients after PCI, thereby offering potential implications for clinical practice. As more evidence related to the benefits and safety of CHMs emerges from large-scale and long-term trials, CHMs may serve as an adjunctive therapy to conventional treatment for ACS after PCI in the future.

In conclusion, this study demonstrated that CHMs in combination with conventional treatment further reduced cardiovascular events in patients with ACS after PCI without an increased risk of major bleeding.

References

[1] Iqbal J, Fox KAA. Epidemiological trends in acute coronary syndromes: understanding the past to predict and improve the future. Archives of Medical Science, 2010, 6 (1): S3-S14.

[2] Kolansky DM. Acute coronary syndromes: morbidity, mortality, and pharmacoeconomic burden. The American Journal of Managed Care, 2009, 15 (2): S36-S41.

[3] Norgardand NB, Abu-Fadel M. Comparison of prasugrel and clopidogrel in patients with acute coronary syndrome undergoing percutaneous coronary intervention. Vascular Health and Risk Management, 2009, 5: 873-882.

[4] Wiviott SD, Braunwald E, McCabe CH, et al. Prasugrel versus clopidogrel in patients with acute coronary syndromes. The New England Journal of Medicine, 2007, 357 (20): 2001-2015.

[5] Yusuf S, Zhao F, Mehta SR, et al. Effects of clopidogrel in addition to aspirin in patients with acute coronary syndromes without ST-segment elevation. The New England Journal of Medicine, 2001, 345 (7): 494-502.

[6] Li YQ, Jin M, Qiu SL. Effect of Chinese herbal medicine for benefiting qi and nourishing yin to promote blood circulation on ventricular wall motion of AMI patients after revascularization. Zhongguo Zhong Xi Yi Jie He Za Zhi, 2009, 29 (4): 300-304.

[7] Qiu SL, Jin M, Zhu TG, et al. Effect of replenishing Qi and nourishing Yin to promote the blood circulation on 103 patients with acute myocardial infarction after reperfusion. Journal of Capital Medical University, 2009, 30 (4): 426-428.

[8] Sheng GY, Niu DM, Wu SB. Influence of complex Chuanxiong capsule on the blood fat of coronary and the heart function. Journal of Chinese Modern Medicine, 2009, 6 (6): 401-404.

[9] Zhang W. Clinical Study of Fufang Chuanxiong capsule on angina pectoris. Medical Innovation of China, 2011, 8 (11): 57-58.

[10] World Medical Association declaration of Helsinki. Recommendations guiding physicians in biomedical research involving human subjects. Journal of the American Medical Association, 1997, 277: 925-926.

[11] Chinese Society of Cardiology of Chinese Medical Association, Editorial Board of Chinese Journal of Cardiology. Guideline for diagnosis and treatment of patients with unstable angina and non-ST-segment elevation myocardial infarction. Chinese Journal of Cardiology, 2007, 35 (4): 295-304.

[12] Antman EM, Hand M, PW Armstrong, et al. 2007 Focused update of the ACC/AHA 2004 guidelines for the management of patients with ST-elevation

myocardial infarction: a report of the American College of Cardiology/American Heart Association task force on practice guidelines. Circulation, 2008, 117 (2): 296-329.

[13] Li Y, Torguson R, Syed AI, et al. Effect of drug-eluting stents on frequency of repeat revascularization in patients with unstable angina pectoris or non-st-elevation myocardial infarction. American Journal of Cardiology, 2009, 104 (12), 1654-1659.

[14] Spaulding, Henry P, Teiger E, et al. Sirolimus-eluting versus uncoated stents in acutemyocardial infarction. The New England Journal of Medicine, 2006, 355 (11): 1093-1104.

[15] Chen KJ, Shi DZ, Xu H, et al. S0601 reduces the incidence of restenosis: a prospective study of 335 patients undergoing percutaneous coronary intervention in China. Chinese Medical Journal, 2006, 119 (1): article 6.

[16] Cui XY, Wu Y, Nong YB, et al. Effect of Liangxue Shengji recipe on incidence of post-percutaneous coronary intervention restenosis and adverse cardiovascular events. Zhongguo Zhong Xi Yi JieHe Za Zhi, 2010, 30 (1): 30-32.

[17] Lu XY, Shi DZ, Xu H. Clinical study on effect of Xiongshao capsule on restenosis after percutaneous coronary intervention. Zhongguo Zhong Xi Yi Jie He Za Zhi, 2006, 26 (1): 13-17.

[18] Shang QH, Xu H, Lu XY, et al. A multi-center randomized double-blind placebo controlled trial of Xiongshao Capsule in preventing restenosis after percutaneous coronary intervention: a subgroup analysis of senile patients. Chinese Journal of Integrative Medicine, 2011, 17 (9): 669-674.

[19] Wang CL, Shi DZ, Yin HJ. Effect of panax uinquefolius saponin on angiogenesis and expressions of VEGF and bFGF in myocardium of rats with acute myocardial infarction. Zhongguo Zhong Xi Yi Jie He Za Zhi, 2007, 27 (4): 331-334.

[20] Karmazyn M, Moey M, Gan XT. Therapeutic potential of ginseng in the management of cardiovascular disorders. Drugs, 2011, 71 (15) : 1989-2008.

[21] Qi LW, Wang CZ, Yuan CS. Ginsenosides from American ginseng: chemical and pharmacological diversity. Phytochemistry, 2011, 72 (8): 689-699.

[22] Zhang HT, Jia ZH, Zhang J, et al. No-reflow protection and long-term efficacy for acute myocardial infarction with Tongxinluo: a randomized double-blind placebo-controlled multicenter clinical trial (ENLEAT trial). Chinese Medical Journal, 2010, 123 (20): 2858-2864.

[23] Nordmann AJ, Briel M, Bucher HC. Mortality in randomized controlled trials comparing drug-eluting vs. bare metal stents in coronary artery disease: a meta-analysis. European Heart Journal, 27 (23): 2784-2814.

第三章

Analysis on Outcome of 3537 Patients with Coronary Artery Disease: Integrative Medicine for Cardiovascular Events*

GAO Zhu-ye   QIU Yu   JIAO Yang   SHANG Qing-hua   XU Hao   SHI Da-zhuo

1. Introduction

According to research, the risk factors like hypertension, diabetes mellitus, dyslipidemia and smoking has a positive correlation with CAD. If the numbers of risk factors reduced, the incidence of CAD will decrease significantly. European Society of Cardiology (ESC), American Heart Association (AHA), American College of Cardiology (ACC), Chinese Medical Association have published in succession clinical guidelines on angina pectoris, myocardial infarction, hypertension and dyslipidemia, which have played an important role in improving secondary prevention of CAD. However, the implementation of the above mentioned guidelines in clinical practice IM hospitals in China and the potential benefit of IM therapy in improving CAD prognosis remain unclear. The previous study showed that the treatment of IM can prevent restenosis after PCI [1] and potentially decrease the incidence of cardiovascular events [2]. In this study, we performed a prospective research for CAD patients who were hospitalized in cardiovascular department in twelve hospitals in Beijing from Sep 2009 to May 2011 for analyzing the secondary prevention status of CAD. We also investigate the one-year following incidence of cardiovascular events with the purpose of the problem of secondary prevention and the potential role of IM.

2. Materials and Methods

2.1　Patients

3537 patients were recruited from 12 hospitals in Beijing, China. The research followed guidelines of the Declaration of Helsinki and Tokyo for humans, and was approved by the institutional human experimentation committee, and that informed consent was obtained. The source of patients was shown in Table 1.

2.2　Inclusion and Diagnostic Criteria

Inclusion criteria

① In hospital with CAD (angina pectoris or myocardial infarction or heart failure or arrhythmia);

② Comply with one of the following conditions:

• old myocardial infarction

• acute myocardial infarction diagnosed in hospital

• coronary artery stenosis > 50% confirmed by coronary angiography

2.3　Evaluation Methods

The diagnostic and therapeutic status of CAD patients was evaluated based on relevant clinical guidelines including Guidelines for the Diagnosis and Treatment of Chronic Unstable Angina Pectoris and Myocardial Infarction [3] published by Chinese Medical Association Cardiovascular Society, Guidelines for Diagnosis and Treatment of Unstable Angina Pectoris [4] and Guidelines for Diagnosis and Treatment of myocardial infarction [5] published by American Heart Association (AHA) and American College of Cardiology (ACC), and clinical guidelines about heart failure [6,7], Guidelines for Diagnosis

* 原载于 Evidence-Based Complementary and Alternative Medicine，2013，Article ID 162501

Table 1　Source of Patients

Hospital	Case (male/female)	Percentage of total
Dongzhimen Hospital affiliated to Beijing University of Chinese Medicine	178 (111/67)	5.03%
Guanganmen Hospital affiliated to China Academy of Chinese Medical Science	564 (363/201)	15.95%
Huairou Hospital of Traditional Chinese Medicine	121 (77/44)	3.42%
Beijing Hospital of Traditional Chinese Medicine	220 (142/78)	6.22%
People's Hospital affiliated to Beijing University	107 (72/35)	3.03%
Tongzhou Hospital of Traditional Chinese Medicine	160 (98/62)	4.52%
Tongren Hospital affiliated to Capital University of Medical Sciences	260 (162/98)	7.35%
Wangjing Hospital affiliated to China Academy of Chinese Medical Science	93 (58/35)	2.63%
Xiyuan Hospital affiliated to China Academy of Chinese Medical Science	462 (304/158)	13.06%
China-Japan Friendship Hospital	632 (425/207)	17.87%
Beijing Hospital of Integrated Traditional Chinese with Western Medicine	124 (80/44)	3.51%
Anzhen Hospital affiliated to Capital University of Medical Sciences	616 (422/194)	17.42%

and prevention of Proposal and Guidelines for hypertension[8,9], Diagnosis and prevention of dyslipidemia and National Cholesterol Education Program (NCEP) Expert Panel on Detection, Evaluation, and Treatment of High Blood Cholesterol in Adults (Adult Treatment Panel Ⅲ)[10,11].

2.4　Definition of cardiovascular events

Death due to any cause;

Acute myocardial infarction;

Revascularization is needed;

2.5　Materials

2.5.1　Data collection　Research process in accordance with the subject of the investigator's brochure. The clinical researchers were all trained and pass the examination. The clinical data collected by an integrative platform of clinical and research was analyzed after clearing up. The treatment of IM mean the patient accept the treatment of conventional treatment of modern medicine and the treatment of herbal medicine including both herbal-based injection and Chinese patent medicine, as well as decoction at least 7 days in-hospital or 3 months out of hospital.

2.5.2　Follow-up　The follow-up was mainly through telephone. Home visit will implement if cannot contact patients with telephone. The latest clinical data will use if the patient lost to follow-up.

2.5.3　Observation index　Demographic data, general clinical condition, drug use, outcome of follow-up were observed.

2.5.4　Statistics　Statistical analysis of the experimental data was carried out using SPSS (version 11.0). Patients' demographic and clinical characteristics were analyzed with descriptive analytic method and the chi-square test for categorical variables. Continuous variables were presented as mean with standard deviation and categorical variables were expressed as frequencies with percentages. Logistic regression analysis using fractional polynomial modeling was conducted to determine the association between demographic and clinical information and mortality in MACEs. The criterion for statistical significance was at $P < 0.05$.

3. Results

3.1　Demographics and Clinical Characteristics

3537 consecutive hospitalized CAD patients were enrolled into the study, which was approved by the local ethic committee. The average age in patients was 64.88 ± 11.97 years (range 24-96). The number of male is 2314, accounting for

155

65.42%. 795 patients had a history of smoking, accounting for 22.5%. The average history of smoking was 30.93 ± 12.54 years (range 1-70). 327 patients had a history of drinking.

3.2 Subtype of CAD and Complicating Disease

The 3537 patients were divided into four groups through the first diagnosis which contain angina pectoris, acute myocardial infarction, arrhythmia and heart failure. The group of angina pectoris is 2212 patients, accounting for 62.54%. The group of acute myocardial infarction is 836 patients, accounting for 23.92%. The group of arrhythmia is 244 patients, accounting for 6.90%. The group of heart failure is 235 patients, accounting for 6.64%. The status of complicating diseases was shown in Table 2.

Table 2 Status of Complicating Disease

Complicating disease	Number	Percentage of total
Hypertension	2398	67.80%
Diabetes mellitus	1162	32.85%
Dyslipidemia	1161	32.82%
Old myocardial infarction	741	20.95%
Stroke	496	14.02%
Chronic obstructive pulmonary Disease (COPD)	397	11.22%
Peripheral vasculopathy	165	4.66%
Chronic kidney disease	154	4.35%

3.3 Status of Treatment

Displayed in Table 3 are the numbers and rates of each medications, coronary artery revascularization and Chinese herbal medicine which patients had received treatment of IM.

3.4 Prognostic Analysis

3.4.1 Prognostic Status 312 patients were loss for follow-up, accounting for 8.82%. The average age was 70.25 ± 10.93 (range 30-90) in the 469 patients with cardiovascular events, accounting for 14.54%. The male is 289, accounting for 61.62%.

Table 3 Status of Treatment

Treatment	Number	Percentage of total
IM therapy	1459	41.25%
PCI or CABG	1425	40.29%
Anti-platelet agents	3253	91.97%
Statins	2959	83.66%
Nitrate medications	2709	76.59%
β-receptor blockers	2566	72.55%
Heparin	1905	53.86%
ACEI and ARB	2084	58.92%
Calcium channel blockers	1137	32.15%
Insulin	471	13.32%

3.4.2 Single Factor Analysis Table 4 displayed the result of single factor analysis, in which myocardial infarction, heart failure, stroke, arrhythmia, LDL-C elevating, age $\geqslant$ 65 years and diabetes mellitus were signi-ficantly higher in event-group, meanwhile, TG elevating and TC elevating were significantly higher in Non-event group.

Table 4 Single Factor Analysis

Variable	Non-event group	Event-group	P
Myocardial infarction	39.15%	47.97%	< 0.001
Heart failure	6.91%	20.47%	< 0.001
Stroke	4.63%	8.53%	0.001
Arrhythmia	18.71%	24.73%	0.003
TG elevating	38.90%	30.79%	0.001
LDL-C elevating	22.27%	27.39%	0.028
TC elevating	23.97%	17.57%	0.004
Age $\geqslant$ 65 years	49.28%	68.87%	< 0.001
Diabetes mellitus	16.36%	20.68%	0.024
β-receptor blockers	73.11%	68.87%	0.059
Insulin	12.91%	15.99%	0.068
Anti-platelet agents	92.28%	89.98%	0.1
IM therapy	40.9%	43.5%	0.291

3.4.3　Logistic Regress Analysis　Based on measured indexes which $P < 0.1$ in the former analysis and IM therapy, a multiple regression equation was generated between cardiovascular events and indexes. Table 5 displayed the result of logistic stepwise regress analysis, in which heart failure, age ≥ 65 years and myocardial infarction were the independent negative prognostic factors for cardiovascular events, while TG elevating was the independent protective factors.

Table 5　Analysis of Prognostic Factors Using Multivariate Logistic Stepwise Regress

Variables	β	P	OR	95% CI
Heart failure	1.310	< 0.001	3.707	2.756-4.986
Age $\geq$ 65 years	0.697	< 0.001	2.007	1.587-2.539
Myocardial infarction	0.500	< 0.001	1.649	1.322-2.057
TG elevating	−0.259	0.02	0.754	0.595-0.956

Table 6 displayed the result of logistic regress analysis, in which IM therapy showed potential tendency of decreasing the incidence of cardiovascular events.

4. Discussions

It is shown that the range of the majority hospitalized CAD patients' age is from 60 years old to 74 years old, accounting for 41.93% in this study. Event rate of one-year follow-up of hospitalized CAD patients is 14.54% (469 cases), the average age is (70.25 ± 10.93) years (range 30-90). The probability of recurrent cardiovascular events in patients whose age are greater than 65 years old is 2.4 times of the age lower than 65 years old patients (18.5% vs 7.6%). It is also suggesting that age is an important affecting factor of the prognosis of CAD which can't be changed. Other studies have confirmed that age is an independent risk factor for CAD prognosis; the rate of CAD incidence and mortality is increasing with age [12-14].

Epidemiological and clinical studies have demonstrated that hypertension, diabetes,

Table 6　Analysis of Prognostic Factors Using Multivariate Logistic Regress

Variables	β	P	OR	95% CI
IM therapy	−0.227	0.09	0.797	0.613-1.036
Myocardial infarction	0.386	0.001	1.471	1.172-1.847
Heart failure	1.308	< 0.001	3.7	2.737-5.002
Stroke	0.392	0.095	1.48	0.935-2.342
Arrhythmia	0.084	0.536	1.088	0.833-1.42
Anti-platelet agents	−0.115	0.591	0.892	0.587-1.355
β-receptor blockers	−0.077	0.548	0.926	0.72-1.19
Insulin	0.333	0.056	1.396	0.991-1.966
TG elevating	−0.208	0.099	0.812	0.635-1.04
LDL-C elevating	0.036	0.846	1.036	0.722-1.487
TC elevating	−0.255	0.206	0.775	0.522-1.15
Age $\geq$ 65	0.574	< 0.001	1.775	1.384-2.278
Different hospital	0.295	0.16	1.343	0.89–2.026
Diabetes mellitus	0.072	0.647	1.075	0.789-1.465

dyslipidemia, smoking and obesity and other risk factors can aggravate atherosclerosis and increase the morality of CAD [15]. It is shown that hypertension, diabetes, dyslipidemia, cerebrovascular disease and COPD are common complications of CAD and with the development of CAD and the increasing of age and complications are more and more serious. One research from abroad show that once artery atherosclerosis form, only a simple monitoring of risk factors cannot fully control the progression of disease [16]. The correlative guidelines of CAD also recommend that patients with CAD should insist long-term drug therapies that include β-receptor blockers, anti-platelet agents and statin. Overall treatment modalities in this study was similar with the suggestion of relevant guidelines. Although the treatment rate of statins, β-blocker, ACEI/ARB are more than 50%, neither of these treatment show beneficial effects to decrease the incidence of cardiovascular events. This result is different from previous RCTs, it may be related to the type of design and cases as well as too short follow-up period.

Therefore, as to CAD patients who also get complication should pay more attention to the treatment of secondary prevention drugs and to control the complications in the long-term, for reaching the maximum limit to decrease the incidence of cardiovascula r events [17].

Diabetes mellitus was a CAD risk equivalent[18,19]. It is shown diabetes and injection of insulin may be attributed to more incidences of cardiovascular events. It may contribute to serious complex illness and poor glycemic control usually accompanying CAD patients who also contract diabetes. It is certificated that the rate of cardiovascular events such as morality in CAD. Complicating diabetes patients is greater than non-diabetes ones in interrelating reach.

It was found that patients in normal left ventricular ejection fraction group and lower left ventricular ejection fraction group have similar prognosis in previous epidemiological investigations and observational studies [20]. But most of those experiment objects are dilated cardiomyopathy and hypertensive heart disease patients take low proportion in patients with CAD. As well as most of the clinical trials will be usually exclude patients with heart failure whose left ventricular ejection fraction is normal. CAD is one of the important cause of heart failure and persistent coronary ischemia will further aggravate heart failure. This study also showed that heart failure can increase the incidence of endpoint events. It is important to effectively prevent HF readmissions and improve over all outcomes [21].

In recent years, the combination of medicine rise extensively in the world-wide and it is be used increasingly in clinical application. IM is an unique discipline in China, it also have a wide range of applications in china[22]. This study shows that from the results of one-year follow-up, although IM have no statistical significance in affecting incidence of cardiovascular events, IM therapy showed the tendency of decreasing incidence of cardiovascular events. This also shows that a single drug or treatment could not to prevent multiple factors disease such as CAD. IM have advantages to improve the clinical symptoms especially for CAD patients combine with diabetes, high blood pressure, lung infection, kidney disease. It was shown that have greater advantages in improving the quality of life for patients in previous studies [23,24]. There are many people willing to adopt for the IM treatment for cardiovascular disease [25].

In this study, a lengthways study design was adopt, using traditional Chinese medicine clinical research integrated research platform to investigate and analogize the clinical information and cardiovascular events in patients with CAD from cardiovascular department of 12 hospitals in Beijing. This research reflects objectively and accurately the treatment and independent prognostic factors of hospitalized CAD patients in Beijing. There are many complications of CAD high incidence of clinical events and a gap between clinical drugs and guidelines. Therefore, we should strengthen secondary prevention degree and health education for patients with CAD. Control multiple risk factors and intervene complete complex situation to reduce the incidence of complication and the rate of endpoint events.

For the limiting of follow-up time, this research could not make new diseases as the endpoint, such as new-onset diabetes, new-onset kidney disease and new-onset heart failure. In the view of IM treatment of coronary artery disease have advantages of multidimensional and multi-target. Further research can be evaluated synthetically combining with the quality of life of patients, the degree of symptom improvement and the situation of cases occurred to define the adaptation flock of Integrative Medicine treatment and then to draw up intervening program of IM treatment for coronary artery disease.

References

[1] Xu H, Chen KJ. Integrative medicine: the experience from China. J Altern Complement Med, 2008, 14 (1): 3-7.

[2] Gao ZY, Xu H, Shi DZH, et al. Analysis on outcome of 5284 patients with coronary artery disease: the role of integrative medicine. J Ethnopharmacol, 2012, 141 (2): 578-583.

[3] Chinese Society of Cardiology of Chinese Medical Association, Editorial Board of Chinese Journal of Cardiology. Guideline for diagnosis and treatment of patients with unstable angina and non-ST-segment elevation myocardial infarction. Chinese Journal of Cardiology, 2007, 35 (4): 295-304.

[4] Anderson JL, Adams CD, Antman EM, et al. ACC/AHA 2007 guidelines for the management of patients with unstable angina/non-ST-Elevation myocardial infarction: a report of the American College of Cardiology/American Heart Association Task Force on Practice Guidelines. J Am Coll Cardiol, 2007, 50 (7): e1-e157.

[5] Canadian Cardiovascular Society; American Academy of Family Physicians, American College of Cardiology, et al. 2007 focused update of the ACC/AHA 2004 guidelines for the management of patients with ST-elevation myocardial infarction: a report of the American College of Cardiology/American Heart Association Task Force on Practice Guidelines. J Am Coll Cardiol, 2008, 51 (2): 210-247.

[6] Hunt SA; American College of Cardiology, American Heart Association, et al. ACC/AHA 2005 guideline update for the diagnosis and management of chronic heart failure in the adult: a report of the American College of Cardiology/American Heart Association Task Force on Practice Guidelines. J Am Coll Cardiol, 2005, 46 (6): e1-82.

[7] Chinese Society of Cardiology of Chinese Medical Association, Editorial Board of Chinese Journal of Cardiology. Guidelines for the diagnosis and management of chronic heart failure. Chinese Journal of Cardiology, 2007, 35 (12): 1076-1095.

[8] The Drafting Committee of Chinese Guidelines for Hypertension Prevention and Treatment. A draft of Chinese guidelines for prevention and treatment of hypertension. Chinese Journal of Hypertension, 2000, 8 (1), 94-102.

[9] The Drafting Committee of Chinese Guidelines for Hypertension Prevention and Treatment. 2009 Community Version of Chinese Hypertension Prevention Guideline. Chinese Journal of Hypertension, 2010, 18 (1): 11-30.

[10] Joint committee for developing Chinese guidelines on prevention and treatment of dyslipidemia in adults. Chinese guidelines on prevention and treatment of dyslipidemia in adults. Chinese Journal of Cardiology, 2007, 35 (5): 390-419.

[11] National Cholesterol Education Program (NCEP) Expert Panel on Detection, Evaluation, and Treatment of High Blood Cholesterol in Adults (Adult Treatment Panel III). Third report of the National Cholesterol Education Program (NCEP) Expert Panel on Detection, Evaluation, and Treatment of High Blood Cholesterol in Adults (Adult Treatment Panel III) final report. Circulation, 2002, 106: 3143-3421.

[12] Jiang G, Wang D, Li W, et al. Coronary heart disease mortality in China: age, gender, and urban-rural gaps during epidemiological transition. Rev Panam Salud Publica, 2012, 31 (4): 317-324.

[13] Gao YL, Su JT, Wei ZH, et al. Characteristics of out-of-hospital acute coronary heart disease deaths of Beijing permanent residents at the age of 25 or more from 2007 to 2009. Zhonghua Xin Xue Guan Bing Za Zhi, 2012, 40 (3): 199-203.

[14] Levine BS, Kannel WB. Coronary heart disease risk in people 65 years of age and older. Prog Cardiovasc Nurs, 2003, 18 (3): 135-140.

[15] Ebrahim S, Taylor F, Ward K, et al. Multiple risk factor interventions for primary prevention of coronary heart disease. Cochrane Database Syst Rev, 2011, (1): CD001561.

[16] Spence JD, Hackam DG. Treating arteries instead of risk factors: a paradigm change in management of atherosclerosis. Stroke, 2010, 41: 1193-1199.

[17] Hofmann T. Risk management of coronary artery disease——pharmacological therapy. Wien Med Wochenschr, 2004, 154 (11-12): 266-281.

第三章

第三章

[18] Daniels LB, Grady D, Mosca L, et al. Is diabetes mellitus a heart disease equivalent in women? results from an international study of postmenopausal women in the Raloxifene Use for the Heart (RUTH) trial. Circ Cardiovasc Qual Outcomes, 2013, 6 (2): 164-170.

[19] Chiha M, Njeim M, Chedrawy EG. Diabetes and coronary heart disease: a risk factor for the global epidemic. Int J Hypertens, 2012, 2012: 697240.

[20] Miyagishima K, Hiramitsu S, Kimura H, et al. Long term prognosis of chronic heart failure: reduced *vs* preserved left ventricular ejection fraction. Circ J, 2009, 73: 92 -99.

[21] Gheorghiade M, Vaduganathan M, Fonarow GC, et al. Rehospitalization for heart failure: problems and perspectives. J Am Coll Cardiol, 2013, 61 (4): 391-403.

[22] Wang J, Xiong X. Current situation and perspectives of clinical study in integrative medicine in china. Evid Based Complement Alternat Med, 2012; 2012: 268542.

[23] Yang QY, Lu S, Sun HR. Clinical effect of Astragalus granule of different dosages on quality of life in patients with chronic heart failure. Chin J Integr Med, 2011, 17 (2): 146-149.

[24] Wang L, Zhang M, Guo L, et al. Clinical pathways based on integrative medicine in chinese hospitals improve treatment outcomes for patients with acute myocardial infarction: a multicentre, nonrandomized historically controlled trial. Evid Based Complement Alternat Med, 2012, 2012: 821641.

[25] Prasad K, Sharma V, Lackore K, et al. Use of complementary therapies in cardiovascular disease. Am J Cardiol, 2013, 111 (3): 339-345.

The Effect of Sodium Tanshinone IIA Sulfate and Simvastatin on Elevated Serum Levels of Inflammatory Markers in Patients with Coronary Heart Disease: Study Protocol for a Randomized Controlled Trial*

SHANG Qing-hua WANG Han-jay LI Si-ming XU Hao

1. Background

Cardiovascular disease is the worldwide leading cause of death. Globally in 2008, over 17 million people died from cardiovascular diseases, representing 30% of total deaths around the world[1]. Among all cardiovascular diseases, coronary heart disease (CHD) is responsible for the greatest mortality, accounting for 7.3 million deaths worldwide in 2008 [1].

CHD involves narrowing of the arteries supplying oxygen to the heart, most often due to buildup of atherosclerotic plaque in the coronary vessels. The ultimate rupture of atherosclerotic plaque may lead to the onset of acute coronary syndrome (ACS), a medically emergent manifestation of CHD involving unstable angina or myocardial infarction.

The formation of atherosclerotic plaque is an inflammatory response, usually associated with elevated levels of low-density lipoprotein cholesterol (LDL-C) in the blood[2]. To this end, statins have served as a notably successful

* 原载于 Evidence-Based Complementary and Alternative Medicine, 2013, Article ID 756519

pharmacologic intervention against CHD from the standpoint of Western medicine. One meta-analysis study found that the average statin regimen reduces LDL-C levels by 35%, leading to a 60% decrease in ischemic cardiac events such as those of ACS[3]. Remarkably, as demonstrated by the PRINCE study, statins also moderate the atherosclerotic inflammatory response by reducing levels of C-reactive protein (CRP) [4], a robust marker of systemic inflammation whose concentration in the blood strongly correlates with the patient's cardiovascular risk[5]. Nevertheless, a multicenter study involving over 4,000 ACS patients showed that 22.4% of patients receiving intensive statin therapy suffered a serious cardiovascular or cerebrovascular event within two years of initiating treatment [6], indicating that although statins may be one of Western medicine's most effective agents for CHD, the toll of this disease remains significantly high.

At East-West integrative medical centers in Asia, cardiovascular diseases may also be evaluated according to the principles of Traditional Chinese Medicine (TCM). Among patients with the Western diagnosis of CHD, the TCM diagnosis of blood stasis syndrome (BSS) is exceedingly common, and the treatment for these CHD-BSS patients via TCM frequently involves herbal therapies using the root of Salvia miltiorrhiza (丹参, danshen) [7].

The danshen root contains tanshinone ⅡA, an active biochemical compound that has been shown to possess a multitude of anti-atherosclerotic properties [8]. Most noteworthy is the ability of tanshinone ⅡA to decrease the levels of numerous inflammatory mediators associated with the progression of atherosclerosis, such as CRP, interleukin-6 (IL-6), tumor necrosis factor alpha (TNFα), vascular cell adhesion molecule-1 (VCAM-1), CD40, monocyte chemotactic protein-1 (MCP-1), and matrix metalloproteinase-9 (MMP-9) [8,9]. A recent clinical trial demonstrated that giving simvastatin in combination with intravenous sodium tanshinone ⅡA sulfate (STS), the most widely used clinical formulation of tanshinone ⅡA in China, significantly decreased the levels of CRP, cholesterol, and plaque buildup in patients with peripheral vascular disease [10]. Notably, the integrative therapy was safer and more effective in treating this form of atherosclerosis than simvastatin alone. Whether there is potential for synergy between STS and statins in treating CHD, however, remains unknown.

Here, we present the protocol for a randomized, controlled clinical study that applies East-West integrative medicine to the treatment of CHD. Using standard Western therapy involving simvastatin as a foundation, we aim to explore the potential of further dampening the atherosclerotic inflammatory reaction in CHD-BSS patients through the concomitant addition of STS, utilizing the compound's potent anti-inflammatory properties as a supplement to simvastatin. In addition, we also aim to assess the integrative therapy's safety, and its efficacy in improving angina and BSS symptoms relative to the simvastatin regimen without STS. Overall, this study offers an entry point for understanding and verifying the clinical applications of STS-statin integrative therapy in treating patients with CHD.

2. Methods/Design

2.1 Setting and Design

This trial is a monocentric, parallel-design, randomized, controlled, clinical pilot study that will be conducted at Xiyuan Hospital, China Academy of Chinese Medical Sciences in Beijing, China. Subject recruitment is scheduled to begin in August 2012. This study will involve 72 patients with the diagnoses of CHD and BSS according to Western medicine and TCM, respectively. The 72 participants will be randomized 1 : 1 into a standard Western therapy (control) group and an East-West integrative therapy (experimental) group. For 14 days, all 72 patients will be treated with a standard Western therapy involving simvastatin, and patients in the experimental group will additionally receive intravenous STS. Data will be collected before initiating treatment, immediately after the 14-day treatment period, and 30 days posttreatment. Serum CRP levels measured by high-sensitivity CRP (hs-CRP) testing will serve as the primary outcome parameter, whereas the levels of other inflammatory markers, the improvement of angina and BSS symptoms, and safety will serve as secondary outcome parameters.

The study design is illustrated in Figure 1 and described in detail below according to the CONSORT 2010 statement[11].

2.2 Diagnostic Criteria

The diagnosis of CHD will be based on the standardized criteria established in "Nomenclature and criteria for diagnosis of ischemic heart disease", a joint report published by the International Society and Federation of Cardiology and the World Health Organization[12]. In addition, following the current practice of CHD clinical research, we will require subjects to either have a previous history of myocardial infarction or have at least one coronary artery stenosis ≥ 50% confirmed by coronary angiography in order to ensure the diagnosis of CHD.

The TCM diagnosis of BSS will follow the principles described in "Criteria for TCM syndrome differentiation of patients with coronary heart disease", published by the China Society of Integrated Traditional Chinese and Western Medicine[13].

2.3 Subject Inclusion and Exclusion

To participate in this study, subjects must be 35 to 75 years of age, and must either have a previous history of myocardial infarction or have at least one coronary artery stenosis ≥ 50% confirmed by coronary angiography. In addition, subjects must currently be hospitalized with either unstable angina or an acute non-ST segment elevation myocardial infarction and have taken statin medicine for at least 1 months. From a TCM perspective, study participants must have the diagnosis of BSS. Finally, subjects must have a serum hs-CRP level between 3 mg/L and 15 mg/L.

The criteria for exclusion includes infection, fever, trauma, burn injury, or surgery within one month prior to recruitment; a concomitant diagnosis of cancer, sexually transmitted diseases, tuberculosis, or rheumatoid arthritis or other autoimmune diseases; or a history of serious pulmonary, hepatic, renal, neurological, psychiatric, or hematological diseases. In addition, subjects must not have previously undergone or currently be planning to undergo surgical intervention for CHD. Patients with severe heart failure indicated by an ejection fraction < 35% will be excluded, as will those with a reduced platelet count or a tendency to bleed or hemorrhage. Study participants must not currently be taking antibiotics or using TCM preparations that relieve fever or clear internal heat. Finally, patients who may become noncompliant

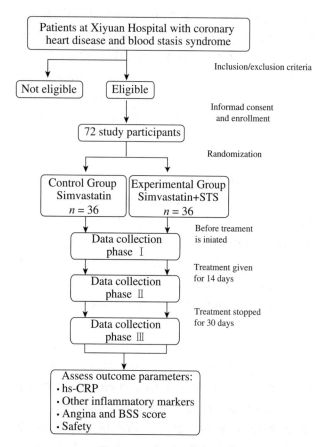

Figure 1　Study flowchart

or may participate in other clinical trials will be excluded.

During the course of the study, a subject may be excluded if (1) it is discovered that a subject was misdiagnosed for either BSS or CHD, or was otherwise inappropriately accepted for participation in the trial; (2) if a subject misses a significant number of treatments or is missing significant records of data; (3) if a subject's blood samples from the first two phases of the study (see Data Collection Phases, below) are contaminated or damaged in any way such that reliable data cannot be obtained; or (4) if for any reason (e.g. onset of a mid-study nosocomial infection), a patient's inflammatory marker levels may not accurately reflect atherosclerotic inflammation.

2.4　Sample Size Estimation

Because the data required to perform an a prior sample size calculation for this study is not available, we have adopted the sample size of a comparable trial for use in this pilot study. The comparable trial investigated the effects of TCM on unstable angina patients undergoing percutaneous coronary intervention, and involved 60 subjects randomized into two treatment groups of 30 each [14]. For our pilot study, we will recruit 72 patients to begin the trial, assuming conservatively that 20% of the participants in each treatment group will ultimately not complete the study.

2.5　Randomization and Blinding

A member of the Good Clinical Practice (GCP) Clinical Center of Xiyuan Hospital who is independent of the study will use SAS 9.2 software to perform a block randomization, generating a sequence of 72 random numbers in 1 : 1 allocation between the two groups. In order to conceal the generation, the outcomes will be conducted by another member of GCP Clinical Center using a central randomization, once a patient meet to all the critria, a random number will then be delivered by telephone to the clinical researchers. unblinding only after data is collected for the first phase of the study (see Data Collection Phases, below). The number delivered by telephone will determine whether the subject receives the control or experimental therapy.

Because the color of the STS solution given to the experimental group is unique and challenging to emulate, blinding will be difficult to achieve at the physician and patient levels. In order to minimize biases as much as possible, all other potential sources of information that may reveal treatment allocation to patients (e.g. contents of case report form, patient's random number) will be judiciously guarded. Additionally, the details of treatment allocation will not be disclosed to any patient until the study has concluded, and all study participants will be discouraged from discussing with one another their involvement in the trial. Finally, the clinical researchers will strictly abide by the study's random design and will interact with the patients in each group with as few differences as possible.

Blinding will be maintained at the level of outcome assessment. The individuals performing laboratory blood analyses, data management, and statistical analyses will be independent of the clinical component of the study, and will not be provided with any information that may reveal treatment allocation details.

2.6　Ethics

This trial has been approved by the local institutional ethics committee (Xiyuan Hospital, China Academy of Chinese Medical Sciences, Beijing, China; (2012XL022-2)) and is registered at the Chinese Clinical Trial Registry (ChiCTR-TRC-12002361). All aspects of our study will be conducted with adherence to the current version of the Declaration of Helsinki, the guidelines established by the International Conference on Harmonization of Good Clinical Practice, and the laws of China. Informed written consent will be required of all study participants, none of whom will be denied a standard, accepted therapy.

2.7 Treatment

Each patient in the standard Western therapy (control) group will receive 20 mg simvastatin orally once per evening, in addition to any other oral or IV Western medications or TCM preparations (aside from those listed as exclusion criteria, above) that are deemed appropriate for a standard treatment of the patient's individual condition. These other medications will be prescribed by physicians who are not associated with the trial.

In addition to receiving the treatments described above for the control group, each patient in the East-West integrative therapy (experimental) group will also receive a daily intravenous dose of 80 mg STS (10 mg per ampoule, Jiangsu Carefree Pharmaceutical Co., Ltd., national drug approval number: H31022558), diluted with 250 mL 0.9% NaCl solution.

All study participants will receive treatment as indicated above for 14 consecutive days.

2.8 Outcome Parameters

Serum hs-CRP level will serve as the primary outcome parameter in this study. The levels of other inflammatory mediators, including IL-6, TNFα, VCAM-1, CD40 and soluble CD40 ligand (sCD40L), MCP-1, and MMP-9, as measured by enzyme-linked immunosorbent assay (ELISA), will constitute secondary outcome parameters. Additional secondary parameters will include safety and the extent of improvement in angina and BSS symptoms.

To assess safety, patients will be asked to report any side effects or changes in feelings that they have noticed since the previous phase of data collection. In addition, the results of routine blood, urine, and stool tests, liver and kidney function tests, coagulation tests, and electrocardiogram tests will also be considered in the evaluation of safety. Finally, the clinical researchers will carefully monitor all patients for the potential onset of adverse events, the most severe of which may include arrhythmias, heart failure, recurrent myocardial infarction, myocardial rupture, cerebral infarction, cerebral hemorrhage, sudden cardiac death, and all-cause death.

To assess improvement in angina symptoms, a scoring system will be applied based on the frequency, duration, and intensity of angina episodes[15-16]. Similarly, a scoring system will also be used to evaluate BSS based on changes in signs and symptoms such as angina, a pulse of choppy or knotted nature, ecchymoses, dark purple tongue, lips, and gums, and expanded sublingual veins [17].

2.9 Data Collection Phases

Table 1 indicates the data to be collected at each phase of the study. At Phase I, before treatment for the trial is initiated, each patient's full medical history will be recorded, along with vital signs, symptoms of present illness, and all current medications. Tongue and pulse examination will be performed by experienced TCM physicians. Laboratory tests will include routine blood, urine, and stool tests, an electrocardiogram, an hs-CRP test, and various other tests measuring cardiac markers (creatine kinase, CK-MB; troponin T, cTnT; troponin I, cTnI), liver and kidney function, blood lipid and glucose, and coagulation. A 10 mL blood sample will also be collected from each patient, centrifuged, and stored at −80 ℃ for subsequent measurement of other inflammatory mediators (IL-6, TNFα, VCAM-1, CD40, sCD40L, MCP-1, and MMP-9) at the end of the study. Finally, the severity of each patient's angina and BSS symptoms will be quantitatively scored.

Phase II marks the end of the 14-day treatment period, at which time the medications specific to this study (i.e. simvastatin and STS) will be discontinued and the patients reassessed. Again, vital signs, symptoms of present illness, tongue and pulse exam results, and all current medications will be recorded. Angina and BSS scoring will be repeated, along with all Phase I laboratory tests aside from those measuring cardiac markers and blood lipid and glucose. As in Phase I, a blood sample from each patient

Table 1　Data Collection Phases and Scheme

Data collection phase		Phase I: Pre-treatment 0 day	Phase II: Post-treatment 14 days	Phase III: Post-treatment 30 days
Inclusion/exclusion criteria		✓		
Signed informed consent		✓		
Patient interview	General health	✓		
	Past medical history	✓		
	Signs and symptoms of present illness	✓	✓	✓
	Current medications	✓	✓	✓
Physical exam	Tongue and pulse examination	✓	✓	✓
	Heart rate and blood pressure	✓	✓	✓
Laboratory tests	Routine blood, urine, and stool (+occult blood)	✓	✓	
	Liver and kidney function	✓	✓	
	Blood lipid and glucose	✓		
	Coagulation	✓	✓	
	High-sensitivity CRP	✓	✓	✓
	Cardiac markers: CK-MB, cTnT, cTnI	✓		
	Electrocardiogram	✓	✓	
	Inflammatory markers*	✓	✓	✓
Assessment using TCM and Western medicine		✓	✓	✓
Angina and BSS score		✓	✓	✓
Randomization into treatment groups		✓		
Overall evaluation	Evaluation of efficacy		✓	✓
	Evaluation of compliance		✓	✓
	Evaluation of safety and side effects		✓	✓

*NOTE: Blood sample will be stored for analysis at the end of the study. Inflammatory markers include interleukin-6 (IL-6), tumor necrosis factor alpha (TNFα), vascular cell adhesion molecule (VCAM-1), CD40 antigen and CD40 ligand (sCD40L), monocyte chemo-tactic protein-1 (MCP-1), and matrix metalloproteinase-9 (MMP-9)

will be collected and preserved for subsequent analysis of secondary inflammatory factors at the end of the study. A preliminary, non-statistical evaluation of treatment safety and efficacy will also be performed by the data collectors.

30 days after simvastatin and STS are discontinued, Phase III data will be recorded, including level of hs-CRP, angina and BSS scores, vital signs, symptoms of present illness, tongue and pulse exam results, and all current medications. As before, a blood sample for analysis of secondary inflammatory factors will be collected, and treatment safety and efficacy will again be preliminarily evaluated.

2.10　Data Management

The principal investigator of this study will

collaborate with the director of the GCP Clinical Center of Xiyuan Hospital to schedule and coordinate this clinical trial. The GCP Clinical Center will be responsible for randomizing subjects into treatment groups, monitoring research progress, managing the data, and performing statistical analyses. All those involved in these aspects of the trial will remain blind to the details of treatment allocation.

All patient data will be recorded by trained clinical researchers using a standardized, preprinted, paper case report form (CRF). Collection, transportation, and preservation of all blood samples will be performed by trained staff using a standardized procedure. The Laboratory of Cardiovascular Diseases at Xiyuan Hospital will analyze all blood samples and report all results to the clinical researchers for documentation. At the conclusion of the study, CRFs will be delivered to the GCP Clinical Center and examined for completeness by an individual unassociated with the data collection process. If complete, the CRF will be closed to further revision in preparation for data entry.

At the GCP Clinical Center, a data manager uninvolved with subsequent statistical analysis for the study will be responsible for overseeing data entry. To ensure the reliability of the recorded data, two individuals under the data manager will each independently input a copy of the CRF data into a special database (EpiData 3.1 software, http: //www. epidata. dk/). If any data in the CRF is unclear, the data manager will submit a clarification form to the principal investigator of the study, who will then issue an inquiry for the clinical researchers to resolve as soon as possible. The data manager will confirm the correct data according to the clinical researchers' response.

A third individual under the data manager will proofread the two independently completed database records to ensure that they are identical and accurately represent the data in the CRF. If the database records are not identical, the data in

question will be confirmed from the original CRF. Once complete, the database records will be locked to further revision.

2.11 Statistical Analysis

Statistical analyses will be performed using SPSS 15.0 software (SPSS, Inc., Chicago, IL, USA). A student's t test or Wilcoxon Rank-sum test was used, as appropriate, for the analyses of intergroup differences of measurement data; χ^2 test or Fisher exact test if necessary was used for comparison of enumeration data. All tests were two tailed and a statistical probability of < 0.05 was considered significant.

3. Discussion

Despite recent advances in the treatment and prevention of cardiovascular diseases, CHD remains a significant threat to global health. The use of intensified lipid-lowering therapy involving statins and other Western medications has been proposed in an effort to reduce residual cardiovascular risk [18]. The multinational JUPITER trial, however, clearly demonstrated that patients with healthy LDL-C levels according to standard guidelines may still be at elevated risk due to inflammation associated with atherosclerosis, as measured by hs-CRP[19]. Controlling inflammation may therefore be critically important in the treatment of CHD, and to this end, our study will explore the effect of an East-West integrative therapy involving STS and simvastatin on elevated levels of inflammatory markers in CHD patients.

The inflammatory process of atherosclerosis begins when excess LDL particles accumulate in the arterial intima and undergo oxidative modification [20,21], resulting in recruitment of circulating monocytes via factors including MCP-1 and VCAM-1 [22-24]. In the vascular subendothelium, the monocytes differentiate into macrophages and then become foam cells after endocytosis of the oxidized LDL complexes [25]. Expansion of the inflammatory reaction occurs as these lipid-laden foam cells form the necrotic core of the developing atherosclerotic lesion and release proinflammatory cytokines such as TNFα that recruit additional monocytes, dendritic cells, mast cells, and T cells to the area [26]. The extensive crosstalk of cytokines induces vascular smooth muscle cells to produce IL-6, resulting in CRP release by the liver via the acute-phase response [27]. The activated smooth muscle cells also migrate into the arterial intima and lay down fibrous deposits [28], ultimately forming the atherosclerotic plaques that contribute to the development of CHD. As the disease progresses, CD40L-mediated stimulation of MMP-9 expression by vascular smooth muscle cells plays a major role in plaque destabilization [29], altogether increasing the risk of plaque rupture and the onset of complications such as ACS.

Elevated levels of the inflammatory mediators mentioned above may serve as useful tools for gauging a patient's disease state and cardiovascular risk. CRP is widely regarded as the most useful biomarker for assessing atherosclerotic diseases, not only because of its ease and reliability of measurement, its wide and dynamic range of concentrations, and its remarkable stability, but also because its degree of elevation in the blood correlates significantly with the level of risk for future adverse cardiovascular events associated with advanced atherosclerosis, such as myocardial infarction and ischemic stroke [27,30]. Notably, CRP level is not related to the risk of developing venous thrombosis, a vascular condition typically independent of atherosclerosis [30]. Moreover, Liuzzo et al. found that although CRP levels are significantly increased in patients with unstable angina, which is usually caused by CHD due to atherosclerosis, the biomarker's concentration is not elevated in patients with variant angina, which is caused not by atherosclerosis but by vasospasms of the coronary arteries [31]. These observations altogether suggest that, in the context of cardiovascular disease, the extent of CRP elevation predicts the extent of atherosclerotic inflammation, thereby making CRP level a suitable primary outcome parameter for our study.

The levels of IL-6, TNFα, VCAM-1, CD40, sCD40L, MCP-1, and MMP-9 were selected as secondary outcome parameters in this trial, as these inflammatory markers are less effective indicators of atherosclerotic disease status compared to CRP. Tayebjee et al. found that levels of sCD40L and MMP-9 are significantly higher in stable CHD patients than in healthy controls, but also that these markers may not strongly predict the severity of CHD [32]. In addition, although Biasucci et al. found that elevated IL-6 levels predict worse prognosis in patients with unstable angina, the authors were able to detect IL-6 in only 61% of their unstable angina group [33]. Nevertheless, the analysis of these inflammatory markers in addition to CRP provides a broader perspective of the inflammatory state of each patient, allowing us to examine and interpret the effect of STS-simvastatin integrative therapy on inflammation reduction with greater depth.

It is possible that the biomarker concentrations measured in our study may reflect systemic inflammation due to a cause other than atherosclerosis. Indeed, CRP is an acute phase protein released by the liver as part of the body's immune response to non-specific disturbances, including infection, autoimmune disorders, trauma or surgery, and cancer [34]. To diminish the effect of this possibility, we will carefully consider the past and present medical histories of all eligible patients before enrollment and exclude any patients in whom inflammatory markers may not accurately reflect the state of CHD. Additionally, we will also monitor all study participants during the course of the trial for changes that may confound interpretation of biomarker data, such as acquisition of a nosocomial infection.

The mechanisms by which tanshinone ⅡA and statins inhibit the inflammatory process of atherosclerosis are diverse, numerous, and

第三章

in many cases shared [reviewed in 8 and 35]. Using STS and simvastatin in combination may yield an additive, supplementary effect not only in the reduction of internal inflammation, but also in the improvement of external symptoms associated with CHD. In this trial, we will examine the therapeutic efficacy of a STS-simvastatin integrative therapy in CHD patients by quantitatively scoring each study participant's angina and BSS symptoms and examining for any changes over the course of the trial.

There is a risk for negative interactions in any combination drug therapy, but integrative treatments involving STS appear to be relatively safe. In a systematic review of 25 randomized controlled trials, Qiu et al. found that integrative therapies involving STS for unstable angina may produce fewer side effects than the component Western therapies alone [36]. Side effects that were associated with the integrative therapies included flushing, dizziness, bruising, gum bleeding, blood in the sputum, and swelling at the STS injection site, but none were considered severe and none resulted in discontinuation of treatment. Another clinical study, which used STS and simvastatin in combination to treat peripheral vascular disease, also found the integrative treatment to be safer than the statin therapy alone [10]. Our study will continue to monitor the short- and long - term side effects of STS-simvastatin integrative therapy and verify the safety observations reported by previous trials.

Several limitations affect the strength of our study design. Due to the unavailability of data needed to perform an a prior calculation, we determined the sample size for this study by adopting the number used in a comparable trial that we previously completed [14]. As a result, it is possible that our current study design may have insufficient power to reveal statistical significance at the level we desire. In addition, because the color of the STS solution makes double-blinding difficult, our study will be subject to potential expectation biases from both the clinical researchers and the study participants. We will attempt to minimize these biases by maintaining blinding at the patient level to the fullest extent possible, and by having clinical researchers interact with all subjects as similarly as possible. Full blinding will be maintained at the data analysis level. Finally, our project represents a single-center study and our results may not be wholly generalizable due to a possible selection bias. In the future, multicenter double blinded, randomized controlled trials are necessary in order to faithfully establish the potential of STS-statin integrative therapy in treating CHD.

Nevertheless, the results of this trial are expected to clarify the potential of an East-West integrative therapy involving STS and simvastatin in reducing atherosclerotic inflammation in CHD patients. Our results will additionally confirm the safety and efficacy of this integrative therapy in treating CHD. Finally, the protocol of our study will also provide a methodological foundation upon which future clinical studies of integrative medicine may develop.

Trial Status

This trial has begun to recruit patients from November 2012, there has been 10 volunteers up to February 2013.

Abbreviations Used

ACS, acute coronary syndrome; BSS, blood stasis syndrome; sCD40L, soluble CD40 ligand; CHD, coronary heart disease; CK-MB, creatine kinase; CRF, case report form; CRP, C-reactive protein; hs-CRP, high-sensitivity C-reactive protein; ELISA, enzyme-linked immunosorbent assay; GCP, Good Clinical Practice; IL-6, interleukin-6; LDL-C, low-density lipoprotein cholesterol; MCP-1, monocyte chemotactic protein-1; MMP-9, matrix metalloproteinase-9; STS, sodium tanshinone IIA sulfate; TCM, traditional Chinese medicine; TNFα, tumor necrosis factor alpha; cTnI, troponin I; cTnT, troponin T; VCAM-1, vascular cell adhesion molecule-1.

Competing Interests

This trial received financial support from the Jiangsu Carefree Pharmaceutical Co., Ltd. The company is not involved in developing the study design, collecting or interpreting the data, writing the manuscript, or publishing the results related to this trial.

Authors' Contributions

QS: design of the study, registration of the trial, and drafting of the manuscript. HW: design of the study, and drafting of the manuscript. HX: conceptualization and design of the study, and revision of the manuscript. SL: execution of the study. All authors read and discussed the manuscript, and all gave approval for the publication of this protocol.

Authors' Information

QS is a physician of the Department of Cardiovascular Diseases at Xiyuan Hospital, China Academy of Chinese Medical Sciences in Beijing, China, and she is also a doctorate student at the Beijing University of Chinese Medicine in Beijing, China. HW is a medical student from Columbia University's College of Physicians and Surgeons in New York, NY, USA, who is a summer research intern at Xiyuan Hospital, China Academy of Chinese Medical Sciences in Beijing, China. SL is a doctorate student at the Beijing University of Chinese Medicine in Beijing, China. HX is the chief physician and director of the Department of Cardiovascular Diseases at Xiyuan Hospital, China Academy of Chinese Medical Sciences in Beijing, China.

References

[1] World Health Organization. Cardiovascular diseases. Fact sheet No317, 2011. [http://www.who.int/mediacentre/factsheets/fs317/en/index.html]

[2] Hansson GK. Inflammation, atherosclerosis, and coronary artery disease. N Engl J Med, 2005, 352 (16): 1685-1695.

[3] Law MR, Wald NJ, Rudnicka AR. Quantifying effect of statins on low density lipoprotein cholesterol, ischaemic heart disease, and stroke: systematic review and meta-analysis. BMJ, 2003, 326 (7404): 1423-1429.

[4] Albert MA , Danielson E, Rifai N, et al. Effect of statin therapy on C-reactive protein levels. The pravastatin inflammation/CRP evaluation (PRINCE): a randomized trial and cohort study. JAMA, 2001, 286 (1): 64-70.

[5] Paffen E, DeMaat MP. C-reactive protein in atherosclerosis: a causal factor? Cardiovasc Res, 2006, 71 (1): 30-39.

[6] Cannon CP, Braunwald E, McCabe CH, et al. Intensive versus moderate lipid lowering with statins after acute coronary syndromes. N Engl J Med, 2004, 350 (15): 1495-1504.

[7] Gao ZY, Xu H, Shi DZ, et al. Analysis on outcome of 5284 patients with coronary artery disease: the role of integrative medicine. J Ethnopharmacol, 2012, 141 (2): 578-583.

[8] Ga S, Liu Z, Li H, et al. Cardiovascular actions and therapeutic potential of tanshinone IIA. Atherosclerosis, 2012, 220 (1): 3-10.

[9] Wang QL, Deng XJ, Li XQ, et al. Effect of sodium tanshinone injection on CRP and D-dimer level in patients with unstable angina. Journal of New Chinese Medicine, 2007, 39 (7): 16-17.

[10] Wang WL, Ma BR, Hu XS, et al. The effect of tanshinone IIA and simvastatin treating the legs atheromatosis. Chinese Journal of Arteriosclerosis, 2010, 18 (11): 897-899.

[11] Schulz KF, Altman DG, Moher D, et al. CONSORT 2010 statement: updated guidelines for reporting parallel group randomised trials. Trials, 2010, 11: 32.

[12] Nomenclature and criteria for diagnosis of ischemic heart disease. Report of the Joint International Society and Federation of Cardiology/World Health Organization task force on standardization of clinical nomenclature. Circulation, 1979, 59 (3): 607-609.

[13] Subcommittee of Cardiovascular Diseases of China Society of Integrated Traditional Chinese and Western Medicine. Criteria for TCM syndrome differentiation of patients with coronary heart disease. Chinese Journal of Integrated Traditional and Western Medicine, 1991, 11 (5), 257-258.

[14] Chen H, Gao ZY, Shi HXDZ, et al. Clinical study of unstable angina patients undergoing percutaneous coronary intervention treated with Chinese medicine for activating blood circulation and detoxification. Chinese Journal of Integrative Medicine on Cardio/

第三章

cerebrovascular Disease, 2009, 7 (10): 1135-1137.

[15] Bureau of Drug Administration of the People's Republic of China. New Medicine (Western Medicine) Clinical Research Guiding Principles. 1993.

[16] Zheng XY, Ren DQ. Chinese herbal medicine clinical research guiding principles (for trial implementation). Chinese Medicine and Technology Publishing House, 2002.

[17] Chen KJ. Study and clinical practice of methods for activating blood to resolve stagnation. Beijing: Beijing Medical University and Peking Union Medical College Press, 1993.

[18] Evans M, Roberts A, Davies S, et al. Medical lipid-regulating therapy: current evidence, ongoing trials, and future developments. Drugs, 2004, 64 (11): 1181-1196.

[19] Ridker PM, Danielson E, Fonseca FA, et al. Rosuvastatin to prevent vascular events in men and women with elevated C-reactive protein. N Engl J Med, 2008, 359 (21): 2195-2207.

[20] Nievelstein PF, Fogelman AM, Mottino G, et al. Lipid accumulation in rabbit aortic intima 2 hours after bolus infusion of low density lipoprotein. A deep-etch and immunolocalization study of ultrarapidly frozen tissue. Arterioscler Thromb Vasc Biol, 1991, 11 (6): 1795-1805.

[21] Palinski W, Rosenfeld ME, Yla-Herttuala S, et al. Low density lipoprotein undergoes oxidative modification in vivo. Proc Natl Acad Sci USA, 1989, 86 (4): 1372-1376.

[22] Berliner JA, Territo MC, Sevanian A, et al. Minimally modified low density lipoprotein stimulates monocyte endothelial interactions. J Clin Invest, 1990, 85 (4): 1260-1266.

[23] Cushing SD, Berliner JA, Valente AJ, et al. Minimally modified low density lipoprotein induces monocyte chemotactic protein 1 in human endothelial cells and smooth muscle cells. Proc Natl Acad Sci USA, 1990, 87 (13): 5134-5138.

[24] Huo Y, Ley K. Adhesion molecules and athero-genesis. Acta Physiol Scand, 2001, 173 (1): 35-43.

[25] Goldstein JL, Ho YK, Basu SK, et al. Binding site on macrophages that mediates uptake and degradation of acetylated low density lipoprotein, producing massive cholesterol deposition. Proc Natl Acad Sci USA, 1979, 76 (1): 333-337

[26] Hansson GK, Libby P, Schönbeck U, et al. Innate and adaptive immunity in the pathogenesis of atherosclerosis. Circ Res, 2002, 91 (4) : 281-291.

[27] Packard RR, Libby P. Inflammation in atheros-clerosis: from vascular biology to biomarker discovery and risk prediction. Clin Chem, 2008, 54 (1): 24-38.

[28] Raines EW, Ferri N. Cytokines affecting endothelial and smooth muscle cells in vascular disease. J Lipid Res, 2005, 46 (6): 1081-1092.

[29] Schönbeck U, Mach F, Sukhova GK, et al. Regulation of matrix metalloproteinase expression in human vascular smooth muscle cells by T lymphocytes: a role for CD40 signaling in plaque rupture？ Circ Res, 1997, 81 (3): 448-454.

[30] Ridker PM, Cushman M, Stampfer MJ, et al. Inflammation, aspirin, and the risk of cardiovascular disease in apparently healthy men. N Engl J Med, 1997, 336 (14): 973-979.

[31] Liuzzo G, Biasucci LM, Rebuzzi AG, et al. Plasma protein acute-phase response in unstable angina is not induced by ischemic injury. Circulation, 1996, 94 (10): 2373-2380.

[32] Tayebjee MH, Lip GY, Tan KT, et al. Plasma matrix metallo proteinase-9, tissue inhibitor of metallo proteinase-2, and CD40 ligand levels in patients with stable coronary artery disease. Am J Cardiol, 2005, 96 (3): 339-345.

[33] Biasucci LM, Vitelli A, LiuzzoG, et al. Elevated levels of interleukin-6 in unstable angina. Circulation, 1996, 94 (5): 874-877.

[34] Gruys E, Toussaint MJM, Niewold TA, et al. Acute phase reaction and acute phase proteins. J Zhejiang Univ Sci B, 2005, 6 (11): 1045-1056.

[35] Rosenson RS. Pluripotential mechanisms of cardioprotection with HMG-CoA reductase inhibitor therapy. Am J Cardiovasc Drugs, 2001,1 (6): 411-420.

[36] Qiu X, Miles A, Jiang X, et al. Sulfotanshinone sodium injection for unstable angina pectoris: a systematic review of randomized controlled trials. Evid Based Complement Alternat Med, 2012: 715790.

第三章

第二节　中西医结合防治心肌梗死及介入术后干预

益气养阴活血中药对急性心肌梗死患者血运重建后心室壁运动的影响 *

李永强　金枚　仇盛蕾　朱天刚　边红　王承龙　刘红旭　姚立芳　史大卓

经皮冠状动脉介入治疗（percutaneous coronary intervention，PCI）、静脉溶栓或冠状动脉旁路移植术可使急性心肌梗死（acute myocardial infarction，AMI）罪犯血管再通，恢复缺血心肌血供，已成为目前 AMI 治疗的主要方法。然而，血运重建后部分患者心肌灌注并不完全，甚至存在无再灌注现象（no-reflow），严重影响了 AMI 患者的预后[1]。以往研究表明，益气养阴活血中药结合西医常规治疗具有降低 AMI 住院病死率和并发症发生率的作用[2]。本研究采用多巴酚丁胺负荷状态的多普勒超声技术（dobutamine stress echocardiography，DSE），随机双盲、安慰剂对照观察益气养阴活血中药对 AMI 患者血运重建后心室壁运动和心肌收缩功能的影响。

1. 资料与方法

1.1　诊断标准

西医诊断参照"AMI 诊断和治疗指南"中 AMI 的诊断标准[3]，中医诊断参照"胸痹心厥急症诊疗规范"标准[4]。

1.2　纳入标准

（1）心电图显示 ST 段抬高的首次 AMI 患者，经冠状动脉造影或静脉溶栓血管再通标准[5]证实罪犯血管再通的患者。（2）行静脉溶栓后直接 PCI 的患者。（3）年龄≤75 岁。（4）Killip 分级属Ⅰ～Ⅲ级者。

1.3　排除标准

（1）年龄＞75 岁的患者。（2）合并严重肝、肾、造血系统、神经系统等原发性疾病。（3）患有精神病、恶性肿瘤患者。（4）患者拒绝签署知情同意书，或估计依从性较差，随访可能性较小者。（5）妊娠期或哺乳期妇女。（6）参加其他临床试验的患者。

1.4　一般资料

选择中国中医科学院西苑医院、首都医科大学附属北京中医医院、北京大学人民医院及首都医科大学同仁医院共 4 家医院 2005 年 3 月—2006 年 6 月治疗的 AMI 患者 80 例，根据 SAS 软件数字表随机分为西药常规治疗加心悦胶囊及复方丹参片组（简称中药组）和西药常规治疗加安慰剂组（对照组）。

中药组 40 例，男性 33 例，女性 7 例；平均年龄（56.34±11.12）岁；前壁 AMI 23 例，下壁 AMI 17 例；就诊到血运重建的时间为（6.22±2.67）h，其中即刻行 PCI 术 39 例，静脉溶栓术 1 例。PCI 术后梗死相关血管前向血流达 TMI Ⅲ级者占 98.36%，静脉溶栓者按标准[4]证实血管再通。入选时心功能 Kilip Ⅰ级 21 例，Killp Ⅱ级 16 例，Killp Ⅲ级 3 例；有吸烟史 26 例，合并高血压病 16 例，糖尿病 12 例，血脂异常 18 例，脑梗死 2 例。

* 原载于《中国中西医结合杂志》，2009，29（4）：300-304

对照组 40 例，男性 35 例，女性 5 例；平均年龄（55.76±12.09）岁。前壁 AMI 22 例，下壁 AMI 18 例，就诊到血运重建的时间（6.31±1.72）h，其中行即刻 PCI 术 38 例，静脉溶栓术 2 例。PCI 术后梗死相关血管前向血流达 TMI Ⅲ 级者占 97.88%，静脉溶栓者均证实血管再通。入选时心功能 Killip Ⅰ 级 22 例，Killip Ⅱ 级 13 例，Killip Ⅲ 级 5 例；有吸烟史 29 例，合并高血压病 18 例，糖尿病 16 例，血脂异常 15 例，脑梗死 3 例。两组患者临床资料经统计学处理，差异无统计学意义（$P > 0.05$）。

1.5 治疗方法

AMI 患者行 PCI 术或静脉溶栓治疗，经冠状动脉造影或静脉溶栓血管再通标准[5]判断罪犯血管再通后，中药组在按照指南[3]进行西医规范治疗（在没有药物使用禁忌证和不良反应的情况下，抗血小板治疗：给予阿司匹林 100mg/d 终身服用；氯吡格雷 75mg/d，植入药物涂层支架者服用至少 1 年，植入金属裸支架者服用至少 1 个月；尽早使用 β- 受体阻断剂、血管紧张素、转换酶抑制剂或血管紧张素、转换酶受体拮抗剂，并逐渐加至目标剂量；继续使用他汀类降脂药、硝酸酯类药物）基础上，加心悦胶囊（每粒胶囊含西洋参茎叶总皂苷 50mg，由吉林省集安益盛药业股份有限公司生产，批号为 030073）2 粒，3 次 / 日；复方丹参片（每片含丹参 450mg、三七 141mg、冰片 8mg，由吉林省集安益盛药业股份有限公司生产，批号：030073）3 片，3 次 / 日。对照组在西医规范治疗的基础上，加模拟心悦胶囊安慰剂 2 粒，3 次 / 日；模拟复方丹参片安慰剂 3 片，3 次 / 日（两者成分均为淀粉，包装、外形、颜色等与中药组完全相同，均由吉林省集安益盛药业股份有限公司生产，批号均为 041102）。安慰剂和中药治疗药物均自入选后当日口服，连续服药 3 个月或达临床研究终点。

1.6 观察指标及方法

1.6.1 多巴酚丁胺负荷状态超声方法 各中心均应用美国 GE 公司生产的 VIVID 7 型彩色多普勒仪，对研究人员进行培训，统一操作标准。患者取左侧卧位，M3S 探头，频率 1.7 ～ 3.4MHz，按照实时心肌灌注能量多普勒模式，自心尖四腔、心尖二腔和心尖长轴取样，范围包括整个左心室。经肘部浅静脉连续泵入多巴酚丁胺，剂量依次为每分钟 5、10、20μg/kg，各持续 3min，最终泵入剂量为

每分钟 20μg/kg。负荷态（每分钟 20μg /kg）下，采集左室长轴、左室短轴、心尖四腔、心尖二腔图像。分别于患者入选后 14 天及 3 个月各进行 1 次。

1.6.2 左室射血分数（LVEF） 采用改良 Simpson 法[6]测定。

1.6.3 室壁运动计分指数和正常心肌百分比 参照 1987 年美国超声心动图学会推荐的 16 节段室壁运动计分方法[6]，根据室壁运动增厚率进行计分：1 分为正常室壁运动（增厚率 ≥ 25%）；2 分为室壁运动减弱（增厚率 < 25%）；3 分为室壁运动消失（增厚率 =0）；4 分为矛盾运动或局部室壁膨出。室壁运动计分指数 = 计分总和 / 总节段数。所有的室壁评分完成后，VIVID7 型彩色多普勒仪自带软件可以自动计算正常心肌百分比。

1.6.4 各节段收缩期纵向峰值应变力（longitudinal systolic peak strain，LSPS）及应变率峰值（longitudinal systolic peak strain rate，LSPSR） LSPS 指因收缩期心肌适应力变化而产生的局部组织最大形状变化，LSPSR 测量收缩期单位时间内应变力的最大变化，它描述的是心肌组织的变形速率。两者均反映心肌收缩做功的大小，负向值越大，心肌收缩功能越强。LSPS 和 LSPSR 按照文献[6]方法，运用美国 GE 公司 EchoPac 工作站进行图像处理和分析，对心尖长轴切面分别进行心内膜边界描记，工作站图像处理软件自动计算出心尖长轴的收缩期应变力峰值及应变率峰值。

1.7 统计学方法

应用 SPSS 13.0 软件处理数据，计数资料用 χ^2 检验，计量资料用 t 检验，$P < 0.05$ 为差异有统计学意义。

2. 结果

试验过程中，中药组脱落 3 例，其中 1 例原因为不能按时服用试验药物，2 例因不同意进行超声检查；对照组脱落 2 例，其中 1 例因不能按时服用试验药物，1 例为入组后病情不宜行负荷超声检查，并于 3 周时死亡。不能进行最终疗效评价。本研究共 75 例完成试验，其中中药组 37 例，对照组 38 例。

2.1 益气养阴活血中药对 AMI 患者心功能、正常心肌百分比及室壁运动的影响（表 1）

AMI 患者血运重建后 14 天负荷态超声显示，LVEF 值和正常心肌百分比中药组较对照组明显增

加（$P < 0.05$，$P < 0.01$）。血运重建 3 个月与 14 天比较，中药组正常心肌百分比、LVEF 值、正常心肌百分比均有所增加，室壁运动计分指数有一定程度下降，但差异无统计学意义（$P > 0.05$）。

表 1　益气养阴活血中药对 AMI 患者心功能、正常心肌百分比及室壁运动的影响（$\bar{x} \pm s$）

组别	例数	时间	LVEF（%）	正常心肌百分比（%）	室壁运动计分指数
对照	38	14 天	60.40±13.40	79.95±12.14	1.62±0.59
		3 个月	68.48±8.48	88.11±11.70	1.32±0.33
中药	37	14 天	66.09±8.36*	86.87±8.77**	1.60±0.48
		3 个月	70.73±6.55	89.26±9.91	1.23±0.21

注：与对照组同期比较，*$P < 0.05$，**$P < 0.01$

2.2　益气养阴活血中药对 AMI 患者左室前壁心肌节段 LSPS 及 LSPSR 的影响（表 2）

血运重建后 14 天负荷态超声显示，中药组心尖段 LTS、LSPSR，基底段、中间段 LSPSR 较对照组负向值明显增加（$P < 0.01$，$P < 0.05$）；血运重建后 3 个月负荷态超声显示，中药组心尖段 LSPS、LSPSR 较对照组负向值明显增加（$P < 0.05$）；血运重建后 3 个月与 14 天比较，中药组心尖段 LSPS 负向值明显增加（$P < 0.05$）。

2.3　益气养阴活血中药对 AMI 患者左室下壁心肌节段 LSPS 及 LSPSR 影响（表 3）

血运重建后 14 天负荷态超声显示，中药组基底段 LSPS 较对照组负向值明显增加（$P < 0.05$），基底段和中间段 LSPSR 较对照组负向值明显增加（$P < 0.01$）；血运重建后 3 个月负荷态超声显示，中药组基底段 LSPS 和 LSPSR 较对照组负向值明显增加（$P < 0.05$）；血运重建后 3 个月和 14 天比较，中药组基底段 LSPSR 负向值明显增加（$P < 0.05$）。

3. 讨论

AMI 血运重建后 slow-flow 或 no-reflow 现象的病理过程十分复杂，涉及血栓形成、内膜损伤、氧化应激反应和炎症反应等多个方面[7]。这些病理改变与传统中医学的"心脉痹阻"、"心脉不通"多有相似之处，属于"血瘀证"的范畴。有研究认为 AMI 血运重建后中医病机多为本虚标实，本虚以气虚或气阴两虚为主，标实则多以血瘀、痰浊或痰瘀互结、蕴而化毒为主[8,9]。20 世纪 70—80 年代，中国中医科学院西苑医院心血管病中心联合北京地区 4 家医院在西医常规治疗基础上，进行益气养阴活血药物干预 AMI 的临床观察，证明益气养阴活血制剂结合西医常规治疗具有降低 AMI 住

表 2　益气养阴活血中药对 AMI 患者左室前壁心肌节段 LSPS 及 LSPSR 的影响（$\bar{x} \pm s$）

组别	例数	时间	LSPS（%）			LSPSR（s⁻¹）		
			基底段	中间段	心尖段	基底段	中间段	心尖段
对照	18	14 天	−13.00±4.95	−12.21±5.81	−9.55±4.17	−0.68±0.24	−0.67±0.28	−0.64±0.29
		3 个月	−13.92±4.95	−12.37±6.37	−12.68±3.73	−0.75±0.31	−0.83±0.31	−0.75±0.29
中药	16	14 天	−15.16±6.04	−13.26±5.68	−14.12±5.79△△	−0.94±0.40△	−0.87±0.33△	−0.96±0.43△△
		3 个月	−16.00±5.99	−13.57±4.04	−15.97±5.87*△	−0.95±0.41	−0.92±0.34	−0.98±0.42△

注：与本组 14 天比较，*$P < 0.05$，与对照组同期比较，△$P < 0.05$，△△$P < 0.01$

表 3　益气养阴活血中药对 AMI 患者左室下壁心肌节段 LSPS 及 LSPSR 的影响（$\bar{x} \pm s$）

组别	例数	时间	LSPS（%）			LSPSR（s⁻¹）		
			基底段	中间段	心尖段	基底段	中间段	心尖段
对照	18	14 天	−10.21±4.34	−9.35±3.92	−12.92±4.37	−0.41±0.09	−0.63±0.31	−0.80±0.36
		3 个月	−11.41±3.85	−10.83±4.43	−14.56±3.28	−0.58±0.26	−0.85±0.33	−0.93±0.39
中药	16	14 天	−14.03±5.82△	−10.62±4.68	−14.77±6.28	−0.62±0.27△	−0.99±0.43△	−0.89±0.40
		3 个月	−15.15±6.56△	−11.71±5.10	−15.15±6.23	−0.75±0.09△	−1.02±0.08	−0.95±0.40

注：与本组 14 天比较，*$P < 0.05$，与对照组同期比较，△$P < 0.05$，△△$P < 0.01$

院病死率和并发症发生率的作用[3]。研究表明，益气养阴活血中药配伍具有促进梗死及缺血区血管新生、调节糖脂代谢、抗氧化、抗心肌缺血、改善左室重构等作用[10,11]。本研究选用益气养阴中药心悦胶囊和活血化瘀中药复方丹参片对 AMI 血运重建后进行综合干预。两药均为国内上市的治疗冠心病的常用有效制剂，两者联合应用，以奏益气养阴活血之效。运用多巴酚丁胺负荷状态的多普勒超声技术观察益气养阴活血中药制剂对 AMI 血运重建后室壁运动和心肌收缩功能的影响。

应变力和应变率成像技术是近年来迅速发展的多普勒超声心动图技术，其原理是基于灰阶成像的定向追踪技术，以各方向运动的心肌组织回声信号为追踪对象，其不受角度限制，在整个心动周期跟踪心内膜运动变化，分辨率达 3.7ms，较传统评价方法可更客观、准确地评价心肌活性和运动状态[12,13]，结合多巴酚丁胺试验则可增加其特异性[14]。

由于 AMI 患者血运重建后患者即刻进行多巴酚丁胺负荷超声检查增加心肌氧耗而存在一定的危险、且患者也不宜挪动，国内多数医院又缺乏可靠敏感的 14 天床旁超声检查设备，本研究未能于 AMI 血运重建后即刻进行心脏功能和室壁节段性运动状况评价。本研究对两组病例进行了梗死部位、Killip 分级等影响因素的比较，未显示出统计学差异，说明两组患者 AMI 后的心功能状况具有可比性。AMI 后 14 天，病情基本达到初步稳定阶段，冬眠心肌、顿抑心肌或未重新获得充分血液灌注的梗死相关动脉支配心肌皆得到了一定的恢复或修复，此时进行超声检查，基本可反映药物的干预效应。因此，本研究选择 AMI 血运重建后 14 天和 3 个月作为临床超声观察的时间点。

本研究运用 VIVID 7 型彩色多普勒仪，在多巴酚丁胺负荷状态下通过实时观察对 75 例 AMI 患者血运重建 14 天和 3 个月左室收缩功能、室壁运动计分指数、正常心肌百分比进行观察，整体评价心脏功能和室壁运动情况；分别对前壁和下壁心肌梗死病例左室相关节段的 LSPS 及 LSPSR 进行比较，评价心肌梗死相关节段的室壁运动。结果表明，血运重建后 14 天 AMI 患者整体收缩功能和梗死相关节段室壁运动皆有一定程度的改善。中药组 AMI 患者左室收缩功能、正常心肌百分比、前壁 AMI 患者左室前壁各节段 LSPS 和 LSPSR 均有改善，以心尖段最为明显，下壁 AMI 患者左室下壁基底段和中间段最为明显。血运重建后 3 个月，

前壁 AMI 患者左室前壁心尖段 LSPS 和 LSPSR，下壁 AMI 患者左室下壁基底段仍有明显改善。分析相关节段的改善可能与入选病例的梗死部位及侧支循环的分布有关。结果表明益气养阴活血中药结合西医常规治疗有进一步改善 AMI 血运重建后心功能和室壁运动的作用，显示有良好的临床应用前景。

本研究在西医常规治疗的基础上服用益气养阴活血中药治疗，临床观察仅 3 个月，时间偏短，其对 AMI 血运重建后长期预后的作用如何？尚待扩大样本量和远期随访研究进一步评价。但 AMI 血运重建后的心功能、室壁运动状况和长期预后密切相关，因此有理由推测益气养阴活血中药对 AMI 患者的长期预后可能具有一定的有益作用，值得进一步临床验证。

参考文献

[1] Centurin OA. The open artery hypothesis beneficial effects and long-term prognostic importance of patency of the infarct-related coronary artery. Angiobgy, 2007, 58 (1): 34-44.

[2] 中国中医研究院西苑医院内科等. 以"抗心梗合剂"为主治疗急性心肌梗塞 118 例疗效分析. 中华内科杂志, 1976, 4 (1): 212-215.

[3] 中华医学会心血管分会. 急性心肌梗死诊断和治疗指南. 中华心血管病杂志, 2001, 29 (12): 705-720.

[4] 胸痹协作组. 胸痹心厥（冠心病心肌梗塞）急症诊疗规范. 中国中医急症, 1995, 4 (4): 183-185.

[5] 中华心血管杂志编委会. 急性心肌梗塞溶栓疗法参考方案. 中华心血管病杂志, 1996, 24 (5): 328-329.

[6] 周永昌, 郭万林. 超声医学. 第 5 版. 北京: 科学技术文献出版社. 2008: 440-448.

[7] Lee KW, Nore II MS. Management of "no-reflow" complicating reperfusion therapy. Acute Card Care, 2008, 10 (1): 5-14.

[8] 陈可冀, 史大卓. 中医药防治冠状动脉内手术后再狭窄的思路与方法. 中国中医药信息杂志, 1996, 5 (3): 35.

[9] 张敏州, 王磊. 邓铁涛对冠心病介入术后患者的辨证论治. 中国现代中药, 2006, 5 (2): 32-33.

[10] 王承龙, 史大卓, 殷惠军, 等. 西洋参茎叶总皂苷对急性心肌梗死大鼠心肌 VEGF、bFGF 表达及血管新生的影响. 中国中西医结合杂志, 2007, 27 (4): 331-334.

[11] 季海刚, 司亮. 丹参对心肌缺血再灌注损伤保护作用的研究进展. 光明中医, 2006, 21 (3): 52-53.

[12] Thbault H, Gomez L, Donal E, et al. Acute myocardial infarction in mice assessment of transmurality by strain rate imaging. Am J Physiol Heart Circ Physiol, 2007, 293: 496-502.

[13] Vartdal T, Brunvand H, Pethrsen E, et al. Early prediction of infarct size by strain Doppler echocardiography after coronary reperfusion. J Am Coll Cardiol, 2007, 49 (16): 1715-1721.

[14] Reant P, Lab rousse L, Lafitle S, et al. Experimental validation of circum ferential, longitudinal, and radial 2-dimensional strain during dobutamine stress echocardio-graphy in ischemic conditions. J Am Coll Cardiol, 2008, 51 (2): 149-157.

Protective Effect of Chinese Herbs for Supplementing Qi, Nourishing Yin and Activating Blood Circulation on Heart Function of Patients with Acute Coronary Syndrome after Percutaneous Coronary Intervention*

LIU Hong-ying　WANG Wei　SHI Da-zhuo　GE Jun-bo　ZHANG Lei　PENG Juan
WANG Cheng-long　WANG Pei-li

Acute coronary syndrome (ACS) is a series of pathological states from unstable angina (UA) to acute non-ST segment elevation myocardial infarction (NSTEMI) and ST segment elevation myocardial infarction (STEMI). ACS is a main cause of cardiovascular mortality and morbidity. With the development of percutaneous coronary intervention (PCI) techniques and materials, the prognosis of patients with ACS has been significantly improved[1]. However, heart damage caused by acute myocardial ischemia, especially the impacts of acute myocardial necrosis on heart function for patients with acute myocardial infarction (AMI), will be remained after revascularization of culprit-related vessel. Ventricular remodeling (VR) and heart failure are still the key deleterious factors for long-term prognosis[2]. Therefore, how to improve heart function and prognosis of ACS patients is still the central issue in clinical practice.

ACS belongs to "chest stuffiness and precordial pain" and "syncopal precordialgia"

in Chinese medicine (CM). ACS often manifests the syndrome of deficiency in both qi and yin and blood stasis in the diagnosis of CM differentiation. Accordingly, supplementing qi, nourishing yin and activating blood circulation can be used as a treatment principle. Recently, the pharmacological studies have shown that Chinese herbs for supplementing qi, nourishing yin and activating blood circulation have some favorable effects on the treatment of ACS, such as reducing myocardial oxygen consumption, regulating myocardial metabolism, increasing myocardial perfusion, reducing ischemic damage and infarct size, and inhibiting VR[3]. Xinyue capsule with effects of supplementing qi, nourishing yin and Chuanxiong capsule with effects of activating blood circulation are both widely used in the treatment of coronary heart disease (CHD). The main component of Xinyue capsule is panax quinquefolius saponin, while the Chuanxiong capsule is composed of *Rhizoma Ligustici wallichii* and *Radix Angelicae*

* 原载于 Chinese Journal of Intergrative Medicine, 2012, 18 (6): 423-430

Sinensis; the two capsules together play a role in supplementing qi, nourishing yin and activating blood circulation according to CM theory.

In the present clinical study, the efficacy of Xinyue capsule and Chuanxiong capsule on patients with ACS after successful PCI were observed in a prospective, randomized, controlled, valuator and data handler-blinded design, which mainly focused on the heart function and the incidence of major adoerse cardiovascular events (MACE) after PCI.

1. Methods

1.1 Diagnostic Criteria

Unstable angina and acute myocardial infarction were diagnosed with reference to the diagnostic criteria by Chinese Society of Cardiology in Chinese Medical Association and Editorial Board of Chinese Journal of Cardiology[4,5]. CM symptom scores and blood stasis syndrome scores were diagnosed with reference to the diagnostic criteria documented by Committee of Cardiovascular Disease and by Committee of Activating Blood Circulation, respectively, in China Society of Integrated Traditional Chinese and Western Medicine[6,7]. New York Heart Association (NYHA) heart functional class was evaluated with reference to the diagnostic criteria published by New York Heart Association[8].

1.2 Inclusion Criteria

Patients fulfilled the diagnostic criteria of ACS; aged 40 to 75; treated with successful PCI (complete revascularization in target vessel, thrombolysis in myocardial infarction (TIMI) 3) 12 h after ACS; providing written informed consent.

1.3 Exclusion Criteria

Patients treated with thrombolytic therapy before emergent PCI; with serious liver and renal dysfunction, hematological or neurological diseases, mental illness, or malignancy; continued with mechanical assistant device after successful emergent PCI; pregnant or lactating women; and

patients participated in other studies.

1.4 Baseline Characteristics

100 patients with ACS after successful PCI in Zhongshan Hospital of Fudan University (Shanghai) from July to December in 2008 were randomly assigned using consecutively numbered envelopes and the randomization sequences were blinded for clinical investigators. Randomization blocks of size 50 were generated by the SPSS statistical software (13.0 soft version). The WMG and CMG groups had similar baseline characteristics ($P > 0.05$). The details are listed in Table 1. The program of the present study was approved by the Ethics Committee of Xiyuan hospital affiliated to China Academy of Chinese Medical Sciences (approved document number: 2007XL005).

1.5 Quality Control

The present study was a prospective, randomized, and parallel controlled clinical trial. Quality control personnel trial was responsible for reviewing any documentation in this clinical trial. All data were inputted and statistically analyzed by specialized person who did not participate in the clinical trial.

1.6 Medication

WMG: After successful PCI, patients with ACS were given conventional western medicine treatment including anti-ischemic therapy (nitrates, β blockers, calcium antagonists, ACEI or ARB), anti-platelet therapy (clopidogrel plus aspirin or aspirin alone), anti-coagulant therapy (heparin or low molecular weight heparin) and statins.

CMG: After successful PCI, patients with ACS took orally Chuanxiong capsule (two capsules, three times a day) and Xinyue capsule (two capsules, three times a day) for 6 months in addition to the conventional western treatment.

Chuanxiong capsule consists of Rhizoma *Ligustici Wallichii* and *Raidx Angelicae Sinensis*, while Xinyue capsule is made from the total saponin of stem and leaves of Genseng. Both

Xinyue capsule and Chuanxiong capsule have been approved by state food and drug administration as the Chinese herbal patents for CHD patients for more than 5 years and listed in Chinese Pharmacopoeia. In the present study, Xinyue capsules were provided by Yisheng Pharmaceutical Company, Jilin Province, China, 0.3g per capsule (approved document number:

Table 1 Comparison of Baseline Characteristics between Groups

Items	CMG (50 cases)	WMG (50 cases)	P value
Sex (Male/female)	45/5	44/6	0.75
Smoking (cases)	32	28	0.54
CHD family history (cases)	13	11	0.64
Hypertension history (cases)	34	37	0.51
Hyperlipidemia history (cases)	17	21	0.41
Diabetes history (cases)	12	14	0.65
Stoke history (cases)	7	5	0.64
UA (cases)	19	18	0.84
STEMI (cases)	26	25	0.85
NSTEMI (cases)	5	7	0.54
NYHA Ⅰ (cases)	15	16	0.83
NYHA Ⅱ (cases)	20	18	0.68
NYHA Ⅲ (cases)	12	14	0.65
NYHA Ⅳ (cases)	3	2	0.65
Single coronary artery vessel disease (cases)	7	6	0.77
Double coronary artery vessel disease (cases)	24	22	0.69
Multiple vessel disease (cases)	19	22	0.54
Intervention of LAD in PCI (cases)	25	27	0.69
Intervention of LCX in PCI (cases)	9	11	0.62
Intervention of RCA in PCI (cases)	15	12	0.50
Intervention of left main coronary in PCI (cases)	1	0	0.31
Wall motion abnormality (cases)	28	27	0.84
Mean age (yr)	61.68±7.64	62.78±8.60	0.50
Height (cm)	169.50±10.25	168.78±12.49	0.90
Weight (kg)	74.58±13.25	79.77±9.86	0.41
CK-MB (U/L)	135.29±19.33	129.38±28.17	0.22
cTnT (ng/mL)	4.97±3.32	4.34±2.98	0.32
TC (mmol/L)	4.26±1.07	4.21±1.01	0.79
TG (mmo/L)	1.53±0.83	1.85±1.53	0.20
LDL (mmol/L)	2.50±0.96	2.30±0.89	0.31
ALT (U/L)	38.98±3.40	35.88±3.60	0.53
AST (U/L)	116.84±22.10	84.57±18.47	0.26
Cr (mmol/L)	75.16±21.44	82.28±34.57	0.22
UA (mmol/L)	356.67±83.97	351.82±79.15	0.77

第三章

第三章

Z20030073); Chuanxiong capsules were provided by Fenghuang Pharmaceutical Corporation, Shandong Province, China, 0.37g per capsule (approved document number: Z20000035).

1.7 Items of Investigation

CM symptom scores and blood stasis syndrome scores: the scores were calculated at baseline, 6 months and 1 year after PCI. According to the medical history, symptoms, tongue and pulse, three experienced clinicians did syndrome differentiation and scores, and then the average scores were taken into analysis.

Heart function: NYHA functional class and UCG were recorded at baseline, 6 months and 1 year after PCI. The NYHA functional class of the patients was classified by three experienced clinicians to get unanimous conclusion. Data of UCG for the patients were collected by fixed technician using Siemens Sequia 512 color ultrasound diagnostic apparatus with the probe frequency in 4.25 MHz. Standard four chambers of heart and left ventricular long axis views were measured in the method of Simposon[9]. Systolic and diastolic amplitude of the left ventricular and left ventricular end-diastolic (LVEDD) were measured with digital recorder. Left ventricular end-diastolic volume (LVEDV) , left ventricular end-systolic volume (LVESV) , inter-ventricular septal thickness (IVST) , left ventricular posterior wall thickness (LVPWT) were detected by area-length. Wall motion were analyzed with the method of 16 segment recommended by the United States Institute of UCG[10]. Regional wall motion abnormality scores were calculated as described previously[11].

N-terminal pro-brain natriuretic peptide (NT-proBNP) and hyper-sensitivity C-reactive protein (hs-CRP) : the levels of NT-proBNP and hs-CRP in plasma were measured at baseline, 6 months and 1 year in the present study. The 3 mL peripheral venous blood from median cubital vein was immediately placed in EP tubes; subsequently the EP tubes were put in the centrifugal machine (Sigma3k-30) and were centrifuged for 15 minutes with 3000 rpm. After that, the supernatants were drawn into the new EP tubes and were placed in $-70\,^{\circ}\text{C}$ refrigerator for the measurement. In accordance with the instructions of the NT-proBNP-ELISA (F00232, the ShangHai Xi Tang Corporation) and hs-CRP-ELISA (F00451, the ShangHai Xi Tang Corporation) , serum concentrations of NT-proBNP and hs-CRP were detected with double-antibody sandwich ABC-ELISA.

1.8 Definition of Major Adverse Cardiovascular Events

The MACE was defined in the present study as cardiovascular death, recurrent AMI, recurrent angina, revascularization, cardiogenic shock, heart failure, malignant arrhythmia and stroke. Telephone and outpatient follow-up were performed for the MACE with once a week and once a month, respectively.

1.9 Statistical Analysis

Analysis of data for all enrolled patients were performed in use of SPSS (version 13.0) software. Continuous variables were presented as mean ± standard deviation, and compared in use of Student's t-test in normal distribution, corrected t-test or rank sum test in abnormal distribution. Categorical variables were presented as constituent rate or ratio and were compared with the use of Chi-square test. A two-side alpha level of 0.05 was used for all testing. P-values of less than 0.05 were considered to indicate statistical significance.

2. Results

2.1 Comparisons of NYHA Functional Class between Groups

There were no significant difference in cases of NYHA functional class in both groups at baseline, 6 months, and 1 year follow-up ($P > 0.05$). It was notable that P value was 0.054 when comparing cases of NYHA functional class between CMG and WMG at 1 year with the use of Chi-square test, which suggested that there was a more improved tendency of NYHA functional class in CMG than that in WMG (Table 2).

Table 2 Comparisons of NYHA Function Class between Groups (Cases)

Group	Cases	Time	NYHA function class			
			I	II	III	IV
CMG	50	Baseline	15	2	12	3
		6 months	38	11	0	1
		1 year	45	4	0	1
WMG	50	Baseline	16	18	14	2
		6 months	27	20	1	2
		1 year	36	11	2	1

2.2 Comparisons of CM Symptom Scores and Blood Stasis Syndrome Scores between Groups

CM syndrome scores and blood stasis scores of the patients in both groups at 6 months and at 1 year follow-up were less than that at the baseline ($P < 0.01$). There were no significant difference in CM syndrome scores and blood stasis scores of the patients in both groups between at 6 months and at 1 year follow-up ($P > 0.05$). CM syndrome scores and blood stasis scores of the patients in CMG were less than that in WMG at 6 months and at 1 year follow-up ($P < 0.01$) (Table 3).

Table 3 Comparisons of CM Symptom Scores and Blood Stasis Syndrome Scores between Groups ($\bar{\chi} \pm s$)

Group	Cases	Time	Scores	
			Symptom	Blood stasis
CMG	50	Baseline	20.82 ± 5.88	22.98 ± 7.40
		6 months	$2.45 \pm 1.89^{*\triangle}$	$5.67 \pm 2.33^{*\triangle}$
		1 year	$1.92 \pm 0.90^{*\triangle}$	$4.98 \pm 2.07^{*\triangle}$
WMG	50	Baseline	19.00 ± 6.14	19.94 ± 10.42
		6 months	$4.86 \pm 3.85^{*}$	$8.47 \pm 5.09^{*}$
		1 year	$3.53 \pm 2.97^{*}$	$7.25 \pm 4.11^{*}$

Notes: *$P < 0.01$, compared with the baseline; $\triangle P < 0.01$, compared with the WMG

2.3 Comparisons of Heart Function Indexes of UCG between Groups

LVEDV、LVESV and VWM of the patients determined by UCG in both groups at 6 months and at 1 year follow-up were lower than that at the baseline ($P < 0.01$). There were no significant difference in LVEDV, LVESV and VWM in both groups between at 6 months and at 1 year ($P > 0.05$). LVEDV, LVESV and VWM in CMG were lower than that in WMG at 6 months and at 1 year follow-up ($P < 0.05$). LVEF of the patients in both groups at 6 months and at 1 year follow-up were higher than that at the baseline ($P < 0.01$). There was no significant difference in LVEF in both groups between at 6 months and at 1 year follow-up ($P > 0.05$). LVEF in CMG was higher than that in WMG at 6 months and at 1 year follow-up ($P < 0.01$) (Table 4).

2.4 Comparisons of the Serum Levels of NT-proBNP and hs-CRP between Groups

The serum levels of NT-proBNP and hs-CRP of the patients in both groups at 6 months and at 1 year were lower than that at the baseline ($P < 0.01$). There were no significant difference in the serum levels of NT-proBNP and hs-CRP in both groups between at 6 months and at 1 year follow-up ($P > 0.05$). The serum levels of NT-proBNP and hs-CRP of the patients in CMG were lower than that in WMG at 6 months and at 1 year follow-up ($P < 0.05$) (Table 5).

2.5 Comparisons of the Incidence of MACE between Groups

At 1-year follow-up, there was no case of death or cardiogenic shock, three patients had recurrent myocardial infarction, three cases recurrent angina pectoris, five cases of heart failure, two cases of malignant arrhythmia, 1 case of stroke. There was no significant difference of single events between two groups ($P > 0.05$); however, the overall MACE rate in CMG was significantly lower than that in WMG ($P < 0.05$); the relative risk (RR) was 0.2727, and 95% confidence interval (CI) was 0.0899-0.8276, $P = 0.0218$ (Table 6).

Table 4 Comparisons of Heart Function Indexes of UCG between Groups ($\bar{\chi} \pm s$)

Group	Cases	Time	LVEDV (mm)	LVESV (mm)	IVST (mm)	LVPWT (mm)	LVEF (%)	VWMI
CMG	50	Baseline	61.77±6.58	40.44±5.22	9.90±1.45	9.71±1.11	49.17±8.81	5.52±1.03
		6 months	50.62±7.89*△	32.34±3.57*△	9.74±2.01	9.47±2.37	65.62±5.15*△△	3.89±1.67*△
		1 year	48.30±8.43*▲	30.88±4.30*▲	9.88±2.44	9.55±2.03	67.88±6.97*▲▲	3.01±2.77*▲
WMG	50	Baseline	62.25±6.50	41.86±6.84	10.11±4.68	9.84±1.50	49.43±9.11	5.47±1.21
		6 months	53.67±7.33*	35.78±4.10*	9.98±3.76	9.78±2.48	58.45±6.47*	4.56±1.93*
		1 year	51.24±5.70*	33.76±6.78*	9.89±4.01	9.86±2.17	60.98±4.01*	3.97±1.04*

Notes: *$P < 0.01$, compared with the baseline at 6 months and 1 year; △$P < 0.05$, △△$P < 0.01$, compared with the WMG at 6 months; ▲$P < 0.05$, ▲▲$P < 0.01$, compared with the WMG at 1 year

Table 5 Comparisons of the Serum Level of NT-proBNP and hs-CRP between Groups ($\bar{\chi} \pm s$)

Group	Cases	Time	NT-proBNP (pg/mL)	hs-CRP (mg/L)
CMG	50	Baseline	661.69±445.39	18.87±8.24
		6 months	225.37±176.54*△	6.60±3.12*△
		1 year	169.27±129.88*△	5.51±2.77*△
WMG	50	Baseline	715.43±409.01	19.34±7.53
		6 months	302.12±189.03*	8.32±4.38*
		1 year	223.32±116.54*	6.87±3.21*

Notes：*$P < 0.01$，compared with the baseline；△$P < 0.01$, compared with the WMG

Table 6 Comparisons of the Incidence of MACE between Groups [Cases（%）]

MACE	CMG	WMG	P value
Cardiovascular death	0	0	—
Recurrent myocardial infarction	0	3（6）	0.08
Recurrent angina pectoris	1（2）	2（4）	0.56
Heart failure	1（2）	4（8）	0.17
Malignant arrhythmia	1（2）	1（2）	1.00
Cardiogenic shock	0	0	—
Stoke	0	1（2）	0.32
Others	0	0	—
Total	3（6）	11（22）	0.02

3. Discussion

Heart function is an important prognostic factor for ACS patients; heart failure may result in a significant increase of risk of MACE such as cardiovascular death, cardiogenic shock, recurrent myocardial infarction and malignant arrhythmia. The main reasons which seriously influence heart function in patients with ACS after successful PCI are no-reflow (NR) phenomenon or VR pathological process. Some studies have found that about 5% to 50% of STEMI patients received coronary artery reperfusion in epicardium but had no myocardial reperfusion, and the proportion of occurring heart failure in these patients increased significantly[12, 13]. A growing body of evidence also demonstrated that long-term VR after successful revascularization commonly leads to heart dysfunction[14]. Thus, how to effectively protect heart function from ischemic injury is a key problem for improving prognosis in patients with ACS.

LVEF is the most widely used as the indicator of heart function. Lang, et al[15]. found that LVEF < 45% was associated with the incidence of MACE in patients with ACS. Wall motion abnormality is a sensitive index reflecting myocardial ischemia, analysis of which is commonly used to evaluate the heart function. Naresh et al[16]. found that 68% of the patients had wall motion abnormality in the clinical trial that enrolled 226 patients with ACS. The higher VWMI was, the worse the heart function of the patients and the greater risk of occurring MACE. A study that enrolled 767 patients with AMI found that VWMI is an independent predictor of death and hospitalization due to heart failure, being similar with LVEF, cTnT and CK-MB in prognosis[17]. BNP is a peptide hormone which mainly originated from the ventricles and has a high specificity and sensitivity to the left ventricular function. NT-proBNP is a precursor of BNP's N-terminal and commonly examined for patients to represent the BNP level due to its more stability, longer half-life and better reflecting the activation of natriuretic peptide pathway. The elevated NT-proBNP level is in accordance with the severity of myocardial injury and cardiac dysfunction. Several clinical studies such as OPUS-TIMI 16, TACTICS-TIMI 18, FRISC- Ⅱ, and PRISM found that the serum levels of BNP or NT-proBNP suggested an accurate predictor for the death or heart failure of patients with ACS[18-20]. hs-CRP is the CRP detecting with ultra-sensitive technique. CRP is a strong biomarker of inflammation to predict cardiovascular events in patients with ACS and it is also directly involved in the pathological process of ACS. The elevated CRP level is related to the complex and multi-vessel lesions[21]. A meta-analysis by Li-ping He showed that the rates of MACE in ACS patients with CRP 3.1-10.0 mg/L and > 10.0 mg/L were 1.40 times and 2.18 times respectively more than that in patients with CRP ≤ 3.0 mg/L, which showed that the CRP level was a sensitive predictor of prognosis in patients with ACS[22].

Our previous studies have shown that Chinese herbal medicine for supplementing qi, nourishing yin and activating blood circulation had a beneficial treatment effect on myocardial ischemia and its metabolism[23]; however, there have been rare reports about whether it could improve heart function and the prognosis of patients with ACS in combination with routine western medicine treatment. The present study recruited 100 patients with ACS after successful PCI to investigate the effects of Xinyue capsule and Chuanxiong capsule in addition to the conventional western medicine. During 1-year follow-up, the study showed that CM symptom score, blood stasis score, heart function index of UCG, and serum levels of NT-proBNP and hs-CRP were all improved from the baseline ($P < 0.05$, $P < 0.01$) in CMG and its effects were better than that in WMG ($P < 0.05$). In addition, primary endpoints defined the total incidence of MACE in CMG was significantly lower than that in WMG ($P < 0.05$). Although there was no significant difference in NYHA functional class between both groups at all follow-up time point, which has a trend at 1 year follow-up ($P = 0.054$), it implied that improvement of NYHA functional class in CMG was better than WMG. Analysis of RR showed that MACE rate was related with the combination treatment of Chinese herbal medicine for supplementing qi, nourishing yin and activating blood circulation which suggested that treatment with Xinyue capsule and Chuanxiong capsule in addition to conventional western medicine could significantly improve heart function and the clinical symptoms, and reduce the incidence of MACE in patients with ACS during 1 year after PCI. The present clinical study was conducted in a prospective, randomized, controlled valuator and data handler-blinded design, which is the first clinical trial about the treatment with Chinese herbal medicine (Xinyue capsule and Chuanxiong capsule) for supplementing qi, nourishing yin and activating blood circulation in addition to conventional western medicine and showed beneficial effects on improvement of 1-year prognosis in patients with ACS after PCI; therefore, our present clinical study provided certain evidence for guiding further clinical practice.

During the 1-year follow-up, secondary endpoints such as recurrent myocardial infarction or angina, heart failure, arrhythmia, cardiogenic shock, and stroke that happened in two groups had no significant difference ($P > 0.05$), which may be relevant to the short follow-up period and small sample size. Furthermore, the recruited patients of the present study were limited in the region of Shanghai, which may have regional bias.

References

[1] Antman EM, Anbe DT, Armstrong PW, et al. ACC/AHA guidelines for the management of patients with ST-elevation myocardial infarction—executive summary. A report of the American College of Cardiology/American Heart Association Task Force on Practice Guidelines (Writing Committee to revise the 1999 guidelines for the management of patients with acute myocardial infarction). J Am Coll Cardiol, 2004, 44: 671-719.

[2] Ferrari R. Perindopril and Remodeling in Elderly with Acute Myocardial Infarction Investigators. Effects of angiotensin-converting enzyme inhibition with perindopril on left ventricular remodeling and clinical outcome: results of the randomized perindopril and remodeling in elderly with acute myocardial infarction (PREAMI) study. Arch Intern Med, 2006, 166: 659-666.

[3] Su CL, Shen SG. Modern cardiology of CM. BeiJing: Beijing Science and Technology Press, 1997, 61-65.

[4] Chinese Society of Cardiology in Chinese Medical Association, Editorial Board of Chinese Journal of Cardiology. Diagnosis and treatment recommendations of unstable angina. Chin J Cardiol, 2000, 28: 409-412.

[5] Chinese Society of Cardiology in Chinese Medical Association, Editorial Board of Chinese Journal of Cardiology, Editorial Board of Chinese Journal of Circulation. Diagnosis and treatment recommendations of acute myocardial infarction. Chin J Cardiol, 2001, 29: 705-720.

[6] Committee of Cardiovascular Disease in China Society of Integrated Traditional Chinese and Western Medicine. Standard of syndrome differentiation of coronary heart disease in Chinese medicine. Chin J Integr Tradit West Med, 1991, 11: 257.

[7] Wang J, Chen KJ, Weng WL, et al. Research on the diagnostic criteria of blood-stasis symptom-complex. Chin J Integr Tradit West Med, 1988, 10: 580-585.

[8] Chen ZJ, Gao RL. Studies on clinical coronary heart disease. BeiJing: People's Medical Publishing House, 2002: 381-405.

[9] Wang XF. Ultrasound echocardiography. BeiJing: People's medical publishing house, 2002: 456-458.

[10] Eigenbaum H. Echocardiography. Ed 4. Philadelphia: Lea and Febiger, 1986, 462-513.

[11] Møller JE, Hillis GS, Oh JK, et al. Wall motion score index and ejection fraction for risk stratification after acute myocardial infarction. Am Heart J, 2006, 151: 419-425.

[12] Shereif H. Rezkalla, Robert AK. No-reflow phenomenon. Circulation, 2002, 105: 656-662.

[13] Gong X, Yang J, Fang YM. No-reflow phenomenon following reperfusion in acute myocardial infarction. Medical Recapitulate, 2006, 12: 480-482.

[14] Dzavík V, Buller CE, Lamas GA, et al. Randomized trial of percutaneous coronary intervention for subacute infarct-related coronary artery occlusion to achieve long-term patency and improve ventricular function: the Total Occlusion Study of Canada (TOSCA) -2 trial. Circulation, 2006, 114: 2449-2457.

[15] Lang RM, Bierig M, Devereux RB, et al. Recommendations for chamber quantification. Eur J Echocardiogr, 2006, 7: 79-108.

[16] Ranjith N, Pegoraro RJ, Naidoo DP, et al. The role of echocardiography and its comparison with NT-proBNP measurements in patients with acute myocardial infarction. Med Sci Monit, 2007, 13: CR574-578.

[17] Biagini E, Galema TW, Schinkel AF, et al. Myocardial wall thickness predicts recovery of contractile function after primary coronary intervention for acute myocardial infarction. J Am Coll Cardiol, 2004, 43: 1489-1493.

[18] Olsen MH, Wachtell K, Nielsen OW, et al. N-terminal brain natriuretic peptide predicted cardiovascular events stronger than high-sensitivity C-reactive protein in hypertension: a LIFE substudy. J Hypertens, 2006, 24: 1531-1539.

[19] Jernberg T, Stridsberg M, Venge P, et al. N-terminal pro brain natriuretic peptide on admission for early risk stratification of patients with chest pain and no ST-segment elevation. J Am Coll Cardiol, 2002, 40: 437-445.

[20] FRISC-II Study Group. Invasive compared with non-invasive treatment in unstable coronaryartery disease: FRISC II prospective randomised multicentre study. Fragmin and fast revascularisation during instability in coronary artery disease Investigators. Lancet, 1999, 354: 708-715.

[21] Abbate A, Biondi-Zoccai GG, Brugaletta S, et al. C-reactive protein and other inflammatory biomarkers as predictors of outcome following acute coronary syndromes. Semin Vasc Med, 2003, 3: 375-384.

[22] He LP, Tang XY, Ling WH, et al. Early C-reactive protein in the prediction of long-term outcomes after acute coronary syndromes: a meta-analysis of longitudinal studies. Heart, 2010, 96: 339-346.

[23] Li YQ, Jin M, Qiu SL, Wang PL, et al. Effect of Chinese drugs for supplementing Qi, nourishing Yin and activating blood circulation on myocardial perfusion in patients with acute myocardial infarction after revascularization. Chin J Integr Med, 2009, 15: 19-25.

Clinical Outcomes and Cost-Utility after Sirolimus-Eluting versus Bare Metal Stent Implantation[*]

ZHAO Fu-hai　LÜ Shu-zheng　LI Hui　NING Shang-qiu　YUAN Fei　SONG Xian-tao　JIN Ze-ning　ZHOU Yuan　CHEN Xin　LIU Hong　TIAN Rui　MENG Kang　LI Hong　HAN Feng

Lately drug-eluting stent (DES) has dramatically reduced restenosis rate and need for repeated revascularization in a wide subset of lesions and patients, and it nearly becomes the default selection for most of the percutaneous coronary intervention (PCI) procedure[1]. However, a rising amount of reports concerning DES describe the occurrence of late or very late in-stent thrombosis, even restenosis after the conventional follow-up[2-4]. Still published study showed that insignificant difference of major cardiac adverse events (MACE) occurred irrespective of whether DES or bare metal stent (BMS) implanted[5]. The decision to use DES has large economic implication. Studies showed that the use of sirolimus-eluting stent (SES) was associated with a significant incremental cost along with prolonged clopidogrel therapy.

Moreover, data suggested compared with medication, a comparable improvement in several scales of health-related quality of life (HRQOL) on patients who underwent PCI occurs[6]. Given the repeated findings of little or no difference in mortality outcomes between PCI with or without stent and coronary artery bypass graft surgery, it is necessary to assess HRQOL outcomes between DES and BMS.

Currently few data concern about clinical outcomes, HRQOL and cost in angina pectoris patients who implanted SES or BMS. We conducted a prospective, multi-center trial to address this important issue for the treatment of native *de novo* coronary artery lesion in China.

1. Methods

1.1　Study Design and Patient Population

* 原载于 Chinese Medical Journal，2010，123（20）：2797-2802

183

This was a prospective, nonrandomized, multi-center registry study. This study evaluated data collected from 1241 patients who participated in the study of PCI *status quo* for coronary heart disease and reimbursement method by basic medical insurance fund implanted SES, and patients who implanted BMS from two tertiary hospitals. The study protocol conforms to the principles of the Declaration of Helsinki and was approved by the Ethics Committee. Patients who were at least 18 years old and less than 75 years old were eligible for coronary revascularization if they had stable angina (Canadian Cardiovascular Society class), unstable angina (Braunwald's class), or silent ischemia, and the lesion located in the different major epicardial vessel with diameter ranging from 2.25 mm to 4.0 mm. All the DES exclusively was SES (Cypher, Cordis, Johnson & Johnson, USA), and BMS had no special assignment.

1.2　Exclusion Criteria

Patients with left ventricular dysfunction (ejection fraction < 30%), recent non-Q and Q-wave myocardial infarction (MI) (< 1month), history of renal insufficiency (serum creatinine level 2.5 mg/dL), left main stenosis, in-stent restenosis, coagulation disorders, thrombopenia, hypersensitivity or allergy to aspirin and/or clopidogrel, short life expectancy (< 2 years) were excluded.

1.3　Definition and Endpoints

The aim of our study was to determine composite cumulative MACE. The primary endpoints include death from any causes, acute MI, in-stent thrombosis, recurrent angina and cardiovascular rehospitalization. The second endpoints include HRQOL and costs after PCI procedure. Non-Q-wave MI was defined according to World Health Organization definition: increase of total creatine kinase (CK) two times or more the upper limit of normal range with an elevated MB isoform level without development of new Q waves. A Q-wave MI was present when, in addition to CK elevation, there were new Q waves in at least two leads. In all patients, CK and CK-MB were evaluated two times after the procedure or until normalization if they were elevated. All end points were reviewed by an independent clinical events committee that was blinded to treatment assignment.

1.4　Procedure and Post-intervention Medications

All interventions were performed according to current standard guidelines, and the final interventional strategies were left entirely to the discretion of the operator. All patients were advised to maintain lifelong aspirin 100 mg per day use. Clopidogrel 75 mg daily was to be started at least 24 hours before the procedure, if the time to procedure less than 6-8 hours, 300 mg loaded dosage was prescribed, less than 2 hours, 600 mg loaded, and lasted for at least 9 months for whom implanted SES, and 3 months for those implanted BMS. Concomitant medication such as beta-blockade, statins, angiotensin-converting enzyme inhibitor (ACEI) and nitrates were prescribed according to the American College of Cardiology (ACC) /American Heart Association (AHA) recommended guidelines.

1.5　Assessment of HRQOL

HRQOL was assessed by using the physical and mental health summary scales of the medical outcomes study short-form survey (SF-36). This survey contains 36 questions to measure eight health constructs. Physical component summary (PCS) reflecting overall physical status, consists of physical functioning, physical role functioning, bodily pain and general health; mental component summary (MCS) reflecting overall mental health status, consists of vitality, social functioning, emotional role functioning and mental health. Higher scores indicated better health.

1.6　Cost Methodology

We adopted a health service perspective and calculated total cost for PCI procedure and overheads, post-procedure services and follow-up expenditure. Pre-PCI costs were excluded. Variable and fixed direct costs were obtained for each care area according to the activity-based costing methodology and included stent, medication, disposables, medical equipment utilization and clinical support services such as nursing care, therapeutic cost, radiology and laboratory services. Follow-up cost was also calculated to include any medication, laboratory test, revascularization and readmission within 12 months' investigation. Cost unit was calculated as Yuan (Renminbi, RMB).

1.7 Follow-up

Clinical follow-up was obtained by direct phone-call with the subject or subject's visit at one, three, six, nine and twelve months. Baseline and nine-month HRQOL were evaluated by the professional staff. Angiographic follow-up was not assigned after stenting unless clinically indicated or at the patient's request.

1.8 Statistical Analysis

Continuous variables are expressed as mean ± standard deviation or median. Categorical variables are expressed as frequencies and percentages. Fisher's exact test was used for discrete variables and analysis of variance (ANOVA) for continuous variables. Baseline and follow-up SF-36 scores were compared using repeated measurement variables analysis of variance. Kaplan-Meier analysis was used to estimate the cumulative rate of survival. Groups were compared by the log-rank test. All tests of significance were two-tailed. We chose a significance level of 0.05. All the data were analyzed using SPSS statistical packagel 3.0 (SPSS Inc., USA).

2. Results

2.1 Baseline Characteristics

Enrollment was started from May 2005, and 1241 patients with *de novo* native lesions undergoing PCI met the inclusion criteria, and signed the written informed consent. In total, 609 patients underwent placement of a BMS and 632 patients for SES. The study finished in July 2007. Follow-up was completed in 1205 (97.1%) patients. The baseline characteristics

of the patients in the two groups were similar except for a higher prevalence of prior PCI in the SES group. Moreover the BMS group had higher body mass index (BMI), total cholesterol (TC), low density lipoprotein-cholesterol (LDL-C) level and larger left ventricular end diastolic diameter (LVEDD) compared to that of SES patients (Table 1).

2.2 Concomitant Medical Therapy

The hospitalization medication usage was similar in the two groups, except for higher rates of heparin and ACEI in the SES group and low molecular weight heparin in the BMS group. Dual anti-platelet therapy with aspirin and clopidogrel was prescribed to more than 99% of successful PCI patients in the two groups (Table 2). However, clopidogrel was used for 57% patients in the SES group and 3% in those of BMS patients at 12-month follow-up, aspirin 78% and 76% in the SES and BMS group, $P = 0.37$, respectively during 12-month follow-up (Table 2).

2.3 Angiographic and PCI Procedure Data

Total of 1570 stents were implanted for 1334 lesions. The involved target vessel, lesion type, access site of artery, contrast medium, proportion of complete revascularization were similar in the two groups, except for a higher PCI procedure time in the BMS group (the BMS group *vs.* the SES group (62.74 ± 33.27) minutes *vs.* (52.15 ± 33.43) minutes, $P = 0.001$) (Table 3).

2.4 Primary Outcome

The primary outcomes for all patients are shown in Table 4, Figure 1 and Figure 2. Rates of MI, death from both cardiovascular and non-cardiovascular causes were similar between the two groups. Angiography confirmed stent thrombosis was found in 3 (0.48%) and 5 (0.79%) in the BMS and SES group respectively ($P = 0.09$). Significant difference was found at cardiovascular rehospitalization (136 (22.4%) *vs.* 68 (10.76%), $P = 0.001$) and recurrent angina (149 (24.5%) *vs.* 71 (11.3%), $P = 0.001$) between the BMS and SES groups. The 1-year cumulative survival for death was similar in the two groups (log rank=3.288, P=0.07). No significant difference of the 1-year

Table 1 Baseline Demographic and Clinical Characteristics

Variables	BMS group (n=609)	SES group (n=632)	P value
Age (mean (SD))	58.97 (10.09)	59.41 (10.28)	0.591
Male (n (%))	465 (76.3)	501 (79.2)	0.394
Current smoke (n (%))	294 (48.3)	307 (45.8)	0.517
Prior hypertension (n (%))	369 (60.6)	365 (57.8)	0.484
Prior diabetes mellitus (n (%))	140 (23.0)	123 (19.5)	0.278
Prior hypertriglycerin (n (%))	213 (35.0)	185 (29.2)	0.116
Prior hypercholesterol (n (%))	192 (31.5)	162 (25.6)	0.096
Prior cerebral infarction (n (%))	48 (7.9)	30 (4.8)	0.111
Prior renal failure (n (%))	2 (0.3)	8 (1.3)	0.214
Prior angina pectoris (n (%))	356 (58.4)	396 (62.6)	0.274
Prior CABG (n (%))	0 (0)	10 (1.6)	0.453
Prior PCI (n (%))	46 (7.6)	97 (15.3)	0.002
Old myocardial infarction (n (%))	92 (15.1)	111 (17.6)	0.410
BMI (mean (SD))	25.61 (3.71)	24.89 (3.91)	0.019
SBP (mmHg，mean (SD))	132.36 (19.08)	131.26 (18.55)	0.462
DBP (mmHg，mean (SD))	79.65 (12.60)	79.48 (11.61)	0.866
Heart rate (beats/min，mean (SD))	72.25 (11.64)	73.72 (11.24)	0.109
Creatinine (5mol/L，mean (SD))	86.89 (34.77)	87.63 (27.84)	0.479
Blood glucose (mmol/L，mean (SD))	6.22 (2.40)	6.30 (11.70)	0.909
Total cholesterol (mmol/L，mean (SD))	4.78 (1.11)	4.48 (l.16)	0.001
LDL-cholestcrol (mmol/L，mean (SD))	2.99 (1.00)	2.63 (0.924)	0.010
HDL-cholesterol (mmol/L，mean (SD))	1.06 (0.25)	1.07 (0.42)	0.609
Ejection fraction (mean (SD))	0.61 (0.08)	0.62 (0.11)	0.347
LVEDD (mm，mean (SD))	48.09 (15.41)	44.78 (16.39)	0.002

CABG: coronary artery bypass graft; PCI: percutaneous coronary intervention; BMI: body mass index; SBP: systolic blood pressure;DBP: diastolic blood pressure; LVEDD: left ventricular end diastolic diameter

cumulative survival for MI was observed in the SES and BMS group (log rank=1.776, P = 0.188).

2.5 Secondary Outcomes

2.5.1 HRQOL Data. There was no significant difference in baseline characteristics between the two groups in SF-36 score, except for body pain in the BMS and SES group (51.3±20.0 vs. 52.6±23.0, P = 0.015), and social functioning (61.1±26.1 vs. 63.3±26.2, P = 0.003) during baseline investigation. At 9-month follow-up, dramatic improvement occurred in every item of SF-36 score, but no significant difference was found between the two groups. When compared the baseline and follow-up score intra-group, significant difference was found either in the SES or BMS group ($P < 0.001$, Table 5).

2.5.2 Cost Data Except for the total cost of revascularization (BMS vs. SES: 62 546.0 vs. 78 245.0 Yuan, P=0.001), index stent cost (24 150.0 vs. 43 345.0 Yuan, P=0.0001), at discharge, there was no significant difference in other index hospitalization cost between the two groups. The follow-up total expenditure was remarkably higher in the BMS group than that for the SES group (13 412.00 vs. 8812.00 Yuan, P = 0.000). The median medicine cost in the BMS group was 3280.00

Table 2 Medication on Hospitalization and Follow-up

Variables	BMS group (n=609)	SES group (n=632)	P value
In hospitalization (n (%))			
Nitrate	527 (86.5)	523 (82.7)	0.189
Aspirin	603 (99.0)	626 (99.0)	0.984
Clopidogrel	603 (99.0)	626 (99.0)	0.984
Beta-blockade	460 (75.6)	463 (73.2)	0.502
Calcium antagonism	196 (32.2)	200 (31.7)	0.904
Heparin	21 (4.5)	126 (20.9)	0.000
LM WH	478 (78.5)	399 (64.7)	0.001
Statin	533 (87.5)	562 (88.9)	0.268
Oral hypoglycemic agent	127 (20.9)	97 (15.3)	0.071
ACEI	319 (52.4)	381 (60.3)	0.048
GP IIb/IIIa	74 (12.1)	55 (8.7)	0.165
12-month follow-up (n (%))			
Aspirin	463 (76)	493 (78)	0.431
Clopidogrel	18 (3)	360 (57)	0.000

ACEI: angiotensin-converting enzyme inhibitor; LMWH: low molecular weight heparin; GP IIb/IIIa: glycoprotein IIb/IIIa blockers

Table 3 Baseline Angiographic Characteristics and Procedure

Variables	BMS group (n=609)	SES group (n=632)	P value
Reference vessel diameter (mm)			
LAD (mean (SD))	3.1 (1.5)	3.3 (3.0)	0.395
LCX (mean (SD))	2.7 (0.4)	2.9 (2.0)	0.391
RCA (mean (SD))	3.1 (0.5)	3.5 (0.7)	0.57
Single vessel lesion (n (%))	238 (39.1)	262 (41.4)	0.63
Two vessel lesion (n (%))	208 (34.1)	235 (37.1)	0.26
Triple vessel lesion (n (%))	163 (26.7)	175 (27.6)	0.23
Long lesion (n (%))	294 (48.3)	303 (47.9)	0.911
Bifurcation lesion (n (%a))	108 (17.8)	102 (16.1)	0.578
Chronic total occluded lesion (n (%))	118 (19.4)	119 (18.8)	0.849
Femoral artery access (n (%))	441 (72.4)	442 (70.0)	0.52
Radial artery access (n (%))	186 (30.6)	190 (30.0)	0.45
Average stent number (mean (SD))	1.61 (1.05)	1.58 (0.76)	0.15
Complete revascularization (n (%))	487 (80.0)	512 (81.0)	0.745
Procedure time (minutes，mean (SD))	62.74 (33.27)	52.15 (33.43)	0.001
Volume of contrast medium (L，mean (SD))	176.94 (69.40)	175.29 (78.58)	0.808

LAD: left anterior descending; LCX: left circumflex branch; RCA: right coronary artery

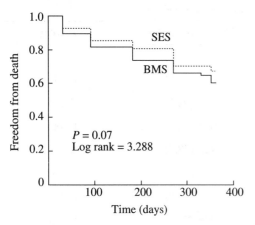

Figure 1 Kaplan-Meier Survival Curves for Patients' Freedom from Death Who Received a SES and Those Who Received a BMS

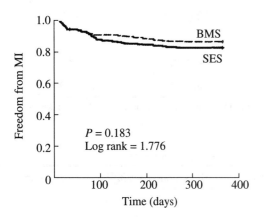

Figure 2 Kaplan-Meier Survival Curves for Patients' Freedom from MI Who Received a SES and Those Who Received a BMS

Table 4 Incidences of Death, Myocardial Infarction, Stent Thrombosis and Cardiac Rehospitalization after 365 Days of Follow-up [n (%)]

Endpoints	BMS group (n=609)	SES group (n=632)	P value
Death	7 (1.15)	6 (0.95)	0.07
Cardiac death	4 (0.66)	4 (0.63)	0.21
Non-cardiac death	3 (0.49)	2 (0.32)	0.13
MI	19 (3.12)	20 (3.16)	0.183
Angiographic confirmed stent thrombosis	3 (0.48)	5 (0.79)	0.09
Cardiovascular rehospitalization	136 (22.4)	68 (10.76)	0.001
Recurrent angina	149 (24.5)	71 (11.3)	0.001

Yuan, while 5831.00 Yuan in the SES group ($P = 0.000$, Table 6).

3. Discussion

In this study, we found equivalent clinical outcomes irrespective of BMS or SES in MACE except for higher cardiovascular rehospitalization and recurrent angina rates in the BMS group during 12-month follow-up. A numerous clinical trials investigated clinical outcomes and stent thrombosis (ST) included 3513 patients randomly assigned to DES or BMS. The 4-year target vessel revascularization rates were markedly reduced irrespective of whether SES or PES was used. In addition, the rate of death or infarction was not significantly different between DES and BMS. Of interest was the finding that although overall ST through 4 years was not different with DES versus BMS, beginning after 1 year ST was more frequent after DES. No significant differences in death or MI were observed[7-9]. In the BASKET LATE study, between 7 and 18 months of follow-up, the rates of nonfatal infarction and death were increased in the DES group although the absolute frequency was low[10]. An analysis of a large registry using propensity scores for stent type used comparing DES with BMS concluded that only high-risk patients had a marked benefit from DES[11,12]. Although no coronary angiographic follow-up, we deduced the higher proportion of cardiac rehospitalization and recurrent angina in BMS resulted from its inherited higher restenosis rate. However, published studies were performed in a very select patient group and substantial uncertainties remained regarding the safety and utility of DES in the "real-world" clinical practice.

The second endpoint of this study was to compare baseline and 9-month HRQOL outcomes for patients with angina who were implanted with SES versus BMS. Multiple previous studies have demonstrated improvements in HRQOL from pre- to post-procedure for both PCI and

Table 5　Comparison of SF-36 Between Baseline and 9-month Follow-up (mean (SD))

Variables	Baseline			9-month follow-up		
	BMS group (n=609)	SES group (n=632)	P value	BMS group (n=609)	SES group (n=632)	P value
PF	63.4 (25.2)	67.3 (31.9)	0.365	86.9 (11.6)	84.5 (12.4) [+]	0.339
RP	39.4 (44.1)	42.9 (47.6)	0.075	91.5 (22.0)*	89.6 (29.4) [+]	0.365
BP	51.3 (20.0)	52.6 (23.0)	0.015	83.9 (14.9)*	82.4 (15.3) [+]	0.635
GH	56.0 (17.9)	55.7 (21.3)	0.531	65.7 (16.7)*	64.1 (17.4) [+]	0.561
VT	59.9 (23.5)	57.4 (25.1)	0.324	77.5 (13.2)*	75.5 (12.8) [+]	0.208
SF	61.1 (26.1)	63.3 (26.2)	0.003	83.9 (17.6)*	82.8 (17.6) [+]	0.100
RE	61.8 (45.6)	67.3 (49.7)	0.400	94.5 (21.7)*	91.2 (27.1) [+]	0.394
MH	66.5 (23.8)	67.1 (26.0)	0.229	83.8 (9.5)*	82.5 (9.8) [+]	0.264
PCS	54.0 (19.9)	55.3 (24.3)	0.113	81.0 (11.2)*	79.0 (11.8) [+]	0.452
MCS	60.9 (22.1)	62.1 (23.8)	0.166	81.0 (10.8)*	79.2 (11.3) [+]	0.244

PF: physical functioning: RP: physical role functioning; BP: bodily pain; GH: general health; VT: vitality; SF: social functioning; RE: emotional role functioning; MH: mental health；PCS: physical component summary; MCS: mental component summary. *Notified intra-BMS group comparison, $P < 0.001$; [+]Notified intra-SES group comparison, $P < 0.001$

Table 6　Discharge and Follow-up Cumulative Cost in Two Groups

Variables	BMS group	SES group	P value
Index hospitalization			
Hospitalization day (mean (SD))	8.60 (4.59)	9.20 (5.33)	0.129
X-ray cost (Yuan，median)	570.00	585.00	0.17
Theraputic cost (Yuan，median)	239.95	239.61	0.594
Drug cost (Yuan，median)	3432.42	3430.89	0.629
Lab cost (Yuan，median)	584.00	591.00	0.42
Disposable material cost (Yuan，median)	15 009.07	14 128.91	0.059
Stent cost (Yuan，median)	24 150.00	43 345.00	0.0001
Total hospitalization cost (Yuan，median)	62 546.00	78 245.00	0.001
Follow-up			
Total cost (Yuan，median)	13 412.00	8812.00	0.000
Medication cost (Yuan，median)	3280.00	5831.00	0.000

CABG surgery[13-19]. The results of this study are consistent with the previously published trials when comes to the baseline and 9-month follow-up SF-36 score. In this study we found that both SES and BMS were effective in alleviating body pain and improvement of HRQOL during 9-month follow-up for known reasons. By hypothesis we know DES dramatically decreases the rate of restenosis and target vessel/lesion revascularization. Nevertheless the equivalent improvement of HRQOL was observed in the two groups. Interpreting this difference needed further clinical investigation.

We found that although the initial hospital cost was higher for the SES group, there was a significant difference in follow-up costs that favored the SES group. The median stent cost for SES is nearly 19 000 Yuan higher than that of BMS on discharge. Calculated costs for initial hospitalization, follow-up, and total costs for the SES in our study were similar to those reported in previously published analyses[20,21] that compared costs associated with use of DES and BMS. These studies found reasonable balance between costs and effects for SES as compared with BMS for both simple and complex coronary lesions. Basically, both previous studies analyzed all the resources used during initial interventions and at follow-up, including hospitalization days, different fees, and use of medical and other materials. In our study we focused on the MACE, initial and follow-up cost, but did not intend to analyse the target vessel/lesion revascularization rate. So we judiciously deduced that the increased cost in the BMS group was related to repeated revascularization during follow-up. On the other hand, the higher rate of cardiovascular rehospitalization and angina in this study was also attributed to increased cost in BMS.

There are several limitations needed to be mentioned in this study. First, as with any clinical trial, the results of our study may not be generalizable to the full population of PCI patients. Of particular, we did not analyze the relation of target lesion diameter and clinical outcomes. The performance of angiographic follow-up was not planned initially. So the proportion of revascularization in two groups was unknown. Second, our analysis was limited to a 1-year follow-up period. It seems that the cost-utility of SESs would be unfavorable with longer follow-up on account of very late in-stent thrombosis events. Third, we just simply compared the detailed costs in two groups, the cost utility and inflation-deflation factors were not considered. So our results may be compromised by the above limitations.

In conclusion, despite these limitations, the findings of the present analysis may have important implication. We prudently concluded there were no significant differences on death, in-scent thrombosis, MI irrespective of stent type within 12-month follow-up. SES was superior to BMS on improvement of life quality. SES showed more cost-utility compared with BMS.

References

[1] Maisel WH. Unanswered questions—drug-eluting stents and the risk of late thrombosis. N Engl J Med, 2007, 356: 981-984.

[2] Ong AT, McFadden EP, Regar E, et al. Late angiographic stent thrombosis (LAST) events with drug-eluting stents. J Am Coll Cardiol, 2005, 45: 2088-2092.

[3] Pfisterer M, Brunner-La Rocca HP, Buser PT, et al. for the BASKET-LATE Investigators. Late clinical events after clopidogrel discontinuation may limit the benefit of drug-eluting stents: an observational study of drug-eluting versus bare-metal stents. J Am Coll Cardiol, 2006, 48: 2584 -2591.

[4] Wessely R, Kastrati A, Schomig A. Late restenosis in patients receiving a polymer-coated sirolimus-eluting stent. Ann Intern Med, 2005, 143: 392-394.

[5] Quizhpe AR, Feres F, de Ribamar Costa J Jr, et al. Drug-eluting stents vs bare metal stents for the treatment of large coronary vessels. Am Heart J, 2007, 154: 373-378.

[6] Pocock SJ, Henderson RA, Clayton T, et al. Quality of life after coronary angioplasty or continued medical treatment for angina: three-year follow-up in the RITA-2 trial. J Am Coll Cardiol, 2000, 35: 907-914.

[7] Mauri L, Hsieh WH, Massaro JM, et al. Stent thrombosis in randomized clinical trials of drug-eluting stents. N Engl J Med, 2007, 356: 1020-1029.

[8] Stone GW, Moses JW, Ellis SGT, et al. Safety and efficacy of sirolimus and paclitaxel-eluting coronary stents. N Engl J Med, 2007, 356: 998-1008.

[9] Spaulding C, Daemen J, Boersma E, et al. A pooled analysis of data comparing sirolimus-eluting stents with bare-metal stents. N Engl J Med, 2007, 356: 989-997.

[10] Pfisterer M, Brunner-La Rocca HP, Buser PT, et al. Late clinical events after clopidogrel discontinuation may limit the benefit of drug-eluting stents: an observational study of drug-eluting versus bare-metal stents. J Am Coll Cardiol, 2006, 48: 2584-2591.

[11] Marzocchi A, Piovaccari G, Manari A, et al. Comparison of utility of sirolimus-eluting stents versus bare metal stents for percutaneous

coronary intervention in patients at high risk for coronary restenosis or clinical adverse events. Am J Cardiol, 2005, 95: 1409-1414.

[12] Brunner-La Rocca HP, Kaiser C, et al. Targeted stent use in clinical practice based on evidence from the Basel Stent Cost Utility Trial (BASKET). Eur Heart J, 2007, 28: 719-725.

[13] Strauss WE, Fortin T, Hartigan P, et al. A comparison of quality of life scores in patients with angina pectoris after angioplasty compared with after medical therapy. Veterans Affairs Study of Angioplasty Compared to Medical Therapy investigators. Circulation, 1995, 92: 1710-1719.

[14] Kiebzak GM, Pierson LM, Campbell M, et al. Use of the SF36 general health status survey to document health-related quality of life in patients with coronary artery disease: effect of disease and response to coronary artery bypass graft surgery. Heart Lung, 2002, 31: 207-213.

[15] Seto TB, Taira DA, Berezin R, et al. Percutaneous coronary revascularization in elderly patients: impact on functional status and quality of life. Ann Intern Med, 2000, 132: 955-958.

[16] Duits AA, Boeke S, Taams MA, et al. Prediction of quality of life after coronary artery bypass graft surgery: a review and evaluation of multiple, recent studies. Psychosom Med, 1997, 59: 257-268.

[17] Ayanian J, Guadagnoli E, Cleary P. Physical and psychosocial functioning of women and men after coronary artery bypass surgery. JAMA, 1995, 274: 1767-1770.

[18] Rumsfeld JS, Magid DJ, O' Brien M, et al. Changes in health-related quality of life following coronary artery bypass graft surgery. Ann Thorac Surg, 2001, 72: 2026-2032.

[19] Lii S, Liu W, Song X, et al. Effects of different therapies on coronary artery diseasese. Chin Med J, 2003, 116: 1341-1344.

[20] Cohen DJ, Bakhai A, Shi C, et al. Cost-utility of sirolimuseluting stents for treatment of complex coronary stenoses: results from the Sirolimus-Eluting Balloon Expandable Stent in the Treatment of Patients With De Novo Native Coronary Artery Lesions (SIRIUS) trial. Circulation, 2004, 110: 508-514.

[21] van Hout BA, Serruys PW, Lemos PA, et al. One year cost utility of sirolimus eluting stents compared with bare metal stents in the treatment of single native de novo coronary lesions: an analysis from the RAVEL trial. Heart, 2005, 91: 507-512.

第三章

A Multi-Center Randomized Double-Blind Placebo-Controlled Trial of Xiongshao Capsule in Preventing Restenosis after Percutaneous Coronary Intervention: A Subgroup Analysis of Senile Patients*

SHANG Qing-hua   XU Hao   LU Xiao-yan   WEN Chuan   SHI Da-zhuo   CHEN Ke-ji

Percutaneous coronary intervention (PCI), including percutaneous transluminal coronary angioplasty (PTCA) and intracoronary stent implantation, has become an effective method in the treatment of CHD. However, restenosis after PCI has been one of the major factors limiting the longterm efficacy of PCI. Studies in recent years show that drug-eluting stents could significantly lower the restenosis rate. However, it's not as optimistic as we expected for PCI patients in a "real-world" setting with regard to the clinical outcomes[1]. The elderly CHD patients often recover much slower after PCI operation, partly due to their complicated coronary lesions and comorbid conditions such as diabetes, and suffer from recurrent angina more frequently. Therefore, comprehensive intervention on the older post-PCI population needs to be further strengthened. In view of the pathologic process, restenosis falls into the category of "obstruction of heart vessel" and "stasis of blood circulation" in Chinese medicine (CM) theory. As our earlier experimental and clinical studies show, Xiongshao Capsule (芎芍胶囊 , XS), a Chinese herbal preparation with the effect of activating blood circulation (ABC), exhibited a beneficial effect on inhibiting restenosis after PCI[2-6]. On the basis of these preliminary results, we conducted a multicenter randomized double-blind placebo-controlled trial in accordance with the principle of evidence-based medicine (EBM) to further

demonstrate the efficacy and safety of the combination therapy of routine Western medicine and XS in preventing post-PCI restenosis[7]. This paper conducts a subgroup analysis of senile CHD patients in this clinical trial so as to provide evidences for the combination therapy of CM and Western medicine in the elderly CHD patients after PCI.

1. Methods

1.1 Diagnostic Standard

The diagnostic standard of CHD is formulated and referred to the report of Nomenclature and Criteria for Diagnosis of Ischemic Heart Disease issued by Joint International Society and Federation of Cardiology/World Health Organization task force on standardization of clinical nomenclature[8].

The successful PCI was defined as dilatation of the lesions with less than 50% residual stenosis and a more than 20% decrease in percent diameter stenosis with no major complications after PCI. Lesion specific classification of coronary artery referred to the standard formulated by ACC/AHA in 1988[9].

1.2 Patients Selection

1.2.1 Inclusion Criteria. Patients were included if they met all of the following criteria simultaneously: (1) 35 to 75 years old; (2) objective evidence of angina pectoris and/or myocardial ischemia; (3) at least one significant

* 原载于 Chinese Journal of Integrative Medicine，2011，17（9）：669-674

(> 50%) stenosis that was documented on a recent coronary angiogram; (4) patients treated successfully with PCI.

1.2.2 Exclusion Criteria. Patients were excluded if they met any of the following criteria: (1) restenosis lesion or graft vessel lesion; (2) chronic total occlusion lesion (> 3 months) ; (3) severe left main artery lesion; (4) severe heart failure (EF < 35%); (5) uncontrolled level Ⅲ hypertension; (6) severe valvular heart disease; (7) insulin-dependent diabetes mellitus; (8) diseases of hepatic, renal, hematologic and neurologic systems, psychological abnormalities, and malignancies; (9) patients who refuse to sign an informed consent form, or with expected poor compliance, and who are unlikely to participate angiographic follow-up; (10) participants of other clinical trials, and (11) women in pregnancy and lactation.

1.3 Sample Estimation

As previously described[7], to obtain the result of XS treatment with a statistically significant difference (two-side test, α = 0.05; β = 0.20) in 6 months, a minimum of 136 patients in each group would be needed. A total of 396 patients (198 in each group) were estimated for the study considering the exclusion of patients who failed to participate in angiographic follow-up and those who drop out of the trial.

1.4 General Information

A randomized double-blind, placebo-controlled trial was conducted at 5 hospitals, including Beijing Anzhen Hospital Affiliated to Capital Medical University, Beijing Tongren Hospital Affiliated to Capital Medical University, China-Japan Friendship Hospital, The Second Affiliated Hospital of Guangzhou University of Chinese Medicine, and Xiyuan Hospital of China Academy of Chinese Medical Sciences. With the aid of SAS software, 396 random numbers (001-396) were generated for randomized arrangement to 396 cases (treated or controlled), and medicine was issued based on the visit sequence of the subjects. To ensure an equal distribution of treatments in each center, a block randomization procedure on a site basis was used. All the subjects came from hospitalized patients. From June 2002 to December 2003, 335 patients were recruited and randomly assigned to either the XS group (regular treatment plus XS, 166 cases) or the placebo group (regular treatment plus placebo, 169 cases). During the period of 6-month clinical observation, 308 patients finished the trial as previously described [7], among which a total of 152 cases of elderly patients over 60 years old were included (73 cases in the XS group and 79 cases in the placebo group). There was no significant difference between the two groups with regard to general information, clinical history, diagnosis, and location and classification of coronary artery lesion. See Table 1 and 2 as follows.

1.5 Treatment Protocol

The clinical trial was conducted with the approval of the ethics committees of relevant hospitals and in strict accordance with the principles stipulated in Declaration of Helsinki and Guidelines for Good Clinical Practice.

1.5.1 PCI Procedure and Angiographic Analysis. The operation was conducted through femoral artery with routine methods. The coronary angiograms and PCI electronic data of all patients were preserved for further analysis. The imaging data collected were independently assessed in a blind fashion and analyzed with a computer-assisted quantitative coronary angiographic (QCA) analysis system (Cardio 500, Kontron Elektronik, Eching, Germany).

1.5.2 Drug Regimens. All patients received aspirin, ticlopidine, ditiazem, herbesser, nitroglycerin, heparin, etc., as routine administration before, during, and after the operation. Then the XS (consisting of Chuangxiongol and paeoniflorin) and the placebo were initiated on the day of PCI for both groups, taking 250 mg 3 times per day for 6 months. The patients participating in this trial had to sign informed consent forms and withdraw all the other Chinese herbal decoctions and

第三章

Table 1　General Information between the XS and the Placebo Group before PCI（%）

Item	XS group	Placebo group	P value
Cases	73	79	
Age (Year)	67.79 ± 4.77	66.70 ± 4.16	> 0.05
Male (%)	50 (68.5)	52 (65.8)	> 0.05
Height (cm)	165.03 ± 7.57	164.92 ± 7.30	> 0.05
Weight (kg)	70.33 ± 11.49	68.09 ± 9.98	> 0.05
Heart rate (times/min)	74.62 ± 10.94	73.86 ± 13.70	> 0.05
Systolic pressure (mmHg)	135.23 ± 20.85	134.03 ± 20.91	> 0.05
Diastolic pressure (mmHg)	80.89 ± 11.80	80.00 ± 11.12	> 0.05
Hypertension history (%)	47 (64.4)	48 (60.8)	> 0.05
Hyperlipidemia history (%)	16 (21.9)	17 (21.5)	> 0.05
Diabetes history (%)	19 (26.0)	20 (25.3)	> 0.05
Myocardial infarction history (%)	27 (37.0)	33 (41.8)	> 0.05
Diagnosis			
Stable angina	3 (4.1)	2 (2.5)	> 0.05
Unstable angina	48 (65.8)	47 (59.5)	> 0.05
Acute myocardial infarction	22 (30.1)	30 (38.0)	> 0.05

Table 2　Angiographic Data between the XS and the Placebo Group before PCI（%）

Item	XS group	Placebo group	P value
Vessel Distribution			
Right dominant pattern	61 (83.6)	63 (79.7)	> 0.05
Left dominant pattern	4 (5.5)	5 (6.3)	> 0.05
Balanced pattern	8 (11.0)	11 (13.9)	> 0.05
Number of vessels involved			
Single vessel lesion	32 (43.8)	33 (41.8)	> 0.05
Double vessel lesion	29 (39.7)	28 (35.4)	> 0.05
Triple vessel lesion	12 (16.4)	18 (22.8)	> 0.05
Coronary artery involved	100	108	
LAD	41 (41)	54 (50)	> 0.05
LCx	27 (27)	24 (22.2)	> 0.05
RCA	32 (32)	30 (27.8)	> 0.05
Types of vessel lesion*	123	125	
A	19 (15.4)	19 (15.2)	> 0.05
B1	62 (50.4)	73 (58.4)	> 0.05
B2	26 (21.1)	23 (18.4)	> 0.05
C	16 (13.0)	10 (8.0)	> 0.05
Stenosis (%)	86.97 ± 10.30	87.19 ± 10.36	> 0.05
Stenosis > 90%	73 (59.3)	76 (60.8)	> 0.05
PCI	127	134	
Stent implantation	113	126	> 0.05
Drug-eluting stent	10	14	> 0.05
PTCA	14	8	> 0.05

Notes: LAD: left anterior descending; LCx: left circumflex artery; RCA: right coronary artery

*Lesion-specific classification of coronary artery referred to the standard formulated by ACC/AHA in 1988

Chinese patent medicines. Patient compliance was monitored depending on the empty medicine bottles provided by the patients during the monthly clinic reexamination.

1.6 Clinical and Angiographic Endpoints

The angiographic endpoint of this study was restenosis defined as a residual stenosis of < 50% after angioplasty and subsequent aggravation to ≥ 50% during follow-up. The minimum lumen diameter (MLD) before and immediately after PCI as well as in the angiographic follow-up was also compared between the XS and the placebo group. The clinical end points were the combined incidence of death, nonfatal target lesion myocardial infarction, coronary artery bypass graft surgery (CABG), or repeat target-vessel angioplasty.

1.7 Clinical Follow-up

The clinical follow-ups were scheduled every month after PCI in clinic examination or through the telephone to determine the incidence of recurrent angina and adverse reactions. The safety indices including routine blood, urine and stool test, electrocardiogram, hepatic function (glutamic-pyruvic transamine, GPT) and renal function tests (blood urea nitrogen and creatine) were scheduled before and 6 months after PCI. An additional follow-up up to 12 months after PCI was conducted to assess the incidence of clinical endpoints.

1.8 Statistic Analysis

Statistical analysis was performed with SAS 6.12 software, and a statistical probability of < 0.05 was considered statistically significant. t test was used for comparison of measurement data; χ^2 test or Fisher exact test if necessary was used for comparison of enumeration data. Ridit and Wilcoxon tests were used for interclass ranked data and in-group ranked data, respectively.

2. Results

2.1 Comparison of the Angiographic Restenosis

Among the 152 cases that completed the clinical follow-up, 68 cases (44.74%) received an angiographic follow-up. The average angiographic follow-up duration was 218.41 ± 56.91 days in the XS group (37 cases) and 223.94 ± 76.40 days in the placebo group (31 cases, $P > 0.05$). Fewer patients who received XS treatment experienced restenosis (24.32%) in comparison to those who received placebo (38.71%) with no statistically significant difference ($P > 0.05$). The per lesion restenosis rate in the XS group also showed a decreasing tendency although without significant difference as compared with that in the placebo group (23.08% in the XS group *vs.* 31.91% in the placebo group, $P > 0.05$). The result was shown in Table 3.

Table 3　Comparison of the Angiographic Restenosis Rates

Group	Cases	Per patient restenosis (68)		Per lesion restenosis (112)	
		Cases	Restenosis rate (%)	Lesion	Restenosis rate (%)
XS	37	9	24.32	15	23.08
Placebo	31	12	38.71	15	31.91

2.2 Comparison of the MLD in Affected Vessels

There was no significant difference in the MLD before or immediately after PCI between the XS group and the placebo group (0.93 ± 0.59 mm *vs.* 0.95 ± 0.58 mm and 2.94 ± 0.59 mm *vs.* 2.88 ± 0.63 mm, respectively, $P > 0.05$). However, a significantly improved MLD was noted in the XS group at the follow-up measurement as compared with that in the placebo group (2.15 ± 0.84 mm *vs.* 1.73 ± 0.91 mm, $P < 0.05$), as shown in Table 4.

Table 4　Comparison of MLD in Affected Vessels (mm, $\bar{\chi} \pm s$)

Time	XS group	Placebo group
Before the PCI	0.93 ± 0.59	0.95 ± 0.58
Immediately after PCI	2.94 ± 0.59	2.88 ± 0.63
Follow-up	2.15 ± 0.84*	1.73 ± 0.91

Note: *$P < 0.05$, compared with the placebo group

2.3 Comparison of Recurrent Angina

As shown in Figure 1, as the follow-up time progressed, the incidence of recurrent angina increased in both the XS and placebo groups, but with a faster pace in the latter. One month after PCI, the incidence of recurrent angina in the XS group (4.11%) tended to be lower than that in the placebo group (8.86%), although there was no significant difference ($P > 0.05$). At three months after PCI, the incidence in the XS group was significantly lower than that in the placebo group (4.11% *vs.* 17.22%, $P < 0.01$). The significant difference continues to 6 months after PCI, when recurrent angina occurred in 9 cases (12.33%) in the XS group compared with 34 cases (43.04%) in the placebo group ($P < 0.01$).

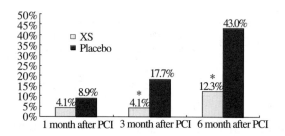

Figure 1   The Incidence of Recurrent Angina during the Follow-up Period

Note：*$P < 0.01$, compared with the placebo group

2.4 Comparison of Clinical Endpoints

As shown in Table 5, no death and acute myocardial infarction was found in either the XS or the placebo group. Target lesion revascularization was performed in 5 patients and no patient underwent CABG in the XS group, whereas 8 patients performed target lesion revascularization and 1 patient underwent CABG to the target lesion in the placebo group. There was no significant difference as for the combined incidence of clinical endpoint events between the XS and placebo groups (6.85% *vs.* 11.39%, $P > 0.05$).

2.5 Safety Analysis

During the follow-up period, blood pressure, heart rate, routine tests of blood, urine and

Table 5   Comparison of Clinical Endpoint Events

Endpoints	XS group		Placebo group	
	Cases	(%)	Cases	(%)
Death	0	0.00	0	0.00
Nonfatal acute myocardial infarction	0	0.00	0	0.00
Target lesion revascularization	5	6.85	8	10.13
Target lesion CABG	0	0.00	1	1.27

stool, as well as liver and kidney functions did not differ from that measured at the beginning of the study in both XS and placebo groups. Out of a total of 152 senile patients enrolled in this study, one in the XS group experienced gastric discomfort, which was alleviated without interruption of XS treatment. Granulocytopenia occurred in one patient in the placebo group, which was considered to be related to administration of Western medicine.

3. Discussion

In September 1977, Gruntzig conducted the first PTCA in the world, opening up an important era in the interventional cardiology. In more than three decades afterwards, PTCA and subsequent developed endovascular stent implantation were popularized rapidly all over the world and became one of the major effective therapies for CHD. Although coronary artery revascularization can be realized without thoracotomy, restenosis has become a major factor limiting the long-term efficacy of PCI, usually occurring in 6 to 9 months after PCI. The restenosis rate was even up to 30% to 50% in the era of PTCA alone. Although endovascular stent implantation made a milestone progress, the post-PCI restenosis rate remained at the level of 20% to 35%. In recent years, application of drug-eluting stents has significantly reduced the restenosis rate in high-risk patients and contributes greatly to the prevention of restenosis. However, whether it will increase the incidence of long-term thrombus remains disputable[10,11]. Furthermore, the restenosis rate of drug-eluting stents in real-world practice still needs to be further improved.

The mechanism of restenosis was thought to be related to arterial vascular wall injury induced by balloon dilation or stents implantation, and subsequent adherence and aggregation of platelets, release of growth factors, migration and proliferation of vascular smooth muscle cells, accumulation of extracellular matrix (ECM), as well as intimal hyperplasia and vascular remodeling. This pathologic process is similar to the theory of "obstruction of heart vessel" and "stasis of the blood circulation" in CM. Our previous studies indicated that there is a relationship between restenosis and blood-stasis syndrome, and the concentrated Xuefu Zhuyu Pill (血府逐瘀浓缩丸) a classic formula for activating blood circulation, could inhibit the formation of restenosis, reduce the recurrent angina after PCI, and alleviate the symptoms of blood stasis. However, there was no significant difference between the XS group and the placebo group as for restenosis rate, which was probably due to a small sample size[12,13]. On that basis, we further simplified the prescription into XS, consisting of Chuangxiongol and paeoniflorin, by optimizing the dosage ratio according to the orthogonal design method. The experimental study showed that XS could significantly inhibit the intimal hyperplasia and vascular remodeling in a porcine coronary injury model[2,5]. In consideration of these promising results, a multi-center, randomized, double-blind, placebo-controlled trial was conducted and demonstrated the efficacy and safety of XS in reducing restenosis in post-PCI patients[7].

The treatment for elderly CHD patients is often difficult and complicated due to comorbidities of such diseases as hyperlipidemia, hypertension, diabetes and cerebrovascular disease. Meanwhile, multivessel involved, complicated and diffused coronary lesions are prevalent in coronary angiography of senile patients. Furthermore, slower recovery and higher recurrent angina after PCI demand intensified comprehensive interventions among this population. We have conducted an investigation of diagnosis and treatment status for 1864 senile hospitalized CHD patients and then followed up one-year clinical events after discharge; the results showed that the therapy of integrative Chinese and Western medication could reduce the incidence of clinical endpoint events in the elderly CHD patients[14], which was coincident with the concept of multifactorial complicated intervention. However, the specific intervention protocols, course of treatment and their efficacy for different subgroups of senile CHD patients still need further research. Along with the popularization of PCI, whether intervention with the combined therapy of CM and Western medicine in senile post-PCI CHD patients is beneficial has been drawing more and more attention. In view of this, we conducted a subgroup analysis for the elderly CHD patients in the multi-center, randomized, double-blind and placebo-controlled trial mentioned above. The results showed that XS combined with routine Western medicine could significantly reduce the recurrence of angina and to some extent inhibit the formation of restenosis after PCI in the elderly CHD patients, indicating a wide application prospect. Nevertheless, whether this combined therapy can improve the long-term prognosis and reduce the incidence of clinical endpoints in elderly post-PCI patients still needs to be further demonstrated.

References

[1] Nienaber CA, Akin I, Schneider S, et al. Clinical outcomes after sirolimus-eluting, paclitaxel-eluting, and bare metal stents. Am J Cardiol, 2009, 104: 1362-1369.

[2] Xu H, Shi DZ, Chen KJ, et al. Effect of Xiongshao Capsule on vascular remodeling in porcine coronary balloon injury model. Chin J Integr Tradit West Med, 2001, 21: 591-594.

[3] Xu H, Shi DZ, Chen KJ, et al. Effect of Xiongshao Capsule on proliferation and apoptosis of vascular smooth muscle cells in rabbits observed by serum pharmacological method. Chin J Integr Tradit West Med, 2000, 20: 757-760.

[4] Xu H, Shi DZ, Chen KJ, et al. Clinical effect of Xiongshao Capsule on preventing restenosis post-PTCA or/and stenting. Chin J Integr Tradit West Med, 2000, 20: 494-497.

[5] Xu H, Shi DZ, Chen KJ, et al. Effect of XS0601 on apoptosis and gene expression of p53 and bcl-2 in neointima of porcine coronary artery after balloon injury. Chin J Intervent Cardiol, 2001, 9: 152-154.

[6] Xu H, Chen KJ, Shi DZ, et al. Clinical study of Xiongshao Capsule in preventing restenosis after coronary interventional treatment. Chin J Integr Med, 2002, 8: 162-166.

[7] Chen KJ, Shi DZ, Xu H, et al. XS0601 reduces the incidence of restenosis: a prospective study of 335 patients undergoing percutaneous coronary intervention in China. Chin Med J, 2006, 119: 6-13.

[8] Nomenclature and criteria for diagnosis of ischemic heart disease. Report of the Joint International Society and Federation of Cardiology/World Health Organization task force on standardization of clinical nomenclature. Circulation, 1979, 59; 607-609.

[9] Ryan TJ, Faxon DP, Gunnar RM, et al. Guidelines for percutaneous transluminal coronary angioplasty. A report of the American College of Cardiology/American Heart Association Task Force on Assessment of Diagnostic and Therapeutic Cardiovascular Procedures (Subcommittee on Percutaneous Transluminal Coronary Angioplasty). Circulation, 1988, 78: 486-502.

[10] Maisel WH. Unanswered questions-drug-eluting stents and the risk of late thrombosis. NEJM, 2007, 356: 981-984.

[11] Curfman GD, Morrissey S, Jarcho JA, et al. Drug-eluting coronary stents-promise and uncertainty. NEJM, 2007, 356: 1059-1060.

[12] Shi DZ, Li Jing, Ma XC, et al. Clinical observation of concentrated Xuefu Zhuyu Pill in preventing restenosis of patients with coronary heart disease after percutaneous transluminal coronary angioplasty. J TCM, 1997, 38: 27-29.

[13] Yu B, Chen KJ, Mao JM. Clinical study on effect of Concentrated Xuefu Zhuyu Pill on restenosis of 43 cases coronary heart disease after intracoronary scenting. Chin J Integr Tradit West Med, 1998, 18: 585-589.

[14] Xu H, Gao ZY, Chen KJ. A prospective study on the diagnositic and therapeutic status and prognosis of the 1864 elderly patients with coronary heart disease. Chin J Geriatr, 2008, 27: 617-622.

Clinical Efficacy of Traditional Chinese Medicine on Acute Myocardial Infarction—A Prospective Cohort Study[*]

DUAN Wen-hui   LU Fang   LI Li-zhi   WANG Cheng-long   LIU Jian-gang   YANG Qiao-ning   GU Feng   ZHANG Lei   SHI Da-zhuo

Acute myocardial infarction (AMI) is a leading cause of death and physical disability for coronary heart disease (CHD) patients. Although a great progress has been achieved in revascularization and secondary prevention in recent years, the cardiovascular event in one year after AMI-related coronary artery revascularization reached about 18%[1]. In 1970s, Xiyuan Hospital affiliated to China Academy of Chinese Medical Sciences, Guang'anmen Hospital affiliated to China Academy of Chinese Medical Sciences, and

* 原载于 Chinese Journal of Integrative Medicine, 2012, 18 (6): 1-7

Beijing Dongzhimen Hospital and Xuanwu Hospital treated AMI with Chinese medicine (CM) for nourishing qi and activating blood circulation in combination with western medicine, the results showed that the mortality and the complications (such as hypotension, shock, and heart failure) in the combined treatment group was much lower than that in the western medicine group[2]. It has been proven by the recent researches that CM has certain advantages in improving myocardium perfusion, reducing the reperfusion injury[3, 4], improving the patient's heart function[5], and improving the life quality after AMI[6] . However, the clinical trials without large samples and randomized, blinded, controlled design lead to suspicious clinical results of the treatment with CM. In previous clinical trials, the effects of single CM preparation or treatment method were often used to evaluate the effects of CM on AMI, while the overall effects of CM has rarely been reported. Therefore, how to comprehensively evaluate the effects of CM on AMI were explored in this prospective cohort study.

1. Methods

1.1　Study Design

A prospective cohort study was designed on CM intervention including treatment based on syndrome differentiation and treatment with CM patent medicines as the single intervention factor to evaluate the clinical effects of CM. A total of 348 AMI patients from Xiyuan Hospital affiliated to China Academy of Chinese Medical Sciences, China-Japan Friendship Hospital and Beijing Anzhen Hospital affiliated to Capital University of Medical Sciences from January 2007 to March 2009 were enrolled. The patients treated with combined CM (decoction of herbal medicine or CM patent medicine) for at least one month and western medicine were regarded as the treatment group; those with western medicine were regarded as the control group.

This study had been approved by Medical ethics committee of Xiyuan Hospital, China-Japan

Friendship Hospital, and Beijing Anzhen Hospital.

1.2　Diagnostic Criteria

The diagnostic criteria of AMI referred to the Guide to Diagnosis and Treatment of Acute Myocardial Infarction in China[7]. The differentiation criteria of CM refered to CM Syndrome Standards for Coronary Heart Disease[8]. The CM syndrome scores refered to National Standards for CM Industry of People's Republic of China-CM Syndrome Part[9], which involved 9 symptoms including chest pain, chest stuffiness, palpitation, short of breath, hypodynamia, extreme chilliness, ache and weak at waist and knee, spontaneous perspiration and insomnia. The diagnostic criteria of blood stasis syndrome consulted the criteria formulated by Speciality Committee of Promoting Blood Circulation to Remove Stasis in Chinese Association of Integrated Chinese and Western Medicine[10]. The symptoms and signs of blood stasis including angina, purple and dark tongue or with ecchymosis, purple and dark lip and gum, sublingual varices, uneven pulse or slow pulse with regular or irregular intervals were scored according to methods introduced by literature[11]. CM syndrome scoring criteria was seen in Table 1.

1.3　Inclusion and Exclusion Criteria

Patients eligible for the study were 35 to 75 years old, who are diagnosed as AMI and signed the informed consent form. Patients were excluded if they met any of the following criteria: presence of (1) serious diseases of liver, kidney, hematopoietic system and nervous system, etc., and metal diseases, malignant tumor, serious chronic obstructive pulmonary diseases, pulmonary heart diseases or respiratory failures; (2) refusal to sign the informed consent forms or the estimated poor compliance and little possibility of follow-up visits of the patients; (3) women at pregnancy or lactation; (4) partici-pation in other researches; (5) valvular heart disease or cardiomyopathy; (6) cardiogenic shock or requiring continuous mechanical adjuvant

Table 1　Criteria for CM Syndrome Scores

Syndrome	Slight (1 score)	Moderate (2 score)	Severe (3 score)
Chest pain	Slight, relieves easily	Obvious, relieves after taking medicine	Serious, or continuous
Chest stuffiness	Slight	Obvious, often sighs	Severe, sighs frequently
Short of breath	Short breath when moderate exercises	Short breath when mild exercises	Short breath even in rest
Palpitation	Occurs occasionally	Occurs often, and lasts for a relatively long time	Occurs frequently and continuously
Hypodynamia	Tiredness, but can insist on ordinary work	Tiredness, difficult to insist on ordinary work	Exhausted, even in rest
Extreme chilliness	Chilliness in limbs	Chilliness in limbs, always wears more clothes	Chilliness of the whole body, can not relieve when wearing more clothes
Soreness and weakness in waist and knees	Soreness and weakness of waist and knees, can insist on ordinary work	Soreness and weakness of waistand knees, difficult to insist on ordinary work	Soreness and weakness of waist and knees, can not do ordinary work
Spontaneous sweating	Slight sweat on the skin, sweating on exertion	Mild sweat on the skin, sweating when mild exercises	Severe sweat on the skin, sweating even in rest
Insomnia	Slight disorder in sleeping, no impact on daily life	Sleepless than 4 hours every night, impact on daily life	Sleepless whole night

treatments.

The losing follow-up was defined as: (1) not completed the clinical investigating protocols; (2) missing the visits, and (3) ordered off by the doctor due to their poor compliance.

1.4　Items of Observation

CM symptom scores and blood stasis syndrome score were observed when admitted in hospital and at 6-month, the occurrence of endpoint was observed at 6-month. The primary endpoint criteria in the present study was defined as death, MI and revascularization (including the percutaneous coronary intervention and coronary artery bypass graft). The secondary endpoint criteria included stroke, rehospitalization due to angina recurrence (above angina grade III of the Canada Society of Cardiology), heart dysfunction (above New York Heart Association grade II) and shock.

1.5　Statistical Analysis

Statistical analysis was performed with SPSS 13.0 software. The values were expressed as mean $\pm$ standard deviation ($\bar{x} \pm s$). Continuous variables were analyzed using the independent samples t-test and categorical variables using the chi-square test or Fisher's exact test. Kaplan-Meier method was used for the survival analysis. The multifactor analysis was analyzed by Cox proportional hazards regression.

2. Results

Of the 348 cases, 14 (4.0%) lost during the follow-up. The total completed cases in this clinical trial were 334 cases, 169 in the treatment group and 165 in the control group.

2.1　Baseline Demographic and Clinical Characteristics

The baseline clinicial characteristics in the two groups showed no significant differences (Table 2).

2.2　Comparison of CM Symptom Scores

CM symptom scores of the two groups were 11.53 ± 2.39 and 11.58 ± 2.33 respectively ($P > 0.05$) when admitted in hospital, whereas the scores of the treatment group at the end of the 6-month follow-up were lower than that of

Table 2　Baseline Demographic，Medical History and Clinical Characteristics of the Two Groups

Characteristics		Treatment group (169 cases)	Control group (165 cases)	P
Age [Year $\bar{\chi} \pm s$]		64.61±7.39	63.42±8.51	0.175
Male [Cases (%)]		114 (67.46)	110 (66.67)	0.878
Smoking [Cases (%)]		100 (59.17)	97 (58.79)	0.943
Hypertension [Cases (%)]		108 (63.91)	102 (61.82)	0.693
Hyperlipidaemia [Cases (%)]		39 (23.08)	41 (24.85)	0.704
Diabetes [Cases (%)]		49 (28.99)	47 (28.48)	0.918
History of MI [Cases (%)]		35 (20.71)	33 (20.00)	0.872
Area of infarction	Antero-septal [Cases (%)]	15 (8.88)	19 (11.52)	0.425
	Anterior [Cases (%)]	32 (18.93)	39 (23.64)	0.294
	Extensive anterior [Cases (%)]	8 (4.73)	6 (3.64)	0.617
	Anterolateral [Cases (%)]	4 (2.37)	6 (3.64)	0.496
	Inferior [Cases (%))	28 (16.57)	31 (18.79)	0.595
	Two or more walls [Cases (%)]	11 (6.51)	8 (4.85)	0.512
	NSTEMI [Cases (%)]	71 (42.01)	56 (33.94)	0.129
Heart function (Killip Class)	Class Ⅰ [Cases (%)]	107 (63.31)	98 (59.39)	0.462
	Class Ⅱ [Cases (%)]	55 (32.54)	58 (35.15)	0.615
	Class Ⅲ [Cases (%)]	7 (4.14)	9 (5.45)	0.574
Treatment	PCI [Cases (%)]	118 (69.82)	121 (73.33)	0.477
	Aspirin [Cases (%)]	163 (96.45)	162 (98.18)	0.328
	Clopidogrel [Cases (%)]	164 (97.04)	162 (98.18)	0.496
	ACEI/ARB [Cases (%)]	131 (77.51)	128 (77.58)	0.989
	β-adrenoceptor antagonists [Cases (%)]	134 (79.29)	123 (74.55)	0.303
	Statin [Cases (%)]	153 (90.53)	154 (93.33)	0.348
	Nitrates [Cases (%)]	152 (89.94)	151 (91.52)	0.620

the control group (3.86±1.68 *vs.* 4.32±1.79, P=0.018). The difference was mainly shown in three symptoms of chest pain, spontaneous perspiration and insomnia (Table 3).

2.3　Comparison of Blood Stasis Syndrome Score

The blood stasis syndrome score was 27.50±6.25 in the treatment and 27.30±6.46 in the control group ($P > 0.05$) before treatment. At the end of the 6-month follow-up, the score was significantly lower in the treatment group than the control group (11.48±4.33 *vs* 13.79±5.29, $P < 0.01$).

2.4　Comparison of Clinical Endpoint

The events of the endpoints of the treatment group was significantly lower than that of the control group (11.24% *vs.* 23.64%, $P < 0.01$) during the 6-month follow-up. Rehospitalization due to angina of the treatment group was significantly lower than that of the control group (2.96% *vs.* 7.88%, $P < 0.05$) during 6 months (Table 4).

The survival curve revealed that the nonrehospitalization due to angina of the treatment group was significantly higher than that of the control group during the 6-month (Log Rank

Table 3　Comparison of CM Symptom Scores of the Two Groups（score, $\bar{\chi} \pm s$ ）

Group	Time	Chest pain	Chest stuffiness	Palpitation	Short of breath	Hypo-dynamia	Extreme chilliness	Soreness and weakness of waist and knees	Spontaneous sweating	Insomnia	Total scores
Treatment (169 cases)	Before treatment	2.57 ±0.88	2.50 ±0.77	1.86 ±0.59	0.93 ±0.95	1.15 ±1.02	0.57 ±0.72	0.64 ±0.72	0.37 ±0.66	0.80 ±0.85	11.53 ±2.39
	6-month follow-up	0.60 ±0.50*	0.66 ±0.57	0.33 ±0.50	0.38 ±0.57	0.49 ±0.54	0.29 ±0.46	0.36 ±0.56	0.31 ±0.47**	0.45 ±0.63*	3.86 ±1.68**
Control (165 cases)	Before treatment	2.53 ±0.80	2.53 ±0.72	1.86 ±0.69	0.78 ±0.94	1.03 ±0.96	0.69 ±0.72	0.58 ±0.65	0.37 ±0.67	0.67 ±0.84	11.58 ±2.33
	6-month follow-up	0.75 ±0.60*	0.66 ±0.59	0.36 ±0.49	0.38 ±0.57	0.50 ±0.50	0.26 ±0.44	0.38 ±0.56	0.43 ±0.52**	0.61 ±0.69+	4.32 ±1.79++

Note：*P=0.013, **P=0.042, +P=0.036, ++P=0.018, compared with the control group

Table 4　Comparison of Endpoint of the Two Groups（Cases（%））

Group	Primary endpoint			Secondary endpoint			Total events
	Death	Non-fatal myocardial infarction	Revascularization	Stroke	Rehospitalization due to angina	Heart dysfunction	
Treatment (169cases)	3 (1.78)	1 (0.59)	9 (5.33)	0	5 (2.96) *	1 (0.59)	19 (11.24)**
Control (165cases)	5 (3.03)	3 (1.82)	11 (6.67)	3 (1.82)	13 (7.88)	4 (2.42)	39 (23.64)

Note：*P < 0. 05, **P < 0. 01, compared with the control group

Statistic=4.700, P=0.30, Figure 1).

2.3　Cox Regression Analysis

A total number of 22 items were applied to analyze the relationship between the related factors and endpoints, including gender, age, smoking, heart dysfunction, hypertension, hyperlipidaemia, diabetes, old myocardial infarction, CM, percutaneous coronary intervention (PCI), early use of angiotension-converting enzyme (ACE) inhibitors, β-adrenoceptor antagonists, clopidogrel, aspirin, statin, nitrates, antero-septal myocardial infarction, anterior myocardial infarction, extensive anterior myocardial infarction, inferior myocardial infarction, high lateral myocardial infarction and two or more walls myocardial infarction. Analize-Survival-Cox Regression modle was used to choose variables with P < 0.05 to enter into the Cox proportional hazards regression analysis, which including CM, heart dysfunction, diabetes, PCI and early use of ACE inhibitors. Wherein, heart dysfunction and diabetes were hazard factors to endpoint; whereas CM, PCI and early use of ACE inhibitors were protective factors of endpoints (Table 5).

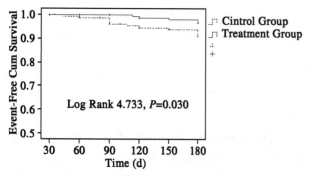

Figure 1　Survival Analysis of the Rehospitalization due to Angina during 6 Months

Table 5 Predictive Factors for Endpoint at the 6-Month

Factor	HR	95% CI	P
Heart dysfunction	1.601	1.084-2.364	0.018
Diabetes	1.755	1.031-2.989	0.038
Diabetes	0.405	0.231-0.712	0.002
PCI	0.352	0.204-0.607	0.000
Early use of ACE inhibitors	0.541	0.313-0.936	0.028

3. Discussion

The studies on prevention and treatment of AMI with CM and western medicine in recent years indicated that CM had a certain favour effects on improving myocardial perfusion, reducing the damages from reperfusion and enhancing the heart function of the patients with AMI[5,12]. Multi-center, double-blind, randomized, placebo-controlled studies showed that CM was effective in reducing restenosis after PCI in the patients with acute coronary syndrome (ACS) [6,13]. However, there were no reports on clinical studies to taking several kind of intervention method with CM including decoction of herbal medicine or CM patent medicine as one factor to evaluate the effects of CM on AMI. Moreover, most of the effectiveness was taken from the laboratory examination indexes or ultrasonic cardiography indexes, with few observations on the clinical endpoint.

As for the cohort study, the main shortage was bias and confounding factor, which influences the reliability of the study. In present study, the two groups had a good match in clinical general conditions possibly affecting the prognosis, such as gender, age, hypertension, diabetes, history of myocardial infarction, heart function, infarction area, PCI and drug intervening and so on. Moreover, the missing followup rate is only 4.0% in the present study. So it is reasonable to believe that the present clinical trial had a well controlled confounding bias, which indicated the results had good reliability and credibility.

3.1 Influence of CM on the CM Symptoms Scores and Blood Stasis Syndrome Score

According to CM theory, the pathogenesis of AMI was related to two aspects (excessive and deficiency), the main excessive factors were blood stasis, phlegm turbidity, cold obstruction and qi stagnation; while the main deficiency factors were deficiency of qi and yang. Thus, in the aspect of CM syndrome scores, besides chest pain, tightness and palpitation, other six symptoms of shortness of breath, fatigue, extreme chilliness, ache and weak at waist and knee, spontaneous perspiration and sleeplessness were also chosen as investigation index for this study, which could well cover the main clinical symptoms of AMI patients. The study found that the CM syndrome scores of the treatment group at 6-month follow-up was obviously lower than that of the control group, and the differences were mainly in three symptoms including chest pain, spontaneous perspiration and insomnia. The treatment methods of CM for AMI in the present study mainly aimed at invigorating the circulation of blood, reducing phlegm, regulate the flow of qi, nourishing qi and (or) warming heart yang, which demonstrated that it could not only relieve chest pain, but also improve deficiency of qi and yang.

The pathogenic factor of blood stasis was throughout the AMI course. It was found that 88.3% of AMI patients have blood stasis syndrome[14]. In this study, the blood stasis syndrome score was regarded as one of the index used to evaluate the effect of CM, which including angina, tongue nature, sublingual varices, lips color and others. The follow-up during 6-month demonstrated that treatment with CM could significantly reduce the blood stasis syndrome score of AMI patients comparing with treatment with only western medicine.

3.2 Influence of CM on Endpoint

The result of this clinical trial illustrated that CM could reduce the rehospitalization due to angina of AMI patients during 6 months

(HR 33.8%, 95% CI=0.176–0.649, *P*=0.001), which indicated that CM was a beneficial protective factor for the 6-month prognosis. The occurrence of endpoints including death, non-fatal myocardial infarction, revascularization, stroke and heart failure in the treatment group during the 6-month follow-up had a decreased trend compared with the control group, with no significant difference between the two groups, the reasons might be: (1) medicines including CM for secondary prevention of coronary artery disease need to be administered for lifelong, however the patients in this study were those who have just taken CM for not less than one month. Thus, the relatively short period of CM taking may affect the clincial effect to some extent; (2) the follow-up period of this study was relatively short and the amount of cases was relatively small.

3.3 Factors Affecting the AMI Prognosis

The study screened out factors affecting AMI prognosis by using the Cox hazard proportion regression model (Table 5), which included heart dysfunction, diabetes mellitus, early use of ACE inhibitors, PCI, CM and others. Among which, the CM, PCI and early use of ACE inhibitors were protective factors of the 6-month prognosis, while heart dysfunction and diabetes were the risk factors of the 6-month prognosis. A retrospective cohort study[15]showed that age (HR 2.021, 95% CI=1.347–3.032, *P*=0.001), heart failure (HR 1.863, 95% CI=1.280–2.711, *P*=0.001), diabetes (HR 4.039, 95% CI=1.627–10.031, *P*=0.003) were risk factors of the long-term prognosis; While the use of ACE inhibitors was the protective factor (HR 0.141, 95% CI=0.054–0.369, *P* < 0.001). A study involved 1437 AMI patients with an average follow-up of 4.2 years showed that the cardiac mortality of patients who treated with PCI was 5.4%, while the cardiac mortality of those patients who received the conservative treatment was 17.7%. For those patients with a high risk, the risks of 30-day and long-term cardiac death

to patients having received emergency PCI were 27% (95% CI=0.18–0.44, *P* < 0.001) and 40% (95% CI=0.22–0.73, *P*=0.0032) of risks to patients not receiving PCI[16]. The results of the present study were in accordance with the previous results, which indicated to some extent the reliability of this study.

The study showed that CM had some advantages in reducing the 6-month CM syndrome scores and blood stasis syndrome score of the AMI patients and reducing the occurrence of rehospitalization due to angina during 6-month. As the study was a prospective cohort study, and had a relative small sample size, multi-center, large sample, randomized, controlled trial are needed in the further to provide higher-level evidences.

References

[1] Spaulding C, Henry P, Teiger E, et al. Sirolimus-eluting versus uncoated stents in acute myocardial infarction. N Engl J Med, 2006, 355: 1093-1104.

[2] Xiyuan Hospital under Institute of Traditional Chinese Medicine, et al. The "anti-infarct mixture" for acute myocardial infarction clinical analysis of 118 cases. Chin J Intern Med, 1976, 1: 212-215.

[3] Yin HJ, Wang XG, Shi DZ. Effects of GSTT on release of TNF-α and IL-1 β in rats with myocardial ischemia reperfusion injury. Med J Chin PLA, 2006, 31: 986-987.

[4] Shang LZ, Wei DW, Wang F. Effects of ligustrazine on expression of HSP25 and p38MAPK proteins in rats with myocardial ischemia reperfusion injury. CJTCMP, 2008, 23: 882-884.

[5] Li YQ, Jin M, Qiu SL, et al. Effects of Chinese herbal medicine for benefiting qi and nourishing yin to promote blood circulation on ventricular wall motion of AMI patients after revascularization. Chin J Integr Tradit West Med, 2009, 29: 300-304.

[6] Lu XY, Shi DZ, Xu H, et al. Clinical study on effect of Xiongshao Capsule on restenosis after percutaneous coronary intervention. Chin J Integr Tradit West Med, 2006, 26: 13-16.

[7] Chinese Society of Cardiology of Chinese Medical Association, Editorial Board of Chinese Journal of

Cardiology. Guide to diagnosis and treatment of acute myocardial infarction in China. Chin J Cardiol, 2001, 29: 710-725.

[8] Cardiovascular Institute of Traditional Chinese Medicine Professional Committee. Coronary heart disease diagnostic criteria. Chin J Integr Tradit West Med, 1991, 11: 257-260.

[9] National Standards for CM Industry of Peopled's Republic of China-CM Syndrome Part. Clinic terminology of traditional Chinese medical diagnosis and treatment-Syndromes (GB/T 16751. 2-1997).

[10] Chinese Association of Integrative Medicine, Professional Committee of Blood Circulation Research. Diagnosis standard of blood stasis synrome. Chin J Integr Tradit West Med, 1987, 7: 129-131.

[11] Wang J. Study on diagnostic criteria of blood stasis syndrome. Research and clinical application of promoting blood circulation and removing blood stasis. Beijing: Beijing Medical University and Peking Union Medical College Press, 1993, 7.

[12] Qiu SL, Jin M, Zhu TG, et al. Effect of replenishing qi and nourishing yin to promote the blood circulation on 103 patients with acute myocardial infarction after reperfusion. J Capital Med University, 2009, 30: 426-429.

[13] Chen KJ, Shi DZ, Xu H, et al. XS0601 reduces the incidence of restenosis: a prospective study of 335 patients undergoing percutaneous coronary intervention in China. Chin Med J, 2006, 119: 6-13.

[14] Duan WH, Li LZ, Wang CL, et al. Study on correlation between heart function and Chinese medicine syndrome distribution of acute myocardial infarction. Beijing J Tradit Chin Med, 2010, 29: 4-6.

[15] Lin Q, Nong YB, Duan WH. Retrospective study on influence of Chinese herbal drugs on long-term prognosis of acute myocardial infarction. J Beijing University Tradit Chin Med, 2006, 29: 419-421.

[16] Ryo K, Nobuhisa H, Hiroshi K, et al. Primary percutaneous coronary intervention vs conservative treatment for acute ST elevation myocardial infarction short- and long-term follow-up according to disease severity. Circ J, 2008, 72: 1391-1396.

Effect of Chinese Drugs for Supplementing Qi, Nourshing Yin and Activating Blood Circulation on Myocardial Perfusion in Patients with Acute Myocardial Infarction after Revascularization[*]

LI Yong-qiang　JIN Mei　QIU Sheng-lei　WANG Pei-li　ZHU Tian-gang　WANG Cheng-long
LI Tian-chang　LIU Hong-xu　BIAN Hong　YAO Li-fang　SHI Da-zhuo

Revascularization (RV), including intravenous thrombolysis, percutaneous coronary intervention (PCI) and coronary bypass, is the first choice of treatment for acute myocardial infarction (AMI) at present, could evidently improve short- and long-term prognosis of patients. However, it was found by current studies that even if the blood flow of the criminal vessels after vascular recanalization reaches thrombolysis in myocardial infarction (TIMI) grade Ⅲ, perfect blood flow in myocardial tissue level fails in about 25% of the patients, which results in no-reflow or slow-flow phenomenon. There has been no ideal solution for this puzzling problem so far, and

* 原载于 Chinese Journal of Integrative Medicine，2009，15（1）：19-25

so it has become a focus in modern research on prevention and treatment of coronary heart disease (CHD) [1,2].

With randomized, double-blinded, controlled method, using myocardial contrast echocardiography (MCE), and dobutamine stress echocardiography (DSE) adopted, Chinese drugs for supplementing qi, nourishing yin and activating blood circulation (abbr. as SQNYAB), in combination with conventional Western medical therapy was adopted to observe their effects on blood perfusion at the myocardial tissue level in this study in post-RV patients of AMI.

1. Methods

1.1　Diagnostic Standard

Western medical diagnosis was made according to the diagnostic criteria for AMI from "Guidance on diagnosis and treatment of acute myocardial infarction" [3] issued by Chinese Society of Cardiovascular Diseases, Chinese Medical Association and the Editorial Committee of Chinese Journal of Cardiology, 2001. Meanwhile traditional Chinese medical diagnosis was made in reference to the "Norm for Emergent Diagnosis and Treatment of Xiongbi and Xinjue" [4] formulated by the Department of Medical Administration, State Administration of Traditional Chinese Medicine, 1995.

1.2　Criteria for Inclusion

Included were patients of primary AMI with elevated ST segment of ECG, who had vascular recanalization of criminal vessel confirmed by coronary arteriography and met the standard issued from the Editorial Committee of Chinese Journal of Cardiology, 1996[5], who had received intravenous thrombolytic treatment or direct PCI; aged ≤ 75 years and with heart functions of Killip grade I-III.

1.3　Criteria for Exclusion

Patients who were with any of the following conditions were excluded: (1) complicated by severe primary diseases of liver, kidney, hematopoietic system or nervous system; (2) with

tumor or mental diseases; (3) refusing to sign the informed consent or estimated as with poor compliance and low possibility for follow-up; (4) in pregnancy or lactating; (5) participating in other clinical trials at that time.

1.4　General Materials

Eighty AMI patients hospitalized between March, 2005 to November, 2006 were selected from four hospitals, including the Xiyuan Hospital, China Academy of Chinese Medical Sciences, Beijing Hospital of Traditional Chinese Medcine Affiliated to the Capital Medical University, the People's Hospital of Peking University and Tongren Hospital Affiliated to the Capital Medical University. The patients were assigned equally, by the randomized digital table of the SAS software, to the treated group and the control group.

The 40 patients in the treated group were 33 males and 7 females. Their mean ages were 56.34 ± 11.12 years. Twenty-three were with anterior wall AMI and 17 with inferior wall AMI. Thirty-five had received immediate PCI and 98.36% of them had their forward blood flow in infarction related vessels reaching TIMI grade III, with the other 1 having received intravenous thrombolysis that was confirmed to have vascular recanalization which met the standard[5]. The time from hospitalization to RV was 6.22 ± 2.67 h. At the time of enrolment, the heart function was classified as Killip grade I in 21 patients, as grade II in 16 and as grade III in 3. Twenty-six patients had a history of smoking, 16 were complicated with hypertension, 12 with diabetes mellitus, 18 with blood lipid abnormality and 2 with cerebral infarction.

The 40 patients in the control group were 35 males and 5 females with a mean age of 55.76 ± 12.09 years. Twenty-two were with anterior wall AMI and 18 with inferior wall AMI. Thirty-eight had received immediate PCI with 97.88% having forward blood flow reaching TIMI grade III. Two were proven to have vascular recanalization after intravenous thrombolysis. The time from hospitalization to RV was

6.31±1.72 h. Heart function at the time of enrolment was Killip grade Ⅰ in 22, grade Ⅱ in 13 and grade Ⅲ in 5. Twenty-nine patients had a history of smoking. Eighteen were complicated with hypertension, 16 with diabetes mellitus, 15 with blood lipids abnormality and 3 with cerebral infarction. The basic clinical materials in the two groups were similar, showing no significant difference ($P > 0.05$).

1.5 Treatment

After being treated with PCI or intravenous thrombolysis, and with vascular recanalization of the criminal vessels conforming to the standard[3], all AMI patients enrolled were treated with conventional Western medical (WM) therapy according to the Norm[5] in combination with scheduled test drugs medications, respectively. For the treated group, the scheduled medication consisted of 2 capsules of Xinyue Capsule (心悦胶囊 , XYC, each capsule contains 50 mg of total saponin of American ginseng stem and leaf) and 3 tablets of Composite Salvia Tablet (CST, each tablet contains red sage root 450 mg, notoginseng 141 mg and borneol 8 mg), given orally 3 times per day. For the control group, mimetic placebos of XYC and CST, i. e. capsule/tablet containing starch only but in similar packages, shape and color to XYC/CST, were administered with the dose and specification the same as those given to the treated group. The medication of both test drugs and placebos were started from the day of enrolment, and continued for 3 successive months or until the patients died.

Both the test drugs and the placebos were produced by the Ji'an Yisheng pharmarceutical Co., Ltd., Jilin province, China. The batch number of placebo was 041102 and that of test drugs 030073.

1.6 Method for Stress Echocardiography

A color Doppler's echocardiography type VIVID 7 produced by GE Company (USA) with M3S detector and a frequency of 1.7-3.4 MHz was used. Patients were required to lie on the left lateral position. ECG images were sampled from views of apex-4-chamber, apex-2-chamber and apex-long axis, involving the whole left ventricular area. Sonovisc freeze dried powder (sulfur hexafluoride micro bubble, produced by the BRACCO Company, Italy batch number J20030117) 250 mg was diluted by 5.0 mL of normal saline on standby. Dobutamine was pumped successively in the dose order of 5, 10 and 20μg/(kg·min) to the cubital superficial vein, every dose lasting for 3 min. Prepared Sonovisc solution (2mL) was injected slowly in the stress test (20μg/(kg·min)), and the images from the four views were collected when the echo of myocardial contrast medium was basically stabilized. DSE was performed on every patient two times, i. e., on the 14th day and at the end of the 3rd month of the observation (abbr. as 14-day DSE and 3-month DSE).

The steady-state peak echo value of contrast medium, named b value, could reflect the extent of local blood perfusion. The perfusion speed of contrast medium, named k value, could reflect the speed of myocardial perfusion. The product of the two, b×k, reflects the volume of local myocardial blood flow. All the results of myocardial perfusion was semi-quantitatively assessed adopting the 16 segment analysis[6] recommended by American Society of Echocardiography (ASE), with the myocardial acoustic image analyzing software provided by the Doppler apparatus. The wash-in time image was taken for analyzing the myocardial microcirculation perfusion in affected segments under dobutamine 20μg/(kg·min) stress.

1.7 Statistical Analysis

SPSS 13.0 software was applied for data management and the enumeration data were tested by Chi-square test. The measurement data were tested by the t-test. A $P < 0.05$ was regarded as having statistical meaning.

2. Results

The trial was finally completed in 75 patients as 5 patients (3 in the treated group and 2 in the control group) dropped out during the observation period. The causes for dropping out were poor tolerance to duly take the test drug in 2 (1 in each group), refusing to receive ultrasonic examination in 2 (in the treated group), and one in the control group died at the 3rd week of observation. The basic characteristics of patients enrolled actually in both group showed no significant difference ($P > 0.05$).

2.1 Effect on the Myocardial Perfusion of Various Segments of Left Anterior Ventricular Wall in Patients with Anterior Wall AMI

The 14-day DSE shows that the b value and k × b of mid and apex segments, as well as the k value of apex segment in the treated group were higher than those in the control group, respectively ($P < 0.05$ or $P < 0.01$). The 3-month DSE shows that the b value of apex segment and k × b value of basal, mid and apex segments were higher in the treated group than those in the control group, respectively ($P < 0.05$). And comparison of the two DSE shows that the apex segment b value markedly increased in the period from the 14th day to the end of the 3rd month after RV ($P < 0.05$, Table 1). The apex segment perfusion areas on the 14th day and at the time of the 3rd month in the treated group were higher than that in the control group respectively, and the area increased in the period from the 14th day to the 3rd month (Figure 1).

2.2 Effect on the Myocardial Perfusion of Various Segments of Left Inferior Ventricular Wall in Patients with Inferior Wall AMI

The 14-day DSE shows that the b value, k

value and k × b of basal segment in the treated group were significantly higher than those in the control group, respectively ($P < 0.05$ or $P < 0.01$). The 3-month DSE shows that the b value and k × b of basal segment in the treated group were significantly higher than those in the control group, respectively ($P < 0.05$). Comparison of the 14-day DSE with the 3-month DSE in the treated group shows a significant increase of k × b of apex and mid segments ($P < 0.05$, Table 2). The apex segment perfusion on the 14th day and at the time of the 3rd month in the treated group is higher than those in the control group, respectively. The area increased in the period from the 14th day to the 3rd month (Figure 2).

3. Discussion

RV in treatment of AMI, a landmark development in the therapeutic history of CHD, is an effective approach widely applied. But due to the existence of capillary endothelial function disorder induced by such causes as microthrombi formation in the recanalized criminal vessels, fragments of atherosclerosis plaques drifting along with blood stream to the distal end of vessels, after reperfusion production of oxygen free radicals, calcium overloading and activation of inflammatory factors, no-reflow and slow-flow phenomena on myocardial tissue level could be brought about in 25% of patients even if their blood flow may reach TIMI grade III after RV, which would have a severe impact on the patients' prognosis, so it has become the focus

Table 1　Effect on the b, k and k × b Values of Left Anterior Ventricular Wall in Patients with Anterior Wall AMI ($\bar{x} \pm s$)

Group	Cases	Time	b value (bp)			k value (s-1)			k × b value (db/s)		
			Basal	Mid	Apex	Basal	Mid	Apex	Basal	Mid	Apex
Control	20	14-day	5.64±1.77	4.43±1.02	4.58±0.86	1.74±0.17	1.66±0.18	1.49±0.13	9.77±3.20	7.31±1.87	6.88±1.68
		3-month	5.78±1.74	5.02±0.59	5.52±0.54	1.83±0.14	1.80±0.26	1.62±0.13	10.55±3.25	8.99±1.53	8.96±1.17
Treated	21	14-day	5.99±1.86	5.31±1.03**	5.54±0.75**	1.78±0.14	1.76±0.21	1.59±0.14*	10.65±3.33	9.29±1.96**	8.81±1.42**
		3-month	6.77±1.67	5.43±0.75	5.90±0.44*△	1.86±0.10	1.88±0.25	1.66±0.08	12.58±3.02*	10.19±2.02**	9.81±0.88*

Notes: *$P < 0.05$, **$P < 0.01$, compared with the control group at the same time points; △$P < 0.05$, compared with the 14-day in the same group

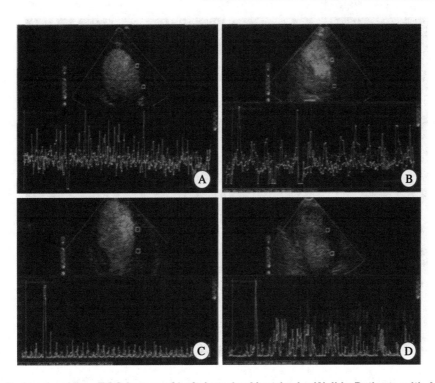

Figure 1 Apex 2-chamber View ECG Image of Left Anterior Ventricular Wall in Patients with Anterior Wall AMI

Notes: A: on the 14th day in the treated group; B: at the time of the 3rd month in the treated group; C: on the 14th day in the control group; D: at the time of the 3rd month in the control group. The round marks in red, yellow and blue color showed the apex, mid and basal segment perfusion areas of left anterior ventricular wall, respectively.

Table 2　Effect on the b, K and K × b Values of Left Inferior Ventricular Wall in Patients with Inferior Wall AMI ($\bar{\chi} \pm s$)

Group	Cases	Time	b value (bp)			k value (s-1)			k × b value (db/s)		
			Basal	Mid	Apex	Basal	Mid	Apex	Basal	Mid	Apex
Control	18	14-day	4.16±0.54	4.77±0.88	4.54±1.03	1.21±0.21	1.49±0.19	1.52±0.23	5.07±1.16	7.12±1.76	6.87±1.80
		3-month	4.28±0.55	5.26±0.54	5.11±1.16	1.47±0.22	1.54±0.15	1.67±0.25	6.32±1.26	8.12±1.39	8.63±2.68
Treated	16	14-day	4.64±0.57*	5.10±0.49	4.82±1.05	1.45±0.24**	1.54±0.26	1.69±0.27	6.72±1.51**	7.83±1.49	8.12±2.22
		3-month	4.77±0.77*	5.42±0.57	5.59±1.31	1.61±0.18	1.62±0.13	1.75±0.28	7.73±1.74*	8.80±1.26△	9.67±2.59△

Notes: *$P < 0.05$, **$P < 0.01$, compared with the control group at the same time points; △$P < 0.05$, compared with 14 day in the same group

and nidus in the field of modern prevention and treatment of CHD[7,8].

Some researchers hold that the TCM pathogenesis of most AMI patients after intervention is due to deficiency in origin and excess in superficiality. The former mainly dominated as qi-deficiency or qi-yin deficiency, and the latter mostly as blood stasis, phlegm-turbidity or cementation of phlegm and stasis accumulation so as to produce toxin[9, 10]. A clinical observation on the intervention of AMI with SONYAB was conducted at the cardiovascular center in Xiyuan Hospital in the 1970s and 1980s in cooperation with four other hospitals in Beijing. Results of the observation have proven that the mortality and complication incidence of AMI during hospitalization could be reduced by using these drugs in combination with WM[11]. But studies concerning the question "whether the treatment plays its role through improving the perfusion at the myocardial tissue level" have never been reported so far. From this view, this study was designed to observe the effects of intervention on AMI at the myocardial perfusion level by using the combined therapy of XYC (a Chinese herbal medicine for supplementing

第三章

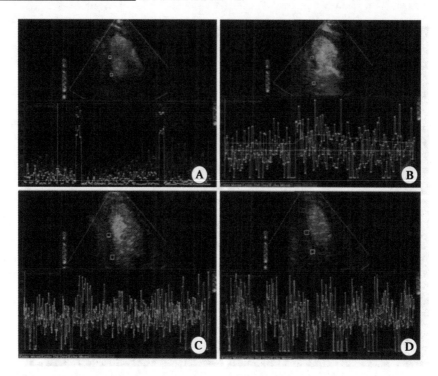

Figure 2　Apex 2-chamber View ECG Image of Left Inferior Ventricular Wall in Patients with Inferior Wall AMI

Notes: A: on the 14th day in the treated group; B: at the time of the 3rd month in the treated group; C: on the 14th day in the control group; D: at the time of the 3rd month in the control group. The round marks in red, yellow and blue color showed the apex, mid and basal segment perfusion areas of left inferior ventricular wall, respectively

qi and nourishing yin), CST (a Chinese herbal preparation for activating blood circulation to remove stasis) and WM to intervene in post-RV AMI, with the MCE and DSE technique adopted.

XYC and CST are commonly used patent Chinese market drugs effective in treating CHD. The main component of XYC is the total saponin of American ginseng stem and leaf, which is considered by TCM as effective in supplementing qi and nourishing yin. CST consists of red sage root and notoginseng, and has the action for activating blood circulation to remove stasis and relieving pain. Combined use of the two could be effective in supplementing qi, nourishing yin and activating blood circulation to remove stasis. Previous studies illustrated that Chinese preparations of this kind have functions of promoting vascular regeneration in the infarcted and ischemic area, anti-lipid-peroxidation injury, anti-myocardial ischemia, improving left ventricle reconstruction, and so on[12, 13].

MCE is a modern technique rapidly developed in the latest ten years for determining the velocity of ventricular wall motion, which could be used to evaluate the level of myocardial reperfusion. As compared with traditional methods such as corrective clinical trial for thrombolysis of myocardial infarction by frame counting and coronary blood flow determination, MCE could better reflect the status of post-RV myocardial perfusion in AM[14, 15]. Following the truth that sound wave could produce strong reflection for gases, MCE could determine the myocardial perfusion extent through the back scatter signal enhancement and video gray scale enhancement of contrast medium, by injecting microbubble-containing solution into blood vessels, which, acting as a tracer, drifts along with the blood stream to the myocardial tissue area administered by these vessels. Then, the status and extent of post-RV myocardial blood perfusion could be evaluated by the scope of myocardial image as well as the emptying velocity of acoustic contrast medium from myocardium and the intensity of gray scale. It has been illustrated that the emptying velocity from the myocardium and the strength of perfusion of Somovisc acoustic contrast medium are of important meaning for the risk level of AMI[16].

Immediate post-RV DSE in AMI was not performed on AMI patients in this study because it could be dangerous to some extent to patients due to the increase of myocardial oxygen consumption. Moreover, difficulty in moving patients and lack of reliable sensitive bedside ultrasonic apparatus in most hospitals in China should also be taken into consideration. Comparisons between groups in the infarcted position and the TIMI grade of forward blood flow in infarction related vessels were performed remedially in this study, and the results showed no statistical difference, which illustrated indirectly that the perfusion states in the two groups were comparable.

Two weeks after AMI, when the condition of the disease is basically stabilized, all hibernant myocardium, stunned myocardium or myocardium supplied by the infarction related arteries which failed to be perfused sufficiently were restored or repaired to certain extent. Conducting ultrasonographic examination at this time could reflect the intervening effect of drugs. Therefore, 2 weeks and 3 months after RV of AMI are selected as the two due time points for DSE in this study.

In this study, comparative analysis of under stress perfusion on left ventricular infarction related segment on the 14th day and at the end of the 3rd month in patients with anterior wall infarction or inferior wall infarction were carried out and the results show that mean flow velocity, perfusion intensity and local myocardial blood flow in the related segments of the treated group at 14-day post-RV were all higher than those in the control group, respectively, and the

improved segment was also extended. Besides, the improvements in mean flow velocity and local myocardial flow were advanced at the time point of the 3rd month and were also superior to those in the control group. These results indicated that the intervention in AMI by using SQNYAB in combination with WM could induce significant improvement on post-RV myocardial perfusion either on the 14th day or at the time of the 3rd month, which was especially significant in the early stage (the 14th day).

Post-RV myocardial tissue perfusion state in AMI is closely related with the apoptosis of cardiac muscle cells, fibrosis of myocardial tissues and ventricular reconstruction after AMI, and has a direct impact on the remote prognosis of post-RV patients. This study proved that combined therapy of SQNYAB and WM could improve the perfusion at the myocardial tissue level. So, it is reasonable to believe that the therapy is helpful for mid- and long-term prognosis of patients. However, a credible conclusion was not arrived at by this study due to its limited size of samples and time of research. Further approval by large samples and multi-centered, randomized controlled long-term clinical trials is expected.

References

[1] Tanaka A, Kawarabayashi T, Nishibori Y, et al. No-reflow phenomenon and lesion morphology in patients with acute myocardial infarction. Circulation, 2002, 105: 2148-2152.

[2] Lee KW, Norell MS. Management of "no-reflow" complicating reperfusion therapy. Acute Card Care, 2008, 10: 5-14.

[3] Chinese Society of Cardiovascular Diseases, Chinese Medical Association and the Editorial Committee of Chinese Journal of Cardiology. Guidance on diagnosis and treatment of acute myocardial infarction. Chin J Cardiol, 2001, 29: 705-720.

[4] Cooperation Group of Xiongbi and emergency. Norm for emergent diagnosis and treatment of

Xiongbi and Xinjue (coronary artery disease and myocardial infarction). J Emerg Tradit Chin Med, 1995, 4: 183-185.

[5] Editorial Committee of Chinese Journal of Cardiology. Reference proposal of thrombolytic therapy on acute myocardial infarction. Chin J Cardiol, 1996, 24: 328-329.

[6] Zhou YC, Guo WL, eds. Ultrasonic medicine. 5th ed. Beijing: Scientific and Technical Documents Publishing House, 2006, 401-402.

[7] Brosh D, Assali AR, Mager A, et al. Effect of no-reflow during primary percutaneous coronary intervention for acute myocardial infarction on six month mortality. Am J Cardiol, 2007, 99: 442-445.

[8] Stone GW, Webb J, Cox DA, et al. Distal microcirculatory protection during percutaneous coronary intervention in acute ST-segment elevation myocardial infarction: a randomized controlled trial. JAMA, 2005, 293: 1063-1072.

[9] Chen KJ, Shi DZ. Thinking and methods of traditional Chinese medicine for treatment and prevention of restenosis after coronary artery stenting. Chin J Inform Tradit Chin Med, 1996, 5: 35.

[10] Zhang MZ, Wang L. Deng tie-tao's TCM syndrome differentiation for patients of coronary heart disease after coronary artery bypass graft. J Tradit Chin Med, 2006, 5: 32-33.

[11] Xiyuan Hospital, China Academy of Chinese Medicine. Efficacy analysis of Kangxingeng Mixture on the treatment of 118 patients with acute Myocardial infarction. Chin J Intern Med, 1976, 4: 212-215.

[12] Wang CL, Shi DZ, Yin HJ, et al. Effect of Panax quinquefolius saponin on angiogenesis and expressions of VEGF and bFGF in myocardium of rats with acute myocardial infarction. Chin J Integr Tradit West Med, 2007, 27: 331-334.

[13] Ji HG, Si L, Si XC, et al. Progress on protection of salvia miltiorrhiza on cardiac ischemia-reperfusion injuries. Guangming Tradit Chin Med, 2006, 21: 52-53.

[14] Wang H, Huang L, Jin J, et al. Comparing evaluative methods on myocardial reperfusion after percutaneous coronary intervention. Chin J Intervent Cardiol, 2006, 14: 327-330.

[15] Guo SZ, Shu XH, Pan CZ, et al. Relationship between myocardial perfusion and contractile function by use of dobutamine stressing realtime myocardial contrast echocardiography. Chin J Ultrasonography, 2005, 14: 485-489.

[16] Baskot B, Obradovic S, Ristic-Angelkov A, et al. Myocardial damage size assessment in the zone of infarction for indicating rescue percutaneous coronary intervention. Vojnosanil Preg, 2008, 65: 61-63.

Appraisal of the Prognosis in Patients with Acute Myocardial Infarction Treated with Primary Percutaneous Coronary Intervention[*]

MA Xiao-juan   YIN Hui-jun   CHEN Ke-ji

Percutaneous coronary intervention (PCI) is a landmark advance in the therapeutic history of acute myocardial infarction (AMI), which could reduce inpatient mortality and incidence of complications. But the existence of restenosis, in-stent thrombosis and so on increases the risk for recurrence of cardiovascular events in post-PCI patients[1]. Along with the development of drug eluting stents (with drugs for anti-inflammation, anti-transportation, anti-proliferation, pre-

* 原载于 Chinese Journal of Integrative Medicine，2009，15（1）：236-240

treatment, etc.), the nuisance of restenosis was somewhat alleviated, and its immediate effect has been affirmed by some randomized controlled trials. But the long-term effectiveness and safety of the revolutionary technique remains a vexing problem[2]. Therefore, the evaluation and intervention in the post-PCI associated risk factor is one of the foci in clinical studies that attracted much attention from all over the world in the recent years. Some explicit factors valuable for clinical prognosis and affirmed by current research, include C-reactive protein (CRP), tumor necrosis factor-α (TNF-α), brain natriuretic peptide (BNP) and atrial natriuretic peptide (ANP) as well as Chinese medicine (CM) syndromes with regarding to their correlation with the condition and course of AMI patients. These are discussed in this thesis, and their values for clinical prognosis evaluated.

1. C-reactive Protein

CRP is a kind of protein discovered by Pearson, et al[3] which is synthesized and secreted by hepatocytes and is capable of binding with cell wall C-amylose of pneumococci. As a nonspecific inflammation marker, its concentration in blood is positively proportionate with the degree of tissue damage. In case that other inflammatory factors have been excluded, the level of CRP could present the intensity of inflammatory reaction in coronary lesions. Hypersensitive CRP (hs-CRP) is a new independent forecasting index for coronary heart disease (CHD), with the strongest forecasting effect of all the 12 markers for cardiovascular diseases.

Research by Li, et al[4] shows that in ST-segment elevation AMI patients after emergent PCI, left ventricular ejection fraction (LVEF) was lower and peak values of WBC count and creatine kinase isozyme were higher in patients with raised hs-CRP than in those with normal hs-CRP. One hundred and eighty days after PCI, the incidence of cardiac adverse events in the former was significantly higher than in the latter. Multiple factor analysis displayed that the hs-CRP level determined on the very day of hospitalization is the main independent factor for forecasting adverse cardiac events in ST-segment elevation AMI patients 180 days after emergeni PCI. But the research conducted by Gach, et al[5] shows that post-PCI transient elevation of hs-CRP could forecast the main malignant cardiac events more strongly than the pre-PCI or post-PCI high hs-CRP level.

Anzai, et al[6] indicated that in patients who experienced one Q-wave AMI, the peak value of CRP is a key factor for forecasting short- and long- term prognosis. The peak was rather lower in non-senile patients, presenting angina before myocardial infarction or with successful recanalization, while irregular elevation of CRP level was often revealed in patients with heart rupture. The possibility of heart rupture, ventricular aneurysm and cardiogenic death within one year would be greatly increased in case of CRP ≥ 20 mg/dL. A study by Smit, et al[7] illustrated that in patients with ST-elevated PCI, the pre-PCI high CRP level shows obvious correlation with reinfarction rate and mortality within one year after PCI.

Some research displayed that CRP level is raised after AMI and the degree of which is related with the infarcted area to a certain extent[8, 9]. PCI could result in temporal elevation of CRP levels, which might be related with the stimulation of stent on plaque, endothelial injury, plaque rupture and aggravation of local inflammatory reaction. From this it could be seen that since the degree of inflammation, which could be represented by CRP level, is an important cause for post-PCI restenosis, CRP level should definitely be of value in forecasting the occurrence of restenosis.

2. Tumor Necrosis Factor-α

TNF-α is a kind of pre-inflammatory cytokine mainly produced by activated mononuclear macrophage, as well as an important and negatively regulatory factor for growth. It could promote the adhesion between endothelial cells and white blood cells, stimulate endothelial cells to secrete inflammatory mediators, activate the blood coagulation system, suppress fibrinolysis, increase inflammatory exudation and oxygen free radical production, and accelerate the release of interleukin-1, -6 and -8 by mononuclear macrophage, etc. so as to promote the occurrence and development of inflammation[10,11]. TNF-α is the key factor in triggering and promoting "cascade amplification" induced excessive inflammatory reaction, and thus, plays an important role in the pathophysiologic development process of myocardial ischemia/reperfusion injury[12]. Studies in recent years show TNF-α could be secreted also by mature cardiac muscle cells and vascular endothelium is one of its important targets[13,14]. Therefore, TNF-α induced vascular endothelial injury is of vital meaning in the pathogenesis of many cardiovascular diseases.

It has been shown by Li, et al[15] that the serum level of TNF-α is escalated along with the exacerbation of myocardial ischemia, i. e. that in AMI patients pectoris > in patients with unstable angina > in patients with stable angina pectoris > in normal persons. Thus, it can be regarded as a fine index for myocardial ischemia.

Animal experiments have proven that the myocardial infarct area, vascular endothelial injury, endothelin release and lipid peroxidation injury of cells in patients could be reduced significantly by effectively neutralizing plasma TNF-α with its own mono-antibody[16]. It was also proven by Kubica, et al[17] that the inflammatory activation degree in the peri-operative stage could influence the long-term prognosis of post-PCI patients. The level of TNF-α is significantly related with the re-infarction rate and incidence of adverse cardiovascular events in patients.

Another report[18] shows that in the course of AMI, the evident rise of plasma TNF-α with earlier peaking is a clue for severe conditions and bad prognosis in the near future. It has been found that the patients' peripheral plasma level of TNF-α that was determined 4-8 weeks after they were discharged from hospital (hospitalized for CHD events, including post-AMI angina pectoris, reinfarction, heart failure and even sudden death) was significantly higher than in those without CHD events, suggesting that the persistent post-AMI high level of TNF-α expression might be of definite significance in predicting post-AMI recurrence of CHD events.

Observation by Théroux, et al[19] found that the mortality and incidence of cardiac shock in elevated ST-segment AMI patients after PCI would be high if they presented high TNF-α level post-PCI. High levels of inflammatory reaction in 72 h after PCI were evidently correlated with the mortality of patients within 90 days. However, for post-PCI prognosis evaluation, the value of TNF-α level is inferior to that of CRP level.

Many studies illustrated that in AMI patients, the level of TNF-α is correlated with the course and severity of the illness to a definite extent, as it could evidently rise after PCI, which could be taken as an index for post-PCI adverse event forecasting. This is of great significance in evaluating short- and long-term prognosis of AMI patients. It has been displayed in a study[1] that the gene type of TNF-α could be regarded as a risk forecasting factor for occurrence of restenosis in post-PCI patients and suppressing the secretion of TNF-α may be a new way of thinking for restenosis prevention in clinical practice.

3. Brain Natriuretic Peptide

BNP is a polypeptide hormone composed of 32 amino acids and a cardiac neuropeptide hormone secreted from the ventricle during dilatation of the ventricular cavity with increased pressure load. The amount of its secretion is regulated by the tension of the ventricle wall, and positively correlated with the severity of left heart dysfunction. Therefore, the peripheral blood level of BNP could reflect the BNP secretion rate of ventricle and the condition of heart function.

This is due to infarction related artery block with corresponding myocardial ischemia and necrosis, which could lead to increase of ventricular tension. This is especially evident in the junctional area between ischemic area and normal area. Moreover, the hemodynamic changes induced by neuro-humoral factors would influence the tension of the cardiac cavity and ventricular wall, and thus, to cause rapid elevation of peripheral BNP level[20, 21].

By observing the change of BNP in 72 patients with acute coronary syndrome after PCI, Wu, et al[22] found that the level of BNP raised significantly immediately after PCI, reached peak 3 h later and recovered gradually to the baseline 12 h later, demonstrating a transient elevation of BNP level. Yildirir A, et al[23] indicated that for patients with stable CHD, the BNP level 24 h after PCI could be taken as an independent forecasting factor for adverse cardiovascular events 12 months after PCI.

Liang, et al[24] found that the change of BNP levels in AMI patients who underwent emergent PCI (the test group) differed from that in patients treated with non-reperfusion treatment (the control group). On the first day after hospitalization, BNP levels raised in both of them, showing insignificant difference. Seven days after that, it lowered significantly in the test group but remained unchanged in the control group. Thirty days afterward, in the test group, it was significantly lower as compared with that in the control group, though the levels in both groups were reduced. Moreover, the changes in plasma BNP levels were different when emergent PCI was applied on different vessels associated with infarction, and the lowering of BNP was more significant after the anterior descending branch intervention than that after intervention on the right coronary artery or on the circumflex branch. And the changes of LVEF and left ventricular end diastolic diameter correspond to the change in BNP level.

The observation of 76 AMI patients performed by Li, et al[25] show that plasma BNP concentrations in patients who underwent emergent PCI on the 1st, 7th and 28th day after hospitalization were lower than those in the patients treated with non-reperfusion, though the BNP levels at the time of hospitalization were similar. And it was displayed[26] that higher incidence of heart failure and mortality would occur in patients with high levels of BNP (> 80 pg/mL) than in those with normal level of BNP.

Research[27] shows that BNP is superior to cardio-ultrasonic examination in evaluating post-AMI heart function, ventricular rebuilding, morbidity and prognosis. The higher the BNP level, the worse the clinical prognosis. Intervention therapy could induce transient elevation of BNP, but the level of BNP was lowered more significantly and recovered more quickly in patients after PCI.

4. Atrial Natriuretic Peptide

ANP was discovered by DeBold, et al[28] in 1984, which was secreted mainly by left atrial cardiac myocytes, and possesses a potent effect in sodium discharging, diuresis, vascular dilatation and blood pressure lowing, and its secretion is jointly regulated by cardiac hemodynamics and neuro-hormones.

A lot of studies have proven that anoxia, acute increased blood volume, auricular muscle stretching, augmentative right auricular pressure, etc. could all promote the release of ANP, while limiting intake of sodium and water, decreased venous return blood, etc. could reduce it. Some reports[29] have indicated that the apparently elevated plasmal level of ANP in AMI patients might be mainly correlated with the change of ventricular compliance, cardiac insufficiency and myocardial damage.

Research by Li, et al[30] showed that the elevation of ANP appeared twice, i. e. 1 h and 12 h after AMI, the first time due to heart function disturbance, which could induce the release of ANP secretive granules in the atrium, which in turn comes earlier and quicker than the elevation of creatine kinase isoenzyme B, and the second, caused by the accelerated resynthesis and release of plasmal ANP in atrial and ventricular muscle cells, is meaningful for the estimation of heart function and clinical prognosis of patients.

Zhao, et al[31] found that ANP level may be reduced in AMI patients of Killip grade II after PCI, as PCI can effectively open up coronary arteries, retrieve agonal cardiac muscle cells and turning away ventricular reconstruction, and thereby improve heart function and reduce synthesis and secretion of ANP. So, the existence of post-PCI cardiac functional insufficiency could be found out by monitoring ANP level before and after the operation, and could be used for therapeutic guidance and estimation on both short-and long-term prognosis.

However, a different result was reported by Peng, et al[32], they found the level of ANP was obviously higher than the normal range in AMI patients at the very time of hospitalization, reaching the peak after 24 h reperfusion, then decreasing gradually, but remaining a high level on the 7th day after reperfusion, illustrating that the pattern and course of ANP release curve is not changed by PCI intervention. It is held that the post-PCI release of ANP is mainly due to the elevation of atrial pressure induced by myocardial necrosis and heart failure, and there is definite relationship between ANP level and scope of myocardial infarction. Besides, a 1-year follow-up study found that ANP level in patients with heart failure was obviously higher than those in patients without heart failure. The level of ANP could be used as an index for long-term prognosis forecasting in AMI patients after emergent coronary intervention.

Although the post-PCI trend of ANP is still disputable, the close correlation between ANP level and heart function in AMI patient surely exists, and its value in evaluating the clinical prognosis of AMI patients after PCI is quite clear.

5. CM Syndrome

Syndrome means generalization of the pathologic essence at a certain stage in the genesis and development process of disease, which could reflect the evolution rule and trend of the disease to a certain degree. In AMI patients, their CM syndromes show definite relation with clinical prognosis, and the relationship of syndrome types with the condition, course and prognosis of AMI have been proven by studies. Li, et al[33] reported that myocardial injury in AMI patients of yin-deficiency syndrome types was rather more severe, their time of hospitalization longer, mortality higher and prognosis worse. This might be correlated to the vigorous function of sympathetic-epinephrine system and enhanced activity of aldosterone in patients. Yin, et al[34] proposed that in AMI patients, the order of CM syndrome types in the descending sequence of constituent proportion was of the turbid-phlegm obstruction type, qi-stagnant with blood-stasis type, both qi-yin deficiency type, and yang-qi deficiency type, while the order in descending sequence of occurrence of such complications as arrhythmia, heart failure and cardiac shock were of the turbid-phlegm obstructive type, both qi-yin deficiency type and yang-qi deficiency type, among which the least mortality was shown in patients of the yang-qi deficiency type. Zhang, et al[35] discovered that the use of CM syndrome typing could help express and forecast the clinical severity and prognosis of acute coronary syndrome more authentically than that of coronary arteriography. However, due to the limited results of research, an universally applicable and clinically guidable norm for syndrome differentiation in AMI patients has not been formulated so far, and post-PCI syndrome specificities associated with prognosis are waiting for further studies.

Besides the above-mentioned chief forecasting factors, there are several indices valuable for AMI prognosis evaluation in clinical practice, such as creatine kinase isozyme, troponin, myoglobin, etc., which could reflect the degree of myocardial necrosis. TIMI myocardial perfusion grading and the falling percent of the total elevation of ST-segment in EGG are two methods for evaluating myocardial perfusion that have received much attention. Besides, cardiovascular ultrasonic examination, radionuclide examination, coronary CT imaging, etc. are all of definite value for post-PCI clinical prognosis forecasting in AMI patients.

For AMI, a leading cause for cardiovascular diseases to induce crippling and death, PCI could significantly reduce its inpatient mortality and incidence of complications, but could not cut down post-PCI recurrence of cardiovascular events, times of repeated hospitalization, the crippling rate, or mortality. Therefore, to perfect the evaluation system of post-PCI associated risk factor and prognosis and to provide a theoretical basis for early application of intervention on high risk patients in clinical practice will be quite beneficial in improving short- and long-term prognosis and living quality of patients. In as much as current studies on post-PCI prognosis evaluation in AMI patients are limited to a single or a few indices of correlation analysis, it is necessary for the comprehensive analysis of relevant risk factors and scientific evaluation method establishment.

References

[1] Monraats PS, Pires NM, Schepers A, et al. Tumor necrosis factor-alpha plays an important role in restenosis development. FASEB J, 2005, 19: 1998-2004.

[2] Raja SG, Berg GA. Safety of drug eluting stents: current concerns and controversies. Curr Drug Saf, 2007, 2: 212-219.

[3] Pearson TA, Mensah GA, Alexander RW, et al. Markers of inflammation and cardiovascular disease: application to clinical and public health practice: a statement for healthcare professionals from the Centers for Disease Control and Prevention and the American Heart Association. Circulation, 2003, 107: 499-511.

[4] Li L, Guo YH, Wang GS, et al. Value of hypersensitive C-reactive protein for predicting the prognosis of patients after emergent percutaneous coronary intervention. Chin J Minim Invas Surg, 2006, 6: 483-485.

[5] Gach O, Legrand V, Biessaux Y, et al. Long-term prognostic significance of high-sensitivity C-reactive protein before and after coronary angioplasty in patients with stable angina pectoris. Am J Cardiol, 2007, 99: 31-35.

[6] Anzai T, Yoshikawa T, Shiraki H, et al. C-reactive protein as a predictor of infarct expansion and cardiac rupture after a first Q-wave acute myocardial infarction. Circulation, 1997, 96: 778-784.

[7] Smit JJ, Ottervanger JP, Slingerland RJ, et al. Comparison of usefulness of C-reactive protein versus white blood cell count to predict outcome after primary percutaneous coronary intervention for ST elevation myocardial infarction. Am J Cardiol, 2008, 101: 446-451.

[8] Versaci F, Gaspardone A, Tomai F, et al. Predictive value of C-reactive protein in patients with unstable angina pectosis undergoing coronary artery stent implantation. Am J Cardiol, 2000, 85: 92-95.

[9] Zhang M, Huang TG, Zhou LJ, et al. Serum CRP, SAA, IL-6 in patients with acute myocardial infarction and effective of PCI on them. South Chin J Cardiol Dis, 2004, 10: 412-415.

[10] Chen L, Li JJ. The relativity between tumor necrosis factor-α and chronic congestive heart failure. J Chin Microcirc, 2004, 14: 56-58.

[11] Chen BY, Li XQ, Chen XL. Study in the serum TNF-α, IL-1β and IL-6 patient with congestive heart failure. J Clin Inter, Med, 2006, 23: 184-185.

[12] Ke JJ, Wang YL, Li JG, et al. Pretreatment effect of adenosine on activation of NF-kappa B and level of TNF-α during myocardial ischemia and reperfusion in rats. Chin J Traumatol, 2004, 7: 25-27.

[13] Lv JP, Wang SR, Ma ZC, et al. Proteomic analysis of the effects of tumor necrosis factor-α on endothelial cells. Chin J Pathophysiol, 2004, 20: 1121-1125.

[14] Kang YJ. Molecular and cellular mechanisms of cardiotoxicity. Environ Health Perspect , 2001, 109: 27-34.

[15] Lin ZJ, Pan H. The role of IL-10 and TNF-α in acute coronary syndrome. Prev Treat Cardio Cereb Vas

Dis, 2006, 6: 297-299.

[16] Liu D, Zhao L. Dynamic Change of tumor necrosis factor-α in patients of acute myocardial infarction. Chin J Inter Med, 2000, 39: 499.

[17] Kubica J, Kozinski M, Krzewina-Kowalska A, et al. Combined peri-procedural evaluation of CRP and TNF-alpha enhances the prediction of clinical restenosis and major adverse cardiac events in patients undergoing percutaneous coronary interventions. Int J Mol Med, 2005, 16: 173-180.

[18] Pan XM, Wu ZG, Huang Z, et al. The influence of elevated TNF-α levels on prognosis after AMI. Chin Heart J, 2004, 16: 39-40.

[19] Théroux P, Armstrong PW, Mahaffey KW, et al. Prognostic significance of blood markers of inflammation in patients with ST-segment elevation myocardial infarction undergoing primary angioplasty and effects of pexelizumab, a C5 inhibitor: a substudy of the COMMA trial. Eur Heart J, 2005, 26: 1964-1970.

[20] Maisel AS, Krishnaswamy P, Nowak RM, et al. Rapid measurement of B-type natriuretic peptide in the emergency diagnosis heart failure. N Engl J Med, 2002, 347: 161-167.

[21] Maisel AS. Practical approaches to treating patients with acute decompensated heart failure. J Cardiac Fail, 2001, 7: 13-17.

[22] Wu ZD, Wang MH, Yu XD, et al. Effects of percutanious coronary intervention on plasma brain natriuretic peptide level in patients with acute coronary syndrome. Fujian Med J, 2006, 2: 101-102.

[23] Yildirir A, Acikel S, Ertan C, et al. Value of pert-procedural B-type natriuretic peptide levels in predicting cardiac events after elective percutaneous coronary intervention. Acta Cardiol, 2008, 63: 47-52.

[24] Liang JO, Zhou XX, Huang YG, et al. Effect of primary percutaneous coronary intervention on plasma B-type natriuretic peptide in patients with acute myocardial infarction. J First Milit Med Univ, 2005, 25: 1555-1557.

[25] Li G, Gong YC, Chen S, et al. Effect of urgent percutaneous coronary intervention on brain natriuretic peptide level in patients with acute myocardial infarction. Chin J Cardiol Med, 2006, 11: 119-120.

[26] Ahmed W, Zafar S, Alam AY, et al. Plasma levels of B-type natriuretic peptide in patients with unstable angina pectoris or acute myocardial infarction: prognostic significance and therapeutic implications. Angiology, 2007, 58: 269-274.

[27] Du TX, Wang ZZ, Wang SK, et al. Clinical analysis of the changes of plasma BNP, ET, CRP and ANP levels in patients with acute myocardial infarction. J Radioimmunol, 2004, 17: 6-7.

[28] Sun JB, Lu XG, Zhang L, et al. Study and progress of cardionatrin in medical science and sports medicine. Chin J Clin Rehabil, 2005, 9: 198-199.

[29] Xiao YY, Jia WJ, Liu ZW, et al. Comparison of plasma level of artrial natriuretic factor in patients with acute myocardial infarction before and after treatment. Labeled Immunoassays Clin Med, 1999, 6: 152-154.

[30] Liu XZ, Xu JP, Zhao KO, et al. Measurement of the plasma ANP and serum CK-MB in patients with acute myocardial infarction. J Zhengzhou Univ, 2004, 39: 633-636.

[31] Zhao HL, Li L, Wang Y. Plasma levels of atrial natriuretic peptide and brain natriuretic peptide in patients with acute myocardial infarction in Killip classes II underwent percutaneous coronary intervention. Chin J Cardiol Med, 2005, 10: 109-110.

[32] Peng JJ, Wu Y, Hu DY, et al. Serial changes and prognostic significance of atrial natriuretic polypeptide in patients with acute myocardial infarction undergoing emergency coronary intervention. Chin J Med Guide, 2004, 6: 340-342.

[33] Li NY, Li YY, Hong CX, et al. Exploration on the relationship between pathogenesis for yin-deficiency of acute myocardial infarction and immediate prognosis as well as its mechanism. Chin J Integr Tradit Chin West Med, 2004, 24: 400-403.

[34] Yin KC, Luo Y, Zhang BP, et al. Characteristics of differentiating symptoms and signs and prognosis analysis on 65 cases of acute myocardial infarction. J Pract Tradit Chin Med, 2001, 17: 3-4.

[35] Zhang BT, YAN QL, Yan DX, et al. Study on the number of vulnerable vessels, level of coronary artery stenosis, integral of Braunwald clinical grades and their correlation among different traditional Chinese medcine syndromes in patients with acute coronary syndromes. J Emerg Tradit Chin Med, 2005, 14: 147-149.

第三章

第三节 中西医结合防治高血压

病证结合治疗高血压病[*]

马晓昌

陈可冀老师是最早对高血压病进行病证结合研究的学者之一。早在 1959 年他就开始注重中西医结合研究工作，阐明了高血压弦脉与儿茶酚胺代谢水平的相关性。陈可冀老师自 20 世纪 50 年代末开展高血压病的临床研究以来，在诊治方案上，先后经过了：（1）辨证施治 - 辨证定方，随证加减、分证治疗。（2）辨病制定基本治则，并辨证加减。（3）专方专药治疗，以现代的中药药理作用为依据。（4）综合治疗等。其中在辨病的基础方上根据具体证型加减配伍最能体现辨病与辨证相结合的论治特色，适应中医临床实际，符合病证结合的中西医结合最佳诊疗模式，具有优异的症状疗效，能较好地调整高血压病患者内在失调的生理功能，达到温和降压的目的，阻止或延缓病情的发展。现将陈可冀老师对高血压病的中医病证结合治疗经验总结如下。

1. 对病因、病机的认识

高血压病可因情志刺激，五志过极，忧郁恼怒惊恐，思虑过度，持续性精神紧张；或饮食不节，嗜食肥甘辛辣，纵情饮酒；或劳欲过度，精气内伤；或体质禀赋偏盛、偏虚，如过瘦、过肥等多种因素及其相互作用所致，且总以内因为发病的基础。当其发病之后，由于素体及原始病因的不同，疾病先后阶段的演变发展可以表现多种病理变化及不同证候。

1.1 肝、肾、心的气血阴阳失调为主要病理变化

审证求因，高血压病虽然表现为肝经病候为主，但因脏腑之间的整体关系，往往与肾、心密切相关，早期多以肝为主，以后常见与肾、心同病，且可涉及脾，但其间又有主次的不同。由于脏腑阴阳的不平衡，表现为阳亢与阴虚两个方面的病变为多。阳亢主要为心肝阳亢，但久延可致阴伤，发展为肝肾阴虚；而肝肾（心）阴虚，阴不制阳，又可导致心肝阳亢。两者之间互为联系、演变，故其病理中心以"阴虚阳亢"为主，表现为"下虚上实"之候。从其病程经过而言，一般病初及中青年患者以阳亢居多，逐渐发展为阴虚阳亢，久病不愈又可见阴虚为主。阳亢为标，多属暂时性，阴虚是本，常为重要的后果，标实与本虚对立而又联系。脏腑阴阳的正常功能活动是生化气血并主宰运行的基础，脏腑阴阳失调也必然引起气血运行的反常。而气血运行的紊乱又可加重脏腑阴阳的失调，如《妇人大全良方》在论述中风病时指出："皆因阴阳不调，脏腑气偏，荣卫失度，气血错乱"。提示气血失调是高血压病发展至中风的病理基础，它是阴阳失调的具体表现。

1.2 风、火、痰、瘀、虚为主要病理因素

在脏腑阴阳失调的基础上，不但阳亢与阴虚互为因果，且可导致化火、动风、生痰、夹瘀、助虚，五者又可相互转化、并存，表现为"火动风生""风助火势""痰因火动""痰郁化火""风动痰

* 原载于《中国中西医结合杂志》，2012，32（8）：1134-1136

升"等。在不同个体及病的不同阶段，又有主次先后之分。风、火、痰、瘀临床可各有侧重，且每多和正虚并存，有偏实、偏虚的不同。凡属肝肾不足、阴虚阳亢化风，而致心肝火盛、蒸液成痰、气滞血瘀者属实，久延伤阴，则由实转虚，因阴虚而致虚风内动、虚火上炎，气不化津，气虚血瘀者属因虚致实，表现为本虚标实（虚中夹实）之证。

1.3 气血逆乱为主要病理转归

如病延日久，或病情急剧发展，虚实向两极分化，阴虚于下，阳亢于上，肝风痰火升腾，冲激气血，气血逆乱，可见气升血逆，甚至阻塞窍络，突发昏厥卒中之变，或风痰入络，气血郁滞，血瘀络痹，而致肢体不遂，偏枯僻，或因心脉瘀阻而见胸痹、心痛。《素问·调经》云："血与之气，并走于上，则为大厥，厥则暴死，气复反则生，不反则死"，即系指高血压病发展转归为中风的后果而言。

2. 诊治特色

2.1 辨治要点

（1）辨清病理性质：掌握阳亢与阴虚、标实与本虚的主次，予以潜阳、滋阴、活血、益气，阴虚及阳者又当温养。（2）区别病理因素：标实为主者，辨别风、火、痰、瘀的主次、兼夹，予以熄风、清火、化瘀、活血。（3）审察脏腑病机：本虚为主者，鉴别肝、肾心的重点，予以柔肝、滋肾、养心。

2.2 治疗方法

2.2.1 肝阳上亢证 症状：头晕目眩，头胀头痛，或颠顶掣痛，面赤升火，头筋跃起，脑响耳鸣，烦躁，肢麻肉瞤，口干口苦，苔薄黄，舌质红，脉弦数。治疗：平肝熄风，潜阳清热方。苦丁茶 15～30g、钩藤 15～30g（后下）、天麻 15g、决明子 15g、野菊花 15g、罗布麻叶 15g、珍珠母 30g（先煎）、玄参 15g、车前草 15g、桑叶 15g。加减：肢麻不利加臭梧桐、豨莶草；头晕痛甚加白蒺藜、蝉衣；面红、目赤、鼻衄、便结加龙胆草、黑山栀或大黄。

2.2.2 痰火内盛证 症状：头晕重痛，咳吐黏痰，胸闷，神烦善惊，形体多肥，身重肢麻，语謇多涎，口干苦或黏，舌苔黄腻、舌尖红，脉弦滑数。治疗：清热化痰方。半夏 10g、胆南星 6g、炒黄芩 10g、夏枯草 12g、僵蚕 10g、海藻 10g、牡蛎 30g（先煎）、泽泻 15g、鲜竹沥 10～20mL。加减：心烦梦多加黄连、莲子心、茯神；神情异常

加郁金、天竺黄；胸闷、痰多、便秘加栝蒌、石菖蒲。

2.2.3 气血失调证 症状：头痛头胀，或痛处如针刺，面色黯红，时有烘热，胸部有紧压感，或胸痛如刺，间有心悸，肢体窜痛或顽麻，妇女月经不调，口干、苔薄，舌质偏黯，或有紫斑、瘀斑，脉或细、或涩、或结代。治疗：调气和血方。丹参 12g、川芎 10g、大（小）蓟 15g、怀牛膝 10g、夜交藤 12g、生槐米 10g、广地龙 10g、代赭石 30g。加减：头昏加白蒺藜；颈项强痛加葛根；胸闷、胸痛加栝蒌皮、元胡；肢麻不利加鸡血藤、红花；胸胁满胀或窜痛加柴胡、青木香；妇女月经不调加茺蔚子、女贞子、旱莲草。

2.2.4 肝肾阴虚证 症状：头昏晕痛，目涩视糊，耳鸣，遇劳则面赤升火，肢麻，腰酸腿软，口干，舌红少苔，脉细弦或细数。治疗：滋阴柔肝益肾方。生地 30g、枸杞子 10g、炙女贞子 10g、制首乌 12g、桑寄生 12g、生石决明 30g（先煎）、菊花 10g、白蒺藜 10g。加减：头眩面色潮红加牡蛎、鳖甲；烦热加知母、黄柏；肢麻加白芍；失眠多梦加枣仁、夜交藤、合欢皮。

2.2.5 阴虚及阳证 症状：头晕，目花，视物模糊，面白少华，间有烘热，神疲气短，腰酸腿软，肢清足冷，夜尿频数，舌淡红或淡白、质胖，脉沉细。治疗：温补肝肾方。仙茅 10g、仙灵脾 10g、肉苁蓉 10g、当归 10g、生熟地各 15g、甘杞子 15g、灵磁石 30g、黄柏 6g。加减：头昏目花加潼蒺藜；心悸气短加生黄芪、五味子；倦怠大便不实加党参、淮山药；祛寒、足肿加制附子、白术、车前草。加减一般不超过 3 味药。

3. 规律总结

3.1 辨治规律

陈可冀老师根据高血压发病的不同病因及不同年龄阶段，总结了独具特色辨证规律和辨病与辨证相结合的证治特点。针对老年期高血压病，根据近年来的研究，健康老年人存在阴虚、肾虚，实证主要表现为痰浊、血瘀。临床上老年高血压病患者以肝肾亏虚、阳亢、血瘀最为多见，常以补肾为主的复方治疗。而中、青年期高血压病患者，多数属起病伊始，病程较短，以肝郁化火，火热上冲较为多见，肝阳上亢者亦不少见，适用清热降火、平肝潜阳的复方治疗。此外，陈可冀老师还十分重视妊娠期高血压的防治。妊娠期高血压危害严重，早期

预防、早期发现、早期治疗甚为重要。由于妊娠期的生理特点是阴血不足，所以临床亦常见妊娠高血压患者以肝肾阴血亏损和肝阳上亢同时并见，常多选用滋阴养血药治疗。

3.2　常用药物分类及临床应用特点

陈可冀老师根据临床辨证将常用药物归纳为以下 10 类：（1）滋阴药，如玄参、白芍、知母等；（2）潜镇药，如石决明、牡蛎、珍珠母等；（3）清热药，如龙胆草、夏枯草、黄连、黄芩等；（4）补益肝肾药，如熟地、枸杞子、龟版等；（5）平肝熄风药，如天麻、钩藤、菊花、羚羊角等；（6）祛风通络药，如地龙、牛膝、秦艽、桑枝等；（7）养心安神药，如茯苓、夜交藤、酸枣仁等；（8）豁痰药，如半夏、南星、贝母、竹茹等；（9）化瘀药，如川芎、桃仁、益母草、鸡血藤等；（10）温阳药，如杜仲、续断、仙茅、仙灵脾等。

复方治疗高血压病经过临床系列研究的众多方剂中，机制较为明确、疗效亦较可靠的，陈可冀老师常据证选用的有：天麻钩藤饮，对头晕、耳鸣、肢麻、头重足轻等肝风患者有效；二仙汤或二仙合剂，对阴虚阳亢患者尤为适合，而并不只适用于女性冲任不调之阴虚阳亢证型；六味地黄汤加味及其衍变方，用于阴虚阳亢者，如杞菊地黄汤、知柏地黄汤等，每每获效；桂附二味汤或桂附地黄汤加味，针对阳虚型或阴阳两虚型的高血压病患者，均为多用而有效的方剂。另外，对许多降压有效的中成药或小复方，也常常据证使用，亦常嘱轻症患者用小复方代茶饮，也是其临证特色之一。不仅如此，许多单味药经过现代药学、药理学及临床研究证明确有降压疗效者，在辨证的前提下，亦常常加减使用或单味应用。如：汉防己、罗布麻、葛根、元胡、臭梧桐、土青木香、钩藤、天麻、长春花、地龙、旱芹菜、黄连、黄芩、黄柏、三棵针、野菊花、杜仲、牛膝、萝芙木、牡丹皮、莲子心等。

4.　博采众长，自创新方

陈可冀老师通过几十年的临床实践研究证明，高血压以肝肾阴虚、肝阳上亢类型为多见，约占高血压病的 90% 以上。凡辨证属于肝肾阴虚、肝阳上亢者，常采用自拟的经验方清眩降压汤治疗。

方用苦丁茶 30g、天麻 30g、钩藤 30 ~ 60g（后下）、黄芩 10g、川牛膝 10g、生杜仲 10g、夜交藤 30g、鲜生地 30g、桑叶 15g、菊花 15g，每日 1 剂，水煎，分 2 次口服。方中以苦丁茶散肝风、清头目、活血脉，天麻、钩藤平肝潜阳熄风为主，辅以杜仲补益肝肾，夜交藤搜风通络、养心安神，黄芩、桑叶、菊花清肝热、平肝阳，佐以牛膝祛瘀通络、引血下行以折其阳亢，更助苦丁茶等活血通脉之力，鲜生地清热养阴以滋肾水，诸药合用，共奏益肝肾、清肝热、平肝阳之功效。纵观全方配伍，药精力专，可直中肝肾阴虚、肝阳上亢之病机所在。若眩晕、耳鸣、头痛重者，可加羚羊角粉 3 ~ 4.5g，分 2 次药液冲服，以凉肝熄风镇惊。羚羊角粉虽属血肉有情之品，并非补益。

5.　典型病例

患者，女，50 岁，因"头晕、头痛 4 年，加重伴胸痛半年"收住院。主诉：头晕、头痛、耳鸣，烦躁易怒，口干口苦，胸闷，大便干，舌红苔薄黄，脉弦。既往发现高血压病史 4 年，血压最高 160/100mmHg。常服硝苯地平 10mg，每日 3 次，血压控制在（140 ~ 150）/（85 ~ 95）mmHg。查体：血压 140/90mmHg，心率 75 次/分，律齐，主动脉第二音亢进，双肺未闻干、湿啰音，双下肢不肿。西医诊断：高血压病 Ⅱ 级；中医诊断：眩晕（肝肾阴虚，肝阳上亢型）。予清眩降压汤治疗，服药第二天，血压即降至 120/80mmHg，服药 5 剂后头晕、头痛减轻，但自觉时有烘热，加知母 12g、黄柏 12g、生石决明 30g 养阴清热，平肝潜阳。再服 4 剂，患者诸证明显减轻，血压平稳，24h 动态血压监测，血压最高为 136/80mmHg。

对该病例陈可冀老师在第一次应用中药方剂时，即首选辨病，予清眩降压汤治疗，服药第二日即见收效，继服几日后根据患者时有烘热的症状，辨证为阴虚内热，即在原方基础上再加用知母、黄柏等养阴清热之药，之后症状缓解明显，同时血压稳定，此病例证实了辨病与辨证结合治疗高血压的良好效果。

波动性高血压与血小板活化及其中西医结合干预策略 *

刘 玥 张京春 史大卓 陈可冀

《中国心血管病报告2011》[1]指出，目前中国有2亿左右的高血压患者，且中国脑卒中的发病率及致死、致残率显著高于欧美等发达国家，而降低高血压患者的血压能够有效减少卒中事件的发生，因此对于高血压的积极控制应该放在心脑血管疾病危险因素防控的首要地位。对血压波动性的病理生理特点及其与血小板活化、中医血瘀证之间的关系进行深入探讨，有利于提高对高血压靶器官损害发病机制的认识，同时可为中西医结合干预策略的制定提供新的思路。

1. 波动性高血压

人的血压受生理、病理、精神状态以及环境等因素的影响而处在不断的波动当中，这种在24h内自发性的波动被定义为"血压波动性"或"血压变异性"（blood pressure variability，BPV），根据观察时间分为短时变异与长时变异，前者指24h之内，后者指数天、数周、数月甚至数年[2, 3]。BPV超过正常范围即称为"BPV增高"或"波动性高血压"，引起BPV异常升高的机制尚不明确，可能与神经、体液和血管等因素密切相关[4]。

临床研究发现，阵发性高血压病患者虽然平均动脉血压控制良好，但仍然存在很高的心脑血管事件发生风险[5]。由于受到饮食、运动、环境、情绪、药物、治疗不当等诸多因素的干扰，临床许多高血压病患者处于BPV增高状态，因此"波动性高血压"的描述应该更符合临床实际。晨峰高血压以及夜间血压升高均是波动性高血压的重要表现形式，前者与晨起交感神经和肾素-血管紧张素-醛固酮系统的激活以及血液流变学的异常改变密切相关，已证实晨峰高血压可以加重靶器官损害，是心脑血管事件发生的独立危险因素之一[6]，而后者多由阻塞性睡眠呼吸暂停引起的慢性间歇性低氧导致。自从2010年Rothwell PM[7]在《柳叶刀》（The Lancet）撰文系统阐述了平均动脉血压的临床局限性，以及波动性高血压在预测心脑血管事件发生中存在重要作用的观点后，近年来有关波动性

高血压的相关研究层出不穷。目前已有研究表明，相对于动脉血压平均值，BPV尤其是长时BPV升高是脑卒中事件发生的独立危险因素，同时也是心血管事件的强预测因子[5, 8]。大量临床研究已经证实，波动性高血压（特别是波动性收缩压增高）相对于稳定性高血压（平均动脉压增高）更能促进高血压病患者靶器官损害的发生、发展与恶化，血压波动幅度越大，急性心脑血管事件的发生率越高、预后也越差[9-11]。近年来对于波动性高血压及其靶器官损害的防治已成为全球高血压病研究领域的热点和难点问题之一，而重视降低增高的BPV则成为高血压治疗的重要目标[12]。

2. 波动性高血压与血小板活化

血管内皮功能受损被认为是高血压病靶器官损害的重要病理生理基础，BPV增高在血流动力学上造成的异常主要是血流不稳定，从而改变了血流的切应力，切应力的改变可使血管结构异常化，以致血管平滑肌细胞增生、管壁肥厚，继而大血管壁张力和切力降低，同时可增加脂蛋白在管壁上的不断沉积，日久可以损害血管内皮功能，加速血管平滑肌细胞的内膜增生，同时脂质不断浸润血管壁都会加速动脉粥样硬化斑块的形成，因此高血压病患者较常见血栓栓塞性靶器官损害[13]，这个过程中血小板活化必然也起到了关键作用，但具体机制尚不明确。血小板不仅在止血与血栓形成中发挥重要作用，在动脉粥样硬化的发生发展中也扮演了极为重要的角色。血小板氧化应激能够导致血小板活化，增加对血管内皮细胞的黏附以及血栓的形成，影响血管内皮细胞的功能，刺激泡沫细胞生成从而加速动脉粥样硬化的发生发展以及后续心脑血管事件的发生[14]。

近年来，有关波动性高血压与血小板活化方面的研究日益引起学者的关注。我国学者通过建立体外单纯血流波动模型，观察了单纯血流波动对血小板黏附聚集功能的影响，同时观察了体外血流波动模型中压力波动性增高对血小板的活化作用，结

* 原载于《中国中西医结合杂志》，2013，33（7）：869-8720

果发现单纯的血流波动状态引起的血小板对胶原的黏附率较单纯的低血流量或高血流量状态时均明显升高，且流式细胞检测到血小板 P- 选择素水平显著升高，表明压力波动性增高可以活化血小板，波动的血流更能够增加血栓的形成[15]。同时在体实验借助单纯 BPV 增高动物模型——去窦弓神经（SAD）大鼠，观察到 SAD 大鼠血小板黏附聚集功能增强，血小板 P- 选择素表达增加，进一步证实了波动性高血压能够导致血小板活化[16]。动物实验研究还表明，BPV 增高早期可以导致左心室微循环异常，以血管内皮细胞损害、血液黏度增加和毛细血管密度减少为特征，随后可出现左心室肥厚，而血小板活化参与了 BPV 增高导致微循环障碍的发生[17]。临床研究也发现，波动性高血压特别是收缩压波动性增高与血小板活化水平以及颈动脉粥样硬化程度密切相关[18-22]。由上可知，在波动性高血压状态下，机体已经出现了血栓前状态（prethrombotic state，PST），即以血小板活化为突出特征的易致血栓形成伴随血管内皮功能障碍的病理状态[23]，日久必然加速血管管腔内的血栓形成，进一步导致靶器官损害的发生。

3. 干预策略

BPV 增高伴随血栓前状态这一病理特征的发现，可能为临床中西药物联合使用预防高血压靶器官损害提供了一个非常重要的干预策略，即在降低 BPV 的同时改善 PST（抑制血小板活化）。

不同种类的西医降压药物对 BPV 增高的影响各有差异。一项旨在比较不同降压药物在随访期间对收缩压波动水平影响的荟萃分析[24]显示，长效钙离子拮抗剂（CCB）和利尿剂均分别能够明显降低收缩压的波动水平，因此卒中发生的风险也相对较小，而血管紧张素转换酶抑制剂（ACEI）、血管紧张素 Ⅱ 受体拮抗剂（ARB）、β 受体阻滞剂等对 BPV 的降低效果较差。推测其原因可能与 CCB、利尿剂都属于容量型降压药（作用于降压最末端，受影响因素较少），而其他三类药物属于肾素 - 神经递质系统抑制剂（受人体自身影响因素较多）有关[12]。在联合用药方面，Matsui Y 等[25]完成了一项临床随机对照的药效研究，比较了 ARB 分别与 CCB 以及利尿剂联用时对高血压人群 BPV 以及动脉硬化程度的干预效应。研究结果发现，对于平均收缩压的降低两组间差异无统计学意义，但是 ARB 与 CCB 联用能够显著降低随访期

间收缩压的波动水平，同时发现该组患者血管硬化程度亦明显降低。此研究结果提供了一个可能的临床优化处方，即 CCB 与 ARB 类药物联合使用在降低平均动脉收缩压之外还显著降低增高的 BPV 水平，这可能与其改善高血压病患者血管硬化程度密切相关。西药在改善高血压血小板活化方面，主要还是应用传统的抗血小板药物为主，但随着抗血小板药物广泛、长期的临床应用，其胃肠道及神经系统出血风险及抗血小板药物抵抗事件也在不断增加，这就促使我们在传统中医药中寻求更加安全有效的干预药物，开展高血压病中西医结合研究[26]。

近年来随着补充与替代医学（Complementary and Alternative Medicine，CAM）在全球的不断升温[27]，中医中药防治理论[28,30]与传统非药物疗法[31,32]也在逐渐走进对波动性高血压及其血栓前状态的干预中来。既往对于高血压病的中医辨证多集中在"肝肾"以及"阴阳"的角度，补益肝肾或平肝潜阳成为中医药治疗高血压病的主流治法，但这远远不能涵盖和解释高血压病西医发病机制的复杂性和产生不良脑血管事件的严重性。值得注意的是已有学者对此作出了不一样的探索，早在 20 世纪 80 年代袁肇凯等[33]就提出了高血压病患者存在血瘀证候，其后临床研究表明血瘀证是高血压病中医常见证型之一，并可能贯穿高血压病的始终[34]，并且发现 BPV 增高可能是高血压病血瘀证中医辨证标准之一[35]，高血压病血瘀证患者收缩压波动性增高与血小板活化及胰岛素抵抗密切相关[36]。有学者从基因多态性的角度研究了高血压血瘀证患者的易患基因[37]。有学者采用量化的中医学血瘀证目征积分的方法，发现高血压病患者 BPV 水平与血瘀证目征量化积分呈高度正相关[38]。同时学者们逐渐尝试用活血化瘀药物治疗严重的高血压病患者，并取得了一定的临床疗效[39,40]，亦对活血化瘀方药抗高血压的机制做了初步研究[41,42]，发现其可以降低异常增高的 BPV 水平，但具体作用机制及靶点目前尚不明确。中医学血瘀证与血小板活化状态密切相关，已有大量临床及基础研究表明活血化瘀方药体内、体外均可以抑制血小板活化水平，改善血液流变学异常[43]，阻断 PST 的发展。

4. 展望

综上所述，波动性高血压与血小板活化密切相关，两者均可明显导致高血压靶器官的损伤及急性血管事件的发生。活血化瘀方药可能在降低高血

压病患者增高的 BPV 同时还可明显抑制血小板活化水平，改善其导致的血栓前状态，在高血压靶器官损害的防治方面具有重要的应用价值。值得注意的是，目前对于应用活血化瘀方药联合西药干预波动性高血压以及血栓前状态的疗效尚缺乏临床研究证据，未来应该开展大样本、多中心、随机对照的临床研究，合理评价其临床疗效，为其广泛应用提供高质量的临床证据。同时，对活血化瘀中药的单体（有效成分）或复方对 BPV 干预作用机制进行深入探讨，特别是 BPV 增高对血小板活化的病理学意义以及活血化瘀方药的干预效应方面，同时加强对其作用信号通路、分子靶点的相关基础实验研究，相信这些研究会不断丰富对波动性高血压时血小板活化现象的深入认识，为高血压血栓栓塞性并发症的防治提供新的思路。

参考文献

[1] 卫生部心血管病防治研究中心. 中国心血管病报告 2011. 北京：中国大百科全书出版社，2012：1.

[2] Mancia G, Grassi G. Mechanisms and clinical implications of blood pressure variability. J Cardiovasc Pharmacol, 2000, 35 (7 Suppl 4)：S15-S19.

[3] 张维忠. 血压变异研究进展和临床意义. 中华心血管病杂志，2011，39 (1)：23-24.

[4] 苏定冯，缪朝玉. 血压波动性的研究. 高血压杂志，2005，13 (7)：394-397.

[5] Rothwell PM, Howard SC, Dolan E, et al. Prognostic significance of visit-to-visit variability, maximum systolic blood pressure, and episodic hypertension. Lancet, 2010, 375 (9718)：895-905.

[6] Kario K, Picketing TG, Umeda Y, et al. Morning surge in blood pressure as a predictor of silent and clinical cerebrovascular disease in elderly hypertensive：a prospective study. Circulation, 2003, 107 (10)：1401-1406.

[7] Rothwell PM. Limitations of the usual blood-pressure hypothesis and importance of variability, instability, and episodic hypertension. Lancet, 2010, 375 (9718)：938-948.

[8] Rothwell PM, Howard SC, Dolan E, et al. Effects of beta blockers and calcium-channel blockers on within individual variability in blood pressure and risk of stroke. Lancet Neurol, 2010, 9 (5)：469-480.

[9] Muntner P, Shimbo D, Tonelli M, et al. The relationship between visit-to-visit variability in systolic blood pressure and all-cause mortality in the general population：findings from NHANES III, 1988 to 1994. Hypertension, 2011, 57 (2)：160-166.

[10] Rothwell PM. Does blood pressure variability modulate cardiovascular risk? Curr Hypertens Rep, 2011, 13 (3)：177-186.

[11] Yokota K, Fukuda M, Matsui Y, et al. Impact of visit-to-visit variability of blood pressure on deterioration of renal function in patients with non-diabetic chronic kidney disease. Hypertens Res, 2013, 36 (2)：151-157.

[12] Dolan E, O'Brien E. Blood pressure variability：clarity for clinical practice. Hypertension, 2010, 56 (21)：179-181.

[13] Gkaliagkousi E, Douma S, Zamboulis C, et al. Nitricoxide dysfunction in vascular endothelium and platelets：role in essential hypertension. J Hypertens, 2009, 27 (12)：2310 -2320.

[14] 赵晓民，秦树存. 血小板氧化应激和动脉粥样硬化. 生理科学进展，2011，42 (1)：33-38.

[15] Zhao XM, Wu YP, Cai HX, et al. The influence of the pulsatility of the blood flow on the extent of platelet adhesion. Thromb Res, 2008, 121 (6)：821-825.

[16] 赵晓民，韩继举，焦鹏，等. 血压波动性增高对血小板聚集功能的影响. 中国病理生理杂志，2010，26 (10)：1957.

[17] 赵晓民. 血压波动性增高致微循环异常和左心室肥厚及其机理的实验研究. 济南：山东大学，2008：69.

[18] Alexandru N, Popov D, Dragan E, et al. Platelet activation in hypertension associated with hyper-cholesterolemia：effects of irbesartan. J Thromb Haemost, 2011, 9 (1)：173-184.

[19] Preston RA, Coffey JO, Materson BJ, et al. Elevated platelet P-selectin expression and platelet activation in high risk patients with uncontrolled severe hypertension. Atherosclerosis, 2007, 192 (1)：148-154.

[20] 李剑，孙宝玲，杨光敏，等. 高血压患者和正常血压者血压波动程度与血栓前状态的关系. 中国心血管病杂志，2011，16 (4)：267-270.

[21] 刘傲亚，余振球，王文化，等. 高血压病患者颈动脉粥样硬化与血压变异性的相关性. 中华心血管病杂志，2011，39 (6)：484-487.

[22] 杜江川，赵洛沙，李阳，等. 老年高血压病患者血压变异性对血小板体积、高敏 C 反应蛋白的影响. 中国循证心血管医学杂志，2011，3 (5)：359-361.

[23] Chan MY, Andreotti F, Becker RC. Hypercoagulable states in cardiovascular disease.

Circulation，2008，118（22）：2286-2297．

[24] Webb AJ，Fischer U，Mehta Z，et al．Effects of antihypertensive-drug class on interindividual variation in blood pressure and risk of stroke：a systematic review and meta-analysis．Lancet，2010，375（9718）：906-915．

[25] Matsui Y，O'Rourke MF，Hoshide S，et al．Combined effect of angiotensin Ⅱ receptor blocker and either a calcium channel blocker or diuretic on day-by-day variability of home blood pressure：the Japan combined treatment with Olmesartan and a calcium-channel blocker versus Olmesartan and diuretics randomized efficacy study．Hypertension，2012，59（6）：1132-1138．

[26] 陈可冀．关于高血压病的中西医结合研究．中国中西医结合杂志，2010，30（5）：453．

[27] Xu H，Chen KJ．Complementary and alternative medicine：is it possible to be mainstream? Chin J Integr Med，2012，18（6）：403-404．

[28] 黄烨，殷惠军，陈可冀．心主血脉与血栓前状态．中华中医药杂志，2011，26（4）：633-636．

[29] 于泓，王海云，徐凤芹．从"调整阴阳，以平为期"干预高血压病血压变异性．中西医结合心脑血管病杂志，2012，10（6）：744-745．

[30] 陈懿宇，张京春．高血压血管内皮机制的中西医研究现状．中国老年学杂志，2010，20（30）：3010-3013．

[31] 李会娟，申鹏飞．针刺降低血压变异性．吉林中医药，2011，31（1）：53-54．

[32] 马丽，尚玉红，何佳．耳穴贴压辅助疗法对老年高血压病患者血压变异性的影响．江苏中医药，2011，43（11）：56-58．

[33] 袁肇凯，郭振球．高血压病血瘀辨证与舌尖微观变化的初步研究．中医杂志，1982，23（11）：65-67，81．

[34] 王文智，徐树楠，徐伟超．高血压病血瘀证机理研究述评．中医杂志，2007，48（6）：560-562．

[35] 陈健，陈治卿．原发性高血压血瘀证患者动态血压变化特点的临床研究．世界中西医结合杂志，2008，3（10）：600-602．

[36] 陈健，陈治卿，梁立新，等．原发性高血压血瘀证患者活化血小板、胰岛素抵抗及动态血压变化特点．中国临床康复，2006，10（15）：14-16．

[37] 骆杰伟，陈慧，吴小盈，等．去甲肾上腺素转运体基因启动子多态性及单倍体型与高血压病血瘀证的相关性研究．中国中西医结合杂志，2010，30（5）：458-462．

[38] 吴锐，吴波，余淑娇，等．高血压病血瘀证目征与血压变异性关系的临床研究．江苏中医药，2010，42（4）：30-31．

[39] 徐贵成，张流成．活血降压方治疗高血压病102例．北京中医，1994，13（2）：26-27．

[40] 林桂珍．银丹心脑通软胶囊对高血压患者血压变异性的影响．中西医结合心脑血管病杂志，2011，9（10）：1163-1164．

[41] 李伟，王德忠，朱京涛，等．白花丹参对清醒自发性高血压大鼠血压及血压波动性的影响．中国老年学杂志，2010，30（2）：200-202．

[42] 程少冰，周永红，陈利国．血府逐瘀汤对高血压血瘀证患者血清致内皮功能障碍的影响．中国老年学杂志，2011，31（6）：971-973．

[43] Liu Y，Yin HJ，Shi DZ，et al．Chinese herbs and formulas for promoting blood circulation and removing blood stasis and anti-platelet therapies．Evid Based Complement Alternat Med，2012：184503．

清眩调压方治疗更年期女性高血压病的临床研究 *

陶丽丽　马晓昌　陈可冀

　　高血压是一种常见多发病，也是心脑血管病最重要的危险因素。因此积极降压，减少心脑血管疾病的发病风险是我国高血压防治的主要目标。清眩调压方是陈可冀院士根据数十年临床经验，针对高血压病的病机特点，以清肝热、平肝阳、益肝肾为法，创立的治疗肝肾阴虚、肝阳上亢证高血压的有效经验方。本研究重点观察清眩调压方对更年期女性高血压病的临床疗效。

* 原载于《中国中西医结合杂志》，2009，29（8）：680-684

1. 资料与方法

1.1 诊断标准

高血压病诊断和分级标准按照1999年《中国高血压防治指南》[1]。中医证候诊断标准按照2002年《中药新药临床研究指导原则》[2]中高血压病阴虚阳亢证标准。更年期诊断参照《实用中西医结合妇产科学》[3]及《新编妇产科疾病诊疗学》[4]标准，拟定诊断标准为：临床具有潮热汗出、感觉异常、失眠、易激动、抑郁、眩晕、头痛、疲乏、心悸、皮肤蚁走感、泌尿系统症状和骨、关节肌肉痛中1种以上，且查血 $FSH > 40U/L$，$E_2 < 150pmo1/L$。

1.2 纳入标准

凡符合高血压病诊断标准，高血压分级属1～2级者，中医辨证属阴虚阳亢证的更年期女性，年龄40～60岁。

1.3 排除标准

（1）继发性高血压；（2）收缩压（SBP）≥180mmHg或舒张压（DBP）≥110mmHg者；（3）合并有肝、脑、心、肾疾患和参加其他临床试验的患者；（4）对本汤药不能耐受、过敏者。

1.4 临床资料

87例患者均为2006年9月—2008年1月在中国中医科学院西苑医院心血管中心的病房及门诊的高血压病患者，按照随机数字表法分组，其中对照组43例，试验组44例。两组患者年龄、病程、体重指数、血压及高血压分级比较（表1），无统计学意义（$P > 0.05$）。

1.5 方法

1.5.1 治疗方法 试验组给予培哚普利片1片[每片4mg，由施维雅（天津）制药有限公司生产，批号：X960273]加清眩调压方颗粒剂（由苦丁茶30g、天麻30g、钩藤30g、黄芩10g、川牛膝10g、杜仲10g、夜交藤30g、生地30g、桑叶15g、菊花15g组成，江苏江阴药业有限公司生产，每剂由单味中药免煎颗粒剂组成），对照组给予培哚普利片1片加中药模拟剂（麦芽颗粒，由中国中医科学院西苑医院药厂提供，性状、包装与

清眩调压方颗粒剂相同）。培哚普利片每天早上8点口服，中药颗粒剂／中药模拟剂每日2次，每次1剂冲服。4周为1个疗程，连续观察2个疗程，每2周进行1次临床症状记录，治疗过程中出现的任何不适或症状均按不良反应记录。

1.5.2 观察指标及方法 （1）两组患者均在治疗前后行动态血压检测（采用美国Spacelabs Medical公司生产的9027-ABP型24h动态血压记录仪测量），记录24h血压、心率的测定值；（2）观察治疗前后相关症状（眩晕、头痛、腰酸、膝软、五心烦热、心悸、耳鸣、健忘）改善情况，每例症状积分之和为该例症状总积分值；（3）治疗前后空腹采肘静脉血检查血脂（TC、TG、HDL-C、LDL-C、VLDL-C，采用日立7600全自动生化分析仪测定，试剂盒：Cholestest STD和APO Control，由日本第一化学生产提供）、血清雌二醇（E_2，采用Cohase 601型全自动分析仪测定，试剂盒采用Cohas Estradiol试剂盒）、血浆超敏C反应蛋白（hs-CRP）、同型半胱氨酸（HCY）、血管紧张素Ⅱ（Ang Ⅱ）水平（采用日立7600全自动生化分析仪测定，试剂盒由中生北控生物科技股份有限公司代理的瑞士BUHLMANN公司提供）。

1.5.3 疗效判定标准

1.5.3.1 血压疗效判定标准 按照《中药新药临床研究指导原则》[2]有关标准。显效：（1）舒张压下降≥10mmHg并达到正常范围；（2）舒张压虽未降至正常但已下降20mmHg。有效：（1）舒张压下降<10mmHg但已达到正常范围；（2）舒张压较治疗前下降10～19mmHg但未达到正常范围；（3）收缩压较治疗前下降≥30mmHg。须具备其中一项。无效：未达到以上标准者。

1.5.3.2 症状积分疗效评定标准 参照《中药新药临床研究指导原则》[2]中症状量化标准，采用4级记分法进行评分：无症状记0分；轻度记2分；中度记4分；重度记6分。根据专家论证及预试验结果的统计学分析，证明此量化标准确实可行。疗

表1 两组一般资料比较

级别	例数	年龄（岁，$\bar{\chi} \pm s$）	病程（年，$\bar{\chi} \pm s$）	体重指数（kg/m², $\bar{\chi} \pm s$）	高血压分级（例）		SBP	DBP
					1	2	(mmHg, $\bar{\chi} \pm s$)	
对照	43	47.55±5.36	7.85±4.33	26.45±3.56	22	18	156.75±10.58	87.62±10.22
试验	44	48.03±3.77	8.11±3.58	27.44±4.01	22	20	160.24±12.3	90.07±10.32

效评价按照尼莫地平法[2]。显效：临床症状、体征明显改善，症状积分减少＞70%。有效：临床症状、体征均有好转，症状积分减少30%～70%。无效：临床症状、体征无明显改善，甚或加重，症状积分减少＜30%。

1.5.3.3　血压变异性（blood pressure variability，BPV）疗效评定标准　参照文献[5]，以24h动态血压监测得到的血压标准差（SD）作为BPV的指标。血压变异的正常参考值：24h SBP血压变异性＜15.1mmHg，DBP血压变异性＜13.6mmHg，白天SBP血压变异性＜13.3mmHg，DBP血压变异性＜12.6mm Hg，夜间SBP血压变异性＜12.5mmHg，DBP血压变异性＜9.7mmHg。

1.5.4　统计学方法　用SPSS 10.0软件统计分析，计量资料用t检验、ANOVA检验，计数资料采用$\bar{\chi}$检验，等级资料用秩和检验。

2. 结果

试验过程中，对照组脱落2例，因不能耐受干咳，剔除1例，因动态血压数据不足；试验组脱落2例，因不能耐受干咳。本研究共82例完成试验，其中对照组40例，试验组42例。

2.1　血压疗效

2.1.1　两组治疗前后不同时间血压变异性比较（表2）　治疗后两组BPV均明显下降，具有统计学意义，且试验组优于对照组（$P<0.05$）。

2.1.2　降压疗效　治疗后对照组、试验组的降压总有效率分别为87.5%（35/40）、90.5%（38/42），显效率分别为45.0%（18/40）、59.5%（25/42）。经秩和检验，两组间差异有统计学意义（$P<0.05$）。

2.1.3　两组治疗前后夜间血压下降率比较（表3）治疗后两组夜间血压下降率均明显上升，试验组优于对照组，差异有统计学意义（$P<0.05$）。

2.2　两组治疗前后心率比较（表3）

两组治疗后心率明显下降，且试验组优于对照组，差异有统计学意义（$P<0.05$）。

表3　两组治疗前后夜间血压下降率及心率变化比较（$\bar{\chi}\pm s$）

组别	例数	时间	夜间血压下降率（%）	心率（次/分）
对照	40	治疗前	6.68±1.65	80.54±6.88
		治疗后	10.11±1.64*	70.24±8.45*
试验	42	治疗前	6.21±1.61	81.23±5.71
		治疗后	13.61±1.07*△	65.02±7.98*△

注：与本组治疗前比较，*$P<0.05$；与对照组治疗后比较，△$P<0.05$

2.3　两组治疗前后单项症状积分比较（表4）

两组治疗后各症状均有明显改善，与治疗前比较，差异有统计学意义（$P<0.01$），试验组对头痛、腰酸、膝软、失眠改善优于对照组，差异亦有统计学意义（$P<0.05$）。

2.4　两组治疗前后血脂水平变化比较（表5）

两组治疗后HDL-C水平均明显提高，且试验组在降低TC、LDL-C方面明显优于对照组，差异有统计学意义（$P<0.05$）。

2.5　两组治疗前后血清E_2变化比较（表6）

两组治疗后血清E_2水平均上升，且试验组治疗后差异有统计学意义（$P<0.05$）。

2.6　两组治疗前后血浆hs-CRP、HCY及AngⅡ水平比较（表6）

两组治疗后血浆hs-CRP水平均明显下降，且试验组优于对照组，差异有统计学意义（$P<0.05$）；两组血浆HCY水平均有不同程度的改善，但差异无统计学意义（$P>0.05$）；两组血浆AngⅡ水平均有一定程度的下降，且试验组优于对照组，差异

表2　两组治疗前后不同时间血压变异性比较（mmHg，$\bar{\chi}\pm s$）

组别	例数	时间	SBP			DBP		
			24h	白天	夜间	24h	白天	夜间
对照	40	治疗前	25.57±9.46	23.78±8.05	20.44±8.25	17.56±6.55	15.64±7.65	13.75±6.14
		治疗后	15.49±12.11*	13.76±9.07*	12.36±6.35*	13.22±5.45*	11.96±7.34*	10.34±6.39*
试验	42	治疗前	21.03±7.97	24.42±8.99	20.56±8.11	17.88±7.26	16.07±6.47	14.01±8.45
		治疗后	10.14±8.09*△	11.26±6.35*△	9.75±7.35*△	9.98±6.73*△	8.13±6.23*△	7.54±7.42*△

注：与本组治疗前比较，*$P<0.05$；与对照组治疗后比较，△$P<0.05$

表4 两组治疗前后单项症状积分比较（分，$\bar{\chi} \pm s$）

症状	时间	对照组（40例）	试验组（42例）
眩晕	治疗前	3.16±1.25	3.21±1.32
	治疗后	1.19±0.21*	1.13±0.24*
头痛	治疗前	3.54±1.04	3.48±1.12
	治疗后	0.96±1.19*	0.70±1.08*△
腰酸	治疗前	3.33±1.45	3.57±1.16
	治疗后	0.99±1.13*	0.54±1.01*△
膝软	治疗前	3.63±1.50	3.62±1.20
	治疗后	1.41±1.70*	1.13±1.46*△
五心烦热	治疗前	3.88±1.34	3.79±1.47
	治疗后	1.24±1.44*	1.32±1.46*
心悸	治疗前	1.22±0.54	1.34±0.48
	治疗后	0.77±0.33*	0.56±0.78*
失眠	治疗前	1.68±0.35	1.59±0.57
	治疗后	0.75±0.44*	0.49±0.71*△
耳鸣	治疗前	1.76±0.77	1.59±0.56
	治疗后	1.03±0.63*	0.91±0.55*
健忘	治疗前	1.17±0.39	1.20±0.26
	治疗后	0.38±0.66*	0.27±0.44*

注：与本组治疗前比较，*$P < 0.01$；与对照组治疗后比较，△$P < 0.05$

有统计学意义（$P < 0.05$）。

3. 讨论

高血压病属于中医学"眩晕""头痛""肝风""肝阳"等范畴。研究表明[6-8]，肝肾阴虚、肝阳上亢证不仅是高血压病的主要证型，更是更年期女性高血压的主要证型。专家认为 JNG-7 提出的"高血压前期"多已有"肝阳偏亢"证候的表现[9]，清眩调压方是陈可冀院士针对肝肾阴虚、肝阳上亢证的病机特点，以清肝热、平肝阳、益肝肾为法，创立的治疗高血压的有效方剂。本研究结果显示清眩调压方对更年期女性高血压病有良好的临床疗效。

清眩调压方以苦丁茶散肝风、清头目、活血脉，天麻、钩藤平肝潜阳熄风为主，辅以杜仲补益肝肾，夜交藤搜风通络、养心安神，黄芩、桑叶、菊花清肝热、平肝阳，佐以牛膝祛瘀通络，引血下行以折其阳亢，鲜生地清热养阴以滋肾水，诸药合用，共奏益肝肾、清肝热、平肝阳之功。现代药理学研究表明，上述诸药其有效成分多有不同程度的扩血管、降压及抗炎作用。苦丁茶是我国南方的常用中草药，具有清热解毒、生津止渴、活血脉、提神醒脑等功效，其有效成分苦丁茶总皂苷有扩血管作用，可对抗去甲肾上腺素所致的血管收缩[10]。天麻的有效成分之一天麻素已被证明有镇痛、镇静

表5 两组治疗前后血脂水平变化比较（mmlo/L，$\bar{\chi} \pm s$）

组别	例数	时间	TC	TG	HDL-C	LDL-C	VLDL-C
对照	40	治疗前	5.78±0.97	2.24±1.08	1.04±0.68	3.44±1.20	1.05±0.89
		治疗后	5.48±0.66	1.96±1.52	1.51±0.41*	3.27±1.55	0.88±0.57
试验	42	治疗前	5.69±1.02	2.18±1.13	1.10±0.74	3.28±1.53	0.99±0.97
		治疗后	4.96±0.75△	1.59±0.94	1.63±0.53*	2.81±0.99△	0.50±0.25

注：与本组治疗前比较，*$P < 0.01$；与对照组治疗后比较，△$P < 0.05$

表6 两组治疗前后 E_2、hs-CRP、HCY 及 Ang Ⅱ 水平比较（$\bar{\chi} \pm s$）

组别	例数	时间	E_2（pmol/L）	hs-CRP（mg/L）	HCY（μmol/L）	Ang Ⅱ（μg/L）
对照	40	治疗前	18.36±3.41	2.87±0.65	17.77±2.31	15.01±10.25
		治疗后	107.98±10.23*	1.69±0.54*	16.81±1.78	9.80±6.44*
试验	42	治疗前	20.17±3.64	2.85±0.51	19.37±1.93	18.00±15.86
		治疗后	214.62±11.65*△	0.69±0.58*△	15.89±2.01	6.88±9.42*△

注：与本组治疗前比较，*$P < 0.05$；与对照组治疗后比较，△$P < 0.05$

及增加脑血流量，减少脑血流阻力的作用[11]；钩藤可通过直接或间接抑制血管运动中枢而导致周围血管扩张；杜仲可作用于血管平滑肌，使外周血管扩张，降低外周阻力。其中清热解毒类中药通过降血脂、拮抗内皮素、抑制平滑肌细胞增殖和抑制血小板聚集达到消炎的目的，因而具有防治动脉粥样硬化的功效[12]。

近年来，一些研究结果表明在高血压患者中，不仅血压平均值，而且血压变异的程度也独立并显著地与高血压引起的靶器官损害有关[13, 14]。清眩调压方合用培哚普利降低高血压患者血压变异性优于单用培哚普利组，提示中西药合用在降低血压变异性方面有优势。中西药合用除降压外，可能通过多环节、多途径，如影响交感神经、迷走神经活性，调整肾素 - 血管紧张素系统活性而改善血压情况。清眩调压方在改善高血压相关临床症状、提高患者生活质量方面较单纯西药降压有优势，提示了中医、中西医结合辨证治疗高血压病的优势所在。

血脂异常和高血压是一组相互关联的心血管疾病危险因素。本研究结果提示，清眩调压方有调节血脂代谢的作用，可能与组方中苦丁茶、桑叶和黄芩等的有效成分有降脂作用有关。本方滋补肝肾、平肝潜阳的功效，从整体上调整阴阳气血的平衡，使肾精得充，肝火得降，气血流通。

绝经后女性心脑血管病的发生率迅速上升，如果生育期女性由于其他原因切除双侧卵巢，又没有接受雌激素替代治疗，也会导致绝经女性冠心病发生率的明显上升[15]，这提示雌激素具有维持血管正常功能的作用。因此，推测绝经后女性脑血管病发生率上升是由于失去了内源性雌激素的保护作用。清眩调压方在与西药合用降压之外，能够升高围绝经期妇女的内源性雌激素水平，提示清眩调压方能够调整女性性激素水平，在辅助降压之外，减少心血管事件的发生。

有研究发现 hs-CRP 浓度随着血压级别的增加而增加，在排除高血压的其他危险因素后，C 反应蛋白仍与原发性高血压病高度相关，提示炎症反应参与了原发性高血压的发生发展[16]。清眩调压方组降低 hs-CRP 的优势，可能与其组方中清热解毒类中药通过降血脂、拮抗内皮素、抑制平滑肌细胞增殖和抑制血小板聚集达到消炎的作用有关。肾素 - 血管紧张素 - 醛固酮系统（RAAS）在心血管活动调节中起着十分重要的作用，清眩调压方降低血浆 Ang Ⅱ水平，不只是抑制 Ang Ⅱ生成，这可能与其从多方面、多靶点抑制血管活性物质的生成、储存、传递和表达，更全面地抑制 RAAS 活性有关。

总之，清眩调压方在临床运用中证明对更年期女性轻、中度高血压病患者具有良好的降压作用，能降低更年期女性高血压的血压变异性，改善患者更年期综合征症状、血脂代谢及血清 E_2 及血浆 hs-CRP、Ang Ⅱ水平，以减少其心脑血管疾病的发病风险。现代研究认为血压达标是治疗高血压的基本目标，如何进一步防治其靶器官损害是治疗的关键。中医药的历史悠久，大力发掘传统医药的优势和特长，在平稳降压的同时可减少患者的临床症状，改善生活质量，减少心脑血管疾病的发病风险，是中西医结合治疗高血压病的优势所在。清眩调压方是一个含有复杂成分的中药复方，经过临床验证疗效可靠，其作用机制可能与调节交感 - 迷走神经功能、神经 - 内分泌 - 免疫功能及抑制循环 RAAS 活性有关，使机体恢复自身功能，达到防病治病的目的。

参考文献

[1] 中华医学会心血管病分会. 心血管病治疗指南和建议. 北京：人民军医出版社，2005：279-281.

[2] 中华人民共和国卫生部制定颁布. 中药新药临床研究指导原则. 北京：中国医药科技出版社，2002：73-77.

[3] 俞瑾. 实用中西医结合妇产科学. 北京：北京医科大学、中国协和医科大学联合出版社，1997：114.

[4] 刘元姣，曹来英. 新编妇产科疾病诊疗学. 北京：人民卫生出版社，2002，1039-1040.

[5] 上官新红，张维忠. 血压变异参数的正常参照值. 国外医学. 心血管分册，1997，24（5）：35-37.

[6] 蔡光先，朱克俭，韩育明. 高血压病常见症候临床流行病学观察. 中医杂志，1999，40（8）：492-493.

[7] 王清海，李桂明，李典鸿. 高血压病中医证型分布规律的临床研究. 新中医，2005，37（11）：26-27.

[8] 任敏之，符德玉，颜乾麟. 高血压病患者中医证型与靶器官损害关系的临床研究. 四川中医，2006，24（9）：47-48.

[9] 陈可冀，马晓昌，张京春. 关于美国新高血压指南（JNG-7）的积极意义. 中西医结合心脑血管病杂志，2003，6（1）：311.

[10] 王志祺，田育望，杜方龘. 苦丁茶皂苷类物质对家兔离体胸主动脉条影响的实验研究. 湖南中医学院学报，2002，22（2）：29-31.

[11] 何晶. 天麻素的药理作用及临床应用. 天津药学，2006，18（5）：62-63.

[12] 范秀珍. 清热解毒类中药抗动脉粥样硬化作用机制的研究进展. 中国动脉硬化杂志, 2004 (3): 246-248.

[13] Parati G, Ravagi A, Frattola A, et al. Blood pressure variability. Clinical impication and effects of antihypertensive treatment. J Hypertens, 1994, 12 (5):35-40.

[14] Mancia G, Parati G, Bib G, et al. Assessment of long-term antihypertensive treatment by clinic and ambulatory blood pressure data from the European Lacidipine Study on Atheroselerosis. J Hypertens, 2007, 25 (5):1087-1094.

[15] 赵智深. 雌激素对女性心血管系统的保护作用. 国外医学·内科学分册, 1998, 25 (9): 371-374.

[16] 高文静, 郝冰, 吴寿岭. C-反应蛋白与原发性高血压的关系研究. 中国综合临床, 2005, 21 (3): 209-211.

补肾清肝方不同剂型对高血压阴虚阳亢证患者血压及血管紧张素Ⅱ水平的干预效应 *

邬春晓　张京春　刘　玥　陈　静　陈懿宇　赵莹科

Ang Ⅱ 作为肾素 - 血管紧张素 - 醛固醇系统（renin-angiotension-aldosterone，RAAS）中一种主要多功能活性肽，通过特异受体结合，对血流动力学及心血管结构、功能产生重要影响[1]。已有大量研究比较了中药配方颗粒剂与传统中药饮片的有效成分及干预效应，但研究结果一直存在争议。部分认为颗粒剂的使用符合中医理论且患者依从性更好，另一种观点则认为传统中药均应复方共煎，否则疗效将发生改变[2]。本文在以往临床研究初步证明补肾平肝类中药复方预防高血压靶器官损伤有效的基础上[3]，采用随机、安慰剂对照的研究方法，进一步评价了补肾清肝方不同剂型对高血压阴虚阳亢证患者血压平均值及血浆 Ang Ⅱ 水平的干预效应，为中药复方治疗高血压的临床应用提供研究证据。

1. 资料与方法

1.1　诊断标准

1.1.1　高血压诊断标准　参照 2003 年 WHO/ISH 高血压防治指南及 2005 年《中国高血压防治指南》[4]。

1.1.2　中医辨证标准　参照卫生部 2002 年《中药新药临床研究指导原则》高血压阴虚阳亢证标准[5]。

1.2　入选标准

年龄 18 ～ 75 岁；符合高血压诊断标准及中医阴虚阳亢辨证分型标准，高血压病程在 3 个月以上，未用药或已服用降压药但经 2 周洗脱期后达到上述标准；原发性高血压，过去未用降压药或经洗脱期后 1 周内不同日 3 次测压，达到诊断标准者。

1.3　排除标准

3 级高血压或顽固性高血压；半年内有心肌梗死或明显脑卒中史；合并严重心、肝、肾、造血系统、神经系统等原发性疾病及精神病、恶性肿瘤患者；妊娠或哺乳期妇女；拒绝签署知情同意书或 3 个月内参加其他临床试验者。

1.4　一般资料

选择 2010 年 1 月—2012 年 5 月中国中医科学院西苑医院门诊就诊的高血压患者 139 例，脱落 2 例，随机、平行安慰剂对照。按照病例脱落率不超过 20% 原则，运用 SAS 统计软件产生受试者所接受处理（颗粒剂、煎剂和安慰剂）的随机安排，即列出药物流水编号所对应的治疗分配，按照受试者就诊顺序发给相应编号的药。三组患者年龄、性别等一般资料经统计学分析，差异均无统计学意义（$P > 0.05$），具有可比性。

1.5　研究方法

1.5.1　研究流程　记录符合纳入标准患者的 24h 动态血压、身高、体重、理化检查指标、中医症状积分、生活质量量表等，服药前后检查肝肾功能、

---

* 原载于《中国老年医学杂志》，2013，33（8）：1753-1755.

血脂、血常规、尿常规、心电图等安全性指标。所有患者在西药治疗基础上，分别加补肾清肝方颗粒剂、煎剂或安慰剂干预2个月后，检查相关指标，评价疗效。

1.5.2　药物治疗　常规应用氨氯地平5mg Qd，辉瑞制药有限公司提供，国药准字H10950224。补肾清肝方组成为：天麻30g、钩藤30g、杜仲30g、黄芩15g、苦丁茶15g。煎剂组药物采用传统煎煮方法制为汤剂。颗粒剂组药物采用颗粒剂冲服，批号为100718206。对照安慰剂与颗粒剂外观及包装完全相同，均由四川新绿色药业科技发展股份有限公司制备。三组患者在西药常规治疗的基础上，于入组当天分别加服补肾清肝方颗粒剂、煎剂、安慰剂，均为每日2次，与西药间隔0.5h后口服，连续服用2个月。所有试验病例在试验期间不得合并使用其他西药降压药、中药汤剂和中成药制剂。

1.5.3　观察指标及方法

1.5.3.1　24h动态血压监测（ABPM）　治疗前后均采用美国SP（a）celabs Medical公司生产的9027-ABP型24h动态血压记录仪测量。

1.5.3.2　血压平均值　通过24h动态血压检测结果记录各组患者治疗前后24h、日间、夜间收缩压及舒张压的平均值。

1.5.3.3　血浆Ang Ⅱ水平　直接采用放射免疫方法检测，试剂盒由北京华英生物技术研究所提供，严格按说明书操作程序进行。

1.6　统计方法

采用SPSS 12.0统计软件进行分析，计量资料以$\bar{x}\pm s$形式表示，组内比较采用配对t检验，组间比较用单因素方差分析。

2.　结果

2.1　治疗前后血压平均值比较

结果见表1。与本组治疗前相比，煎剂组治疗后24h收缩压平均值，三组治疗后日间平均收缩压均下降（$P<0.05$或$P<0.01$）；治疗后组间比较，日间平均收缩压煎剂组较安慰剂组明显降低，差异有统计学意义（$P<0.05$），颗粒剂组与安慰剂组比较无效（$P>0.05$）。治疗后24h、夜间平均收缩压及24h、日间、夜间平均舒张压颗粒剂组、煎剂组与对照组比较，均没有统计学差异（$P>0.05$）。

2.2　治疗前后血浆Ang Ⅱ水平的比较

结果见表2。与本组治疗前相比，颗粒剂组、煎剂组血浆Ang Ⅱ水平均显著下降（$P<0.05$），而安慰剂组无明显变化（$P>0.05$）。治疗后组间比较，颗粒剂组、煎剂组血浆Ang Ⅱ含量均明显低于安慰剂组（$P<0.05$），颗粒剂组与煎剂组血浆Ang Ⅱ比较无统计学意义（$P>0.05$）。

3.　讨论

肾素-血管紧张素-醛固酮（RAAS）系统的激活以及血管活性物质均参与高血压发病过程[6]。RAAS主要通过Ang Ⅱ实现其对血压的调节。现已明确，Ang Ⅱ通过结合受体，增加细胞内钙离子浓度，促进血管收缩和刺激醛固酮分泌，增加水、钠潴留[7]。Ang Ⅱ除影响血流动力学外，仍是重

表1　治疗前后血压平均值的变化（mmHg）

指标		安慰剂组（n=45）	颗粒剂组（n=45）	煎剂组（n=47）
24h收缩压平均值	治疗前	135.06±13.25	136.93±12.49	138.55±11.02
	治疗后	130.37±14.16	129.22±9.71	127.57±12.15[2)]
日间收缩压平均值	治疗前	146.46±7.43	147.75±9.03	144.19±11.87
	治疗后	133.35±15.24[1)]	132.44±10.55[2)]	129.23±12.28[2) 3)]
夜间收缩压平均值	治疗前	127.60±12.41	127.66±14.59	125.49±10.96
	治疗后	122.40±13.01	122.93±12.91	120.89±13.31
24h舒张压平均值	治疗前	84.08±8.92	84.22±9.89	83.36±10.69
	治疗后	79.84±10.85	77.60±10.55	78.38±9.58
日间舒张压平均值	治疗前	86.44±9.04	86.48±9.83	85.49±11.32
	治疗后	81.86±11.40	79.75±11.12	80.79±10.56
夜间舒张压平均值	治疗前	77.37±9.58	78.04±10.70	75.85±10.43
	治疗后	72.82±9.93	71.13±10.53	73.17±10.37

与本组治疗前比较：[1)] $P<0.05$，[2)] $P<0.01$；与安慰剂组比较：[3)] $P<0.05$

表 2　治疗前后血浆 Ang Ⅱ 水平的比较

指标		安慰剂组（*n*=45）	颗粒剂组（*n*=45）	煎剂组（*n*=47）
Ang Ⅱ（pg/mL）	治疗前	71.79±9.78	70.40±9.26	69.54±12.38
	治疗后	69.24±7.79	65.38±7.74[1) 2)]	63.96±10.941[2)]

与本组治疗前比较：[1)] $P < 0.05$；治疗后，与安慰剂组比较：[3)] $P < 0.05$

要的生长因子，诱导心肌细胞肥大，心脏成纤维细胞增殖，诱导心肌细胞凋亡[8]。补肾清肝方两种剂型与安慰剂相比均能有效地抑制 Ang Ⅱ，提示中药或可抑制高血压的进一步发展及其引起的靶器官损伤。与对照组相比，中药组（煎剂组和颗粒剂组）明显抑制 Ang Ⅱ，而对血压平均值无显著影响，仅煎剂组疗后日间收缩压平均值较对照组明显降低，提示或应延长研究观察周期，并进一步扩大样本量。

高血压以肝肾气血阴阳失调为主要病理变化，临床尤以肝肾阴虚类型多见。补肾清肝方用天麻、钩藤、黄芩、杜仲、苦丁茶，滋肾阴以摄纳，平肝阳以熄风。天麻、钩藤平肝潜阳熄风，辅以杜仲补益肝肾；黄芩清肝热、平肝阳，更助苦丁茶活血通脉。本次研究发现补肾清肝方不同剂型具有改善患者血压的趋势，并能有效抑制 Ang Ⅱ，预防靶器官损伤。现代药理实验亦有效揭示了这一作用机制。钩藤生物碱具备抑制血管平滑肌细胞增殖、改善动脉病理组织学损害的功能[9]；黄芩茎叶总黄酮证明对心肌细胞凋亡有保护作用[10]；杜仲提取物经过多年临床实验证实具有降压活性[11]，且杜仲中微量元素钙和锌含量较高，可能通过补充阴虚证型高血压患者的锌含量而达到降压效果。

目前对中药配方颗粒与传统煎剂的作用及疗效还存在争议，临床及药理研究结果不尽相同[12-15]，为进一步探索两种剂型的特点，本研究对补肾清肝方颗粒剂、煎剂进行了疗效评价。中药配方颗粒由于服用方便，具有医从性好的优点，并且避免传统中药手抓、秤称所致的剂量误差。中药合煎过程中，能产生一系列物理化学变化，以达到增强疗效、解毒和缓和药性的作用。配方颗粒由于单味提取，故不具备药物相互作用的优势。近年日本政府近年提出"标准汤剂"概念，即为制定标准汤剂化学基准、生物学基准，要求提供其他剂型中药制剂的生产工艺过程细节及其在化学、生物学上与标准汤剂具有同一性的研究资料，以确保在化学（指标成分）及生物学（药理作用）上与标准汤剂具有同一性[16]。本研究结果提示补肾清肝方颗粒剂、煎剂对高血压阴虚阳亢证患者血压平均值及血浆 Ang Ⅱ 水平两组间比较无显著差异，但有待采用两者有效成分与药理机制多角度结合的方法进一步验证。

参考文献

[1] Weir MR. Effects of renin-angiotensin system inhibition on end-organ protection: can we do better？ Clinical Therapeutics, 2007, 29 (9): 1803-1824.

[2] 周嘉琳. 中药单煎与共煎利弊分析. 中医杂志, 2007, 48（8）：745.

[3] 张京春, 陈懿宇, 陈静, 等. 清眩颗粒对伴及不伴睡眠呼吸暂停高血压患者内皮功能的影响. 中国老年学杂志, 2012, 32（4）：672-675.

[4] 中华人民共和国卫生部. 中国高血压防治指南（2005年修订版）. 2005.

[5] 郑筱萸. 中药新药临床研究指导原则. 北京：中国医药科技出版社, 2002：73-77.

[6] Dielis AW, Smid M, Spronk HM, et al. The prothrombotic paradox of hypertension: role of the renin-angiotensin and kallikrein-kinin systems. Hypertension, 2005, 46 (6):1236-1242.

[7] Tsai CT, Chiang FT, Chen W P, et al. Angiotensin Ⅱ induces complex fractionated electrogram in a cultured atrial myocyte monolayer mediated by calcium and sodium-calcium exchanger. Cell Calcium, 2011, 49 (1): 1-11.

[8] Gassanov N, Brandt MC, Michels G, et al. Angiotensin Ⅱ-induced changes of calcium sparks and ionic currents in human atrial myocytes：potential role for early remodeling in atrial fibrillation. Cell Calcium, 2006, 39 (2):175-186.

[9] 戴国华, 孙敬昌, 齐冬梅等. 钩藤生物碱对自发性高血压大鼠胸主动脉成纤维细胞凋亡/增殖及 FN、LN 的影响. 中国中西医结合杂志, 2012, 32（9）：1233-1237.

[10] 周晓慧, 龚明玉, 杨鹤梅, 等. 黄芩茎叶总黄酮对缺氧/复氧诱导心肌细胞凋亡的影响. 中国中西医结合

杂志，2011，31（6）：803-806.

[11] 管淑玉，苏薇薇. 杜仲化学成分与药理研究进展. 中药材，2003，26（2）：124-129.

[12] 王育红，张志清，李仲兴，等. 5种中药煎剂与颗粒剂对临床分离菌株的体外抑菌作用比较. 中国药房，2005，16（17）：1354-1356.

[13] 冯少华，张春红，廖惠芳. 苦参颗粒与苦参煎剂药效及毒性的对比性研究. 中华中医药学刊，2007，25

（8）：1602-1604.

[14] 陈自雅，蒋荣民. 坤宁汤治疗围绝经期综合征68例疗效观察. 上海中医药杂志，2012，46（4）：40-41.

[15] 肖锦仁，吴红娟，邱赛红，等. 银翘散煎剂与颗粒剂药效学作用的比较研究. 中药材，2002，25（2）：114-117.

[16] 刘瑞新. 中药剂型选择及制剂等效性研究概况. 中医杂志，2007，48（1）：83-85.

清眩颗粒对伴及不伴睡眠呼吸暂停高血压患者内皮功能的影响 *

张京春　陈懿宇　陈　静　刘建刚　邬春晓　马　玲

阻塞性睡眠呼吸暂停（obstructive sleep apnea，OSA）为高血压的独立危险因素，对高血压合并OSA患者进行内皮损伤机制及药物干预的研究，将对探索降压机制、靶器官的保护，进而预防心脑血管事件产生积极的意义[1]。本研究拟在常规降压治疗基础上，对伴OSA的高血压患者和不伴OSA的高血压患者予以中药干预，从而观察血管内皮功能相关指标的变化，为探讨高血压伴OSA患者的内皮损伤机制，选择适宜的中药干预提供科学依据。

1. 资料与方法

1.1 研究对象

2010年1月至2010年12月中国中医科学院西苑医院门诊就诊的高血压患者，根据是否合并OSA分为伴OSA和不伴OSA两个亚组。

1.2 诊断标准

1.2.1 高血压诊断标准　参照2003年WHO/ISH高血压防治指南[2]，以及2005年《中国高血压防治指南》[3]。

1.2.2 中医证候诊断标准　参照卫生部2002年《中药新药临床研究指导原则》中高血压阴虚阳亢证标准[4]。

1.2.3 睡眠呼吸暂停低通气OSA诊断标准　参照2002年4月中华医学会呼吸病学分会睡眠呼吸疾

病学组制定的《阻塞性睡眠呼吸暂停低通气综合征诊疗指南（草案）》[5]和《睡眠呼吸暂停与心血管专家共识》[6]。

1.2.4 病例纳入标准及排除标准　高血压患者纳入标准：（1）符合1级和2级高血压患者诊断标准和中医阴虚阳亢之辨证分型标准。（2）原发性高血压，过去未用降压药或经洗脱后1周内不同日三次测压，血压达到诊断标准。（3）未用药，或已服用降血压药物但经2周洗脱期后血压达到上述标准者。（4）1级高血压病程在3个月以上者。（5）年龄在18～75岁。（6）知情同意并签署知情同意书者。排除标准：（1）妊娠，或近期准备妊娠，或哺乳期妇女。（2）继发性高血压。（3）收缩压（SBP）≤140mmHg或≥180mmHg，舒张压（DBP）≤90mmHg或≥110mmHg。（4）3级高血压或单纯收缩期高血压者。（5）合并有精神病。（6）半年内有心肌梗死或明显脑卒中史。（7）过敏体质或对多种药物过敏者。（8）近3个月内接受过其他新药临床试验者。（9）洗脱期结束后未达到高血压诊断标准者。（10）合并心、脑、肾等严重脏器损害者。（11）因中枢神经系统脑部外伤疾病及先天颌面结构畸形而致打鼾患者。（12）有颌面结构发育障碍及单纯性耳鼻喉科疾病引起打鼾者。病例的剔除标准：（1）病例选择不符

* 原载于《中国老年学杂志》，2012，32（4）：672-675

合纳入标准，符合排除标准，本不应当进行随机化。（2）未曾使用研究用药。（3）在随机化之后没有任何数据。资料统计分析前，由统计人员及主要研究者讨论判断研究病例是否剔除。

1.3 方法

本试验严格遵照《赫尔辛基宣言》进行，并经中国中医科学院西苑医院伦理委员会批准。采用分层随机双盲安慰剂对照法。

1.3.1 研究流程 本研究为分层随机双盲、安慰剂对照试验。将纳入的符合高血压诊断标准的患者，详细记录血压、治疗情况、心率、身高、体重、颈围、颈长、腰围、臀围、理化检查指标、中医症状积分、Epworth 量表、生活质量量表等，检查肝功能、肾功能、血脂、尿常规、血常规、心电图等安全性指标。洗脱期 2 周。根据便携式睡眠仪检查得到的患者 OSA 情况，按是否伴有 OSA 分层，运用 SAS 9.2 统计软件，按伴 OSA 和不伴 OSA 两个亚组的病例分配数及随机比例生成随机数字分组表，将每个亚组的患者随机分为试验组和对照组。所有患者在西药治疗（氨氯地平）的基础上，再加中药清眩颗粒或安慰剂干预 2 个月后，检查相关指标，评价疗效。对于需要持续正压通气治疗（continuous positive airway pressure，CPAP）的中重度 OSA 患者，在结束 2 个月药物治疗后，再推荐使用 CPAP 治疗。

1.3.2 观察药物 清眩颗粒：杜仲 30g、钩藤 30g、天麻 30g、黄芩 15g、苦丁茶 15g，由四川新绿色药业科技发展股份有限公司提供。中药安慰剂：安慰颗粒剂在外观、气味、包装等方面和清眩颗粒相同，由四川新绿色药业科技发展股份有限公司提供。氨氯地平（络活喜）5mg，由辉瑞制药有限公司提供。

1.3.3 观察指标及方法

1.3.3.1 便携式多导睡眠仪 在治疗前患者均接受便携式多导睡眠仪（采用美国凯迪泰公司 SW-SM2000CB 便携型多导睡眠分析诊断系统）记录鼻气流、鼾声、胸式呼吸、腹式呼吸、血氧、脉率、体位等。对于诊断有 OSA 的高血压患者，在治疗结束后再复查。OSA 相关指标包括：最长暂停时间、平均暂停时间、睡眠呼吸暂停低通气指数（apnea hypopnea index，AHI）、睡眠呼吸暂停指数（apnea index，AI）、低通气指数（hypopnea index，HI）、最低 SaO_2%、平均 SaO_2%、氧减指数。

1.3.3.2 内皮依赖性血管舒张功能（flow mediated

dilation，FMD）参照 Celermajer 等介绍的方法进行 [7]。被检者在安静遮光的房间中平卧 15min 以上开始检查，使用 7.5MHz 的 15L8W 线阵探头（西门子 ACUSON Sequola 512 型超声诊断仪）。受试者取仰卧位，右上肢充分暴露，外展 15°，手心向上，在右肘窝上方 2～5cm 处显示肱动脉长轴图像然后冻结，测量同步心电图 R 波顶点时，即肱动脉在心室舒张末期基础内径（D1），取 3 个心动周期的平均值，在检测部位皮肤上作标记以便重复操作。在测定 D1 后进行反应性充血实验，以袖带血压计缚于右上肢前臂，充气加压至 200mmHg，维持 4min 后迅速放气，60～90s 内在原来同一部位超声检测肱动脉内径（D2），记录加压放气后舒张期肱动脉内径值（D2），与静息时基础内径相减，以百分率表示肱动脉变化率，加压放气后肱动脉内径增宽即血流介导的 FMD。以 FMD（%）大小判断肱动脉 FDM。FMD（%）=（D2–D1）/D1×100%。

1.3.3.3 血管活性物质检查 （1）ET-1：非平衡放射免疫方法；PRA：放射免疫方法测定；Ang Ⅱ：直接测定放射免疫方法；ALD：采用放射免疫学检测法。以上指标所用的放射免疫测定试剂盒均由北京华英生物技术研究所提供，操作过程严格按说明书操作程序进行。（2）NO：硝酸还原酶法测定，操作过程严格按说明书操作程序进行。

1.4 统计学方法

用 SAS 8.1 软件统计分析，计量数据以 $\bar{x}\pm s$ 表示，计量资料采用 t 检验，计数资料采用 χ^2 检验。在本研究中，治疗后各效应指标上升或下降的差值，除了和所接受的药物不同有关，还受到治疗前各指标基线水平不同的影响，也受到是否伴有 OSA 的影响，故本文采用广义线性模型来分析这些因素对结果的影响。其中将是否接受试验组用药设为因素 a，是否伴有 OSA 设为因素 b，各指标治疗前基线水平设为因素 c，这些因素共同影响治疗后各指标变化的差值（设为应变量 Y），所有实际差值需转化为修正均数 D（即最小二乘均数）再比较大小。

2. 结果

2.1 患者一般资料

90 例阴虚阳亢型轻中度高血压患者中伴 OSA 者 46 例（51.11%），不伴 OSA 者 44 例（48.89%）。年龄 31～75 岁，平均（55.11±10.07）岁。男

性34例，其中伴OSA者21例（61.67%）：女性56例，伴OSA者25例（44.64%），男性高血压患者OSA比例高于女性高血压患者。90例患者平均腰围（93.43±10.244）cm，平均臀围（105.088±7.89）cm，腰/臀0.88±0.06，平均颈围（38.38±7.28）cm，平均颈长（8.75±2.16）cm，平均BMI（26.34±3.36）kg/m²。

伴中重度OSA患者和轻度OSA的高血压患者比较，FMD%、NO、NO/ET、ET-1、PRA、Ang Ⅱ、ALD水平没有统计学差异（$P > 0.05$）。伴中重度OSA患者和不伴OSA的高血压患者相比，FMD%、NO、NO/ET比值较低，ET-1、PRA、Ang Ⅱ、ALD水平更高，差异均有统计学意义（$P < 0.05$）。伴轻度OSA患者和不伴OSA的高血压患者相比，FMD%、NO、NO/ET比值较低，Ang Ⅱ、ALD水平较高，有统计学差异（$P < 0.05$）。见表1。

2.2　治疗前后相关指标的比较

2.2.1　治疗前后内皮功能的改变

2.2.1.1　治疗前后内皮依赖性血管舒张功能改变　各组均比治疗前本组FMD升高（$P < 0.05$）；总体患者、不伴OSA患者的FMD试验组比治疗后对照组高（$P < 0.05$）。总体患者FMD升高幅度试验组D（-2.04）大于对照组D（-0.31）

（$P_{(a)} =0.013$）；是否伴有OSA影响FMD的升高（$P_{(b)} =0.0027$），伴OSA患者D（-0.08）升高幅度低于不伴OSA患者D（-2.33）。亚组内分析，不伴OSA者FMD的升高幅度试验组D（-2.95）高于对照组D（0.04）（$P < 0.05$），伴OSA的高血压患者试验组和对照组D比较没有统计学差异（$P > 0.05$）。见表2。

2.2.1.2　治疗前后血管活性物质测定　与本组治疗前比较，各试验组ET-1值下降，且不伴OSA组和总体患者中试验组比治疗后对照组ET-1值低（$P < 0.05$）。NO/ET比值各试验组均比本组治疗前升高（$P < 0.05$），且试验组比治疗后对照组NO/ET比值高（$P < 0.05$）。Ang Ⅱ各试验组均比本组治疗前Ang Ⅱ降低（$P < 0.05$），且试验组比治疗后对照组低（$P < 0.05$）。总体患者试验组和对照组相比（$P_{(a)}$），能增加ET、NO/ET比值、Ang Ⅱ的下降或升高幅度。伴OSA和不伴OSA患者相比（$P_{(b)}$），OSA能减弱NO、NO/ET、PRA、Ang Ⅱ、ALD的下降或升高幅度。亚组内分析：不伴OSA的患者：ET-1下降幅度试验组D（3.80）高于对照组D（-1.38）（$P < 0.05$）；NO/ET比值升高幅度试验组D（-0.14）均大于对照组D（-0.01）（$P < 0.05$）；Ang Ⅱ下降幅度试

表1　根据AHI分组后的各组血管活性物质比较（$\bar{x} \pm s$）

指标	不伴OSA组（n=44）	伴轻度OSA组（n=28）	伴中重度OSA组（n=18）
FMD%	6.2±3.89[1) 2)]	4.17±2.31	3.83±3.27
NO（μmol/L）	62.93±17.14[1) 2)]	51.91±9.04	51.71±7.87
ET-1（pg/mL）	62.94±8.22[2)]	66.85±9.91	68.71±3.37
NO/ET	1.02±0.33[1) 2)]	0.79±0.20	0.76±0.14
PRA[ng/（mL·h）]	0.78±0.11[2)]	0.84±0.12	0.89±0.13
Ang Ⅱ（pg/mL）	68.31±9.38[1) 2)]	72.98±9.89	74.99±7.23
ALD（pg/mL）	84.16±15.90[1) 2)]	94.28±18.93	100.42±29.16

与伴轻度OSA组比较：[1)] $P < 0.05$；与伴中重度OSA组比较：[2)] $P < 0.05$

表2　治疗前后FMD比较（$\bar{x} \pm s$，%）

时间	亚组				总体	
	伴OSA		不伴OSA			
	试验组（n=23）	对照组（n=23）	试验组（n=22）	对照组（n=22）	试验组（n=45）	对照组（n=45）
治疗前	4.02±2.58	3.88±3.25	6.39±4.41	6.19±3.89	5.20±3.78	4.94±3.41
治疗后	5.59±3.05[1)]	4.55±4.3[1)]	9.34±3.12[1) 2)]	7.63±3.30[1)]	7.16±3.62[1) 2)]	5.34±3.67[1)]
差值	-1.56±2.63	-0.66±4.30	-3.14±5.17[2)]	-0.11±4.38	-1.95±4.10[2)]	-0.4±4.2

与本组治疗前比较：[1)] $P < 0.01$；与治疗后对照组比较：[2)] $P < 0.05$

验组 D（3.88）高于对照组 D（0.90）（$P < 0.05$）。伴 OSA：NO/ET 比值升高幅度试验组 D（-0.15）均大于对照组 D（-0.05）；Ang Ⅱ 下降幅度试验组 D（7.69）高于对照组 D（2.55）。见表 3。

2.2.2 治疗前后 OSA 患者相关指标的变化　对 46 例伴 OSA 患者的睡眠呼吸暂停相关指数进行分析，OSA 患者试验组的 HI 比治疗前降低，差异有统计学意义（$P < 0.05$）。其他睡眠相关指标比治疗前有改善的趋势，但无显著差异（$P > 0.05$）；试验组与治疗后对照组比无显著差异（$P > 0.05$）。见表 4。

3. 讨论

治疗前伴 OSA 的高血压患者 FMD 明显低于不伴 OSA 的高血压患者，可见伴 OSA 的高血压患者内皮依赖性血管舒张功能损伤比不伴 OSA 的高血压患者更为严重。治疗后不伴 OSA 的高血压患者试验组 FMD 高于对照组，差异有统计学意义；而伴 OSA 的高血压患者试验组和对照组之间没有差异。可见 OSA 引起内皮依赖性血管舒张功能损伤更为严重，中药清眩颗粒可以改善损伤较轻的患者，对损伤较为严重的 OSA 患者则没有显著作用。本研究对治疗前后 FMD 的差值进行协方差分析，结果显示 OSA 影响 FMD 的改善，同时试验组 FMD 增加的幅度高于对照组，提示清眩颗粒可以改善血管内皮功能。

动物研究发现清眩胶囊对自发性高血压大鼠（SHR）和二肾一夹（2KIC）大鼠具有一定降压作

表 3　治疗前后血管活性物质比较（$\bar{\chi} \pm s$）

指标	亚组				总体	
	伴 OSA		不伴 OSA			
	试验组（$n=23$）	对照组（$n=23$）	试验组（$n=22$）	对照组（$n=22$）	试验组（$n=45$）	对照组（$n=45$）
NO（μmol/L）						
治疗前	51.60±6.78	51.96±10.11	61.85±19.65	64.01±14.58	56.61±15.30	57.86±13.77
治疗后	56.52±11.49	53.32±10.33	69.01±16.80	64.90±15.91	62.63±15.51	58.98±14.47
差值	−4.92±13.07	−1.34±12.05	−7.16±27.27	−0.89±24.00	−6.01±21.02	−1.12±18.64
ET-1（pg/mL）						
治疗前	68.38±9.58	66.78±9.12	64.04±8.43	61.84±8.05	66.26±9.20	64.37±8.88
治疗后	60.72±6.99[1)	65.13±9.12	59.19±5.34[1) 3)	64.27±8.64	59.97±6.21[1) 3)	64.71±9.35
差值	7.66±10.62	1.64±10.82	4.84±8.203	−2.42±12.60	6.28±9.51[3)	−0.34±11.77
NO/ET						
治疗前	0.77±0.16	0.79±0.20	0.98±0.37	1.05±0.30	0.87±0.30	0.92±0.28
治疗后	0.94±0.22[1) 3)	0.83±0.23	1.17±0.30[1)3)	1.03±0.29	1.05±0.28[2) 3)	0.93±0.27
差值	−0.17±0.29[3)	−0.04±0.27	−0.18±0.51[3)	0.03±0.45	−0.17±0.41[3)	−0.006±0.37
PRA [ng/（mL·h）]						
治疗前	0.86±0.13	0.86±0.12	0.77±0.11	0.80±0.10	0.82±0.13	0.83±0.12
治疗后	0.80±0.10	0.82±0.10	0.76±0.07	0.78±0.095	0.78±0.093	0.80±0.10
差值	0.057±0.18	0.033±0.16	0.01±12.46	0.01±0.16	0.034±0.15	0.023±0.16
Ang Ⅱ（pg/mL）						
治疗前	72.49±8.67	75.04±9.1	68.22±9.55	68.40±9.42	70.40±9.26	71.79±9.78
治疗后	66.29±7.60[1) 3)	71.00±8.09	64.43±7.96[1) 3)	67.40±7.18	65.38±7.74[1) 3)	69.24±7.79
差值	6.20±12.64[3)	4.04±13.27	3.78±12.44[3)	0.99±12.71	5.02±12.46[3)	2.55±12.94
ALD（pg/mL）						
治疗前	96.75±28.09	96.62±18.07	83.36±17.24	84.97±14.81	90.20±24.13	90.92±17.39
治疗后	91.96±21.14	92.13±18.54	80.14±21.39	83.59±21.56	86.18±21.86	87.95±20.31
差值	4.78±25.84	4.49±27.09	3.22±26.19	1.38±29.85	4.02±25.73	2.97±28.19

与本组治疗前比较：[1)] $P < 0.05$；[2)] $P < 0.01$；与治疗后对照组比较：[3)] $P < 0.05$

表4　治疗前后伴 OSA 患者相关指标的变化（$\bar{x} \pm s$）

指标		试验组	对照组
最长暂停时间	治疗前	51.22±26.03	52.40±31.02
	治疗后	48.33±25.58	51.95±30.84
平均暂停时间	治疗前	27.56±11.66	27.23±9.94
	治疗后	26.80±11.08	26.62±9.73
AHI	治疗前	14.59±10.60	16.61±14.40
	治疗后	13.87±9.88	16.07±14.06
HI	治疗前	8.94±6.25	8.88±6.46
	治疗后	7.27±6.62[1]	8.69±6.04
AI	治疗前	5.70±6.24	7.66±10.99
	治疗后	6.60±5.67	7.33±10.91
最低 SaO$_2$%	治疗前	83.43±5.25	82.73±7.61
	治疗后	85.08±4.91	82.91±7.11
氧减指数	治疗前	14.31±13.97	17.48±15.77
	治疗后	13.29±12.73	17.75±16.00

与本组治疗前比较：[1] $P < 0.05$

用，其中清眩胶囊对 2KIC 大鼠降压有剂量依赖性；清眩胶囊的降压机制可能与抑制循环 RAAS 活性、纠正 ET/CGRP 紊乱有关[8]。本次临床研究发现总体患者试验组和对照组相比，清眩颗粒能增加 Ang Ⅱ 和 ET-1 的下降幅度，以及 NO/ET 比值的上升幅度，从而推测其可能可以降低 RAAS 活性，调整 NO/ET 比值使其平衡，与上述动物实验结论相似。

本研究选用的药物清眩颗粒主要是在清眩胶囊的基础上简化方药制成，主要包括杜仲 30g、钩藤 30g、天麻 30g、黄芩 15g、苦丁茶 15g，用以平肝潜阳。其中以天麻、钩藤平肝潜阳熄风，苦丁茶散肝风、清头目、活血脉为主，辅以杜仲补益肝肾，黄芩清肝热、平肝阳，共奏益肝肾、清肝热、滋肝阴、平肝阳之功。现代药理学研究证实如上药物具有明确的降压作用，未出现明显的不良反应。其中杜仲主要通过促进内皮细胞释放 NO 舒张血管，还可以通过抑制血管平滑肌细胞的 Ca^{2+} 通道等途径舒张血管，对血管紧张素 Ⅱ（Ang Ⅱ）生成亦有持久的抑制作用。钩藤提取物可以抑制血管内皮细胞生成自由基，保护内皮功能，对早期高血压可能有血管保护作用。天麻的主要成分天麻多糖对 RHR 大鼠具有良好的降压作用，其作用机制为

促进内源性舒血管物质 NO 的生成，抑制内源性缩血管物质 ET 和 Ang Ⅱ 的释放，最终恢复二者拮抗效应的平衡[7]。黄芩对血管内皮细胞的钙通道具有阻滞作用，这可能与其扩张血管、降压作用机制有关。苦丁茶提取液能增加心脑血流量，降低血管的阻力和压力，对血管有一定的扩张作用，能调整血管功能，对于治疗高血压病有较好的疗效[9]。

同时为观察清眩颗粒对 OSA 的影响，本研究将 46 例伴 OSA 的高血压患者治疗前后 OSA 情况进行了比较，发现 OSA 患者试验组的低通气指数 HI 比治疗前降低，差异有统计学意义。其他睡眠相关指标比治疗前都有改善的趋势，但没有统计学意义；治疗后试验组和对照组比较，差异也没有统计学意义。可见对伴 OSA 的高血压患者用氨氯地平不会加重其 OSA 的病情，加上中药清眩颗粒以后，可以改善 OSA 患者的低通气次数，这在临床上是值得进一步关注的。

参考文献

[1] Ramar K, Caples SM. Vascular changes, cardiovascular disease and obstructive sleep apnea. Future Cardiol, 2011, 7: 241-249.

[2] Whitworth JA, World Health Organization, International Society of Hypertension Writing Group. 2003 World Health Organization (WHO)/International Society of Hypertension (ISH) statement on management of hypertension (Guidelines and recommendations). J Hypertens, 2003, 21: 1983-1992.

[3] 中华人民共和国卫生部. 中国高血压防治指南（2005 年修订版）. 2005.

[4] 郑筱萸. 中药新药临床研究指导原则. 北京：中国医药科技出版社，2002：73-77.

[5] 中华医学会呼吸病学分会睡眠呼吸疾病学组. 阻塞性睡眠呼吸暂停低通气综合征诊治指南（草案）. 中华结核和呼吸杂志，2002，25（3）：195-198.

[6] 睡眠呼吸暂停与心血管疾病专家共识组. 睡眠呼吸暂停与心血管专家共识. 中华内科杂志，2009，48（12）：1059-1067.

[7] 缪化春，沈业寿. 有关天麻多糖的降压作用. 高血压杂志，2006，14（7）：531-533.

[8] 卢全生，雷燕，陈可冀. AT1R 基因多态性与原发性高血压中医证型及降压中药疗效的关系. 中国中西医结合杂志，2005，25（8）：682-685.

[9] 苏金平，刘干中，彭继道. 五种中草药对钙通道阻滞作用的初步研究. 中药药理与临床，2006，22（6）：45-46.

第三章

第四节　中西医结合防治其他心血管病

慪性心力衰竭病证结合与临床治疗初探 *

苗阳　王鹏军

慪性心力衰竭（简称心衰）发病率高，病死率高，成为 21 世纪危害人类健康的主要疾病之一。现代医学治疗心衰虽然取得了明显进步，但在治疗上带来的不良反应不容忽视，如利尿剂引起的电解质、代谢紊乱，ACEI 引起的干咳，加之长期吃药造成的对胃的刺激等。随着中医药研究的不断深入，尤其是病证结合思想的深入，在中医传统辨证分型的基础上，进行西医病的辨证，使得中医药治疗心衰具有独特的优势。兹从慪性心衰疾病分期与中医证候演变规律方面作一简述，希望能抛砖引玉，引起学术争鸣。

慪性心衰是一种进行性、逐渐恶化的临床综合征，中医病机属本虚标实，以心之气阳虚衰为本，血脉瘀滞、水饮内停、痰浊不化为标，心气虚是心力衰竭的病理基础，心阳虚是心气虚的发展，血瘀是心力衰竭的重要病理环节，水停是心力衰竭的必然结果 [1, 2]。其中气虚、血瘀贯穿本病发展的始终，随着病情的发展，中医证候演变规律主要表现为气阴两虚、心血瘀阻→气虚血瘀水停→心肾阳虚、水饮泛滥。病位则主要在心，随着病情进展可涉及肺、脾、肝、肾其他诸脏 [3]。

1. 心衰早期，病证结合，辨证为气阴两虚、心血瘀阻证

慪性心衰初期时，肺循环淤血，心室舒张和（或）收缩功能开始降低，心功能大多处于 I 到 II 级（NY-HA）[1, 4]，N 端 B 型钠尿肽（NT-proBNP）

及 BNP 轻度升高，射血分数尚可达正常水平，临床上主要表现是心悸气短，活动后明显或加重，伴胸闷气喘、乏力、腰膝酸软、两颧潮红、自汗盗汗、口干欲饮、舌暗红苔少、脉细数无力或结代等。

此期中医辨证多属心肺气阴两虚、瘀血内停证。相关研究表明心功能 II 级的患者中医证型主要为气阴两虚、心血瘀阻证 [5]，比较该证型与其他证型 NT-proBNP 水平表明，该证型 NT-proBNP 分泌轻度升高，与心衰初期 NT-proBNP 的变化水平相一致 [6]，BNP 水平也表现为类似的规律 [7-9]。心气亏虚，气不行血，瘀血内停，而致心悸。气血瘀滞，气机不畅，故见胸闷憋气；心气不足，日久及肺，肺气亏虚，故见"少气而喘"之气短。劳则耗气，故活动后明显或加重。慪性心衰患者多为老年人，肝肾已亏，筋骨失养，故见腰膝酸软；自汗盗汗、舌暗红苔少、脉细数无力或结代均是气阴两虚、瘀血内停之征。

心衰早期病证结合辨证多属气阴两虚、瘀血内停，病位主要在心、肺，涉及肝、肾，临证以生麦散合六味地黄汤加减：党参 15～30g、黄芪 30～60g、麦冬 10～15g、五味子 5～10g、生地 15～30g、山萸肉 10～15g、玉竹 15～20g、茯苓 15～30g、泽兰 15～20g、丹参 20～30g、益母草 15～30g、车前子（包）15～30g。临床对症加减，肺气虚而出现恶寒、易感冒者加白术、防风；肺淤血较重、舌暗明显者加川芎、赤芍，咳

* 原载于《中国中西医结合杂志》，2011，31（10）：1306-1308

喘较重者，加葶苈子、苏子、大枣，气虚乏力明显者合四君子汤；高血压心脏病左室肥厚者加红花、地龙、三七粉冲服[4]。

2. 心衰中期，病证结合，辨证属气虚血瘀水停证

心衰中期，在左心衰竭的基础上，右心功能逐渐减退，体循环淤血，心功能发展至Ⅱ到Ⅲ级（NYHA）[1,4]，NT-proBNP及BNP中度升高，神经内分泌因子升高，射血分数正常水平或轻度降低。临床主要表现为心悸胸闷、腹胀痞满、纳呆、双下肢水肿明显、颈部青筋暴露，甚则胁下痞块疼痛，舌淡暗苔白润，脉沉缓或滑。

中医辨证多属气虚血瘀水停证，病位主要涉及肝、脾。研究表明心功能Ⅲ级的患者中中医证型主要为气虚血瘀水停证[5]，该证型NT-proBNP分泌中度升高，与心衰中期NT-proBNP的变化水平相一致[6]。BNP水平也呈现类似的变化规律[7-9]。心病日久，累及肝脾。心血亏虚，肝失荣养，藏血不能，故见心悸怔忡；肝血亏虚，肝体失养，疏泄失职，气不行血，故见瘀血内停，胁下痞块疼痛；血行不畅，水饮内生，随气而至，故见肝经循行之处水肿明显。"土得木而达"，肝失疏泄，木不疏土，故土气壅滞，腹胀纳呆。舌淡暗苔白润、脉沉缓或滑均是气虚血瘀水停之征。

心衰中期病证结合辨证多属气虚血瘀水停证，病位主要涉及肝、脾，临证时以保元汤合五苓散加减：党参15～30g、黄芪30～60g、桂枝10～15g、生姜10～15g、炙甘草10～15g、茯苓15～30g、猪苓15～30g、白术15～30g、泽泻12g、泽兰15g、益母草20～40g、丹参20～30g、红花6～15g。临证时对症加减，食欲不振、纳差者，加入鸡内金、焦三仙；干呕、呕吐明显者加入姜半夏、砂仁、陈皮；中焦虚寒、胃痛明显者，加入干姜、吴茱萸；结合中药药理，可加入柏枣仁、远志、琥珀等调节神经内分泌系统的药物[1]。

3. 心衰晚期，病证结合属心肾阳虚、水饮泛滥

心衰晚期，全心衰竭，体循环和肺循环瘀血明显，心功能明显降低，大多属Ⅳ级（NYHA）[1,4]，NT-proBNP及BNP重度升高，神经内分泌因子明显升高，射血分数明显降低，临床主要表现为喘息不能平卧，端坐呼吸，动则喘甚，伴见心悸怔忡、口唇青紫、全身水肿、肝脾肿大、甚则腹大如鼓、面色苍白、形寒肢冷、少尿或无尿、舌嫩苔白滑、脉细微欲绝。此属危急重症，如治疗不及时，可导致阴竭阳脱，阴阳离决而亡。

中医辨证多属心肾阳虚、水饮泛滥。研究表明心功能Ⅳ级的患者中中医证型主要为心肾阳虚、水饮泛滥证[5]，该证型NT-proBNP分泌重度升高，与心衰晚期NT-proBNP的变化水平相一致[6]，BNP水平也呈现类似的变化规律[7-9]，且该证型射血分数明显低于气阴两虚组[5]。肾阳为五脏阳之本，气虚日久，肾阳亏虚，纳气失司，故患者喘促明显，动则喘甚；膀胱气化不利，开阖失司，故见小便短少，甚则无尿；肾阳亏虚，水失蒸化，火不暖土，中阳不足，土不制水；子病及母，肺失通调，津液布散失常，故见患者全身水肿明显，甚则腹大如鼓；肾水上行于肺，则患者表现为喘息不得平卧，端坐呼吸；形寒肢冷、面色苍白、舌嫩苔白滑、脉细微欲绝均是心肾阳虚、水饮泛滥之征。

心衰晚期病证结合，临床辨证多属心肾阳虚、水饮泛滥证，病位主要涉及心、肾，旁及肝、脾、肺诸脏，临证治疗以真武汤合防己黄芪汤加减：制附片10～15g（先煎）、桂枝、10～15g、茯苓15～30g、白术15～30g、赤芍15～20g、干姜10～15g、黄芪30～60g、党参15～30g、防己15～20g、益母草15～30g、泽兰15～30g、丹参20～30g。临证时对症加减，喘憋重者加人参，肝、脾大甚者加三棱、莪术、合上鳖甲煎丸；小便点滴而出者合滋肾通关丸[10]；腹大如鼓者合疏凿饮子，并用黑白丑末吞服[1]；若病情严重，正虚喘脱时，急服参附汤送服黑锡丹，并中西医结合治疗。

综上所述，从病证结合角度分析，可使心衰的临床辨治化繁为简，并能显著提高临床疗效。然而，临床证治错综复杂，不可能简单地将其按照病程发展分为几个证型，应当更加深刻地探讨心衰的病证结合规律，从而提高心衰的临床疗效。

参考文献

[1] 苗阳，段文慧，吴梦玮，等. 中国中医科学院西苑医院名老中医治疗心力衰竭学术经验. 北京中医药杂志，2010，29（7）：502-505.

[2] 苗阳，赵文静，荆鲁，等. 中西医结合治疗慢性心力衰竭的回顾性分析. 中国中西医结合杂志，2008，28

（5）：406-409.

[3] 赵文静，苗阳，马晓昌. 慢性充血性心力衰竭的辨证论治. 中西医结合心脑血管病杂志，2008，7（6）：816-817.

[4] 李立志. 陈可冀治疗充血性心力衰竭经验. 中西医结合心血管病杂志，2006，4（2）：136-137.

[5] 段文慧，郑思道，苗阳，等. 慢性心力衰竭中医证型与心功能关系探讨. 中西医结合心血管病杂志，2010，8（5）：511-513.

[6] 李立志，王承龙，苗阳，等. 慢性心力衰竭中医证型与 N 端 B 型钠尿肽关系探讨. 中西医结合心血管病杂志，2008，6（8）：883-885.

[7] 张艺英，李长生. 充血性心力衰竭辨证分型与血浆 BNP、血清 CRP 相关性研究. 山东医药，2008，48（13）：53-54.

[8] 潘光明，邹旭，林晓忠，等. 心力衰竭患者脑钠肽与中医辨证分型相关性的临床研究. 新中医，2006，38（4）：33-35.

[9] 朱红俊，龚少愚，邹逊，等. 脑利钠肽与中医证型及 NY-HA 分级的相关性研究. 辽宁中医杂志，2006，33（4）：385-386.

[10] 史大卓，张昱. 实用中医内科病证结合治疗. 北京：人民卫生出版社，2007：38-39.

中西医结合治疗心源性休克 1 例 *

董国菊　李立志　史大卓

心源性休克多为急性心肌梗死严重泵衰竭所致，住院病死率大多在 80% 以上，是目前急性心肌梗死患者住院死亡的主要原因之一。笔者运用中西医结合疗法成功救治心源性休克 1 例，现报道如下。

病例介绍　患者，女，80 岁，病历号：0119367，因"阵发胸闷气短半个月，加重 3 天"于 2009 年 12 月 04 日急诊入院。患者半个月前反复于活动或休息时出现胸闷气短，每次持续 0.5h 左右，若含服硝酸甘油 10min 左右缓解，曾在我院门诊查心电图提示 ST-T 改变，建议住院，患者拒绝。3 天前，患者无明显诱因上述症状加重，持续时间最长达 2h 左右，入院前 3h 无明显诱因再次出现胸闷憋气，伴汗出，于我院急诊就诊，查心电图示广泛胸前导联 ST 段压低（图 1A），心肌损伤标志物：肌酸激酶同工酶（CK-MB）：9.8mmol/L；肌钙蛋白 I（TnI）：3.14mmol/L，考虑急性非 ST 段抬高心肌梗死，予以急诊介入，急诊冠状动脉造影见左主干（LM）末端至左前降支（left anterior descending coronary，LAD）开口处 60% 狭窄，心肌梗死溶栓试验（thrombolysis in myocardial infarction，TIMI）血流 3 级；LAD 中端 100% 闭塞，TIMI 血流 0 级；左回旋支

（LCX）近端 100% 闭塞，TIMI 血流 0 级；右冠状动脉（RCA）全程弥漫性狭窄，最窄 90%。RCA 的后降支（PDA）向 LAD 逆向供血；左房旋支向 LCX 近端形成侧支循环。术中患者血压下降至 60mmHg，烦躁。考虑心源性休克，置入主动脉内球囊反搏泵（intra-aortic balloon pump，IABP）转入病房。既往有高血压病史 40 余年，脑梗死病史 13 年，诊断糖耐量异常 1 周。患者有长期习惯性便秘史，已 4 天未解大便。

入院后查体：体温 36.7℃，脉搏 113 次/分，呼吸 23 次/分，血压 120/60mmHg（IABP 支持下）。神志清，精神萎靡，高枕卧位，呼吸急促，说话、翻身时加重。颈静脉无怒张，双肺呼吸音粗，双中下肺可闻及湿啰音，心界不大，心率 113 次/分，律齐，未闻及杂音及心包摩擦音，肝、脾不大，双下肢轻度水肿。舌质暗红，苔黄燥少津，脉弦细。

辅助检查：心电图（图 1B）：窦性心律，电轴正常，STV_3 ~ V_6 压低 0.3 ~ 0.4mV；心肌梗死三项：肌钙蛋白 T（cTnT）：32.8ng/dL；肌红蛋白（MYO）：536ng/dL；CK-MB：78.0mmol/L；心脏超声：左心室心肌弥漫性收缩运动减低，左心室舒张末径：60mm，左心室射血分数（LVEF）：

* 原载于《中国中西医结合杂志》，2011，31（2）：1701-1702

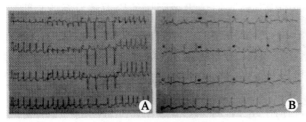

图1 患者的心电图

注：A为急诊心电图；B为入院心电图

31%。血常规：白细胞：$11.8 \times 10^9/L$；中性粒细胞：91%。

1. 治疗过程

入院第1天

病情分析：中医诊断：喘证，证属气虚血瘀、痰浊互阻，西医诊断为急性非ST段抬高心肌梗死，危险评估：TIMI评分7分、全球急性冠状动脉事件注册（GRACE）评分192分，均属于极高危，病死率在80%以上，拟定心源性休克合并有肺部感染为治疗原则。治疗方案：中医针对患者喘憋动则加重、大便秘结、舌苔黄厚少津、舌质暗红、脉弦细的主要症状，考虑患者属于正虚邪实，以邪实为主。正虚为气血亏虚，邪实属瘀毒互结，以瘀为主，治以益气活血、化浊通腑，方选陈可冀院士经验方愈梗通瘀汤加减：党参15g、生黄芪20g、紫丹参30g、当归尾10g、延胡索10g、川芎10g、广藿香10g、佩兰10g、陈皮10g、半夏10g、生大黄10g、肉苁蓉30g。每天1剂浓煎，分3次鼻导管饲入。西医予IABP作循环支持，积极抗炎，强化抗凝，抗血小板。考虑患者为急性心肌梗死泵衰竭，未用β-受体阻断剂。

入院第3天

IABP因故障被迫撤除。患者气促加重，端坐位，咳痰，痰无力咳出，大便在服用汤药情况下可以顺利排出，舌暗红苔薄黄少津，脉细数。血压（90～110）/（50～60）mmHg，心率116次/分，双肺呼吸音粗，可闻及湿啰音，双下肢轻度水肿，指尖血氧为96%。病情分析：目前循环尚不稳定，IABP应重新置入，但患者及家属均拒绝。热毒笃势已见消，现气阴不足之象。治疗方案：充分发挥中医药优势，益气强心，养阴复脉，予生脉注射液（由华润三九医药股份有限公司生产）60mL静脉滴注，每天1次；抗心梗合剂增甘寒养阴之品：太子参20g、生炙黄芪各20g、丹参30g、黄精20g、赤芍15g、郁金15g、肉苁蓉30g、大黄

10g，每天1剂，水煎200ml，分2～3次服用。西医治疗以最大限度减轻心脏前后负荷为主，静脉泵入硝普钠（由北京双鹤药业生产，50mg/支）50～100μg/min，监测血压，使收缩压不低于80mmHg；静脉入壶呋塞米（由郑州羚锐制药生产，每支20mg），每天40mg（如出量偏少，每天临时追加，每天最大用量80mg），保证出入量为负平衡，嘱患者静息与保持情绪稳定，避免大、小便用力。

入院第5天

患者仍感到喘憋，静息心率在100次/分左右，说话、翻身、吃饭等活动时心室率在110～120次/分；床旁心脏超声结果：左心室舒张末内径：62mm；LVEF：38%。患者目前大便已通，静息时憋气好转，动则加重。治疗方案同前。

入院第10天

患者胸闷憋气好转，夜间可高枕卧，自汗，口干，静息心率在90次/分左右，吃饭、交谈后心率可以上升至100次/分左右，舌红苔薄黄，脉弦细。查体：双肺仍可闻及湿啰音，较前略有减少。双下肢不肿。治疗方案：患者目前正虚为主，兼有痰浊血瘀，在上方基础上加益气养阴的太子参30g，去党参，加五味子以生津敛汗；患者心功能逐渐恢复，静息心率有时可以维持在80次/分左右，停用硝普钠泵入，呋塞米减为20mg入壶，每天1次。

入院第16天

患者胸闷气短明显好转，夜间可以平卧安睡，仍倦怠乏力，盗汗，咽干口燥，偶有咳嗽，舌红少苔，脉弦细。静息心率进一步回降至80次/分左右。双肺呼吸音清。治疗方案：患者目前中医主证以气阴两虚为主，方以生脉散加减：太子参30g、麦冬15g、五味子10g、生黄芪20g、丹参20g、三七粉3g（冲服）、肉苁蓉30g。西药停用静脉利尿剂，改呋塞米20mg口服，每天1次，停用抗生素；开始从极小量加用β-受体阻断剂，予美托洛尔（倍他乐克）（阿斯利康，每片25mg）6.25mg，口服，每天2次，根据情况逐渐递加剂量。

入院第22天

患者无明显不适，已下床活动，美托洛尔已调至12.5mg，每天2次。复查心脏超声：左心室舒张末内径：62mm；LVEF：41%。好转出院，嘱门诊随访治疗。

2. 讨论

该患者为非血运重建适应证的高龄急性心肌梗死患者，合并肺部感染、糖耐量异常、脑梗死病史、高血压病史，发生急性泵衰竭致心源性休克，心功能极差，病情危重，预后凶险。笔者在运用中西医结合方法救治过程中有以下几点体会。

IABP 在心脏收缩期通过抽空主动脉内球囊气体，造成负压，可以有效减少心脏负荷；在心脏舒张期通过给球囊充气，可以提升主动脉根部压力，保证冠状动脉供血，能够代替心脏一部分泵功能，为发挥中西医结合的治疗优势赢得了治疗时间。

2.1 充分发挥中医药优势

2.1.1 分期治疗 该患者急性期标实为主，主要表现为因瘀致毒，毒邪内盛，故治疗应清解热毒，活血透毒；但患者处于休克状态，即存厥脱之象，故在苦寒与甘寒之品之中应注意中病即止，以免正气损耗而致厥脱加重。恢复期邪实已去，以本虚为主，治以补气养阴为主，调补为治。

2.1.2 活血化瘀贯穿始终 梗死相关动脉内存在不稳定斑块，加之急性心肌梗死患者血小板易于活化、黏附、聚集，释放诸多生物活性物质，临床在辨证治疗的同时，应始终不忘活血化瘀。

2.1.3 通便是关键 大部分心肌梗死患者因为大便秘结，在排便过程中因用力而发生猝死。患者高龄、正气亏虚，又长期卧床，解决便秘至关重要。急性期选用通腑力度大的大黄。大黄不仅可通腑解毒，还有活血化瘀的功效。缓解期选用活血润肠通便的肉苁蓉，避免患者因排便用力诱发新的心肌缺血。

2.1.4 中药注射剂与口服汤剂相得益彰 在此类正虚邪实的急危重患者中，生脉注射液、参附注射液、丹参注射液、痰热清注射液等具有活血固脱解毒作用的注射剂可酌情选用，配合汤剂口服有协同增效之功。但应用过程中，应注意患者出入量的负平衡问题。

2.2 遵循指南，不拘泥于指南

在治疗过程中，西药的起始应用剂量、增减剂量，要根据患者临床情况个体化调整，遵循指南，但不拘泥于指南。比如倍他乐克的起用是在入院后 16 天，患者病情比较稳定时才考虑的，与指南尽早应用有一定的出入，原因是基于患者心功能极差，动则喘憋，早期应用可能加重心功能恶化。

2.3 细节决定成败

急性心肌梗死合并心源性休克的患者心脏功能差，随时会因为一个诱因加重泵衰竭，也随时可能会因为抢救无效而死亡，所以要特别注意细枝末节，不能因小失大。比如出入量的问题，呋塞米常规给量之外，是否需要临时再加？不能等患者喘憋加重才想起再追加呋塞米，而是要在患者白天出入量统计的基础上决定是否需要追加；再比如电解质的问题，患者进食量少，每天还应有大量利尿剂排钾，血钾水平肯定会低，不能等血钾低了再补，而要提前补、同时补，动态查，确保电解质水平的平衡。

第四章

中医药防治心血管疾病的药理研究

第一节 中医药防治心肌缺血/再灌注损伤的研究

西洋参茎叶总皂苷通过抑制过度内质网应激减轻大鼠心肌缺血/再灌注损伤 *

王 琛 刘 蜜 孙 胜 宋丹丹 刘秀华 史大卓

西洋参茎叶总皂苷（*Panax quinquefolium* sapopins，PQS）是西洋参茎叶中主要的活性成分。以往实验研究表明，PQS 具有减轻缺血/再灌注（ischemia/reperfusion，I/R）诱导的心肌细胞凋亡和心律失常、改善梗死后心室重构等作用[1-3]，其机制可能与增强抗氧化酶活性、维持细胞内 Ca^{2+} 稳态等有关[4]。

内质网（endoplasmic reticulum，ER）是细胞加工蛋白质和贮存 Ca^{2+} 的主要场所。缺血缺氧、葡萄糖/营养物质匮乏、ATP 耗竭、大量自由基产生及 Ca^{2+} 稳态破坏等均可引起 ER 功能障碍，触发内质网应激（endoplasmic reticulum stress，ERS），表现为 ERS 标志分子葡萄糖调节蛋白 78（glucose-regulated protein 78，GRP78）和钙网蛋白（calreticulin，CRT）的表达。持续而严重的 ERS 可诱导 ERS 相关细胞凋亡途径如 CCAAT/增强子结合蛋白同源蛋白（CCAAT/enhancer-binding protein homologous protein，CHOP）和 caspase-I2 的激活，加重 I/R 损伤[5-6]。我们前期研究表明 PQS 可通过抑制 ERS 相关细胞凋亡而减轻离体培养乳鼠心肌细胞缺氧/复氧损伤[7]。PQS 对大鼠心肌缺血/再灌注模型是否具有相同的作用，其机制是否与抑制过度 ERS 有关，尚缺少研究。因此本研究旨在证明 PQS 是否通过抑制过度 ERS 而减轻大鼠心肌 I/R 损伤。

1. 材料和方法

1.1 药品和试剂

PQS 粉由吉林省集安益盛药业股份有限公司提供；TUNEL 试剂盒购自 Promaga；氯化三苯基四氮唑（2，3，5-triphenyltetrazolium chloride，TTC）和伊文思蓝均购自 Sigma；蛋白电泳分子量为 7 ~ 175，为 Bio-Rad 产品；兔抗人 CRT、caspase-12 和 GRP78 多克隆抗体均购自 Stressgen；兔抗人 GAPDH 单克隆抗体、小鼠抗人 CHOP 单克隆抗体、兔抗人 Bax 和 Bcl-2 多克隆抗体均购自 Cell Signal；增强化学发光（ECL）试剂盒购自 Millipore；辣根过氧化酶标记山羊抗兔和山羊抗小鼠 IgG 均购自 Santa Cruz。

1.2 动物模型建立

清洁级健康 SD 大鼠，雌雄各半，体重（150±20）g，购自军事医学科学院实验动物中心[许可证号为 SCXK-（军）2007-004]，适应性喂养 1 周。术前禁食 12h，自由饮水，以 2% 戊巴比妥钠（2.3mL/kg）腹腔注射麻醉后固定于鼠台，气管插管，采用微型动物呼吸机（浙江大学医疗器械厂生产）支持呼吸，频率 50 ~ 60 次/分，潮气量 4 ~ 6mL。连接 SMUP-PC1 型生物信号处理系统，以 MFL Lab200 心电软件（复旦大学医学院生理教研室研制）记录标准导联心电图。按照既往

---

* 原载于《中国病理生理杂志》，2013，29（1）：20-27

报道方法[8]复制心肌 I/R 模型：胸骨正中切口，钝性分离皮下组织及肌肉，在胸骨左缘第 3、4 肋间开胸暴露心脏。打开心包膜，揭开脂肪垫，暴露左心耳后，持 7 号针线，在肺动脉圆锥和左心耳之间冠状动脉左前降支（left anterior descending coronary，LAD）处穿一缝合线，将充水（0.5mL）的球囊垫于血管与结扎线之间，结扎造成心肌缺血。心电图监测显示进行性心肌缺血变化后证明造模成功，45min 后，抽出球囊，关胸，再灌注 24h。结束实验时，动脉取血，用于血清肌钙蛋白（cardiac troponin，cTnT）测定，按照不同检测指标分别留取心肌组织标本迅速液氮冷冻后置于 –80℃ 冰箱保存备用，用于制备组织切片或进行心肌梗死面积测定。

1.3　实验分组

随机分为 3 组，每组 15 只。（1）假手术（sham）组：与药物组等量饮用水灌胃，每天 1 次，连续 6 周，开胸后穿线，但不结扎冠状动脉左前降支。（2）I/R 组：与药物组等量饮用水灌胃，每天 1 次，连续 6 周，开胸后可逆性结扎冠状动脉左前降支致心肌缺血 45min，再灌注 24h；（3）药物预处理（PQS+I/R）组（根据预实验结果）：270mg/（kg·d）PQS 水溶液灌胃，每天 1 次，连续 6 周后进行与 I/R 组相同的干预。

1.4　观察指标

1.4.1　心率（heart rate，HR）、平均动脉压（mean arterial pressure，MAP）和左心室压上升、下降最大速率（$\pm dp/dt_{max}$）测定　实验结束时，大鼠称重，2% 戊巴比妥腹腔麻醉，固定后分离右侧颈总动脉，将 PE-50 导管插入颈总动脉经压力传感器与 SMUP-PC1 型生物信号处理系统相连。稳定 10min 后，描计颈动脉波形，再将导管送入左心室，描计左心室压力曲线。以 MFL Lab200 心功能软件记录 HR、MAP 和 $\pm dp/dt_{max}$。

1.4.2　血清心肌损伤标志物 cTnT 含量测定　经动脉插管抽取血液约 5mL，肝素抗凝，1000r/min 离心 10min，收集血清，液氮速冻，–80℃ 保存。以全自动生化分析仪（日立公司）测定血清 cTnT 的含量。

1.4.3　心肌梗死面积测定　按照文献[9]报道方法，实验结束后原位结扎左冠状动脉前降支，经主动脉逆行灌注 1% 伊文思蓝 2mL，将非缺血区蓝染，显示出缺血区心肌。取出心脏，去除左右心房，置于 –20℃ 冷冻 20min，垂直其长轴横切为 5 片厚约

2mm 的心肌片，按顺序置入 2% TTC 磷酸缓冲液中，避光 37℃ 孵育 10min，此时梗死区为灰白色，即坏死面积（area of necrosis，AN）；缺血非梗死区呈砖红色，缺血区面积（area at risk，AAR）为灰白区与砖红色区之和，正常区为蓝色。扫描仪扫描成像，以 Image-Pro Plus 图像分析软件（Version 4.1）分别计算各部分面积，缺血心肌用 AAR 与左心室（left ventricle，LV）面积之比表示，梗死范围以 AN 与 AAR 之比表示。

1.4.4　心肌细胞凋亡测定　经颈动脉取血后，取出心脏，将缺血区心肌组织（左心室前壁中间段）剪下，4% 甲醛固定 1 周，常规石蜡包埋，制备 3μm 切片。采用 TUNEL 法，按照试剂盒说明进行心肌组织切片细胞凋亡的原位检测。共聚焦显微镜观察，正常心肌细胞核呈蓝色，凋亡细胞核呈深浅不一的绿色。每张切片于凋亡细胞分布区域随机取 5 个高倍视野，计算平均每个视野中的凋亡细胞数占总细胞数的百分比（%），以凋亡指数（apoptotic index，AI）表示。

1.4.5　心肌病理学观察　采用 HE 染色，将心肌组织样本固定于 4% 甲醛 1 周后，梯度乙醇脱水，二甲苯透明，石蜡包埋，切片厚度 3μm，脱蜡至水，Harris 苏木素染核，70% 盐酸乙醇分化，1% 乙醇伊红染色，梯度乙醇脱水，二甲苯透明，中性树胶封固，光镜观察并摄像。

1.4.6　Western blotting 分析　按文献报道方法[10]，提取心肌组织总蛋白，Bradford 法蛋白定量后，–80℃ 保存。取上述蛋白提取液上清（含蛋白 150μg）进行聚丙烯酰胺凝胶电泳（SDS-PAGE，12% 分离胶）。将电泳分离后的蛋白质电转移至硝酸纤维素（nitrocellulose，NC）膜，5% BSA 封闭 40min 后分别加入 Bcl-2、Bax、CRT、GRP78 和 caspase-12 多克隆抗体（均为 1∶500）和 CHOP 单克隆抗体（1∶500）4℃ 过夜孵育，1×TBS-T 洗膜后，以相应的 II 抗孵育 1.5h，并以 GAPDH（1∶500）单克隆抗体重复上述实验过程，作为上样对照。化学发光 ECL 显示，采用 Image-Pro Plus（Version 4.1）软件分析蛋白条带的积分吸光度值（integrated absorbance，IA=A× 面积），以靶蛋白 IA 值 /GAPDH IA 值的比值反映靶蛋白水平。

1.5　统计学处理

采用 SAS 8.2 统计软件对实验数据进行分析，数据均用均数 ± 标准差（mean±SD）表示，采

用单因素方差分析（One-way ANOVA）进行多组间比较，采用 q 检验进行多组间两两比较，以 $P < 0.05$ 为差异有统计学意义。

2. 结果

2.1 PQS 对大鼠心肌 I/R 损伤的影响

2.1.1 平均动脉压和左心室压上升、下降最大速率 术中假手术组大鼠状态良好，I/R 组和 PQS+I/R 组分别死亡大鼠 3 只和 4 只，死亡原因包括感染、严重心律失常或麻醉致死。各组大鼠心率无显著差异（$P > 0.05$）。与 sham 组比较，I/R 组 MAP 高 55%（$P < 0.05$），左室（$\pm dp/dt$max）分别低 42% 和 43%（$P < 0.05$）。PQS 干预后可明显改善 I/R 大鼠心功能，表现为 PQS+I/R 组 MAP 较 I/R 组低 32%（$P < 0.05$），$\pm dp/dt$max 分别较 I/R 组高 64% 和 35%（$P < 0.05$），见表 1。

2.2 PQS 对血清 cTnT 含量的影响

I/R 组血清 cTnT 含量较 sham 组显著升高，为 sham 组的 3.9 倍（$P < 0.05$）。PQS 干预可明显减少 I/R 大鼠血清 cTnT 的含量，PQS+I/R 组血清 cTnT 含量较 I/R 组低 53.3%（$P < 0.05$），见图 1。

2.3 PQS 对大鼠心肌梗死面积的影响

伊文思蓝和 TTC 双染评价心肌梗死面积，结果显示，sham 组大鼠无心肌梗死，sham 组、I/R 组和 PQS+I/R 组的缺血区面积分别为（49.8±3.4）%、（50.2±2.2）% 和（50.1±1.3）%，各组间无显著差异（$P > 0.05$）；I/R 组 AN/AAR 百分比为（44.2±1.4）%，PQS 明显缩小心肌梗死面积，PQS+I/R 组 AN/AAR 百分比为（15.3±4.2）%，较 I/R 组降低 65.5%（$P < 0.05$），见图 2。

2.4 PQS 对心肌细胞凋亡的影响

Sham 组心肌细胞凋亡指数为（8.2±0.6）%，I/R 可致心肌细胞凋亡显著增加，I/R 组心肌细胞凋亡指数为（56.9±6.0）%，是 sham 组的 7.0

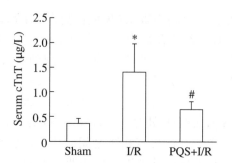

图 1 PQS 对血清 cTnT 含量的影响
Mean ± SD. $n=8$. $^*P < 0.05$ vs sham；$^\#P < 0.05$ vs I/R

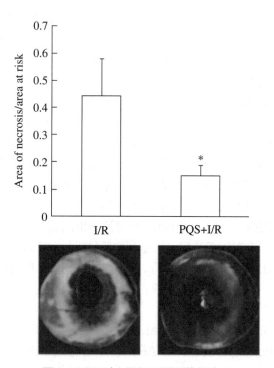

图 2 PQS 对心肌梗死面积的影响
I/R：ischemia/reperfusion；PQS：*Panax quinquelium* saponins. Mean ± SD. $n=3$. $^*P < 0.05$ vs I/R

倍（$P < 0.05$），PQS 可显著减轻 I/R 所致的心肌细胞凋亡，PQS+I/R 组心肌细胞凋亡指数为（25.7±5.1）%，较 I/R 组低 54.9%（$P < 0.05$），见图 3。

表 1 PQS 对大鼠血流动力学的影响

Group	MAP（mmHg）	HR（次/分）	$+dp/dt_{max}$（mmHg/s）	$-dp/dt_{max}$（mmHg/s）
Sham	60.9±7.2	422.6±15.1	1147.5±294.6	1067.6±253.0
I/R	94.3±15.2*	441.0±32.0	652.9±170.3*	620.1±179.0*
PQS+I/R	64.1±15.0#	445.8±18.5	1069.0±288.0#	839.7±151.9#

I/R：ischemia/reperfusion；PQS：*Panax quinquefolium* saponins. $^*P < 0.05$ vs sham；$^\#P < 0.05$ vs I/R

第四章

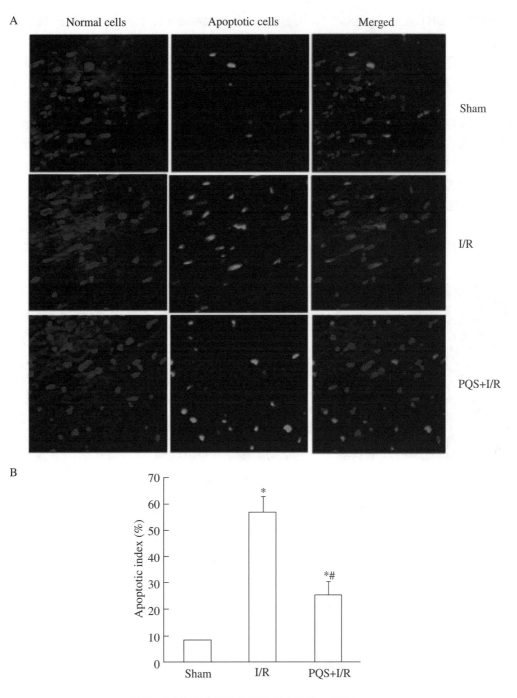

图 3 **PQS** 对大鼠心肌细胞凋亡指数的影响
Mean ± SD. *n*=3. *P < 0.05 *vs*. sham；#P < 0.05 *vs*. I/R

2.5 心肌组织病理形态学改变

　　光镜检查结果显示，sham 组心肌组织形态学无明显改变，肌纤维完整，排列规则；I/R 组心肌纤维排列不规则，结构紊乱，局部横纹消失，呈断裂坏死融合；PQS+I/R 组病理变化程度较 I/R 组减轻，未见明显的心肌纤维断裂、溶解、坏死，见图 4。

2.5.1 凋亡相关因子 Bcl-2、Bax 蛋白的表达 结果显示，与 sham 组比较，I/R 组 Bcl-2 蛋白表达

低 54.9%（*P* < 0.05），Bax 蛋白表达是 sham 组的 3.9 倍（*P* < 0.05）。PQS 可显著诱导抗凋亡蛋白 Bcl-2 的表达，PQS+I/R 组 Bcl-2 蛋白表达是 I/R 组的 2.1 倍（*P* < 0.05）；抑制促凋亡蛋白 Bax 的表达，Bax 蛋白表达较 I/R 组低 47.8%（*P* < 0.05），见图 5。

2.6 PQS 对 I/R 心肌组织内质网应激相关分子蛋白表达的影响

2.6.1 GRP78 和 CRT 蛋白的表达 结果显示，I/R 可明显诱导 GRP78 和 CRT 蛋白的表达，与 sham 组比较，I/R 组 GRP78、CRT 蛋白表达水平显著增加，分别为 sham 组的 3.1 倍和 3.0 倍（$P < 0.05$）；PQS 可抑制 I/R 诱导的 CRT 过表达，较 I/R 组低 43.4%（$P < 0.05$），见图 6。

2.6.2 CHOP 蛋白表达的变化和 caspase-12 的活化 I/R 可明显诱导 CHOP 蛋白表达，为 sham 组的 3.4 倍（$P < 0.05$）。PQS 抑制 I/R 诱导的 CHOP 蛋白表达，较 I/R 组降低 38.6%（$P < 0.05$），见图 7。

采用可同时识别 caspase-12 酶原（pro-caspase-12，分子量 48～50）和剪切后的 caspase-12（cleaved caspase-12，分子量为 36）的特异性抗体，进行免疫印迹检测，结果显示，I/R 可明显诱导 caspase-12 蛋白剪切活化，剪切后的 caspase-12 的蛋白表达是 sham 组的 2.5 倍（$P < 0.05$）；PQS 抑制 I/R 后 caspase-12 蛋白活化，PQS+I/R 组剪切后 caspase-12 蛋白表达较 I/R 组降低 23.7%（$P < 0.05$），见图 7。

3. 讨论

冠状动脉结扎法建立大鼠心肌 I/R 损伤模型，为目前评价药物心肌缺血保护最常用的模型之一。

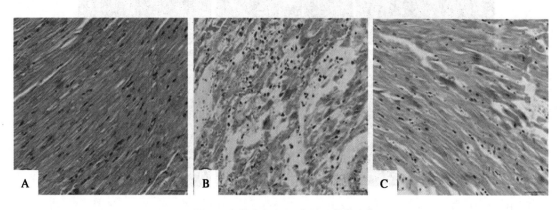

图 4 大鼠心肌组织病理形态学改变

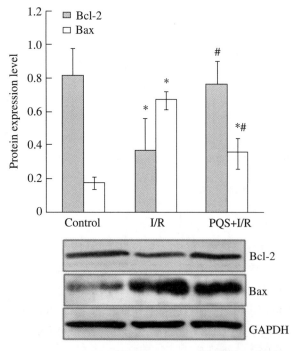

图 5 PQS 对 I/R 心肌 Bcl-2 和 Bax 蛋白表达的影响
Mean ± SD. *n*=6 *$P < 0.05$ vs control; #$P < 0.05$ vs I/R

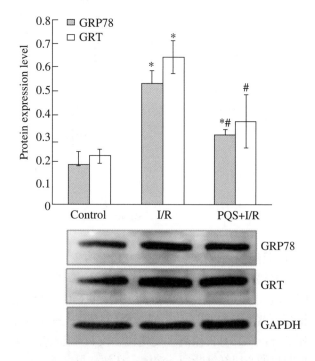

图 6 PQS 对 I/R 心肌 GRP78 和 CRT 蛋白表达的影响
Mean ± SD. *n*=6. *$P < 0.05$ vs control; #$P < 0.05$ vs I/R

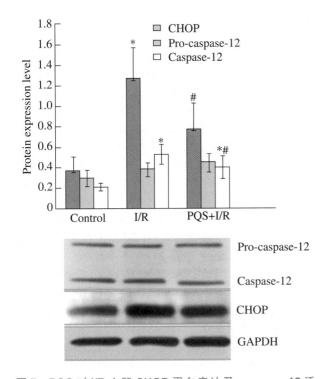

图7　PQS 对 I/R 心肌 CHOP 蛋白表达及 caspase-12 活化的影响

Mean ± SD. $n=6$. $*P < 0.05$ vs control; $\#P < 0.05$ vs I/R

因实验大鼠品系纯正、组间差异小、冠状动脉侧支循环少、易结扎、操作简单等特点，成为首选 I/R 动物模型。本研究采用 SD 大鼠，建立 I/R 损伤模型，肉眼观察可见模型组左心室前壁心肌颜色变淡甚至苍白，而假手术组无明显改变。心肌组织病理学染色与心肌梗死面积测定既是反映组织损伤最直观的指标，亦是反映药物治疗缺血性损伤有效性的客观证据。本实验采用心肌组织病理 HE 染色观察心肌的组织病理变化，结果显示模型组细胞核固缩，间质水肿，心肌纤维排列紊乱、断裂；假手术组未见明显改变；PQS 组心肌组织病理变化程度较 I/R 组减轻。采用伊文思蓝、TTC 双染评价心肌梗死面积，结果显示各组缺血区无显著差异，说明各组结扎部位一致，不存在因结扎部位的不同而造成的人为误差；模型组心肌梗死面积较假手术组明显增加，PQS 可显著减少 I/R 导致的心肌梗死面积；平均动脉压是一个心动周期中持续地推动血液向前流动的平均推动力，更精确地反映心脏和血管的功能状态，每一心动周期由于舒张期时程长于收缩期，故平均动脉压不是收缩压与舒张压的平均数，而是更靠近于舒张压，平均动脉压升高说明血管壁弹性减少，顺应性下降。本研究发现模型组平均动

脉压较假手术组明显升高，反映左室舒张及收缩功能的 $\pm dp/dt_{max}$ 显著降低，PQS 能显著降低 I/R 引起的平均动脉压升高，增加左室 $\pm dp/dt_{max}$；心肌损伤标志物 cTnT 是目前诊断心肌损伤的特异性标志物，心肌急性缺血（氧）时，细胞膜损伤，通透性增加，cTnT 大量漏出。本研究发现缺血 45min、再灌注 24h 后，血清 cTnT 含量明显增加。与模型组相比，PQS 组血清 cTnT 显著减少。以上均提示 PQS 可保护 I/R 心肌损伤，表现为减轻心肌坏死、改善心功能、减轻心肌细胞膜损伤等。

细胞凋亡是心肌 I/R 损伤的一个重要特征，在心肌 I/R 损伤过程中发挥重要作用[11]。Gottlieb 等[12]利用家兔离体心脏灌流模型首次发现 I/R 中存在心肌细胞凋亡。Musat-Marcu 等[13]研究发现离体灌流大鼠心脏再灌注早期即可发生心肌细胞凋亡。TUNEL 法测心肌细胞凋亡，既可定性又可定量，可准确定位，且灵敏度高。本研究利用此方法发现，与假手术组比较，模型组心肌细胞凋亡指数显著增加，PQS 可显著降低 I/R 引起的细胞凋亡，提示 PQS 可通过抑制 I/R 心肌细胞凋亡，减轻心肌 I/R 损伤。抗凋亡基因 bcl-2 与促凋亡基因 bax 参与心肌 I/R 损伤细胞凋亡的调控[14-16]，抑制细胞凋亡的发生和发展是促进心肌 I/R 损伤后心功能恢复和减轻心肌致死性损伤的一条重要途径。本研究采用 Western blotting，检测凋亡相关因子 Bcl-2 和 Bax 的蛋白表达，发现模型组促凋亡因子 Bax 蛋白表达较假手术组显著升高，抗凋亡因子 Bcl-2 的表达明显降低，PQS 可明显降低 I/R 诱导的 Bax 蛋白表达，升高 Bcl-2 蛋白表达。提示 PQS 可通过调节凋亡相关因子的表达，调控心肌细胞凋亡过程，减轻心肌损伤。

I/R 发生的主要病理环节是氧自由基产生和钙超载。ER 是调节 Ca^{2+} 和蛋白质合成的重要场所，ER 理化环境改变和 ER 过负荷等因素导致的 ERS 在 I/R 损伤的发生发展过程中具有重要意义[17]。GRP78 为内质网标志分子，早期 ERS 时 GRP78 与 ER 内误折叠及未折叠蛋白结合，减轻 ER 负荷，恢复其稳态，因此，GRP78 的表达标志 ERS 的发生。Shibata 等[18]发现，小鼠大脑缺血 1h 后 GRP78 表达升高。Flores-Diaz 等[19]报道，心肌缺血/缺氧可诱导内质网分子伴侣 GRP78、CRT 表达上调。本研究采用 Western blotting 方法检测内质网分子伴侣 GRP78 的蛋白表达，发现各处理组 GRP78 的蛋白表达均明显高于假手术组，提示

第四章

I/R 诱发了 ERS，与文献[20] 报道一致。PQS 通过调节 ERS，维持细胞内环境稳态，从而增加心肌抗 I/R 损伤的能力；CRT 是 ER 中主要钙结合伴侣蛋白，在维持细胞 Ca^{2+} 稳态、协助蛋白质正确折叠及调节细胞凋亡等方面发挥重要作用。Ihara 等[21] 利用 H9c2 成心肌细胞研究证实高表达的 CRT 可促进细胞凋亡。本研究亦发现 I/R 诱导 CRT 蛋白表达水平显著升高，与文献报道一致[22]。PQS 可减轻 I/R 诱导的 CRT 过表达，表明 PQS 可通过调节 CRT 蛋白表达，减少 I/R 引起的细胞凋亡。

I/R 诱导细胞凋亡，除经典的死亡受体途径和线粒体途径外，ERS 相关凋亡途径引起广泛关注[23-26]。持续或严重的 ERS 通过激活凋亡信号分子 CHOP、caspase-12 和 JNK 启动 ERS 相关凋亡途径，诱导细胞凋亡。CHOP 又称生长停滞及 DNA 损伤诱导蛋白 153（growth arrest and DNA damage-inducible protein 153，GADD153），是 CCAAT/ 增强子结合蛋白（C/EBP）转录因子家族成员，为 ERS 相关凋亡途径的特异性标志物。严重 ERS 时，CHOP 通过直接调节核内靶基因，增加细胞对 ERS 介导凋亡的敏感性[27]。研究表明，缺血 / 缺氧可诱导 CHOP 表达显著增加，破坏了 Bcl-2 家族促凋亡与抗凋亡基因之间的平衡，促进细胞凋亡[28]。本研究发现，与假手术组相比，I/R 显著诱导了 CHOP 蛋白表达，PQS 可显著抑制 I/R 诱导的 CHOP 蛋白表达，提示 PQS 可能通过抑制过度 ERS 介导的细胞凋亡起到心肌保护作用。Caspase-12 定位于 ER 外膜，以无活性的酶原形式存在，是 ERS 相关凋亡途径的特异性分子，持续或严重的 ERS 引起 caspase-12 激活，活化的 caspase-12 进一步激活 casepase-9，接着激活 caspase-3，最终导致细胞凋亡[29-30]。本研究发现，I/R 可明显诱导剪切后 caspase-12 的蛋白表达，提示 ERS 相关凋亡途径在 I/R 损伤中具有重要作用，与文献[22] 报道一致。PQS 可显著抑制 I/R 诱导的 caspase-12 活化，PQS 抑制 I/R 引起的细胞凋亡也与其抑制 caspase-12 活化有关。

综上所述，PQS 具有抗大鼠心肌 I/R 损伤的作用，其机制可能通过抑制过度 ERS 引起的细胞凋亡有关，表现为降低 I/R 诱导的 CRT 过表达，抑制 CHOP、caspase-12 等内质网应激凋亡通路激活，其下游信号通路有待进一步探索。

参考文献

[1] 曹霞，谷欣权，陈燕萍，等. 西洋参茎叶三醇组皂甙对缺血再灌注损伤心肌的保护作用. 中国老年学杂志，2004，7（24）：654-655.

[2] 殷惠军，张颖，蒋跃绒，等. 西洋参叶总皂甙对急性心肌梗死大鼠心肌细胞凋亡及凋亡相关基因表达的影响. 中国中西医结合杂志，2005，25（3）：232-235.

[3] 关利新，衣欣，杨世杰，等. 西洋参茎叶皂甙对大鼠心肌细胞 Ca^{2+} 内流的影响. 中国药理与临床，2004，20（6）：8-9.

[4] 鞠传静，张志国，赵学忠，等. 西洋参叶二醇组皂甙对大鼠实验性心室重构的保护作用. 中国老年学杂志，2007，27（22）：2173-2175.

[5] Boya P, Cohen I, Zamzami N, et al. Endoplasmic reticulum stress-induced cell death requires mitochondrial membrane permeabilization. Cell Death Differ, 2002, 9 (4): 465-467.

[6] Breckenridge DG, Gennain M, Mathai JP, et al. Regulation of apoptosis by endoplasmic reticulum pathways. Oncogene, 2003, 22 (53): 8608-8618.

[7] Wang C, Li YZ, Wang XR, et al. *Panax quinquefolium* saponins reduce myocardial hypoxia/reoxygenation injury by inhibiting excessive endoplasmic reticulum stress. Shock, 2012, 37 (2): 228-233.

[8] 赵秀梅，孙胜，刘秀华. 垫扎球囊法复制大鼠在体心肌缺血 / 再灌注模型. 中国微循环，2007，11（3）：206-208.

[9] Liu XH, Grund F, Kanellopoulos GK, et al. Myocardial extracellular signal regulatory kinases are activated by laser treatment. J Cardiovasc Surg (Torino), 2003, 44 (1): 1-7.

[10] Xu FF, Liu XH, Cai LR. Role of hypoxia-inducible fac-tor-1α in the prevention of cardiomyocyte injury induced by hypoxic preconditioning. Acta Physiol Sin, 2004, 56 (5): 609-614.

[11] Zhao ZQ, Vinten-Johansen J. Myocardial apoptosis and ischemic preconditioning. Cardiovasc Res, 2002, 55 (3): 438-455.

[12] Gottlieb RA, Burleson KO, Kloner RA, et al. Reperfusion injury induces apoptosis in rabbit cardiomyocytes. J Clin Invest, 1994, 94 (10): 1621-1628.

[13] Musat-Marcu S, Gunter HE, Jugdutt BI, et al. Inhibition of apoptosis after ischemia-reperfusion in rat myocardium by cycloheximide. J Mol Cell Cardiol, 1999, 31 (5): 1073-1082.

[14] Fliss H, Gattiuger D. Apoptosis in ischemic and

reperfused rat myocardium. Circ Res, 1996, 79 (5): 949-956.

[15] Borutaite V, Brown GC. Mitochondria in apoptosis of ischemic heart . FEBS Lett, 2003, 541 (1-3): 1-5.

[16] 姚震，焦解歌，冯建章 . 心肌缺血再灌注损伤与细胞凋亡关系的实验研究 . 海南医学院学报，2000, 6 (3): 129-133.

[17] Vilatoba M, Eckstein C, Bilbao G, et al. Sodium 4-phe-nylbutyrate protects against liver ischernia reperfusion injury by inhibition of endoplasmic reticulum stress mediated apoptosis. Surgery, 2005, 138 (2): 342-351.

[18] Shibata M, Hattori H, Sasaki T, et al. Activation of caspase-12 by endoplasmic reticulum stress induced by transient middle cerebral artery occlusion in mice. Neuroscience, 2003, 118 (2): 491-499.

[19] Flores-Diaz M, Higuita JC, Florin I, et al. A cellular UDP-glucose deficiency causes overexpression of glucose oxygen-regulated proteins independent of endoplasmic reticulum stress elements. J Biol Chem, 2004, 279 (21): 21724-21731.

[20] Szegezdi E, Duffy A, O' Mahoney ME, et al. ER stress contributes to ischemia-induced cardiomyocyte apoptosis. Biochem Biophys Res Commun, 2006, 349 (4): 1406-1411.

[21] Ihara Y, Urata Y, Goto S, et al. Role of calreticulin in the sensitivity of myocardiac H9c2 cells to oxidative stress caused by hydrogen peroxide. Am J Physiol Cell Physiol, 2006, 290 (1): C208-C221.

[22] Liu XH, Zhang ZY, Sun S, et al. Ischemic postconditioning protects myocardium from ischemia/reperfusion injury through attenuation endoplasmic reticulum stress. Shock, 2008, 30 (4): 422-427.

[23] Hayashi T, Saito A, Okuno S, et al. Damage to the endoplasmic reticulum and activation of apoptotic machinery by oxidative stress in ischemic neurons. J Cereb Blood Flow Metab, 2005, 25 (1): 41-53.

[24] Matindale JJ, Fernandez R, Thuerauf D, et al. Endoplasmic reticulum stress gene induction and protection from ischemia/reperfusion injury in the hearts of transgenic mice with a tamoxifen-regulated from of ATF6. Circ Res, 2006, 98 (9): 1186-1193.

[25] 王琛，李玉珍，王晓礽，等 . 西洋参茎叶总皂苷通过抑制过度内质网应激减轻大鼠心肌细胞缺氧 / 复氧损伤 . 中国病理生理杂志，2012, 28 (1): 22-28.

[26] 刘颖，纪超，吴伟康 . 附子多糖保护缺氧 / 复氧乳鼠心肌细胞及其抗内质网应激的机制研究 . 中国病理生理杂志 , 2012, 28 (3): 459-463.

[27] Oyadomari S, Mori M. Roles of CHOP/GADD153 in endoplasmic reticulum stress. Cell Death Differ, 2004, 11 (4): 381-389.

[28] McCullough KD, Martindale JL, Klotz LO, et al. Gadd153 sensitizes cells to endoplasmic reticulum stress by down-regulating Bcl-2 and perturbing the cellular redox state. Mol Cell Biol, 2001, 21 (4): 1249-1259.

[29] Szegezdi E, Fitzgerald U, Samali A. Caspase-12 and ER-stress-mediated apoptosis: the story so far. Ann N Y Acad Sci, 2003, 1010: 186-194.

[30] Nakagawa T, Zhu H, Morishima N, et al. Caspase-12 mediates endoplasmic-reticulum-specific apoptosis and cytotoxicity by amyloid-β. Nature, 2000, 403 (6765): 98-103.

第
四
章

西洋参茎叶总皂苷通过抑制过度内质网应激减轻大鼠心肌细胞缺氧/复氧损伤 *

王　琛　李玉珍　王晓初　吕振嵘　史大卓　刘秀华

20世纪90年代以来我国对西洋参茎叶的化学成分和药理学作用进行了大量研究，表明其化学成分包括皂苷类、氨基酸类、糖类、挥发油类、无机元素类和脂肪酸类等，西洋参茎叶总皂苷（*Panax quinquefolium* saponin，PQS）是从西洋参茎叶中提取出的活性成分。研究显示，PQS具有抗缺血/再灌注（ischemia/reperfusion，I/R）心肌细胞凋亡、抗心律失常、改善梗死后心室重构、增强抗氧化酶活性、减轻缺血所致的游离脂肪酸代谢紊乱和乳酸堆积、维持细胞内Ca^{2+}稳态等作用[1-4]。内质网（endoplasmic reticulum，ER）是细胞加工蛋白质和贮存Ca^{2+}的主要场所，缺血缺氧、葡萄糖或营养物质匮乏、ATP耗竭、大量自由基的产生及Ca^{2+}稳态破坏等均可引起ER功能障碍，触发内质网应激（endoplasmic reticulum stress，ERS）。持续而严重的ERS可通过钙超载、影响线粒体功能等加重细胞凋亡和I/R损伤[5-6]，表现为ERS标志分子葡萄糖调节蛋白78（glucose-regulated protein 78，GRP78）、钙网蛋白（calreticulin，CRT）的表达及ERS相关细胞凋亡途径[C/EBP同源蛋白（C/EBP homologous protein，CHOP）、caspase-12等]的激活。PQS是否通过抑制过度的ERS，发挥抗心肌I/R损伤的作用，以往尚缺乏研究。本研究利用乳鼠心肌细胞缺氧/复氧（hypoxia/reoxygenation，H/R）模型，观察PQS对心肌细胞损伤的保护作用，并通过ERS探讨PQS抗心肌缺血再灌注损伤的相关保护机制。

1. 材料和方法

1.1 动物与试剂

清洁级SD 24h内新生乳鼠由军事医学科学院实验动物中心提供；PQS粉由吉林省集安益盛药业股份有限公司提供；DMEM培养基购自Gibco；新生牛血清（newborn calf serum，NCS）购自

PAA；胰蛋白酶（trypsin）购自Amresco；蛋白酶抑制剂购自Sigma；Annexin V-FITC细胞凋亡检测试剂盒购自南京凯基生物工程公司；乳酸脱氢酶（lactate dŴydogenase，LDH）测试盒购自南京建成生物工程研究所；TRNzol-A⁺总RNA提取试剂、$2×$Taq PCR Master Mix和电泳级琼脂糖购自北京天根生化科技有限公司；cDNA第1链合成试剂盒购自北京全式金生物技术有限公司；PCR引物由北京三博远志生物技术有限责任公司合成；蛋白电泳分子量（7～175）标记为Bio-Rad产品；兔抗人CRT、caspase-12和GRP78多克隆抗体购自Stressgen；兔抗人GAPDH单克隆抗体、小鼠抗人CHOP单克隆抗体和兔抗人Bax、Bcl-2多克隆抗体均购自Cell Signal；增强化学发光（ECL）试剂盒购自Millipore；辣根过氧化酶标记山羊抗兔和山羊抗小鼠IgG购自Santa Cruz。

1.2 乳鼠心肌细胞培养

参照Simpson等[7]加以改进，无菌操作取出生后24h内SD新生乳鼠心尖部组织，剪碎成$1mm×1mm×1mm$大小，加入适量0.15%胰蛋白酶，37℃水浴下轻柔搅动、反复消化，制备心肌细胞悬液，差速贴壁。用含15%新生牛血清的DMEM培养液，调整细胞浓度为每瓶$3×10^6$，接种于底面积为$75cm^2$的培养瓶，置CO_2孵箱进行原代培养。

1.3 实验分组

取原代培养心肌细胞，置于CO_2孵箱常规培养24h，换无新生牛血清的DMEM培养液同步化24h后，进行如下2个部分研究。为证明PQS对H/R心肌细胞的保护作用分为以下3组：正常对照（control）组：细胞置CO_2孵箱37℃，常规培养至实验结束；H/R组：按Li等[8]将细胞置于缺氧仓内，通入95%N_2-5%CO_2混合气，缺氧4h后放回CO_2孵箱，37℃常规继续培养12h结束实验；PQS+H/R组：以PBS缓冲液稀释PQS原粉，配

---

* 原载于《中国病理生理杂志》，2012，28（1）：22-28

成浓度分别为 20、40、80、160g/L 的储存液，过滤除菌，4℃保存，应用时将储存液 1000 倍稀释并加入心肌细胞培养液中，培养 24h，进行 H/R 操作，根据预实验结果（见图 1），选取终浓度为 160mg/L 为最佳给药浓度。为进一步探讨 PQS 对 H/R 心肌细胞保护作用的机制，又分为以下 4 组：正常对照组、H/R 组和 H/R+PQS 组，处理同上；PQS 组，细胞置 CO_2 孵箱 37℃常规培养 16h，然后加入 160mg/L 的 PQS 水溶液，继续培养 24h。

1.4　凋亡率、LDH 漏出及细胞存活率测定

实验结束时，收集各组细胞培养液，用 0.25% 胰蛋白酶 +0.02%EDTA 消化液制备单细胞悬液，按照测试盒方法分别加入染料 Annexin V 和溴化丙啶（propidium Iodide，PI），室温下孵育 5～15min，以流式细胞仪（BD FACScalibur，Becton-Dickinson）检测细胞凋亡情况，以台盼蓝排斥实验[9]测定细胞存活率，按 LDH 测试盒方法检测细胞培养液中 LDH 活性。

1.5　RT-PCR 测定

TRNzol-A+ 提取总 RNA，紫外分光光度计测定 RNA 含量。按 cDNA 第 1 链合成试剂盒操作步骤将 RNA 反转录成 cDNA，进行 PCR 扩增。各目的基因上、下游引物见表 1。采用 Image-Pro Plus 4.1 软件分析条带平均吸光度值（A），以目的片段和 GAPDH 的平均光密度比值反映目的基因 mRNA 水平。

1.6　Western blotting 分析

按 Liu 等[10]报道方法提取心肌细胞总蛋白，Bradford 法蛋白定量后分装，–80℃保存取上述细胞蛋白提取液上清（含蛋白 80μg）进行聚丙烯酰胺凝胶电泳（SDS-PAGE，12% 分离胶），将电泳分离后的蛋白质电转移至硝酸纤维素膜上，用 5%BSA 封闭 40min 后分别加入 CRT、GRP78、caspase-12、Bcl-2、Bax 多克隆抗体（均为 1∶500）、CHOP 单克隆抗体（1∶500）4℃过夜孵育，用 1×TBS-T 洗膜后，以相应的Ⅱ抗孵育 1.5h，并以 GAPDH（1∶500）单克隆抗体重复上述实验过程，作为上样对照。化学发光 ECL 显示，采用 Image-ProPlus 4.1 软件分析蛋白条带的积分吸光度值（integrated A value，IA，平均吸光度值 × 面积），以靶蛋白 /GAPDH IA 比值反映靶蛋白水平。

1.7　统计学处理

采用 SAS 8.2 统计软件对实验数据进行分析，数据用均数 ± 标准差（$\bar{x} \pm s$）表示，采用单因素方差分析（One-way ANOVA）进行多组间比较，采用 q 检验进行多组间两两比较，两变量相关性采用 Pearson 相关分析，以 $P < 0.05$ 为差异有统计学意义。

2.　结果

2.1　西洋参茎叶总皂苷对 H/R 心肌细胞的保护作用

2.1.1　心肌细胞凋亡率　正常对照组细胞生长状

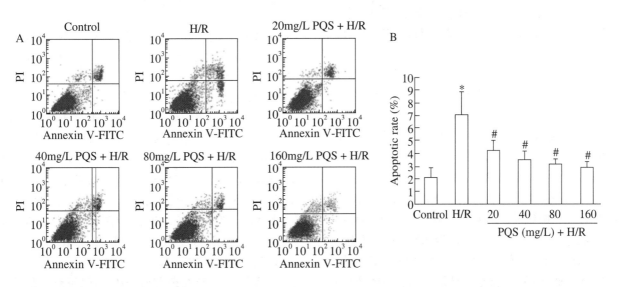

图 1　流式细胞术分析 PQS 对 H/R 诱导心肌细胞凋亡的影响

A：flow cytometric images；B：apoptotic rates of cardiomyocytes in different groups. $\bar{x} \pm s$. n=3. *P < 0.05 *vs* control；#P < 0.05 *vs* H/R

表 1 PCR 反应中目的片段引物

Gene	Primer sequence	Tm（℃）	Length（bp）
CRT	P1：5′-CAAGGATATCCGGTGTAAGGA-3′	58.01	445
	P2：5′-CATAGATATTCGCATCGGGG-3′	57.80	
GRP78	P1：5′-TCTGGTTGGCGGATCTACTC-3′	59.85	345
	P2：5′-TCTTTTGTCAGGGGTCGTTC-3′	57.80	
CHOP	P1：5′-AGCTGGAAGCCTGGTATGAG-3′	59.85	256
	P2：5′-GACCACTCTGTTTCCGTTTC-3′	57.80	
Bcl-2	P1：5′-AATTTCCTGCATCTCATGCC-3′	55.75	279
	P2：5′-AGCCCCTCTGTGACAGCTTA-3′	59.85	
Bax	P1：5′-TTCATCCAGGATCGAGCAG-3′	57.56	234
	P2：5′-CCAGTTGAAGTTGCCATCAG-3′	57.80	
GAPDH	P1：5′-TGCTGAGTATGTCGTGGAG-3′	61.12	496
	P2：5′-GTCTTCTGAGTGGCAGTGAT-3′	60.07	

态良好，细胞凋亡率为 2.12%；H/R 组细胞凋亡率为 7.09%（$P < 0.05$）；分别以 20、40、80、160mg/L PQS 培养细胞 24h，细胞凋亡率分别为 4.2%、3.5%、3.2% 和 2.9%，$P < 0.05$，呈剂量依赖性，见图 1。

2.1.2 细胞培养液 LDH 活性 正常对照组细胞生长状态良好，细胞培养液 LDH 活性为 113.4U/L，H/R 组细胞膜通透性增高，培养液 LDH 活性较对照组升高约 6 倍（$P < 0.05$），以 160mg/L PQS 培养液培养细胞 24h，其细胞培养液 LDH 活性较 H/R 心肌细胞培养液降低了 66.58%（$P < 0.05$），见表 2。

2.1.3 细胞存活率 台盼蓝排斥实验结果显示，正常对照组细胞存活率为 96.3%，H/R 组细胞存活率较对照组降低 21.7%（$P < 0.05$），以 160mg/L PQS 培养液孵育细胞 24h，其细胞存活率较 H/R 心肌细胞升高了 21.1%（$P < 0.05$），见表 2。

2.1.4 凋亡相关蛋白 Bax、Bcl-2 mRNA 和蛋白的表达 RT-PCR 的结果显示，H/R 组 Bcl-2mRNA 的表达较对照组降低 44.5%（$P < 0.05$），Bax mRNA 的表达较对照组升高 86.9%（$P < 0.05$），提示 H/R 可诱导抗凋亡蛋白 Bcl-2 和抑制促凋亡蛋白 Bax mRNA 的表达。PQS 可诱导 H/R 后抗凋亡蛋白 Bcl-2 mRNA 表达，PQS+H/R 组心肌细胞 Bcl-2 mRNA 表达较 H/R 组升高 30.9%（P

表 2 PQS 预处理对 H/R 后细胞存活率及 LDH 活性的影响（$\bar{\chi} \pm s$，$n=4$）

组	Cell survival rate（%）	LDH activity（U/L）
Control	96.29±0.79	113.40±11.87
H/R	75.36±2.32*	671.33±46.62*
160mg/L PQS+H/R	95.47±0.53#	224.33±22.57*#

*$P < 0.05$ vs control；#$P < 0.05$ vs H/R，H/R：hypoxia/reoxygenation；PQS：Panax quinquelium saponin

< 0.05）；抑制促凋亡蛋白 Bax mRNA 的表达，Bax mRNA 表达较 H/R 组降低 39.7%（$P < 0.05$），见图 2A、B。

Western blotting 的结果显示，H/R 组 Bcl-2 蛋白表达较对照组降低 58.3%（$P < 0.05$），Bax 蛋白表达较对照组升高 167.0%（$P < 0.05$），提示 H/R 可诱导抗凋亡蛋白 Bcl-2 和抑制促凋亡蛋白 Bax 蛋白表达。PQS 可诱导 H/R 后抗凋亡蛋白 Bcl-2 的表达，PQS+H/R 组心肌细胞 Bcl-2 蛋白表达较 H/R 组升高 48.0%（$P < 0.05$）；抑制促凋亡蛋白 Bax 的表达，较 H/R 组降低 48.4%（$P < 0.05$），见图 2C、D。

2.2 西洋参茎叶总皂苷对 H/R 心肌细胞内质网应激相关分子表达的影响

2.2.1 GRP78、CRT mRNA 和蛋白表达的变化

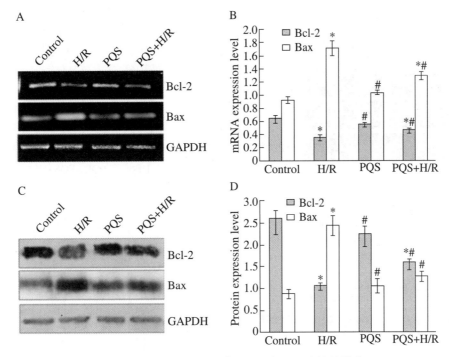

图2　PQS 对 H/R 心肌细胞 Bcl-2 和 Bax 表达的影响
A：The levels of Bcl-2 and Bax mRNA were examined by RT-PCR. GAPDH was used as a normalization control. B：Bar chart of densitometry of the bands shown in A. C：The levels of Bcl-2 and Bax protein were examined by Western blotting. GAPDH was used as a normalization control. D：Bar chart of densitometry of the bands shown in C. $\bar{x} \pm s.$ n=3. $^{*}P < 0.05$ vs control；$^{\#}P < 0.05$ vs H/R

RT-PCR 的结果显示，H/R 可明显诱导 GRP78 和 CRT mRNA 的表达，较对照组分别高 380.0% 和 96.0%（$P < 0.05$）；PQS 可抑制 H/R 诱导的 GRP78 和 CRT mRNA 的表达，PQS+H/R 组较 H/R 组分别降低 61.6% 和 35.7%（$P < 0.05$）。Western blotting 的结果显示，H/R 可明显诱导 GRP78 和 CRT 蛋白的表达，较对照组分别升高 142.0% 和 312.0%（$P < 0.05$）；PQS 可抑制 H/R 诱导的 GRP78 和 CRT 蛋白表达，较 H/R 组分别降低 37.7% 和 52.2%（$P < 0.05$），见图3。

2.2.2　CHOP mRNA 和蛋白表达的变化　RT-PCR 的结果显示，H/R 可明显诱导心肌细胞 CHOP mRNA 的表达，较对照组高 311.0%（$P < 0.05$）；PQS 可抑制 H/R 后的 CHOP mRNA 的表达，PQS+H/R 组心肌细胞 CHOP mRNA 表达较 H/R 心肌细胞降低 57.0%（$P < 0.05$）；Western blotting 结果显示，H/R 可明显诱导 CHOP 蛋白表达，较对照组升高 219.0%（$P < 0.05$）；PQS 抑制 H/R 后的 CHOP 蛋白的表达，PQS+H/R 组心肌细胞 CHOP 蛋白表达较 H/R 组降低 51.7%（$P < 0.05$），见图4A、B。

2.2.3　Capase-12 蛋白表达的变化　采用可同时识别 caspase-12 酶原（pro-caspase-12，分子量 48～50kD）和剪切后的 caspase-12（cleaved caspase-12，分子量 36kD）的特异性抗体，进行免疫印迹检测，结果显示 H/R 可明显诱导 caspase-12 蛋白剪切活化，较对照组升高 180.0%（$P < 0.05$）；PQS 抑制 H/R 后 caspase-12 蛋白活化，以 160mg/L PQS 培养液培养 24h，剪切后 caspase-12 蛋白表达较 H/R 心肌细胞降低 34.9%（$P < 0.05$），见图4C、D。

2.3　CHOP 蛋白表达与凋亡调节因子 Bcl-2、Bax 蛋白表达的相关性分析

相关性分析显示，ERS 凋亡分子 CHOP 蛋白表达与促凋亡因子 Bax 蛋白表达显著正相关（$r = 0.956$，$P < 0.05$），与抗凋亡因子 Bcl-2 蛋白表达显著负相关（$r = -0.967$，$P < 0.05$）。

3. 讨论

缺血再灌注（ischemia/reperfusion，I/R）损伤指缺血一定时间的心肌恢复灌流后，组织损伤反而进行性加重，心肌细胞从可逆损伤转变为不

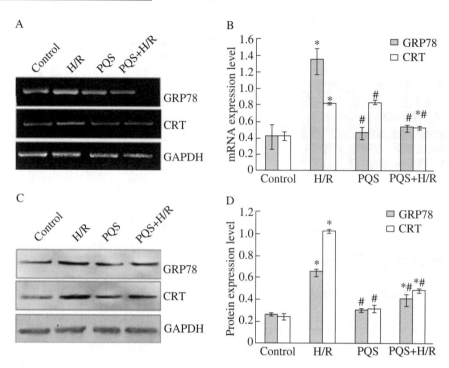

图3　PQS 对 H/R 心肌细胞 GRP78、CRT 表达的影响

A：The levels of GRP78 and CRT mRNA were examined by RT-PCR．GAPDH was used as a normalization control．**B**：bar chart of densitometry of the bands shown in A．**C**：The levels of GRP78 and CRT protein were examined by Western blotting．GAPDH was used as a normalization control．**D**：Bar chart of densitometry of the bands shown in C．$\bar{x}\pm s$．n=3．*$P < 0.05$ vs control；#$P < 0.05$ vs H/R

可逆损伤的现象。心肌细胞坏死和凋亡是心肌 I/R 损伤的特征之一[11]。Musat-Marcu 等[12] 在离体灌流大鼠心脏上发现，再灌注早期即可发生心肌细胞凋亡。其中抗凋亡蛋白 Bcl-2 与促凋亡蛋白 Bax 参与了心肌 I/R 损伤中细胞凋亡的调控[13]。本研究利用乳鼠心肌细胞 H/R 模型，采用 LDH 活性检测法、台盼蓝排斥实验、流式细胞术以及 RT-PCR 和 Western blotting 方法，证实 PQS 能明显减轻 H/R 诱导的心肌细胞损伤和凋亡。H/R 前以 160mg/L PQS 培养液培养细胞 24h，与 H/R 心肌细胞相比，细胞凋亡率、LDH 活性以及促凋亡蛋白 Bax mRNA 和蛋白的表达均明显降低，而细胞存活率及抗凋亡蛋白 Bcl-2 mRNA 和蛋白的表达显著升高。

I/R 发生的主要环节是氧自由基产生和钙超载，其机制尚未完全阐明，ER 是调节 Ca^{2+} 和蛋白质合成的重要场所，因此 ER 理化环境改变和 ER 过负荷等因素导致的 ERS 在 I/R 损伤的发生发展中具有重要意义[14-15]。ERS 是细胞对刺激的适应性反应，一定程度的 ERS 诱导 GRP78、CRT 等内质网伴侣分子表达上调[16]，增强 ER 处理未折叠蛋白的

能力，促进 ER 功能恢复。但 H/R 触发的严重 ERS 可显著增加 GRP78 和 CRT 的蛋白表达[17-18]，诱导 CHOP、caspase-12 等促凋亡因子的表达及活化，触发 ERS 相关凋亡途径，诱导细胞凋亡和组织损伤[19-20]。本研究发现 H/R 前以 160mg/L 的 PQS 培养液培养心肌细胞 24h，可显著抑制 H/R 诱导的 GRP78、CRT mRNA 和蛋白表达，提示 PQS 可能通过减轻 H/R 诱导的严重 ERS 触发的细胞凋亡，起到心肌保护作用；CHOP 通过直接调节核内靶基因，增加细胞对 ERS 介导凋亡的敏感性，促进细胞凋亡[21]。CHOP 介导的凋亡信号通路与线粒体凋亡途径有密切联系，CHOP 可通过下调 Bcl-2 蛋白表达而促进细胞凋亡，并导致 Bax 从胞浆内向线粒体内易位[22]。本研究发现，H/R 前以 160mg/L 的 PQS 培养液培养心肌细胞 24h，可显著抑制 H/R 诱导的 CHOP mRNA 和蛋白表达；在此基础上对 CHOP 蛋白表达与凋亡调节因子 Bcl-2、Bax 蛋白表达之间进行相关分析，发现 CHOP 蛋白表达与 Bax 蛋白表达呈正相关，与 Bcl-2 蛋白表达呈负相关，提示 CHOP 介导的凋亡信号通路可能通过抑制 Bcl-2 和促进 Bax 蛋

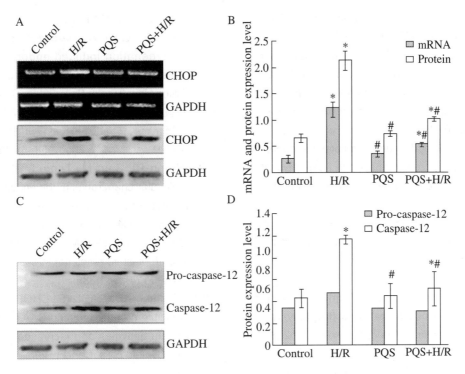

图 4　PQS 对 H/R 心肌细胞后 CHOP 表达的影响

A：The levels of CHOP mRNA and protein were examined by RT-PCR and Western blotting. GAPDH was used as a normalization control. B：Bar chart of densitometry of the bands shown in A. C：Western blotting analysis of caspase-12 activation in cardiomyocytes. GAPDH was used as a normalization control. D：Bar chart of densitometry of the bands shown in C. $\bar{\chi} \pm s$. n=3. $^*P < 0.05$ *vs* control；$^\#P < 0.05$ *vs* H/R

白表达，引起细胞凋亡，与以往文献报道一致 [23-24]，由此推测 PQS 可能通过抑制过度 ERS 介导的细胞凋亡起到心肌保护作用；caspase-12 是内质网膜上的组成性蛋白，以无活性酶原形式存在于 ER 膜胞浆侧，在 ERS 时被剪切激活，cleaved caspase-12 通过激活 caspase-9、caspase-3 引起细胞凋亡 [25]，因而 caspase-12 被认为是内质网凋亡信号通路的关键分子。本研究发现，H/R 明显诱导心肌细胞 cleaved caspase-12 蛋白表达并引起细胞凋亡，与以往文献报道一致 [26]。H/R 前以 160mg/L PQS 培养液培养 24h，可显著抑制 H/R 诱导的 cleaved caspase-12 的蛋白表达，提示 PQS 可能通过抑制 caspase-12 介导的内质网相关凋亡发挥心肌保护作用。

综上所述，我们认为 PQS 通过抑制过度 ERS 发挥抗心肌细胞 H/R 损伤作用，表现为降低 H/R 诱导的 GRP78、CRT mRNA 和蛋白表达，抑制 CHOP、caspase-12 等内质网凋亡通路激活。但 PQS 对在体大鼠心肌缺血 / 再灌注损伤的心肌保

护作用尚待进一步研究。

参考文献

[1] 曹霞，谷欣权，陈燕萍，等. 西洋参茎叶三醇组皂苷对缺血再灌注损伤心肌的保护作用. 中国老年学杂志，2004，24（7）：654-655.

[2] 殷惠军，张颖，蒋跃绒，等. 西洋参叶总皂苷对急性心肌梗死大鼠心肌细胞凋亡及凋亡相关基因表达的影响. 中国中西医结合杂志，2005，25（3）：232-235.

[3] 关利新，衣欣，杨世杰，等. 西洋参茎叶皂苷对大鼠心肌细胞 Ca^{2+} 内流的影响. 中国药理与临床，2004，20（6）：8-9.

[4] 鞠传静，张志国，赵学忠，等. 西洋参叶二醇组皂苷对大鼠实验性心室重构的保护作用. 中国老年学杂志，2007，27（22）：2173-2175.

[5] Boya P, Cohen I, Zarnzarni N, et al. Endoplasmic reticulum stress induced cell death requires mitochondrial membrane permeabilization. Cell Death Differ, 2002, 9 (4): 465-467.

[6] Breckenridge DG, Germain M, Mathai JP, et al.

Regulation of apoptosis by endoplasmic reticulum pathways. Oncogene, 2003, 22 (53): 8608-8618.

[7] Simpson P, Savion S. Differentiation of rat myocytes in single cell cultures with and without proliferating nonmyocardial cells. Cross-striations, ultrastructure, and chronotropic response to isoproterenol. Circ Res, 1982, 50 (1): 101-116.

[8] Li YZ, Liu XH, Rong F. Puma mediates the apoptotic signal of hypoxia/ reoxygenation in cardiomyocytes through mitochondrial pathway. Shock, 2011, 35 (6): 579- 584.

[9] Rabkin SW, Kong JY. Nitroprusside induces cardiomyocyte death: interaction with hydrogen peroxide. Am J Physiol Heart Circ Physiol, 2000, 279 (6): H3089-H3100.

[10] Liu X, Wu X, Han Y, et al. Signal pathway of cardioprotection induced by monophosphoryl lipid A in rabbit myocardium. Pathophysiology, 2002, 8 (3): 193-196.

[11] Fliss H, Gattinger D. Apoptosis in ischemic and reperfused rat myocardium. Circ Res, 1996, 79 (5): 949-956.

[12] Musat-Marcu S, Gunter HE, Jugdutt BI, et al. Inhibition of apoptosis after ischemia-reperfusion in rat myocardium by cycloheximide. J Mol Cell Cardiol, 1999, 31 (5): 1073- 1082.

[13] Borutaite V, Brown GC. Mitochondria in apoptosis of ischemic heart. FEBS Lett, 2003, 541 (1-3): 1-5.

[14] Shihata M, Hattori H, Sasaki T, et al. Activation of caspase-12 by endoplasmic reticulum stress induced by transient middle cerebral artery occlusion in mice. Neuroscience, 2003, 118 (2): 491-499.

[15] Vilatoba M, Eckstein C, Bilbao G, et al. Sodium 4-phenylbutyrate protects against liver ischemia reperfusion injury by inhibition of endoplasmic reticulum stress-mediated apoptosis. Surgery, 2005, 138 (2): 342-351.

[16] Kaufman RJ. Stress signaling from the lumen of the endoplasmic reticolum: coordination of gene transcriptional and translational controls. Gene, 1999, 13 (10): 1211-1233.

[17] Ma QB, Gao W, Guo YH, et al. Hypoxia/ reoxygenation induced endoplasmic reticulum stress in cultured neonatal rat cardiomyocyte. J Pwing Univ (Health Sci) , 2005, 37 (4): 386-388.

[18] 祝筱梅, 刘秀华, 蔡莉蓉, 等. P38 丝裂素活化蛋白激酶介导低氧预处理诱导的内质网应激相关的心肌细胞保护. 生理学报, 2006, 58 (5): 463-470.

[19] Zhang PL, Lun M, Teng J, et al. Preinduced molecular chaperones in the endoplasmic reticulum protect cardiomyocytes from lethal injury. Ann Clin Lab Sci, 2004, 34 (4): 449- 457.

[20] Oyadomari S, Mori M. Roles of CHOP/GADD153 in endoplasmic reticulum stress. Cell Death Differ, 2004, 11 (4): 381-389.

[21] Friedman AD. GADD153/CHOP, a DNA damage-inducible protein, reduced CAAT/enhancer binding protein activities and increased apoptosis in 32D c13 myeloid cells. Cancer Res, 1996, 56 (14): 3250-3256.

[22] McCullough KD, Martindale JL, Klotz LO, et al. Gadd153 sensitizes cells to endoplasrnic reticulum stress by down-regulating Bcl- 2 and perturbing the cellular redox state. Mol Cell Biol, 2001, 21 (4): 1249-1259.

[23] Nieto-Miguel T, Fonteriz RI, Vay L, et al. Endo-plasmic reticulum stress in the proapoptotic action of edelfosine in solid tumor cells. Cancer Res, 2007, 67 (21): 10368- 10378.

[24] Gotoh T, Terada K, Oyadomari S, et al. hsp70-DnaJ chaperone pair prevents nitric oxide-and CHOP -induced apoptosis by inhibiting translocation of Bax to mitochondria. Cell Death Differ, 2004, 11 (4): 390-402.

[25] Nakagawa T, Zhu H, Morishirna N, et al. Caspase-12 mediates endoplasmic-reticulum-specific apoptosis and cytotoxicity by amyloid-β. Nature, 2000, 403 (6765): 98- 103.

[26] 祝筱梅, 刘秀华, 蔡莉蓉. 缺氧后处理对缺氧/复氧心肌细胞的保护作用及其机理研究. 中国微循环, 2007, 11 (4): 223-230.

第四章

丹参、红花水溶性组分及配伍对大鼠心肌缺血/再灌注损伤作用的实验研究 *

刘剑刚 张大武 李 婕 丰加涛 杨小平 史大卓 梁鑫淼

中药的药对配伍是中药复方的核心，也是中药研究中最简单的形式。丹参和红花是传统活血化瘀药中应用最早且药理作用最为广泛的药对之一，丹参和红花提取物配伍在临床上得到广泛应用并取得了较好的疗效，尤其在治疗心肌缺血疾病方面有显著治疗作用 [1]。丹参为唇形科鼠尾草属植物丹参（*Salvia miltiorrhiza* Bunge）的干燥根及根茎，其主要水溶性有效成分包括丹参素、原儿茶醛和丹酚酸类成分，其中含量最高的 2 个成分丹酚酸 A（Sal A）和丹酚酸 B（Sal B）活性最强。近年的药理研究表明，丹酚酸在抗氧化应激损伤、抗动脉粥样硬化及心肌缺血等方面具有显著活性 [2-3]。红花为菊科植物红花（*Carthamus tinctorius* L.）的筒管状花冠，红花的化学成分主要为黄酮和脂肪油两大类，其中查耳酮类化合物红花黄色素（safflor yellow，SY）为红花的主要有效成分，是含有多种成分的水溶性混合物，其中羟基红花黄色素 A（hydroxysafflor yellow A，HSYA）为红花黄色素中含量较高的成分，具有扩张冠状动脉、改善心肌缺血、减少 AMI 范围的作用 [4-5]。

丹参和红花 2 味药物水溶性组分是复杂的水溶性混合物，其水溶性部位化学成分的研究有一定难度且化学成分不稳定，因此基于定量指纹图谱技术对丹参、红花进行定性、定量化学质量控制，对其水溶性的多个目标成分尤其是有效成分进行准确定量，提高其生药含量，并使得 2 味中药所对应的化学组成更加清晰和稳定性可靠 [6]。本实验研究将丹参、红花水溶性有效组分（丹酚酸 B 和羟基红花黄色素 A）含量提高后进行配伍，观察其对大鼠实验性心肌缺血/再灌注损伤（ischemia-reperfusion injury，IRI）的作用。

1. 材料

1.1 动物

SD 大鼠 70 只，体重 180～200g，雌雄各半，清洁级，动物许可证号 SCXK（京）2007-0001，由北京维通利华实验动物技术有限公司提供。清洁级动物房饲养，定时给予全价营养饲料喂食，室温 22～25℃，湿度 50%～70%。

1.2 药物与试剂

丹参水溶性组分注射液（丹酚酸 B 49g/L，约相当于生药 104g/mL），红花水溶性组分注射液（羟基红花黄色素 A 31.76g/L，约相当于生药 80.87g/mL），丹参红花水溶性组分配伍注射液（丹酚酸 B 34.3g/L，羟基红花黄色素 A 22.21g/L）由中国科学院大连化学物理研究所提供；丹红注射液（原儿茶醛 0.05g/L，约相当于生药 1g/mL），由山东济南步长制药有限公司生产，批号 060904。肌钙蛋白 T（cardiac troponin T，cTnT）试剂盒由美国 Rapid Bio Lab 公司生产，由北京莱博特利生物医学科技公司提供，批号 08060502；肌酸激酶同工酶（CK-MB）试剂盒，由北京中生北控生物科技股份有限公司提供，批号 070181；硝基四氮唑蓝（NBT），由上海前进试剂厂生产，批号 060509。血栓素（TXB_2）和 6-酮-前列腺素 $F_{1\alpha}$（6-keto-$PGF_{1\alpha}$）放射免疫试剂盒，由北京普尔伟业生物技术有限公司提供，批号 20070607；二磷酸腺苷（adenosine diphosphate，ADP），由美国 CHRONO-LOG 公司生产，北京现代威士达医疗器械有限公司提供，批号 3368，浓度 0.2mmol/L。

1.3 仪器

SC-3 人工呼吸机（上海医疗设备厂）；ECG-6511 心电图机（上海光电仪器有限公司）；RX-2000 全自动生化仪（美国 Technicon 公司）；LBY-NJ2 血小板聚集仪（北京普利生公司）；SN-682 放射免疫γ计数仪（上海核辐射仪器有限公司）。

2. 方法

2.1 动物模型制作

20% 氨基甲基乙酯（乌拉坦）腹腔注射麻醉

* 原载于《中国中药杂志》，2011，36（2）：189-194

（0.7mL/kg），将大鼠固定在专用木板上，气管插管，人工呼吸（潮气量为20mL/kg，呼吸频率为50次/分钟）吸入室内空气，开胸，剪开心包膜，轻轻挤压大鼠胸腔右侧壁，将心脏挤出。在左心耳下缘，肺动脉圆锥左缘与左心耳之间进针，以冠状静脉主干为标志，左心耳下方2～3mm处用丝线结扎（垫1个半圆形硅胶管）冠状动脉前降支，造成大鼠心肌缺血。心电监护显示结扎冠状动脉成功（持续2min）后10min经股静脉注射给药。假手术组只穿线不结扎，注射等剂量生理盐水；模型组结扎后，给予等剂量生理盐水。实验过程中动物处置方法符合动物伦理学要求标准。

2.2 动物分组

实验分为假手术（空白对照）组：只穿刺不结扎，注射等量生理盐水；模型组：注射等剂量生理盐水；阳性药物对照：丹红注射液，给药剂量为0.36mL/kg，约合生药1.8g/kg；丹参水溶性有效组分组：给药量为0.30mL/kg，约合生药30.68g/kg；红花水溶性有效组分组：给药量为0.22mL/kg，约合生药17.87g/kg；丹参红花水溶性有效组分配伍（按生药量3:1配制）低剂量组：给药量0.42mL/kg，约合生药24.28g/kg；丹参红花水溶性有效组分配伍高剂量组：给药量0.82mL/kg，约合生药48.56g/kg。所有注射药液均用生理盐水稀释，按10mL/kg给予动物注射。

2.3 标本采集

大鼠造模缺血后40min，剪断丝线再灌注120min。记录结扎前、结扎后10min、40min及剪开丝线后（再灌注）30min、60min、120min Ⅱ导心电图。观察120min后，腹主动脉取血，一部分放入3.8%枸橼酸钠溶液1:9抗凝真空管和异山梨酯（消心痛）+2% EDTANa$_2$溶液抗凝管后离心，测定血小板聚集性和TXB$_2$，6-keto-PGF$_{\alpha 1}$含

量。另一部分不抗凝，放入真空管后离心测定血清cTnT、CK-MB含量。然后，取出心脏，生理盐水冲洗，称量全心重，在心脏结扎线以下，平行于冠状沟均匀地将左心室部分横断切成5片，置于NBT溶液37℃染色15min。用Delta Pix（丹麦）图像分析系统测量每片心肌面积、心室面积和梗死区面积，然后求出梗死区占心室和全心区面积的百分比。

2.4 指标检测方法

放射免疫法测定TXB$_2$、6-keto-PGF$_{\alpha 1}$；全自动生化仪电化学发光法和速率法测定测定cTnT、CK-MB；比浊法测定血小板聚集率，诱导剂为ADP，浓度为0.2mmol/L，取其1、3、5min及最大聚集率。

2.5 统计学方法

所有数据用 $\bar{\chi} \pm s$ 表示，组间比较为单因素方差分析，组间比较采用LSD方法，$P < 0.05$ 为差异有统计学意义，采用SPSS 12.0软件包进行统计学处理。

3. 结果

3.1 丹参、红花组分及配伍对大鼠MI面积和I/R损伤后CK-MB和cTnT的影响

大鼠心肌I/R损伤后，血清CK-MB活性明显升高，和假手术组比较有显著差异（$P < 0.01$）。模型组cTnT水平亦有一定升高，但与假手术组比较无显著差异，穿刺对心肌组织也是一种损伤。与模型组比较，丹参组分、红花组分、丹参红花组分低、高剂量组均能显著降低动物血清CK-MB水平和cTnT含量（$P < 0.01$）。与模型组比较，丹红注射液、丹参组分、红花组分、丹参红花组分低、高剂量组的心肌梗死面积分别下降了14.28%、31.96%、21.45%、25.98%、39.82%，梗死面积下降百分比=（模型组心肌梗死面积－药物组心肌

表1 丹参、红花组分及配伍对大鼠MI面积和I/R损伤后CK-MB和cTnT的影响（$\bar{\chi} \pm s$，n=10）

组别	剂量（g/kg）	心肌梗死面积（%）	cTnT（mg/L）	CK-MB（U/L）
假手术	–	–	0.97 ± 0.17	437.17 ± 154.82 [2)]
模型	–	29.13 ± 3.18	1.04 ± 0.14	1268.17 ± 256.50
丹红注射液	1.80	24.97 ± 5.94 [1)]	0.63 ± 0.14 [2)]	386.39 ± 107.71 [2) 3)]
丹参水溶性组分	30.68	19.85 ± 6.74 [2)]	0.53 ± 0.18 [2)]	904.18 ± 156.44 [1)]
红花水溶性组分	17.87	22.88 ± 3.24 [1)]	0.64 ± 0.15 [2)]	805.65 ± 118.94 [1)]
丹参红花组分配伍	27.48	21.56 ± 2.08 [2)]	0.74 ± 0.14 [2)]	762.92 ± 118.55 [2)]
	54.96	17.53 ± 7.65 [2)]	0.62 ± 0.18 [2)]	385.32 ± 117.05 [2) 3)]

注：与模型组比较 [1)] $P < 0.05$，[2)] $P < 0.01$；与假手术组比较 [3)] $P < 0.01$

梗死面积）/ 模型组心肌梗死面积 × 100%，见表 1。

3.2 丹参、红花组分及配伍对大鼠心肌 I/R 损伤 Ⅱ 导心电图 ST-T 改变的影响

结扎动物冠状动脉后，各组大鼠 Ⅱ 导心电图 ST-T 皆有一定的升高。剪开丝线后 30min 时，丹红注射液组、丹参组分、丹参红花组分配伍低、高剂量组 ST-T 升高幅度有一定的降低，和模型组比较有显著差异（$P < 0.05$），120min 时，还有同样的效果，见表 2。

3.3 丹参、红花组分及配伍对大鼠心肌 I/R 损伤后血小板聚集性、6-keto-PGF$_{1\alpha}$ 和 TXB$_2$ 的影响

大鼠再灌流 120min 后取血测定血小板聚集性，与模型组比较，丹参组分及其配伍高、低剂量均能显著降低血小板最大聚集率（$P < 0.01$，$P < 0.05$）。心肌缺血 / 再灌注损伤后模型组大鼠血浆 6-keto-PGF$_{1\alpha}$ 含量下降，但和假手术组比较无显著差异。丹参红花组分配伍高、低剂量能明显升高 6-keto-PGF$_{1\alpha}$ 含量，和模型组比较有显著差异（$P < 0.05$），升高幅度和丹红注射液比较有显著差异（$P < 0.01$）。丹红注射液、丹参组分和丹参

红花组分配伍大剂量组能降低 TXB$_2$ 含量，和模型组比较有显著差异（$P < 0.01$），见表 3。

4. 讨论

虽然早期、及时再灌注心脏是防止心肌组织缺血造成进一步损害的有效方法，但缺血组织恢复血流灌注时，往往导致再灌注区域心肌细胞及局部血管网显著的病理变化，而这些改变的共同作用可导致进一步的组织损伤即缺血再灌注损伤（ischemic-reperfusion injury，IRI）。临床上所见的心肌无复流、心肌顿抑、再灌注心律失常、心肌组织坏死和微血管功能障碍相关现象均证实了血管开通后 I/R 损伤的存在。再灌注损伤导致不可逆转的组织损伤和细胞坏死是心肌缺血引发的直接结果[7]。再灌注损伤的基本病理生理学机制尚未完全阐明，影响其发病机制涉及自由基损伤、钙超载、细胞损伤、血小板等方面，应用氧自由基清除剂、抗血小板聚集剂、抑制炎症反应等是潜在的药理学治疗靶标，同时补充能量腺苷等药物

表 2　丹参、红花组分及配伍对大鼠心肌 I/R 损伤 Ⅱ 导心电图 ST-T 改变的影响（单位：mV）（$\bar{x} \pm s$，n=10）

组别	剂量（g/kg）	结扎前	结扎冠状动脉后		剪开结扎线后		
			10min	40min	30min	60min	120min
假手术	—	0.16±0.04	0.22±0.10	0.20±0.09[1]	0.28±0.13	0.20±0.08	0.18±0.09
模型	—	0.20±0.01	0.25±0.10	0.34±0.05	0.36±0.06	0.34±0.05	0.30±0.05
丹红注射液	1.80	0.16±0.03	0.27±0.13	0.31±0.05	0.20±0.09[1]	0.24±0.10[1]	0.21±0.07[1]
丹参水溶性组分	30.68	0.18±0.06	0.32±0.11	0.30±0.16	0.24±0.16[1]	0.22±0.14[1]	0.14±0.02[1]
红花水溶性组分	17.87	0.17±0.07	0.30±0.17	0.39±0.14	0.41±0.14	0.41±0.14	0.37±0.23
丹参红花组分配伍	27.48	0.18±0.09	0.23±0.13	0.28±0.13	0.25±0.09[1]	0.25±0.13	0.20±0.04[1]
	54.96	0.18±0.04	0.24±0.11	0.27±0.14	0.24±0.12[1]	0.22±0.07[1]	0.19±0.06[2]

注：与模型组比较 [1] $P < 0.05$，[2] $P < 0.01$

表 3　丹参、红花组分及配伍对大鼠心肌 I/R 损伤后血小板聚集性、6-keto-PGF$_{1\alpha}$ 和 TXB$_2$ 的影响（$\bar{x} \pm s$，n=10）

组别	药物剂量（g/kg）	血小板最大聚集率（%）	6-keto-PGF$_{1\alpha}$（ng/L）	TXB$_2$（ng/L）	6-keto-PGF$_{1\alpha}$/TXB$_2$
假手术	—	64.65±16.11	159.43±43.93	147.90±30.58	1.09±0.24
模型	—	77.32±14.96	142.16±22.25	203.90±43.38	0.80±0.24
丹红注射液	1.80	40.78±5.11[2]	137.87±42.62	120.65±20.89[2]	1.43±0.54[1]
丹参水溶性组分	30.68	49.37±9.96[1]	187.22±32.08	103.75±24.06	1.79±0.61[2]
红花水溶性组分	17.87	61.00±14.79	153.67±40.54	230.23±38.71	0.75±0.29
丹参红花组分配伍	27.48	53.95±9.91[1]	213.65±32.22[2]	184.69±42.66	1.76±0.43[2]
	54.96	44.12±12.96[2]	279.40±43.61[2][4]	85.26±8.46[2][3]	2.54±0.36[2][4]

注：与模型组比较 [1] $P < 0.05$，[2] $P < 0.01$；与假手术组比较 [3] $P < 0.05$，[4] $P < 0.01$

能明显减轻组织的再灌注损伤。临床研究表明中药可通过多层次、多靶点抑制组织氧化反应、炎症细胞浸润、抗血小板聚集等多种途径干预心肌I/R，以保护再灌注损伤的心脏，而发挥独特作用的优势[8]。缺血损伤心肌导致心肌细胞膜通透性改变，细胞内 CK-MD 漏出增加，检测血清 CK-MD 活性是临床常用的生化指标之一。心肌酶谱诊断急性心肌梗死（AMI）的敏感性与发病时间长短有关。临床研究表明 AMI 患者的 CK-MB 在 2～4h 内升高，24h 达到峰值[9]。实验造成大鼠急性再灌注损伤后，其血清 CK-MB 活性明显升高，2h 后取血测定，虽然没有达到峰值，但较假手术组上升了 65.52%，而心肌特异性的 cTnT 是心肌损伤的敏感生化指标。假手术组大鼠 cTnT 因穿刺心肌组织造成损伤而升高，并早于 CK-MB（假手术组大鼠 CK-MB 略高于正常值），cTnT 阴性基本可以排除 AMI，其特异性和时间窗优于 CK-MB[10]。PGI_2/TXA_2 失衡是加剧缺血心肌损伤的重要原因，PGI_2 能抑制血小板聚集，增强一氧化氮的释放而舒张血管，保护心肌组织。TXA_2 则促进血小板聚集，收缩血管，加重缺血组织损伤。心肌再灌注损伤后导致 PGI_2/TXA_2 平衡失调，激活中性粒细胞释放炎症因子，导致再灌注损伤发生。

IRI 是缺血损伤的延续，在缺血期及早使用药物干预，可以减轻心肌细胞的缺血性损伤，增强心肌细胞对 IRI 的抵抗能力。结扎冠状动脉造成大鼠心肌再灌注损伤，120min 时假手术组和模型组大鼠的 cTnT 含量增高明显，模型组 CK-MB 活性比假手术组升高显著（$P < 0.01$）。各给药组均能显著降低大鼠 cTnT 水平（$P < 0.01$）。对 CK-MB 活性，各给药组亦有不同程度的降低作用（$P < 0.05$，$P < 0.01$）。而丹参红花组分配伍在减少大鼠心肌梗死面积较丹红注射液提高了 45.03%，显示了丹参、红花的有效组分含量提高后的配伍优势。实验首先从模型组开始，因手法原因导致模型组结扎前的 ST 幅度增高，和其他组比较尚无统计学差异。丹参红花组分配伍高、低剂量组可明显降低大鼠心电图 ST-T 升高的幅度，改善心肌缺血程度，一直持续到 120min，和模型组比较差异显著。实验研究发现，手术穿刺对大鼠的心肌也造成一定的应激和损伤，模型组的血小板聚集和 TXB_2 指标明显升高，但和假手术组比较无显著差异。丹参红花组分能降低 TXB_2 含量，升高 6-keto-$PGF_{1\alpha}$ 含量，同时纠正 PGI_2/TXA_2 平衡失调。丹参红花

组分对机体的血小板聚集性作用最为显著，丹参组分亦有明显降低血小板聚集性的作用。实验结果表明，丹参、红花侧重面亦有所不同，其配伍显示了疗效的优势，显著抑制血栓烷的生成，防治血栓的形成和改善心肌微循环及心肌缺血状态。

人们对丹参和红花的水溶性成分研究较晚但发展迅速，先后分离得到了一系列水溶性化合物，并得到广泛的应用。丹酚酸是从丹参中提取的一类既有咖啡酰缩酚酸结构又有新木脂素骨架的水溶性成分[11]。现代药理研究表明，丹参水溶性提取物具有增强冠状动脉血流量、抗脂质过氧化、抑制血栓形成及抗血栓、改善微循环等作用[12]。红花在我国仅有一种，红花有效部位的药理研究主要集中在查尔酮类化合物 SY。SY 是一种复杂的水溶性混合物，而 HYSA 是 SY 中的主要成分。现代研究表明，红花水溶性提取物具有抗心肌缺血、抑制血小板聚集、抗氧化、改善神经系统障碍等作用[13]。

传统中药多采用水煎剂型，其化学成分含有大量的强极性组分，这些强极性组分的物质基础及药理药效的研究是新的中药研究领域[14]。采用中药指纹图谱技术与多指标成分定量分析相结合的中药质量控制模式，将丹参定量组分中的水溶性有效组分原儿茶醛、迷迭香酸、丹酚酸 B 成分含量提高，使其成分的含量总和大于 50%，且质量标准得到有效的控制。而红花应用亲水色谱分离模式、新型色谱固定相和二维液相色谱分离系统等联用技术，对强极性、水溶性物质进行分离和质量控制，解决强极性物质和高效分离等难点问题，使红花的水溶性成分得以有效控制[15]。当然作为注射剂而言，两者配伍后其澄清度、稳定性还有待提高。丹参和红花是传统活血化瘀药物，配伍的临床疗效明确。应用活性导向的中药标准组分物质基础研究模式将丹参红花水溶性有效组分含量提高后，结果表明其可以抗心肌缺血、抑制血小板聚集及血栓形成，具有防止和减轻再灌注后心肌损伤的作用。

参考文献

[1] 李艳丽，孟智宏. 丹红注射液治疗急性冠脉综合征 48 例. 实用中医内科杂志，2008，22（3）：22.

[2] Wang SB, Tian S, Yang F, et al. Cardioprotective effect of salvianolic acid A on isoproterenol-induced myocardial infarction in rats. Eur J Pharmacol, 2009, 615 (1/3): 125.

[3] 柳丽，张洪泉. 丹参活性成分的现代中药药理研究进展. 中国野生植物资源，2003，22（6）：3.

[4] Ye SY, Gao WY. Hydroxysafflor yellow A protects neuron against hypoxia injury and suppresses inflammatory responses following focal ischemia reperfusion in rats. Arch Pharm Res, 2008, 31 (8):1010.

[5] 李中原，涂秀华. 红花黄色素的药理研究进展. 中药新药与临床药理，2005，16（2）：153.

[6] 刘艳芳，刘艳明，董军，等. 中药物质基础的高效液相色谱分离分析方法研究. 中国科学，B辑：化学，2009，39（8）：678.

[7] Park JL, Lucchesi BR. Mechanisms of myocardial reperfusion injury. Ann Thorac Surg, 1999, 68 (5): 1905.

[8] 黄烨，王宗仁. 中药干预心肌缺血/再灌注炎症反应的研究进展. 心脏杂志，2009，21（4）：592.

[9] 朱妙章，袁文俊，吴博威，等. 心血管生理学与临床.

北京：高等教育出版社，2004：293.

[10] 章华础，萧祥熊. 心肌肌钙蛋白检测的临床评价. 放射免疫学杂志，2002，15（4）：193.

[11] 徐德然，王康才，王峥涛，等. 丹参中丹参素、原儿茶醛来源的初步研究. 中国天然药物，2005，3（3）：147.

[12] Wang SB, Tian S, Yang F, et al. Effects of salvianolic acids on oxidative stress and hepatic fibrosis in rats. Toxicol Appl Pharmacol, 2010, 242 (2):155.

[13] Sai MK, Lin YL, Huang YT. Cardioprotective effect of salvianolic acid A on isoproterenol-induced myocardial infarction in rats. T Eur J Pharmacol, 2009, 615 (1/3):125.

[14] 王艳萍，丰加涛，金郁，等. 中药物质基础研究的思路与方法. 中国天然药物，2009，7（1）：13.

[15] 丰加涛，金郁，王金成，等. 基于定量指纹图谱技术的中药质量控制. 色谱，2008，26（2）：180.

益气活血中药联合缺血后适应保护缺血/再灌注大鼠心肌的机制研究 *

张大武　张　蕾　刘剑刚　王承龙　史大卓　陈可冀

　　益气活血是目前中医治疗急性心肌梗死（acute myocardial infarction，AMI）的主要治法。20世纪70年代，中国中医科学院西苑医院联合北京4家医院在西医常规治疗的基础上采用益气活血法治疗AMI，证明具有降低住院死亡率和减少并发症发生率的作用[1]。近年来研究[2,3]表明，益气活血中药治疗心肌梗死后再灌注损伤有促进缺血心肌血管新生、抑制炎症反应、改善AMI后心肌缺血和能量代谢，对心肌缺血再灌注（ischemic reperfusion，I/R）损伤的多个病理环节有调控作用。

　　缺血后适应（ischemic postconditioning，IPoC）由Zhao等[4]在2003年提出，在恢复组织血流灌注前给予反复几次短暂的再灌注/缺血循环，可明显减轻再灌注损伤导致的心肌组织损伤和功能障碍；随后的实验和小样本临床研究[5,6]皆证明IPoC能减少心肌梗死面积，改善AMI早期再灌

治疗患者的心脏功能。益气活血中药能否增加后适应对I/R损伤心肌的保护作用，目前尚无研究报道。本研究采用益气中药心悦胶囊（西洋参茎叶总皂苷）和活血化瘀中药芎芍胶囊（川芎总酚和赤芍总苷）体现益气活血的效用，进行益气活血中药联合缺血后适应保护缺血/再灌注大鼠心肌的疗效观察和机制研究。

1. 材料与方法

1.1 实验动物

　　SD大鼠，清洁级，75只，雌雄兼用，体重180～200 g，由北京维通利华实验动物技术有限公司提供，动物许可证号为SCXK（京）2007-0001。适应性饲养3d后进行实验。动物自由摄水，室温控制23～25 ℃，湿度为50%～70%，光照12h，黑暗12h。

* 原载于《中西医结合学报》，2010，8（5）：465-471

1.2 药物和试剂

芎芍胶囊，由川芎、赤芍的有效部位川芎总酚和赤芍总苷组成，每粒胶囊0.25g，每克药粉约合生药30g，由北京国际生物制品研究所提供，批号为200094；心悦胶囊，每粒0.3g，主要成分是西洋参茎叶总皂苷（每粒50mg），由吉林省集安益盛药业股份有限公司生产，批号为国药准字Z20030073；福辛普利钠（fosinopril sodium）每粒10mg，批号0804087，由中美上海施贵宝制药有限公司生产。心肌肌钙蛋白T（cardiac troponin T，cTnT）试剂盒，由美国RapidBio Lab公司生产，批号08060502。肌酸激酶同工酶MB（creatine kinase-MB，CK-MB）试剂盒，由北京中生北控生物科技股份有限公司提供，批号为070181；白细胞介素1β（interleukin-1，IL-1β）、白细胞介素6（interleukin-6，IL-6）酶联免疫吸附测定（enzyme-linked immunosorbant assay，ELISA）试剂盒，由美国RD公司生产；考马斯亮蓝蛋白测定试剂盒，由南京建成科技有限公司生产，批号为090828；氯化硝基四氮唑蓝（nitroblue tetrazolium chloride，NBT），由美国R&D（R&D systems）公司生产。Toll样受体2（Toll-like receptor 2，TLR2）抗体试剂盒，Toll样受体4（Toll-like receptor 4，TLR4）抗体试剂盒，由北京博奥森生物技术有限公司提供。浓缩型二氨基联苯胺试剂盒和免疫组织化学试剂盒，由北京中杉金桥生物技术有限公司提供。

1.3 实验仪器

ECG-6511型心电图机，由上海光电仪器有限公司生产；DW-2000型动物人工呼吸机，由上海嘉鹏科技有限公司生产；Multiskan MK3型酶标仪，由荷兰雷勃生物医学有限公司生产；SN-682型γ计数器，由上海核福光仪器有限公司生产；7020型全自动生化仪，由日本日立公司生产；DpxView Pro型显微彩色图像处理系统，由丹麦DeltaPix公司生产；Imagepro-Plus 6.0图像分析系统，由美国Media Cybernetics公司生产。

1.4 动物分组及用药

大鼠随机分为5组，每组15只。即假手术组开胸后冠状动脉前降支下置线不结扎；I/R组予结扎冠状动脉前降支30min后，持续灌注1h；IPoC组结扎30min，然后给予3次10s再灌注-缺血循环，再持续灌注1h；福辛普利钠+IPoC组，福辛普利钠根据成人剂量，折合成大鼠剂量：0.9mg/（kg·d），建立I/R模型，过程中给予IPoC干预；益气活血+IPoC组，将成人剂量折合成大鼠剂量，心悦胶囊0.162mg/（kg·d）+芎芍胶囊0.135mg/（kg·d），药物均用蒸馏水稀释后，按10mL/kg体重灌胃。假手术组、I/R组和IPoC组每日均给予等量的蒸馏水灌胃，所有动物均灌胃14d，于末次灌胃2h后手术。

1.5 大鼠心肌I/R模型制作及标本采集

大鼠20%氨基甲酸乙酯（乌拉坦，6mL/kg）腹腔麻醉，将已麻醉的大鼠置于解剖台上，仰卧位固定，记录Ⅱ导联心电图。颈部、胸骨左侧、腹部消毒，并剪毛备用。剪开颈部皮肤，暴露气管并插管，连接动物呼吸机（潮气量30mL/kg体重，呼吸频率为50次/分钟），沿胸骨左缘3～4肋间开胸，暴露心脏，剪开心包膜，左冠状动脉前降支上1/3处穿3/0缝合线，缝合线两端共穿过一直径为1.5mm的硅胶软管，拉线推管，用蚊式止血钳固定以阻断前降支血流。结扎后行Ⅱ导联心电图，示ST段明显抬高或T波高尖，结扎线下左室前壁呈暗红色为结扎成功。30min后松开蚊式止血钳，放松缝合线，以恢复冠状动脉血流，给予再灌注60min。后适应操作是在结扎30min结束后，立即给予3次10s的再灌注-缺血循环，松开蚊式止血钳放松缝合线为再灌注，拉线推管用止血钳夹紧硅胶管为缺血，共60s[7]。之后完全打开缝合线再灌注60min，然后腹主动脉取血并分离血清，取出大鼠心脏，用生理盐水冲洗干净后，每组按随机数字表检测心肌组织指标，5只做NBT染色以测量大鼠左室心肌梗死面积，5只于−80℃冰箱保存，用于组织ELISA检测，5只用10%中性甲醛溶液中保存，用于免疫组织化学检测。实验中假手术组因灌胃死亡1只，I/R组造模中死亡4只，其余三组死亡各2只，后均予相应补充。

1.6 血清CK-MB和cTnT含量测定

比色法测定血清CK-MB和cTnT的含量。

1.7 心肌梗死面积的测量

将取下的大鼠心脏用生理盐水冲洗干净，用滤纸吸除多余水分，以房室沟为平行线，均匀切成5片，放入NBT染色液中，置于37℃水箱中温浴，温浴过程中观察心肌组织颜色。当非梗死区变成蓝色，梗死区为红色后，取出放置在滤纸上，用Canon IXUS 90IS数码相机微距拍摄后，使用DpxView Pro型显微彩色图像处理系统计算出心肌切片中横切面上总的左室梗死面积（%），计算公式为左室心肌梗死面积 / 左室面积 × 100%。

1.8 免疫组织化学法检测心肌组织 TLR 蛋白表达

将心肌标本用 10% 中性缓冲甲醛液固定 18h。脱水、透明、浸蜡、石蜡包埋。连续切片约 5 μm 厚，捞片于多聚赖氨酸防脱处理过的载玻片上。根据 SABC 试剂盒说明书操作，大鼠心肌切片常规脱蜡，封闭内源性过氧化物酶，10% 正常山羊血清封闭。分别滴加一抗 TLR2 抗体（1∶200）和 TLR4 抗体（1∶800），37℃孵育 1h，PBS 冲洗；滴加二抗生物素化山羊抗小鼠 IgG，室温 20min，PBS 溶液冲洗；滴加 SABC 复合物，室温 20min，PBS 溶液冲洗；DAB-H_2O_2 显色，苏木素轻度复染；乙醇脱水、透明、中性胶封片，选取同批染色切片进行光学显微镜下观察。每张切片随机选取 3 个不重叠的视野（×200），每只共计 15 个视野，以心肌炎症部位的胞浆染成棕褐色为阳性细胞标志，采用 Imagepro-Plus 6.0 图像分析系统测定每只动物心肌组织 TLR-2、4 阳性细胞的积分光密度（integral optical density，IOD）值，以 IOD 值反映组织切片中相应阳性物质的表达程度。

1.9 ELISA 检测心肌组织 IL-1β 和 IL-6 表达

每组 5 只心脏，取前降支结扎线下 2mm 至心尖部左室缺血心肌组织 100mg，加入 2mL 低温生理盐水（0℃），T18 高速分散机匀浆后，离心取上清液，于 –80℃保存待测。所有标本 ELISA 检测的操作过程严格按说明书操作程序进行。同时用考马斯亮蓝蛋白测定检测每个标本的蛋白含量，得出数值后，将每毫升匀浆液中的细胞因子含量换算成每毫克心肌蛋白中的细胞因子含量。

1.10 统计学方法

所有计量资料数据以 $\bar{x} \pm s$ 表示，使用 SPSS 14.0 进行统计学分析。单因素方差分析各组别之间的差异，组间两两比较采用 LSD-t 法，$P < 0.05$ 表示差异有统计学意义。

2. 结果

2.1 各组大鼠血清心肌损伤标志物和心肌梗死范围

与假手术组比较，各组血清心肌损伤标志物 CK-MB 活性和 cTnT 含量均显著升高（$P < 0.01$）；与 I/R 组比较，IPoC 组血清 CK-MB 活性和 cTnT 含量显著降低（$P < 0.01$）；与单纯 IPoC 比较，福辛普利钠和益气活血药在 IPoC 前预处理可减少大鼠血清中 CK-MB 活性（$P < 0.05$，$P < 0.01$），但对血清中 cTNT 含量无明显影响。见表 1。

I/R 组左室梗死面积为（35.28±3.85）%，IPoC 组左室梗死面积减少到（21.02±2.29）%，两组梗死面积比较，差异有统计学意义（$P < 0.01$）；与 IPoC 组比较，福辛普利钠 +IPoC 组和益气活血 +IPoC 心肌梗死范围进一步缩小（$P < 0.05$，$P < 0.01$），分别为（17.17±3.12）% 和（15.53±3.02）%。益气活血 +IPoC 组心肌梗死范围虽较福辛普利钠 +IPoC 组有所降低，但差异无统计学意义。见图 1。

2.2 各组大鼠心肌组织 TLR2、4 的表达

假手术组可见少量棕褐色颗粒，I/R 组心肌内棕褐色颗粒明显增多。与假手术组比较，各组心肌组织 TLR2、4 的表达均有显著升高（$P < 0.05$，$P < 0.01$）；与 I/R 组比较，各组大鼠心肌组织 TLR 2、4 表达显著降低（$P < 0.01$）；与 IPoC 组比较，益气活血 +IPoC 能进一步抑制 TLR2、4 表达（$P < 0.01$），福辛普利钠 +IPoC 组虽能降低 TLR 2、4 表达，但差异无统计学意义；与福辛普利钠 +IPoC 组比较，益气活血 +IPoC 能进一步抑制 TLR 2、4 表达（$P < 0.05$，$P < 0.01$）。见表 2、图 2 和图 3。

表 1 各组大鼠血清 CK-MB 活性和 cTnT 含量（$\bar{x} \pm s$）

Group	n	CK-MB（IU/L）	cTNT（ng/mL）
Sham-operated	14	693.64±114.85	0.015±0.01
I/R	11	1635.30±229.20**	4.41±0.93**
IPoC	13	1222.39±188.16** △△	2.53±0.51** △△
Fosinopril sodium plus IPoC	13	1047.61±223.13** △△ ▲	2.36±0.96** △△
NQABC plus IPoC	13	967.10±222.99** △△ ▲▲	2.34±0.60** △△

**$P < 0.01$，vs sham-operated group；△△$P < 0.01$，vs I/R group；▲$P < 0.05$，▲▲$P < 0.01$，vs IPoC group

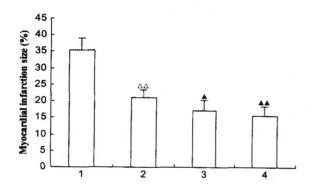

Figure 1　Changes of Myocardial Infarction Size in Different Groups

1：I/R group（*n*=5）；2：IPoC group（*n*=5）；3：Fosinopril sodium+IpoC group（*n*=5）；4：NQABC+IPoC group（*n*=5）. Data were represent as $\bar{\chi} \pm s$. $^{\triangle\triangle} P < 0.01$, *vs* I/R group；$^{\blacktriangle} P < 0.05$, $^{\blacktriangle\blacktriangle} P < 0.01$, *vs* IPoC group

2.3　各组大鼠心肌组织 IL-1β 和 IL-6 水平

与假手术组比较，I/R 组、IPoC 组和福辛普利钠 +IPoC 组大鼠心肌组织促炎性细胞因子 IL-1β 和 IL-6 含量均显著增高（$P < 0.05$，$P < 0.01$），益气活血 +IPoC 组 IL-1β 含量也显著升高（$P < 0.05$），IL-6 含量虽有升高，但差异无统计学意义；与 I/R 组比较，各干预组 IL-1β 和 IL-6 含量显

著降低（$P < 0.05$，$P < 0.01$）；与 IPoC 组比较，益气活血 +IPoC 能进一步降低 IL-1β 和 IL-6 含量（$P < 0.05$），而福辛普利钠 +IPoC 干预后 IL-1β 和 IL-6 含量虽有所降低，但差异无统计学意义。见表3。

3.　讨论

心肌 IPoC 是指在恢复持续冠状动脉血流灌注前给予反复几次短暂再灌注 / 缺血循环的一种机械性辅助治疗方法，这种方法已被大量实验研究和小样本临床研究证实可以减小心肌梗死面积，保护 I/R 心肌[5,6]。本实验发现，IPoC 能减轻 I/R 心肌损伤标志物 CK-MB 和 cTNT 的水平，在缩小心肌梗死范围方面，与既往研究结果[4]相符。在此基础上我们发现，益气活血中药预处理则能进一步减少 IPoC 处理后大鼠的心肌梗死面积，降低血清 CK-MB 活性，表明益气活血中药联合 IPoC 能更好地保护再灌注损伤心肌的作用。以往尚未见有相关报道，这为临床应用益气活血法治疗心肌梗死提供了实验依据。

局部和全身的炎症反应是心肌 I/R 损伤的重要机制之一，严重影响了心肌梗死后心脏功能的恢复。在 I/R 过程中，免疫反应被诱导活化，其中

表2　各组大鼠心肌 TLR2、4 表达水平变化（$\bar{\chi} \pm s$）

Group	n	TLR2	TLR4
Sham-operated	5	4763.99±694.09	5 166.78±1 487.01
I/R	5	23452.49±4817.16**	23 306.79±5 268.56**
IPoC	5	14362.93±3223.33**△△	13 336.19±3 274.79**△△
Fosinopril sodium+IPoC	5	12699.40±2167.25**△△	11 843.54±2 312.79**△△
RQAB+IPoC	5	7725.51±1558.97*△△▲▲□□	8 802.69±2 879.51**△△▲▲□

$^*P < 0.05$, $^{**}P < 0.01$, *vs* sham-operated group；$^{\triangle\triangle}P < 0.01$, *vs* I/R group；$^{\blacktriangle\blacktriangle}P < 0.01$, *vs* IPoC group；$^{\square}P < 0.05$, $^{\square\square}P < 0.01$, *vs* fosinopril sodium+IPoC group

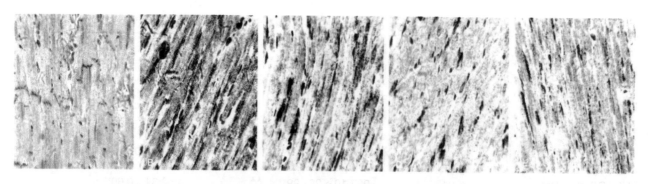

图2　免疫组织化学法检测各组大鼠心肌 TLR2 表达（光学显微镜，×200）
A：Sham-operated group；B：I/R group；C：IPoC group；D：Fosinopril sodium+IPoC group；E：RQAB+IPoC group

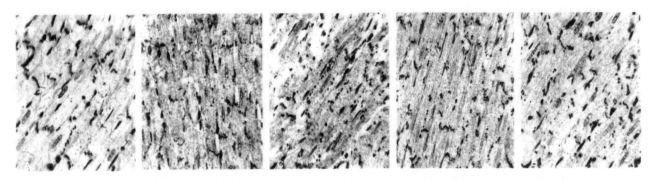

图 3　免疫组织化学法检测各组大鼠心肌 TLR4 表达（光学显微镜，×200）

A：sham-operated group；B：I/R group；C：IPoC group；D：Fosinopril sodium+IPoC group；E：NQABC+IPoC

表 3　各组大鼠心肌 IL-1β 和 IL-6 含量（$\bar{\chi}\pm s$, pg/mg）

Group	n	IL-1β	IL-6
Sham-operated	5	14.57±3.72	14.10±1.23
I/R	5	44.61±7.70**	24.78±3.47**
IPoC	5	33.67±7.59** △	20.57±1.95** △
Fosinopril sodium+IPoC	5	24.88±7.13* △	19.17±2.44** △△
RQAB+IPoC	5	24.33±6.14* △△▲	16.78±1.39 △△▲

*$P<0.05$, **$P<0.01$, vs sham-operated group；△$P<0.05$, △△$P<0.01$, vs I/R group；▲$P<0.05$, vs IPoC group

TLR 介导的炎症信号通路日益受到重视。TLR 是一组 I 型跨膜受体，通过与内、外源性配体结合，激发天然免疫和获得性免疫应答，启动与免疫和炎症相关的细胞因子 IL-1β、IL-6 等基因的转录和蛋白的表达 [8]。有研究发现，I/R 过程中 TLR4 的表达在再灌注 1h 达高峰，并与其下游炎性细胞因子 IL-1β、IL-6 等细胞因子的水平呈正相关 [9]。本实验研究发现，心肌 I/R 后心肌组织 TLR4 表达增加，IL-1β 和 IL-6 水平升高，与上述文献报道 [9,10] 一致。

近年来研究表明，缺血后适应保护 I/R 损伤心肌的作用主要与减轻再灌注氧化应激损伤 [4]、减少线粒体钙超载 [11]、改善内皮功能 [4]、激活再灌注损伤保护激酶通路、开放线粒体 ATP 敏感钾离子通道和抑制线粒体渗透孔道的开放 [6] 等机制有关，其保护作用是否与抑制 TLR 2、4 的表达有关，目前尚无研究报道。有研究将小鼠 TLR 4 基因敲除后建立心肌 I/R 损伤模型，发现其与同种野生型小鼠相比心肌梗死范围减少、炎症反应减轻、心肌梗死后的不良重塑改善 [12,13]。Sakata 等 [14] 同样也发现 TLR 2 缺陷小鼠遭受心肌 I/R 损伤后左心室舒张末压较同种野生型小鼠下降，促炎性细胞因子 IL-1β 水平降低。还有研究发现给予 TLR 4 的抑制剂 eritoran 干预后，I/R 后心肌梗死面积减少，心肌组织核转尿因子 κB 和促炎性细胞因子 IL-1β、

IL-6 和 TNF-α 水平降低 [10]。以上研究均表明抑制 TLR 2、4 的表达可保护 I/R 损伤心肌。我们实验研究发现，IPoC 干预再灌注损伤大鼠心肌后 TLR 2、4 表达降低，心肌内 IL-1β 和 IL-6 含量也下降，表明 IPoC 抑制 TLR 2、4 的表达可能是其保护 I/R 心肌的一个重要途径。给予益气活血中药预处理后，TLR 2、4 的表达进一步降低，心肌内 IL-1β 和 IL-6 含量也有显著下降，表明益气活血联合 IPoC 能更好地抑制 TLR 2、4 的表达和促进炎性细胞因子的分泌。

芎芍胶囊由活血化瘀代表药物川芎、赤芍的有效作用部位川芎总酚和赤芍总苷制成。现代药理研究表明，川芎总酚和赤芍总苷具有改善心肌缺血缺氧、抑制血小板聚集及血栓形成、保护血管内皮功能和抑制炎症反应等作用 [15,16]。心悦胶囊由西洋参茎叶中提取的西洋参茎叶总皂苷组成，主要含有人参二醇组及人参三醇组，具有抗心肌缺血、改善心肌能量代谢和促进血管新生等作用 [17,18]。本实验采用西洋参茎叶总皂苷联合芎芍胶囊，体现中医益气活血的效用，在 IPoC 的基础上进行 2 周预处理，可减少 I/R 大鼠心肌梗死面积，降低血清 CK-MB 活性，其机制可能与降低 I/R 心肌 TLR 2、4 以及炎性细胞因子 IL-1β、IL-6 的表达有关。应用血管紧张素转化酶抑制剂类药物福辛普利钠作为

阳性对照药物，发现益气活血中药与福辛普利钠有着基本相似的保护 I/R 心肌作用，但益气活血中药在抑制 TLR 表达方面的优势更加明显，在一定程度上表明益气活血代表药物心悦胶囊联合芍苓胶囊具有更好的保护 I/R 损伤心肌的作用。

本实验研究观察了益气活血中药（心悦胶囊和芍苓胶囊）对 IPoC 后 I/R 大鼠心肌损伤的作用，未分别对益气和活血中药进行研究，它们在 I/R 损伤方面作用机制有何不同，两者联合是否具有协同作用，皆有待于进一步研究。

参考文献

[1] 中国中医研究院西苑医院内科，东直门医院内科，广安门医院内科，北京宣武医院内科．以"抗心梗合剂"为主治疗急性心肌梗塞 118 例疗效分析．中华内科杂志，1976，1（4）：212-215．

[2] 侯霄雷，李白翎，赵雷，等．血府逐瘀胶囊对急性心肌梗死再灌注后心肌及内皮素 -1、一氧化氮 / 一氧化氮合酶体系影响的实验研究．中西医结合学报，2008，6（4）：381-386．

[3] 贺运河，古继红，陈光贤，等．益气活血法对大鼠心肌缺血再灌注损伤保护作用的实验研究．中西医结合心脑血管病杂志，2007，5（8）：707-708．

[4] Zhao ZQ, Corvera JS, Halkos ME, et al. Inhibition of myocardial injury by ischemic postconditioning during reperfusion: comparison with ischemic preconditioning. Am J Physiol Heart Circ Physiol, 2003, 285 (2): H579-H588.

[5] Thibault H, Piot C, Staat P, et al. Long-term benefit of postconditioning. Circulation, 2008, 117 (8): 1037-1044.

[6] Dow J, Bhandari A, Kloner RA. The mechanism by which ischemic postconditioning reduces reperfusion arrhythmias in rats remains elusive. J Cardiovasc Pharmacol Ther, 2009, 14 (2): 99-103.

[7] Zatta AJ, Kin H, Lee G, et al. Infarct-sparing effect of myocardial postconditioning is dependent on protein kinase C signalling. Cardiovasc Res, 2006, 70 (2): 315-324.

[8] Boyd JH, Mathur S, Wang Y, et al. Toll-like receptor stimulation in cardiomyoctes decreases contractility and initiates an NF-kappa B dependent inflammatory response. Cardiovasc Res, 2006, 72 (3): 384-393.

[9] Yang J, Yang J, Ding JW, et al. Sequential expression of TLR4 and its effects on the myocardium of rats with myocardial ischemia-reperfusion injury. Inflammation, 2008, 31 (5): 304-312.

[10] Shimamoto A, Chong AJ, Yada M, et al. Inhibition of Toll-like receptor 4 with eritoran attenuates myocardial ischemia-reperfusion injury. Circulation, 2006, 114 (1): I270-I274.

[11] Sun HY, Wang NP, Kerendi F, et al. Hypoxic postconditioning reduces cardiomyocyte loss by inhibiting ROS generation and intracellular Ca^{2+} overload. Am J Physiol, 2005, 288 (4): H1900-H1908.

[12] Oyama J, Blais C Jr, Liu X, et al. Reduced myocardial ischemiareperfusion injury in toll-like receptor 4-deficient mice. Circulation, 2004, 109 (6): 784-789.

[13] Riad A, Jager S, Sobirey M, et al. Toll-like receptor-4 modulates survival by induction of left ventricular remodeling after myocardial infarction in mice. J Immunol, 2008, 180 (10): 6954-6961.

[14] Sakata Y, Dong JW, Vallejo JG, et al. Toll-like receptor 2 modulates left ventricular function following ischemia-reperfusion injury. Am J Physiol Heart Circ Physiol, 2007, 292 (1): H503-H509.

[15] 李立志，刘剑刚，马鲁波，等．芍苓胶囊对兔动脉粥样硬化模型脂质代谢及血小板聚集的影响．中国中西医结合杂志，2008，28（12）：1100-1103．

[16] 阮金兰，赵钟祥，曾庆忠，等．赤芍化学成分和药理作用的研究进展．中国药理学通报，2003，19（9）：965-970．

[17] 丁涛，徐惠波，孙晓波，等．西洋参茎叶总皂苷对心肌缺血的保护作用．中药药理与临床，2002，18（4）：14-16．

[18] 王承龙，史大卓，殷惠军，等．西洋参茎叶总皂苷对急性心肌梗死大鼠心肌 VEGF、bFGF 表达及血管新生的影响．中国中西医结合杂志，2007，27（4）：331-334．

急性心肌梗死后大鼠缺血心肌胶原蛋白的表达及益气养阴活血和解毒活血中药的干预作用 *

徐伟 石 萌 刘剑刚 王承龙

急性心肌梗死（acute myocardial infarction，AMI）后，神经内分泌系统的激活引起心肌结构、功能和表型的变化以及心肌细胞外基质组成和量的变化，导致心室重构（ventricular remodeling，VR），最终失代偿，出现心力衰竭。心力衰竭的治疗目标是防止和延缓心肌重塑的发展[1]。前期研究表明，应用益气养阴活血中成药（复方芪丹液）可调节心肌局部细胞因子分泌，限制胶原过度沉积，改善AMI后血流动力学并对动物早期AMI后VR有明显的减轻作用[2]。临床研究中，AMI患者经皮冠状动脉介入术后，在西药常规治疗下加用益气养阴、活血化瘀制剂，能改善AMI患者的临床症状及心功能[3]。常规西药联合养阴活血解毒中药能缓解冠心病患者的临床症状，改善患者的冠状动脉内皮炎症反应、内皮功能和心功能储备能力[4]。本文探讨益气养阴活血和解毒活血中药组分配伍对AMI后VR的影响及对Ⅰ、Ⅲ型胶原蛋白表达的干预作用。

1. 材料与方法

1.1 实验材料

1.1.1 实验动物 雄性8周龄Wistar大鼠120只，清洁级，体重180～220g，由北京维通利华实验动物技术有限公司提供，合格证号为SCXK（京）2007-0001。

1.1.2 实验药物 培哚普利片（培哚普利叔丁胺盐），4mg/片，施维雅（天津）制药有限公司生产（批号：7M 0434）；生脉胶囊（红参、麦冬、五味子），每粒0.3g，每克相当于生药4.40g，正大青春宝制药有限公司生产（批号：0803004）；复方川芎胶囊（川芎、当归），每粒0.37g，每克相当于生药3.64g，山东凤凰制药股份有限公司生产（批号：0802205）；黄连提取物（黄连生物碱），每克相当于生药6.25g，由北京同仁堂制药有限公司提供。

1.1.3 实验主要试剂和仪器 抗Ⅰ型、抗Ⅲ型胶原抗体试剂盒，由北京博奥森生物技术有限公司提供。浓缩型二氨基联苯胺（diaminobenzidine tetrahydrochloride substrate，DAB）试剂盒，浓缩型脱氧核糖核酸酶亲和素标记复合体（strept avidin biotin complex，SABC）免疫组织化学试剂盒，由北京中杉金桥生物技术有限公司提供。Ⅲ型前胶原试剂盒、Ⅳ型胶原试剂盒，由上海海军医学研究所生物技术中心提供。Multiskan MK3型酶标仪，由芬兰Thermo Labsystems公司生产；SN-682型γ计数器，由上海核福光仪器有限公司生产；DpxView Pro型显微彩色图像处理系统，由丹麦DeltaPix公司生产。

1.2 实验方法

1.2.1 造模方法 大鼠术前禁食12h以上，称体重后用乙醚麻醉，通过角膜反射判断麻醉是否充分。左侧胸部备皮，消毒后剪开皮肤，于3～4肋间钝性分离肌肉组织，开胸快速挤出心脏，于左心耳与动脉圆锥下（心大静脉为体表标志）1～2mm处结扎左冠状动脉前降支，造成AMI模型，然后迅速将心脏放回胸腔后缝合[5]。记录Ⅱ导联心电图，ST段弓背抬高且持续2min以上表示AMI形成。术后给予青霉素4万U腹腔注射，每日1次，连续3天。假手术组只穿刺不结扎，其他手术步骤同上。手术成功率40%左右。

1.2.2 动物分组与用药 24h后存活大鼠视为造模成功大鼠，共40只，随机（采用Excel生成随机数字法）分为4组，每组10只。模型组大鼠20mL/kg生理盐水灌胃，其余各组大鼠根据成人用药量按体表面积进行用药量换算[6]：培哚普利组大鼠0.36mg/kg培哚普利片水溶液灌胃，益气养阴活血（Yiqi Yangyin Huoxue，YQYYHX）组0.24g/kg生脉胶囊和0.40g/kg复方川芎胶囊水溶液灌胃。解毒活血（Jiedu Huoxue，JDHX）组

* 原载于《中西医结合学报》，2010，8（11）：1041-1047

0.40g/kg 复方川芎胶囊和 0.16g/kg 黄连生物碱水溶液灌胃。所有药物按临床有效剂量换算，灌胃量同模型组。另设正常对照组 10 只，假手术组 10 只，生理盐水灌胃剂量同上。术后第 2 天开始灌胃，每日 1 次，连续 4 周。

1.2.3 血样及病理组织处理 4 周后大鼠腹腔注射 20% 氨基甲基乙酯（乌拉坦，7mL/kg）麻醉，经腹主动脉取血，放射免疫法检测血清Ⅲ型前胶原、Ⅳ型胶原含量（参照试剂盒说明）。无菌条件下剥离心脏组织，生理盐水冲洗，滤纸吸干，称取质量，沿房室交界处剪去左、右心房及大血管，去除右心室游离壁，称取余下的左心室质量，记录并计算左室质量指数（left ventricular mass index，LVMI）。每组用随机数字法（运用 SPSS 13.0 软件生成随机数字）随机取 5 只心脏标本并以 10% 中性甲醛磷酸缓冲液固定，常规苏木精 - 伊红（hematoxylin-eosin，HE）染色法观察。取结扎部位以下左室缺血心肌组织，常规石蜡包埋，均匀间断切片，厚度约 5μm，普通光镜及 Dpx View Pro 型显微彩色图像分析系统下观察大鼠心肌组织的形态结构。

1.2.4 免疫组织化学检测 根据 SABC 试剂盒说明书操作。每组随机数字法（采用 Excel 生成随机数字）随机取 5 只大鼠的心脏切片，常规脱蜡，封闭内源性过氧化物酶，10% 正常山羊血清封闭。滴加一抗（1∶800）Ⅰ型胶原染色用抗Ⅰ型胶原抗体，37℃孵育 1h，PBS 溶液冲洗。滴加二抗生物素化山羊抗小鼠 IgG，室温 20min，PBS 溶液冲洗。滴加 SABC 复合物，室温 20min，PBS 溶液冲洗。DAB-H_2O_2 显色，苏木精轻度复染；乙醇脱水、透明、中性胶封片，选取同批染色切片进行显微镜观察。抗Ⅲ型胶原抗体（1∶400）如上操作。每张切片随机（运用 SPSS 13.0 软件生成随机数字）选取 3 个不同视野（根据病理画面等位置角度三个画面），每组共计 15 个视野，以心肌纤维染成棕褐色为阳性细胞标志，经病理图像计算机分析系统半定量分析大鼠心肌组织中的阳性表达，以阳性细胞面积占所有细胞面积百分比表示结果。

1.3 统计学方法

用 SPSS 13.0 软件处理数据，以 $\bar{x}\pm s$ 表示。正态性检验及方差齐性检验后，多组间比较用单因素方差分析，两两比较用 q 检验，$P < 0.05$ 为差异有统计学意义。

2. 结果

2.1 益气养阴活血和活血解毒中药组分对大鼠缺血心肌组织病理的影响

与假手术组比较，模型组心脏标本可见梗死区心脏与胸壁粘连，室壁呈灰白色，室壁扩张，常有室壁瘤形成。纵向切开心脏，可见梗死区心室壁变薄。HE 染色后观察显示，正常对照组、假手术组大鼠心肌细胞排列整齐紧密，细胞核饱满；模型组大鼠心肌细胞疏松、肥大，心肌坏死区域较多，心肌纤维排列不齐；各给药组大鼠心肌细胞排列尚整齐紧密，心肌纤维增粗不明显，坏死区域较少，缺血组织病理变化有显著改善。见图 1。

2.2 益气养阴活血和解毒活血中药组分对大鼠血清Ⅲ型前胶原、Ⅳ型胶原的影响

造模成功后因心肌坏死面积较大、心功能不全，模型组、益气养阴活血组和解毒活血组死亡大鼠数分别为 3、1、1 只，因灌胃不当致正常对照组、假手术组死亡大鼠分别为 1、2 只，最终成活数如表 1 所示。与假手术组比较，模型组大鼠的Ⅲ型前胶原含量增加明显（$P < 0.01$）。与模型组比较，3 组治疗组大鼠的Ⅲ型前胶原含量明显降低（$P < 0.01$，$P < 0.05$）。各给药组对血清Ⅳ型胶原含量的影响比较差异无统计学意义。见表 1。

2.3 益气养阴活血和解毒活血中药组分对大鼠左室质量和 LVMI 的影响

和假手术组比较，造模组大鼠 4 周后左心室质量和 LVMI 明显增加（$P < 0.01$，$P < 0.05$）。和模型组比较，造模 4 周后益气养阴活血组和解毒活血组大鼠左心室质量和 LVMI 均明显降低（$P < 0.01$，$P < 0.05$）。各给药组之间比较差异无统计学意义。见表 2。

2.4 益气养阴活血和解毒活血中药组分对大鼠缺血心肌Ⅰ、Ⅲ型胶原蛋白的影响

4 周后，和假手术组比较，模型组大鼠的Ⅰ型、Ⅲ型胶原蛋白含量明显增加（$P < 0.01$）。和模型组比较，3 组治疗组大鼠的Ⅰ型、Ⅲ型胶原蛋白含量均明显降低（$P < 0.01$）。与培哚普利组比较，解毒活血组Ⅲ型胶原蛋白含量明显减少（$P < 0.01$），益气养阴活血组Ⅲ型胶原蛋白含量亦有减少，但差异无统计学意义。各给药组对Ⅰ型胶原蛋白含量的影响比较差异无统计学意义。见图 2、图 3 与表 3。

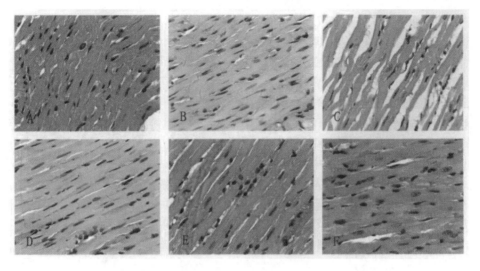

图 1　AMI 后各组大鼠缺血心肌的病理状态（HE 染色，光学显微镜，×400）

A：Normal control group；B：Sham-operated group；C：Untreated group；D：Perindopril group；E：YQYYHX group；F：JDHX group

表 1　AMI 后各组大鼠血清中 Ⅲ 型前胶原和 Ⅳ 型胶原含量

（$\bar{\chi} \pm s$，μg/L）

Group	n	Procollagen Type Ⅲ	Collagen Type Ⅳ
Normal control	9	47.61±7.25	52.30±5.56
Sham-operated	8	44.16±5.44	53.94±4.90
Untreated	7	55.96±8.86**	56.27±8.64
Perindopril	10	45.61±3.23△△	48.38±6.77
YQYYHX	9	47.61±7.26△	52.30±5.56
JDHX	9	46.47±8.58△	49.33±3.10

**$P < 0.01$, vs sham-operated group；$^{\triangle}P < 0.05$，$^{\triangle\triangle}P < 0.01$, vs untreated group

表 2　AMI 后各组大鼠的左心室质量及 LVMI（$\bar{\chi} \pm s$）

Group	n	Left ventricle Weight (mg)	LVMI (mg/g)
Normal control	9	744.44±42.46	2.55±0.13
Sham-operated	8	857.50±51.48	2.69±0.22
Untreated	7	1018.57±108.85**	3.32±0.66*
Perindopril	10	706.00±115.30△△	2.55±0.34△△
YQYYHX	9	881.11±127.81△	2.91±0.23△
JDHX	9	846.67±149.33△△	2.81±0.43△△

*$P < 0.05$，**$P < 0.01$, vs sham-operated group；$^{\triangle}P < 0.05$，$^{\triangle\triangle}P < 0.01$, vs untreated group

3. 讨论

AMI 后，由于血流动力学变化，交感系统和肾素-血管紧张素-醛固酮系统被激活，在神经内分泌因子的作用下，导致心肌细胞的肥大与凋亡以及心肌纤维的增生，产生 VR，最终形成进行性的心功能减退，导致患者死亡。如何有效地干预 AMI 后 VR，是现代冠心病防治领域普遍关注的难题。VR 包括心室大小、形状、质量变化，LVWI 是衡量心室重构的敏感指标。VR 是发生于细胞水平的变化（包括心肌细胞和非心肌细胞），表现为心脏成纤维细胞大量增生，合成和分泌大量胶原纤维沉积于心肌间质[7,8]。胶原蛋白包括 Ⅰ、Ⅲ、Ⅳ、Ⅴ、Ⅵ 五种。Ⅰ 型约占心肌胶原总数的 55%，抗拉强度高，而伸展性和回缩性小，决定心肌舒张收缩的僵硬度；Ⅲ 型约占 11%，纤维较细，具有良好的弹性[9]。Ⅰ、Ⅲ 型胶原的含量及比值增加可导致心脏僵硬度增加，顺应性变小，心脏舒张、收缩功能障碍。Ⅲ 型前胶原是 Ⅰ 型和 Ⅲ 型胶原的前体，被认为是胶原合成速率的一个可靠指标[10]。

研究证明生脉胶囊可降低慢性心力衰竭大鼠心肌胶原容积分数和 Ⅰ、Ⅲ 型胶原的含量，并具有减轻心室重构的作用[11]。人参总皂苷和黄连小檗碱对慢性心力衰竭大鼠血流动力学异常、血浆 B 型尿钠肽、心肌细胞内钙超载有良好的改善作用，并可增加心肌细胞内肌球蛋白重链 α mRNA 表达，降低肌球蛋白重链 β mRNA 表达，从而改善心功能和心室重构[12,13]。现代药理研究表明，生脉胶囊中人参皂苷 Rbl 可抑制血管紧张素 Ⅱ

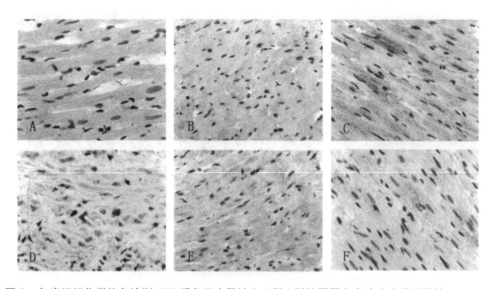

图 2　免疫组织化学染色检测 AMI 后各组大鼠缺血心肌 I 型胶原蛋白表达（光学显微镜，×400)

A: Normal control group; B: Shame-operated group; C: Untreated group; D: Perindopril group; E: YQYYHX group; F: JDHX group. Brown color in the picture refers to the expression of type Ⅰ collagen protein in myocardium

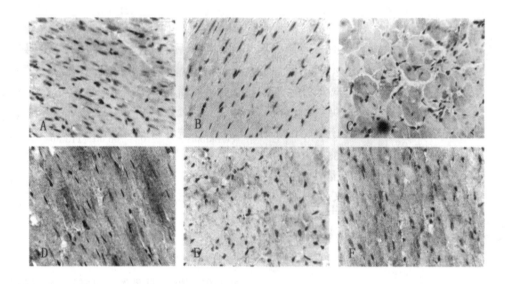

图 3　免疫组织化学染色检测 AMI 后各组大鼠缺血心肌Ⅲ型胶原蛋白表达（光学显微镜，×400 ）

A：Normal control group；B：Sham-operated group；C：Untreated group；D：Perindopril group；E：YQYYHX group；F：JDHX group. Brown color in the picture refers to the expression of type Ⅲ collagen protein in myocardium

（angiotension Ⅱ，Ang Ⅱ）诱导的细胞肥大[14]；麦冬多糖可以抗心肌缺血，增加心肌血流量，减少心肌细胞的受损[15]；五味子乙素具有明显的清除自由基和抑制脂质过氧化作用[16]。川芎嗪具有扩张冠状动脉、抗脂质过氧化、抑制平滑肌细胞增生等功能[17]。临床观察显示川芎嗪能改善缺血性心肌病和心功能不全患者的心功能分级[18]。川芎和当归中的阿魏酸具有抑制巨噬细胞活化、抑制花生四烯酸代谢、抗组胺、降低血管通透性、抗氧化和清除自由基、抑制由 Ang Ⅱ诱导的血管内皮细胞

增生等药理作用[19]。以上有效组分共同作用，可能从多个方面调节心肌细胞的代谢和细胞因子的分泌，抑制心肌胶原增生，改善心功能。

心肌间质重构是指成纤维细胞增生、纤维化、血管结构改变以及细胞外基质胶原网的量和组成的变化。本研究表明，益气养阴活血组、解毒活血组中药制剂均能降低 AMI 后大鼠血清Ⅲ型前胶原，减少缺血心肌Ⅰ、Ⅲ型胶原蛋白的表达，从而减轻VR，表明它们抑制 VR 的机制与抑制胶原增生有关，且解毒活血组中药对Ⅲ型胶原蛋白的作用优于

表3 AMI后各组大鼠心肌组织中Ⅰ、Ⅲ型胶原蛋白含量
$(\bar{x} \pm s, \%)$

Group	n	Area of positive cells	
		Type Ⅰ collagen	Type Ⅲ collagen
Normal control	5	2.61 ± 1.70	1.86 ± 0.28
Sham-operated	5	4.59 ± 3.94	1.31 ± 0.90
Untreated	5	32.02 ± 15.77**	28.00 ± 5.54**
Perindopril	5	$14.02 \pm 5.50^{\triangle\triangle}$	$12.42 \pm 0.70^{\triangle\triangle}$
YQYYHX	5	$9.66 \pm 4.79^{\triangle\triangle}$	$8.32 \pm 4.36^{\triangle\triangle}$
JDHX	5	$17.23 \pm 8.92^{\triangle\triangle}$	$6.49 \pm 3.10^{\triangle\triangle}$▲▲

**$P < 0.01$, vs sham-operated group；$^{\triangle\triangle}P < 0.01$, vs untreated group；▲▲$P < 0.01$, vs perindopril group

培哚普利。中医认为脏腑功能和气血运行失常，病理产物不能及时排出，蕴积体内，可化生毒邪，造成疾病难治不愈。发生 AMI 时，心肌的坏死，心肌间质充血、水肿，炎症细胞浸润和血管活性物质的过度释放等，均可看成是毒邪，解毒治疗及其机制研究可以为冠心病 AMI 后的中西医结合治疗提供新的思路和结合点。现代心力衰竭的防治要求由短期血流动力学改变转为长期的、修复性的策略，以防止和延缓心室重构的发展。本实验为中医益气养阴活血法、解毒活血法治疗 AMI，抑制胶原沉积，改善心肌病理组织结构提供了药理依据，值得进一步研究，以期更加明确益气养阴活血、解毒活血中药组分防治心室重构的机制。

参考文献

[1] 戴闺柱. 慢性收缩性心力衰竭治疗建议. 中华心血管病杂志，2002，30（1）：7-23.

[2] 史大卓，马鲁波，刘剑刚，等. 复方芪丹液对中国小型猪急性心肌梗死后早期心室重构的影响. 中国中西医结合杂志，2008，28（1）：43-46.

[3] 仇盛蕾，金玫，易京红，等. 急性心肌梗死直接经皮冠状动脉介入术后应用益气养阴活血法治疗的效果：随机对照试验. 中西医结合学报，2009，7（7）：616-621.

[4] 谢雄伟，庄汉屏，唐凤英，等. 养阴活血解毒法对冠心病患者心功能储备及内皮功能的影响. 中医杂志，2009，50（2）：133-135.

[5] 陈奇. 中药药理研究方法学. 北京：人民卫生出版社.
1993：495.

[6] 徐淑云，卞如濂，陈修. 药理实验方法学. 3版：北京：人民卫生出版社. 2001：283.

[7] Dez J, Ertl G. A translational approach to myocardial remodelling. Cardiovasc Res, 2009, 81(3):409-411.

[8] Spinale FG. Myocardial matrix remodeling and the matrix metalloproteinases：influence on cardiac form and function. Physiol Rev, 2007, 87 (4): 1285-1342.

[9] Miner EC, Miller WL. A look between the cardiomyocytes: the extracellular matrix in heart failure. Mayo Clin Proc，2006，81 (1): 71-76.

[10] Li G, Yan QB, Wei LM. Serum concentrations of hyaluronic acid, procollagen type Ⅲ NH2-terminal peptide, and laminin in patients with chronic congestive heart failure. Chin Med Sci J，2006，21 (3): 175-178.

[11] 邓元江，梁伟雄，刘卫英，等. 生脉胶囊对压力超负荷心衰大鼠心肌胶原纤维的影响. 中华中医药学刊，2009，27（3）：483-484.

[12] 李永民，陈晓春，刘华，等. 人参总皂苷合黄连小檗碱对慢性心衰大鼠血浆 BNP、心肌细胞内钙离子浓度的影响. 中国中药杂志，2009，34（3）：324-327.

[13] 李永民，陈晓春，罗飞，等. 人参总皂苷合黄连小檗碱对慢性心衰大鼠心肌肌球蛋白重链的影响. 第四军医大学学报，2009，30（14）：1281-1284.

[14] 陈小文，黄燮南，吴芹. 人参皂苷 Rbl 抑制 Ang Ⅱ诱导的心肌细胞肥大. 遵义医学院学报，2008，31（5）：457-460.

[15] 周跃华，徐德生，冯怡，等. 麦冬提取物对小鼠心肌营养血流量的影响. 中国实验方剂学杂志，2003，9（1）：22-24.

[16] Chiu PY, Mak DH, Poon MK, et al. Role of cytochrome P-450 in schisandrin B-induced antioxidant and heat shock responses in mouse liver. Life Sci, 2005, 77(23): 2887-2895.

[17] 陈可冀，张之南，梁子钧，等. 血瘀证与活血化瘀研究. 上海：上海科学技术出版社. 1990:514-516.

[18] 徐丽娟. 川芎嗪对缺血性心肌病和心功能不全的疗效观察. 实用心脑血管病杂志，2009，17（4）：306.

[19] Hou YZ, Yang J, Zhao GR, et al. Ferulic acid inhibits vascular smooth muscle cell proliferation induced by angiotensin Ⅱ. Eur J Pharmacol, 2004, 499 (1-2): 85-90.

第四章

芎芍胶囊联合缺血后适应对大鼠缺血/再灌注心肌 MCP-1 及 TNF-α 的影响 *

张大武　张　蕾　刘剑刚　王承龙　史大卓　陈可冀

大量实验和小样本临床研究[1, 2]表明，缺血后适应（ischemic postconditioning，IPoC）能减少心肌梗死面积和心肌损伤标志物的水平，保护缺血/再灌注（ischemic reperfusion，I/R）损伤心肌，这为临床改善急性心肌梗死早期再灌注治疗后患者的心脏功能提供了依据。芎芍胶囊（Xiongshao Capsule，XSC）由川芎总酚和赤芍总苷组成，在改善冠心病患者心绞痛症状、血液流变学以及抑制炎症反应等方面有较好疗效[3,4]。本实验研究采用芎芍胶囊预处理联合 IPoC 干预再灌注损伤大鼠心肌，观察芎芍胶囊是否有增强 IPoC 保护 I/R 心肌的作用，并从心肌组织炎性细胞因子——单核细胞趋化蛋白-1（monocyte chemoattractant protein-1，MCP-1）、肿瘤坏死因子-α（tumor necrosis factor-α，TNF-α）水平和炎性细胞浸润方面探索其作用机制。

1. 材料与方法

1.1 材料

1.1.1　动物　SD 大鼠，清洁级，75 只，雌雄兼用，体重 180～200g，由北京维通利华实验动物技术有限公司提供，合格证号：SCXK（京）2007-0001。适应性饲养 3 天后进行实验。

1.1.2　药物　XSC，由川芎、赤芍的有效部位川芎总酚和赤芍总苷组成，每粒 0.25g，北京国际生物制品研究所提供，批号：200094；福辛普利钠片，每粒 10mg，中美上海施贵宝制药有限公司生产，批号：0804087。

1.1.3　试剂　肌钙蛋白T（cardiac troponin T，cTnT）试剂盒由美国 RapidBio Lab 公司生产，北京莱博特利生物医学科技公司提供，批号：08060502；肌酸激酶同工酶（creatine kinase-MB，CK-MB）试剂盒，由北京中生北控生物科技股份有限公司提供，批号：070181；MCP-1、TNF-α 酶联免疫吸附测定（enzyme-linked immunosorbant assay，ELISA）试剂盒，由美国 R&D 公司生产；考马斯亮蓝蛋白测定试剂盒，由南京建成科技有限公司生产，批号：090828；氯化硝基四氮唑兰（nitro blue tetrazolium chloride，NBT），由美国 R&D 公司生产。

1.1.4　仪器　ECG-6511 型心电图机，由上海光电仪器有限公司生产；DW-2000 型动物人工呼吸机，由上海嘉鹏科技有限公司生产；Multiskan MK3 型酶标仪，由荷兰雷勃生物医学有限公司生产；7020 型全自动生化仪，由日本日立公司生产；Dpx View Pro 型显微彩色图像处理系统，由丹麦 DeltaPix 公司生产。

1.2 方法

1.2.1　分组及用药方法　将大鼠随机分为 5 组，每组 15 只，即假手术组：开胸冠状动脉前降支下置线不结扎。I/R 组：结扎冠状动脉前降支 30min，持续灌注 1h。IPoC 组：结扎冠状动脉前降支 30min，然后给予 3 次 10s 再灌注/缺血循环，再持续灌注 1h。福辛普利钠加 IPoC 组：福辛普利钠，每天 0.9mg/kg，用等量蒸馏水稀释后灌胃，建立 I/R 模型，过程中给予 IPoC 干预。XSC 加 IPoC 组：芎芍胶囊每天 0.135g/kg，方法同福辛普利钠加 IPoC 组。假手术组、I/R 组和 IPoC 组每天均给予等量生理盐水灌胃，所有动物均灌胃 14 天，于末次灌胃 2h 后手术。

1.2.2　大鼠 I/R 模型制作及标本采集　20% 氨基甲酸乙酯（6mL/kg）腹腔麻醉大鼠，仰卧位固定于解剖台上，记录 II 导联心电图。颈部、胸骨左侧、腹部消毒，并剪毛备用。剪开颈部皮肤，暴露气管并插管，连接动物呼吸机（潮气量 3mL/100g 体重，呼吸频率为 50 次/min），沿胸骨左缘 3～4 肋间开胸，暴露心脏，剪开心包膜，左冠状动脉前降支上 1/3 处穿 3/0 缝合线，缝合线两端共穿过一直径为 1.5mm 的硅胶软管，拉线推管，用蚊式止血钳固定以阻断前降支血流。结扎后 II 导联心

* 原载于《中国中西医结合杂志》，2010，30（12）：1279-1289

电图示 ST 段明显抬高或 T 波高尖，结扎线下左室前壁呈暗红色为结扎成功。30min 后松开蚊式止血钳放松缝合线以恢复冠状动脉血流，给予再灌注 60min。后适应操作是在结扎 30min 结束后，立即给予 3 次 10s 的再灌注 / 缺血循环，松开蚊式止血钳放松缝合线为再灌注，拉线推管用止血钳夹紧硅胶管为缺血。完全打开缝合线，再灌注 60min，然后腹主动脉取血并分离血清，取出大鼠心脏，用生理盐水冲洗干净后，每组按随机数字表检测心肌组织指标，5 只做 NBT 染色，测量大鼠左室心肌梗死面积，5 只在 -80℃ 冰箱保存，用于组织 ELISA 检测，5 只在 10% 中性甲醛溶液中保存，用于苏木精和伊红（hematoxylin and eosin，HE）染色。实验中假手术组因灌胃死亡 1 只，I/R 组造模中死亡 4 只，其余 3 组死亡各 2 只，后均予相应补充。

1.2.3　血清 CK-MB 和 cTnT 的含量测定　采用 7020 型全自动生化仪测定。

1.2.4　左心室梗死面积的测量　将取下的大鼠心脏用生理盐水冲洗干净，用滤纸吸除多余水分，均匀切成 5 片，放入 NBT 染色液中，置于 37℃ 水箱中温浴，温浴过程中观察心肌组织颜色，当非梗死区变成蓝色，梗死区为红色后，取出放置在滤纸上，用 Canon IXUS 90IS 数码相机微距拍摄后，使用 Dpx View Pro 型显微彩色图像处理系统计算出左心室梗死面积（%），用心肌梗死面积 / 左室面积 ×100% 表示。

1.2.5　HE 染色观察心肌组织浸润的炎性细胞数　心肌组织用 10% 中性甲醛液固定后，石蜡包埋。连续切片厚约 5μm，放置于多聚赖氨酸防脱处理过的载玻片上，进行常规脱蜡，HE 染色，脱水、透明、封片后在光学显微镜（×400 倍）下观察，每张切片随机选取 3 个连续的视野，根据文献[5]将 3 个视野中浸润的炎性细胞（单核 / 巨噬细胞和淋巴细胞）数量求和，得出 3 个视野总的浸润细胞数。

1.2.6　ELISA 检测心肌组织细胞因子表达　每组 5 只心脏，取前降支结扎线下 2mm 至心尖部左室缺血心肌组织 100mg，加入 2mL 低温生理盐水（0℃），T18 高速分散机匀浆后，离心取上清液，于 -80℃ 保存待测。所有标本均采用 ELISA 法检测，操作过程严格按说明书操作程序进行。同时用考马斯亮蓝蛋白测定法检测每个组织标本的蛋白含量，得出数值后，将每毫升匀浆液中的细胞因子含量换算成每毫克蛋白中的细胞因子含量。

1.2.7　统计学方法　所有数据以 $\bar{x} \pm s$ 表示，使用 SPSS 14.0 进行统计学分析。多组间比较采用单因素方差分析，组间两两比较采用 LSD 法，相关性采用 Pearson 相关分析。$P < 0.05$ 表示差异有统计学意义。

2. 结果

2.1　各组大鼠血清心肌损伤标志物和心肌梗死面积比较（表 1）

与假手术组比较，I/R 组心肌损伤标志物 CK-MB 和 cTnT 及左心室梗死面积均显著升高（$P < 0.01$）；与 I/R 组比较，IPoC 组、福辛普利钠加 IPoC 组及 XSC 加 IPoC 组 CK-MB 和 cTnT 及左心室梗死面积显著降低（$P < 0.01$）；与 IPoC 组比较，福辛普利钠加 IPoC 组、XSC 加 IPoC 组能进一步降低心肌细胞 CK-MB 的释放及左心室梗死面积，差异均有统计学意义（$P < 0.05$）。

2.2　各组大鼠心肌组织 MCP-1 及 TNF-α 水平比较（表 2）

与假手术组比较，I/R 组心肌组织炎性细胞因子 MCP-1 及 TNF-α 含量显著增高（$P < 0.01$）；与 I/R 组比较，IPoC 干预能显著降低心肌 MCP-1 及 TNF-α 水平（$P < 0.05$，$P < 0.01$）；在此基础上，芎芍胶囊能进一步降低 IPoC 心肌 MCP-1

表 1　各组大鼠血清心肌损伤标志物和心肌梗死面积比较（$\bar{x} \pm s$）

组别	CK-MB（IU/L）	cTnT（ng/mL）	左心室梗死面积（%）
假手术	693.64±114.85（14）	0.02±0.01（14）	0
I/R	1635.30±229.20（11）*	4.41±0.93（11）*	35.28±3.85（5）*
IPoC	1222.39±188.16（13）△	2.53±0.51（13）△	21.02±2.29（5）△
福辛普利钠加 IPoC	1047.61±223.13（13）△▲	2.36±0.96（13）△	17.17±3.12（5）△△▲
XSC 加 IPoC	1043.00±231.50（13）△▲	2.18±0.58（13）△	16.01±3.26（5）△△▲

注：与假手术组比较，*$P < 0.01$；与 I/R 组比较，△$P < 0.01$；与 IPoC 组比较，▲$P < 0.05$，▲▲$P < 0.01$；（ ）内数据为样本数

及 TNF-α 含量（$P < 0.05$，$P < 0.01$）。

表2 各组大鼠心肌 MCP-1 及 TNF-α 水平比较（pg/mg，$\bar{x} \pm s$）

组别	n	MCP-1	TNF-α
假手术	5	12.60±3.68	3.00±0.19
I/R	5	39.27±7.55*	6.55±0.30*
IPoC	5	29.97±2.29△	4.71±0.27△△
福辛普利钠加 IPoC	5	25.50±4.50△△	4.21±0.32△△▲▲
XSC 加 IPoC	5	21.12±8.27△△▲	4.11±0.16△△▲▲

注：与假手术组比较，*$P < 0.01$；与 I/R 组比较，△$P < 0.05$，△△$P < 0.01$；与 IPoC 组比较，▲$P < 0.05$，▲▲$P < 0.01$

2.3 各组大鼠缺血心肌组织炎性细胞的浸润情况比较（表3，图1）及与 MCP-1 的相关性分析（图2）

HE 染色结果显示，与假手术组比较，I/R 组浸润的炎性细胞数显著增加（$P < 0.01$）；与 I/R 组比较，IPoC 组浸润细胞数显著降低（$P < 0.01$）；与 IPoC 组比较，XSC 加 IPoC 组炎性细胞的浸润进一步减少（$P < 0.01$）。对 I/R 组和 IPoC 组两组大鼠心肌 MCP-1 含量与浸润细胞数进行相关性分析，表明两组均呈显著正相关（$r1=0.966$，

$r2=0.998$，$P < 0.01$）。

表3 各组大鼠缺血心肌组织炎性细胞浸润情况比较（$\bar{x} \pm s$）

组别	n	浸润细胞数（个）
假手术	5	7.00±2.73
I/R	5	43.40±11.13*
IPoC	5	24.80±4.44△
福辛普利钠加 IPoC	5	22.60±4.88△
XSC 加 IPoC	5	16.00±3.24△▲

注：与假手术组比较，*$P < 0.01$，与 I/R 组比较，△$P < 0.01$，与 IPoC 组比较，▲$P < 0.05$

3. 讨论

2003 年，Zhao ZQ 等[6] 研究发现，将开胸的犬冠状动脉结扎 60min 后予以重复开通 30s、再结扎 30s，连续 3 次循环，然后恢复冠状动脉血流，结果较未予 IPoC 处理的心脏降低了 40% 的梗死面积，这种机械性辅助治疗方法即 IPoC。本实验研究表明，IPoC 能够减轻 I/R 心肌损伤标志物 CK-MB 和 cTnT 的释放，减小心肌梗死的范围，与既往研究报道[2] 相符。同时本研究也显示芍药胶囊预处理能进一步减小 IPoC 大鼠心肌梗死面积，降低血清 CK-MB 的含量，表明芍药胶囊能更

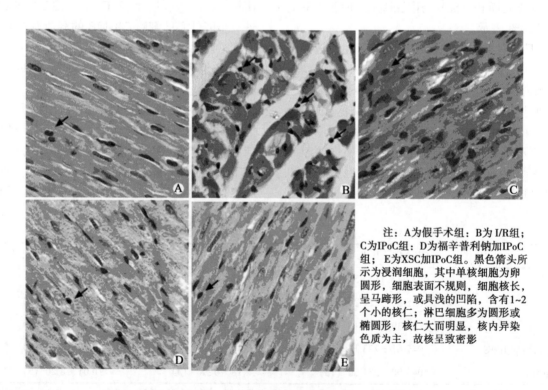

注：A为假手术组；B为I/R组；C为IPoC组；D为福辛普利钠加IPoC组；E为XSC加IPoC组。黑色箭头所示为浸润细胞，其中单核细胞为卵圆形，细胞表面不规则，细胞核长，呈马蹄形，或具浅的凹陷，含有1~2个小的核仁；淋巴细胞多为圆形或椭圆形，核仁大而明显，核内异染色质为主，故核呈致密影

图1 各组大鼠缺血心肌组织浸润细胞数的变化（HE 染色，×400）

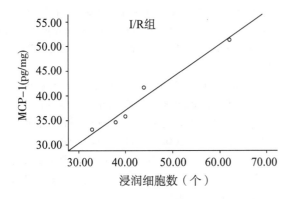

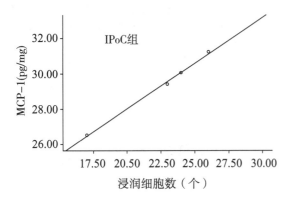

图 2　I/R 组及 IPoC 组大鼠心肌 MCP-1 含量与浸润细胞数的相关性分析

好地保护 IPoC 心肌免于 I/R 的损伤。

MCP-1 是趋化因子家族成员之一，心肌缺血再灌注时 MCP-1 表达增加，趋化和激活单核 / 巨噬细胞、T 淋巴细胞、嗜碱性粒细胞和自然杀伤细胞等免疫细胞，引发一系列的炎症反应，加重心肌的损伤。有研究表明，将 MCP-1 特异性受体 CC 类趋化因子受体（CCR2）基因敲除后，小鼠缺血再灌注心肌炎性细胞浸润显著降低，心肌梗死面积缩小[7]。同样，转染家兔 MCP-1 抑制剂 7ND 基因抑制 MCP-1 活性后，再建立心肌 I/R 损伤家兔模型，结果显示心肌炎性细胞浸润减少，促炎性细胞因子 TNF-α 和 IL-1β 水平降低，家兔心脏功能明显改善，表明抑制 MCP-1 活性是保护 I/R 心肌的重要环节之一[5]。本实验研究观察缺血再灌注后心肌中浸润细胞，主要以淋巴细胞和单核 / 巨噬细胞为主，且随着 MCP-1 表达增加，炎性细胞的浸润也明显增加。给予 IPoC 干预后，MCP-1 含量和炎性细胞浸润均显著降低。相关性分析显示，两者呈显著正相关，表明在缺血再灌注过程中心肌中炎性细胞浸润与 MCP-1 水平密切相关。

Herskowits A 等[8] 和 Formigli L 等[9] 研究表明，I/R 损伤中浸润的单核 / 巨噬细胞是心肌组织内炎性细胞因子的主要来源，促炎性细胞因子 TNF-α 主要由单核 / 巨噬细胞产生，在再灌注早期即大量表达，血管内皮细胞、血管平滑肌细胞和心肌细胞在再灌注损伤后也产生 TNF-α，大量产生的 TNF-α 可抑制心肌收缩力和加速缺血心肌细胞的凋亡[10]。同时，TNF-α 可以启动激活转录因子 NF-kappaB 的信号通路，使单核 / 巨噬细胞进一步激活，并分泌包括 TNF-α 在内的多种促炎性细胞因子，引发细胞因子级联反应，导致炎症反应的扩大。本实验研究显示，IPoC 能够降低心肌组织 MCP-1 和 TNF-α 含量，这可能是其保护 I/R 损伤心肌的机制之一。IPoC 基础上应用芎芍胶囊干预能进一步降低心肌组织 MCP-1、TNF-α 水平和炎性细胞浸润，表明芎芍胶囊增加 IPoC 对 I/R 心肌的保护作用与抑制缺血再灌注心肌 MCP-1、TNF-α 含量和炎性细胞浸润有关。

芎芍胶囊是在传统活血化瘀代表方剂血府逐瘀汤的基础上，采用其主要药物川芎、赤芍的有效部位川芎总酚和赤芍总苷制成。现代药理研究表明，川芎和赤芍具有扩张冠状动脉、改善心肌缺血缺氧、抑制血小板聚集及血栓形成、减弱氧化应激和炎症反应等作用[11-13]。本实验研究显示芎芍胶囊能更好地保护 IPoC 心肌免于 I/R 的损伤，这为血运重建时代应用活血化瘀药物治疗急性心肌梗死提供了实验依据。

参考文献

[1] Thibault H, Piot C, Staat P, et al. Long-term benefit of postconditioning. Circulation, 2008, 117 (8): 1037-1044.

[2] Dow J, Bhandari A, Kloner RA. The mechanism by which ischemic postconditioning reduces reperfusion arrhythmias in rats remains elusive. J Cardiovasc Pharmacol Ther, 2009, 14 (2): 99-103.

[3] 徐凤芹，陈可远，马晓昌，等. 芎芍胶囊治疗冠心病心绞痛的临床观察. 中国中西医结合杂志，2003，23（1）：16-18.

[4] 徐浩，文川，陈可冀，等. 川芎、赤芍及其有效部位配伍对载脂蛋白 E 基因缺陷小鼠动脉粥样硬化斑块稳定性影响的研究. 中国中西医结合杂志，2007，27（6）：513-518.

[5] Kajihara N, Morita S, Nishida T, et al. Transfection with a dominant-negative inhibitor of monocyte chemoattractant protein-1 gene improves cardiac

function after 6 hours of cold preservation. Circulation, 2003, 108 (Suppl 1): Ⅱ 213- Ⅱ 218.

[6] Zhao ZQ, Corvera JS, Halkos ME, et al. Inhibition of myocardial injury by ischemic postconditioning during reperfusion: comparison with ischemic preconditioning. Am J Physiol Heart Circ Physiol, 2003, 285 (2): H579-H588.

[7] Hayasaki T, Kaikita K, Okuma T, et al. CC chemokine receptor-2 deficiency attenuates oxidative stress and infarct size caused by myocardial ischemia-reperfusion in mice. Circ J, 2006, 70 (3): 342-351.

[8] Herskowits A, Choi S, Ansari AA, et al. Cytokine mRNA expression in postischemic /reperfused myocardium. Am J Pathol, 1995, 146 (2): 419-428.

[9] Formigli L, Manneschi LI, Nediani C, et al. Are macrophages involved in early myocardial reperfusion injury? Ann Thorac Surg, 2001, 71 (5): 1596-1602.

[10] Frangogiannis NG. The immune system and cardiac repair. Pharmacol Res, 2008, 58 (2): 88-111.

[11] 王艳萍，李文兰，范玉奇. 川芎嗪药理作用的研究进展. 药品评价，2006，3（2）：144-146.

[12] 梁日欣，肖永庆，高伟. 川芎内酯A预处理对大鼠离体心脏缺血再灌注损伤的保护作用. 中药药理与临床，2004，20（6）：1-3.

[13] 阮金兰，赵钟祥，曾庆忠，等. 赤芍化学成分和药理作用的研究进展. 中国药理学通报，2003，19（9）：965-970.

益气养阴活血配伍对缺血心肌差异基因表达的影响 *

殷惠军　郭春雨　史大卓

第四章

急性心肌梗死（acute myocardial infarction，AMI）引起的心肌缺血过程存在着心肌细胞的能量代谢障碍[1]，虽然 AMI 发生的确切病理机制尚有待进一步的阐明，但大量研究证明，由心肌细胞急性缺血、缺氧引发的心肌能量耗竭是多种原因诱导引起 AMI 心肌损伤的共同基础。深入研究缺血心肌能量代谢改变的分子机制，并干预这些机制中的分子靶点，成为世界范围内心血管基础和临床研究领域关注的焦点。

缺血、缺氧引起心肌收缩功能减退、能量储备下降等，表现为心前疼痛、乏力、气短等，符合中医气虚血瘀特点，益气养阴活血治法是目前中医临床治疗 AMI 的主要方法。多项研究证明，采用益气养阴、活血及其配伍结合西医常规治疗 AMI，可明显减少 AMI 患者住院死亡率及并发症发生率[2]。心悦胶囊（西洋参茎叶总皂苷）具有益气阴之效，是目前国内治疗冠心病的有效中药。本课题组前期研究显示，心悦胶囊可改善心肌缺血、调整糖脂代谢、促进缺血心肌血管新生[3]。丹参片是目前国内治疗冠心病最为普及的活血化瘀制剂。大量研究表明，该药可以改善心肌缺血、扩张冠状动脉，对 AMI 后左心室重构亦有一定作用，与心悦胶囊有机结合可充分体现传统中医益气养阴活血治法。

本课题组前期应用长标签基因表达系列分析（Long SAGE）方法，构建了 AMI 后大鼠缺血心肌基因差异表达谱。对其进行生物信息学分析后发现，以正常心肌 LongSAGE 谱为对照，得到缺血心肌组织显著性差异基因 142 个（$P < 0.05$），其中大部分差异基因在缺血心肌组织特异性表达，有 20 个基因与氧化磷酸化、ATP 合成、糖酵解 / 糖异生等能量代谢通路相关，提示 AMI 发生后能量代谢相关基因表达调控的改变是诱发缺血心肌损伤的一个主要原因[4]。

益气养阴、活血及其配伍治法是否通过调控能量相关靶基因来发挥促进心肌血供，保护存活心肌的作用？其作用机制如何呢？由此，本研究选取线粒体氧化磷酸化作为目标通路，以表达差异较大的通路关键基因细胞色素 C 氧化酶 5a （Cox5a）

* 原载于《科学通报》，2009，54（16）：2325-2328

和 ATP 合酶 5e（ATP5e）基因为目标基因，观察益气养阴、活血及其配伍中药对 2 个基因 mRNA 表达和蛋白酶活性的影响，为益气养阴、活血及其配伍治疗 AMI 提供分子生物学依据。

1. 材料和方法

1.1 材料

健康 Wistar 大鼠 140 只，雄性，体重（160±20）g，清洁级，由北京维通利华实验动物技术公司提供，经适应性喂养 1 周后开始实验。倍他乐克（酒石酸美托洛尔）由阿斯利康制药有限公司生产，规格每片 25mg，批号 0707012；心悦胶囊由吉林省集安益盛药业公司生产，每粒含西洋参茎叶总皂苷 50mg，批号 Z20030073；复方丹参片由广州白云山中药厂生产，每粒含丹参酮 Ⅱ A0.44mg，丹参素 193mg，批号 030435；荧光定量 PCR（real time fluorescence quantitative PCR，Q-PCR）试剂盒购自 BioEasy 公司；细胞色素 C 氧化酶（CCO）及 ATP 合成酶（ATPase）活性试剂盒购自美国 GENMED 公司。

1.2 动物模型建立

参照文献[5]建立大鼠 AMI 模型：钝性分离肌肉，打开胸腔，轻挤出心脏，在肺动脉圆锥与左心耳交界处下 1～2mm 用无创手术线结扎左冠状动脉前降支，以结扎部位下心肌组织变白和体表心电图肢体 Ⅱ 导联出现 ST 段弓背向上抬高，持续半小时以上为模型成功的标志。假手术组开胸后，在造模对等位置只穿线不结扎。

1.3 实验分组及给药

造模成功后，将大鼠随机分为 7 组，术后第 2 日开始灌胃给药，药物剂量换算依 70kg/d 用量，换算出大鼠的日用量，制成一定浓度水溶液灌胃。分组及给药情况见表 1。

表 1 实验分组及给药情况

分组	给药 [n = 20，20mL/（kg·d）]
正常对照组	常规饲养
假手术组	常规饲养
模型对照组	常规饲养
美托洛尔组	美托洛尔水溶液
益气养阴组	心悦胶囊水溶液
活血组	复方丹参片水溶液
益气养阴活血组	心悦胶囊和丹参片水溶液

1.4 样本的取得、分离、制备

以上各组大鼠分别于手术 7d 后麻醉剪开胸腔，迅速取出心脏，截取左室游离壁和心尖部，生理盐水冲洗后，一部分以 10% 甲醛溶液固定，一部分 –80℃ 保存备用。

1.5 病理切片观察

心肌组织由 10% 甲醛溶液固定后，进行常规切片、染色、脱水、包埋等处理，用 i50 型 Nikon 光学显微镜观察组织学病理改变。

1.6 *Cox5a* 及 *ATP5e* 相对表达量检测

将各组心肌组织制备成 10% 的组织匀浆，按照 Trizol 试剂（美国 Invitrogen 公司）操作说明，一步法提取总 RNA。分别将各组组织总 RNA 充分混合，各取 200μg 进行纯度鉴定。甲醛变性琼脂糖凝胶电泳鉴定 RNA 的完整性，紫外分光法确定 RNA 的量和纯度。利用 Q-PCR 技术检测 2 个差异基因在各组总 RNA 混合样品中的相对表达量。以 *β-actin* 作为内参基因，每个基因重复 3 次实验。

1.7 CCO 及 ATPase 活性检测

将心肌组织制备成 10% 的组织匀浆，应用 GENMED 试剂盒提取组织线粒体并定量蛋白含量。利用化学比色法，参照 GENMED 公司试剂盒说明书，波长在 550nm 处，并设置 0s 和 60s 各测读 1 次，分别记为 *A1* 和 *A2*，$\Delta A = A1 - A2$。CCO 比色活性（U/mg）=（ΔA 样品 $-\Delta A$ 背景）/[取样量中线粒体蛋白毫克数 ×21.84（毫摩尔吸光系数）]。ATPase 活性检测方法同 CCO。

1.8 统计方法

采用 SPSS 13.0 软件进行统计分析，所有数据用均数 ± 标准差（$\bar{x} \pm s$）表示，计量资料用单因素方差分析，组间比较用 q 检验，$P < 0.05$ 认为有统计学意义。

2. 结果

2.1 各组大鼠心肌组织病理形态学观察

HE 染色后，光学显微镜下观察心肌组织。与空白对照组相比，其他各组可见缺血区心肌肿胀、炎症细胞浸润，部分心肌细胞出现空泡样变性，细胞溶解，梗死的心肌可见纤维化等病理改变，以模型组表现最为明显。各用药组的损伤程度介于空白组与模型组之间。具体见图 1。

2.2 目标差异基因 mRNA 表达检测结果

应用 Q-PCR 技术检测 *COX5a*、*ATP5e* mRNA

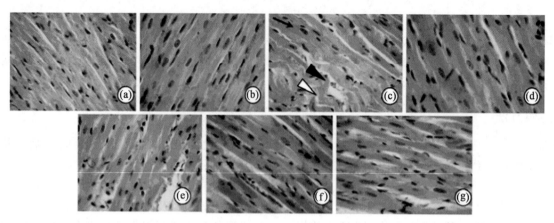

图1　各组大鼠心肌组织病理切片光学显微镜照片（×400）

（a）正常对照组；（b）假手术组；（c）模型组；（d）美托洛尔组；（e）活血组；（f）益气养阴组；（g）益气养阴活血组。以模型组病理切片为例，→，心肌细胞；▲，炎性细胞等浸润；▽，屈曲变形的心肌纤维

的相对表达丰度。检测结果进行标准曲线分析，得出 C_t 值，计算 2 个目标基因的 C_t 值与 *β-actin* 的 C_t 值的差值 $\triangle C_t$，以 $2^{-\triangle Ct}$ 作为 *Cox5a* 及 *ATP5e* mRNA 的相对含量。然后以正常组作为对照样品，以 $2^{-\triangle\triangle Ct}$ 为各处理组样品中检测到的相对基因表达量 [6,7]。*COX5a*、*ATP5e* 基因表达结果见表 2。与正常组相比，模型组、假手术组及各药物组基因表达出现明显下调趋势，其中以模型组下调最显著；与模型组比较，各个用药组目标基因 mRNA 均出现明显上调趋势，其中以益气养阴活血组基因上调较为明显。

表2　样品中 *COX5a*、*ATP5e* 基因表达量比较（ $2^{-\triangle\triangle C_t}$ ）

分组	COX5a	ATP5e
正常对照组	1	1
假手术组	0.88	0.75
模型对照组	0.26	0.56
美托洛尔组	0.95	0.62
活血化瘀组	0.80	0.63
益气养阴组	0.78	0.72
益气养阴活血组	0.92	0.91

2.3　目标基因翻译蛋白酶活性检测结果

应用试剂盒进行细胞色素 C 氧化酶、ATP 合酶活性检测。与正常组相比，各用药组 CCO 酶活性均未见显著性差异。从检测的数值趋势发现，模型组、假手术组 CCO 活性有所下降，其中以模型组下降最明显。与模型组相比，ATPase 酶活性在正常组和益气养阴活血组出现显著下降（ $P < 0.05$ ），具体见表 3。

表3　样品中 CCO、ATPase 酶活性比较（单位：U/mg）

分组	n	CCO	ATPase[a]
正常对照组	20	1.15±0.26	2.16±0.42*
假手术组	20	0.83±0.40	1.88±0.37
模型对照组	20	0.81±0.33	1.25±0.23
美托洛尔组	20	1.18±0.22	1.49±0.36
活血化瘀组	20	0.90±0.24	1.54±0.41
益气养阴组	20	0.89±0.22	1.90±0.45
益气养阴活血组	20	1.00±0.31	2.12±0.34*

a)*，与模型组比较， $P < 0.05$

3.　讨论

AMI 是严重危害人类健康的重大疾病之一，具有发病率和死亡率高的特点。能量的耗竭是 AMI 引起的心肌组织最初和最直接损伤的原因。目前认为线粒体是缺血性损害的亚细胞目标，线粒体功能障碍是导致心肌组织缺血、损伤和坏死的主要原因，同时也是启动细胞凋亡的关键因素 [8,9]。*COX5a* 和 *ATP5e* 是存在于线粒体氧化磷酸化通路上的显著差异基因，它们的表达量及酶活性变化直接影响整个呼吸链的功能发挥。有研究报道，*COX5a* 的转录水平与凋亡机制的启动密切相关，在小鼠卵母细胞中应用 RNA 干扰（RNA interference，RNAi）技术使 *COX5a* 等 3 个 CCO 亚基基因表达沉默，能够导致细胞内 Caspase-3 等凋亡前因子水平升高，促使大量细胞凋亡 [10,11]。ATPase 是线粒体进行氧化磷酸化合成和水解 ATP 的关键酶，在能量代谢中有至关重要的作用。发生 AMI 时，为了满足缺血心肌对能量的需要，线粒体 ATPase 活性应激性升高，以产生更多的 ATP，维持心肌能量的供需平衡[12,13]。有学者对酵母中的 ATP5 亚基功能进行研究，结果提示 ATP5 亚基是构成 ATPase 的关键部分，ATP5 翻译蛋白能固定在线粒体内膜 N 端，以稳定 ATPase 的二聚结构，从而发挥影响 ATPase 表达的作用[14]。

既往研究表明，西洋参茎叶总皂苷和丹参酮具有促进心肌血管新生、抗氧化损伤、增加氧供的心肌保护作用[15,16]。本研究将益气养阴药物西洋参茎叶总皂苷制剂和活血化瘀常用药物丹参制剂有机配伍治疗 AMI 模型大鼠。结果显示，与正常组相比，COX5a 基因的表达与 CCO 酶活性在模型组明显下调。AMI 后，缺血心肌 COX5a 表达发生下调，使其翻译蛋白 CCO 活性降低，引发了部分缺血心肌细胞凋亡机制的启动。与模型组比较，各个用药组 COX5a 基因的表达及 CCO 酶活性均有所上调，其中以美托洛尔组和益气养阴活血组上调最为明显。同时，研究发现，在 AMI 后缺血心肌中，ATP5e 基因的表达和 ATPase 酶活性均发生了下调，其中 ATPase 酶活性出现显著下降（$P < 0.05$），表明益气养阴活血配伍能够通过降低线粒体 ATPase 活性的应激性升高，减轻心肌氧化应激损伤，进一步抑制细胞凋亡。综上所述，西洋参茎叶总皂苷和丹参酮可能通过提升 CCO 及 ATPase mRNA 及蛋白活性，增加 ATP 生成的速率，减少无氧酵解和乳酸产生，抑制钙离子超载，最终达到促进缺血心肌供能、减轻氧化应激损伤的目的，其效果比单纯应用益气养阴或活血化瘀中药更加显著。

目前，AMI 的治疗在血运重建、强化降脂和抗血小板活性等方面取得了较大进展，但如何改善 AMI 后心肌组织能量代谢障碍一直没有理想的治疗对策。本研究通过能量代谢相关基因的研究，为靶向性干预缺血心肌能量代谢变化提供了一定的实验依据。同时，为大规模筛选抗心肌损伤的药物建立了一个初步的基因水平技术平台。

参考文献

[1] Wolff AA, Rotmensch HH, Stanley WC, et al. Metabolic approaches to the treatment of ischemic heart disease: the clinicians' perspective. Heart Fail Rev, 2002, 7: 187-203.

[2] 汤益明，杨宁. 从冠心病中医防治的若干进展探讨结合点. 中国中西医结合杂志，2002，22：863-865.

[3] 邵南齐，朱萱萱. 心肌缺氧缺血的药理学研究进展. 实用中医内科杂志，2007，21：3-4.

[4] 郭春雨，殷惠军，蒋跃绒，等. 梗死后大鼠缺血心肌基因差异表达谱构建. 科学通报，2008，53：1657-1663.

[5] 张润峰，王继生. 建立大鼠心肌梗死模型的若干问题探讨. 山西医科大学学报，2004，35：13-15.

[6] Livak KJ, Schmittgen TD. Analysis of relative gene expression data using real-time quantitative PCR and the 2 (-Delta Delta C (T)). Methods, 2001, 25:402-408.

[7] Arocho A, Chen B, Ladanyi M. Validation of the 2-DeltaDelta Ct calculation as an alternate method of data analysis for quantitative PCR of BCR-ABL P210 transcripts. Diagn Mol Pathol, 2006, 15: 56-61.

[8] Zhang J, Liem DA, Mueller M, et al. Altered proteome biology of cardiac mitochondria under stress conditions. J Proteome Res, 2008, 7: 2204-2214.

[9] Sammut IA, Burton K, Balogun E, et al. Time-dependent impairment of mitochondrial function after storage and transplantation of rabbit kidneys. Transplantation, 2000, 69: 1265-1275.

[10] 张铭，周胜华. 心肌缺血的能量代谢障碍治疗进展. 心脏杂志，2006，18：467-469.

[11] Lee SD, Kuo WW, Lin JA, et al. Effects of long-term intermittent hypoxia on mitochondrial and Fas death receptor dependent apoptotic pathways in rat hearts. Int J Cardiol, 2007, 116: 348-356.

[12] Cui XS, Li XY, Jeong YJ, et al. Gene expression of Cox5a, 5b, or 6b1 and their roles in preimplantation mouse embryos. Biol Reprod, 2006, 74: 601-610.

[13] Weinberg JM, Venkatachalam MA, Roeser NF, et al. Mitochondrial dysfunction during hypoxia/reoxygenation and its correction by anaerobic metabolism of citric acid cycle intermediates. Proc Natl Acad Sci USA, 2000, 97: 2826-2831.

[14] 梁晚益，唐立新，杨宗城，等. 大鼠严重烧伤早期心肌线粒体 F0F1-ATPase 活性变化及其对能量代谢的影响. 第三军医大学学报，2001，23：780-782.

[15] 殷惠军，张颖，杨领海，等. 西洋参茎叶总皂苷对胰岛素抵抗脂肪细胞葡萄糖转运、GLUT-4 转位和 CAP 基因表达的影响. 中国药理学通报，2007，23：1332-1337.

[16] 殷惠军，张颖，蒋跃绒，等. 西洋参叶总皂苷对急性心肌梗死大鼠心肌细胞凋亡及凋亡相关基因表达的影响. 中国中西医结合杂志，2005，25：232-235.

第四章

莪术组分涂层支架预防猪冠状动脉再狭窄的研究 *

赵福海　刘剑刚　王　欣　张大武　王培利　张　蕾　杜建鹏　史大卓

药物洗脱支架主要通过抑制内膜增生，降低支架内再狭窄的发生，进而减少以靶病变血运重建为主的不良心脏事件。然而，无论是西罗莫司（雷帕霉素）还是紫杉醇药物洗脱支架，都有发生晚期支架内血栓的风险。研究显示，中药莪术的提取物有抑制血管平滑肌细胞迁移、增殖以及抑制二磷酸腺苷诱导的血小板聚集作用[1]。以金属裸支架（BMS）为平台，以高分子聚合物材料为载体，制成莪术组分中药涂层支架（ZES），但其具体作用如何，目前鲜见报道。我们以实验用球囊损伤小型猪为模型，旨在观察 ZES 的体内生物学特性。

1. 材料与方法

1.1 实验动物与分组

采用普通级中华实验用小型猪 18 头，由中国农业大学动物科技推广中心提供，雌雄不限，体重 25 ~ 30kg，随机分为 ZES 组、雷帕霉素涂层支架组（SES 组）和 BMS 组，每组 6 头。

1.2 ZES 制备

以 316L 不锈钢 BMS 为基体，表面涂覆莪术组分和高分子载体混合涂层，将支架预装在快速交换型球囊导管上组成。所有支架长度为 15mm，直径 2.5 ~ 3.0mm，采用 ^{60}Co 辐照灭菌。ZES 和 SES 均采用高分子材料涂层控制药物释放，所有支架均由乐普医疗器械公司制备和提供。

1.3 实验过程

术前 3d 开始给予阿司匹林 300mg/d、氯吡格雷 50mg/d。建立静脉通路，称重后，采用肌内注射戊巴比妥 0.5mg/kg 及氯胺酮 10mg/kg 静脉注射复合麻醉。冠状动脉造影以 Seldinger 法穿刺猪股动脉并置入 6F 动脉鞘，经鞘管给予肝素 200U/kg，行选择性冠状动脉造影。置入支架直径与靶血管直径比为 1.2：1，分别在左前降支、左回旋支及右冠状动脉置入同一种支架各 1 枚。如左回旋支直径较小，则将 2 枚支架置入右冠状动脉内，术中连续心电监护。术后单笼普通谷物饲料喂养观察，

给予阿司匹林 100mg/d、氯吡格雷 50mg/d，直至处死。

1.4 标本制备

处死小型猪后，立即开胸取出心脏，将心脏放入含 25 000U 肝素、60mg 罂粟碱的 1000mL 生理盐水中，从升主动脉伸入 7F 扩张管分别至左、右冠状动脉开口，用该液冲洗冠状动脉 3 ~ 4 次。将游离的心脏经升主动脉伸入 7F 扩张管至左心室。用止血钳封扎心脏各出口，压力监测下用加压装置以 100mmHg（1mmHg=0.133kPa）的压力连续灌注 15min。分离左前降支、左回旋支、右冠状动脉支架置入处血管段，取材标本包括支架以及支架两侧 5mm 内区域。近段标本经 2.5% 戊二醛固定 24h 后，用 1/15 mol/L 磷酸缓冲液冲洗 3 次，用 1% 锇酸固定 2h，分别用 30%、50%、70%、90% 乙醇和 90% 乙醇丙酮各脱水 10min，脱水后行电镜观察。远段标本经 10% 中性缓冲甲醛加压灌注固定 24h 后，行塑料包埋后，制成 5μm 厚的连续切片，常规 HE 染色后行光镜观察。

1.5 病理观察分析

（1）切片用 HE 染色后，用 LEIKA DFC300 FX 光学显微镜观察支架段血管炎症、血栓、内膜增殖情况。（2）血管壁炎性反应采用炎症积分：0 分，无炎性细胞；1 分，散在炎性细胞；2 分，25% ~ 50% 血管周径内的支架点被炎性细胞包绕 50%；3 分，25% ~ 50% 血管周径内的支架点被炎性细胞完全包绕。（3）血管壁损伤程度应用损伤积分：0 分，内弹力膜完整；1 分，内弹力膜损伤；2 分，内弹力膜和中膜损伤；3 分，外弹力膜损伤。（4）内皮化积分：1 分，25% 管腔表面有内皮覆盖；2 分，25% ~ 75% 管腔表面有内皮覆盖；3 分，> 75% 管腔表面有内皮覆盖[2-3]。（5）采用 lightlab 光学相干断层成像（optical coherence tomography，OCT）系统进行血管内扫描成像，测量血管腔和血管外膜直径，计算直径狭窄率和面积狭窄率，定性评价支架内皮修复和支架内血栓。

* 原载于《中华老年心血管病杂志》，2012，14（6）：859-862

1.6　统计学方法

采用 SPSS 13.0 统计软件，所有计量数据采用 $\bar{\chi} \pm s$ 表示，计量资料组间比较采用 ANOVA 分析，计数资料采用中位数或百分位数表示，计数资料采用 χ^2 检验，$P < 0.05$ 为差异有统计学意义。

2.　结果

2.1　各组 OCT 形态学比较

30d 时，与 BMS 组比较，ZES 组和 SES 组平均管腔直径、平均管腔面积明显增大（$P < 0.05$）；直径狭窄率、面积狭窄率明显减小（$P < 0.05$）。ZES 组与 SES 组各项指标比较，差异无统计学意义（$P > 0.05$，表1）。

表 1　各组 OCT 形态学比较（$\bar{\chi} \pm s$）

项目	ZES 组 （6 头）	SES 组 （6 头）	BMS 组 （6 头）
参考血管直径 （mm）	2.38 ± 0.25	2.39 ± 0.24	2.36 ± 0.31
平均管腔直径 （mm）	2.00 ± 0.41[a]	1.93 ± 0.38[a]	1.43 ± 0.31
平均外膜直径 （mm）	2.61 ± 0.32	2.54 ± 0.19	2.60 ± 0.16
直径狭窄率 （%）	21.42 ± 22.31[a]	24.51 ± 12.93[a]	43.21 ± 14.03
平均管腔面积 （mm²）	2.94 ± 1.13[a]	2.85 ± 0.88[a]	1.92 ± 0.63
平均外膜面积 （mm²）	4.79 ± 1.39	4.87 ± 0.71	5.01 ± 0.56
面积狭窄率 （%）	27.73 ± 23.95[a]	26.83 ± 16.81[a]	47.12 ± 15.18

注：与 BMS 组比较，[a]$P < 0.05$

2.2　各组组织病理学比较

30d 时，光镜及 OCT 观察显示，ZES 组和 BMS 组内膜均有不同程度增生，以 BMS 组支架内膜增生明显，未见内膜下出血及附壁血栓形成，无动脉瘤形成及血管正性重构。OCT 显示，SES 组可见部分支架横梁裸露在血管腔。扫描电镜显示，ZES 组和 BMS 组内皮覆盖完整，未见血栓形成及白细胞、嗜酸性粒细胞聚集。SES 组可见部分支架横梁无内皮覆盖，并有白细胞、嗜酸性粒细胞和少量淋巴细胞聚集（图 1 ~ 3）。

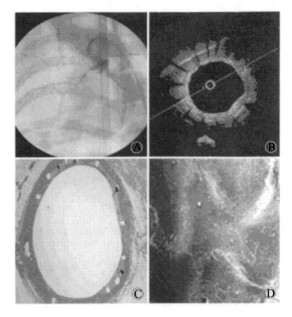

图 1　电镜（×50）、光镜（低倍）和 OCT 显示 ZES 组内皮覆盖完整，未见明显内膜增生

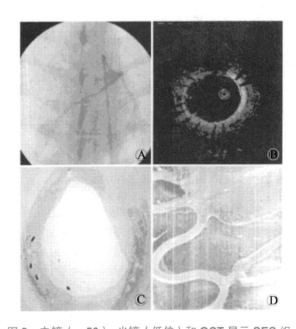

图 2　电镜（×50）、光镜（低倍）和 OCT 显示 SES 组部分内皮化不全

2.3　各组 30d 各项积分比较

30d 时，与 SES 组比较，ZES 组和 BMS 组炎症积分明显降低，内皮化积分明显升高（$P < 0.05$）。3 组损伤积分比较，差异无统计学意义（$P > 0.05$，表 2，图 4）。

3.　讨论

本研究表明，30d 观察时，ZES 组不但具有

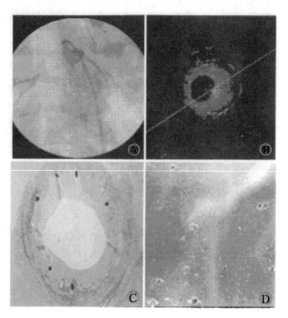

图3 电镜（×50）、光镜（低倍）和 OCT 显示 BMS 组内膜明显增生

表2 各组 30d 各项积分比较（$\bar{x}\pm s$，n=12）

项目	ZES 组	SES 组	BMS 组
炎症积分	0.93±0.41[a]	1.23±0.82	1.01±0.41[a]
损伤积分	2.36±0.63	2.33±0.52	2.19±0.75
内皮化积分	3.00±0.00[a]	2.69±0.42	3.00±0.00[a]

注：与 SES 组比较，[a]$P < 0.05$

第四章

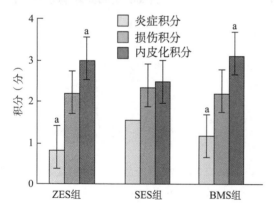

图4 各组 30d 时各项积分比较
注：与 SES 组比较，[a]$P < 0.05$

明显抑制内膜增生的作用，而且能促进内皮愈合，未见明显的支架内血栓事件。

莪术为姜科植物蓬莪术、广西莪术和温郁金的干燥根茎。其有效成分主要有莪术二酮、莪术醇、β 榄香烯、α 蒎烯、樟烯、姜黄素等[4]。研究表明，莪术对 L615 白血病细胞有直接细胞毒作用，可致肿瘤细胞变性坏死。体外可明显抑制小鼠 CT26 结肠癌细胞生长，其浓度与细胞生长抑制率呈正比，且可抑制 S180 肉瘤瘤体内血管内皮生长因子、碱性成纤维细胞生长因子的表达[5-6]。本研究以 BMS 为平台，以高分子聚合物材料为载体制成 ZES。30d 的组织形态学分析结果表明，ZES 组和 BMS 组可明显减少晚期管腔丢失，表现出良好的抑制内膜增生的作用，其抑制新生内膜增殖的作用与 SES 相似。动物研究也显示，莪术具有抑制细胞生长和诱导细胞凋亡、抗炎、抗血栓形成、抑制球囊损伤后血管内膜增生和胶原合成等作用，可干预球囊扩张后血管内膜增生多个病理环节[7-8]。该研究结果与我们的研究结果相似，具体机制还需进一步深入研究。

无论是 SES，还是紫杉醇药物洗脱支架，临床试验皆观察到置入后支架节段内皮化延迟，甚至出现晚期支架内血栓的发生，有可能导致死亡、心肌梗死等严重后果。Cook 等[9]研究发现，发生极晚期支架内血栓的患者，血栓抽吸和血管内超声有 73% 的患者有血管壁正性重构、支架贴壁不全、内皮化不全，且有白细胞和嗜酸性粒细胞浸润。一项包括 12 374 例患者的注册研究显示，药物洗脱支架发生极晚期支架风险明显高于 BMS（RR=2.89，95% CI：1.48～5.65），表明 DES 有增加晚期支架内血栓的风险。其血栓形成机制可能与血管内皮化延迟或缺乏内皮化，血管壁对聚合物的超敏反应有关，但现有动物研究结果并不完全支持这一论点[10-13]。

本研究结果发现，支架置入后 30d 时，无论 OCT、病理、电镜扫描均可见 ZES 支架内皮覆盖完整，未见明显炎性细胞浸润，未见支架内血栓形成及血管正性重构，提示 ZES 有促进内皮愈合的作用。动物实验表明，莪术醇具有抑制血管平滑肌细胞迁移和增殖作用，莪术二酮有抑制二磷酸腺苷诱导的血小板聚集作用[1, 14]。ZES 可能是通过抑制二磷酸腺苷诱导的血小板聚集，降低了支架内血栓事件的发生。

本研究尽管采用了球囊扩张的小型猪冠状动脉模型，与小型动物如大鼠、家兔等相比有一定的优势，但仍存在一定的局限性：（1）本研究应用球囊扩张再狭窄冠状动脉模型，其新生内膜增殖的机制不完全等同于冠状动脉粥样硬化过程，因此，该动物模型无法真正模拟人体冠状动脉病变。（2）研究中使用高分子聚合物材料作为药物载体，是否会出现人冠状动脉支架置入后，极晚期由于对聚合物高敏反应而发生的管壁正性重构甚至动脉瘤现象，仍需要研究证实。（3）研究周期较短，需观察更长时间有无发生支架内血栓的风险。

虽然存在上述局限性，但 ZES 支架在置入后 30d 时表现出显著抑制血管内膜增殖的作用，同时表现出良好的体内生物学相容性，值得进一步研究，以为临床应用提供可靠的依据。

参考文献

[1] 夏泉，董婷霞，詹华强，等. 莪术二酮对 ADP 诱导的兔血小板聚集的抑制作用. 中国药理学通报，2006，22：1151-1152.

[2] Schwartz RS, Huber KC, Murphy JG, et al. Restenosis and the proportional neointimal response to coronary artery injury: results in a porcine model. J Am Coll Cardiol, 1992, 19: 275-277.

[3] Suzuki T, Kopia G, Hayashi S, et al. Stent-based delivery of sirolimus reduces neointimal formation in a porcine coronary model. Circulation, 2001, 104: 1183-1193.

[4] 王琰，王慕邹. 莪术的质量研究. 药学学报，2001，36：849-853.

[5] 李传伟，徐英萍，苗芳，等. 莪术油抗小鼠结肠癌效应的实验研究. 泰山医学院学报，2005，26：89-91.

[6] 施广霞，于丽华，刘金友，等. β-榄香烯抗肿瘤作用的实验研究 I：β-榄香烯体外对 L615 白血病细胞直接作用的实验研究. 大连医学院学报，1994，16：137-139.

[7] 赵军礼，孙宝贵，温沁竹，等. 莪术油洗脱支架防治犬冠状动脉支架术后再狭窄的实验研究. 中国中西医结合杂志，2008，28：326-329.

[8] Jang HS, Nam HY, Kim JM, et al. Effects of curcumin for preventing restenosis in a hyperchole-sterolemic rabbit iliac artery stent model. Catheter Cardiovasc Interv, 2009, 74: 881-888.

[9] Cook S, Ladich E, Nakazawa G, et al. Correlation of intravascular ultrasound findings with histopathological analysis of thrombus aspirates in patients with very late drug-eluting stent thrombosis. Circulation, 2009, 120: 391-399.

[10] Jensen LO, Tilsted HH, Thayssen P, et al. Paclitaxel and sirolimus eluting stents versus bare metal stents: long-term risk of stent thrombosis and other outcomes. From the Western Denmark Heart Registry. Euro Intervention, 2010, 5: 898-905.

[11] Chin-Quee SL, Hsu SH, Nguyen-Ehrenreich KL, et al. Endothelial cell recovery, acute thrombogenicity, and monocyte adhesion and activation on fluorinated copolymer and phosphorylcholine polymer stent coatings. Biomaterials, 2010, 31: 648-657.

[12] Kang KW, Ko YG, Shin DH, et al. Impact of positive persistent vascular remodeling after sirolimus-eluting and paclitaxel-eluting stent implantation on 5-year clinical outcomes. Circ J, 2012, 76: 1102-1108.

[13] Rober L, Magro M, Stefanini GG, et al. Very late coronary stent thrombosis of a newer-generation everdlimus-eluting stent compared with early-generation drug-eluting stents: a prospective cohort study. Circulation, 2012, 125: 1110-1121.

[14] Mayanglambam A, Dangelmaier CA, Thomas D, et al. Curcumin inhibits GPVI-mediated platelet activation by interfering with the kinase activity of Syk and the subsequent activation of PLC gamma 2. Platelets, 2010, 21: 211-220.

福辛普利钠预处理结合缺血后适应保护大鼠心肌缺血/再灌注损伤的研究[*]

张大武　张蕾　刘剑刚　王承龙　史大卓　陈可冀

　　尽早给予急性心肌梗死患者再灌注治是挽救濒死心肌、恢复心脏功能最为有效的治疗方法，但再灌注损伤却减弱了早期再灌注带来的益处。再灌注损伤的诸多因素如活性氧产生、多形核中性粒

* 原载于《中华心血管病杂志》，2010，38（7）：633-637

细胞聚集、钙超载和血管内皮功能受损等，在再灌注开始几分钟内即可发生，导致严重的心肌组织损伤和功能障碍。2003年，Zhao等[1]提出了缺血后适应（ischemic postconditioning，IPoC）的概念，研究发现结扎犬冠状动脉前降支60分钟，恢复持续冠状动脉血流灌注前给予反复几次短暂缺血可明显减轻再灌注损伤。此后多项研究证实，后适应对大鼠、兔、猪等动物心肌缺血/再灌注（ischemic reperfusion，I/R）损伤有相似的心肌保护作用[2,3]。药物预处理对I/R损伤心肌的保护也有较多报道，其中血管紧张素转化酶抑制剂（angiotensin converting enzyme inhibitors，ACEI）对I/R心肌的保护作用尤为突出[4]，但ACEI预处理是否具有增加IPoC对I/R损伤心肌的保护作用，目前尚无报道。本实验观察ACEI制剂福辛普利钠预处理结合IPoC对再灌注损伤心肌的保护作用，并从氧化应激及促炎性细胞因子水平研究其作用机制。

1. 材料与方法

1.1 实验动物

SD（Spragu-Dawley）大鼠，清洁级，60只，雌雄兼用，体重180～200g，由北京维通利华实验动物技术有限公司提供，合格证号：SCXK（京）2007-0001。适应性饲养3d后进行实验，动物自由摄水，室温控制在23～25℃，湿度为50%～70%，光照12h，黑暗12h。

1.2 药物和试剂

福辛普利钠片（商品名：蒙诺），每粒10mg，批号：0804087，由中美上海施贵宝制药有限公司生产；肌钙蛋白T（cardiac troponin T，cTnT）试剂盒由美国RapidBio Lab公司生产，由北京莱博特利生物医学科技公司提供，批号：08060502；肌酸激酶同工酶（creatine kinase-MB，CK-MB）试剂盒由北京中生北控生物科技股份有限公司提供，批号：070181；白细胞介素-1β（interleukin-1β，IL-1β）、白细胞介素-6（interleukin-6，IL-6）、肿瘤坏死因子-α（tumor necrosis factor-α，TNF-α）放射免疫试剂盒，由北京北方生物技术公司生产；超氧化物歧化酶（superoxide dismutase，SOD）试剂盒，批号：090310，丙二醛（malondialdẂyde，MDA）试剂盒，批号：090312，由南京建成科技有限公司

生产；氯化硝基四氮唑兰（nitroblue tetrazolium chloride，NBT），由美国Amresco公司生产；IL-1β、IL-6和TNF-α酶联免疫吸附测定（enzyme-linked immunosorbant assay，ELISA）试剂盒，由美国R&D（R&D systems）公司生产；考马斯亮蓝蛋白测定试剂盒，由南京建成科技有限公司生产，批号：090828。

1.3 实验仪器

心电图机，型号：ECG-6511，由上海光电仪器有限公司生产；动物人工呼吸机，型号：DW-2000，由上海嘉鹏科技有限公司生产；Ultra Turrax T18高速分散机，由德国IKA公司生产；7020型全自动生化仪，由日本日立公司生产；Multiskan MK3型酶标仪，由荷兰雷勃生物医学有限公司生产；DpxView Pro型显微彩色图像处理系统，由丹麦DeltaPix公司生产。

1.4 动物分组及用药

大鼠随机分为4组，每组15只：（1）假手术组：开胸冠状动脉前降支下置线不结扎。（2）I/R组：冠状动脉前降支结扎30min，再灌注1h，建立I/R损伤模型。（3）IPoC组：建立I/R模型中予以3次10s的再灌注/缺血循环，（4）福辛普利钠＋IPoC组，福辛普利钠，0.9mg/（kg·d），用等量蒸馏水稀释后灌胃14天，于末次灌胃2h后建立I/R模型，过程中给予IPoC干预。各组（除福辛普利钠+IPoC组外）均给予等量生理盐水灌胃14d。

1.5 大鼠I/R模型的建立及标本采集

大鼠以20%氨基甲酸乙酯（乌拉坦）6mL/kg腹腔麻醉，置于解剖台上仰卧位固定，记录Ⅱ导联心电图。颈部、胸骨左侧、腹部消毒，并剪毛备皮。剪开颈部皮肤，暴露气管并插管，连接动物呼吸机（潮气量3mL/100g体重，呼吸频率为60次/min），沿胸骨左缘3～4肋间开胸，暴露心脏，剪开心包膜，在左心耳的下缘、肺动脉圆锥的左缘之间穿刺进针，围绕左冠状动脉前降支上1/3处穿3-0缝合线，缝合线两端穿过一直径为1.5mm的硅胶软管，拉线推管，蚊式止血钳固定以阻断左冠状动脉血流。结扎后Ⅱ导联心电图示ST段明显抬高或T波高尖，结扎线下左室前壁呈暗红色为结扎成功。30min后松开蚊式止血钳放松缝合线，恢复冠状动脉血流再灌注60min。后适应操作在结扎30min结束后，立即给予3次10s的再灌注/缺血

循环（松开蚊式止血钳放松缝合线为再灌注，拉线推管用止血钳夹紧硅胶管为缺血）。完全松开缝合线再灌注 60min 结束后，腹主动脉取血并分离血清，取出大鼠心脏生理盐水冲洗干净后，每组 5 只心脏做 NBT 染色测量大鼠左室心肌梗死面积，将另 5 只心脏快速放入液氮中，然后移入 –80℃ 冰箱保存，用于组织 ELISA 检测。在灌胃和造模过程中，大鼠死亡 9 只，共有 51 只大鼠进入实验。

1.6　血清学检测指标

全自动生化仪测定 CK-MB 和 cTnT 的水平，放射免疫法测定 IL-1β、IL-6 和 TNF-α 水平，比色法测定 SOD 含量，硫代巴比妥酸法测定 MDA 含量。

1.7　左心室梗死面积测量

将取下的大鼠心脏用生理盐水冲洗干净，用滤纸吸除多余水分，均匀切成 5 片，放入 NBT 染色液中，置于 37℃ 水箱中温浴 5 分钟，温浴过程中观察心肌组织颜色。当非梗死区显示蓝色，梗死区为红色时，取出放置在滤纸上，用 Canon IXUS 90IS 数码相机微距拍摄后，使用 DpxView Pro 型显微彩色图像处理系统计算出左心室梗死面积（%），用心肌梗死面积 / 左心室面积 ×100% 表示。

1.8　心肌组织细胞因子水平的检测

每组 5 只心脏，取前降支结扎线下 2mm 至心尖部左心室缺血心肌组织 100mg，加入 2mL 低温生理盐水（0℃），T18 高速分散机匀浆后，离心取上清液，于 –80℃ 保存待测。所有标本均采用 ELISA 法检测，操作过程严格按说明书操作程序进行。同时用考马斯亮蓝蛋白测定法检测每个组织标本的蛋白含量，得出数值后，将每毫升匀浆液中的细胞因子含量换算成每毫克蛋白中的细胞因子含量。

1.9　统计学分析

所有数据以 $\bar{x}±s$ 表示，使用 SPSS 14.0 软件进行统计学分析。用单因素方差分析各组别之间的差异，组间两两比较采用 LSD 法，$P < 0.05$ 表示差异有统计学意义。

2.　结果

2.1　各组大鼠血清心肌损伤标志物和左心室梗死范围

I/R 组、IPoC 组以及福辛普利钠 +IPoC 组心肌损伤标志物 CK-MB 和 cTnT 水平均高于假手术组（P 均 < 0.01）。IPoC 组 CK-MB 和 cTnT 水平均低于 I/R 组（P 均 < 0.01）。福辛普利钠 +IPoC 组 CK-MB 水平低于 IPoC 组（$P < 0.05$）。见表 1。

表 1　各组大鼠心肌损伤标志物水平（$\bar{x}±s$）

组别	鼠数（只）	CK-MB（IU/L）	cTNT（ng/mL）
假手术组	14	693.64±114.85	0.02±0.01
I/R 组	11	1635.30±229.20[a]	4.41±0.93[a]
IPoC 组	13	1222.39±188.16[b]	2.53±0.51[b]
福辛普利钠 +IPoC 组	13	1047.61±223.13[bc]	2.36±0.96[b]

注：与假手术组比较，[a]$P < 0.01$；与 I/R 组比较，[b]$P < 0.01$；与 IPoC 组比较，[c]$P < 0.05$

I/R 组左心室心肌梗死面积为 35.28%±3.85%，IPoC 组为 21.02%±2.29%，$P < 0.01$。福辛普利钠 + IPoC 组为 17.17%±3.12%，进一步小于 IPoC 组，$P < 0.05$，见图 1、2。

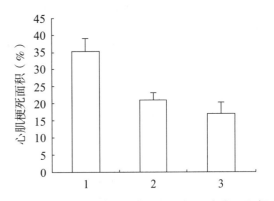

图 1　福辛普利钠预处理结合 IPoC 对 I/R 大鼠心肌梗死面积的影响（$\bar{x}±s$）

1：I/R 组，2：IPoC 组，3：福辛普利钠 +IPoC 组（每组 5 只）；与 I/R 组比较，[a]$P < 0.01$；与 IPoC 组比较，[b]$P < 0.05$

2.2　各组大鼠血清 SOD 和 MDA 含量

与假手术组比较，I/R 组血清 SOD 含量显著降低，MDA 含量显著增高（$P < 0.05$，$P < 0.01$）；与 I/R 组比较，IPoC 组能明显增加 SOD 含量，减少 MDA 含量（$P < 0.01$）；福辛普利钠 +IPoC 组与 IPoC 组比较，能显著增加 SOD 含量（$P < 0.05$），见表 2。

2.3　各组大鼠血清 IL-1β、IL-6 和 TNF-α 含量

与假手术组比较，I/R 组血清促炎性细胞因子 IL-1β、IL-6 和 TNF-α 水平显著增高（$P < 0.01$）；与 I/R 组比较，IPoC 干预能显著降低 IL-1β、IL-6 和 TNF-α 水平（$P < 0.05$，$P < 0.05$，$P < 0.01$）；与 IPoC 比较，福辛普利钠 +IPoC 组能进一步降低血清 IL-6 水平（$P < 0.05$），见表 3。

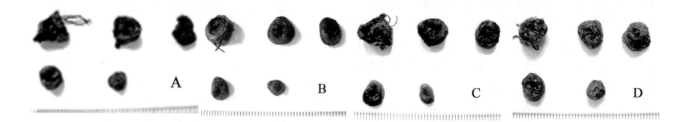

图 2　各组大鼠心肌梗死面积大体观

A：假手术组，B：I/R 组，C：IPoC 组，D：福辛普利钠 +IPoC 组（心脏由心底到心尖等分为五层，按从左至右、从上而下顺序依次排列）

表 2　福辛普利钠预处理结合 IPoC 对心肌 I/R 大鼠血清
SOD、MDA 的影响（$\bar{\chi} \pm s$）

组别	n	SOD（ng/mL）	MDA（nmol/mL）
假手术组	14	48.55±6.24	7.45±0.84
I/R 组	11	37.85±6.54[a]	9.01±0.60[b]
IPoC 组	13	53.23±7.73[c]	8.17±0.59[c]
福辛普利钠 +IPoC 组	13	61.26±8.63[cd]	8.10±0.56[c]

注：与假手术组比较，[a]$P < 0.05$，[b]$P < 0.01$；与 I/R 组比较，[c]$P < 0.01$；与 IPoC 组比较，[d]$P < 0.05$

表 3　福辛普利钠预处理结合 IPoC 对心肌 I/R 大鼠血清
IL-1β、IL-6 和 TNF-α 的影响（$\bar{\chi} \pm s$）

组别	n	IL-1β（ng/ml）	IL-6（pg/ml）	TNF-α（ng/ml）
假手术组	14	0.31±0.87	129.33±31.7	1.48±0.91
I/R 组	11	0.55±0.13[a]	288.31±45.53[a]	2.73±0.42[a]
IPoC 组	13	0.44±0.09[b]	243.13±37.68[b]	1.78±0.73[c]
福辛普利钠 +IPoC 组	13	0.43±0.15[b]	201.88±59.67[cd]	1.70±0.58[c]

注：与假手术组比较，[a]$P < 0.01$；与 I/R 组比较，[b]$P < 0.05$，[c]$P < 0.01$；与 IPoC 组比较，[d]$P < 0.05$

2.4　各组大鼠缺血心肌组织 IL-1β、IL-6 和 TNF-α 水平

　　与假手术组比较，I/R 后缺血心肌细胞因子 IL-1β、IL-6 和 TNF-α 水平显著增高（P 均< 0.01）；与 I/R 组比较，IPoC 能降低 IL-1β、IL-6 和 TNF-α 水平（$P < 0.05$，$P < 0.01$）；与 IPoC 比较，福辛普利钠 +IPoC 组能进一步降低组织 TNF-α 水平（$P < 0.01$），结果见表 4。

3.　讨论

　　IPoC 能减轻再灌注氧化应激损伤[1]，减少线粒体钙超载、减缓凋亡细胞的死亡[5]，激活再灌注

表 4　福辛普利钠预处理结合 IPoC 对 I/R 大鼠心肌 IL-1β、
IL-6 和 TNF-α 的影响（$\bar{\chi} \pm s$）

组别	n	IL-1β（pg/mg）	IL-6（pg/mg）	TNF-α（pg/mg）
假手术组	5	14.57±3.72	14.10±1.23	3.00±0.19
I/R 组	5	44.61±7.70[a]	24.78±3.47[a]	6.55±0.30[a]
IPoC 组	5	33.67±7.59[b]	20.57±1.95[b]	4.71±0.27[c]
福辛普利钠 +IPoC 组	5	24.88±7.13[b]	19.17±2.44[c]	4.21±0.32[cd]

注：与假手术组比较，[a]$P < 0.01$；与 I/R 组比较，[b]$P < 0.05$，[c]$P < 0.01$；与 IPoC 比较，[d]$P < 0.01$

损伤抢救激酶通路、线粒体 ATP 敏感钾离子通道和抑制线粒体渗透孔道的开放[6,7] 等，进而减少心肌梗死面积，改善心脏功能。本实验也证实 IPoC 能减少 I/R 大鼠心肌梗死面积和心肌损伤标志物的释放。联合药物治疗是否能提高 IPoC 保护 I/R 心肌的作用，是本实验研究的关键所在。

　　在药物干预 I/R 损伤中，大量研究表明 ACEI 有保护心肌免于 I/R 损伤的作用[4,8,9]。Dogan R 等[8] 报道给荷兰猪灌胃赖诺普利 10 天，证明能减轻 I/R 心肌损伤，保护心脏功能。ACEI 保护 I/R 心肌的机制可能与减少 I/R 过程中大量产生的血管紧张素 Ⅱ 对心肌的损害有关[9]。ACEI 还可使缓激肽生成增多，分解减少，促进前列腺素 I$_2$ 和 NO 生成，用缓激肽受体拮抗剂后，ACEI 抑制再灌注心肌凋亡和减少心肌梗死面积的作用明显减弱[10]。我们的实验研究发现，福辛普利钠预先治疗，可提高 IPoC 保护 I/R 大鼠心肌作用，较单纯 IPoC 可进一步减少心肌损伤标志物 CK-MB 的释放和缩小心肌梗死面积。

　　氧化应激和早期炎症反应是心肌再灌注损伤

的两个主要病理机制，再灌注过程中大量氧自由基和活性氧的产生可产生直接损伤心肌细胞的作用，它们与组成细胞的脂质、蛋白质及核酸等发生直接反应，导致细胞原结构、功能发生改变，引起细胞损伤和死亡[11]。SOD 是一类广泛存在于生物体内的金属酶，它可清除生物体内在利用氧的过程中产生的超氧离子；MDA 是生物膜发生脂质过氧化的重要产物，其含量是衡量氧自由基对细胞损害的标志之一。本实验表明，IPoC 能显著提高心肌 I/R 后血清 SOD 含量，降低血清 MDA 水平；福辛普利钠预处理结合 IPoC，能进一步升高 SOD 含量，增加机体对超氧负离子的清除，保护心肌细胞，表明福辛普利钠预处理能提高 IPoC 抑制再灌注时氧化应激反应对心肌的损害。

再灌注过程中，氧化应激与早期炎症反应的触发有着密切的关系[12]。Kin H 等[13]发现在心肌 I/R 前给予抗氧化剂 N- 乙酰半胱氨酸可明显抑制超氧化物自由基的生成，减少血浆 MDA 的产生和 TNF-α 的释放。促炎性细胞因子 IL-1β、IL-6 和 TNF-α 在 I/R 过程中被大量释放后又可进一步诱导细胞因子的级联反应，上调黏附分子和炎症趋化因子，加速中性粒细胞和单核细胞浸润心肌组织，激活的中性粒细胞和巨噬细胞可引起呼吸爆发，释放大量的氧自由基，导致心肌收缩力减弱和心肌细胞凋亡等不可逆性心肌损伤[14, 15]。本实验研究发现，IPoC 显著降低血清 MDA 水平和升高血清 SOD 含量，抑制了促炎性细胞因子 IL-1β、IL-6 和 TNF-α 的释放，这种对氧化应激和炎性细胞因子的抑制作用与 Kin H 等[13]的报道一致。IPoC 抑制炎症反应是通过抑制氧化应激诱导的早期炎症反应，还是直接抑制炎性细胞因子的释放，有待进一步深入研究。实验中也发现，福辛普利钠 +IPoC 组中血清 IL-6 和心肌组织 TNF-α 的水平较 IPoC 组更低，表明福辛普利钠预处理能增强 IPoC 抑制 I/R 心肌的早期炎症反应。

AMI 早期再灌注治疗，辅以 IPoC 的方法，能够保护心肌免于 I/R 损伤，但 IPoC 是否能改善 AMI 早期再灌注治疗后患者近、远期预后，尚需大规模临床研究证实。炎症反应贯穿在心肌梗死发生发展的全过程，抑制早期的炎症反应对保护心肌，改善长期预后有重要作用[16]。本实验中福辛普利钠预处理结合 IPoC 可以显著减少 I/R 大鼠心肌梗死面积和心肌损伤标志物的释放，升高血清

SOD 含量，抑制血清 IL-6 和心肌组织 TNF-α 的水平，表明福辛普利钠预处理增强 IPoC 对 I/R 心肌的保护作用可能与抑制氧化应激和早期炎症反应有关。因此，福辛普利钠预处理与 IPoC 的联合应用，可能为临床上改善 AMI 早期再灌注治疗后患者的长期预后提供一个重要的干预手段，尤其是对于患有 AMI 高危因素诸如高血压、糖尿病等疾病的患者，ACEI 类药物的应用可能为 AMI 的临床防治开辟一个新的途径。

参考文献

[1] Zhao ZQ, Corvera JS, Halkos ME, et al. Inhibition of myocardial injury by ischemic postconditioning during reperfusion: comparison with ischemic preconditioning. Am J Physiol Heart Circ Physiol, 2003, 285 (2): H579-H588.

[2] Fujita M, Asanuma H, Hirata A, et al. Prolonged transient acidosis during early reperfusion contributes to the cardioprotective effects of postconditioning. Am J Physiol Heart Circ Physiol, 2007, 292 (4): H2004-H2008.

[3] Liu XH, Zhang ZY, Sun S, et al. Ischemic postconditioning protects myocardium from ischemia/reperfusion injury through attenuating endoplasmic reticulum stress. Shock, 2008, 30 (4): 422-427.

[4] Ozer MK, Sahna E, Birincioglu M, et al. Effects of captopril and losartan on myocardial ischemia-reperfusion induced arrhythmias and necrosis in rats. Pharmacol Res, 2002, 45 (4): 257-263.

[5] Sun HY, Wang NP, Kerendi F, et al. Hypoxic postconditioning reduces cardiomyocyte loss by inhibiting ROS generation and intracellular Ca^{2+} overload. Am J Physiol, 2005, 288 (4): H1900-H1908.

[6] Dow J, Bhandari A, Kloner RA. The mechanism by which ischemic postconditioning reduces reperfusion arrhythmias in rats remains elusive. J Cardiovasc Pharmacol Ther, 2009, 14 (2): 99-103.

[7] 张健发, 马依彤, 杨毅宁, 等. 再灌注损伤抢救激酶对小鼠缺血后适应心肌再灌注损伤中的减轻作用. 中华心血管病杂志, 2008, 36 (2): 161-166.

[8] Dogan R, Farsak B, Isbir S, et al. Protective effect of lisinopril against ischemia-reperfusion injury in isolated guinea pig hearts. Cardiovasc Surg (Torino), 2001, 42 (1): 43-48.

[9] Li K, Chen X. Protective effects of captopril and enalapril on myocardial ischemia and reperfusion

第
四
章

damage of rat. J Mol Cell Cardiol, 1987, 19 (9): 909-915.

[10] Wang LX, Ideishi M, Yahiro E, et al. Mechanism of the cardioprotective effect of inhibition of the renin-angiotensin system on ischemia/reperfusion-induced myocardial injury. Hypertens Res, 2001, 24 (2): 179-187.

[11] Dhalla NS, Elmoselhi AB, Hata T, et al. Status of myocardial antioxidants in ischemia-reperfusion injury. Cardiovasc Res, 2000, 47 (3): 446-456.

[12] Wong CH, Crack PJ. Modulation of neuro-inflammation and vascular response by oxidative stress following cerebral ischemia-reperfusion injury. Curr Med Chem, 2008, 15 (1): 1-14.

[13] Kin H, Wang NP, Mykytenko J, et al. Inhibition of myocardial apoptosis by postconditioning is associated with attenuation of oxidative stress-mediated nuclear factor-kappa B translocation and TNF alpha release. Shock, 2008; 29 (6): 761-768.

[14] Finkel MS, Oddis CV, Jacob TD, et al. Negative inotropic effects of cytokines on the heart mediated by nitric oxide. Science, 1992, 257 (5068): 387-389.

[15] Engel D, Peshock R, Armstong RC, et al. Cardiac myocyte apoptosis provokes adverse cardiac remodeling in transgenic mice with targeted TNF overexpression. Am J Physiol Heart Circ Physiol, 2004, 287 (3): H1303-H1311.

[16] Frangogiannis NG. The immune system and cardiac repair. Pharmacol Res, 2008, 58 (2): 88-111.

福辛普利钠预处理对缺血后适应大鼠心肌组织 Toll 样受体表达及炎症因子的影响 *

张大武　张蕾　刘剑刚　王承龙　史大卓

随着现代生活节奏的加快，急性心肌梗死（acute myocardial infarction，AMI）已是严重危害人类健康的世界性问题，其发病通常是在冠状动脉粥样硬化病变的基础上继发斑块破裂，导致血栓形成，阻塞冠状动脉，相应的心肌组织持久的急性缺血所致。因此，建立绿色通道，早期开通患者闭塞的冠状动脉，有效恢复缺血心肌的血流灌注，是限制和缩小心肌梗死面积、改善患者预后的关键措施。近年来的临床研究发现，在冠状动脉再灌注开始时对冠状动脉进行短暂、重复的开通及再闭过程，随后恢复冠状动脉血流，即"缺血后适应"（ischemic postconditioning，IPoC），对缺血再灌注心脏有显著的保护作用[1]。

缺血后适应已被实验和临床研究证实可减轻再灌注损伤心肌的梗死面积，改善心脏功能[2,3]。药物预处理对心肌缺血再灌注（ischemic reperfusion，I/R）损伤心肌的保护也有较多报道，其中血管紧张素转化酶抑制剂（angiotensin converting enzyme

inhibitor，ACEI）对保护 I/R 心肌的作用较为明显[4]，但 ACEI 预处理是否具有增加 IPoC 对 I/R 损伤心肌的保护作用，目前尚无报道。缺血后适应心脏保护作用的机制尚未完全阐明。本实验观察 ACEI 制剂福辛普利钠预处理结合 IPoC 对再灌注损伤心肌的保护作用，并从 Toll 样受体（toll-like receptor，TLR）及促炎性细胞因子水平研究其作用机制。

1. 材料和方法

1.1 实验动物

健康 SD（Spragu-Dawley）大鼠，清洁级，60 只，雌雄兼用，体重 180～200g，由北京维通利华实验动物技术有限公司提供，合格证号：SCXK（京）2007-0001。适应性饲养 3d 后进行实验，动物自由摄水，室温控制 23～25℃，湿度为 50%～70%，光照 12h，黑暗 12h。

1.2 药物和试剂

福辛普利钠片（商品名：蒙诺），每粒

* 原载于《科学通报》，2010，55（24）：2378-2383

10mg，批号：0804087，中美上海施贵宝制药有限公司生产；肌钙蛋白 T（cardiac troponin T，cTNT）试剂盒由美国 RapidBio Lab 公司生产，北京莱博特利生物医学科技公司提供，批号：08060502；单核细胞趋化蛋白 -1（monocyte chemotactic protein-1，MCP-1）、肿瘤坏死因子 -α（tumor necrosis factor-α，TNF-α）、酶联免疫吸附测定（enzyme-linked immunosorbant assay，ELISA）试剂盒、氯化硝基四氮唑兰（nitro blue tetrazolium chioride，NBT），由美国 R&D（R&D systems）公司生产；考马斯亮蓝蛋白测定试剂盒，由南京建成科技有限公司生产，批号：090828；Toll 样受体 2（toll-like receptor 2，TLR2）抗体试剂盒、Toll 样受体 4（toll-like receptor 4，TLR4）抗体试剂盒，由北京博奥森生物技术有限公司提供；浓缩型 DAB 试剂盒和免疫组化试剂盒，由北京中杉金桥生物技术有限公司提供。

1.3　实验仪器

动物人工呼吸机，型号：DW-2000，上海嘉鹏科技有限公司；心电图机，型号：ECG-6511，上海光电仪器有限公司；Ultra Turrax T18 高速分散机，德国 IKA 公司；7020 型全自动生化仪，日本日立公司；Multiskan MK3 型酶标仪，荷兰雷勃生物医学有限公司；DpxView Pro 型显微彩色图像处理系统，丹麦 Delta Pix 公司。

1.4　动物缺血后适应模型的建立

大鼠以 20% 氨基甲酸乙酯（乌拉坦）6mL/kg 腹腔麻醉，置于解剖台上仰卧位固定，记录Ⅱ导联心电图。颈部、胸骨左侧、腹部消毒，并剪毛备皮。剪开颈部皮肤，暴露气管并插管，连接动物呼吸机（潮气量为 3mL/100g 体重，呼吸频率为 60 次 / 分），沿胸骨左缘 3 ~ 4 肋间开胸，暴露心脏，剪开心包膜，在左心耳的下缘、肺动脉圆锥的左缘之间穿刺进针，围绕左冠状动脉前降支上 1/3 处穿 3-0 缝合线，缝合线两端穿过一直径为 1.5mm 的硅胶软管，拉线推管，用蚊式止血钳固定以阻断左冠状动脉血流。结扎后Ⅱ导联心电图示 ST 段明显抬高或 T 波高尖，结扎线下左室前壁呈暗红色为结扎成功。30min 后松开蚊式止血钳放松缝合线，恢复冠状动脉血流，再灌注 60min。后适应操作在结扎 30min 结束后，立即给予 3 次 10s 的再灌注 / 缺血循环（松开蚊式止血钳放松缝合线为再灌注，拉线推管用止血钳夹紧硅胶管为缺血）。

1.5　动物分组及用药

大鼠随机分为 4 组，每组 15 只：（1）假手术组，开胸冠状动脉前降支下置线不结扎；（2）I/R 组，冠状动脉前降支结扎 30min，再灌注 1h，建立 I/R 损伤模型；（3）IPoC 组，建立 I/R 模型中予以 3 次 10s 的再灌注 / 缺血循环；（4）福辛普利钠 +IPoC 组，福辛普利钠，0.9mg/（kg·d），用等量蒸馏水稀释后灌胃 14d，于末次灌胃 2h 后建立 I/R 模型，过程中给予 IPoC 干预。各组（除福辛普利钠 +IPoC 组外）均给予等量生理盐水灌胃 14d。

1.6　动物样本的取材、分离和左室心肌梗死面积测量

完全松开缝合线再灌注 60min 结束后，腹主动脉取血并分离血清，取出大鼠心脏，用生理盐水冲洗干净后，每组按随机数字表检测心肌组织指标，5 只做 NBT 染色测量大鼠左室心肌梗死面积，5 只液氮快速冷冻后，于 -80℃ 冰箱保存，用于组织 ELISA 检测，5 只于 10% 中性甲醛溶液中保存，用于免疫组织化学检测。实验中假手术组因灌胃死亡 1 只，I/R 组造模中死亡 4 只，其余 2 组死亡各 2 只，后均予相应补充。

将取下的大鼠心脏用生理盐水冲洗干净，用滤纸吸除多余水分，均匀切成 5 片，放入 NBT 染色液中，置于 37℃ 水箱中温浴 5min，温浴过程中观察心肌组织颜色，当非梗死区显示蓝色，梗死区为红色时，取出放置在滤纸上，用 Canon IXUS 90IS 数码相机微距拍摄后，使用 DpxView Pro 型显微彩色图像处理系统计算出左室梗死面积（%），用心肌梗死面积 / 左室面积 ×100% 表示。

1.7　血清学指标和心肌组织 MCP-1 和 TNF-α 含量的检测

用比色法测定大鼠血清 cTnT 水平。每组 5 只心脏，取前降支结扎线下 3mm 至心尖部左室缺血心肌组织 100mg，加入 2mL 低温生理盐水（0℃），T18 高速分散机匀浆后，离心取上清液，于 -80℃ 保存待测。所有标本均采用 ELISA 法检测，操作过程严格按说明书操作程序进行。同时用考马斯亮蓝蛋白测定法检测每个组织标本的蛋白含量，得出数值后，将每毫升匀浆液中的细胞因子含量换算成每毫克蛋白中的细胞因子含量。

1.8　心肌组织 TLR 定位和免疫组织化学检测

将心肌标本用 10% 中性缓冲甲醛液固定 18h。脱水、透明、浸蜡、石蜡包埋。连续切片约 5μm 厚，捞片于多聚赖氨酸防脱处理过的载玻片上。根

据 SABC 试剂盒说明书操作,大鼠心肌切片常规脱蜡,封闭内源性过氧化物酶,10% 正常山羊血清封闭。分别滴加一抗 TLR2 抗体（1：200）和 TLR4 抗体（1：800），37℃ 孵育 1h，磷酸缓冲液（PBS）冲洗；滴加二抗生物素化山羊抗小鼠 IgG，室温 20min，PBS 溶液冲洗；滴加 SABC 复合物，室温 20min，PBS 溶液冲洗；DAB-H_2O_2 显色，苏木素轻度复染；乙醇脱水、透明、中性胶封片，选取同批染色切片进行光学显微镜下观察。每张切片随机选取 3 个不重叠的视野（×400），每只共计 15 个视野，以心肌炎症部位的胞浆染成棕褐色为阳性细胞标志，经病理图像计算机分析系统半定量分析大鼠心肌组织阳性细胞的表达，以阳性细胞面积占所有细胞面积百分比表示结果。

1.9 统计学处理

所有数据以均数 ± 标准差（$\bar{x}±s$）表示，使用 SPSS 16.0 软件进行统计学分析。单因素方差分析各组别之间的差异，组间两两比较采用 LSD 法，$P < 0.05$ 表示差异有统计学意义。

2. 结果

2.1 福辛普利钠预处理结合 IPoC 对大鼠血清 cTnT 和心肌梗死范围的影响

与假手术组比较，各组大鼠心肌损伤后 cTnT 有显著升高（$P < 0.01$），与 I/R 组比较，IPoC 组 cTnT 有显著降低（$P < 0.01$）。定量组织学 NBT 染色法显示左室心肌梗死范围，I/R 组左室梗死面积为 35.28%±3.85%，IPoC 组减少到 21.02%±2.29%（$P < 0.01$），福辛普利钠 +IPoC 组和 IPoC 组相比，可进一步缩小心肌梗死面积（17.17%±3.12%，$P < 0.05$）（表 1）。

表 1 各组大鼠血清 cTnT 含量和心肌梗死面积 a)

组别	n	cTNT/（ng/ml）	n	左室梗死区比例（%）
假手术组	14	0.015 ± 0.01	5	0
I/R 组	11	4.41 ± 0.93**	5	35.28 ± 3.85**
IPoC 组	13	2.53 ± 0.51** △△	5	21.02 ± 2.29 △△
福辛普利钠 +IPoC 组	13	2.36 ± 0.96** △△	5	17.17 ± 3.12 △△□

a)**，与假手术组比较，$P < 0.01$；△△，与 I/R 组比较，$P < 0.01$；□，与 IPoC 组比较，$P < 0.05$

2.2 福辛普利钠预处理结合 IPoC 对大鼠心肌组织

TLR 2、4 表达的影响

假手术组可见少量棕褐色颗粒，I/R 组心肌内棕褐色颗粒明显增多。与假手术组比较，I/R 组心肌组织 TLR 2、4 的表达均有显著升高（$P < 0.01$）；与 I/R 组比较，IPoC 组 TLR 2、4 表达显著降低（$P < 0.01$）；与 IPoC 组比较，福辛普利钠 +IPoC 组可进一步抑制 TLR 2、4 表达（$P > 0.05$）（表 2，图 1 和图 2）。

表 2 各组大鼠心肌 TLR 2、4 表达水平变化 a)

组别	n	TLR2（%）	TLR4（%）
假手术组	5	10.92 ± 5.28	12.37 ± 6.64
I/R 组	5	45.12 ± 7.53**	49.33 ± 9.52**
IPoC 组	5	35.89±8.19 △△	38.42±8.16 △△
福辛普利钠 +IPoC 组	5	29.02±6.50 △△□	30.59±7.17 △△□

a)**，与假手术组比较，$P < 0.01$；△△，与 I/R 组比较，$P < 0.01$；□，与 IPoC 组比较，$P < 0.05$

2.3 福辛普利钠预处理结合 IPoC 对大鼠心肌 TNF-α 和 MCP-1 水平以及炎性细胞浸润的影响

与假手术组比较，缺血再灌注后炎性细胞因子 MCP-1 和 TNF-α 显著增高（$P < 0.01$）；与 I/R 组比较，IPoC 干预能显著降低 TNF-α 和 MCP-1（$P < 0.05$，$P < 0.01$）。在此基础上，福辛普利钠能进一步降低 IPoC 心肌 TNF-α 水平（$P < 0.01$），对 MCP-1 有降低趋势，但统计学处理尚不显著。见表 3。

HE 染色结果显示，与假手术组比较，缺血再灌注后浸润的炎性细胞数显著增加（$P < 0.01$）；与 I/R 组比较，IPoC 干预能显著降低浸润细胞数（$P < 0.01$）；福辛普利钠 +IPoC 有进一步减少炎性细胞浸润的趋势，但统计学处理尚不显著（表 3，图 3）。

3. 讨论

在药物干预 I/R 损伤中，大量研究表明 ACEI 有保护心肌免于 I/R 损伤的作用 [4-6]。给荷兰猪灌胃赖诺普利 10d 后，再建立心肌 I/R 损伤模型，结果显示 I/R 荷兰猪心肌损伤明显减轻，心脏功能显著改善 [5]。ACEI 保护 I/R 心肌的机制可能与减少 I/R 过程中大量产生的血管紧张素 Ⅱ 对心肌的损害有关 [6]。ACEI 还可使缓激肽生成增多，分解减少，

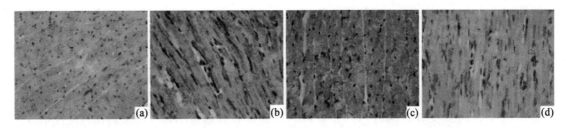

图 1　免疫组织化学法检测各组大鼠心肌 TLR2 表达（光学显微镜，×400）
(a) 假手术组（n=5）；(b) I/R 组（n=5）；(c) IPoC 组（n=5）；(d) 福辛普利钠 +IPoC 组（n=5）

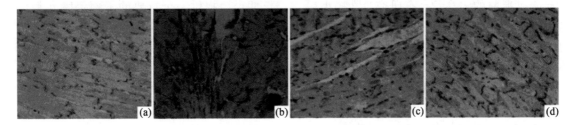

图 2　免疫组织化学法检测各组大鼠心肌 TLR4 表达（光学显微镜，×400）
(a) 假手术组（n=5）；(b) I/R 组（n=5）；(c) IPoC 组（n=5）；(d) 福辛普利钠 +IPoC 组（n=5）

表 3　各组大鼠心肌 MCP-1、TNF-α 水平及炎性细胞浸润的影响（$\bar{\chi} \pm s$）[a]

组别	n	TNF-α（pg/mg）	MCP-1（pg/mg）	浸润细胞数（个）
假手术组	5	3.00±0.19	12.60±3.68	7.00±2.73
I/R 组	5	6.55±0.30**	39.27±7.55**	43.40±11.13**
IPoC 组	5	4.71±0.27△△	29.97±2.29△	24.80±4.44△△
福辛普利钠 +IPoC 组	5	4.21±0.32△△□□	25.50±4.50△△	22.60±4.88△△

a) **，与假手术组比较，$P < 0.01$；△，△△与 I/R 组比较，$P < 0.05$，$P < 0.01$；□□，与 IPoC 组比较，$P < 0.01$

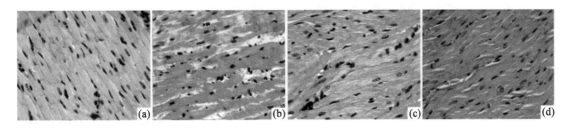

图 3　大鼠心肌 HE 染色浸润细胞数的变化（光学显微镜，×400）
(a) 假手术组（n=5）；(b) I/R 组（n=5）；(c) IPoC 组（n=5）；(d) 福辛普利钠 +IPoC 组（n=5）。黑色箭头所示为浸润细胞，其中单核细胞为卵圆形，细胞表面不规则，细胞核长，呈马蹄形，或具浅的凹陷，含有 1～2 个小的核仁；淋巴细胞多为圆形或椭圆形，核仁大而明显，核内异染色质为主，故核呈密影

促进前列腺素 I₂ 和一氧化氮生成，用缓激肽受体拮抗剂后，ACEI 抑制再灌注心肌凋亡和减少心肌梗死面积的作用明显减弱[7]。

但是对于缺血再灌注损伤而言，其机制涉及活性氧产生、多形核中性粒细胞聚集、钙超载和血管内皮功能受损等诸多因素，以及随之诱导活化的信号级联反应，导致严重的心肌组织损伤和功能障碍。其表现出的是一种多因素、多途径的发病机制，故单纯的药物治疗对于缺血再灌注损伤未显示出有绝对的优势。既往研究也表明，药物治疗干预缺血再灌注损伤仍然停留于动物实验阶段，未能进入大规模临床实验。近年来，IPoC 作为缺血再灌注损伤的辅助性治疗手段被大量报道，它有减少缺血再灌注损伤心肌梗死面积和心肌损伤标志物释放的保护作用。本研究显示，IPoC 能减少缺血再灌注大鼠心肌损伤标志物含量和心肌梗死面积，与既往研究相符，那么药物治疗联合缺血后适应是否能进一步减少心肌梗死面积，改善心脏功能，目前尚未见报道。我们的实验研究表明，福辛普利钠预先治疗，可提高 IPoC 保护 I/R 大鼠心肌作用，较单纯 IPoC 可进一步缩小心肌梗死面积。

TLR 是一组 I 型跨膜受体，通过与内、外源性配体结合，激发天然免疫和获得性免疫应答，启动与免疫和炎症相关的细胞因子 IL-6、TNF-α 等基因的转录和蛋白的表达[8]。有研究[9,10]将小鼠 *TLR4* 基因敲除后建立心肌 I/R 损伤模型，发现其与同种野生型小鼠相比心肌梗死范围减少，炎症反应减轻，心肌梗死后的不良重塑改善。给予 TLR 4 的抑制剂 eritoran 干预后，I/R 后心肌梗死面积减少，心肌组织 NF-kappa B 和促炎性细胞因子 MCP-1 和 TNF-α 水平降低[11]。Sakata 等人[12]同样也发现 TLR2 缺陷小鼠遭受心肌 I/R 损伤后左室舒张末压较同种野生型小鼠下降，促炎性细胞因子 TNF-α 和 IL-1β 水平降低。以上研究均表明抑制 TLR 2、4 的表达可保护 I/R 损伤心肌。我们实验研究发现，IPoC 干预再灌注损伤大鼠心肌后 TLR 2、4 表达降低，心肌内 MCP-1 和 TNF-α 含量也下降，表明 IPoC 抑制 TLR 2、4 的表达可能是其保护 I/R 心肌的一个重要途径。给予福辛普利钠预处理后，TLR 2、4 的表达与 IPoC 组比较，受到进一步抑制和降低。心肌组织 TNF-α 的含量也显著下降，表明福辛普利钠联合 IPoC 可能与抑制 TLR 2、4 的表达和促炎性细胞因子的水平有密切关系。

另外，本实验研究显示心肌缺血再灌注时 MCP-1 表达显著增加，缺血再灌注心肌的炎性细胞浸润也显著增多。有研究[13]表明，将 MCP-1 特异性受体 *CCR2* 基因敲除后，小鼠缺血再灌注心肌炎性细胞浸润显著降低，心肌梗死面积缩小。同样，转染家兔 MCP-1 抑制剂 7ND 基因抑制 MCP-1 活性后，再建立心肌 I/R 损伤家兔模型，结果显示心肌炎性细胞浸润减少，促炎性细胞因子 TNF-α 水平降低，家兔心脏功能明显改善，表明抑制 MCP-1 活性是保护 I/R 心肌的重要环节之一[14]。本研究应用 IPoC 干预 I/R 心肌后，心肌组织 MCP-1 水平显著降低，炎性细胞的浸润也明显减少，表明 IPoC 保护 I/R 心肌的作用与抑制 MCP-1 表达和炎性细胞浸润有关。福辛普利钠联合 IPoC 能进一步降低 MCP-1 水平和炎性细胞浸润，统计

学处理尚不显著，可能和样本量较少有关，今后有待进一步深入研究。

介入治疗技术已成为 AMI 再灌注治疗的重要手段，而缺血后适应的干预手段方法简便，可操作性强，对心肌缺血 I/R 的保护作用如能得以证实并进而在临床应用，可使患者在再灌注治疗中获得最大收益。福辛普利钠预处理与 IPoC 的联合应用，可能为临床上改善 AMI 早期再灌注治疗后患者的长期预后提供一个重要的干预手段，尤其是对有 AMI 高危因素诸如高血压、糖尿病等疾病的患者，预防性应用 ACEI 类药物对于改善 AMI 再灌注损伤的心脏功能具有重要意义。

参考文献

[1] Zhao ZQ, Corvera JS, Halkos ME, et al. Inhibition of myocardial injury by ischemic postconditioning during reperfusion: comparison with ischemic preconditioning. Am J Physiol Heart Circ Physiol, 2003, 285: H579-H588.

[2] Thibault H, Piot C, Staat P, et al. Long-term benefit of postconditioning. Circulation, 2008, 117: 1037-1044.

[3] Laskey WK, Yoon S, Calzada N, et al. Concordant improvements in coronary flow reserve and ST-segment resolution during percutaneous coronary intervention for acute myocardial infarction: a benefit of postconditioning. Catheter Cardiovasc Interv, 2008, 72: 212-220.

[4] Ozer MK, Sahna E, Birincioglu M, et al. Effects of captopril and losartan on myocardial ischemia-reperfusion induced arrhythmias and necrosis in rats. Pharmacol Res, 2002, 45: 257-263.

[5] Doğan R, Farsak B, Isbir S, et al. Protective effect of lisinopril against ischemia-reperfusion injury in isolated guinea pig hearts. Cardiovasc Surg (Torino), 2001, 42: 43-48.

[6] Li K, Chen X. Protective effects of captopril and enalapril on myocardial ischemia and reperfusion damage of rat. J Mol Cell Cardiol, 1987, 19: 909-915.

[7] Wang LX, Ideishi M, Yahiro E, et al. Mechanism of the cardioprotective effect of inhibition of the renin-angiotensin system on ischemia/reperfusion-induced myocardial injury. Hypertens Res, 2001, 24: 179-187.

[8] Boyd J H, Mathur S, Wang Y, et al. Toll-like receptor stimulation in cardiomyoctes decreases contractility and initiates an NF-kappaB dependent inflammatory response. Cardiovasc Res, 2006, 72: 384-393.

［9］ Oyama J, Blais C Jr, Liu X, et al. Reduced myocardial ischemiareperfusion injury in toll-like receptor 4-deficient mice. Circulation, 2004, 109: 784-789.

［10］ Riad A, Jager S, Sobirey M, et al. Toll-like receptor-4 modulates survival by induction of left ventricular remodeling after myocardial infarction in mice. J Immunol, 2008, 180: 6954-6961.

［11］ Shimamoto A, Chong AJ, Yada M, et al. Inhibition of Toll-like receptor 4 with eritoran attenuates myocardial ischemia-reperfusion injury. Circulation, 2006, 114: I270-I274.

［12］ Sakata Y, Dong JW, Vallejo JG, et al. Toll-like receptor 2 modulates left ventricular function following ischemia-reperfusion injury. Am J Physiol Heart Circ Physiol, 2007, 292: H503-H509.

［13］ Hayasaki T, Kaikita K, Okuma T, et al. CC chemokine receptor-2 deficiency attenuates oxidative stress and infarct size caused by myocardial ischemia-reperfusion in mice. Circ J, 2006, 70: 342-351.

［14］ Kajihara N, Morita S, Nishida T, et al. Transfection with a dominant-negative inhibitor of monocyte chemoattractant protein-1 gene improves cardiac function after 6 hours of cold preservation. Circulation, 2003, 108 (Suppl 1): II213-II218.

慢性应激抑郁对心肌梗死大鼠血管活性物质及炎症因子的影响 *

金　星　刘剑刚　史大卓

研究表明，抑郁障碍是心肌梗死（myocardial infarction，MI）患者常见的情绪障碍，并且是心肌梗死患者未来发生心脏事件的独立危险因素[1]。血管内皮功能的改变，特别是一氧化氮（nitric oxide，NO）和内皮素（endothelin，ET）之间平衡关系的破坏以及炎性反应均为冠心病发生、发展进程中重要的病理生理机制。而 NO 和炎症因子异常也常出现在抑郁症患者中[2,3]。因此，探讨血管活性物质和炎症因子在心肌梗死合并抑郁障碍时的病理生理变化及所起的作用显得十分重要。实验性慢性应激抑郁导致的动物行为特征改变、血中神经递质水平上升等均与内源性抑郁症状相似，为此实验在急性心肌梗死（acute myocardial infarction，AMI）大鼠模型上，采用慢性轻度不可预见应激（chronic unpredictable mild stress，CUMS）刺激方法造成抑郁状态，前期观察表明慢性应激可进一步加剧 MI 时的血液流变性异常及增强血小板的活化、聚集[4]，进一步检测大鼠血浆 NO、ET 和炎性因子的含量变化，以探讨心肌梗死后慢性应激抑郁状态下的血管内皮释放血管舒张物质的能力和炎症因子的关系。

1. 材料和方法

1.1 动物

Wistar 大鼠，清洁级，雌雄兼用，体重 220～250g，由北京维通利华实验动物技术有限公司提供，许可证编号：SCXK（京）2007-0001。饲养及实验均在清洁动物房内进行，人工控光（12h 明暗交替，7：00am-19：00pm 光照）、控温（20～23℃）。

1.2 试剂

ET-1 和白细胞介素 -6（interleukin-6，IL-6）试剂盒由解放军总医院放射免疫技术研究所提供；NO 试剂盒由晶美生物工程（北京）有限公司提供，批号为 SA050723；大鼠血清高敏 C- 反应蛋白（high-sensitivity C-reactive protein，hs-CRP）酶联免疫法（ELISA）试剂盒由 Rapid Bio Lab 提供，批号为 08100511。

* 原载于：《中国病理生理杂志》，2010，26（1）：70-74

1.3 动物分组

大鼠适应性饲养 7d，通过旷场实验剔除水平活动和垂直活动总得分小于 30 分和大于 120 分的大鼠，由随机表进行分组。即：正常对照组（control）、慢性应激抑郁模型组（CUMS model）及 AMI 手术组。其中，AMI 手术组待术后存活 1 周后，再随机分为心肌梗死模型（AMI model）组、心肌梗死 + 慢性应激抑郁（AMI+CUMS）组。以上各组雌、雄各 5 只（AMI 组雌、雄各 4 只）。实验过程中共有 5 只大鼠死亡。

1.4 方法

1.4.1 AMI 大鼠模型制备 用乙醚麻醉大鼠，消毒胸前皮肤，经左侧剪开皮肤，于左侧 3～4 肋间钝性分离肌肉组织，打开胸腔，剪开心包膜，快速挤压出心脏，于分支起点处（在肺动脉圆锥和左心耳之间，以左冠状静脉主干为标志）1～2mm 处结扎左冠状动脉前降支，造成 AMI 模型，然后迅速将心脏放回胸腔，随即缝合，术后给予青霉素 40 000U（连续 3d），并记录标准肢导联 II 导（纸速 50/s）心电图 ST 段弓背持续抬高示 AMI 形成。术后常规饲养 7d 后，按下述方法进行处理。

1.4.2 慢性轻度不可预见应激模型（CUMS）制备 参照 Katz 等[5]、Willner 等[6]方法改进。AMI+CUMS 组、CUMS 组动物均单笼饲养，并进行冰水游泳（4℃，5min）、热刺激（45℃，5min）、禁食（24h）、禁水（24h）、夹尾（1min）、昼夜颠倒（24h）、高速水平摇晃（1time/s，5min）、随机配对饲养、频闪灯照射（120 次/min）。上述刺激每天 1 种，半随机安排，连续 28d，每种刺激不超过 3 次。正常对照组、心肌梗死模型组常规饲养，自由饮食，不予应激刺激。第 29d，各实验组大鼠（12h 禁食，不禁水）用 1% 戊巴比妥钠溶液（50mg/kg）腹腔麻醉，腹主动脉取血，按指标要求分离血浆及血清，–40℃存放，分别进行指标的测定。

1.4.3 旷场实验 以大鼠穿越底面方格为水平活动得分（3 爪以上跨入），以直立次数为垂直活动得分（两前肢离地 1cm 以上）。测定 5min 内水平及垂直活动得分。

1.4.4 蔗糖水偏好实验 实验前，训练动物适应含糖饮水。经 24h 的禁食禁水后，同时给予每只大鼠事先定量好的 2 瓶水：1 瓶 1% 蔗糖水，1 瓶纯水，1h 后，取走 2 瓶并称重，计算动物的总液体消耗、糖水消耗、纯水消耗。糖水偏爱 = 糖水消耗（g）/总液体消耗（g）×100%。

1.4.5 血管肽类及炎症因子测定 血浆 ET-1 用放射免疫法（非平衡法）测定，NO 采用硝酸还原酶法测定；血清 IL-6 采用抗原竞争放射免疫法（放射免疫 γ 计数仪，SN-695 型，上海核辐射仪器有限公司）测定；hs-CRP 用双抗夹心 ELISA 法（全自动酶标仪，Wellscan MK3 型，芬兰 Labsystems Dragon）测定，均严格按说明操作方法进行。

1.5 统计学处理

数据符合正态分布时，以均数 ± 标准差（$\bar{\chi} \pm s$）表示；非正态分布时，以中位数 ±4 分位间距表示（M±QR）。同组应激前后旷场实验和蔗糖水偏好实验的比较采用两相关样本的非参数检验（2-related samples test）。血管肽类及炎症因子指标采用二因素析因分析法进行统计学分析。若存在交互作用时，分别用 LSD 和 S-N-K 分析各因素的单独效应（单因素方差分析）。采用 SPSS 11.0 统计软件进行数据的分析处理。

2. 结果

2.1 慢性应激抑郁对大鼠行为学的影响

旷场实验结果表明，正常对照组和 AMI 组大鼠的水平活动及垂直活动得分在施加慢性应激前后均无明显的变化（$P > 0.05$）；而 CUMS 组和 AMI+CUMS 组大鼠的水平活动及垂直活动得分在施加 4 周慢性应激后，均较应激前明显降低，有显著差异（CUMS 组应激后下降了 53.33% 和 62.86%，AMI+CUMS 组应激后下降了 44.19% 和 43.75%，均 $P < 0.05$）。

糖水偏好实验结果表明，正常对照组和 AMI 组大鼠的糖水偏好率在施加慢性应激前后均无明显变化（$P > 0.05$）；而 CUMS 组和 AMI+CUMS 组大鼠的糖水偏好率在施加 4 周慢性应激后，均较应激前出现明显的降低，有显著差异（应激后 2 组分别下降了 16.23% 和 8.42%，均 $P < 0.05$）。

2.2 慢性应激抑郁对 AMI 大鼠血管内皮功能的影响

析因分析结果表明，心肌梗死造模与否对血浆 NO 含量的变化无明显的影响（$P > 0.05$），而施加慢性应激可引起血浆 NO 含量显著升高（$P < 0.01$），且大鼠心肌梗死与施加慢性应激之间存在交互作用（$P < 0.01$）；无论是心肌梗死或慢性应激均对血浆 ET-1 含量无明显影响，见表 1。

表1　慢性应激对 AMI 大鼠血浆 NO、ET 含量的影响（$\bar{x} \pm s$）

AMI model（A）	NO（μmol/L）		ET-1（ng/L）	
CUMS（B）	No（B）	Yes（B）	No（B）	Yes（B）
No（A）	21.59±7.04（9）	34.85±9.76（10）	76.74±9.89（9）	69.06±12.63（10）
Yes（A）	16.50±8.25（8）	48.88±6.79（8）	69.04±11.29（8）	67.44±5.49（8）
A	F=2.352	P＞0.05	F=1.534	P＞0.05
B	F=61.275	P＜0.01	F=1.522	P＞0.05
A*B	F=10.769	P＜0.01	F=0.655	P＞0.05

通过对各因素单独效应的分析，单纯心肌梗死时 NO 含量有降低的趋势（但无显著差异）。慢性应激可使 NO 明显升高（$P < 0.01$）；而心肌梗死合并慢性应激后，NO 的升高更为显著，与单纯的心梗或慢性应激组相比均有显著差异（$P < 0.01$，$P < 0.01$），见表2。

2.3　慢性应激抑郁对 AMI 大鼠 IL-6、hs-CRP 的影响

析因分析表明，无论是心肌梗死造模或施加慢性应激均可引起血浆 hs-CRP 含量显著升高（$P < 0.01$），且心肌梗死造模与施加慢性应激二者之间不存在交互作用（$P > 0.05$）；无论是心肌梗死或是慢性应激均对血清 IL-6 的含量无明显的影响，见表3。

对 hs-CRP 的单因素方差分析表明，无论单纯心肌梗死或慢性应激抑郁或心肌梗死＋慢性应激，均可使 hs-CRP 明显升高（与正常对照组相比 $P < 0.05$）；但单纯心肌梗死与慢性应激组之间相比无显著差异；而心肌梗死合并慢性应激后，hs-CRP 的升高尤为显著，与单纯心肌梗死或慢性应激组相比均有显著差异（$P < 0.01$，$P < 0.01$），见表4。

表2　慢性应激对 AMI 大鼠 NO 含量影响的单因素分析（$\bar{x} \pm s$）

Group	n	NO（μmol/L）	P1	P2	P3	P4	P5	P6
Control	9	21.59±7.04		＜0.01	＞0.05		＜0.01	＞0.05
CUMS model	10	34.85±9.76	＜0.01		＜0.01	＜0.01		＜0.01
AMI model	8	16.50±8.25	＞0.05	＜0.01		＞0.05	＜0.01	
AMI+CUMS	8	48.88±6.79	＜0.01	＜0.01	＜0.01	＜0.01	＜0.01	＜0.01
F					21.961			
P					＜0.01			

P1 vs control（LSD）；P2 vs CUMS model（LSD）；P3 vs AMI model（LSD）；P4 vs control（S-N-K）；P5 vs CUMS model（S-N-K）；P6 vs AMI model（S-N-K）

表3　慢性应激对 AMI 大鼠 IL-6、hs-CRP 含量的影响（$\bar{x} \pm s$）

AMI model（A）	IL-6（μg/L）		hs-CRP（mg/L）	
CUMS（B）	No（B）	Yes（B）	No（B）	Yes（B）
No（A）	221.69±31.36（9）	202.48±23.58（10）	3.01±1.95（9）	5.18±1.73（10）
Yes（A）	223.90±17.06（8）	218.21±23.69（8）	5.01±1.52（8）	9.27±3.74（8）
A	F=0.970	P＞0.05	F=14.343	P＜0.01
B	F=1.867	P＞0.05	F=15.472	P＜0.01
A*B	F=0.550	P＞0.05	F=0.273	P＞0.05

表 4　慢性应激对 AMI 大鼠 hs-CRP 含量影响的单因素分析（$\bar{x} \pm s$）

Group	n	hs-CRP (mg/L)	P1	P2	P3
Control	9	3.01±1.96		< 0.05	< 0.05
CUMS model	10	5.19±1.73	< 0.05		> 0.05
AMI model	8	5.02±1.53	< 0.05	> 0.05	
AMI+CUMS	8	9.28±3.75	< 0.01	< 0.01	< 0.01
F			9.018		
P			< 0.01		

P1 vs control（LSD）；P2 vs CUMS model（LSD）；P3 vs AMI model（LSD）

3. 讨论

目前国内外广泛应用慢性轻度不可预见的应激模拟造成抑郁症的压力源来制作抑郁动物模型，其机制与人类抑郁症发病机制较为接近[7]。本实验结果显示，所采用的慢性应激程式诱导 4 周后可导致大鼠糖水偏爱百分比下降，提示大鼠出现快感缺失。同时施加慢性应激的大鼠还出现反映自主活动和对新鲜环境好奇程度的旷场实验评分减低，以上结果表明实验中采用的 CUMS 程式方法能较好地诱导出大鼠模拟人类的抑郁症状。

NO 与 ET 是人体血管内皮细胞分泌的重要血管调节因子，NO 和 ET 处于动态平衡状态，以维持血管功能的正常。一般认为 NO 升高对心肌梗死患者具有保护作用，而 ET 升高具有促发及加剧心肌梗死的作用，因此 AMI 时出现 NO 降低和 ET 升高[8]。但也有报道急性心肌缺血早期的大鼠心肌组织诱生型一氧化氮合酶（iNOS）蛋白大量表达，高表达的 iNOS 除直接损伤大分子 DNA 外，还诱导心肌细胞的凋亡，导致心功能的损伤[9]。本实验中单纯心肌梗死时 NO 含量虽有降低的趋势，但与正常对照组相比无显著差异，该结果提示可能在不同的实验条件下 NO 产生速率不同和不同类型的 NOS 产生活性作用不同。本实验中 ET 含量无明显变化，可能与心肌梗死后经历时间较长有关，有报道在心肌梗死后 5d，ET 含量即恢复到正常水平[10]。

NO 作为信使分子，能参与调节神经递质释放和血流，还参与神经发育和基因表达调控等多种生理过程[11,12]。故有学者认为，血浆 NO 浓度增加，可能通过影响中枢 5-HT、NE 等神经递质释放并加重脑损伤而诱发抑郁症状[13]。临床观察也发现抑郁症发作期患者血浆 NO 产物水平明显高于缓解期[2]。我们的实验也证实，慢性应激抑郁时，血浆 NO 含量明显升高，进一步支持 NO 与抑郁症发病相关的假设。同时还发现，当心肌梗死合并慢性应激（抑郁）后对血浆 NO 升高的影响有明显的协同促进作用，提示 NO 的异常增加可能是心肌梗死合并抑郁时一个重要的病理生理变化。

冠心病被认为是一种基于血管内皮损伤基础上的慢性炎症反应过程。C-反应蛋白（CRP）是机体非特异性炎症反应的敏感标志物之一。Miller 等[14]研究发现，抑郁症患者血液中 hs-CRP 的含量较健康人增高，提示抑郁可能参与了机体的炎症反应。而 AMI 患者中抑郁者具有较高的炎性活跃倾向[15]。本实验结果表明，无论在心肌梗死模型大鼠或慢性应激抑郁大鼠中，均可出现 hs-CRP 的显著升高（P < 0.01），且在心肌梗死合并慢性应激时，hs-CRP 的升高更为显著（P < 0.01），提示慢性炎症反应可能是抑郁促发及加重冠心病的一个重要的病理生理机制。精神应激或抑郁可能通过改变机体神经-内分泌及免疫系统，从而触发或加重了内皮的损伤以及随后发生的炎症过程[16]，进而诱发、促使冠心病的产生。体内 IL-6 是 CRP 的诱导物，可促进肝合成并分泌 CRP 等急性时相反应产物，因此 CRP 升高时常伴有 IL-6 的升高。但在我们的实验中并未观察到 IL-6 升高的现象，可能与实验样本量小或应激方法等有关，确切的原因还有待进一步的实验来探讨。

能够建立适宜的动物模型来探讨抑郁与冠心病之间共同的病理生理机制，对于防治冠心病合并抑郁具有重要的意义。我们的初步研究结果表明，NO 的变化和炎症反应是心肌梗死合并抑郁时出现的重要的病理生理变化，但它们与心肌梗死后抑郁之间的因果关系还有待于进一步研究探讨。

参考文献

[1] 鲍正宇，毛家亮．抑郁障碍与心肌梗死的研究进展．医学综述，2006，15（2）：921-922．

[2] Suzuki E, Yagi G, Nakaki T, et al. Elevated plasma nitrate levels in depressive states. J Affect Disord, 2001, 63 (1-3): 221-224.

[3] Dentino AN, Pieper CF, Rao MK, et al. Association of interleukin-6 and other biologic variables with depression in older people living in the community. J Am Geriatr Soc, 1999, 47 (1): 6-11.

[4] 金星，刘剑刚，李婕，等．慢性应激对急性心肌梗死大鼠血液流变学的影响．中国血液流变学杂志，2008，18（1）：8-10．

[5] Katz RJ, Roth KA, Carroll BJ. Acute and chronic stress effects on open field activity in the rat implications for a model of depression. Neurosci Biobehav Rev, 1981, 5 (2): 247-251.

[6] Willner P, Towell A, Sampson D, et al. Reduction of sucrose preference by chronic unpredictable mild stress，and its restoration by a tricyclic antidepressant. Psychopharmacology (Berl), 1987, 93 (3):358-364.

[7] Willner P. Validity, reliability and utility of the chronic mild stress model of depression: a 10-year review and evaluation. Psychopharmacology (Berl), 1997, 134 (4):319-329.

[8] 卢萌，罗国荣．冠心病患者治疗前后血 NO/NOS 和 ET 检测的临床意义．放射免疫学杂志，2004，17（6）：435-436．

[9] 石姝梅，陆东风．急性缺血与 L- 精氨酸干预对大鼠心肌组织一氧化氮合酶基因表达的影响．中国老年医学杂志，2008，28（12）：1069-1072．

[10] 公惠萍，张佩珍，王庸晋．急性心肌梗死患者血浆内皮素水平的改变．临床荟萃，2001，16（9）：394-395．

[11] Szabo C. Physiological and pathophysiological roles of nitric oxide in the central nervous system. Brain Res Bull, 1996, 41 (3):131-141.

[12] 孙际童，李洪岩，苏静，等．人参二醇组皂苷（PDS）抑制 NOS 和 p38 减轻 LPS 休克脑损伤．中国病理生理杂志，2008，24（1）：44-46．

[13] 张洪燕，张志君，史家波，等．一氧化氮及内皮型一氧化氮合酶基因 G894T 多态性与抑郁症及抗抑郁疗效相关分析．中国行为医学科学，2007，16（1）：18-20．

[14] Miller GE, Stetler CA, Carney RM, et al. Clinical depression and inflammatory risk markers for coronary heart disease. Am J Cardiol, 2002, 90 (12):1279-1283.

[15] 黄铁军，王雪莱．"后心梗抑郁"与 AMI 患者 IL-6、CRP 水平的关系．放射免疫学杂志，2004，17（4）：262-264．

[16] 吕俊华，钟玲．实验性抑郁症动物模型的评价．中国病理生理杂志，2001，17（9）：916-919．

Panax Quinquefolium Saponins Reduce Myocardial Hypoxia-Reoxygenation Injury by Inhibiting Excessive Endoplasmic Reticulum Stress[*]

WANG Chen　LI Yu-zhen　WANG Xiao-reng　LU Zhen-rong　SHI Da-zhuo　LIU Xiu-hua

1. Introduction

Panax quinquefolium (American ginseng) belongs to the Araliaceous family and is native to the northern United States and southern Canada. It is a popular, nutritional supplement throughout the world, and its leaves and stems exhibit a host of medicinal effects. The chemical compositions of *P. quinquefolium* stem and leaf extracts have been studied for more than a decade, and these analyses have resulted in the identification of

---

* 原载于 Shock，2012，37（2）：228-233

saponins, amino acids, carbohydrates, volatile oils, inorganic elements, and fatty acids that may contribute to these health benefits. The saponins in particular are responsible for numerous pharmacological actions. With the development of modern technology, more than 40 distinct saponin compounds have been isolated and identified, while still a lot is being filtered. Both cell culture and animal models have demonstrated that *P. quinquefolium* saponin (PQS) has potential benefits for the cardiovascular system by chelating transition metal ions, scavenging free radicals, as well as inhibiting the activation of protein tyrosine kinase induced by ischemia-reperfusion (I-R), modifying vasomotor function, and by improving serum lipid profiles. Furthermore, PQS directly exerted preventive effects of myocardial ischemia and reperfusion injury induced by hyperbaric oxygen[1-5]. As a dietary supplement and a tonic, PQS has the unique ability to stimulate the immune system. Pretreatment with PQS can upregulate the ability of treated cardiomyocytes to combat hypoxia-reoxygenation (H-R) injury.

The endoplasmic reticulum (ER) is the main organelle for protein synthesis, protein folding, and intracellular calcium storage. Disordered ER Ca^{2+} homeostasis, ischemia, hypoxia, nutrient deprivation, ATP depletion, oxidative stress, and the accumulation of misfolded proteins all lead to ER stress (ERS). Recent evidence suggests that severe ERS can lead to cell dysfunction following I-R[6]. Moderate ERS upregulates the expression of ERS molecular indicators such as glucose-regulated protein 78 (GRP78) and calreticulin (CRT), enhances degradation of misfolded (mutant or unfolded) proteins, and inhibits protein synthesis to decrease the functional load within the ER. Prolonged and excessive ERS, however, can aggravate I-R injury by reducing ER Ca^{2+} buffering capacity, leading to Ca^{2+} overload and mitochondrial dysfunction[7,8]. Under excessive or prolonged ERS, important mediators of ERS-associated death include the cleavage and activation of ER-associated caspase 12 and increased expression of CCAAT/enhancer-binding protein homologous protein (CHOP), a transcription factor that sensitizes cell to apoptosis.

Excessive ERS is one of the key mechanisms of I-R injury[9]. The aim of the present study was to investigate whether PQS can protect cardiomyocytes against H-R injury by suppressing excessive ERS.

2. Materials and Methods

2.1　Materials

Panax quinquefolium saponins were provided by Yisheng Pharmaceutical Co, Ltd, Jilin, China; other materials adopted in our study were as follows: Dulbecco modified Eagle medium (DMEM; Gibco, Grand Island, NY); newborn calf serum (NCS) (PAA, Pasching, Austria); trypsin (Amresco, Solon, Ohio); protease inhibitor and penicillin/streptomycin (Sigma, St Louis, M); phosphatase inhibitor and bovine serum albumin (Merck, Darmstadt, Germany); an annexin V-fluorescein isothiocyanate apoptosis detection kit (Nanjing Kaiji Biological Engineering Co, Ltd, Nanjing, China); a lactate dŴydrogenase (LDH) detection kit (Nanjing Jiancheng Biological Engineering Institute, Nanjing, China); agarose, TRNzol-A+ RNA extraction reagent, and Taq polymerase (Beijing Tiangen Biochemistry Technique Co, Ltd, Beijing, China); a cDNA first-strand synthesis kit (Beijing Quanshijin Biological Technique Co, Ltd, Beijing, China); the PCR primers (Beijing Sanboyuanzhi Biological Technique Co, Ltd, Beijing, China); rabbit polyclonal antibodies against CRT, GRP78, and caspase 12 (Stressgen, New York); rabbit polyclonal antibodies against Bcl-2 and Bax, a rabbit monoclonal antibody against glyceraldŴyde 3-phosphate dehydrogenase (GAPDH), as well as mouse monoclonal antibody against CHOP (Cell Signaling Technology, Danvers, Mass); an enhanced chemiluminescence kit (Millipore, Mass); and horseradish peroxidase (HRP)-conjugated goat anti-mouse immunoglobulin G (IgG) and anti-rabbit IgG (Santa Cruz Biotechnology, Santa Cruz, Calif).

2.2 Animals

One-day-old male Sprague-Dawley rats were used for cardiomyocyte culture. The investigation conforms to the Guide for the Care and Use of Laboratory Animals published by the US National Institutes of Health (NIH publication 85-23, revised 1996) and approved by the local animal care and use committee.

2.3 Cell Culture and Treatment

Ventricular cardiomyocytes were cultured by Simpson and Savion's[10] method as described with some modifications. Briefly, cardiac ventricles taken from 1-day-old Sprague-Dawley rats were gently minced and enzymatically dissociated using 0.15% trypsin solution in a shaker at 37 ℃. Cells were collected by centrifugation and preplated for 1.5 h in DMEM with 15% NCS and 1% penicillin/streptomycin (100 U/mL) to permit the attachment of noncardiomyocytes. Unattached cells were removed, replated in T-75 flasks with the same medium at a density of 3×10^6 cells per flask, and incubated at 37 ℃ in a cell culture incubator under a humidified atmosphere with 5% CO_2.

After a 24h culturing, cells were transferred to serum-free maintenance medium (DMEM containing 1% penicillin/streptomycin) for 24 h before experimentation. To assess the protective efficacy of PQS against myocardial H-R injury, cells were divided into three groups: (a) normal control group: cells remained in a 5% CO_2 incubator at 37 ℃ for the duration of the experiment; (b) H-R group: cells were transferred to a hypoxic chamber filled with a 95% N_2-5% CO_2 gas mixture for 4 h and then back to the normoxic CO_2 incubator at 37 ℃ for 12 h of reoxygenation; and (c) PQS + H-R group: PQS powder was diluted with phosphate-buffered saline buffer into a concentration of 16 mg/mL (as determined by our pilot experiments), sterile filtrated, and stored at 4 ℃. For application, these stock solutions were diluted 100-fold and added to cardiomyocytes

culture medium at a final concentration of 160μg/mL. Cells were first pretreated with the culture medium containing 160μg/mL PQS for 24 h, then exposed to the 95% N_2-5% CO_2 gas mixture for 4 h and reoxygenated for 12 h without drugs. Above all of these, to elucidate the impact of ERS on H-R-induced cell apoptosis, cells were then divided into four groups: i.e., normal control group, H-R group, PQS + H-R group, and PQS group. The first three groups were treated as described previously. Cells in the PQS group were cultured in the CO_2 incubator at 37 ℃ in the culture medium containing 160μg/mL PQS for 24h in the absence of H-R.

2.4 Cell Viability and LDH Activity

Cell viability was assessed using the trypan blue exclusion technique[11], and viable cell count was calculated by dividing the number of unstained (viable) cells by the total number of the initial cell count. Lactate dehydrogenase activity was determined using a LDH activity detection kit according to the manufacturer's instructions.

2.5 Annexin V and Propidium Iodide Double-Staining Assay

Cardiomyocytes were plated in T-25 flasks at a cell density of 3×10^5 cells per flask. After treatment, the cells were removed from flasks using 0.25% trypsin + 0.02% EDTA and analyzed for apoptosis using an annexin V and propidium iodide apoptosis kit (according to the manufacturer's instructions) on a BD FACScalibur flow cytometer (BD Biosciences, Franklin Lakes, NJ).

2.6 Reverse Transcriptase-Polymerase Chain Reaction

Cardiomyocytes were plated in T-25 flasks at a cell density of 6×10^5 cells per flask. After treatment, total RNA was isolated from cardiomyocytes using TRNzol-A+ reagent. After phenol/chloroform extraction and isopropanol precipitation, total RNA was washed in 75% ethanol and quantified using a spectrophotometer (Unico, St Louis, Mo) at 260 nm. Reverse transcriptasepolymerase chain reaction (RT-

PCR) was performed by a two-step protocol using a cDNA first-strand synthesis kit and Taq polymerase. Primer sequences for RT-PCR analysis of target genes are presented in Table 1. The starting PCR condition was as followed: 5 min predenaturation at 94℃ , 32 cycles of 30-s denaturation at 94 ℃ , 30-s annealing at 55℃ , and 30-s extension at 72℃ , followed by a final extension step for 10 min at 72℃ . The number of cycles and the annealing temperature were adjusted depending on the gene to be amplified. The PCR products were resolved on 1.5% agarose gels, and the GAPDH gene was used as the internal control. The signal intensities of the amplification products were analyzed using the Image-Pro Plus software (Media Cybernetics, Bethesda, Md).

2.7 Western Blot Analysis

Cardiomyocytes were plated in T-25 flasks at a cell density of 1×10^6 cells per flask. After treating, equal amount of protein extracted from cardiomyocytes (80μg/lane as determined by the Bradford method) was separated by 12% sodium dodecyl sulfate-polyacrylamide gels. After electrophoresis, proteins were electrophoretically transferred to nitrocellulose membranes blocked with 5% bovine serum albumin in Tris-buffered saline containing 0.1% Tween 20 (TBS-T) at room temperature for 40 min. Then membranes were probed with primary antibodies against GRP78, CRT, CHOP, caspase 12, Bcl-2, Bax, and GAPDH (all 1 : 500 diluted) at 4℃ overnight. The antibody-tagged membranes were incubated with a secondary antibody solution consisting of either a 1 : 1,000 dilution of HRP-conjugated goat anti-mouse IgG (for CHOP) or a 1 : 1,000 dilution of HRP-conjugated goat anti-rabbit IgG (for GRP78, CRT, caspase 12, Bcl-2, Bax, and GAPDH). An enhanced chemiluminescent detection system was used for immunoblot protein detection. The optical density of the bands (as measured in arbitrary densitometry units) was determined using Image-Pro Plus, and the densitometry of the immunoblots was normalized against GADPH.

2.8 Statistical Analysis

The SAS 8.2 program (Cary, NC) was adopted for statistical analysis. Values are presented as mean (SD). For multiple-group comparisons, oneway analysis of variance followed by Newman-Keuls post hoc analysis was performed. Pearson bivariate correlation analysis was applied to determine the correlation between variables. $P < 0.05$ was considered to be statistically significant.

Table 1　Primer Sequences Used for RT-PCR

Gene name	Primer sequences (rat)	Temperature, ℃	Length, base pairs
CRT	P1: 5′-CAA GGA TAT CCGGTG TAA GGA-3′	58.01	445
	P2: 5′-CAT AGA TAT TCGCAT CGG GG-3′	57.80	
GRP78	P1: 5′-TCT GGT TGG CGG ATC TAC TC-3′	59.85	345
	P2: 5′-TCT TTT GTC AGGGGT CGT TC-3′	57.80	
CHOP	P1: 5′-AGC TGG AAG CCT GGT ATG AG-3′	59.85	256
	P2: 5′-GAC CAC TCT GTTTCC GTT TC-3′	57.80	
Bcl-2	P1: 5′-AATTTCCTGCATC TCATGCC-3′	55.75	279
	P2: 5′-AGCCCCTCTGTG ACAGCTTA-3′	59.85	
Bax	P1: 5′-TTCATCCAGGATC GAGCAG-3′	57.56	234
	P2: 5′-CCAGTTGAAGTTG CCATCAG-3′	57.8	
GAPDH	P1: 5′-TGC TGA GTA TGT CGT GGA G -3′	61.12	496
	P2: 5′-GTC TTC TGA GTG GCA GTG AT -3′	60.07	

3. Results

3.1　Effects of PQS on H-R Injury of Cardio-myocytes

Apoptosis detected by flow cytometry (double-staining with annexin V and PI) at the end of the experiment is shown in Figure 1. The apoptosis rate of control cardiomyocytes was 2%, whereas 7% of cardiomyocytes subjected to H-R were apoptotic ($P < 0.05$). It is revealed that exposure of cardiomyocytes to PQS results in a decrease in apoptosis rate in a dose-dependent (Figure1, A and B) fashion. Therefore, pretreatment with 160 μg/mL PQS 24h before H-R exhibited a significantly lower rate of apoptosis (3%) ($P < 0.05$ vs. the H-R group), and all of the PQS values are not different from the control group ($P > 0.05$).

LDH activity—Lactate dehydrogenase in the culture medium was measured to estimate cell death under the different treatment conditions (Table 2). The LDH leakage from control cardiomyocytes was 113 U/L. Compared with control cardiomyocytes, LDH leakage from cardiomyocytes subjected to H-R was 6-fold higher ($P < 0.05$), whereas PQS-pretreated cardiomyocytes demonstrated a significant 67%

decrease in LDH activity compared with the H-R group ($P < 0.05$).

Cell viability—Cellular viability detected by trypan blue assay is presented in Table 2. The viability of control cardiomyocyte was 96%. Compared with control cardiomyocytes, the viability of cardiomyocytes subjected to H-R was reduced by 22% ($P < 0.05$). Pretreatment with PQS significantly attenuated the H-R injury, and the variability of cardiomyocytes in the PQS + H-R group was 21% higher than that of the H-R group ($P < 0.05$).

3.2　Bcl-2 and Bax Expression

Alterations in mRNA expression of Bax and Bcl-2 in cardiomyocytes were detected by RT-PCR. Hypoxia-reoxygenation reduced the expression of antiapoptotic protein Bcl-2 by 44.5% ($P < 0.05$ vs. control group) and increased the expression of proapoptotic Bax mRNA by 86.9% ($P < 0.05$ vs. control group). Pretreatment with PQS significantly attenuated H-R injury and altered expression of Bcl-2 and Bax. It evoked an in crease in Bcl-2 mRNA expression by 30.9% and a decrease in Bax mRNA expression by 39.7% relative to the H-R group.

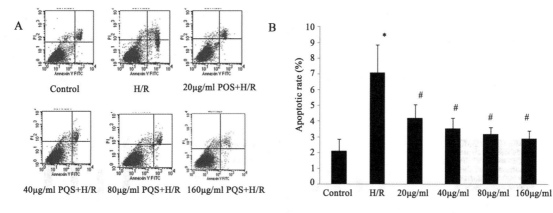

Figure1　PQS Reduce Apoptosis Induced by H-R *in Vitro* as Determined by Flow Cytometric Analysis of Annexin V and Propidium Lodide Double-Stained Cardiomyocytes. A, Cardiomyocytes were pretreated or not with a range dosage of PQS from 20 to 160μg/mL, respectively, for 24 h. Then, cells were exposed to hypoxia for 4 h with 12 h of reoxygenation. Cardiomyocytes were subsequently analyzed by flow cytometry. B, Quantification of flow cytometric counts of apoptotic cells shown in A. Graph showing statistically significant reduction in apoptotic rate in cardiomyocytes pretreated with a range dosage of PQS before H-R (PQS + H-R group) compared with H-R alone and in a dose-dependent fashion. The error bars denote SD (*$P < 0.05$ vs. control, #$P < 0.05$ vs. H-R; $n = 3$)

Table 2　Effect of PQS on Cardiomyocytes' Survival Rates and LDH Activity (*n* = 3)

Group	Cell survival (%)	LDH activity (U/L)
Control	96 (1)	113 (12)
H-R	75 (2)*	671 (47)*
160μg/mL PQS + H-R	95 (1)⁺	224 (23)*⁺

Values are presented as mean (SD)；*$P < 0.05$ *vs.* control；
⁺$P < 0.05$ *vs.* H-R

Alterations in Bcl-2 and Bax protein expression were detected by Western blotting. Hypoxia-reoxygenation reduced expression of Bcl-2 by 58.3% ($P < 0.05$ *vs.* control) and enhanced expression of Bax protein by 167% ($P < 0.05$), whereas PQS pretreatment enhanced Bcl-2 expression by 48% and decreased Bax protein expression by 48.4% compared with H-R alone. Meanwhile, treatment with PQS in the absence of H-R showed no difference from the control group in both mRNA and protein expression ($P > 0.05$) (Figure 2).

3.3　Effects of PQS on Expression of ERS Molecules

GRP78 and CRT expression—We also measured changes in GRP78 and CRT mRNA expression by RT-PCR. Hypoxiareoxygenation evoked a 3-fold increase in GRP78 mRNA and a 96% increase in CRT mRNA relative to the control groups ($P < 0.05$), whereas PQS pretreatment attenuated these H-R-evoked increases in mRNA expression by 61.6% and 35.7%, respectively, compared with H-R alone. In addition, changes in protein expression were qualitatively similar; the H-R-evoked increases in GRP78 and CRT (142% and 312%, $P < 0.05$) were significantly reduced in the PQS + H-R group (by 37.7% and 52.2%, respectively, compared with H-R alone, $P < 0.05$). Meanwhile, treatment with PQS in the absence of H-R showed no difference from the control group in both mRNA and protein expressions of GRP78 and CRT ($P > 0.05$) (Figure 3).

CHOP expression—Hypoxia-reoxygenation enhanced mRNA expression of the proapoptotic factor CHOP by 311% relative to the control groups ($P < 0.05$), whereas PQS pretreatment reduced H-R-evoked CHOP overexpression by 57% compared with H-R alone. Similarly, CHOP protein expression was enhanced by 219% in H-R-treated cardiomyocytes ($P < 0.05$), whereas PQS attenuated H-R-induced CHOP overexpression by 51.7% compared with H-R alone (Figure 4, A and B).

Caspase 12 activity in cardiomy-ocytes-expressions of activated caspase 12 and inactive procaspase 12 were detected by Western blotting (Figure 4, C and D). Expression of the procaspase 12 (48-50 kd) was not significantly different between treatment groups ($P > 0.05$). The level of the 36-kd cleaved (activated) caspase 12 was increased by 1.2-fold in H-R-treated cardiomyocytes compared with the control group ($P < 0.05$), whereas PQS pretreatment reduced 36-kd caspase 12 expression by

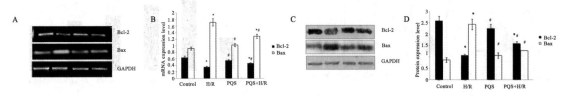

Figure2　PQS Reduced the Expression of Proapoptotic Bax and Increased Expression of Antiapoptotic Bcl-2 in H-R-treated Cardiomyocytes. A, The levels of Bcl-2 and Bax mRNA were examined by RT-PCR. GAPDH was used as a normalization control. Line 1, control group; line 2, H-R group; line 3, PQS group; line 4, PQS + H-R group. B, Histogram of densitometry of the bands shown in A. C, The levels of Bcl-2 and Bax protein were examined by Western blot. GAPDH was used as a normalization control. Line 1, control group; line 2, H-R group; line 3, PQS group; line 4, PQS + H-R group. D, Histogram of densitometry of the bands shown in C. The error bars denote SD (*$P < 0.05$ *vs.* control, #$P < 0.05$ *vs.* H-R; *n* = 3)

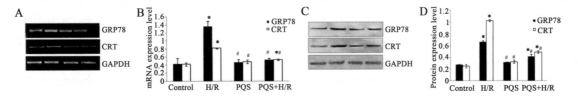

Figure3　Effect of PQS on the Expression of ERS Molecular Indicators of GRP78 and CRT in H-R-treated Cardiomyocytes. A, The levels of GRP78 and CRT mRNA were examined by RT-PCR. GAPDH was used as a normalization control. Line 1, control group; line 2, H-R group; line 3, PQS group; line 4, PQS + H-R group. B, Histogram of densitometry of the bands shown in A. C, The levels of GRP78 and CRT protein were examined by Western blot. GAPDH was used as a normalization control. Line 1, control group; line 2, H-R group; line 3, PQS group; line 4, PQS + H-R group. D, Histogram of densitometry of the bands shown in C. The error bars denote SD (*$P < 0.05$ vs. control, #$P < 0.05$ vs. H-R; $n = 3$)

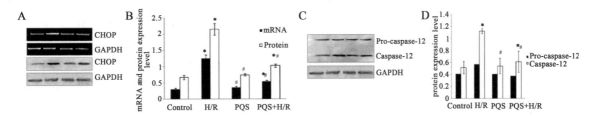

Figure 4　Effect of PQS on the Expression of the ERS-associated Apoptotic Protein CHOP and Activation of the Apoptotic Effector Enzyme Caspase 12 in H-R-induced Cardiomyocytes. A, The levels of CHOP mRNA and protein were examined by RT-PCR and Western blot. GAPDH was used as a normalization control. Line 1, control group; line 2, H-R group; line 3, PQS group; line 4, PQS + H-R group. B, Histogram of densitometry of the bands shown in A. C, Western blot analysis of caspase 12 activation in cardiomyocytes. GAPDH was used as a normalization control. Line 1, control group; line 2, H-R group; line 3, PQS group; line 4, PQS + H-R group. D, Histogram of densitometry of the bands shown in C. The error bars denote SD (*$P < 0.05$ vs. control, #$P < 0.05$ vs. H-R; $n = 3$)

34.9% compared with H-R alone ($P < 0.05$). No significant difference was found in CHOP expression and caspase 12 activation between PQS in the absence of H-R group and control group ($P > 0.05$) (Figure 4, C and D).

3.4　The Correlation Analysis of CHOP and Bcl-2, Bax Protein Expression

The correlation analysis revealed that CHOP expression showed a significant positive correlation with Bax expression ($r = 0.956$, $P < 0.05$) and negative correlation with Bcl-2 expression ($r = -0.967$, $P < 0.05$).

4.　Discussion

Ischemia-reperfusion injury refers to the progressive and irreversible tissue damage caused by ischemia and reperfusion during the return of the blood supply[12]. Apoptosis among cardiomyocytes was first reported by Gottlieb et al.[13]. Increasing evidence suggests that cardiomyocyte apoptosis might contribute to the pathogenesis of I-R injury, and to date, more and more studies focus on the role of ERS in cardiomyocytes apoptosis. Necrosis and apoptosis are distinct mechanisms of cell death. "Necrosis" is often used to describe cell death other than apoptotic cell death. There is no debate that prolonged and severe ischemia alone can kill myocytes by necrosis, and LDH activity is applied to assess the cell injury. When all the cells are lysed, the maximum LDH activity that can be measured is 100%. The percentage of the cells that die by necrosis as indicated by LDH release is less than 20%[14]. However, debate continues over whether the irreversible process culminating in cell death can be initiated by the act of reperfusion itself. Apoptosis as a component of reperfusion injury is a process that is potentially preventable. In the heart, apoptosis is a dominant form of cardiomyocyte death in I-R[15,16].

Musat-Marcu and his colleagues[17] observed apoptotic cells in rat myocardium *in vitro* during the early stage of reperfusion. The Bcl-2 family, composed of both proapoptotic and antiapoptotic members, constitutes a critical intracellular checkpoint for apoptosis within a common cell death pathway[18]. This family includes proteins that predispose cells to apoptosis, such as Bax and proteins that antagonize apoptosis, such as Bcl-2. The antiapoptotic gene Bcl-2 and the proapoptotic gene Bax are involved in the regulation of apoptosis during myocardial I-R injury[19]. As a dietary supplement and a tonic, PQS has the unique ability to stimulate the cellmediated immune system. Pretreatment with PQS can upregulate the ability of treated cardiomyocytes to combat H-R injury. In our study, we show that pretreatment PQS can significantly reduce myocardial H-R injury and apoptosis. Apoptosis rate and LDH activity were all significantly reduced in myocardial cells pretreated with the culture medium containing 160μg/mL PQS for 24 h before H-R; at the same time, cell survival was significantly increased by pretreating with PQS. PQS pretreatment significantly suppressed H-R-induced upregulation of Bax expression, which is similar to that in control group. However, PQS pretreatment showed only a moderate upregulation of Bcl-2 expression, indicating that the PQS's regulatory effect on Bcl-2 expression was lower than its inhibitory effect on upregulation of Bax expression. Our results showed that PQS protected cardiomyocytes from H-R injury mainly by suppressing H-R-induced Bax upregulation.

Oxygen free radicals and calcium overload are critical downstream mediators of I-R injury. Recently, most studies have focused on mitochondrial pathways leading to cell death, whereas the role of the ER has not been extensively studied. The ER is a crucial organelle for intracellular Ca^{2+} transfer and protein synthesis, so ERS resulting from physical and chemical changes of ER is supposed to be a critical pathogenesis for I-R injury[20,21]. Endoplasmic reticulum stress is an adaptive response; moderate ERS induces upregulation of ER chaperones, including GRP78 and CRT [22], which enhance the capacity for processing of unfolded proteins that promote the functional recovery of the ER. However, excessive ERS triggered by H-R leads to overexpression of GRP78 and CRT [23,24] and induces the expression and activation of the proapoptotic factors such as CHOP and caspase 12. Our study demonstrated that PQS suppressed H-R-induced ERS, as shown in decrease in GRP78 and CRT overexpression. Meanwhile, treatment with PQS alone had the tendency of upregulating the expression of GRP78 and CRT, so as to preinduce moderate ERS to protect cardiomyocytes from lethal injury. This agrees with the findings of Zhang et al. [25], who reported that preinduced ERS protects cardiomyocytes from lethal oxidative injury.

The CHOP protein promotes apoptosis through direct regulation of target genes that increase the sensitivity of cells to ERS-mediated apoptosis[26,27]. The CHOP-mediated apoptosis signaling pathway is closely linked to the mitochondrial apoptosis pathway in that CHOP can reduce Bcl-2 protein expression, leading to Bax translocation from cytoplasm to mitochondria [28] and activation of the mitochondrial apoptotic pathway. The present study showed that CHOP overexpression induced by H-R was significantly inhibited in myocardial cells pretreated with the culture medium containing 160μg/mL PQS. Further correlative analysis indicated that CHOP protein expression was positively correlated with Bax protein expression and negatively correlated with Bcl-2 protein expression, suggesting that CHOP-mediated apoptotic signaling may induce apoptosis by inhibiting Bcl-2 and promoting Bax protein expression. These results are consistent with previous literature[29,30]and demonstrate that PQS can protect myocardial cells by inhibiting both ER-mediated and mitochondrial apoptosis pathways.

Procaspase 12 is a constitutively expressed protein located on the cytoplasmic side of the ER membrane. The inactive procaspase 12 zymogens are cleaved and activated by tumor necrosis factor receptor-associated factor 2 [31]. Cleaved caspase 12 causes apoptosis through activation of caspases 9 and 3[32]. Thus, caspase 12 is a key factor of the ER apoptosis pathway and allows ER-mediated apoptosis to act synergistically with the mitochondrial-dependent apoptosis pathway. We found that H-R induced significant cleavage of caspase 12 and apoptosis in cardiomyocytes[33]. Caspase 12 protein expression was significantly inhibited in myocardial cells pretreated with PQS, indicating that PQS inhibited apoptosis by suppressing caspase 12.

The neonatal cardiomyocyte model offers a broad spectrum of experiments. It has been shown that the phenotype of cultured neonatal cardiomyocytes is highly stable, and their contractile profile during H-R is compatible with in situ hearts during I-R [34]. Furthermore, this cardiac cell model of H-R has been successfully used in previous studies[35,36]. We applied this model, therefore, to further investigate the anti-H-R effects of PQS in the present study. We found that PQS has shown a significant cardioprotective effect against H-R injury through inhibiting excessive ERS as evidenced by the reduction in GRP78, CRT, and CHOP overexpression, as well as caspase 12 activation, which is closely associated with reducing ER-related apoptosis of cardiomyocytes. However, the morphology and metabolism of neonatal myocytes are different from in situ adult myocytes, which are able to accommodate higher doses of medicine[37]. Therefore, the efficacy and safety profiles of PQS in adult myocytes and whole-heart tissue remain to be determined.

References

[1] Kitts DD, Wijewickreme AN, Hu C. Antioxidant properties of a North American ginseng extract. Mol Cell Binchem, 2000, 203 (1-2): 1-10.

[2] Dou DQ, Zhang YW, Zhang L, et al. The inhibitory effects of ginsenoides on protein tyrosine kinase activated by hypoxia/reoxygenation in cultured human umbilical vein endothelial cells. Planta Med, 2001, 67 (1): 19-23.

[3] Kang SY, Schini-Kerth VB, Kim ND. Ginsenosides of the protopanaxatriol group cause endothelium-dependent relaxation in the rat aorta. Life Sci , 1995, 56 (19): 1577-1586.

[4] Li JP, Huang M, Teoh H, et al. Interactions between Panax quinquefolium saponins and vitamin C are observed in vitro. Mol Cell Biochem, 2000, 204 (1-2): 77-82.

[5] Maffei Facino R, Carini M, Aldini G, et al. Panax ginseng administration in the rat prevents myocardial ischemia-reperfusion damage induced by hyperbaric oxygen: evidence for antioxidant intervention. Planta Med, 1995, 65 (7): 614-619.

[6] Rao RV, Poksay KS, Castro-Obregon S, et al. Molecular components of a cell death pathway activated by endoplasmic reticulum stress. J Biol Chem, 2004, 279 (1): 177-187.

[7] Boya P, Cohen I, Zamzami N, et al. Endoplasmic reticulum stress induced cell death requires mitochondrial membrane permeabilization.Cell Death Differ, 2002, 9: 465-467.

[8] Breckenridge DG, Germain M, Mathai JP, et al. Regulation of apoptosis by endoplasmic reticulum pathways. Oncogene, 2003, 22: 8608-8618.

[9] Xu C, Bailly-Maitre B, Reed J. Endoplasmic reticulum stress: cell life and death decisions. J Clin Invest, 2005, 115 (10): 2656-2664.

[10] Simpson P, Savion S. Differentiation of rat myocytes in single cell cultures with and without proliferating non-myocardial cells. Cross-striations, ultrastructure, and chronotropic response to isoproterenol. Circ Res, 1982, 50 (1): 101-116.

[11] Rabkin SW, Kong J. Nitroprusside induces cardiomyocyte death: interaction with hydrogen peroxide. Am J Physiol Heart Circ Physiol , 2000, 279 (6): H3089-H3100.

[12] Brawnwald E, Kloned RA. Myocardial reperfusion: a

double edged sword？ J Clin Invest , 1995, 76 (5): 1713.

[13] Gottlieb RA, Burleson KO, Kloner RA, et al. Reperfusion injury induces apoptosis in rabbit cardiomyocytes. J Clin Invest, 1994, 94 (4): 1621-1628.

[14] Kubasiak LA, Hernandez OM, Bishopric NH, et al. Hypoxia and acidosis activate cardiac myocyte death through the Bcl-2 family protein BNIP3. PNAS, 2002, 99 (20): 12825-12830.

[15] Fliss H, Gattinger D. Apoptosis in ischemic and reperfused rat myocardium. Circ Res, 1996, 79: 949-956.

[16] Reeve JL, Duffy AM, Q' Brien T, et al. Don't lose heart-therapeutic value of apoptosis prevention in the treatment of cardiovascular disease. J Cell Mol Med, 2005, 9 (3): 609-622.

[17] Musat-Marcu S, Gunter HE, Jugdutt BI, et al. Inhibition of apoptosis after ischemia-reperfusion in rat myocardium by cycloheximide. J Mol Cell Cardiol, 1999, 31 (5): 1073-1082.

[18] Chao DT, Korsmeyer SJ. Bcl-2 family: regulators of cell death. Ann Rev Immunol, 1998, 16 (1): 395-415.

[19] Borutaite V, Brown GC. Mitochondria in apoptosis of ischemic heart. FEBS Lett, 2003, 541 (1-3): 1.

[20] Shibata M, Hattori H, Sasaki T, et al. Activation of caspase-12 by endoplasmic reticulum stress induced by transient middle cerebral artery occlusion in mice. Neuroscience, 2003, 118 (2): 491-499.

[21] Vilatoba M, Eckstein C, Bilbao G, et al. Sodium 4 phenylbutyrate protects against liver ischemia reperfusion injury by inhibition of endoplasmic reticulum stress mediated apoptosis. Surgery, 2005, 38 (2): 342-351.

[22] Kaufman RJ. Stress signaling from the lumen of the endoplasmic reticulum: coordination of gene transcriptional and translational controls. Gene Dev, 1999, 13 (10): 1211-1233.

[23] Terai K, Hiramoto Y, Masaki M, et al. AMP-activated protein kinase protects cardiomyocytes against hypoxic injury through attenuation of endoplasmic reticulum stress. Mol Cell Biol, 2005, 25 (21): 9554-9575.

[24] Xudong W, Xiuhua L, Xiaomei Z, et al. Hypoxic preconditioning induces delayed cardioprotection through P38 MAPK-mediated calreticulin upregulation. Shock, 2007, 27 (5): 572-577.

[25] Zhang PL, Lun M, Teng J, et al. Preinduced molecular chaperones in the endoplasmic reticulum protect cardiomyocytes from lethal injury. Ann Clin Lab Sci, 2004, 34 (4): 449-457.

[26] Oyadomari S, Mori M. Roles of CHOP/GADD153 in endoplasmic reticulum stress. Cell Death Differ , 2004, 11 (4): 381-389.

[27] Friedman AD. GADD153/CHOP, a DNA damage-inducible protein, reduced CAAT/enhancer binding protein activities and increased apoptosis in 32D c13 myeloid cells. Cancer Res, 1996, 56 (14): 3250-3256.

[28] McCullough KD, Martindale JL, Klotz LO, et al. Gadd153 sensitizes cells to endoplasmic reticulum stress by down-regulating Bcl-2 and perturbing the cellular redox state. Mol Cell Biol, 2001, 21 (4): 1249-1259.

[29] Nieto-Miguel T, Fonteriz RI, Vay L, et al. Endoplasmic reticulum stress in the proapoptotic action of edelfosine in solid tumor cells. Cancer Res, 2007, 67 (21): 10368-10378.

[30] Gotoh T, Terada K, Oyadomari S, et al. Hsp70-DnaJ chaperone pair prevents nitric oxide- and CHOP-induced apoptosis by inhibiting translocation of Bax to mitochondria. Cell Death Differ, 2004, 11 (4): 390-402.

[31] Takunari Y, Kazunori I, Kayoko O, et al. Activation of caspase-12, an endoplasmic reticulum (ER) resident caspase, through tumor necrosis factor receptor-associated factor 2-dependent mechanism in response to the ER stress. J Biol Chem, 2001, 276 (17): 13935-13940.

[32] Nakagawa T, Zhu H, Morishima N, et al. Caspase-12 mediates endoplasmic-reticulum-specific apoptosis and cytotoxicity by amyloid-beta. Nature, 2000, 403: 98-103.

[33] Xiu-Hua L, Zhen-Ying Z, Sheng S, et al. Ischemic postconditioning protects myocardium from ischemia/reperfusion injury through attenuating endoplasmic reticulum stress. Shock, 2008, 30 (4): 422-427.

[34] Yamashita N, Nishida M, Hoshida S, et al. Induction of manganese superoxide dismutase in rat cardiac myocytes increases tolerance to hypoxia 24 hours after preconditioning. J Clin Invest, 1994, 94 (6): 2143-2199.

[35] Liu XH, Wu XD, Cai LR, et al. Hypoxic precondi-

第四章

tioning of cardiomyocytes and cardioprotection phosphorylation of HIF-1 induced by p42/p44 mitogenactivated protein kinases is involved: Pathophysiology, 2003, 9 (4): 201-205.

[36] Li YZ, Liu XH, Rong F. Puma mediates the apoptotic signal of hypoxia/reoxygenation in cardiomyocytes

through mitochondrial pathway. Shock, 2011, 35 (6): 579-584.

[37] Poindexter BJ, Allison AW, Bick RJ, et al. Ginseng: cardiotonic in adult rat cardiomyocytes, cardiotoxic in neonatal rat cardiomyocytes. Life Sciences, 2006, 79 (25): 2337-2344.

Effective Components of *Panax Quinquefolius* and *Corydalis Tuber* Protect Myocardium through Attenuating Oxidative Stress and Endoplasmic Reticulum Stress

XUE Mei　LIU Mei-lin　ZHU Xin-yuan　YANG Lin　MIAO Yu　SHI Da-zhuo　YIN Hui-jun

1. Introduction

Acute myocardial infarction (AMI) is a severe stress condition that causes extensive biochemical changes, which is associated with increasing production of reactive oxygen species (ROS) [1]. The imbalance between ROS production and antioxidant defenses leads to the condition known as oxidative stress. Detrimental effects of ROS are clearly demonstrated by the findings that in transgenic mice in which an antioxidant protein, superoxide dismutase (SOD), is overexpressed, infarct size is markedly reduced [2,3]. There is a growing body of evidence which indicates that oxidative stress plays an important role in the initiation and progression of myocardial infarction (MI) [4-7].

The endoplasmic reticulum (ER) is a multifunctional intracellular organelle responsible for the synthesis and folding of proteins as well as calcium storage and signaling. Various stimuli, such as ischemia, hypoxia, oxidative stress, and inflammatory factors, have been suggested to triggering ER dysfunction, which are designated

as ER stress (ERS) [8,9]. Cells alleviate ERS through the unfolded protein response (UPR). The upregulation of ER chaperones, such as the glucose-regulated protein-78 (GRP78), contributes to the repair of unfolded proteins. However, if stress is sustained, the UPR causes cell death by transcriptional induction of CCAAT/enhancer-binding protein homologous protein (CHOP), the caspase-12 dependent pathway, and activation of the c-Jun NH_2-terminal kinase 1 (JNK1) dependent pathway [10]. Recently, Mitra et al. [11] reported that GRP78, as an ER-resident protein, assisting in protein folding and the most important upstream regulator of the UPR, was exclusively upregulated during MI. Exclusive upregulation of CHOP in MI hearts and nuclear translocation of CHOP in the hypoxic cardiomyocytes signifies induction of ERS-mediated apoptosis (Figure 1) [11]. Further, some data suggest that oxidative stress and ERS reinforce each other in thymic lymphomagenesis and sporadic amyotrophic lateral sclerosis[12-14], while there are very few reports about the mechanisms of them in

* 原载于 Evidence-Based Complementary and Alternative Medicine, 2013, Article ID: 482318

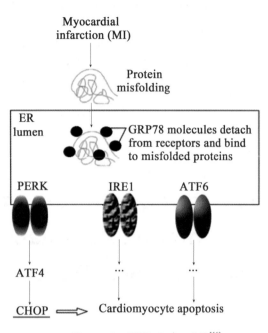

Figure 1　ERS during MI [11]

the progression of MI.

The extracts of *Panax quinquefolius* and Corydalis tuber (EPC), composed of *Panax quinquefolius* saponins and tetrahydropalmatine mainly, showed good effects for the treatment of ischemic cardiovascular diseases in clinic. *Panax quinquefolius* saponins and tetrahydropalmatine have been shown to have protective effects against oxidative stress [15-17]. Recent study demonstrated that *Panax quinquefolius* saponins can also reduce myocardial hypoxia-reoxygenation injury by inhibiting excessive ERS [18]. So we hypothesized that oxidative stress and ERS play important roles in the pathogenesis of MI. And this study was therefore undertaken to investigate whether EPC can protect myocardium against MI by suppressing oxidative stress and excessive ERS, the key proteins—GRP78 and CHOP.

2. Materials and Methods

2.1　EPC Preparation

EPC was provided by Institute of Chinese Materia Medica, China Academy of Chinese Medical Sciences. The main components were shown in Table 1, measured by high perfor-mance liquid chromatogram (HPLC) method.

Table 1　Quality Evaluation of EPC

Major constituent	Content (%)
Ginsenoside Rgl	0.11
Ginsenoside Re	1.88
Ginsenoside Rbl	5.30
Tetrahydropalmatine	0.07

2.2　Animals and Experimental Protocol

A total of 100 male Wistar rats weighing 180 ± 20g were purchased from the Institute of Laboratory Animal Sciences, Chinese Academy of Medical Sciences (Certificate no. SCXK Beijing 2005-0013). The protocol was approved by the animal care and ethics committee of the China Academy of Chinese Medical Sciences. Sham group comprised 10 randomly selected rats, and the remainder was randomly divided into 5 groups, namely, control group, metoprolol group, low-dose EPC group, moderate-dose EPC group, and high-dose EPC group, with 18 rats in each group. The left anterior descending (LAD) coronary artery was ligated in the 5 groups to establish MI model according to Olivetti's methods as described before[19,20]. The rats were anesthetized by intraperitoneal injection of urethane solution (20%) at a dose of 0.6 mL/kg. The rats in sham group did not undergo ligation. Of the surviving rats, metoprolol (AstraZeneca Pharmaceutical Co., Ltd., batch no.: 1012055), EPC were administered to metoprolol group (9 mg/kg), low-dose EPC group (0.54 g/kg), moderate-dose EPC group (1.08 g/kg), and high-dose EPC group (2.16 g/kg) by gastrogavage, respectively, once every 24h for two weeks, and an equal volume of normal saline was given to sham group and control group [21]. One hour after the last administration, the blood samples were collected from the abdominal aorta of rats and kept in a red tube biochemical procoagulant at room temperature for 60 min. The serum was separated by low-speed centrifugation and then was stored at −80℃ for use. The myocardial tissues below the ligature were stored in liquid nitrogen for Western blotting analysis.

2.3　Enzyme-Linked Immunosorbent Assay

The serum levels of malondialdehyde (MDA), SOD, and 8-iso-prostaglandin F2α (8-iso-PGF2α) were detected using enzyme-linked immunosorbent assay (ELISA) according to the manufacturer's instructions. The ELISA kits were provided by Sino-American Biotechnology Co. , Ltd. (Wuhan, China). A Multiskan type 3 microplate reader (Thermo Scientific) was used for detection.

2.4　Quantitative Real-Time Polymerase Chain Reaction (PCR)

Total mRNA was extracted using Trizol reagent (Invitrogen) according to the manufacturer's protocol. The mRNA was reverse transcribed to cDNA using M-MLV reverse transcriptase PCR Kit (TaKaRa). The primer sets for GRP78 (forward 5′-CCTGGTTCTGCTTGATGTGT-3′ and reverse 5′-TCGTTCACCTTCGTAGACCTT-3′), CHOP (forward 5′-CCAGGAAACGAAGAGGAAGA-3′ and reverse 5′-GGTGCTTGTGACCTCTGCT-3′), and glyceraldehydes phosphate dehydrogenase (GAPDH) (forward 5′-CAACTCCCTCAAGATTG TCAGCAA-3′ and reverse 5′-GGCATGGACTGT GGT CATGA-3′) were synthesized by Shanghai Sangon Biotech Co. , Ltd. PCR amplification of GRP78, CHOP, and GAPDH cDNAs was performed with 1.5 μL cDNA in the same parameters. The reverse transcription PCR and analysis were performed using the ABI PRISM 7500 sequence detection system. Reactions were run for optimal cycles with predenaturalization at 94℃ for 15 min; denaturation, annealing, and extension at 94℃ for 15s, 60℃ for 34s, 72℃ for 15 s and repeated for 40 cycles; and lastly extension at 72℃ for 10 min. The housekeeping gene GAPDH was used for internal control. The $2^{-\triangle\triangle CT}$ method [22] was used to analyze the relative changes in gene expression.

2.5　Western Blotting

The myocardium tissues were homogenized and lysed in lysis buffer. Pro-teins were separated by sodium dodecyl sulfate-polyacrylamide gel electrophoresis (SDS-PAGE) and transferred to a polyvinylidene difluoride (PVDF) membrane. The blots were then incubated with the primary antibody against GRP78 (Abcam, USA) and CHOP (Cell Signaling Technology, USA) at 4℃ overnight, and then the membrane was incubated with appropriate secondary antibody. After washing, membranes were exposed to X-ray film. The staining was quantified by scanning the films and the band density was determined with Image-Pro Plus software.

2.6　Statistical Analysis

All data from at least 9 (ELISA results) or 5 (real-time Quantitative PCR and Western blotting analysis) independent experiments were expressed as means ± standard deviation (SD). One-way analysis of variance (ANOVA) was carried out for the comparison of means. All statistical analyses were performed with SPSS version 11.0, and P values of less than 0.05 were considered to be statistically significant.

3. Results

3.1　General Condition

All the survived rats underwent operation exhibited normal physical appearance and behavior during the gavage period of different drugs. The survival outcome after LAD ligation is presented inTable 2.

3.2　Expressions of MDA, SOD, and 8-Iso-PGF2α in Serum.

The serum concentrations of MDA, SOD, and 8-iso-PGF2α are shown in Figure 2. The serum MDA and 8-iso-PGF2α levels in control group were significantly increased, while the serum SOD level decreased, compared to sham group (P < 0.05). Moderate-to-high dose EPC increased SOD, decreased 8-iso-PGF2α, and metoprolol also decreased 8-iso-PGF2α, when, respectively,

Table 2　The Outcome after LAD Ligation

Group	n	Dead rats (n)	Surviving rats (n)
Sham	10	0	10
Control	18	9	9
Metoprolol	18	6	12
Low EPC	18	9	9
Moderate EPC	18	7	11
High EPC	18	8	10

compared with control group ($P < 0.05$).

3.3　EPC Reduces GRP78 and CHOP mRNA Expressions in Infarcted Myocardium

Alterations in mRNA expression of GRP78 and CHOP in infarcted myocardium were detected by quantitative real-time PCR. Compared with sham group, the gene expression of GRP78 and CHOP increased after experimental AMI ($P < 0.05$). Metoprolol and moderate-to-high dose EPC significantly reduced the mRNA expression of GRP78 and CHOP when compared to that of control group ($P < 0.05$). The results are shown in Figure 3.

3.4　EPC Decreases GRP78 and CHOP Protein Expressions in Infarcted Myocardium

Alterations in protein expression of GRP78 and CHOP in infarcted myocardium were detected by Western blotting. As seen in Figure 4, the protein

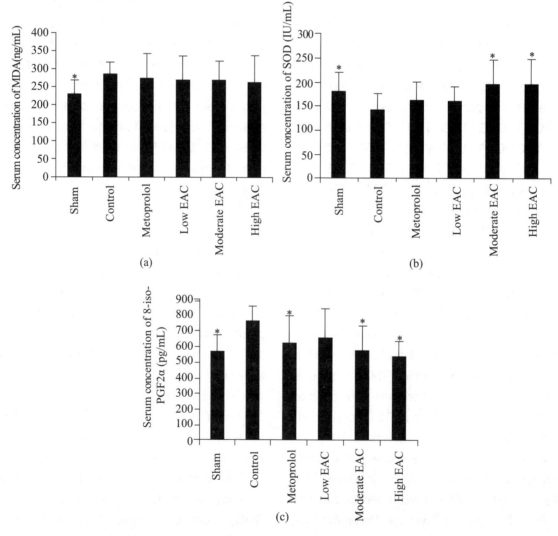

(a)

(b)

(c)

Figure 2　Serum Concentration of MDA (a), SOD (b), and 8-iso-PGF2α (c). The error bars denote SD ($P < 0.05$ compared with control group)

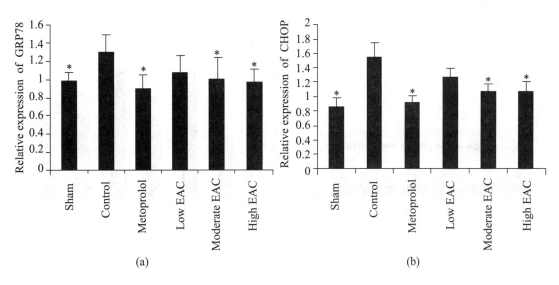

Figure 3　Expressions of GRP78 and CHOP mRNA in Infarcted Myocardium. The gene expressions of GRP78 and CHOP were determined by quantitative real-time PCR. GAPDH was used as a control reference. The error bars denote SD (*$P < 0.05$ compared with control group；n=6)

expression of GRP78 and CHOP increased after experimental AMI ($P < 0.05$). Compared with control group, metoprolol and moderate-to-high dose EPC significantly decreased the protein expression of GRP78 and CHOP ($P < 0.05$).

4. Discussion

In the setting of AMI, ROS has been indicated playing a significant role in tissue necrosis and ischemia-reperfusion injury[23,24]. Several pathways exist to protect against damage induced by ROS, with those best characterized in the heart being the superoxide dismutase. Overexpression of SOD has been shown to reduce infarct size in mice, which supports the contention that SOD is a major defense mechanism against ROS and a critical determinant in the tolerance of the heart to oxidative stress[25]. One method to quantify oxidative injury is to measure lipid peroxidation. MDA, one of the end-products of lipid peroxidation driven by ROS, can contribute significantly to the oxidative damage of proteins as it occurs under conditions of oxidative stress in age-related diseases and ischemic heart disease[26,27]. Quantification of 8-iso-PGF2α derived from the

nonenzymatic oxidation of arachidonic acid provides an accurate assessment of oxidative stress both in vitro and in vivo[28,29], which was also identified as an independent and cumulative risk marker of coronary heart disease[30]. In the present study, the expressions of MDA and 8-iso-PGF2α in control group were increased compared to sham group, while the expression of SOD decreased, which indicats that MI conditions induce oxidative stress.

Perturbations of ER homeostasis affect protein folding and cause ERS. MI conditions induce accumulation of unfolding or misfolding proteins within the ER. ER can sense the stress and then respond to it through translational attenuation, upregulation of the genes for ER chaperones and related proteins, and degradation of unfolded proteins by a quality-control system [31]. GRP78, belonging to the heat shock protein 70 group and widely used as a marker for ERS, plays an important role in many cellular processes, which can contribute to the repair of unfolded proteins [32]. One important component of the ERS-mediated apoptosis pathway is CHOP, which encourages ROS production by depleting the cell

第四章

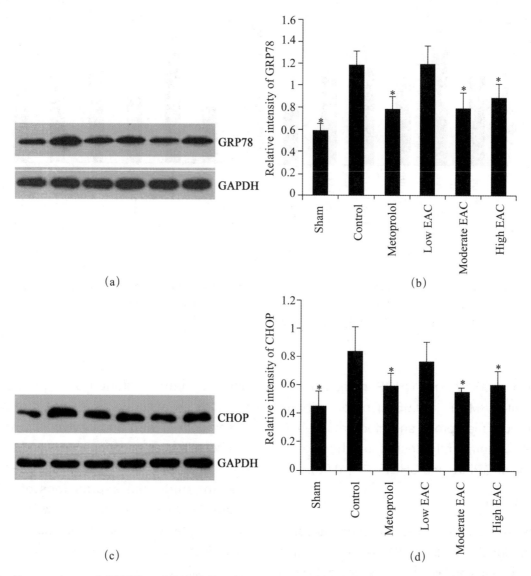

(a)　　　　　　　　　　　　(b)

(c)　　　　　　　　　　　　(d)

Figure 4　Expressions of GRP78 and CHOP Protein in Infarcted Myocardium. The expressions of GRP78 and CHOP protein in infracted myocardium were performed by Western blotting ((a) and (c)). Quantification of protein expressions were shown in (b) and (d). The error bars denote SD ($^*P < 0.05$ compared with control group; n=6)

of glutathione [31]. The results showed that both the gene and protein expressions of GRP78 and CHOP in control group were increased compared to sham group, indicating that MI conditions also induce ERS. Therefore, MI conditions induce both excessive ERS and oxidative stress.

　　Beta-blockers have been used extensively in the last 40 years after AMI as part of primary therapy and in secondary prevention. Metoprolol, a Beta-blocker, as a cornerstone in the therapy of the postinfarct heart, has an important effect

on decreasing mortality in patients after AMI [33]. George et al. reported that metoprolol can significantly improve cardiac function, result in normalized ERS marker, and reduce DNA damage in a coronary embolization model of heart failure [34]. The aforesaid results showed that metoprolol downregulated the expressions of GRP78 and CHOP in myocardium subjected to MI, protecting the myocardium by attenuating ERS. Metoprolol also decreased 8-iso-PGF2α serum level so as to suppress oxidative stress invoked by MI.

Therefore, metoprolol protect myocardium by suppressing excessive ERS and oxidative stress.

EPC, the extracts of *Panax quinquefolius* and *Corydalis tuber*, has been used for the treatment of ischemic cardiovascular diseases for years in clinic. *Panax quinquefolius* saponins and tetrahydropalmatine are the main components of EPC determined by HPLC method. Previous animal experiments and clinical trials have shown that *Panax quinquefolius* saponins have antioxidant effects, and its protective effects may be mostly attributed to scavenging H_2O_2 and hydroxyl radicals, enhancing the activities of superoxide dismutase and catalase, suppressing ROS-induced Jun Nterminal kinase activation[35-37]. Tetrahydropalmatine has been shown to have a protective effect against oxidative stress, which significantly reduced intracellular ROS formation and enhanced the production of intracellular antioxidants—SOD. Wang et al. reported that *Panax quinquefolius* saponins suppressed hypoxia-reoxygenation-induced excessive ERS, as evidenced by reduced caspase 12 activation and decreased GRP78, calreticulin, and CHOP[38]. Our findings presented here confirm and extend findings of the aforesaid works. EPC exhibited significant protective effects against oxidative stress injury in myocardium after MI by increasing SOD and decreasing 8-iso-PGF2α. Moderate-to-high dose EPC significantly decreased the mRNA and protein expressions of GRP78 and CHOP when compared with control group, indicating that EPC could alleviate injury of myocardium subjected to MI by suppressing excessive ERS. Based on our study, ERS and oxidative stress are potential therapeutic targets for human AMI. The beneficial effects of metoprolol on MI are mediated, at least in part, through the prevention of oxidative stress and ERS induced damage. EPC is an effective compound for treatment of MI by suppressing excessive ERS and oxidative stress, which provides experimental evidence for the clinical application of EPC.

5. Conclusions

Metoprolol and EPC protect the myocardium by attenuating oxidative stress and ERS in MI rats, highlighting the ERS pathways as potential therapeutic targets for MI. Further mechanistic study will be necessary to elucidate these interactions fully.

References

[1] Bagatini MD, Martins CC, Battisti V, et al. Oxidative stress versus antioxidant defenses in patients with acute myocardial infarction. Heart and Vessels, 2011, 26 (1) : 55-63.

[2] Hori M, Nishida K. Oxidative stress and left ventricular remodelling after myocardial infarction. Cardiovascular Research, 2009, 81 (3) : 457-464.

[3] Chen Z, Siu B, Ho YS, et al. Overexpression of MnSOD protects against myocardial ischemia/ reperfusion injury in transgenic mice. Journal of Molecular and Cellular Cardiology, 1998, 30 (11) : 2281-2289.

[4] van Deel ED, Lu Z, Xu X, et al. Extracellular superoxide dismutase protects the heart against oxidative stress and hypertrophy after myocardial infarction. Free Radical Biology and Medicine, 2008, 44 (7) : 1305-1313.

[5] Gökdemir MT, Kaya H, Söğüt O, et al. The role of oxidative stress and inflammation in the early evaluation of acute non-ST-elevation myocardial infarction : an observational study. Anatolian Journal of Cardiology, 2013, 13 (2) : 131-136.

[6] Garelnabi M, Gupta V, Mallika V, et al. Platelets oxidative stress in Indian patients with ischemic heart disease. Journal of Clinical Laboratory Analysis, 2010, 24 (1) : 49-54.

[7] Aksoy S, Cam N, Gurkan U, et al. Oxidative stress and severity of coronary artery disease in young smokers with acute myocardial infarction. Cardiology Journal, 2012, 19 (4) : 381-386.

[8] Ron D. Translational control in the endoplasmic reticulum stress response. Journal of Clinical Investigation, 2002, 110 (10) : 1383-1388.

[9] Xu C, Bailly-Maitre B, Reed JC. Endoplasmic reticulum stress: cell life and death decisions. Journal

of Clinical Investigation, 2005, 115 (10) : 2656-2664.

[10] Xin W, Li X, Lu X, et al. Involvement of endoplasmic reticulum stress-associated apoptosis in a heart failure model induced by chronic myocardial ischemia. International Journal of Molecular Medicine, 2011, 27 (4) : 503-509.

[11] Mitra A, Basak T, Datta K, et al. Role of α-crystallin B as a regulatory switch inmodulating cardiomyocyte apoptosis by mitochondria or endoplasmic reticulum during cardiac hypertrophy and myocardial infarction. Cell Death and Disease, 2013, 4 (4): article e582.

[12] Yan M, Shen J, Person MD, et al. Endoplasmic recticulum stress and unfolded protein response in Atm-deficient thymocytes and thymic lymphoma cells are attributable to oxidative stress. Neoplasia, 2008, 10 (2) : 160-167.

[13] Haynes CM, Titus EA, Cooper AA. Degradation of misfolded proteins prevents ER-derived oxidative stress and cell death. Molecular Cell, 2004, 15 (5) : 767-776.

[14] Ilieva EV, Ayala V, Jové M, et al. Oxidative and endoplasmic reticulum stress interplay in sporadic amyotrophic lateral sclerosis. Brain, 2007, 130 (12) A: 3111-3123.

[15] Kim KT, Yoo KM, Lee JW, et al. Protective effect of steamed American ginseng (Panax quinquefolius L.) on V79-4 cells induced by oxidative stress. Journal of Ethnopharmacology, 2007, 111 (3) : 443-450.

[16] Xie JT, Shao ZH, Vanden Hoek TL, et al. Antioxidant effects of ginsenoside Re in cardiomyocytes. European Journal of Pharmacology, 2006, 532 (3) : 201-207.

[17] Li J, Shao ZH, Xie JT, et al. The effects of ginsenoside Rb1 on JNK in oxidative injury in cardiomyocytes. Archives of Pharmacal Research, 2012, 35 (7) : 1259-1267.

[18] Wang C, Li YZ, Wang XR, et al. Panax quinquefolium saponins reduce myocardial hypoxia-reoxygenation injury by inhibiting excessive endoplasmic reticulum stress. Shock, 2012, 37 (2) : 228-233.

[19] Xue M, Yin H, Zhang L, et al. Dynamic expression of the main related indicators of thrombosis, inflammatory reaction and tissue damage in a rat model of myocardial infarction. Molecular Medicine Reports, 2011, 4 (4) : 693-696.

[20] Guo Y, Yin HJ, Shi DZ, et al. Effects of tribuli saponins on left ventricular remodeling after acute myocardial infarction in rats with hyperlipidemia. Chinese Journal of Integrative Medicine, 2005, 11 (2) : 142-146.

[21] Chen Q. Methodological study of chinese herbs pharmacology. People's Medical Publishing House, Beijing, China, 1996.

[22] Livak KJ, Schmittgen TD. Analysis of relative gene expression data using real-time quantitative PCR and the $2^{-\Delta\Delta CT}$ method. Methods, 2001, 25 (4) : 402-408.

[23] Yoshida T, Maulik N, Engelman RM, et al. Targeted disruption of the mouse sod I gene makes the hearts vulnerable to ischemic reperfusion injury. Circulation Research, 2000, 86 (3) : 264-269.

[24] Asimakis GK, Lick S, Patterson C. Postischemic recovery of contractile function is impaired in SOD2+/– but not SOD1+/–mouse hearts. Circulation, 2002, 105 (8) 981-986.

[25] Chen EP, Bittner HB, Davis RD, et al. Extracellular superoxide dismutase transgene overexpression preserves postischemic myocardial function in isolated murine hearts. Circulation, 1996, 94 (Supplement 9) : II412-II417.

[26] Garelnabi M, Gupta V, Mallika V, et al. Platelets oxidative stress in Indian patients with ischemic heart disease. Journal of Clinical aboratory Analysis, 2010, 24 (1) : 49-54.

[27] Refsgaard HHF, Tsai L, Stadtman ER. Modifications of proteins by polyunsaturated fatty acid peroxidation products. Proceedings of the National Academy of Sciences of the United States of America, 2000, 97 (no. 2) : 611-616.

[28] Tacconelli S, Capone ML, Patrignani P. Measurement of 8-iso-prostaglandin F2alpha in biological fluids as a measure of lipid peroxidation. Methods in Molecular Biology, 2010, 644: 165-178.

[29] Milne GL, Sanchez SC, Musiek ES, et al. Quantification of F2-isoprostanes as a biomarker of oxidative stress. Nature Protocols 2007, 2 (no. 1) : 221-226.

[30] Schwedhelm E, Bartling A, Lenzen H, et al. Urinary 8-isoprostaglandin F2α as a risk marker in patients with coronary heart disease: a matched case-control study. Circulation, 2004, 109 (7) : 843-848.

[31] Oyadomari S and Mori M. Roles of CHOP/ GADD153 in endoplasmic reticulum stress. Cell Death and Differentiation, 2004, 11 (4) : 381-389.

[32] Kerri KF, Kroemer G. Organelle-specific initiation of

第四章

cell death pathways. Nature Cell Biology, 2001, 3 (11) : E255-263.

[33] Koenig W, Lowel H, Lewis M. Long-term survival after myocardial infarction: relationship with thrombolysis and discharge medication. Results of the Augsburg myocardial infarction follow-up study 1985 to 1993. European Heart Journal, 1996, 17 (8): 1199-1206.

[34] George I, Sabbah HN, Xu K. β-Adrenergic receptor blockade reduces endoplasmic reticulum stress and normalizes calciumhandling in a coronary embolization model of heart failure in canines. Cardiovascular Research, 2011, 91 (3) : 447-455.

[35] Kim KT, Yoo KM, Lee JW, et al. Protective effect of steamed American ginseng (Panax quinquefolius L.)

on V79-4 cells induced by oxidative stress. Journal of Ethnopharmacology, 2007, 111 (3) : 443-450.

[36] Xie JT, Shao ZH, Vanden Hoŵ TL, et al. Antioxidant effects of ginsenoside Re in cardiomyocytes. European Journal of Pharmacology, 2006, 532 (3) : 201-207.

[37] Li J, Shao ZH, Xie JT, et al. The effects of ginsenoside Rb1 on JNK in oxidative injury in cardiomyocytes. Archives of Pharmacal Research, 2012, 35 (7) : 1259-1267.

[38] Wang C, Li YZ, Wang XR, et al. Panax quinquefolium saponins reduce myocardial hypoxia-reoxygenation injury by inhibiting excessive endoplasmic reticulum stress. Shock, 2012, 37 (2) : 228-233.

Effects of Chinese Herbs Capable of Replenishing Qi, Nourishing Yin and Activating Blood Circulation and Their Compatibility on Differentially Expressed Genes of Ischemic Myocardium[*]

YIN Hui-jun　GUO Chun-yu　SHI Da-zhuo

第四章

Myocardial ischemia caused by acute myocardial infarction (AMI) has been shown to be related to the disorders of energy metabolism in cardiomyocytes[1]. Many investigations suggested that the energy depletion due to acute hypoxia-ischemia in myocardium might play a crucial role in the pathogenesis of AMI, but the exact mechanism still needs to be elucidated. The underlying mechanism and molecular targets in energy metabolism of ischemic myocardium will be a focus of clinical and basic research in the field of cardiovascular diseases.

It is well known that hypoxia-ischemia leads to systolic function decrudescence and energy reserve decrease in myocardium, and the most common symptoms include chest pain, fatigue and shortness of breath in accord with characteristics of qi deficiency and blood stasis syndrome differentiation in Traditional Chinese Medicine (TCM). At present, the principle of replenishing qi, nourishing yin and activating blood circulation is the major therapy for AMI in TCM, and many researches demonstrated that this therapy combined with the routine Western medicine could reduce the mortality and incidence of complications in AMI patients[2]. From the previous study, we found that Xinyue Jiaonang (Panax quinquefolium saponin, PQS), an effective domestic medicine with the function of reinforcing qi and nourishing yin for coronary

* 原载于 Chinese Science Bulletin，2009，54（18）：3278-3282

heart disease, which can improve myocardial ischemia, mediate the carbohydrates and fatty acid metabolism, and promote ischemic myocardial angiogenesis as well[3]. Fufang Danshen Pian (FDP), a popular prescription for promoting blood circulation and removing blood stasis, has been used widely in the field of coronary heart disease. It was reported that FDP could improve myocardial ischemia, dilate coronary arteries, and restrain left ventricular remodeling after AMI. The combination of PQS and FDP may fully embody the principle of replenishing qi, nourishing yin and activating blood circulation in TCM.

In the previous study, we constructed differential gene expression profiles in ischemic and normal myocardium of Wistar rats after AMI by long serial analysis of gene expression (LongSAGE). In the ischemic tissue, 142 genes significantly changed compared to that in the normal tissue ($P < 0.05$), and the majority of them were expressed specifically in myocardium but not other tissues, and 20 genes were considered to be bound up with the biological process of myocardial metabolism, such as oxidative phosphorylation, ATP synthesis and glycolysis or glyconeogenesis, etc. The study hinted that the changes of gene expression involved in energy metabolism pathways after AMI might be the main reason to induce myocardium injury[4].

Then, whether and how Chinese herbs capable of replenishing qi, nourishing yin and activating blood circulation and their compatibility play the roles of promoting myocardial blood flow, preserving survival myocardium by regulating energy metabolism-associated target genes, and how about its mechanism remain to be clarified. In this study, mitochondrial oxidative phosphorylation was selected as the target pathway. Meanwhile, for their significant diversity in the LongSAGE profile, two genes related to energy metabolism, COX5a and ATP5e, were selected as the target genes. The mRNA expression and protease activity of the two genes which were influenced by Chinese herbs capable

of replenishing qi, nourishing yin and activating blood circulation and their compatibility will be determined in order to provide the molecular biological evidence for the compatibility in treatment of AMI.

1. Materials and Methods

1.1 Materials

One hundred and forty healthy Wistar rats of clean grade, weighing 160-180g, male, provided by Beijing Weitong Lihua Experimental Animal Technique Company, were used for this experiment after adaptive feeding for one week. Betaloc (No. 940506, 25 mg/tablet; Metoprolol tartrate tablets) was purchased from AstraZeneca US. Xinyue Jiaonang (No. Z20030073, 50 mg/pill) was from Yisheng Pharmaceutical Co. Ltd. FDP was from Guangzhou Baiyunshan TCM Factory (No. 030435, tanshinonel II A, 0.44 mg/pill; Danshensu, 193 mg/pill). The reagents for Real time fluorescence quantitative PCR (Q-PCR) were from BioEasy. Cytochrome c oxidase (CCO) and ATP synthase (ATPase) kits were from GENMED USA.

1.2 Animal Model

The AMI rat models were established by using the following method[5]: The left anterior descending coronary artery was ligated by non-traumatic thread at 1-2 mm beneath the boundary of pulmonary artery taper and left atria. The model establishment was confirmed by regional cyanosis of myocardial tissue and the elevation of the ST segment in lead II in the electrocardiogram (ECG), which was maintained for at least half an hour. In the sham group, the corresponding myocardinm in modeling was stitched without ligation.

1.3 Grouping and Administration

After operation, the rats were randomly divided into seven groups, and then given medicine by intragastric gavage with corresponding drugs on the 2nd day after operation. The daily dose for the rats in each medication group was converted according to the dosage of an adult weighing 70 kg. The grouping and medication are shown in Table 1.

Table 1　Animal Grouping and Medical Administration

Group	Administration (n= 20, 20 mL /(kg · d)
Normal group	routine
Sham group	routine
Model group	routine
Metoprolol group	metoprolol solution
RN group	PQS solution
AB group	FDP solution
RA group	mixed solution of PQS and FDP

1.4　Sample Collection, Separation and Preparation

All the animals were bred for 7 days. On the 8th day, the rats were sacrificed after 8 h of fasting under deep anesthesia by 20% urethane. Fixing the animals in supine position, the hearts were rapidly harvested, then perfused with normal saline until the fluid was clear. The left ventricle dissociative wall and part of the apex of heart were harvested in each group. Then one part of the tissue was fixed with 10% formaldehyde solution for histopathological assessment, and the other was preserved under –80℃ for further investigation.

1.5　Pathological Observation

Pieces of myocardium were fixed with 10% formalde-hyde solution for 4h. Then the specimens were routinely processed, stained with hematoxylin and eosin (HE) stain, paraffin-embedded and dŴydrated. The histopa-thological changes of myocardial tissues were assessed under an optical system microscope of Nikon 150 type.

1.6　Assay of Relative Expression Levels of *COX5a* and *ATP5e* mRNAs

Ten percent homogenate of myocardium from different groups was prepared, and total RNA was extracted from the frozen tissues using Trizol reagents (Invitrogen, USA) according to the manufacturer's instruction. Total RNA samples in the same group were mixed completely. 200 μg RNA in each group was used for purity identification and the quality of RNA was evaluated by an UV spectrophotometer and formaldehyde denature agarose gel electrophoresis. The relative expression levels of the two differential genes in the mixed samples were measured using Q-PCR. As an internal control, β-actin (a reference gene) amplification was used to normalize the expression levels. All samples were performed three times to achieve reproducibility.

1.7　Assay of CCO and ATPase Activity

Ten percent homogenate of myocardium was used to isolate mitochondria, and the GENMED reagent kit was further used to quantify protein. Activities of correlative functional enzymes, CCO and ATPase were determined by the colorimetric method. The absorbance was read once at 550 nm in 0 and 60 s, marking A1 and A2 respectively and setting △A = A1–A2. The activities of CCO (U/mg) = (sample △A – background △A) /[X (milligrams of mitochondrial protein) × 21.84 (absorbancy index per millimol)]. The activity assay of ATPase was as the same as of CCO.

1.8　Statistical Analysis

Analysis was performed using SPSS13.0 software. All data were expressed as $\bar{x} \pm$ SD. For measurement data, one-way ANOVA was used. As for the comparison in the same group, the q test was used. $P < 0.05$ was considered as significant difference.

2. Results

2.1　Assessment of Myocardium Histopathological Changes

In the normal group, the shapes of cardio-myocytes were regular, the nucleuses were spindle-shaped, and the myocardial fiber was in ordered arrangement. However, in other groups, there were cardiocyte swelling and inflammatory cell infiltration in the ishcemic region, and partial cardiomyocytes showed hydropic degeneration, cytolysis. Some cells showed severe structural changes characterized by vacuolar degeneration, lytic necrosis and myocardial fibrosis, of which the model group changed significantly. In drug medication groups, the injury degree of myocardial tissues showed different changes ranging from that of the normal group to that of the model group (Figure 1).

2.2 mRNA Expressions of the Target Differential Genes

Q-PCR was designed to determine relative quantification of $COX5a$ and $ATP5e$ mRNA, and C_t value was obtained by related the PCR signal to a standard curve. $\triangle C_t$ is the difference between C_t value of mRNA and β-actin, while $2^{-\triangle C_t}$ is considered as the relative quantification of $COX5a$ and $ATP5e$ mRNA[6,7]. In this experiment, $2^{-\triangle\triangle C_t}$ relates the PCR signal of the target transcript in all medication groups to that of the normal control (Table 2). Compared to the normal group, it showed a significantly down-regulated trend in the model group, the sham group and all medication groups, while among them the model group changed significantly. In addition, as compared with the model group, the mRNA expression of the target genes in medication

groups showed a significantly up-regulated trend, and it increased significantly in the RA group.

Table 2　Comparison of mRNA Expression of the Target Genes in Samples ($2^{-\triangle\triangle Ct}$)

Group	COX5a	ATP5e
Normal group	1	1
Sham group	0.88	0.75
Model group	0.26	0.56
Metoprolol group	0.95	0.62
RN group	0.80	0.63
AB group	0.78	0.72
RA group	0.92	0.91

2.3 Proteinase Activity of Target Genes

Activities of CCO in all medication groups showed insignificant difference as compared with that in the normal group. From the trend at measured values, activities of CCO were down-regulated in the sham group and the model group, meanwhile the latter decreased obviously. Compared with the model group, the experiment indicated that activities of ATPase in the normal group and RA group declined significantly ($P < 0.05$; Table 3).

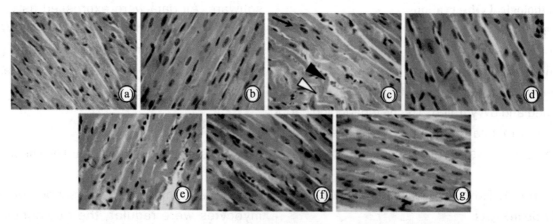

Figure 1　Myocardial Histopathological Changes in Different Groups (×400). (a) The Normal Group; (b) The Sham Group; (c) The Model Group; (d) The Metoprolol Group; (e) The RN Group; (f) The AB Group; (g) The RA Group. Taking the model group for example, →, cardiomyocytes; ▲, inflammatory cells infiltration; ▽, distorted myocardial fibrosis.

Table 3 Comparison of Proteinase Activity Assay of CCO and ATPase (U/mg) [a]

Group	n	CCO	ATPase
Normal group	20	1.15 ± 0.26	2.16 ± 0.42*
Sham group	20	0.83 ± 0.40	1.88 ± 0.37
Model group	20	0.81 ± 0.33	1.25 ± 0.23
Metoprolol group	20	1.18 ± 0.22	1.49 ± 0.36
RN group	20	0.90 ± 0.24	1.54 ± 0.41
AB group	20	0.89 ± 0.22	1.90 ± 0.45
RA group	20	1.00 ± 0.31	2.12 ± 0.34*

a)*, compared with the model group, $P < 0.05$

3. Discussion

AMI, characterized by high incidence and mortality, is one of the most serious diseases which threaten human health. Many studies showed that energy depletion is an initiating agent and may be the direct factor of myocardial injury after AMI. At present, the mitochondrion has become a subunit target in cells, since the dysfunctional mitochondria were reported as the main reason of myocardial ischemia, injury, and necrosis. Meanwhile it was deemed to be closely related to apoptosis starting as well[8,9]. COX5a and ATP5e are significant differential genes expressed in the pathway of mitochondrial oxidative phosphorylation, and their mRNA levels and enzyme activities could directly influence the function of the whole respiratory chain.

In most studies, the transcription level of COX5a was demonstrated to be closely connected with the apoptosis mechanism. It was reported that RNA interference (RNAi) had been used to mice's oocytes to silence three CCO subunits including COX5a, which led to elevation of the levels of pre-apoptosis such as intracellular Caspase-3[10,11].

ATPase, playing an important role in energy metabolism, is a key enzyme of mitochondrial ATP synthesis and hydrolysis on the pathway of oxidative phosphorylation[12,13]. In order to provide more energy for injured myocardium after AMI, more ATP should be produced to ameliorate the impairment of energy metabolism and activity of ATPase should also be increased simultaneously in mitochondria. Another researcher[14] studied the subunit named ATP5 in yeast and ascertained that the subunit was an essential part of ATPase. The subunit could create a uniquely folded N-terminal protein binding domain which might stabilize the structure of ATPase homodimer and promote its translation.

Previous studies confirmed that PQS and tansh-inonel played a certain role in realizing the therapeutic effects such as energy supply, neovascularization and anti-oxidation injury in ischemic myocardium after AMI[15,16]. In the present experiment, compatibility of PQS and tanshinonel was used to treat AMI rats. The results indicated that the mRNA level of COX5a and activity of CCO were significantly down-regulated in the model group than that in the normal group. The down-regulation of COX5a expression after AMI induced low activity of CCO which would activate apoptosis of partial ischemic myocardium. Up-regulation of COX5a expression and increase of CCO activity occurred in all medication groups, specifically in the Metoprolol group and the replenishing qi, nourishing yin and activating blood circulation group. Furthermore, we found that both ATP5e gene expression and ATPase activity decreased in ischemic myocardium after AMI, and the latter was found descended significantly ($P < 0.05$), which showed that Chinese herbs capable of replenishing qi, nourishing yin and activating blood circulation and their compatibility could alleviate oxidation stress injury by inhibiting mitochondria ATPase activity and inhibiting apoptosis further.

In conclusion, combination of PQS and tanshinonel could supply more energy to ischemic myocardium and alleviate oxidation injury. The compatibility could increase ATP generation rate, and reduce anaerobic glycolysis and lactic acid accumulation. Moreover, it could attenuate mitochondrial Ca^{2+} overload via up-regulating mRNA levels and protein activity of *COX5a* and ATPase, the effect of which was better than using Chinese herbs capable of replenishing qi, nourishing yin or activating blood circulation alone.

Up to now, great progress has been made in the treatment of AMI, such as revascularization, intensive lipid-lowering and antiplatelet activity. However, a suitable strategy to improve myocardium energy metabolism after AMI is still in its infancy. In this study, some useful data were presented for the therapeutic target of energy metabolism disorder via investigating these related genes. This may also provide a platform at the gene level for high-throughput screening for drugs in the therapy of myocardium injury after AMI.

References

[1] Wolff AA, Rotmensch HH, Stanley WC, et al. Metabolic approaches to the treatment of ischemic heart disease: the clinicians' perspective. Heart Fail Rev, 2002, 7: 187-203.

[2] Yang YM, Yang N. Discussion of important link from progresses in coronary heart disease therapy with TCM. Chinese J Integr Tradit West Med, 2002, 22: 863-865.

[3] Shao NQ, Zhu XX. Pharmacological progresses in hypoxia-ischemia of myocardium. J Pract Tradit Chinese Intern Med, 2007, 21: 3-4.

[4] Guo CY, Yin HJ, Jiang YR, et al. Differential gene expression profile in ischemic myocardium of Wistar rats with acute myocardial infarction. Chinese Sci Bull, 2008, 53: 2488-2495.

[5] Zhang RS, Wang JS. Discussion of some problems about rat model with myocardial infarction. J Shanxi Med Univ, 2004, 35: 13-15.

[6] Livak KJ, Schmittgen TD. Analysis of relative gene expression data using real-time quantitative PCR and the 2 (-Delta Delta C (T)). Methods, 2001, 25: 402-408.

[7] Arocho A, Chen B, Ladanyi M. Validation of the 2-DeltaDeltaCt calculation as an alternate method of data analysis for quantitative PCR of BCR-ABL P210 transcripts. Diagn Mol Pathol, 2006, 15: 56-61.

[8] Zhang J, Liem DA, Mueller M, et al. Altered proteome biology of cardiac mitochondria under stress conditions. J Proteome Res, 2008, 7: 2204-2214.

[9] Sammut IA, Burton K, Balogun E, et al. Time-dependent impairment of mitochondrial function after storage and transplantation of rabbit kidneys. Transplantation, 2000, 69: 1265-1275.

[10] Zhang M, Zhou SH. Therapy progresses in energy metabolism impairment of myocardial ischemia. Chinese Heart J, 2006, 18: 467-469.

[11] Lee SD, Kuo WW, Lin JA, et al. Effects of long-term intermittent hypoxia on mitochondrial and Fas death receptor dependent apoptotic pathways in rat hearts. Int J Cardiol, 2007, 116: 348-356.

[12] Cui XS, Li XY, Jeong YJ, et al. Gene expression of Cox5a, 5b, or 6b1 and their roles in preimplantation mouse embryos. Biol Reprod, 2006, 74: 601-610.

[13] Weinberg JM, Venkatachalam MA, Roeser NF, et al. Mitochondrial dysfunction during hypoxia/reoxygenation and its correction by anaerobic metabolism of citric acid cycle intermediates. Proc Natl Acad Sci USA, 2000, 97: 2826-2831.

[14] Liang WS, Tang LX, Yang ZC, et al. Changes of myocardial mitochondrial F0F1-ATPase activity and its effects on energy metabolism in early stage of severe burns. Acta Academiae Medicine Militaris Tertiae, 2001, 23: 780-782.

[15] Yin HJ, Zhang Y, Yang LH, et al. The effects of PQS on glucose transport, GLUT4 translocation and CAP mRNA expression of adipocytes. Chinese Pharmacol Bull, 2007, 23: 1332-1337.

[16] Yin HJ, Zhang Y, Jiang YR, et al. Effect of Folium *panax quinquefolium* saponins on apoptosis of cardiac muscle cells and apoptosis-related gene expression in rats with acute myocardial infarction. Chinese J Integr Tradit West Med, 2005, 25: 232-235.

Ischemic Postconditioning through Percutaneous Transluminal Coronary Angioplasty in Pigs: Roles of PI3K Activation

MA Xiao-juan   YIN Hui-jun   GUO Chun-yu   JIANG Yue-rong   WANG Jing-shang   SHI Da-zhuo

1. Introduction

Ischemic postconditioning (IPOC), different from ischemic preconditioning, is a series of mechanical stimulations at the onset of reperfusion, which renders the myocardium more tolerant to lethal ischemic reperfusion (IR) injury [1]. This use of ischemia after a prolonged ischemic period is a simple and logical progression, which theoretically allows unrestricted application in the clinical settings. The mechanisms underlying cardioprotection by IPOC may be multiple. Several studies indicated that IPOC protects the myocardium by activating the phosphatidylinositol 3 kinase (PI3K) /Akt pathway at the onset of reperfusion in an isolated and intact rat or rabbit model [2, 3]. PI3K and its downstream effector, a serine-threonine protein kinase Akt, constitute a key signaling enzyme system implicated in cell survival, growth, migration, and metabolic control in various cell types including cardiomyocytes [4,5]. Most experiments on the activation of PI3K/Akt induced by IPOC were performed in rodents using open-chest models. Apart from species differences, Akt activation by mechanical stimuli [6] during the open-chest procedure may limit these conclusions. Importantly, a recent observation indicated that PI3K activation was not important for IPOC in pigs and was still effective after PI3K blockade [7]. Whether phosphorylation of PI3K is a causal mechanism for protection of the myocardium by IPOC remains controversial. In the present study, we improved the protocol of IPOC by percutaneous transluminal coronary angioplasty (PTCA) in minipigs, which reduced injury caused by the mechanical procedure. Here we showed that cardioprotection by IPOC is preserved in PTCA minipigs and further identified the role of activation of the PI3K/Akt pathway in the protection induced by IPOC.

2. Materials and Methods

2.1 Experimental Model

Chinese minipigs of either sex, weighing20-30kg and free of clinically evident disease, were used for studies in a new IPOC model using PTCA. All procedures were performed in accordance with the regulations of local animal-based research standards and were subjected to local ethical review. Pigs were anesthetized with ketamine (10mg/kg) and pentobarbital (60 mg/kg) and were maintained under anesthesia with pentobarbital by monitoring them using an electrocardiomonitor (TEC-7621C, NihonKohden, Nishiochiai Shinjuku-ku, Tokyo, Japan) and by observing the animal's response to stimuli. Briefly, a preoperation was performed, which involved anterior incision and ligation of the distal right common carotid artery. A 6 Fr sheath was inserted into the right common carotid artery, and heparin (200 U/kg) was administered as an anticoagulant. Under fluoroscopic guidance, a 6 Fr JR3.5 guiding catheter (Cordis, Miami, Florida, USA) was advanced through the sheath into the ostium of the coronary arteries. A left coronary angiography

* 原载于 Coronary Artery Disease，2012，23（4）：245-250

was performed to ensure correct positioning of the catheter. A 2.5-mm angioplasty balloon (Cordis) was then positioned in the mid-distal portion of the left anterior descending (LAD) artery, below the second diagonal branch. Acute myocardial infarction was induced by balloon inflation for 45 min in the LAD artery [8,9]. After the balloon was inflated at 6-8 atm, another coronary angiography was performed to confirm the complete occlusion of the LAD (Figure 1). IPOC was achieved by intermittent reinflation of the balloon at 30 s after deflation of the balloon. This cycle was repeated three times followed by a 24h reperfusion.

2.2 Experimental Protocol

Pigs were assigned to four groups (n= 6/group), as shown in Figure. 2. After the stabilization period, all animals except those in the sham operation group underwent 45 min of coronary artery occlusion. Reperfusion injury animals (IR group) received no further intervention before full reperfusion. Postconditioning (POC group) consisted of three cycles of 30 s of reperfusion followed by 30 s of ischemia and was applied immediately at the onset of reperfusion [10]. One group of pigs (POC+ WORT group) received an intravenous bolus injection of wortmannin (30μg/kg body weight; cat. 38385, Serva Electrophoresis, Heidelberg, Germany) at the onset of the full reperfusion, as

an inhibitor of PI3K [11]. Sham operation animals (SH group) received the intervention only with deflated balloons for 45 min; no treatment with inflated balloons was received until the end.

2.3 Determination of Myocardial Infarct Size

Myocardial infarct size was determined as previously described[12]. After 24h reperfusion, animals were killed using pentobarbital. The heart was rapidly excised and sectioned from the apex to the coronary occlusion spot into six transverse slices in a plane parallel to the atrioventricular groove. The second slice was used for the western blot and real-time PCR. The other five slices were incubated in 0.1 mol/L phosphate buffer (pH 7.4) containing 1% 2,3,5-triphenyl tetrazolium chloride (TTC) at 37℃ for 20 min and then fixed in 10% formalin. For each slice, the area of necrosis was calculated by a multimedia color pathological image analytical system (MPIAS-500, Konghai, Beijing, China), and the infarct size was expressed as a percentage of the total left ventricle area.

2.4 Western Blot Analysis

For analysis of GSK-3β and Akt phosphorylation, left ventricular tissue samples of the second slice were collected 24h after reperfusion, immediately frozen in liquid nitrogen, and stored at -80℃ until further processing. Tissue was homo-

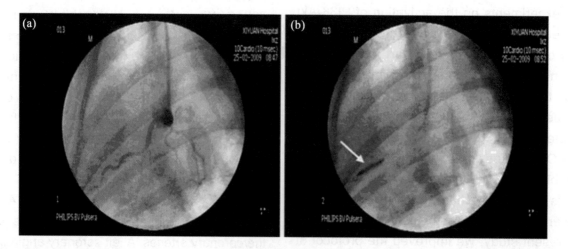

Figure 1　Screenshots of Percutaneous Transluminal Coronary Angioplasty in Minipigs. （a）The normal left anterior descending（LAD）artery was shown by coronary arteriography. （b）A 2.5-mm angioplasty balloon was positioned in the mid-distal portion of the LAD artery. The arrow indicates the location of the inflated balloon

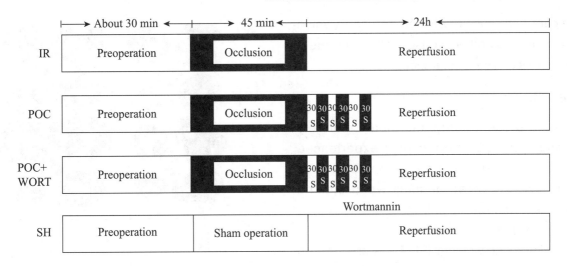

Figure 2 Experimental Protocol of Minipigs. Ischemic reperfusion（IR）: animals were exposed to 45 min of coronary artery occlusion followed by 24 h of reperfusion. Postconditioning（POC）: ischemic postconditioning was induced by three cycles of 30-s reperfusion followed by 30-s ischemia at the onset of reperfusion after 45-min occlusion. POC+WORT: postconditioned animals exposed to the PI3K inhibitor wortmannin（30μg/kg）through the ear vein at the onset of the full reperfusion. SH: sham operation animals underwent the same procedure with IR, except that the balloon was positioned in the LAD artery without inflation for 45 min

genized on ice in protein extraction buffer [50mmol/L Tris-HCl (pH 7.4), 0.25 mol/L NaCl, 1% Nonidet-P40, 1 mmol/L EDTA, 1% protease inhibitor cocktail]. The lysate was centrifuged at 12 000g for 10 min and the supernatant was collected. The supernatant (30μg of protein) was separated by 10% SDS-polyacrylamide gel electrophoresis and then transferred onto a nitrocellulose membrane (Millipore, Bedford, Massachusetts, USA). After blocking, the membranes were probed with primary antibodies (1 : 1000) against phospho-GSK-3β and phospho-Akt (Cell Signaling Technology, Beverly, Massachusetts, USA) at 4 ℃ overnight. Finally, the membranes were hybridized with the secondary antibody peroxidase-conjugated goat anti-rabbit IgG (1 : 2000; Zhongshan Goldenbridge, Beijing, China). β-Actin with a size of 42 kDa was used as a reference protein. Protein expression was detected using an enhanced chemiluminescence detection system (Pierce, Rockford, Illinois, USA).

2.5　Quantitative Real-time PCR

Total RNA was isolated from the myocardium using the TRIzol reagent (Gibco, Invitrogen, Carlsbad, California, USA) and treated with DNaseI (Turbo DNA-free, Ambion, Austin, Texas, USA). Circular DNA was prepared from 500 ng of total RNA with oligo (dT) primers using Moloney murine leukemia virus reverse transcriptase (Promega, Madison, Wisconsin, USA) in a 50μl reaction. The realtime reverse transcriptase-PCR reactions were carried out in a 20μL final volume with LightCycler-FastStart DNA Master SYBR Green I (Roche Applied Science, Meylan, France). Results were normalized to β-actin expression levels. The following primers were used: AKT (AKT1, Gene ID100126861) forward 5'-AGCTCTTCTTCCACCTGTCC-3', reverse 5'-AGCATGAGGTTCTCCAGCTT-3'; GSK-3β (GSK-3β, Gene ID100126852) forward 5'-CTAATGCCGGAGATCGTG-3', reverse 5'-TGACCAGTGTTGCTGAGTGA-3'; β-actin forward 5'-AGCAGATGTGGATCACAAG-3', reverse 5'-GCCAGG GCAAACTTTATTTC-3'.

2.6　Statistical Analysis

All data are reported as mean±SD. Analysis of variance was used to determine significant differences between groups. A value of *P* less than 0.05 was considered to indicate a statistically significant difference.

3. Results

In the present study, the model mortality was about 20%. Some minipigs experienced ventricular fibrillation during the operation. We did not exclude those animals when electric defibrillation was successful.

3.1 Myocardial Infarct Size

To determine whether IPOC has an effect on the protection of the myocardium, we performed an experiment to compare the infarct size by staining the myocardium with TTC 24h after the surgery. The results showed that the infarct size was $36.58 \pm 9.31\%$ in the reperfusion injury animals (IR group), whereas there was no infarct in the animals that underwent sham surgery.

Interestingly, we observed that the animals that accepted IPOC had a significantly reduced infarct size ($26.17 \pm 2.49\%$) in the myocardium after the surgery (Figure 3). There results clearly demonstrated that IPOC has a protective role in the myocardium after reperfusion injury. To test whether PI3K plays a role in the protection of the myocardium, we treated the animals with an inhibitor of PI3K after the IPOC treatment. The results showed that addition of the inhibitor limited the protective effect of IPOC for the infarct size ($34.1 \pm 5.14\%$) compared with the POC group.

3.2 Phosphorylation of AKT and GSK-3β

Western blot analysis was used to evaluate the effect of PI3K phosphorylation, including AKT and GSK-3β phosphorylation. As illustrated in Figure 4, IPOC induced a significant increase in phospho-AKT (ser 473) and phospho-GSK-3β (ser 9; $P < 0.05$). Similarly, the increased phosphorylation of AKT and GSK-3β, stimulated by postconditioning, was significantly inhibited by wortmannin in the POC + WORT group ($P < 0.05$). There were no differences in phosphor-AKT and phospho-GSK-3β expression levels

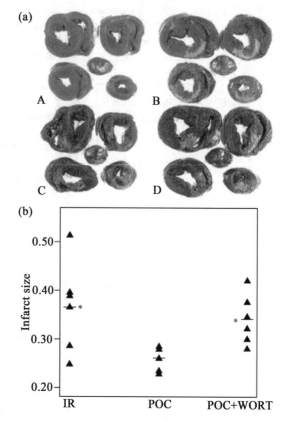

Figure 3 Infarct Size 24 h after Ischemic Postconditioning. (a) Corresponding images of TTC staining to determine the infarct size. A: SH group, B: IR group, C: POC group, D: POC+WORT group. **(b)** The infarct size of each group represented with filled triangles and means. The SH group is not included in (b) because no significant necrotic area was identified. IR group, $36.58 \pm 9.31\%$; POC group, $26.17 \pm 2.49\%$; and POC+WORT group, $34.1 \pm 5.14\%$. $^*P < 0.05$ *vs.* the POC group. IR, ischemic reperfusion; POC, postconditioning; SH, sham operation animals; TTC, 2,3,5-triphenyl tetrazolium chloride; WORT, wortmannin

between IR treatment and sham operation groups ($P > 0.05$).

3.3 mRNA Expression of AKT and GSK-3β

The mRNA levels of AKT and GSK-3β were measured by real-time PCR. As shown in Figure 5, the highest RNA level of AKT in the heart tissue was expressed in the sham operation group, followed by IR, POC, and POC+WORT groups. There was a modestly decreased expression of AKT induced by postconditioning, but this

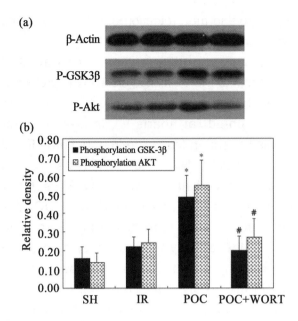

(a)

β-Actin

P-GSK3β

P-Akt

(b)

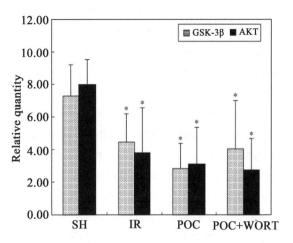

Figure 4　Phosphorylation Status of GSK3β and Akt. (a) GSK3β and Akt phosphorylation shown in an immunoblot. (b) The expression (mean ± SD) of the phosphorylation of GSK3β and phosphorylation of Akt with the protein band intensities normalized for β-actin. n=6 minipigs per group, $^*P < 0.05$ vs. the ischemic reperfusion group and $^\#P < 0.05$ vs. the postconditioning group. IR, ischemic reperfusion; POC, postconditioning; SH, sham operation animals; WORT, wortmannin

Figure 5　mRNA Expression of AKT and GSK-3β by Reverse Transcriptase-PCR. All tests were conducted in six samples of each group and repeated three times. Results were normalized to β-actin expression levels. $^*P < 0.05$ vs. the sham operation animals group (SH group). IR, ischemic reperfusion; POC, postconditioning; SH, sham operation animals; WORT, wortmannin

difference did not reach statistical significance (IR group vs. POC group, $P > 0.05$). The inhibitor wortmannin did not affect the mRNA level of AKT (POC group vs. POC + WORT group, $P > 0.05$). Results of GSK-3β revealed the same tendency.

3.4　Discussion

In 2003, Zhao and colleagues reported an open-chest canine model of LAD artery occlusion and reperfusion to test the hypothesis that brief nonlethal episodes of ischemia during the initial moments of reperfusion would attenuate myocardial injury induced by IR, known as IPOC. They found that infarct size, tissue edema, and postischemic coronary artery endothelial dysfunction in the area of the myocardium at risk were reduced with IPOC to the same extent as that with preconditioning [13]. In the current study, the myocardial infarct size of the POC group was

reduced significantly compared with that of the IR group (26 ± 2 vs. $37 \pm 9\%$), which demonstrated the cardioprotection of IPOC in minipigs. IPOC, use of ischemia after a prolonged ischemic period, is a simple and logical progression that abolishes the limitation of ischemic precondition, translating "conditioning" from a laboratory technique to clinical therapy.

The mechanisms underlying cardioprotection by IPOC may be multiple, involving oxidative stress, mitochondrial calcium accumulation, endothelial function, and inflammation. Interestingly, the reperfusion injury salvage kinase pathways appear to play an important role in IPOC, which activates two pathways implicated in cell survival, namely the PI3K/Akt pathway and the p42/p44 extracellular signalregulated kinase (Erk1/2) pathway [14]. Multiple lines of investigation suggest that activation of PI3K/Akt was especially involved in promoting cardiomyocyte survival and function in models of cardiac injury [6]. On the basis of subunit composition, PI3K members are divided

第四章

into four classes, ⅠA, ⅠB, Ⅱ, and Ⅲ. The PI3K family regulates diverse biological functions in multiple cell lineages by generating lipid second messengers, such as survival, proliferation, differentiation, chemotaxis, and trafficking. Akt, the key downstream effector of PI3K activation, is able to phosphorylate multiple downstream substrates that mediate cell growth, survival, and metabolism. Akt, a serine/threonine kinase, with high homology to protein kinase A and protein kinase C, is also known as protein kinase B, which has three isoforms: Akt1/PKB-α, Akt2/PKB-β and Akt3/PKB-γ[15,16].

Previous evidence shows that IPOC protects the myocardium by activating the PI3K/Akt pathway at the onset of reperfusion in an isolated and intact rat or rabbit model [2,3]. However, these studies were mostly repeated in rodents using open-chest models, which limited the adaptivity of the conclusions to some extent. In addition, Akt activated by multiple stimuli can prevent apoptosis induced by peroxide and hypoxia in the heart and cardiomyocytes. Moreover, mechanical stimuli such as pressure overload and hypoxia also enhance endogenous Akt activation [6]. Thus, Akt activation may be affected by the open-chest procedure, which could be confused with PI3K/Akt activation induced by IPOC. In the present study, we improved the protocol of IPOC by PTCA in minipigs, which reduced injury caused by mechanical procedure. Here we showed for the first time that protection by IPOC is preserved in PTCA minipigs. Our results showed that IPOC induced a significant increase in Akt and downstream target GSK3β phosphorylation compared with the IR group (0.55 ± 0.14 *vs.* 0.24 ± 0.07, 0.48 ± 0.12 *vs.* 0.22 ± 0.05, respectively), which suggested that the PI3K pathway was the mediator of IPOC-induced cardioprotection in pigs. Although we observed an increased tendency for mRNA expression of AKT and GSK-3β by IPOC, the difference did not reach statistical significance. Hence, PI3K/Akt plays a role in the protection of IPOC in proteins and not in genes.

Previous studies have suggested that wortmannin, a PI3K inhibitor, blocked the protective effects of IPOC in in-vivo rat models [17], in isolated hypertrophied rat hearts [18], in in-situ rabbit models [19], and in leukocyte-free, bufferperfused rabbit hearts [20]. Nevertheless, adverse results were observed in the study by Skyschally and colleagues. They found that IPOC was still effective after reperfusion injury salvage kinase blockade by intracoronary coinfusion of wortmannin and U0126 in an open-chest minipig model of 90-min regional myocardial ischemia/120-min reperfusion[5]. Our data, in accordance with the above study, showed that administration of wortmannin abolished the infarct-sparing effect in PTCA minipigs. The infarct size was increased to $34.1\% \pm 5.14\%$ in the POC + WORT group compared with $26.17\% \pm 2.49\%$ in the POC group. In our study, the increased phosphorylation of AKT and GSK-3β induced by IPOC was significantly inhibited by wortmannin, which was different from the results of Skyschally and colleagues' study. Importantly, the present study showed that the PI3K/Akt pathway was involved predominantly as an effector in the cardioprotection of IPOC in PTCA minipigs and that an inhibitor of PI3K did attenuate the potentiated protection induced by IPOC.

In summary, using a new IPOC model with PTCA, we demonstrated the protective effects of brief nonlethal episodes of ischemia during the initial moments of reperfusion in minipigs. Furthermore, we identified that the PI3K/Akt-signaling pathway played an important role in the cardioprotection induced by IPOC.

References

[1] Zhao H. Ischemic postconditioning as a novel avenue to protect against brain injury after stroke. J Cereb Blood Flow Metab, 2009, 29: 873-885.

[2] Hausenloy DJ, Yellon DM. Survival kinases in

ischemic preconditioning and postconditioning. Cardiovasc Res, 2006, 70: 240-253.

[3] Hönisch A, Theuring N, Ebner B, et al. Postconditioning with levosimendan reduces the infarct size involving the PI3K pathway and KATP-channel activation but is independent of PDE-Ⅲ inhibition. Basic Res Cardiol, 2010, 105: 155-167.

[4] Ravingerová T, Matejíková J, Neckár J, et al. Differential role of PI3K/Akt pathway in the infarct size limitation and antiarrhythmic protection in the rat heart. Mol Cell Biochem, 2007, 297: 111-120.

[5] Mocanu MM, Yellon DM. PTEN, the Achilles' heel of myocardial ischaemia/ reperfusion injury? Br J Pharmacol, 2007, 150: 833-838.

[6] Matsui T, Rosenzweig A. Convergent signal transduction pathways controlling cardiomyocyte survival and function: the role of PI3-kinase and Akt. J Mol Cell Cardiol, 2005, 38: 63-71.

[7] Skyschally A, van Caster P, Boengler K, et al. Ischemic postconditioning in pigs: no causal role for RISK activation. Circ Res, 2009, 104: 15-18.

[8] Liu JX, Yu Z, Li XZ, et al. Cardioprotective effects of diltiazem reevaluated by a novel myocardial ischemic model in Chinese miniature swine. Acta Pharmacol Sin, 2007, 28: 52-57.

[9] Bretz B, Blaze C, Parry N, et al. Ischemic postconditioning does not attenuate ischemia-reperfusion injury of rabbit small intestine. Vet Surg, 2010, 39: 216-223.

[10] Loukogeorgakis SP, Panagiotidou AT, et al. Postconditioning protects against endothelial ischemia-reperfusion injury in the human forearm. Circulation, 2006, 113: 1015-1019.

[11] Mozaffari MS, Liu JY, Schaffer SW. Effect of pressure overload on cardioprotection via PI3K-Akt: comparison of postconditioning, insulin, and pressure unloading. Am J Hypertens, 2010, 23: 668-674.

[12] Létienne R, Calmettes Y, Le Grand B. Is postconditioning effective in prevention against long-lasting myocardial ischemia in the rabbit? Physiol Res, 2009, 58: 635-643.

[13] Zhao ZQ, Corvera JS, Halkos ME, et al. Inhibition of myocardial injury by ischemic postconditioning during reperfusion: comparison with ischemic preconditioning. Am J Physiol Heart Circ Physiol, 2003, 285: 579-588.

[14] Oikawa M, Yaoita H, Watanabe K, et al. Attenuation of cardioprotective effect by postconditioning in coronary stenosed rat heart and its restoration by carvedilol. Circ J, 2008, 72: 2081-2086.

[15] Juntilla MM, Koretzky GA. Critical roles of the PI3K/Akt signaling pathway in T cell development. Immunol Lett, 2008, 116: 104-110.

[16] Franke TF. PI3K/Akt: getting it right matters. Oncogene, 2008, 27: 6473-6488.

[17] Bopassa JC, Ferrera R, Gateau-Roesch O, et al. PI 3-kinase regulates the mitochondrial transition pore in controlled reperfusion and postconditioning. Cardiovasc Res, 2006, 69: 178-185.

[18] Peng LY, Ma H, He JG, et al. Ischemic postconditioning attenuates ischemia/reperfusion injury in isolated hypertrophied rat heart. Zhonghua Xin Xue Guan Bing Za Zhi, 2006, 34: 685-689.

[19] Philipp S, Yang XM, Cui L, et al. Postconditioning protects rabbit hearts through a protein kinase C-adenosine A2b receptor cascade. Cardiovasc Res, 2006, 70: 308-314.

[20] Yang XM, Philipp S, Downey JM, et al. Postconditioning's protection is not dependent on circulating blood factors or cells but involves adenosine receptors and requires PI3-kinase and guanylyl cyclase activation. Basic Res Cardiol, 2005, 100: 57-63.

Synergistic Protection of Danhong Injection and Ischemic Postconditioning on Myocardial Reperfusion Injury in Minipigs*

MA Xiao-juan　YIN Shang-jun　JIN Ji-cheng　WU Cai-feng　HUANG Ye　SHI Da-zhuo　YIN Hui-jun

Revascularization, including thrombolytic drugs, percutaneous transluminal coronary angioplasty and coronary artery bypass grafting, can restore ischemic myocardial perfusion rapidly in patients with acute myocardial infarction and rescue the myocardium. It therefore becomes the major therapeutic means in acute myocardial infarction (AMI). Restoration of blood flow to ischemic tissue may promote the damage of cardiomyocytes and vascular network in the reperfused region, which leads to ischemia/reperfusion (I/R) injury and limits the clinical efficacy of revascularization. It has become a study of interest how to alleviate reperfusion injury in the field of prevention and treatment of AMI. Ischemic postconditioning is a clinical treatment measure based on ischemic preconditioning, which refers to the brief intermittent episodes of ischemia and reperfusion, at the onset of reperfusion after a prolonged period of ischemia reduced I/R injury[1]. In recent years, the concept of pharmacologic postconditioning (PPOC) has been proposed[2]. PPOC is stimulated by drugs, or endogenous substances simulation presented cardioprotection on myocardial I/R injury. We have found that some drugs have ischemic postconditioning-like protective effects by promoting the release of endogenous substances or directly triggering mechanisms of endogenous antidamage responses[3]. Danhong Injection (丹红注射液, DHI), a Chinese medicine of activating blood circulation and removing blood stasis, has a role in improving microcirculation, inhibiting thrombosis and alleviating ischemic reperfusion injury [4-6]. The present study explored the synergistic protection of DHI and ischemic postconditioning on myocardial reperfusion injury in minipigs.

1. Methods

1.1　Experimental Animal

Chinese minipigs, weighting 20-30 kg, were purchased from Beijing Kexing Experimental Animal Cultivation Center (No. SYXK 2009-0026). They were housed separately after 1-weŵ quarantine and adaptation of feeding normal diet in animal room before experiments.

1.2　Ischemia Postconditioning Models of Minipigs

The minipigs were sedated by ear intramuscular injection with ketamine hydrochloride (10 mg/kg) after fast for 8 h, minipigs lying and fixed in console, ear vein access established with the trocar, then anaesthesia was induced by 5% pentobarbital (60 mg/kg) and maintained all procedures; the vital signs were monitored during operation. We improved the postconditioning protocol by reference to the acute myocardial infarction model of minipigs by balloon occlusion[7]. A small midline incision was made in the ventral neck, and the right carotid artery was exposed and isolated. A bolus of 200 U/kg heparin was administered intravenously through the sheath (6 French) placed in the carotid artery. An angioplasty balloon was positioned over a

* 原载于 Chinese Journal of Integrative Medicine，2010，16（6）：531-536

guide wire in the left anterior descending coronary artery (LAD) proximal to the second diagonal branch under the C-arm X-ray image intensifier equipment (Philips BV pulsera) perspective. The balloon was inflated at 6 to 8 atm to completely occlude distal flow for 45 min. Then reperfusion was initiated for 30s followed by 30s of reocclusion, repeated for 3 cycles, and preceded the 24 h of reperfusion (Figure 1).

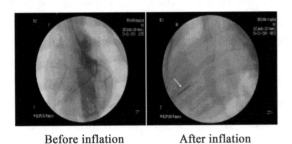

Before inflation   After inflation

Figure 1　Screenshots of Coronary Intervention in Minipigs
Note：The arrow indicated the inflated balloon

1.3　Experimental Protocol

All animals were randomly assigned to four groups: the sham operation group (SH group) involved the same procedures except ischemia and reperfusion; the ischemia/reperfusion group (I/R group), where the LAD was occluded for 45 min, followed by reversal of the occlusion and 24h of reperfusion; the ischemic postconditioning group (POC group), where after 45 min of LAD occlusion, reperfusion was initiated for 30 s followed by 30 s of reocclusion, repeated for three cycles; and DHI combined with ischemic postconditioning group (PAD group), after 45 min of LAD occlusion, and then subjected to the postconditioning protocol of three cycles of 30 s (3×30 s) reperfusion and ischemia, while 20 mL DHI was infused intravenously into the former ear vein (Danhong Injection, major ingredients: Salvia miltiorrhiza and Carthamus tinctorius, Jinan Buchang Pharmaceutical Limited company, SFDA No. Z20026866, production date December 5, 2008).

1.4　Determination of Infarct Size

The TTC method was adopted. After 24-h reperfusion, animals were euthanised by pentobarbital. The heart was rapidly excised and sectioned from apex to the coronary occlusion spot into 5 transverse slices in a plane parallel to the atrioventricular groove; the 5 slices were incubated at 37℃ for 20 min in 1% 2,3,5-triphenyl tetrazolium chloride in 0.1mol/L phosphate buffer adjusted to pH 7.4. The areas at risk were calculated by a multimedia color pathological image analytical system (MPIAS-500, Konghai, Beijing, China), and the myocardial infarct size was expressed as a percent of the area at risk.

1.5　Examination by Light and Electron Microscope

For the light microscopic investigations, tissue samples from the tip of the heart were fixed with 4% paraformaldŴyde solution, dŴydrated in graded alcohol series, and embedded in paraffin. Then we did serial sections along ischemia (UK Shandon 325); the thickness of each slice was 4 μm. Tissue sections were stained with hematoxylin and eosin (H&E) and examined under an Olympus BX51 photomicroscope (Tokyo, Japan).

For the electron microscopic investigations, tissues from the tip of heart (1mm × 1mm × 1mm) were fixed with 2.5% glutaraldehyde, dehydrated in graded alcohol series, and embedded in epoxy resin 618. Then ultrathin sections (Sweden LKB8800) were stained with uranyl acetate and acidum hydrochloricum lead. Changes of the myocardial ultra-structure were observed by a Hitachi H-600 type transmission electron microscope.

1.6　Superoxide Dismutase and Malondial-dehyde Activity in Myocardium

Tissue samples (100 mg) from the tip of the heart were prepared into 10% tissue homogenate on ice for determination of superoxide dismutase (SOD) and malondialdehyde (MDA) activity in myocardium. The activity of SOD and MDA was measured according to the kit instructions (Nanjing Jiancheng Bioengineering Institute, batch No. 20090712, 20090823).

1.7 Statistical Analysis

All data were expressed as mean±standard deviation. Analysis of variance was used to determine significant differences between groups. A value of $P < 0.05$ was considered to indicate a statistically significant difference.

2. Results

2.1 Myocardial Infarction Size

According to the comparison of the myocardial infarction size among groups, the myocardial infarction size was smaller in the POC group than that in the I/R group ($P < 0.05$), and the PAD group displayed a significantly reduced infarction size relative to the I/R group ($P < 0.01$) and the POC group ($P < 0.05$, Table 1 and Figure 2).

Table 1   Comparison of Myocardial Infarction Size
($\bar{x} \pm s$)

Group	n	Infarction Size
SH	6	0
I/R	6	$0.37 \pm 0.09^{\triangle}$
POC	6	$0.26 \pm 0.02^{*}$
PAD	6	$0.14 \pm 0.08^{**\triangle}$

Notes: $^{*}P < 0.05$, $^{**}P < 0.01$, compared with the I/R group, $^{\triangle}P < 0.05$, compared with the POC group

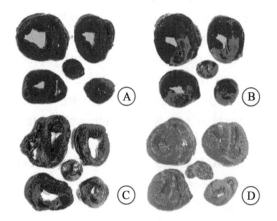

Figure 2   Images of Stained Myocardium
Notes: A: SH group, B: I/R group, C: POC group, D: PAD group

2.2 Results of Light Microscope

In the SH group, myocardial fibers were arranged regularly, and the shape of myocytes was normal. Intercalated disc and nucleus with oval or round shape in the central of the myocardial fibers were observed. In the I/R group, myocardial tissue was significantly damaged, the myocardial fibers were arranged irregularly and the sarcoplasmic reticulum was dissolved with numerous inflammatory cells infiltration. In the PAD group, myocardial tissue injury was significantly reduced as compared to the I/R group. The myocardial fibers were arranged regularly with no or few inflammatory cells, and the morphology of nucleus was almost normal. In the POC group, the arrangement of myocardial fibers was more regular with slight wave as compared to the I/R group. Myocardial cells were swollen slightly with a small amount of inflammatory cells (Figure 3).

2.3 Results of Electron Microscope

In the SH group, the cardiomyocyte ultrastructure was normal, and myocardial fibers were arranged regularly. Myofilament was rich with clear band of light-shade, and mitochondrial integrity was maintained without swelling and vacuolization. In the I/R group, the cardiomyocyte ultrastructure was damaged seriously including disorder arrangement of myocardial fibers, fraction and dissolution of myofilament, mitochondrial swelling, crista fraction, or even vacuolization. In the PAD group, the cardiomyocyte ultrastructure was improved significantly than that in the I/R group. Myocardial fibers were arranged regularly with increased myofilament. The majority of mitochondria have regular morphology with clear cristae. In the POC group, the cardiomyocyte ultrastructure was improved relative to the I/R group. Myocardial fibers were arranged regularly, myofilament was disrupted and some mitochondria were swollen (Figure 4).

2.4 Expression of SOD and MDA in Myocardium

As shown in Figure 5, the analysis revealed a significant increase in SOD of ischemic myocardium in the POC and PAD groups as compared to that in the I/R group (96.96 ± 13.43, 112.25 ± 22.75 vs. 76.32 ± 10.63, $P < 0.05$, P

第四章

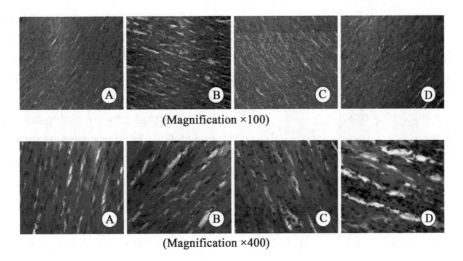

(Magnification ×100)

(Magnification ×400)

Figure 3 Light Microscope Images

Notes: A: SH group; B: I/R group; C: POC group; D: PAD group

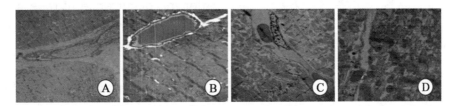

Figure 4 Electron Microscope Images

Notes: A: SH group (×3500); B: I/R group (×5000); C: POC group (×5000); D: PAD group (×4000)

< 0.01). Conversely, MDA was significantly lower in the POC group and the PAD group as compared to the I/R group (1.27 ± 0.19, 1.09 ± 0.21 vs. 1.47 ± 0.16, $P < 0.05$, $P < 0.01$).

3. Discussion

Several experimental animal models have discovered the phenomenon of ischemic precon-ditioning in the 1980s. Endogenous protection against I/R injury, such as improvement in tolerance to secondary ischemia and reduction in reperfusion injury and myocardial infarct size, is obtained by one or more brief preceding episodes of ischemia. With related research in the next decades, molecular and cellular mechanisms of ischemic preconditioning have been interpreted in some aspects, which have brought inspiration to the clinical treatment of AMI. Although a large number of studies have shown that ischemic preconditioning definitely attenuates reperfusion injury, its use as a clinical cardioprotective strategy is limited by the inability to predict the onset of AMI. Zhao, et al[8] reported ligation of LAD in canines for 60 min; repetitive ischemia applied during early reperfusion is cardioprotective by attenuating reperfusion injury significantly. Therefore, the concept of ischemic postconditioning which shows a promising direction in prevention and treatment of I/R injury is put forward. Since then, a number of studies[9-11] confirmed that postconditioning has a similar cardioprotection in rats, rabbits, canines and other animals. Suggested mechanisms of protection include a reduction in neutrophil accumulation and ameliorated coronary artery endothelial

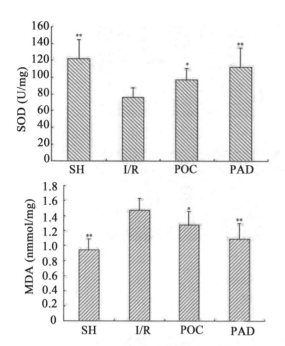

Figure 5 Expression of SOD and MDA in Ischemic Myocardium

Notes：compared with the I/R group，*P < 0.05，**P < 0.01

第四章

function, attenuation of oxidative stress, a reduction in apoptotic cell death, and attenuation of mitochondrial calcium accumulation. Previous studies of postconditioning selected rodents and open-chest models. Our study was modeled in the minipig because this species better approximates human coronary anatomy and responses to reconstruction after AMI. We followed a postconditioning protocol by the method of repetitive brief periods of inflation/deflation of the angioplasty balloon. The results demonstrated that the myocardial infarction size was lower in the POC group than in the I/R group (P < 0.05), and postconditioning ischemia had a cardioprotection against myocardial I/R in minipigs.

Mitochondrial Ca^{2+} overload, excessive production of reactive oxygen species or ATP depletion in the early minutes of reflow triggers opening of the mitochondrial permeability transition pore (mPTP). Opening of mPTP results in the collapse of the membrane potential, uncoupling of the respiratory chain, and

efflux of cytochrome c and other proapoptotic factors that may lead to either apoptosis or necrosis[12,13]. Various studies have indicated that phosphatidylinositol 3 kinase/serine-threonine kinase (P13K/Akt) signaling pathway played an important role in biological functions in cell apoptosis, survival and proliferation, and this signaling pathway is an important signaling exerting a cardioprotection in postconditioning ischemia. Oxidative stress has been demonstrated to participate in the activation of the P13K/Akt signaling pathway to some extent [14]. Modern researches showed that myocardial I/R injury mainly related to the oxidative stress injury, inflammatory response, apoptosis, etc[15]. After the occurrence of reperfusion injury, the production of reactive oxygen species and the antioxidant defense mechanisms lose their dynamic balance, and oxygen free radical scavenging abilities were reduced, such as decreased SOD activity; meanwhile, increased oxygen free radicals trigger MDA production induced by membrane lipid peroxidation. Our study showed that myocardial expression of SOD in the POC group was significantly higher than that in the I/R group (P < 0.05), while the expression of MDA was decreased significantly (P < 0.05). Therefore, postconditioning has a cardioprotection by reducing the myocardial ischemic oxidative stress in minipigs.

The concept of pharmacologic postconditioning has been proposed in clinics recently. PPOC is stimulated by drugs, or endogenous substances simulation presented cardioprotection against myocardial I/R injury. Compared with the mechanical postconditioning, PPOC has better maneuverability and controllability in clinical practice. Nikolaidis, et al [16] reported that when added to percutaneous coronary intervention, Glucagon-like peptide-1 infusion played a cardioprotective role in I/R, which improved left ventricular function, reduced myocardial infarction area and decreased the levels of myocardial enzyme in patients with AMI after successful primary angioplasty. Modern research has shown that [17] isoflurane, insulin, transforming growth factor, granulocyte colony stimulating factor, adenosine receptor agonist, morphine, and statin can produce PPOC; the mechanisms mainly related to Reperfusion Injury Salvage Kinase pathway, mitochondria mPTP, and opening of potassium channel, activation of adenosine and adenosine receptors. As for patients with myocardial ischemia who can not carry out thrombolysis and interventional treatment, effective PPOC can protect myocardium, reduce infarct size and improve the prognosis and quality of life. Therefore, POCC may have the potential to provide a field of interesting medical research in the development of new drugs and new methods of using persisting drugs.

Danhong Injection with the effects of dilating blood vessels, improving microcirculation, reducing inflammation, and protecting against myocardial I/R injury is a Chinese materia medica preparation with definite effects of cardioprotection. Our study revealed that Danhong Injection and ischemic postconditioning showed a synergistic protection on myocardial reperfusion injury in minipigs. This has provided a fundamental evidence of PPOC effects by Chinese medicine.

References

[1] Skyschally A, van Caster P, Iliodromitis EK, et al. Ischemic postconditioning: experimental models and protocol algorithms. Basic Res Cardiol, 2009, 104: 469-483.

[2] Downey JM, Cohen MV. Why do we still not have cardioprotective drugs？ Circ J, 2009, 73: 1171-1177.

[3] Tissier R, Waintraub X, Couvreur N, et al. Pharmacological postconditioning with the phytoestrogen genistein. J Mol Cell Cardiol, 2007, 42: 79-87.

[4] Feng K, Ji XB, Qiu WW, et al. The effect of Danhong injection on cardiovascular event in earlier period and inflammatory reaction of the patients of ACS with PCI. J Chin Microcirculation, 2007, 11: 390-392.

[5] Tian ZQ, Wu L, Yi CH. Clinical observation of Danhong Injection on unstable angina pectoris. Pract J Cardioac Cereb Pneum Vasc Dis, 2008, 16: 19-21.

[6] Xia K, Li JB, Wu JW, et al. Effects of Danhong injection on expression of ICAM-1 in rat kidneys with ischemia reperfusion injury after renal transplantation. J Chongqing Med Univ, 2010, 35: 199-202.

[7] Li XZ, Liu JX, Ren JX, et al. Establishment of coronary heart disease model of phlegm-stasis cementation syndrome type in mini swines. Chin J Integr Tradit West Med, 2009, 29: 228-232.

[8] Zhao ZQ, Corvera JS, Halkos ME, et al. Inhibition of myocardial injury by ischemic postconditioning during reperfusion: comparison with ischemic preconditioning. Am J Physiol Heart Circ Physiol, 2003, 285: 579-588.

[9] Halkos ME, Kerendi F, Corvera JS, et al. Myocardial protection with postconditioning is not enhanced by ischemic preconditioning. Ann Thorac Surg, 2004, 78: 961-969.

[10] Galagudza M, Kurapeev D, Minasian S, et al. Ischemic postconditioning: brief ischemia during reperfusion converts persistent ventricular fibrillation into regular rhythm. Eur J Cardiothorac Surg, 2004, 25: 1006-1010.

[11] Tsang A, Hausenloy DJ, Mocanu MM. Postconditioning: a form of "modified reperfusion" protects the myoicardium by activating the P13k-Akt pathway. Circ Res, 2004, 110: 161-167.

[12] Argaud L, Gateau-Roesch O, Raisky O. Postconditioning inhibits mitochondrial permeability transition. Circulation, 2005, 111: 194-197.

[13] Hausenloy D, Wynne A, Duchen M, et al. Transient mitochondrial permeability transition pore opening mediates preconditioning-induced protection. Circulation, 2004, 109: 1714-1717.

[14] Chen YW, Huang CF, Tsai KS, et al. The role of phosphoinositide 3-kinase/Akt signaling in low-dose mercury-induced mouse pancreatic beta-cell dysfunction in vitro and in vivo. Diabetes, 2006, 55: 1614-1624.

[15] Monassier JP. Reperfusion injury in acute myocardial infarction. From bench to cath lab. Arch Cardiovasc Dis, 2008, 101: 491-500.

[16] Nikolaidis LA, Mankad S, Sokos GG, et al.

Effects of glucagons-like peptide-1 in patients with acute myocardial infarction and left ventricular dysfunction after successful reperfusion. Circulation, 2004, 109: 962-965.

[17] Zhang LN, Wu YL. Protective effect of pharmacologic postconditioning on myocardial ischemia/reperfusion injury. Progress Pharm Sci, 2008, 32: 157-162.

Dynamic Expression of the Main Related Indicators of Thrombosis, Inflammatory Reaction and Tissue Damage in a Rat Model of Myocardial Infarction[*]

XUE Mei   YIN Hui-jun   ZHANG Lu   GUO Chun-yu   JING Yue-rong   WU Cai-feng   LI Xue-feng   CHEN Ke-ji

第四章

1. Introduction

Granule membrane protein-140 (GMP-140), tissue-type plasminogen activator (t-PA), high-sensitivity C-reactive protein (hs-CRP), interleukin (IL) -6, matrix metalloproteinase (MMP)-9 and tissue inhibitors of metallo-proteinase (TIMP)-1 play a significant role in the occurrence and development of acute myocardial infarction (AMI) as the main related indicators of thrombosis, inflammatory reaction and tissue damage[1-7]. For example, previous reports have revealed that GMP-140 reaches its peak expression only 24 h after AMI attack [8]. However, although the dynamic changes of these related indicators have been extremely significant in helping to determine medication and blood sampling time, there are few studies detailing these changes in the acute phase of AMI. Therefore, the present study aimed to evaluate dynamic changes in GMP-140, t-PA, hs-CRP, IL-6, MMP-9 and TIMP-1 in a rat model of AMI.

2. Materials and Methods

2.1 Experimental Protocol.

A total of 276 male Wistar rats weighing 180-200g were purchased from the Institute of Laboratory Animal Sciences, Chinese Academy of Medical Sciences. The protocol was approved by the animal care and ethics committee of the China Academy of Chinese Medical Sciences. The control group comprised 6 randomly selected rats, and the remainder were randomly divided into 18 groups, with 15 rats in each group. The left coronary artery was ligated in 9 of the 18 groups to establish the AMI model according to Olivetti's methods [9,10]. The rats were anesthetized by intraperitoneal injection of urethane solution (20%) at a dose of 0.6 mL/kg. The rats in the remaining 9 groups were shamoperated, and did not undergo ligation. Of the surviving rats, 6 were randomly selected from each myocardial infarction and sham-operated group at 6, 12, 18, 24 and 36h, and at 2, 3, 5 and 7 days after successful modeling. Blood (4-5mL) was drawn from the abdominal aorta after anesthetization with 20% urethane solution, and was centrifuged at 2,000 rpm for 15 min. The serum was collected and preserved at –20°C for further analysis.

2.2 Enzyme-linked Immunosorbent Assay

The serum levels of GMP-140, t-PA, hs-CRP, IL-6, MMP-9 and TIMP-1 were detected using an

* 原载于 Molecular Medicine Reports, 2011, 4: 693-696

enzyme-linked immunosorbent assay (ELISA) according to the manufacturer's instructions. The ELISA kit, GMP-140, t-PA, hs-CRP, IL-6, MMP-9 and TIMP-1 were all provided by R&D Systems Co. (USA), subpackaged by Shanghai Boatman Biological Technology Co., Ltd. A Multiskan type 3 microplate reader (Thermo Scientific) was used for detection.

2.3 Statistical Analysis

Data are presented as the mean $\pm$ SD. The student's t-test was used for the measurement of paired group data. The general linear model was used for comparison of the same index at various time points. $P < 0.05$ was considered statistically significant.

3. Results

3.1 Thrombosis-Related Indicators

Dynamic Changes in Serum GMP-14. The serum GMP-140 levels were significantly increased at various time points in the model groups compared to the sham-operated groups ($P < 0.05$, $P < 0.01$) (Figure 1). The serum GMP-140 levels were higher in the 6 h to day 7 model groups compared to the control group, higher in the 18 h and day 2 model groups compared to the 6 h group ($P < 0.05$, $P < 0.01$), and higher in the day 2 model group compared to the 12 h and day 3 model groups ($P < 0.05$, $P < 0.01$). Differences at other time points were not significant ($P < 0.05$). The serum GMP-140 levels continually increased, reaching their first peak at 18 h and the maximum peak at day 2. They then decreased slightly, but remained higher than those of the control group.

Dynamic changes in serum t-PA. The serum t-PA levels were significantly decreased in the 6 h to day 3 model groups compared to the sham-operated groups ($P < 0.05$) (Figure 2) The serum t-PA levels were lower in the 6 h to day 3 model groups compared to the control group. However, in the day 5 and day 7 model groups ($P < 0.05$) they were increased, though without significance compared to the control group ($P < 0.05$). The

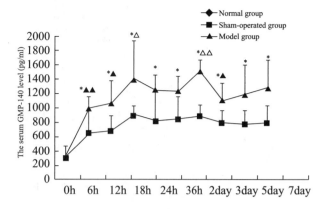

Figure 1 Dynamic Changes in Serum GMP-140 at Various Time Points. $^{*}P < 0.05$, $^{**}P < 0.01$ compared to the sham-operated group; $^{\triangle}P < 0.05$, $^{\triangle\triangle}P < 0.01$ compared to the 6 h model group; $^{\blacktriangle}P < 0.05$, $^{\blacktriangle\blacktriangle}P < 0.01$ compared to the day 2 model group. Data are expressed as the mean $\pm$ SD

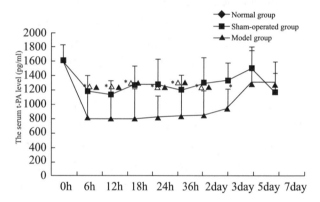

Figure 2 Dynamic Changes in Serum t-PA at Various Time Points. $^{*}P < 0.05$, $^{**}P < 0.01$ compared to the sham-operated group; $^{\triangle}P < 0.05$, $^{\triangle\triangle}P < 0.01$ compared to the 5 day model group; $^{\blacktriangle}P < 0.05$, $^{\blacktriangle\blacktriangle}P < 0.01$ compared to the day 7 model group. Data are expressed as the mean $\pm$ SD

serum t-PA levels significantly decreased and were restored to baseline by day 5.

3.2 Inflammatory Reaction-related Indicators

Dynamic changes in serum hs-CRP. The serum hs-CRP levels were significantly increased at various time points in the model groups compared to the sham-operated groups ($P < 0.05$, $P < 0.01$) (Figure 3). The serum hs-CRP levels were higher in the 6h to day 7 model groups compared to the control group, and higher in the 18h model group compared to the 6 and 36h, day 3 and day 5 model groups, respectively ($P < 0.05$). Differences in comparison to the

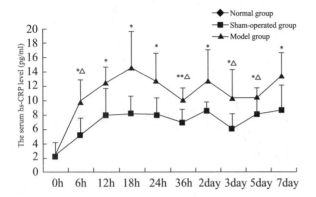

Figure 3 Dynamic Changes in Serum hs-CRP at Various Time Points. $^*P < 0.05$, $^{**}P < 0.01$ compared to the sham-operated group; $^{\triangle}P < 0.05$, $^{\triangle\triangle}P < 0.01$ compared to the 18 h model group. Data are expressed as the mean ± SD

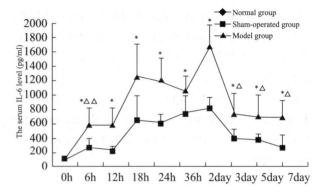

Figure 4 Dynamic Changes in serum IL-6 at Various Time Points. $^*P < 0.05$, $^{**}P < 0.01$ compared to the sham-operated group; $^{\triangle}P < 0.05$, $^{\triangle\triangle}P < 0.01$ compared to the 18, 24 and 36 h and day 2 model groups. Data are expressed as the mean ± SD

remaining model groups were not significant ($P < 0.05$). The serum hs-CRP levels continually increased and reached their first peak at 18 h. They then decreased slightly, but remained higher than those of the control group.

Dynamic changes in serum IL-6. The serum IL-6 levels were significantly increased at various time points in the model groups compared to the sham-operated groups ($P < 0.05$, $P < 0.01$) (Figure 4). The serum IL-6 levels were higher in the 6 h to day 7 model groups compared to the control group, and higher in the 18, 24 and 36 h and day 2 model groups compared to the 6 h, day 3, day 5 and day 7 model groups ($P < 0.05$, $P < 0.01$). Differences in comparison to the remaining model groups were not significant ($P < 0.05$). The serum IL-6 levels continually increased and reached their first peak at 18h. They began to decrease after day 3, but remained higher than those of the control group.

3.3 Tissue Damage-related Indicators

Dynamic changes in serum MMP-9. The serum MMP-9 levels were significantly increased at various time points in the model groups compared to the sham-operated groups ($P < 0.05$, $P < 0.01$) (Figure 5). The serum MMP-9 levels were higher in the 6h to day 7 model groups compared to the control group, significantly higher in the 18, 24 and 36 h, day 2

and day 3 model groups compared to the 6 and 12 h model groups ($P < 0.01$), and significantly higher in the day 2 model group compared to the 6, 12 and 36 h, and day 3, day 5 and day 7 model groups, respectively ($P < 0.05$, $P < 0.01$). The serum MMP-9 levels continually increased, reaching their first peak at 18 h and the maximum peak on day 2. They then decreased slightly, but remained higher than those of the control group.

Dynamic changes in serum TIMP-1. The serum TIMP-1 levels were significantly decreased in the 24 h to day 7 model groups compared to the sham-operated groups ($P < 0.05$, $P < 0.01$) (Figure 6), and were significantly decreased in the 24 h to day 7 model groups compared to the control group ($P < 0.05$, $P < 0.01$). The serum TIMP-1 levels started to decrease as of 24 h, but were maintained until day 7.

4. Discussion

Coronary atherosclerotic plaque rupture and subsequent thrombogenesis may lead to acute occlusion of the coronary arteries, which is the most predominant cause of AMI. Currently, anti-coagulation and anti-platelet therapy are essential treatments for the clinical prevention of re-occlusion of coronary thrombosis[11]. GMP-140, as a member of the selectin family, is only expressed

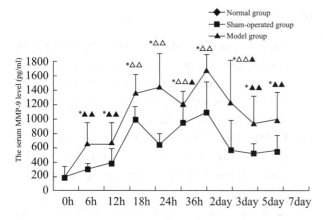

Figure 5 Dynamic Changes in Serum MMP-9 at Various Time Points. $^*P < 0.05$, $^{**}P < 0.01$ compared to the sham-operated group; $^{\triangle}P < 0.05$, $^{\triangle\triangle}P < 0.01$ compared to the 6 and 12 h model groups; $^{\blacktriangle}P < 0.05$, $^{\blacktriangle\blacktriangle}P < 0.01$ compared to the day 2 model group. Data are expressed as the mean ± SD

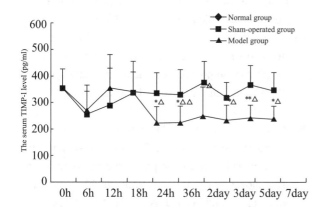

Figure 6 Dynamic Changes in Serum TIMP-1 at Various Time Points. $^*P < 0.05$, $^{**}P < 0.01$ compared to the sham-operated group; $^{\triangle}P < 0.05$. $^{\triangle\triangle}P < 0.01$ compared to the control group. Data are expressed as the mean ± SD

on the degranulated platelet surface. As a marker of late-phase platelet activation and one of the specific indicators presently known to most directly reflect the degree of platelet activation[12], it is closely correlated with thrombosis. A clinical study noted GMP-140 levels to be increased as of 12 h after AMI attack, reaching a peak on day 2[8]. In this study, the serum GMP-140 level in the AMI rats continued to increase 6 h after successful modeling, reaching the first peak at 18 h and the maximum peak on day 2. It then decreased slightly, although it remained increased compared to the control group. After the successful

modeling of AMI, the blood vessels became occluded and the vessel wall was injured, causing platelet aggregation, fibrin deposition and thrombosis. Meanwhile, the t-PA-mediated fibrolysis system was also initiated. Serum t-PA levels significantly decreased, potentially due to their having been exhausted by the activation of the fibrolysis system, which may further promote the occurrence and development of thrombosis. The t-PA levels were restored to baseline levels by day 5. A study on balloon injury to the rabbit iliac artery by More et al. [13]also found that t-PA activation was markedly decreased 2 h after surgery, and remained at a lower level until returning to control group levels 7 days after surgery.

Inflammatory reaction, the main cause of the occurrence and development of atherosclerosis, is one of the primary factors behind the occurrence of AMI [14]. hs-CRP is capable of reliably predicting the risk of cardiovascular diseases. IL-6, with its extensive bioactivities, causes various biological effects in the process of inflammatory reaction, anti-infection and injury[15,16]. The serum levels of hs-CRP and IL-6 were increased in the successfully modeled rats, reaching a peak at 18 h. Afterwards, the serum hs-CRP level decreased somewhat, while the serum IL-6 level did not begin to decrease until day 3. The levels of hs-CRP and IL-6 were increased compared to the control group. The expression of the cytokines GMP-140, t-PA, hs-CRP and IL-6 was significantly increased 6 h after AMI, indicating that platelet activation, fibrolysis and blood clotting system activation, as well as a tissue inflammatory reaction, jointly participated in the process after AMI. Of these, t-PA, which participates in the activation of fibrolysis and the blood clotting system, was the first to be restored to baseline levels, while platelet activation and inflammatory reaction continued throughout the acute phase of MI.

AMI may induce ventricular remodeling. It manifests not only as pachyntic and necrotic myocardial cells, thickening of coronary vessels and insufficient growth of capillaries, but also in the destruction of the dynamic equilibrium between the synthesis and degradation of collagen fibers, which further results in impaired heart function and the occurrence of heart failure. MMP is the main enzyme system to degrade the extracellular matrix. TIMP is the endogenous specific inhibitor of MMP. In this study, serum MMP-9 levels began to increase 6 h after AMI, reaching the first peak after 18 h and the maximum peak by day 2. They then decreased slightly, but remained higher than those of the control group. Serum TIMP-1 levels started to decrease 24 h after successful modeling, but were maintained until day 7. MMP-9 was observed to participate in the reconstitution that occurred in the first several hours to several days after AMI, while changes in the serum TIMP-1 levels lagged slightly behind those of MMP-9. When the relative balance between serum MMP-9 and TIMP-1 is not maintained, it may aggravate tissue damage and the process of ventricular remodeling [17].

Previous studies have revealed that tissue plasminogen activator antigens can be used to predict the occurrence of cardiovascular events after AMI [18], while the fibrolysis and blood clotting system, as well as the metalloproteinases, jointly participate in the pathophysiological process of left ventricular remodeling after AMI [19]. In this study, the expression of t-PA and MMP-9 was increased compared to the control group during the early phase of AMI after successful modeling of rat myocardial infarction.

In conclusion, changes in thrombosis, inflammatory reaction, and tissue damage indicators were observed for 7 days after AMI. Based on the dynamic changes of each indicator, the optimal intervention time may be determined. This provides fundamental reference data for experimental studies. In future studies, more time points will be added and analyzed, and indices such as heart function will be combined.

References

[1] Yip HK, Chang LT, Sun CK, et al. Platelet activity is a biomarker of cardiac necrosis and predictive of untoward clinical outcomes in patients with acute myocardial infarction undergoing primary coronary stenting. Circ J, 2006, 70: 31-36.

[2] Liu WH, Yang CH, YŴ KH, et al. Circulating levels of soluble P-selectin in patients in the early and recent phases of myocardial infarction. Chang Gung Med J, 2005, 28: 613-620.

[3] Ganti AK, Potti A, Yegnanarayan R. Plasma tissue plasminogen activator and plasminogen activator inhibitor-1 levels in acute myocardial infarction. Pathophysiol Haemost Thromb, 2002, 32: 80-84.

[4] Bian Y, Chen YG, Xu F, et al. The polymorphism in aldehyde dehydrogenase-2 gene is associated with elevated plasma levels of high-sensitivity C-reactive protein in the early phase of myocardial infarction. Tohoku J Exp Med , 2010, 221: 107-112.

[5] Kang WQ, Song DL, Guo XG. Relationship between serum vasoactive factors and plaque morphology in patients with acute coronary syndrome. Zhonghua Xin Xue Guan Bing Za Zhi, 2007, 35: 1020-1023.

[6] Miyazaki S, Kasai T, Miyauchi K, et al. Changes of matrix metalloproteinase-9 level is associated with left ventricular remodeling following acute myocardial infarction among patients treated with trandolapril, valsartan or both. Circ J, 2010, 74: 1158-1164.

[7] Dinh W, Füth R, Scheffold T, et al. Increased serum levels of tissue inhibitor of metalloproteinase-1 in patients with acute myocardial infarction. Int Heart J, 2009, 50: 421-431.

[8] He Y, Shen W, Zhao Y, et al. The dynamic changes of platelet P-selectin and glycoprotein V in acute myocardial infarction. Suzhou University of Medical Science, 2006, 26: 777-779.

[9] Abbate A, Salloum FN, Vecile E, et al. Anakinra, a recombinant human interleukin-1 receptor antagonist, inhibits apoptosis in experimental myocardial infarction. Circulation, 2008, 117: 2670-2683.

[10] Olivetti G, Capasso JM, Meggs LG, et al. Cellular basis of chronic ventricular remodeling after myocardial infarction in rats. Cir Res, 1991, 68: 856-869.

[11] Chen Z, Gao R. Coronary heart disease. Beijing: People's Medical Publishing House, 2003, 879-882.

[12] Chen KJ, Xue M, Yin HJ. The relationship between platelet activation and coronary heart disease and blood-stasis syndrome. J Capit Med Univ, 2008, 29: 266-269.

[13] More RS, Underwood MJ, Brack MJ, et al. Changes in vessel wall plasminogen activator activity and smooth muscle cell proliferation and activation after arterial injury. Cardiovasuclar Res, 1995, 29: 22-26.

[14] Napoleão P, Santos MC, Selas M, et al. Variations in inflammatory markers in acute myocardial infarction: a longitudinal study. Rev Port Cardiol, 2007, 26: 1357-1363.

[15] Kishimoto T. Interleukin-6: from basic science to medicine—40 years in immunology. Annu Rev Immunol , 2005, 23: 21.

[16] Ding C, Cicuttini F, Li J, et al. Targeting IL-6 in the treatment of inflammatory and autoimmune diseases. Expert Opin Investig Drugs, 2009, 18: 1457-1466.

[17] Kelly D, Squire IB, Khan SQ, et al. Usefulness of plasma tissue inhibitors of metalloproteinases as markers of prognosis after acute myocardial infarction. Am J Cardiol, 2010, 106: 477-482.

[18] Lowe GD, Danesh J, Lewington S, et al. Tissue plasminogen activator antigen and coronary heart disease. Prospective study and meta-analysis. Eur Heart J, 2004, 25: 252-259.

[19] Weir RA, Balmain S, Steedman T, et al. Tissue plasminogen activator antigen predicts medium-term left ventricular endsystolic volume after acute myocardial infarction. J Thromb Thrombolysis, 2010, 29: 421-428.

第二节　中医药防治心室重构的研究

益气养阴与解毒活血中药对心肌梗死后大鼠早期心室重构心肌 NF-κB 和 PPAR-γ mRNA 表达的影响 *

徐　伟　刘剑刚　王承龙　陈可冀

急性心肌梗死（acute myocardial infarction，AMI）后心室重构（ventricular remodeling，VR）的发生、发展与神经内分泌、细胞因子系统激活等有关。AMI 后的 VR 与预后密切相关，其刺激因素除了缺血缺氧、心室壁张力过高和神经内分泌激素的过度激活外，还有炎症因子的参与。核因子-κB（NF-κB）是近年研究发现的重要核转录因

子，在炎症反应中通过表达炎症介质、黏附分子和生物酶等起作用；而过氧化物酶增殖体激活受体（peroxisome proliferator-actived receptor，PPARs）中受体-γ（PPAR-γ）是一类由配体调节的核激素受体。研究表明 PPAR-γ 激动剂能抑制细胞炎症反应及细胞凋亡等发挥保护作用[1-2]。既往炎症反应与 AMI 后心室重构及药物干预研究较少，前期研

---

* 原载于《北京中医药大学学报》，2010，33(5)：333-338

究表明，益气活血法对动物早期 AMI 后 VR 有明显减轻作用[3]，故从 AMI 后心肌组织 NF-κB 和 PPAR-γ 变化探讨中医益气养阴活血和解毒活血组分对 VR 的影响及可能的作用机制。

1. 材料与方法

1.1 动物

8 周龄雄性 Wistar 大鼠，清洁级，60 只，体重 200 ～ 220g，由北京维通利华实验动物技术有限公司提供，合格证号：SCXK（京）2007-0001。

1.2 药物

生脉胶囊（红参总皂苷、麦冬多糖、五味子总素），每粒 0.3g，正大青春宝制药有限公司生产（批号：0803004）；复方川芎胶囊（川芎嗪、阿魏酸），每粒 0.37g，山东凤凰制药股份有限公司生产（批号：0802205）；黄连提取物（黄连生物碱），每克相当于 6.25g 生药，由北京同仁堂制药有限公司提供；培哚普利片（培哚普利叔丁胺盐），4mg/ 片，由施维雅（天津）制药有限公司生产提供（批号：Batch 7M0434）。

1.3 试剂

白介素 -1β（IL-1β）、白介素 -6（IL-6）放射免疫试剂盒由解放军总医院放射免疫技术研究所提供；超敏 C- 反应蛋白（hs-CRP）试剂盒由美国 E&E Labs 公司生产（批号：03111403）。焦炭酸二乙酯（DEPC）购自美国 Sigma 公司；兔抗人 NF-κB 抗体试剂盒、兔抗人 PPAR-γ 抗体试剂盒由北京博奥森生物技术有限公司提供；辣根生物素标记的山羊抗兔 IgG 由北京中杉金桥生物技术有限公司提供；Taq DNA 聚合酶为美国 Promega 公司产品；RNA 提取剂（Trizol）为 Gibco/BRL 公司产品；反转录 - 聚合酶链反应（RT-PCR）试剂盒、RNA 酶抑制剂（40U/μL）均为日本 TaKaPa 公司产品；扩增 mRNA 引物序列由上海生物工程公司合成。

1.4 实验仪器

Multiskan MK3 型半自动酶标仪，由荷兰雷勃生物医学有限公司生产；SN-682 型 γ 计数器，由上海核福光仪器有限公司生产；BHEC 型显微镜 - 微机彩色图像处理系统，由美国冷泉公司生产；UV-120-02 型紫外分光光度计，由上海光学仪器有限公司生产；UV-VI 型紫外透射分析仪，由北京智源通生物技术研究所生产；Techgene 型基因扩增仪，由英国 Labway Science Development 公司生产；DUR 530 DNA/ 蛋白型检测仪，由美国

BECKMAN 公司生产；VDS 型凝胶成像分析系统，由美国 Pharmacia Biotech 公司生产。

1.5 动物造模方法

动物称重，采用乙醚麻醉。消毒皮肤，经左侧剪开皮肤，于第 3 至 4 肋间钝性分离肌肉组织，开胸，快速挤出心脏，于前降支下 1 ～ 2mm 处结扎左冠状动脉前降支，造成 AMI 模型，然后迅速将心脏放回胸腔，随即缝合。动物稳定后记录标准肢导联 Ⅱ 导心电图（纸速 50mm/s），ST 段弓背抬高示 AMI 形成。术后给予青霉素 4 万单位，连续 3d。假手术组除不结扎冠状动脉外，其余操作同模型组。

1.6 动物分组与用药

造模成功的大鼠随机分为 5 组，每组 10 只，造模后第 2 天灌胃同等体积药物，连续 4 周。假手术组，常规饲养，只穿刺不结扎，喂等量水；模型对照组，喂等量水；阳性药物对照组，灌胃培哚普利片 0.36mg/（kg·d）；益气养阴活血组，灌胃生脉胶囊 0.24g/（kg·d）和复方川芎胶囊 0.40g/（kg·d）；解毒活血组，灌胃复方川芎胶囊 0.40g/（kg·d）和黄连生物碱 0.16g/（kg·d）。另设 10 只正常大鼠作为空白对照组，灌胃等量水。实验过程中因灌胃、结扎部位过高、出血过多等原因，各组大鼠均有死亡：正常组 1 只，假手术组 2 只，模型组 3 只，益气养阴活血组 1 只，解毒活血组 1 只。动物实验过程中严格遵守动物伦理学要求。

1.7 左室重量指数及血清炎症指标测定

灌胃 4 周后，大鼠经腹腔注射 20% 氨基甲基乙酯溶液（7mL/kg）麻醉，腹主动脉取血，按测定指标不同（参照试剂盒说明）加用抗凝剂。无菌条件下快速剥离心脏组织，生理盐水冲洗，用滤纸吸干；沿房室交界处剪去左、右心房及大血管，去除右心室游离壁，称取余下的左心室重量，记录大鼠心脏和左心室重量，计算左心室重量指数（left ventricular mass index，LVMI），即左心室重量（mg）占大鼠体重（g）的比例。另外，每组随机取 6 只缺血区组织迅速放于液氮中冷冻保存，进行分子生物学测定。IL-1β、IL-6 测定用放射免疫法，hs-CRP 检测用酶联免疫（ELISA）法。

1.8 RT-PCR 法检测大鼠心肌组织 PPAR-γ 和 NF-κB mRNA 的表达

心肌组织复溶后进行匀浆，分别加入 Trizol 1.5mL，反复吹吸使组织溶于 Trizol 中。进行 RT-

PCR 测定。引物序列由上海生物工程公司合成，选用 β-Actin 作为内参对照。上游为 5′-AACACC CCAGCCATGTACG3′，下游为 5′-CGCTCAGGA GGAGCAATGA3′。大鼠心肌组织 NF-κBp65m RNA 基因引物，上游为 5′-AAGATCAATGGCT ACACAGG3′，下游为 5′-CCTC AATGTCTTCTTT CTGC3′；大鼠心肌组织 PPAR-γm RNA 基因引物，上游为 5′-GACCACTCC CACTCCTTTGA-3′，下游为 5′-CGACATTCA ATTGCCA TGAG-3′。PCR 反应体系 50μL，其中含提取 RNA 2μL、10×Buffer 5μL、25mmol/L MgCl₂ 23μL、Taq 酶 2.5U、2.5mmol/L 核苷酸（Nucleotide, dNTP）4μL、10μmoL/L 引物各 2μL。组织匀浆，加入 Trizol 1.5mL，反复吹吸使组织溶于 Trizol 中，取 0.5mL 上述液体于 1.5mL 离心管中；加 0.125mL 氯仿，震荡混匀 15min，室温放置 3min；40℃ 12000r/min 离心 15min；取上清，并转移入另 1 只离心管；加入 0.25mL 异丙醇，室温放置 10min；4℃ 12000r/m 离心 5min；去上清，加入 1mL 75% 乙醇；4℃ 7500r/min 离心 5min。弃上清，室温干燥 10min；加 DEPC 水溶解 RNA，电泳鉴定 RNA 条带。PCR 反应条件为 65℃变性 RNA：加入 2.0μL 10×MOPS，3.5μL 甲醛，10μL 甲酰胺，混匀，取 40 ~ 60μg（4.5μL）总 RNA，65℃变性 15min，冰上冷却 2min；加入 2.0μL 上样缓冲液，混匀，50V 预电泳 5min，上样；待染料全部进入凝胶后，电压降为 40V，10min 混合 1 次电泳缓冲液，使电泳液两端的离子浓度趋于一致；待溴酚兰泳动到凝胶底部，停止电泳，照相。

1.9　统计方法

用 SPSS 软件处理数据，计量资料以均数±标准差（$\bar{x}\pm s$）表示。对各组数据指标进行正态性检验和方差齐性检验，多组间比较采用单因素方差分析；方差齐时采用 q 检验（Student-Newman-Keuls），方差不齐采用使用 Dunnett's 法进行多重比较，不符合正态分布采用 Wilcoxon 秩检验。假设检验统一使用双侧检验，给出检验统计量及其对应的 P 值，$P < 0.05$ 为有显著的统计学差异。

2.　结果

2.1　各组大鼠左心室重量及 LVMI 的变化

大鼠造模 4 周后，模型组大鼠的左心室重量增加明显，LVMI 也有增加，和假手术组比较有显著差异（$P < 0.01$，$P < 0.05$）。灌胃不同药物后，

培哚普利组、益气养阴活血组、解毒活血组大鼠的左心室重量和 LVMI 均不同的降低，和模型组比较有显著差异（$P < 0.01$，$P < 0.05$），各给药组之间比较无显著差异（$P > 0.05$）。结果见表 1。

表 1　各组大鼠左心室重量及 LVMI 的比较（$\bar{x}\pm s$）

组别	n	左室重量 (mg)	左室重量指数 (LVMI)
正常组 (Group A)	9	744.44±42.46	2.55±0.13
假手术组 (Group B)	8	857.50±51.48	2.69±0.22
模型组 (Group C)	7	1018.57±108.85**	3.32±0.66*
培哚普利组 (Group D)	10	706.00±115.30▲▲	2.55±0.34▲▲
益气养阴活血组 (Group E)	9	881.11±127.81▲	2.91±0.23▲
解毒活血组 (Group F)	9	846.67±149.33▲▲	2.81±0.43▲
F		9.396	4.915
P		0.000	0.001

注：与假手术组比较 *$P < 0.05$ **$P < 0.01$；与模型组比较 ▲$P < 0.05$，▲▲$P < 0.01$

2.2　各组大鼠血清炎症因子 IL-1β、IL-6、hs-CRP 含量的变化

造模 4 周后，模型组的大鼠血清 IL-6 明显升高，和假手术组比较有显著差异（$P < 0.05$），模型组的血清 IL-1β 和 hs-CRP 含量和假手术组比较无显著变化。给药 4 周后，解毒活血组 IL-6 水平显著下降，和模型组比较有显著差异（$P < 0.05$），与益气养阴活血组比较亦有显著差异（$P < 0.05$），结果见表 2。

2.3　各组大鼠心肌组织 PPAR-γ 和 NF-κB mRNA 的表达

对 Trizol 提取的细胞总 RNA 进行跑胶鉴定，电泳后呈现出明显的 RNA 条带特征。可观察到：28S 条带和 18S 条带，证明 RNA 提取成功，可以满足进行 RT-PCR 的要求，见图 1。在后续实验中，首先用分光光度计将 RNA 定量，然后再进行 RT-PCR 实验。

心肌组织 NF-κB mRNA 的 RT-PCR 结果表明，造模 4 周后，大鼠心肌组织的 PPAR-γ 和 NF-κB mRNA 的表达均显著升高，和假手术组比较有显

表 2　各组大鼠血清 IL-1β、IL-6、hs-CRP 含量的比较（$\bar{\chi} \pm s$）

组别	n	IL-1β(μg/L)	IL-6(ng/L)	hs-CRP(mg/L)
正常组（Group A）	9	0.41 ± 0.08	255.71 ± 91.40	2.59 ± 0.59
假手术组（Group B）	8	0.27 ± 0.06	297.72 ± 122.75	2.51 ± 0.78
模型组（Group C）	7	0.32 ± 0.07	327.12 ± 66.97*	2.71 ± 1.30
培哚普利组（Group D）	10	0.34 ± 0.07	166.56 ± 61.31▲	1.87 ± 0.29▲
益气养阴活血组（Group E）	9	0.44 ± 0.22	387.64 ± 136.29	2.30 ± 0.49
解毒活血组（Group F）	9	0.37 ± 0.11	223.88 ± 30.91▲	2.09 ± 0.75
F		2.251	6.281	1.600
P		0.065	0.000	0.180

注：与假手术组比较，*P < 0.05；与模型组比较 ▲P < 0.05

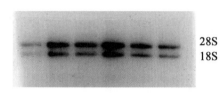

图 1　Trizol 提取的细胞总 RNA 电泳图

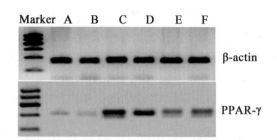

图 2 PPAR-γ 受体 mRNA 的 RT-PCR 扩增产物电泳图
A. 正常组；B. 假手术组；C. 模型组；D. 培哚普利组；E. 益气养阴活血组；F. 解毒活血组

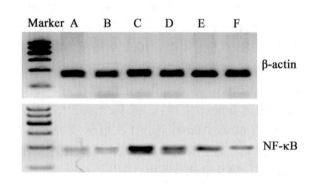

图 3　NF-κB 受体 mRNA 的 RT-PCR 扩增产物电泳图
A. 正常组；B. 假手术组；C. 模型组；D. 培哚普利组；E. 益气养阴活血组；F. 解毒活血组

著差异（P < 0.01）。益气养阴活血组、解毒活血组均有不同程度降低，和模型组比较有显著差异（P < 0.05，P < 0.01），其中对 PPAR-γ mRNA 表达降低的幅度，解毒活血组大于益气养阴活血组，两组比较有显著差异（P < 0.05），结果见图 2、图 3 和表 3。

3. 讨论

AMI 属于中医"真心痛""厥心痛"的范畴。其病机为本虚标实，临床常用的治法有益气养阴、活血化瘀等[4]。细胞因子如肿瘤坏死因子 - α（TNF-α）、IL-1β、IL-6 在心肌缺血损伤后即出现。在 AMI 早期，心肌内细胞因子在梗死区及非梗死区中表达明显增加[5]。因此研究中医治疗 AMI 的常用治法并配伍解毒中药对 AMI 后 VR 和炎症因子的影响，有利于挖掘更有效的临床治疗思路和方法。从病理形态看，各药物组对 VR 均有明显的改善作用。与模型组相比，益气养阴活血组和解毒活血组间 IL-1β、hs-CRP 差异不显著，可能与这些早期升高的炎症因子水平已处于下降阶段有关；4 周时，解毒活血组 IL-6 显著降低；培哚普利对 IL-6、hs-CRP 有一定的抑制作用。

PPARS 是一类由配体激活的核转录因子超家族成员，能调节细胞增殖和炎症反应如细胞因子的表达，减轻左心室重构和心力衰竭的发展[6-7]。NF-κB 能激活 TNF-α、基质金属蛋白酶（matrix metalloproteinases，MMPS）的蛋白合成和基因表达，促进心肌基质胶原纤维降解及心肌纤维化，参与 VR[8]。实验中益气养阴活血与解毒活血中药均可使 NF-κB mRNA 的表达显著降低，减少促炎因子的合成，改善左室重构；还可以明显降低 PPAR-γ mRNA 表达，解毒活血组降低幅度明显大于益气养阴活血组。实验结果 PPAR-γ 的变化与部分文献报道不同，原因可能是炎症因子一方面导致心脏代偿性重构，也可能导致急性心脏破裂或心力衰竭。PPAR-γ mRNA 表达减少，可能与反馈性防止过分抑制有关[9-10]。

表3　各组大鼠心肌 PPAR-γ 和 NF-κB p65mRNA 的表达比较（$\bar{\chi} \pm s$）

组别	n	PPAR-γ	NF-κB
正常组（Group A）	6	0.18 ± 0.06	0.37 ± 0.08
假手术组（Group B）	6	0.22 ± 0.10	0.51 ± 0.12
模型组（Group C）	6	2.66 ± 0.39**	1.66 ± 0.08**
培哚普利组（Group D）	6	1.35 ± 0.09▲	1.22 ± 0.17▲
益气养阴活血组（Group E）	6	1.42 ± 0.14▲	0.86 ± 0.11▲
解毒活血组（Group F）	6	0.65 ± 0.14▲▲	0.82 ± 0.14▲
F		5.261	6.486
P		0.01	0.000

注：与假手术组比较 **$P < 0.01$；与模型组比较▲$P < 0.05$ ▲▲$P < 0.01$

　　生脉胶囊由红参总皂苷、麦冬多糖、五味子总素组成，现代研究表明人参皂苷 Rbl 可抑制 Ang Ⅱ 诱导细胞肥大[11]；麦冬多糖可以抗心肌缺血，增加心肌血流量，减少心肌细胞的受损[12]；五味子乙素具有明显的清除自由基和抑制脂质过氧化作用[13]；川芎嗪具有扩张冠状动脉，抑制血栓素 A_2 的生成和活性，抗脂质过氧化等功能[14]；阿魏酸具有抑制巨噬细胞活化、抑制花生四烯酸（AA）代谢等药理作用[15]。黄连生物碱对大鼠心肌肥厚亦有预防作用[16]。实验表明川芎、当归、黄连配伍的活血解毒中药组分和生脉胶囊、川芎、当归组成的益气活血中药组分，均能抑制 AMI 后大鼠缺血心肌 NF-κB 和 PPAR-γ mRNA 表达。活血解毒与益气活血中药组分可能通过不同途径减轻大鼠 AMI 后炎症因子的表达，从而抑制心室重构，而活血解毒中药组分在改善某些炎性指标方面好于益气活血中药组分，值得今后进一步深入研究。

参考文献

[1] Grip O, Janciausklene S, Lindgren S. Atorvastatin activates PPAR-gamma and attenuates the inflammatory response in human monocytes. Inflamm Res，2002, 51(2): 58-62.

[2] Takata Y, Kitami Y, Yang ZH, et al. Vascular inflammation is negatively autoregulated by interaction between CCAAT/enhancer binding protein delta and peroxisome proliferator activated receptor-gamma. Circ Res, 2002, 91(5): 373-374.

[3] 史大卓，马鲁波，刘剑刚，等．复方芪丹液对中国小型猪急性心肌梗死后早期心室重构的影响．中国中西医结合杂志，2005，28(1)：43-46.

[4] 吴伟，李荣，李建功，等．益气养阴活血法联合不同溶栓剂治疗急性心肌梗死60例．辽宁中医杂志，2006，33(11)：1454-1455.

[5] Deten A, Volah C, Briest W, et al. Cardiac cytokine expression is upregulated in the acute phase after myocardial infarction. Experimental studies in rats. Cardiovasc Res, 2002, 55(2): 329-340.

[6] Shiom IT, Tsutsu IH, Hayash IDAN IS, et al. Pioglitazone，a peroxisome proliferator-activated receptor-gamma agonist, attenuates left ventricular remodeling and failure after experimental myocardial infarction. Circulation, 2002, 106(24): 3126-3132.

[7] Yam Amoto K, Ohkir, Lee RT, et al. Peroxisome proliferator-activated receptor gamm a activators inhibit cardiac hypertrophy in cardiac myocytes. Circulation, 2001, 104(14): 1670-1675.

[8] Bradham WS, Moe G, Wendt KA, et al. TNF-α and Myocardial matrix metalloproteinases in heart failure relationship to LV remodeling. Am J Physiol Heart Circ Physiol, 2002, 97(4):12746-12751.

[9] Suzuk IG, Khana LS, Rastoo IS, et al. Long-term pharmacological activation of PPAR-γ does not prevent left ventricular remodeling in dogs with advanced heart failure . Cardiovasc Drugs Ther, 2007, 21(1): 29-36.

[10] Mudaliar S, Henry RR. New oral therapies for type 2 diabetes mellitus: the glita zones or insulin sensitizers. Ann Rev Med, 2001, 52: 239-257.

[11] 陈小文，黄燮南，吴芹．人参皂苷 Rb Ⅰ 抑制 Ang Ⅱ 诱导的心肌细胞肥大．遵义医学院学报，2008，31(5)：457-460.

[12] 周跃华，徐德生，冯怡，等．麦冬提取物对小鼠心肌营养血流量的影响．中国实验方剂学杂志，2003，9(1)：22.

[13] 李海涛，胡刚．五味子醇甲抑制6羟基多巴胺诱导 PCI 2 细胞凋亡的研究．南京中医药大学学报，2004，20(2)：96-98.

[14] 陈可冀，张之南，梁子钧，等．血瘀证与活血化瘀研究．上海：上海科学技术出版社，1988：311-313.

[15] Hou YZ, Yang J, Zhao GR. Ferulic acid inhibits vascular smooth muscle cell proliferation induced by angiotensin Ⅱ. European Journal of Pharmacology, 2004, 499: 85.

[16] 吴庆玲，周祖玉，徐建国．黄连素对异丙肾上腺素诱导的大鼠心肌肥厚的影响．现代中西医结合杂志，2008，17(13)：1956-1958.

第四章

第三节 中医药促进血管新生的研究

人参和三七提取物在血管生成信号通路上作用靶点的实验研究 *

田 伟 雷 燕 杜雪君 朱凌群 陈可冀

前期的研究证实益气活血中药人参和三七提取物可以促进人脐静脉内皮细胞（human umbilical vein endothelial cell，HUVEC）的增殖，并且促进血管生成信号通路上血管内皮细胞生长因子受体 2（vascular endothelial growth factor receptor 2，VEGFR 2）、Ras、MAPK 蛋白表达[1]，但不清楚中药可能作用的环节和靶点。本研究通过逐级信号阻断的办法，同时加入中药提取物进行干预，观察血管生成下游信号蛋白的表达变化，旨在探究中药提取物在此过程中的作用环节及可能的作用靶点。

1. 材料与方法

1.1 细胞

人脐静脉内皮细胞二代（HUVEC-2C，箱号：C-023-5C，批号：4C0218），购自 Cascade Biologics 公司。

1.2 药物

人参提取物（批号：0609089）和三七提取物（批号：0612051），购自广东一方制药有限公司。

1.3 试剂及仪器

VEGFR-2 抑制剂：SU5416：1，3-Dihydro-3-[（3，5-dimethyl-^{1}H-pyrro1-2-y1）methylene]-^{2}H-indol-2-one；分子式：$C_{15}H_{14}N_2O$；分子量：238.28。Ras 抑制剂：FPP：3，7，11-Trimethyl-2，6，10-

dodecatrien-1-yl pyrophosphate ammonium salt；分子式：$C_{15}H_{37}N_3O_7P_2$；分子量：433.42。抑制剂均购自美国 Sigma 公司。Wellscan MK3 型全自动酶标仪，芬兰 Labsystems Dragon 公司生产；3K30 型高速冷冻离心机，德国 Sigma 公司生产；BioRAD IQ5 型荧光定量 PCR 仪，美国 BioRAD 生产。

1.4 方法

1.4.1 中药提取物制备方法

人参水溶后按吸附树脂层析法提得，三七采用水煎提取和阳离子树脂吸附法分离获得。按 2：1（人参：三七）配比，用时用完全培养基（M200+LSGS）配成所需浓度，经 0.22μm 微孔滤膜过滤除菌，分装，4℃保存。

1.4.2 分组方法

实验用细胞分为 6 组，即：空白对照 I 组（以完全培养基 M200 加 LSGS 作为对照，不加入 SU5416 和中药）、SU5416 组（IC_{50} 的 SU5416：0.04μmol/L[2]）、SU5416 加中药组（IC_{50} 的 SU5416 加生药人参 8/3 mg/mL，生药三七 4/3 mg/mL[1]），以上 3 组检测下游蛋白 Ras 及 MAPK 表达，以及空白对照 II 组（以完全培养基 M200 加 LSGS 作为对照，不加入 FPP 和中药）、FPP 组（IC_{50} 的 FPP：0.1 μmol/L[3-5]）、FPP 加中药组（IC_{50} 的 FPP 加生药人参 8/3mg/mL，生药三七 4/3 mg/mL[1]），

---

* 原载于《中国中西医结合杂志》，2010，30（8）：857-860

以上 3 组仅检测下游蛋白 MAPK 表达。HUVEC 以 1×10^5 个 /mL 密度接种于 75 cm² 培养瓶中，在 37℃，5% CO_2 培养箱培养。接种 24h 后按实验分组加入 SU5416、FPP 和中药，再培养 36h 后分别收集细胞。

1.4.3　Ras、MAPK 蛋白的检测

采用蛋白免疫印迹（Western blot）法。分别收集细胞，加入蛋白提取液并反复吹打，置冰上 15 min，4℃，12 000 r/min 离心 10 min，转移上清至新的 EP 管中。BCA 法测定蛋白浓度。取各蛋白样品 20μL，加入蛋白样品缓冲液变性后将蛋白样品加入 15%（Ras、MAPK）十二烷基磺酸钠（SDS）- 聚丙烯酰胺凝胶中电泳，直至蓝色条带泳出分离胶底部。采用电转移法将蛋白质从 SDS- 聚丙烯酰胺凝胶转移至硝酸纤维素膜，转膜成功后，以 5% 脱脂牛奶 TBS-T 液体封闭硝酸纤维素膜上的非特异蛋白位点，按 1：400 比例加入兔抗人 Ras 多克隆抗体 5μL；1：800 比例加入兔抗人 MAPK 单克隆抗体 5μL，4℃过夜。次日经过洗膜，加入 1：3000 稀释的二抗，再洗膜后，杂交膜显色反应按照 ECL 试剂盒的说明进行，采用数字扫描成像系统分析特异条带的强度。每组实验均重复 3 次。

1.4.4　统计学方法

采用 SPSS 13.0 统计软件，Western blot 数据用 $\bar{x} \pm s$ 表示。进行 One-way ANOVA 分析。

2. 结果

2.1　加入 VEGFR-2 信号转导蛋白抑制剂 SU5416 对下游 Ras 蛋白的影响（图 1，表 1）

各组均有不同程度的 Ras 蛋白表达，SU5416 组 Ras 蛋白表达较空白对照 I 组有明显下降（$P < 0.01$），而 SU5416 加中药组 Ras 蛋白表达较 SU5416 组明显上升（$P < 0.05$）。表明 VEGFR-2 信号转导蛋白抑制剂 SU5416 可以抑制 VEGFR-2 的信号转导，从而下调下游信号蛋白 Ras 的表达；中药可以通过作用于 Ras 蛋白而促进 HUVEC 的增殖。

2.2　加入 VEGFR-2 信号转导蛋白抑制剂 SU5416 对下游 MAPK 蛋白的影响（图 2，表 1）

各组均有不同程度的 MAPK 蛋白表达，SU5416 组 MAPK 蛋白表达较空白对照 I 组明显降低（$P < 0.05$），而 SU5416 加中药组 MAPK 蛋白表达较 SU5416 组明显增加（$P < 0.01$）。表明 VEGFR-2 信号转导蛋白抑制剂 SU5416 可以通

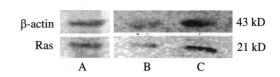

图 1　各组 Ras 蛋白表达条带

注：A：空白对照 I 组；B：SU5416 组；C：SU5416 加中药组

过抑制 VEGFR-2 的信号转导来抑制下游信号蛋白 MAPK 蛋白的表达；中药可以促进 HUVEC MAPK 蛋白的表达。

2.3　加入 Ras 信号转导蛋白抑制剂 FPP 对下游 MAPK 蛋白的影响（图 3，表 1）

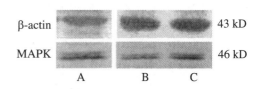

图 2　各组 MAPK 蛋白表达条带

注：A：空白对照 I 组；B：SU5416 组；C：SU5416 加中药组

各组均有不同程度的 MAPK 蛋白表达，空白对照组 II 组的 MAPK 蛋白表达明显高于其他两组，加入 Ras 信号转导蛋白抑制剂 FPP 组，MAPK 蛋白表达较空白对照 II 组明显降低（$P < 0.01$），而 FPP 加中药组下游蛋白 MAPK 蛋白表达较 FPP 组明显增加（$P < 0.05$），说明中药作用于 HUVEC 后促进了 MAPK 蛋白的表达。

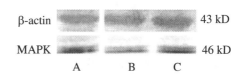

图 3　各组 MAPK 蛋白表达条带

注：A：空白对照 II 组；B：FPP 组；C：FPP 加中药组

表 1　各组蛋白免疫印迹杂交信号强度灰度平均值比较

（$\bar{x} \pm s$）

组别	n	Ras/β-actin	MAPK/β-actin
空白对照 I	3	$0.26 \pm 0.07^{\triangle\triangle}$	$0.40 \pm 0.02^{\triangle}$
SU5416	3	0.13 ± 0.02	0.27 ± 0.04
SU5416 加中药	3	$0.21 \pm 0.05^{\triangle}$	$0.35 \pm 0.02^{\triangle\triangle}$
空白对照 II	3	—	$0.38 \pm 0.11^{**}$
FPP	3	—	0.22 ± 0.02
FPP 加中药	3	—	$0.33 \pm 0.06^{*}$

注：与 FPP 组比较，$^{*}P < 0.05$，$^{**}P < 0.01$；与 SU5416 组比较，$^{\triangle}P < 0.05$，$^{\triangle\triangle}P < 0.01$

3. 讨论

VEGFR-2 是一种受体酪氨酸激酶（receptor protein tyrosine kinase，RPTK），它结合信号分子后，形成二聚体，并发生自磷酸化而活化，活化的 RPTK 激活 Ras，由活化的 Ras 引起蛋白激酶的磷酸化级联反应。Ras 信号途径是一种很常见的细胞分子信号传导途径，也是受体型酪氨酸蛋白激酶（TPK）信号传递中的主要成员。Ras 蛋白是膜结合型蛋白，它活化的第一步就是法尼基化，即法尼基转移酶（FTase）将法尼基焦磷酸中的法尼基基团转移至 Ras 蛋白的 CAAX（C：半胱氨酸；A：脂肪族氨基酸；X：任何氨基酸）的半胱氨酸残基上[6]。FPP 和 Ras 蛋白均为 FTase 的底物，所以 FPP 可以竞争性抑制法尼基转移酶，从而抑制 Ras 信号蛋白的传导[7]。Ras 蛋白与 Raf 的 N 端结构域结合并使其激活，Raf 是丝氨酸/苏氨酸（Ser/Thr）蛋白激酶（又称 MAPKKK），活化的 Raf 结合并磷酸化另一种蛋白激酶 MAPKK，使其活化。MAPKK 又激活有丝分裂原活化蛋白激酶（mito-gen-activated protein kinase，MAPK），MAPK 属丝氨酸/苏氨酸残激酶。活化的 MAPK 进入细胞核，可使许多转录因子活化，促使基因表达的增加，进而促进细胞的增殖和分化。SU5416 是新合成的血管内皮生长因子受体（VEGFR-2/Flk-1/KDR）酪氨酸激酶的抑制剂[5]。实验表明 SU5416 可抑制依赖于血管表皮生长因子刺激的血管内皮细胞增殖[8]，能阻断来自细胞外血管生长刺激信号和已激活信号的转化通路，有效地抑制血管表皮生长因子的活性，从而抑制血管内皮细胞的生长。大量的文献报道主要集中在 SU5416 抑制肿瘤的生长和转移[9-11]。

本实验利用 SU5416 可以阻断 VEGFR-2（KDR）酪氨酸激酶的作用，加入 IC_{50} 的 SU5416，对血管生成信号通路进行阻断。在实验中仅加入 IC_{50} 的 SU5416 主要是防止大剂量的 SU5416 可能过分抑制细胞生长，甚至导致细胞的凋亡或死亡。本实验结果表明，IC_{50} 的 SU5416 部分阻断血管生成通路上的 VEGFR-2 后，下游 Ras 和 MAPK 蛋白的表达较空白组下降，说明 VEGFR-2 在血管生成这个过程中的确影响到信号通路的下游蛋白。

用 IC_{50} 的 SU5416 部分阻断 VEGFR-2 后，下游 Ras 和 MAPK 蛋白表达明显下降，运用益气活血中药人参和三七提取物干预后，两个蛋白表达有明显上升，提示 SU5416 可以阻断血管生成信号通路上的 VEGFR-2，也表明在 IC_{50} 的 SU5416 部分阻断 VEGFR-2 的条件下，中药可以直接作用在 Ras 蛋白这一信号靶点上，并促进信号蛋白 Ras 的表达，但还暂不能肯定中药是否可以直接作用于 MAPK 上，因为上游信号蛋白 Ras 的表达增加或活化，均有可能引发信号的级联反应，促使下游信号蛋白 MAPK 的增加。因此，进行了下一步实验，加入 IC_{50} 的 FPP 部分阻断 Ras 后，同时加入中药进行干预，观察其下游 MAPK 蛋白表达的变化。

用 IC_{50} 的 FPP 部分阻断 Ras 后，下游 MAPK 蛋白表达较空白对照 Ⅱ 组有明显下降，加入益气活血中药人参和三七提取物干预后下游信号蛋白 MAPK 表达有明显上升，提示 FPP 可以阻断血管生成信号通路上的 Ras，而中药可以直接作用在 MAPK 蛋白这一信号靶点上。

综上，本实验表明，益气活血中药人参和三七提取物促进 HUVEC 增殖，最终达到促血管新生作用，主要是影响了 VEGFR-2-Ras-MAPK 这一血管生成信号通路，而中药的有效作用靶点可能正是 VEGFR-2、Ras、MAPK 这三个关键的信号蛋白。这为研究中药复方的作用环节及作用靶标提供了科学依据。

参考文献

[1] 田伟，雷燕，朱凌群，等. 人参、三七组方对 Ras 相关信号蛋白的影响. 中国中西医结合杂志，2009，29（9）：802-805.

[2] Francis JG. Alison TS, Lewis R, et al. SU5416, a small molecule tyrosine kinase receptor inhibitor, has biologic activity in patients with refractory acute myeloid leukemia or myelodysplastic syndromes. Blood, 2003, 102 (3): 795-801.

[3] 屈凌波，郭宗儒. 法尼基转移酶抑制剂的研究进展. 中国药物化学杂志，1998，8（4）：305-310.

[4] Woodward, Julia KL, Coleman, et al. Preclinical evidence for the effect of bisphosphonates and cytotoxic drugs on tumor cell invasion. Anticancer Drugs, 2005, 16 (1): 11-19.

[5] Mendel DB, Laird AD, Smolich BD, et al. Development of SU5146, a selective small molecule inhibitor of VEGF receptor tyrosine kinase activity, as an anti-angiogenesis agent. Anticancer Drug Des, 2000, 15 (1): 29-41.

[6] Lannuzel M, Lamothe M, Schambel P, et al. From pure FPP to mixed FPP and CAAX competitive inhibitors of farnesyl protein transferase. Bioorg Med Chem Lett, 2003, 13 (8): 1459-1462.

[7] 黄文林，朱孝峰. 信号转导. 北京：人民卫生出版社，2005：70-75.

[8] Fong TA, Shawver LK, Sun L, et al. SU5146 is a potent and selective inhibitor of the vascular endothelial growth factor receptor (Flk-1/KDR) that inhibits tyrosine kinase catalysis, tumor vascularization, and growth of multiple tumor types. Cancer Res, 1999, 59 (1): 99-106.

[9] 侍立志，王兆春，陈紫平，等. 血管生成抑制剂 SU5416 对大鼠胰腺癌生长和转移的抑制作用. 中华普通外科杂志，2004，19（7）：404-407.

[10] 张国锋，王元和，王强，等. SU5416 抑制胃癌生长和肝转移的实验研究. 中华消化杂志，2002，22（4）：213-215.

[11] 李万成，刘维佳，李艳萍，等. 血管内皮生长因子受体抑制剂 SU5416 对小鼠肺间质纤维化的影响. 中国呼吸与危重监护杂志，2007，6（1）：55-58.

人参三七川芎提取物延缓衰老小鼠血管老化的实验研究 *

雷　燕　杨　静　赵　浩　杜雪君　刘剑刚　陈可冀

进入 21 世纪，我国老龄化的进程加快，2005 年全国人口调查显示 60 岁以上人口占总人口的 11.03%[1]。老年人群具有心脑血管病发病率高的特点，存在明显血管老化的表现[2]，因此研究随年龄增长出现的血管老化问题成为防治心血管疾病的新靶点。本研究以自然衰老小鼠为模型，观察衰老小鼠血管老化导致的血管壁结构和功能的改变，并探讨益气活血中药人参三七川芎提取物的干预作用。

1. 材料与方法

1.1 动物

美国癌症研究所（Institute of Cancer Researcch，ICR）健康雄性小鼠，14 月龄小鼠 70 只，2 月龄小鼠 14 只，购自北京维通利华公司，许可证号为 SCXK（京）2007-0001。

1.2 药物

人参：Panax ginseng，产自吉林抚松镇；三七：Panax notoginseng（Burk.），产自云南文山；川芎：Ligusticum chuanxiong，产自四川，鉴定均符合《中国药典》[3]2005 年版标准。人参、三七、川芎提取物为醇提物，由中国中医科学院中药研究所提供，含 3.164 g 生药 /g 浸膏；维生素 E 粉购自北京鼎国生物公司。

1.3 试剂盒及仪器

抗超氧阴离子自由基及产生超氧阴离子自由基测试盒（南京建成生物工程研究所，批号 20071218）；血浆血管紧张素 II 放射免疫分析试剂盒（北京科美东雅生物技术有限公司，批号 20080911）；小鼠晚期糖基化终末产物（AGEs）检测试剂盒（31192，WESTINGHOUSEDR-FREMONT，ADLITTERAM DIAGNOSTIC LA-BORATORIES，USA，CA94326，LOT08-06）；小鼠基质金属蛋白酶 -2（MMP-2）ELESA 试剂盒（批号 0809031，货号 F1122，美国 RD 公司）；小鼠 TIMP-2 ELESA 试剂盒（批号 0809033，货号 F1162，美国 RD 公司）。TCS-SP2 激光扫描共聚焦显微镜（Leica，德国）；SIAFRTS Wellscan MK3 型酶标仪（Labsystems Dragon，芬兰）；Wellwash 4 MK2 型洗板机（Labsystems Dragon，芬兰）；T-18 basic 型匀浆机（IKA，德国）；DpxView Pro 型彩色图像处理系统（DeltaPix，丹麦）。

1.4 动物分组及模型制备

14 月龄小鼠采用随机数字表法分为 5 组：衰老模型（模型）组、人参三七川芎（中药）高、中、低剂量组以及维生素 E 组，另设 2 月龄小鼠

---

* 原载于《中国中西医结合杂志》，2010，30（9）：946-951

349

作为青年对照组（对照组），每组 14 只。按照小鼠和人体的体重剂量折算系数关系[4]，中药大、中、小剂量相当于临床用量的 2 倍、1.5 倍、1 倍，分别为 1.42、1.07、0.71 和 0.05 g/（kg·d）。各给药组按上述药物及剂量灌胃给药，每天 1 次，模型组、对照组给予双蒸水灌胃，喂养 3 个月。实验前及实验开始后每月重复测量小鼠体重，并观察小鼠的一般状况。

1.5 观察指标及方法

1.5.1 动物取材 给药 3 个月后，各组小鼠眼球取血，以 EDTA 抗凝，于离心机 3500 r/min，离心 20 min，取上清，置于 −20℃ 保存；小鼠脱颈处死后，开胸，分离心脏及胸主动脉，处理如下：（1）沿主动脉弓下 3 mm 左右剪断血管，取连接心脏的主动脉弓部分血管，以滤纸吸干血液，浸于 10% 中性甲醛固定液以制备石蜡切片；（2）分离腹主动脉部分的血管，从髂动脉分支处剪断，以生理盐水冲洗，滤纸吸干，微量天平称重。以 4℃ 生理盐水制成 10% 的组织匀浆，2000 r/min 离心 15 min，取上清，置于 −80℃ 冰箱备用。

1.5.2 主动脉形态学观察及平滑肌细胞（smooth muscle cells，SMC）、胶原纤维（collagen fibers，CF）相对含量 胸主动脉段固定过夜，常规脱水、透明、浸蜡、包埋，制备石蜡切片，切片厚度 5μm。（1）HE 染色：切片常规脱蜡水化，Harris 苏木素液染色，1% 盐酸乙醇分化，返蓝，乙醇伊红染色，脱水，透明，中性树胶封片，显微镜下观察血管的一般形态。（2）Masson 染色：切片脱蜡水化，地衣红染色，Weigert 铁苏木精染核，磷钼酸水溶液分化，亮绿染色后，脱水，透明，树胶封固。显微镜下观察，胶原纤维染为绿色，肌纤维为红色，胞核为蓝黑色。图像处理系统分别测量血管壁中膜 SMC、CF 的绝对面积，计算不同着色面积与测试区域整体面积之比，计算 SMC、CF 在各血管壁中的相对含量（Aa%）。

1.5.3 血管组织抗超氧阴离子含量测定 检测各组小鼠腹主动脉中抗超氧阴离子自由基活力的含量，反映活性氧水平，取 10% 血管组织匀浆后的上清，依据试剂盒说明操作。

1.5.4 血浆血管紧张素Ⅱ（AngⅡ）含量测定 按照试剂盒说明书放免法检测 AngⅡ。

1.5.5 血管组织晚期糖基化终末产物（advanced glycation end products，AGES）含量测定 采用 ELESA 法，取 10% 组织匀浆后的上清，按照试剂

盒说明进行操作，于酶标仪 450nm 波长处测定各孔的 OD 值。

1.5.6 基质金属蛋白酶（MMP-2）及其抑制剂（TIMPS）比值测定 采用 ELESA 法，取 10% 血管组织匀浆后的上清，按照试剂盒说明进行操作。在酶标仪 450 nm 处测吸光值。

1.6 统计学方法

采用 SPSS 13.0 软件进行统计处理，观察指标以 $\bar{\chi} \pm s$ 表示，各组间计量资料比较采用单因素方差分析。

2. 结果

2.1 各组小鼠一般情况

各组小鼠体质量正常，青年组小鼠体毛白且光泽，行动活泼，反应灵敏；其余各组小鼠被毛较青年组颜色稍暗，动作稍迟缓，尤其模型组小鼠，体毛蓬松，没有光泽，运动减少，动作相对较迟缓。

2.2 各组小鼠主动脉形态学观察结果

2.2.1 各组小鼠主动脉 HE 染色结果比较（图 1）

对照组：内膜较薄，结构完整，中膜 SMC 排列规则，内皮下无脂质沉积；模型组：主动脉内膜增厚、隆起，内皮细胞部分脱落，内皮下间隙增宽，内膜下水肿，有泡沫细胞浸润，SMC 穿过内弹力膜迁移入内皮下，中膜明显增厚，SMC 增生并排列紊乱而垂直于内膜生长，细胞形态改变，细胞增大似成纤维细胞；中药高、中、低剂量组：内膜较薄，部分见隆起，内皮细胞基本完好，未见明显脱落，内皮下间隙未见明显增宽，部分平滑肌细胞迁移至其中，中膜无明显增厚，平滑肌细胞增生不明显，细胞数目接近正常，排列较规则，部分细胞形态改变似成纤维细胞；维生素 E 组：内膜较薄，内皮细胞基本完好，中膜无明显增厚，SMC 增生不明显，细胞数目接近正常，排列较规则。

2.2.2 各组小鼠主动脉 Masson 染色图像分析（表 1，图 2） Masson 染色后平滑肌细胞呈红色，胶原纤维呈绿色。从结果可见，模型组绿色染色区域明显多于对照组与各用药组；与模型组比较，各用药组胶原绿染区域减少。各组 Masson 染色的图像分析得出，模型组小鼠 SMC、CF 相对含量显著升高，与对照组比较差异有统计学意义（$P < 0.05$）。与模型组比较，各给药组 CF 相对含量降低（$P < 0.05$），中药高剂量组和维生

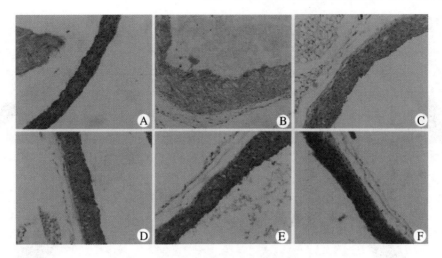

图 1　各组主动脉 HE 染色结果比较（×100）

注：A 为青年对照组；B 为老年衰老模型组；C 为中药高剂量组；D 为中药中剂量组；E 为中药低剂量组；F 为维生素 E 组，下图同

素 E 组 SMC 相对含量降低（$P < 0.05$），中药中、低剂量组 SMC 含量无明显改变，中药各剂量组间 SMC 含量比较差异无统计学意义；中药高剂量组 CF 含量与中、低剂量组比较显著降低（$P < 0.05$），与维生素 E 组比较，差异无统计学意义。

表 1　各组小鼠主动脉 SMC、CF 相对含量比较（Aa%，$\bar{\chi} \pm s$）

组别	n	SMC	CF
对照	14	24.3±0.28	21.6±0.40
模型	14	31.9±0.86*	29.9±0.80*
中药高剂量	14	29.7±1.48△	24.6±0.38△
中剂量	14	30.5±1.46	25.6±0.47△▲
低剂量	14	30.7±2.42	26.1±0.53△▲
维生素 E	14	28.8±1.14△	24.5±0.43△

注：与对照组比较，*$P < 0.05$；与模型组比较，△$P < 0.05$；与中药高剂量组比较，▲$P < 0.05$

2.3　各组抗超氧阴离子、Ang Ⅱ含量比较（表 2）

与对照组比较，模型组血管组织抗超氧阴离子、血浆 Ang Ⅱ含量降低，差异有统计学意义（$P < 0.05$）。与模型组比较，各给药组血管组织抗超氧阴离子含量增高，差异有统计学意义（$P < 0.05$），而血浆 Ang Ⅱ含量差异无统计学意义（$P > 0.05$）。中药高、中、低剂量组血浆 Ang Ⅱ含量两两比较无明显差异；中药高剂量

组抗超氧阴离子含量较中、低剂量组明显增高（$P < 0.05$），与维生素 E 组比较差异无统计学意义。

表 2　各组血浆 Ang Ⅱ含量、血管组织抗超氧阴离子含量的比较（$\bar{\chi} \pm s$）

组别	n	血浆 Ang Ⅱ含量（ng/L）	血管组织抗超氧阴离子（U/L）
对照	14	236.45±31.12	97.06±3.81
模型	14	166.58±28.94*	59.34±4.56*
中药高剂量	14	207.98±44.05	80.61±2.90△
中剂量	14	176.40±45.49	69.16±3.41△▲
低剂量	14	168.61±44.44	65.89±4.03△▲
维生素 E	14	186.84±52.76	81.52±4.31△

注：与对照组比较，*$P < 0.05$；与模型组比较，△$P < 0.05$；与中药高剂量组比较，▲$P < 0.05$

2.4　各组 AGEs、MMP-2、TIMP-2 含量及 MMP-2/TIMP-2 比较（表 3）

与对照组比较，模型组 AGEs、MMP-2 含量及 MMP-2/TIMP-2 增高，TIMP-2 含量降低，差异均有统计学意义（$P < 0.05$）。与模型组比较，各给药组 AGEs、MMP-2 含量及 MMP-2/TIMP-2 降低，TIMP-2 含量增高，差异均有统计学意义（$P < 0.05$）。中药各剂量组 AGEs 含量比较差异均有统计学意义（$P < 0.05$）；中

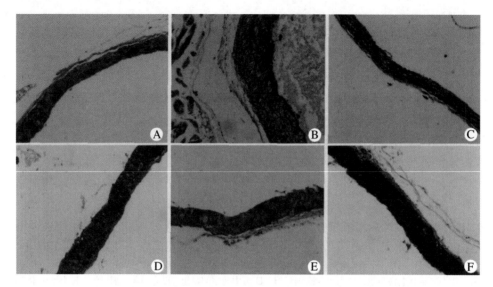

图 2　各组小鼠主动脉 Masson 染色结果比较（×100）

表 3　各组 AGEs、MMP-2、TIMP-2 含量及 MMP-2/TIMP-2 比较（$\bar{\chi} \pm s$）

组别	n	AGEs（ng/mL）	MMP-2（ng/mL）	TIMP-2（ng/mL）	MMP-2/TIMP-2
对照	14	59.55±1.85	180.93±10.46	0.64±0.08	286.50±28.24
模型	14	215.89±1.17*	246.48±5.35*	0.31±0.01*	794.53±25.12*
中药高剂量	14	142.57±1.28△	205.51±10.36△	0.50±0.03△	413.14±30.21△
中剂量	14	152.14±1.52△▲	222.30±6.93△▲	0.39±0.01△▲	565.28±20.41△▲
低剂量	14	170.54±1.66△▲○	224.79±9.54△▲○	0.36±0.01△▲○	628.58±28.17△▲○
维生素 E	14	141.29±1.59△○●	205.19±4.14△○●	0.51±0.01△○●	401.95±9.58△○●

注：与对照组比较，*$P < 0.05$；与模型组比较，△$P < 0.05$；与中药高剂量组比较，▲$P < 0.05$；与中药中剂量组比较，○$P < 0.05$；与中药低剂量组比较，●$P < 0.05$

药高剂量组 MMP-2 含量较中、低剂量组明显降低（$P < 0.05$），与维生素 E 组比较差异无统计学意义；中药各剂量组 TIMP-2 含量、MMP-2/TIMP-2 比较差异均有统计学意（$P < 0.05$），与维生素 E 组比较差异有统计学意义（$P < 0.05$）。

3. 讨论

人参、三七是常见的具有抗衰老作用的天然药物，均富含三萜类达玛烷型皂苷，国内外抗衰老药理学研究均证实此类有效成分与抗衰老作用密切相关[5,6]；川芎主要成分为川芎嗪和阿魏酸，有抗氧化和清除自由基、保护心血管系统的作用[7]。本研究分别从组织病理、生化等多个方面检测血管组织中可直接或间接反映血管老化状况的指标，从而探讨人参三七川芎提取物延缓小鼠血管老化的作用。

随年龄的增长，血管在形态和功能上发生各种衰老变化，结果富有弹性的动脉壁伸展性降低，僵硬血管的组织出现内皮细胞排列紊乱，CF 增生、弹力纤维断裂、SMC、巨噬细胞等浸润，基质金属蛋白酶、转移生长因子 -β 及细胞因子增加，动脉供血功能减退，机体脏器功能逐渐降低，衰老过程开始，这提示血管衰老是人体衰老的关键始发因素。本实验观察了小鼠主动脉形态学的变化，HE 染色发现衰老模型组小鼠血管壁出现典型的衰老表现，而给予中药后的小鼠血管内膜中膜增厚不明显，内皮细胞脱落减少，仅有部分平滑肌细胞向内膜迁移，衰老改变不显著；Masson 染色显示，模型组小鼠血管壁 SMC 和 CF 含量明显增多，给予中药后 CF 增生明显减少，高剂量组可使 SMC 增生明显减少，从血管形态学方面说明给予人参三七川芎提取物后小鼠血管衰老相对减缓。

活性氧学说是血管老化研究中较公认的学说。活性氧水平过高造成的损伤，形成一系列终末产物，如高级蛋白氧化产物、AGEs、高级脂质过氧化终产物等，这些物质引起相关生物学效应，最终可能引起细胞功能失调和衰老[8,9]。研究证实人内乳动脉和冠状动脉活性氧产量很低，但同衰老密切相关[10,11]，因而 ROS 在介导血管衰老中有重要的地位。本实验小鼠给予一定时间中药灌胃后，血管组织抗活性氧生成能力比模型组有一定程度的增强，说明人参三七川芎提取物可能通过减少活性氧的生成来延缓血管老化。

肾素 - 血管紧张素系统（renin–angiotensin system，RAS）与血管老化关系密切，可激活调节许多与细胞生长（凋亡）、纤维化及炎症有关的物质表达，调节血管细胞的凋亡、平滑肌细胞迁移、细胞外基质重建等与血管病理生理有关的过程[12,13]。局部高活性状态的 RAS 通过自分泌、旁分泌、内分泌作用，在高血压、动脉粥样硬化等心血管疾病的发生、发展中起重要作用[14]，而 Ang Ⅱ 作为 RAS 的功能多肽则是这些病理生理改变的中心环节。本研究显示青年组血浆 Ang Ⅱ 含量最高，模型组最低，给予中药后 Ang Ⅱ 含量有所升高但无明显差别。很多研究表明高活性的 Ang Ⅱ 与血管老化密切相关，但本实验模型组 Ang Ⅱ 含量最低，对照组最高，提示血浆中 Ang Ⅱ 含量与血管老化的关系不是很密切。由于局部血管组织的 Ang Ⅱ 与血管重构关系密切[15]，故应进一步检测血管组织中 Ang Ⅱ 的含量，来确定其与血管老化的关系。

AGEs 随增龄在体内逐渐积累，是临床上老年性疾病的病理基础之一[16]。动脉 MMP-2 活性显著增加可能参与与年龄相关的血管重构的发生[17]，TIMP-2 能抑制 MMP-2 的活性，MMP 活性或 MMP/TIMP 比值的调节可以预防和控制血管重构等的发生发展[18]。从结果看出，青年小鼠血管组织中 AGEs 含量相对较少，而老年各组的小鼠 AGEs 含量较多，但给予一段时间人参三七川芎提取物灌胃后，老年小鼠 AGEs 含量有一定程度的降低，这说明中药在一定程度上可能通过减少 AGEs 的形成来降低动脉僵硬程度。模型组小鼠血管组织内 MMP-2 、MMP-2/ TIMP-2 最高，TIMP-2 含量最低，由于 MMP-2 、MMP-2/ TIMP-2 的升高与年龄相关的血管重构关系密切，

表明在衰老小鼠血管组织中已出现年龄相关的血管重构，给予中药灌胃后的各组小鼠 MMP-2、MMP-2/ TIMP-2 指标明显降低、TIMP-2 升高，这表示应用人参三七川芎提取物后可能通过抑制 MMP-2 生成、增强 TIMP-2 活性，减少了细胞外基质的降解，从而达到延缓血管老化的目的。

综上所述，衰老小鼠的血管在结构和功能上都出现了明显的衰老改变，应用人参三七川芎提取物干预后，能够改善衰老小鼠主动脉形态学衰老变化，可能通过降低血管组织中活性氧的生成，减少 AGEs 生成，抑制 MMP-2 的活性，调节 MMP-2/ TIMP-2 的平衡，达到降低衰老小鼠血管僵硬度、减少血管重构的目的，从而延缓了小鼠血管老化的发生。

参考文献

[1] 中华人民共和国国家统计局 . 2005 年全国 1% 人口抽样调查主要数据公报 . 全国人口普查公报，2006，3，16.

[2] 杨静，雷燕 . 细胞衰老与血管老化的关系及其研究进展 . 中国中西医结合杂志，2009，(4)：369-374.

[3] 国家药典委员会 . 中国药典，Ⅰ 部 . 北京：化学工业出版社，2005.

[4] 黄继汉，黄晓辉，陈志扬，等 . 药理试验中动物间和动物与人体间的等效剂量换算 . 中国临床药理学与治疗学，2004，9（9）：1069-1072.

[5] 张嘉麟，徐文安，杨荫康，等 . 三七中人参皂甙对老年鼠血浆脂质及其代谢产物含量的影响 . 昆明医学院学报，2001，22（1）：45-46.

[6] 周晓慧，周晓霞，杨鹤梅 . 三七总皂甙防治动脉粥样硬化的研究进展 . 承德医学院学报，2003，4（20）：350-352.

[7] 周江 . 川芎有效成分及其药理作用研究概况 . 浙江中医杂志，2007，42（10）：615-616.

[8] Droge W. Oxidative stress and aging. Adv Exp Med Biol, 2003, 543 (1): 191-200.

[9] Zhang C, Yang J, Jennings LK. Leukocyte-derived myeloper-oxidase amplifies high-goucose-induced endothelial dysfunction through interaction with high-glucose-stimulated, vascular non-leukocyte-derived reactive oxygen species. Diabetes, 2004, 53 (7): 2950-2959.

[10] Berry C, Hamilton CA, Brosnan MJ, et al. Investigation into the sources of superoxide in human blood vessels: angiotensin Ⅱ increases superoxide production in human internal mammary arteries. Circulation, 2000, 101 (18): 2206-2212.

[11] Csiszar A, Ungvari Z, Edwards JG, et al. Aging-induced phenotypic changes and oxidative stress impair coronary arteriolar function. Circ Res, 2002, 90 (2): 1159-1166.

[12] Ruiz-Ortega, M, Lorenzo O, Ruperez M, et al. Role of renin-angiotensin system in vascular disease. Hypertension, 2001, 38 (6): 1382-1387.

[13] Sotensinadoshima J. Cytokine actions of angiotensin II. Circ Res, 2000, 86 (11): 1187-1189.

[14] 王宏宇. 血管病学. 北京：人民军医出版社，2006：213.

[15] 马宏，张宗玉，童坦君. 衰老的生物学标志. 生理科学进展，2002，33（1）：65-68.

[16] 王宏宇，胡大一. 动脉僵硬的机制、病理生理学及治疗策略（上）. 中国医刊，2006，41（9）：61-62.

[17] Wang MY, Iakatta EG. Altered regulation of matrix metalloproteinase-2 in aortic remodeling during aging. Hypertension, 2002, 39 (4): 865-874.

[18] Galis ZS, Khatri JJ. Matrix metalloproteinases in vascular remodeling and atherogenesis: the good, the bad, and the ugly. Circ Res, 2002, 90 (3): 251-263.

人参、三七提取物对 Ras 相关信号蛋白的影响 *

田　伟　雷　燕　朱凌群　陈可冀

细胞信号通路是细胞应答内外环境信息，经信号网络整合作用调节基因表达及细胞的增殖、分化、发育的途径。细胞的增殖、分化主要与有丝分裂原活化蛋白激酶（mitogen-activated protein kinase，MAPK）途径有关。Ras 是调节细胞生长的重要转导蛋白，通过 Ras-Raf-MAPK 最后产生级联反应。治疗性血管生成是指通过促血管再生因子使缺血部分的侧支循环增加来改善功能，已经成为治疗缺血性疾病的新疗法，近年来研究显示益气活血中药在促血管新生领域前景广阔[1,2]。本研究拟观察人参、三七提取物对血管内皮细胞血管生成信号蛋白的作用，以阐明益气活血中药人参、三七提取物促血管生成信号转导途径。

1. 材料与方法

1.1 仪器

Wellscan MK3 型全自动酶标仪，芬兰 Labsystems Dragon 公司生产；3K30 型高速冷冻离心机，德国 Sigma 公司生产；BIORAD IQ5 型荧光定量 PCR 仪，美国 BIORAD 生产。

1.2 试剂与药物

人脐静脉内皮细胞二代（HU-VEC-2C，箱号：C-023-5C，批号：4C0218），购自 Cascade Biologics 公司。人参（批号：0609089）和三七颗粒剂（批号：0612051）购自广东一方制药有限公司。碱性成纤维生长因子（basic fibrin growth factor，bFGF）购自珠海亿胜生物制药有限公司，产品批号：20070301。

1.3 中药制备

人参水溶后按吸附树脂层析法提取得，三七采用水煎提取和阳离子树脂吸附法分离获得。按 2:1（人参：三七）配比，用时用完全培养基（M200+LSGS）配成所需浓度，经 0.22μm 微孔滤膜过滤除菌，分装，4℃ 保存。

1.4 实验分组

实验用细胞分为 5 组：空白对照组，以完全培养基 M200+LSGS 作为对照；bFGF 组（320U/mL）；中药小剂量组（1mg/mL，含生药人参 0.667mg/mL，生药三七 0.333mg/mL）；中药中剂量组 2mg/mL（小剂量组的 2 倍）；中药大剂量组 4mg/mL（小剂量组的 4 倍）。

1.5 VEGFR-2、Ras 及 MAPK 蛋白的检测

采用 Western Blot 法。分别收集细胞，加入蛋白提取液并反复吹打，置冰上 15min，4℃ 12000r/min 离心 10min，转移上清至新的 EP 管中。BCA 法测定蛋白浓度。取各蛋白样品 20μL，

---

* 原载于《中国中西医结合杂志》，2009，29（9）：802-805

加入蛋白样品缓冲液变性后将蛋白样品加入 7.5%（VEGFR-2）和 15%（Ras、MAPK）十二烷基磺酸钠（SDS）- 聚丙烯酰胺凝胶中电泳，直至蓝色条带泳出分离胶底部。采用电转移法将蛋白质从 SDS- 聚丙烯酰胺凝胶转移至硝酸纤维素膜，转膜成功后，以 5% 脱脂牛奶 TBS-T 液体封闭硝酸纤维素膜上的非特异蛋白位点，按 1：200 比例加入兔抗人 VEG-FR-2 单克隆抗体 20μL；1：400 比例加入兔抗人 Ras 多克隆抗体 5μL；1：800 比例加入兔抗人 MAPK 单克隆抗体 5μL，4℃过夜。次日经过洗膜，加入 1：3000 稀释的二抗，再洗膜后，杂交膜显色反应按照 ECL 试剂盒的说明进行，采用数字扫描成像系统分析特异条带的强度。每组实验均重复 3 次。

1.6　统计学方法

Western Blot 数据的统计方法采用 SPSS 13.0 统计软件，数据用 $\bar{\chi} \pm s$ 表示，进行 One-way ANOVA 分析。

2.　结果

2.1　各组 HUVEC VEGFR-2 蛋白表达比较（图 1，表 1）

各组均有不同程度的 VEGFR-2 蛋白表达，其中中药大剂量组及阳性药对照组（bFGF）VEGFR-2 蛋白表达明显增加，与空白组比较差异有统计学意义（$P < 0.05$），而中药中、小剂量组表达较弱。说明中药大剂量组作用于 HUVEC 后促进了 VEGFR-2 蛋白的表达。

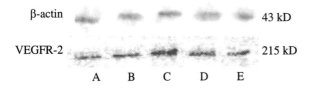

图 1　各组 HUVEC VEGFR-2 蛋白表达比较

注：A 为空白组；B 为 bFGF 组；C 为中药大剂量组；D 为中药中剂量组；E 为中药小剂量组

2.2　各组 HUVEC Ras 蛋白表达比较（图 2，表 1）

各组均有不同程度的 Ras 蛋白表达，其中中药大、小剂量组与 bFGF 组表达最为明显，与空白组比较差异有统计学意义（$P < 0.05$，$P < 0.01$），而中药中剂量组表达较弱。表明中药大、小剂量组均可促进 HUVEC 中 Ras 蛋白的表达。

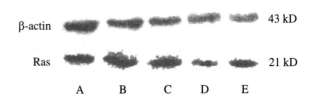

图 2　各组 HUVEC Ras 蛋白表达比较

注：A 为空白组；B 为 bFGF 组；C 为中药大剂量组；D 为中药中剂量组；E 为中药小剂量组

2.3　各组 HUVEC MAPK 蛋白表达比较（图 3，表 1）

各组均有不同程度的 MAPK 蛋白表达，其中 bFGF 组与中药小剂量组 MAPK 蛋白表达明显，与空白组比较差异有统计学意义（$P < 0.05$，$P < 0.01$），而中药大、中剂量组表达较弱。说明中药小剂量组作用于 HUVEC 后促进了 MAPK 蛋白的表达。

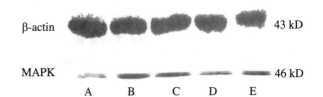

图 3　各组 MAPK 蛋白表达比较

注：A 为空白组；B 为 bFGF 组；C 为中药大剂量组；D 为中药中剂量组；E 为中药小剂量组

表 1　各组蛋白免疫印迹杂交信号强度灰度平均值比较（$n=3$，$\bar{\chi} \pm s$）

组别	VEG FR-2/β-actin	Ras/β-actin	MAPK/β-actin
空白	1.58±0.10	0.28±0.00	0.38±0.11
bFGF	2.11±0.21*	0.42±0.02*	0.58±0.21**
中药大剂量	2.07±0.19*	0.53±0.24**	0.45±0.30
中药中剂量	1.48±0.17	0.34±0.03	0.38±0.22
中药小剂量	1.39±0.26	0.49±0.03**	0.48±0.14*

注：与空白组比较，*$P < 0.05$，**$P < 0.01$

3.　讨论

血管新生是指在原有的血管基础上又产生新的血管。血管新生是一个复杂的过程，新血管形成和调控过程包括内皮细胞的增生和迁移、蛋白溶解酶表达调控、细胞外基质破裂重建和内皮管腔形成的形态发育过程。本实验以人脐静脉内皮细胞为载体，研究中药对血管生成中关键蛋白的作用。

血管内皮生长因子（vascular endothelium growth factor，VEGF）是一类多功能生长因子，由多种细胞分泌，并通过旁分泌机制作用于受体而发挥作用[3]。VEGF 与细胞表面的受体（vascular endothelial growth factor receptor，VEGFR）结合，通过激活酪氨酸激酶信号转导途径发挥功能，其最明显的生物学效应是促使内皮细胞有丝分裂，诱导血管内皮细胞增殖和迁徙。VEGF 的生物学活性主要是通过两个酪氨酸受体所介导的[4-6]，即 VEGFR-1（fms-like tyrosine kinase，Flt-1）及 VEGFR-2（kinase insert domain-containing receptor/fetal liver kinase，KDR/Flk-1）。VEGFR-1 表达主要与鼠胚胎时期血管形成和伤口愈合有关，较少涉及内皮细胞增殖。VEGFR-2 是 VEGF 的主要功能受体，主要分布于内皮细胞表面，VEGF 对内皮细胞的促存活、增殖、分化等作用都是由 VEGFR-2 介导的。Brekken 等[7] 发现 VEGR-2 在 VEGF 所诱导的血管生成和血管通透性中起主要作用。单独使用 KDR 的抑制剂，就能阻断 VEGF 和 bFGF 所诱导的血管生成。

VEGF 刺激内皮细胞 DNA 合成的作用，主要是通过 VEGFR-2 有效激活细胞外信号调节激酶（external-signal regulated kinase，ERK）。ERK 的激活必须依赖 Ras 的激活，其通路可能是 VEGF 通过多种途径（包括 PKC）激活 Ras。Novo 等[8] 研究指出，Ras 能被 VEGF 激活，且是 HUVEC 迁移、增殖及血管形成所必需的。ras 基因可通过直接控制 VEGF 基因的转录，强效刺激血管内皮生长因子的表达[9]。Ras 蛋白为膜结合型的二磷酸鸟苷（GDP）/三磷酸鸟苷（GTP）结合蛋白，定位于细胞膜内侧。Ras 蛋白与 GDP 结合的为失活型，与 GTP 结合的是激活型，在上述两种不同构象之间来回转换，所以 Ras 的功能可视为分子开关。在酪氨酸激酶相关受体的信号转导过程中，生长因子结合蛋白通过 Src 同源区 2 结构域（Src-homology domain 2，SH2）与上游蛋白的磷酸化酪氨酸残基特异性结合，并通过 Src 同源区 3 结构域（Src-homology domain 3，SH3）与鸟苷酸交换因子（G-nucleotide exchange factor，GEF）蛋白 Sos 形成复合物，Sos 蛋白是 Ras 的鸟苷酸解离刺激因子（guaine nucleotide dissociation stimulator，GDS），此复合物可使 GDP-Ras 转化为激活型的 GTP-Ras[10]。

当 Ras 活化后，可使 MAPKK 的丝氨酸/苏氨酸残基磷酸化，从而活化了 MAPKK。MAPKs（MAPK 家族）是一组 Ser/Thr 蛋白激酶，大多数蛋白激酶处于非激活状态，当特定的上游激酶信号诱导其活性时被激活。MAPK 则与之不同，需要对其临近的苏氨酸和酪氨酸残基双位点磷酸化才能使酶具有活性，其磷酸化是由 MAPKK（MAP 激酶的激酶，MEK/MKK）双位点特异性蛋白激酶来完成的[11]。这种双特异性的磷酸化就保证了 MAPK 不被其他蛋白激酶磷酸化，一直保持钝化状态，直至 MAPKK 活化后才能使 MAPK 活化，所以 MAPKK 唯一的底物就是 MAPK。MAPKs 包括胞外信号调节激酶（extracellular signal-regulated kinase，ERK）、Jun 氨基末端激酶（Jun N-terminal kinase，JNK）和 p38，这 3 种激酶能活化 3 条信号传导路径，都参与各种细胞外刺激的信号传导[12]。

本实验通过益气活血中药干预，观察其对血管生成信号通路中信号蛋白 VEGFR-2、Ras 及 MAPK 表达的影响。细胞生长因子首先要与受体结合才能产生生物学效应，所以检测细胞中的 VEGFR-2 的含量变化。结果表明，中药大剂量组 VEGFR-2 蛋白表达明显增加，与空白组比较，差异有统计学意义，说明中药大剂量促进了 VEGFR-2 蛋白的表达。信号由胞外传至胞内，另一个关键的信号蛋白 Ras 起着中继的作用。Western Blot 结果表明，中药大、小剂量组的 Ras 蛋白表达量较空白组明显增高，说明中药的确作用在信号通路的 Ras 蛋白上，促进 Ras 蛋白的表达。这可能与中药干预后，激活胞膜上的 VEGFR-2，受体上磷酸化的酪氨酸又与位于胞膜上的生长因子受体结合蛋白 2（growth factor receptor-bound protein 2，Grb2）的 SH2 结构域相结合，而 Grb2 的 SH3 结构域则同时与鸟苷酸交换因子 Sos 结合，后者使小分子鸟苷酸结合蛋白 Ras 的 GDP 解离而结合 GTP，使 GDP-Ras 转化为激活型的 GTP-Ras，从而产生促进细胞增殖的生物学效应。从下游信号蛋白 MAPK 的表达中，bFGF 及中药小剂量均促进 MAPK 的表达，与空白组比较，差异有统计学意义。不难看出，益气活血中药对上游 Ras 蛋白和下游信号 MAPK 蛋白的表达均有上调作用。

因此推论，益气活血中药人参、三七提取物

可促进血管生成，其机制可能是通过促进血管生成信号通路上关键的信号蛋白 VEGFR-2、Ras 及 MAPK 的表达来影响细胞的增殖和分化。

参考文献

[1] 雷燕，王军辉，陈可冀．黄芪、当归配伍后促鸡胚绒毛尿囊膜血管生成的药效比较研究．中国中药杂志，2003，28（9）：876-878.

[2] 雷燕，王培利，林燕林，等．当归补血汤煎剂对实验性心肌梗死衰老大鼠缺血心肌的促血管生成作用．中国中医基础医学杂志，2005，11（12）：892-894.

[3] Ferrara N, Gerber HP, LeCouter J. The biology of VEGF and its receptors. Nat Med, 2003, 9 (6): 669-676.

[4] Valdés G, Erices R, Chacón C, et al. Angiogenic, hyperpermeability and vasodilator network in uteroplacental units along pregnancy in the Guinea-pig (Cavia porcellus). Reprod Biol Endocrinol, 2008, 27 (6): 13.

[5] La DS, Belzile J, Bready JV, et al. Novel 2, 3-di-hydro-1, 4-benzoxazines as potent and orally bioavailable inhibitors of tumor-driven angiogenesis. J Med Chem, 2008, 51 (6):1695-1705.

[6] Weiss MM, Harmange JC, Polverino AJ, et al. Evaluation of aseries of naphthamides as potent, orally active vascular endothelial growth factor receptor-2 tyrosine kinase inhibitors. J Med Chem, 2008, 51 (6): 1668-1680.

[7] Hata Y, Miura M, Nakao S, et al. Antiangiogenic properties of fasudil, a potent Rho-kinase inhibitor. Jpn J Ophthamlol, 2008, 52 (1): 16-23.

[8] Novo E, Cannito S, Zamara E, et al. Proangiogenic cytokines as hypoxia-dependent factors stimulating migration of human hepatic stellate cells. Am J Pathol, 2007, 170 (6): 1942-1953.

[9] 鲁敏，陈建斌．丝裂原活化蛋白激酶信号通路与白血病的关系．医学综述，2005，11（3）：214-216.

[10] Bhattacharya R, Kwon J, Wang E, et al. Srchomology 2 (SH2) domain containing protein tyrosine phosphatase-1 (SHP-1) dephosphorylatesVEGF receptor-2 and attenuates endothelial DNA synthesis, but not migration. J Mol Signal, 2008, 31 (3): 8.

[11] Yang YH, Wang Y, Lam KS. Suppression of the Raf/MEK/ERK signaling cascade and inhibition of angiogenesis by the carboxyl terminus of angiopoietinlike protein 4. Arterioscler Thromb Vasc Biol, 2008, 28 (5): 835-840.

[12] 许宝青，李继喜，龚兴国．促分裂原活化蛋白激酶磷酸酶．细胞生物学杂志，2005，27（4）：387-390.

Effects of Active Components of Red Paeonia and Rhizoma Chuanxiong on Angiogenesis in Atherosclerosis Plaque in Rabbits*

ZHANG Lu　JIANG Yue-rong　GUO Chun-yu
WU Cai-feng　CHEN Ke-ji　YIN Hui-ju

The rupture of atherosclerosis (AS) unstable plaque is one of the chief causes that induce acute stroke events，and to study and intervene in the pathogenetic mechanism of AS is a meaningful work in clinical practice. Research showed that the pathological newly generated vessels frequently found in AS plaque might advance the development of AS lesion, even induce the occurrence of hemorrhage in plaque and the rupture of plaque, as well as the happening of complications[1]. The effect of Chinese drugs for activating blood circulation and removing stasis (ABCRS) in preventing and treating coronary heart disease has been confirmed, moreover, they

* 原载于 Chinese Journal of Integrative Medicine，2009，15（5）：359-364

also showed definite intervening action on AS. Xiongshao Capsule (芎芍胶囊 , XSC), a Chinese herbal preparation formulated from the classic recipe for ABCRS, Xuefu Zhuyu Decoction (血府逐瘀汤), through extensive simplifying and refining, contains active components from Red Paeonia and Rhizoma chuanxiong, namely total paeony glycoside and Chuanxiongols. The two components have been proved by experimental studies to have AS plaque stabilizing effect [2], but whether they have an influence on angiogenesis in AS plaque or not is still needed to be explored. This study is designed for exploring the acting mechanism of these active components from the view point of angiogenesis in plaque by means of using AS model induced by high fat diet and balloon angioplasty and observing their effects on expressions of vascular endothelial growth factor (VEGF) and factor Ⅷ related antigen (F Ⅷ RAg) in the AS plaque.

1. Methods

1.1 Animals

Healthy male New Zealand rabbits, weighing 1.8 to 2.2 kg, were provided by Beijing Vital River Laboratories Animal Techonlogy Co., Ltd., certification number SCXK (Jing) 2005-0002. High fat diet, i.e. basal forage, containing 2% cholesterol and 5% lard, was produced by the Experimental Animal Center of Military Medical Academy.

1.2 Drugs

Simvastatin, product of Hangzhou Moshadong Pharmaceutical Co., Ltd., China, trade name: Shujiangzhi, batch number: 07432, 40 mg/tablet. XSC, 0.25 g/capsule, provided by Dalian Institute of Physical Chemistry, Chinese Acacemy of Sciences, each capsule containing paeoniflorins $\geqslant$ 28 mg, chuanxiongols $\geqslant$ 34 mg and ferulic acid $\geqslant$ 3.5 mg.

1.3 Modeling and Grouping

Fifty New Zealand rabbits were randomized into 5 groups, the normal group, the model group, and the three medicated groups treated respectively with Simvastatin, low-dose and high-dose XSC, 10 in each group. Rabbits in the normal group were fed with regular diet 100 g per day and un-treated all through the experiment.

As to rabbits in the other 4 groups, after animals were fed with high fat diet 100 g/d for two weeks, they were established into AS model by abdominal aortic balloon angioplasty, which was done, in reference to literature[3], in the following procedures: under anesthesia with 3% sodium pentobarbital 1 mL/kg via auricular marginal vein, the femoral artery was bluntly isolated and sacculus catheter (2.5 mm × 15 mm) inserted into 15-17 cm in depth, the outer end of catheter connected to a force pump for filling the balloon with normal saline and increased the pressure up to 7-8 standard atmospheric pressure, then the balloon was pulled repeatedly for 3 times, the catheter drawn out, and the wound tied up with layered sewing finally. Post-operation muscular injection of gentamycin (80 000 units) was given to prevent infection.

Rabbits at the post-operational period were continuously fed with high fat diet for 6 successive weeks, but to the three treated groups, testing drugs were mixed in the diet correspondingly, i.e. each day, Simvastatin 2.5 mg/kg, XSC 0.24 g/kg, and 0.48 g/kg (equivalent to the human adult dosage and two-fold of it) was respectively given.

1.4 Blood and Tissue Sampling

Blood samples were collected at the end of the 2nd week and the 8th week of the experiment via the auricular marginal vein after 6 h fasting, the serum was separated and preserved under −20℃.

All rabbits were sacrificed at the end of the 8th week, the abdominal aortic tissue at the position with evident pathological changes, that is the balloon wounded position, was taken for analysis through 10% formalin fixation, routine paraffin embedding, intermittent uniform section were done to make slides 4 μm in thickness, and hematoxylin-eosin (HE) or immunohistochemical stain was carried out.

1.5 Items and Methods of Observation

1.5.1 Blood Lipids Measurement

Biochemical methods with the automatic biochemical analyzer type 7600-020 (HITACHI, Japan) were adopted to measure the content of total cholesterol (TC), triglyceride (TG), high- and low-density lipoprotein cholesterol (HDL-C and LDL-C). The level of high sensitivity C-reactive protein (hs-CRP) and tumor necrosis factor α (TNF-α) were detected by ELISA with relevant test kits produced by USCNLIFE Company, USA, batch No. 080527 for hs-CRP and 081014 for TNF-α, which was operated according to the instruction in the kits. Enzyme linked immunosorbent assay apparatus (MULTISKAN EX PRIMARY EIA V.2.3，USA) was used to read the absorbency in various pools at 450 nm. The relevant concentration of the absorbency readings could be checked out from a standard curve drawn in advance by taking the concentration of the standard as X coordinate, and its absorbency detected as Y coordinate.

1.5.2 Patho-morphological Observation of the Plaque Tissue

The HE stained slide was observed under light microscope (Olympus type BX51, Japan) to see the basal constitution of plaque, including such elements as foam cells, fat deposition and cholesterol crystals.

Sizes of AS plaque in various cross sections were analyzed using Image-Pro Plus Version 4.5.1 software (IPP), USA, including the plaque area (PA), plaque circumference (PC) and maximal plaque thickness (MPT), as well as the cross-sectional vascular area (CVA). And the correct plaque area, namely, PA/CVA, was calculated.

1.6 Determination of VEGF and FⅧ RAg Protein Expression in Plaque

Immunohistochemical method was adopted with the first antibody provided by Capital Bio Corporation, batch No. 080501 for VEGF and 080818 for FⅧRAg, with the instruction in the test kits followed. The positive area displayed brown-yellow granular figure, the accumulate positive area was quantitatively measured by imaging processing software IPP, and the percentage of the positive area for VEGF and FⅧRAg in the plaque area was calculated respectively.

1.7 Statistical Analysis

With software SPSS 13.0 adopted, the measurement data were expressed by mean±standard deviation and analyzed by paired t-test, paired comparison among multi-groups was carried out by variance analysis and LSD test.

2. Results

Among all the 50 experimental rabbits, 4 died of balloon angioplasty, 2 died of post-operational infection and 4 were excluded from the study due to inability to take the forage entirely, so, the experiment was accomplished with data obtained in 40 rabbits.

2.1 Pathological Changes of AS Plaque

At the end of the 8th week, pathological examinations on HE stained slides showed that no foam cells and lipodoses was found in the abdominal aortic intima and media of the normal control group; but in that of the model group, markedly abnormal figures could be seen, such as AS plaque formation, thickened intima containing abundant foam cells, cholesterol crystals in sub-endothelium and plaque, and fibrous cap formation. While in the three medicated groups, these pathological changes, such as endothelial cell swelling and degeneration, foam cells and fat deposition, were all lesser than those in the model group (Figure 1).

2.2 Comparison of Blood Lipid Level

At the end of the 2nd week, serum levels of TC, TG and LDL-C were significantly higher in the model group and in the three medicated groups than those in the normal group ($P < 0.01$), though insignificant difference was shown between the 4 groups themselves ($P > 0.05$). But at the end of the 8th week, blood lipid levels did show

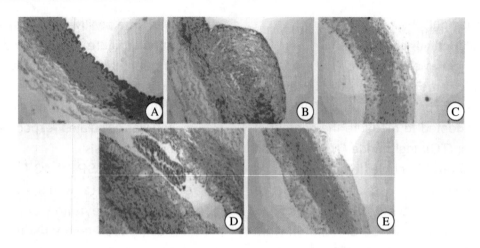

Figure 1　Histological Changes of Abdominal Aortic AS Plaque in Rabbits（HE staining，×200）

Notes：A：normal group；B：model group；C：Simvastatin group；D：low-dose XSC group；E：high-dose XSC group

significant difference when compared the model group with the three medicated groups in TC ($P <$ 0.05 or $P <$ 0.01), and with the Simvastatin group in TG and LDL-C. As for the serum level of HDL-C, excepting that in the high-dose XSC group it was higher than that in the model group ($P <$ 0.05), no significant impact of Simvastatin and low-dose XSC was seen (Table 1).

2.3　Comparison of Changes in Sizes of Plaque

As shown in Table 2, no significant difference was found between the 4 modeled groups in terms of PA and CVA of AS plaque ($P >$ 0.05); PA/CVA and PC were lower in the medicated groups than in the model group ($P <$ 0.05 or $P <$ 0.01), but no difference was shown among the three medicated groups ($P >$ 0.05); besides, MPT was significantly lower in the high-dose XSC group than in the model group ($P <$ 0.01).

Table 1　Comparison of Blood Lipid Levels among Groups（mmol/L，$\bar{\chi} \pm s$）

Group	Time	n	TC	TG	HDL-C	LDL-C
Normal	2nd weŵ	10	1.75±0.81	0.52±0.17	0.37±0.15	0.61±0.39
	8th weŵ	9	1.75±0.47	0.51±0.19	0.43±0.19	0.91±0.08
Model	2nd weŵ	10	15.77±3.97*	1.92±1.04*	0.78±0.15	7.63±2.41*
	8th weŵ	7	30.01±3.11	2.79±0.83	0.81±0.21	14.59±2.38
Simvastatin	2nd weŵ	10	14.65±4.42*	1.75±0.76*	0.88±0.22	7.21±3.62*
	8th weŵ	8	22.51±2.74△△	1.22±0.93△△	0.94±0.21	10.41±2.61△△
Low-dose XSC	2nd weŵ	10	18.63±6.21*	2.18±0.71*	0.91±0.24	7.46±3.09*
	8th weŵ	8	26.98±3.09△	2.36±0.64	1.01±0.23	13.14±2.28
High-dose XSC	2nd weŵ	10	18.91±2.63*	2.20±0.74*	0.95±0.16	6.72±3.43*
	8th weŵ	8	27.11±3.33△	2.16±0.89	1.05±0.31△	15.10±1.02

Notes：*$P <$ 0.01，compared with the normal group at the 2nd weŵ；△$P <$ 0.05，△△$P <$ 0.01，compared with the model group at the 8th weŵ

Table 2　Comparison of Changes in Sizes of Plaques among Groups ($\bar{\chi} \pm s$)

Group	n	PA (mm²)	CVA (mm²)	PA/CVA (%)	MPT (μm)	PC (mm)
Normal	9	–	1.88±0.28	–	–	–
Model	7	0.46±0.23	1.90±0.21	28.48±5.47	64.85±15.87	2.03±0.93
Simvastatin	8	0.29±0.17	1.95±0.17	12.76±3.93**	54.13±17.50	1.00±0.52**
Low-dose XSC	8	0.30±0.16	1.91±0.10	13.03±3.76**	57.27±5.74	1.46±0.64**
High-dose XSC	8	0.32±0.21	1.85±0.92	12.19±2.25**	39.63±13.40**	1.44±0.47*

Notes：*$P < 0.05$, **$P < 0.01$, compared with the model control group

2.4　Comparison of Serum of Levels hs-CRP and TNF-α

The serum levels of hs-CRP and TNF-α were higher in all the modeled groups than in the normal group; after intervention for 6 weŵs, that is at the end of the 8th week, the levels of hs-CRP in the medicated groups were lower than in the model group, while insignificant difference was found between the three groups themselves. As for the level of TNF-α, it was not changed significantly in all the modeled groups, though a lowering trend appeared in the low-dose XSC group ($P > 0.05$, Table 3).

Table 3　Comparison of Serum Levels of hs-CRP and TNF-α among Groups (ug/L, $\bar{\chi} \pm s$)

Group	n	hs-CRP	TNF-α
Normal	9	7.35±0.44△△	0.46±0.08△△
Model	7	9.80±1.39**	0.75±0.17**
Simvastatin	8	8.65±1.33*△	0.69±0.15*
Low-dose XSC	8	8.46±0.78*△	0.67±0.15*
High-dose XSC	8	8.62±0.76*△	0.73±0.12**

Notes: *$P < 0.05$, **$P < 0.01$, compared with the normal group; △$P < 0.01$, compared with the model group

2.5　Comparison of the VEGF and F Ⅷ RAg Positive Area in AS Plaque

Immunohistochemical and imaging analysis showed that the abdominal aortic intima in the normal group was smooth, with no plaque formation, so the positive area percentage could not be calculated. While in the model group, large amount of brown-yellow granules could be seen, especially evident aggregation on the shoulder and basal region of the plaque (Figures 2 and 3). The expression of VEGF and FⅧRAg positive area in the three medicated groups were significantly lessened after intervention, showing significant difference from that in the model group ($P < 0.05$ or $P < 0.01$); while in comparison between the three medicated groups, significant difference was only presented between the low-dose XSC group and the Simvastatin group in positive area of FⅧ RAg ($P < 0.05$, Figures 4 and 5).

3. Discussion

Pathological angiogenesis is frequently presented in AS plaque, which might be an important factor in promoting the progress of AS lesion and for forming instability, even the rupture, of plaques. Animal experiment has proven that angiogenesis suppressive agents could inhibit the neo-genesis of vessels in AS lesion to retard its progress [4]. And drugs of statins could serve to stabilize them.

Besides apparent action in lowering blood lipids levels, Statins showed also an effect of stabilizing AS plaque by way of angiogenesis inhibiting and matrix metalloproteinase secretion reducing and thus identified from therapeutic aspect the promoting effect of angiogenesis on the development of AS and the occurrence of AS complications as well[5].

The physio-pathologic changes presented in the AS forming progress, such as thrombus formation, vascular wall inflammation, cell

第四章

361

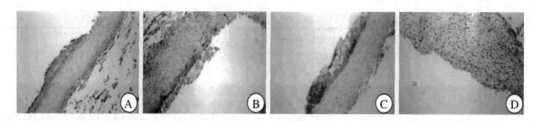

Figure 2   Expression of VEGF Positive Area in AS Plaque (Immunohistochemical staining, ×200)

Notes: A: model group; B: Simvastatin group; C: low-dose XSC group; D: high-dose XSC group

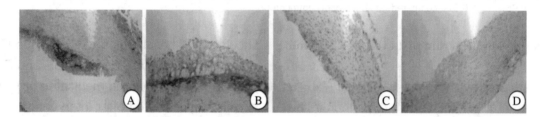

Figure 3   Expression of FⅧRAg Positive Area in AS Plaque (Immunohistochemical staining, ×200)

Notes: A: model group; B: Simvastatin group; C: low-dose XSC group; D: high-dose XSC group

proliferation and matrix accumulation, are recognized by Chinese medicine as internally associated with blood stasis syndrome, and the Chinese medicine drugs for ABCRS are proved to be capable of antagonizing AS by way of anti-platelet, adjusting lipid metabolism, inhibiting smooth muscular cell proliferation, etc.

XSC, a composite preparation for ABCRS, consists of active components from Red Paeonia and Rhizoma chuanxiong, which have been proved by previous studies to have a definite effect in directly or indirectly stabilizing AS plaque by their anti-inflammatory action through multiple paths[2]. On the basis of this, the effect of these components on expressions of VEGF and FⅧRAg in rabbits' AS plaque and the correlation between them with AS formation were observed.

VEGF is a mitotic growth factor, which has been discovered currently to have specificity in promoting the mitosis of vascular endothelial cells. VEGF is highly expressed in AS plaque, which is considered to be able to possibly act to advance the genesis and development of AS plaque[6,7]. FⅧRAg, a kind of glycoprotein extensively existing on the surface of endothelial cells, is a specific marker of neogenerated

vascular endothelium on small capillaries and their un-canalized offsets. It participates in the angiogenesis process, and it is regarded as an index reflecting the adhesive state of vascular endothelial cells[8].

Results of this study showed that the expressions of VEGF and FⅧRAg in the XSC groups, both high-and low-dose, were significantly lower than those in the model group respectively, the lowering in the high-dose group was especially evident; but the two indices in the XSC groups were not significantly different to those in the Simvastatin group. This result suggested that both XSC and Simvastatin could inhibit the angiogenesis in AS plaque. Meantime, pathologic examinations showed that under the same high fat diet feeding, the vascular morphologic figure in the XSC groups was markedly better than that in the model group, which also illustrated that XSC has a certain effect in improving the size of AS plaque and in restraining the genesis and development of AS.

AS is a inflammatory disease. Inflammatory reaction runs all through the developing process, and is the central link of genesis and development of AS. hs-CRP is a sensitive index reflecting the

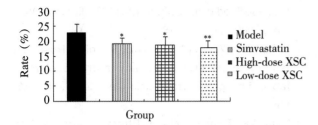

Figure 4　VEGF Positive Area Percentage

Notes: $^*P < 0.05$, $^{**}P < 0.01$, compared with the model group

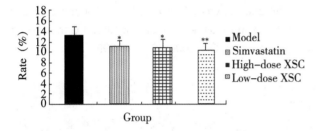

Figure 5　FⅧRAg Positive Area Percentage

Notes: $^*P < 0.05$, $^{**}P < 0.01$, compared with the model group; $^\triangle P < 0.05$, compared with Simvastatin group

inflammatory process of AS[9]. Results of this study showed that the serum level of hs-CRP significantly raised after modeling, but could be reduced by XSC medication, suggesting that the inflammatory process was suppressed. At the same time of suppressing inflammation, XSC could also lower the blood lipids level, which is displayed as reduction of blood TC level in all the three medicated groups.

In sum, both XSC and Simvastatin could inhibit the expressions of VEGF and FⅧRAg in AS plaque, the mechanism might be related with lipids metabolic regulation and inflammatory reaction inhibition. Moreover, XSC could decrease the size of plaque, which is conducive to restraining the development of AS.

Nowadays, the researches concerning angiog-enesis all focus on the treatment of ischemic heart diseases. DAI RH, et al[10] indicated that some Chinese medicine drugs for moving qi and activating blood circulation may have effects of promoting angiogenesis, and therefore it may be helpful to the collateral circulation formation in the heart and could relieve

myocardial ischemia and anoxemia in patients with coronary heart diseases. Nevertheless, current studies have proved that application of some Chinese medicine drugs for ABCRS in treating AS could inhibit neo-genesis of vessels in AS plaque[11-13], and this study has also verified that XSC, a Chinese medicine preparation for ABCRS, could inhibit the expressions of VEGF and FⅧRAg in AS plaque. These facts suggested that Chinese drugs for activating blood might have bi-directional regulative effects, and they might act, on the one hand, to promote neo-genesis of vessels in ischemic myocardium, and on the other hand, to interrupt or even inhibit the angiogenesis in plaque. This is an issue waiting for further studies.

References

[1] Ross JS, Staglian NE, Donovan MJ, et al. Atherosclerosis and cancer: common molecular pathways of disease development and progression. Ann N Y Acad Sci, 2001, 947: 271-292.

[2] Xu H, Wen C, Chen KJ, et al. Study on the effect of Rhizoma Chuanxiong, Radix Paeoniae Rubra and the compound of their active ingredients, Xiongshao Capsule, on stability of atherosclerotic plaque in ApoE-/- mice. Chin J Integr Tradit Chin West Med, 2007, 27: 513-518.

[3] Han XF, Zhang W, Zhao YM. The establishment of the atherosclerosis model in rabbit abdominal aorta by high fat diet and percutaneous transluminal angioplasty. J Clin Exp Med, 2006, 5: 1679-1680.

[4] Moulton KS, Olsen BR, Sonn S, et al. Loss of collagen xⅧ enhances neovascularization and vascular permeability in atherosclerosis. Circulation, 2004, 110: 1330-1336.

[5] Wilson SH, Herrmann J, Lerman LO, et al. Simvastatin preserves the structure of coronary adventitial vasa vasorum in experimental hypercholesterolemia independent of lipid lowering. Circulation, 2002, 105: 415-418.

[6] Caldwell RB, Bartoli M, BŴzadian MA, et al. Vascular endothelial growth factor and diabetic retinopathy: role of oxidative stress. Curr Drug Targets, 2005, 6: 511-524.

[7] Panutsopulos D, Papalambros E, Sigala F, et al.

Protein and mRNA expression levels of VEGF-A and TGF-beta in different types of human coronary atherosclerotic lesions. Int J Mol Med, 2005, 15: 603-610.

[8] Galbusera M, Zoja C, Donadelli R, et al. Fluid shear stress modulates von Willebrand factor release from human vascular endothelium. Blood, 1997; 90: 1558-1564.

[9] Schlager O, Exner M, Mlekusch W, et al. C-reactive protein predicts future cardiovascular events in patients with carotid stenosis. Stroke, 2007, 38: 1263-1268.

[10] Dai HR, Li Y. Therapeutic angiogenesis of myocardial ischemia with coronary artery disease and traditional Chinese Medicine. Chin J Integr Tradit Chin West Med, 2000, 20: 163-164.

[11] Li TQ, Fan WH, Li Y. Effect of Rhodiola Rosea on femoral artery plaque stability in arteriosclerosis rabbit. Shanghai J Tradit Chin Med, 2006, 40: 66-68.

[12] Feng LP, Song T, Xia H. Effect of paclitaxel on atherosclerotic plaque in rats. J Cardiovasc Pulm Dis, 2006, 25: 230-232.

[13] Li TQ, Li Y, Fan WH. Effects of She Xiang Bao Xin Pill and simvastatin on stability of atherosclerotic plaque in rabbit femoral artery. Chin J Geriatr Heart Brain Vessel Dis, 2006, 8: 296-299.

第四节　中医药防治动脉粥样硬化的研究

人参皂苷 Rb1 对氧化型低密度脂蛋白诱导的人单核细胞源树突状细胞免疫成熟的影响 [*]

刘红樱　葛均波　马晓娟　史大卓

树突状细胞（dendritic cells，DCs）是人体内功能最强大的专职抗原递呈细胞，具有独特的诱导和放大免疫效应的功能。目前认为，动脉粥样硬化（atherosclerosis，AS）是一种慢性炎症免疫性疾病，DCs 在 AS 发生、发展过程中具有重要的调控作用。DCs 的成熟是其发挥免疫作用的关键，多个外源性或内源性的抗原如氧化型低密度脂蛋白（oxygenized low density lipoprotein，OX-LDL）、脂多糖、热休克蛋白等均可诱导其成熟。OX-LDL 作为自身抗原通过参与泡沫细胞形成、诱导血管平滑肌细胞增生、加重血管内皮细胞损伤、产生抗 OX-LDL 自身抗体等途径参与 AS 的病理过程 [1-4]。

人参皂苷 Rb1（ginsenoside Rb1，GRb1）为人参的主要活性成分，具有广泛的药理作用。以往对 GRb1 在血管系统作用的研究主要集中于改善微循环、保护血管内皮细胞、抗氧化应激损伤、调节脂质代谢、抑制心肌细胞凋亡等方面 [5]，本研究从调节炎症免疫方面观察 GRb1 对 OX-LDL 诱导的 DCs 成熟的影响，并阐述其抗 AS 的可能机制。

1. 材料与方法

1.1 人单核细胞源 DCs 的分离培养

参考文献 [6] 取健康成人外周血，制成浓缩白细胞悬液，经淋巴细胞分离液（Histopaque1077）密度梯度离心分离出单个核细胞，磷酸盐缓冲液（PBS）洗涤后重悬，加入 CD14+ 磁珠，4 ℃

---

* 原载于《中国中西医结合杂志》，2011，31（3）：350-354

孵育 30min，经分选柱流洗，分选出纯度＞98%的 CD14⁺ 单核细胞，接种于含有 10% 胎牛血清的 RPMI-1640 培养基的细胞培养板中，然后加入含重组人粒细胞-巨噬细胞集落刺激因子（rhGM-CSF）100ng/mL、重组人白细胞介素 4（rhIL-4）20ng/mL，调节细胞浓度为 1×10^5/mL，置于 37℃含 5%CO_2 的培养箱中，每 48h 半量换液 1 次。

1.2　试剂和药物

CD14⁺ 免疫磁珠试剂盒（批号 130-050-201），购自德国 Miltenyi Biotech 公司；rh-GM-CSF（批号 215-GM-010）和 rhIL-4（批号 204-IL-010），购自美国 R&D 公司；OX-LDL（批号 5685-3557），购自英国 AbD 公司；Histopaque 1077（批号 10771）、环格列酮（CIG，批号 GW9662）、异硫氰酸荧光素标记的右旋糖苷（FITC-Dextran，FD10S）、Rb₁（批号 G0777，HPLC ≥ 98%，5mg 溶于 5mL PBS，终浓度 1mg/mL），购自美国 Sigma 公司；单克隆抗人抗体 CD1a、CD40 和 HLA-DR，购自美国 Invitrogen 公司；白细胞介素 -12（IL-12）和肿瘤坏死因子 -α（TNF-α）的 ELISA 检测试剂盒，购自美国 eBioscience 公司；RPMI-1640 培养基和 10% 胎牛血清，购自美国 Hyclone 公司。

1.3　实验仪器

FACS Calibur 流式细胞仪，美国 Becton Dickinson 产品；BX41-32P02 光学显微镜，日本 Olympus 产品；S-520 扫描电镜，日本 Hitachi 产品；5840 台式水平高速离心机，德国 Eppendorf 产品。

1.4　实验分组

分离的单个核细胞培养 5 天，分化成 DCs，随机分组为：(1) PBS 组，加 PBS（与 OX-LDL 相同体积）孵育 24h；(2) GRb₁ 组，加 GRb₁50μg/mL 干预 24h，再加入 PBS 孵育 24h；(3) CIG 组，加 CIG25μg/mL 干预 24h，再加入 PBS 孵育 24h；(4) OX-LDL 组，加 OX-LDL50μg/mL 孵育 24h；(5) GRb₁ 预处理加 OX-LDL 组，加入 GRb₁ 50μg/mL 预处理 24h，再加入 OX-LDL 50μg/mL 孵育 24h；(6) CIG 预处理加 OX-LDL 组，加 CIG 25μg/mL 预处理 24h，再加 OX-LDL 50μg/mL 孵育 24h。收集悬浮细胞，采用台盼蓝染色测定细胞活力。

1.5　DCs 表型检测

收集细胞，调整细胞浓度为 1×10^5/mL，分别加入单克隆抗人抗体 CD1a、CD40 和 HLA-DR，4℃孵育 30min，PBS 洗涤，细胞重悬，用流式细

胞仪 FACS Calibur 检测，WinMDI 2.9 软件分析检测结果。

1.6　DCs 吞噬功能检测

收集细胞，重悬于 RPMI-1640 培养基，调整细胞浓度为 1×10^5/mL，加入 FITC-Dextran，终浓度为 1mg/mL，37℃孵育 1h，PBS 洗涤，用流式细胞仪 FACS Calibur 检测 DCs 吞噬的功能（用吞噬 FITC-Dextran 的 DCs 所占的百分比表示），WinMDI 2.9 软件分析检测结果。

1.7　细胞因子检测

收集细胞培养上清液，按 ELISA 检测试剂盒说明书介绍方法测定 IL-12 和 TNF-α 浓度。试剂盒检测 IL-12 和 TNF-α 的最小检测浓度分别是 ＜ 0.5ng/L 和＜ 3ng/L。

1.8　统计学处理

所有实验结果重复 3 次，采用 SPSS 11.0 软件包进行统计学处理。数据用 $\bar{x} \pm s$ 表示，多组间比较采用单因素方差分析，$P < 0.05$ 为差异有统计学意义。

2.　结果

2.1　DCs 形态学改变（图 1）

CD14⁺ 免疫磁珠分选的单核细胞均匀一致，纯度＞98%。加入 rhGM-CSF 和 rhIL-4 培养第 1 ~ 2 天，可见细胞为类圆形，呈集落样生长，集落逐渐增大，呈半悬浮样。第 4 ~ 5 天可见细胞有少量毛刺形成，具备 DCs 的特征。OX-LDL 刺激 24h 后，可见细胞体积增大，悬浮，并有大量毛刺状突起形成。GRb₁ 预处理组细胞呈半悬浮样生长，毛刺生成较少。

2.2　各组 DCs 表型改变（图 2）

与 PBS 组比较，OX-LDL 组 DCs 表面分子 CD40、CD1a 和 HLA-DR 的表达明显增加（$P <$ 0.01）；与 OX-LDL 组比较，GRb₁ 预处理明显抑制 OX-LDL 诱导的 DCs 表面分子的表达，CD40、CD1a 和 HLA-DR 分别为 67.40±1.62 vs. 145.69±14.86（$P < 0.01$）、79.64±3.04 vs. 159.89±6.09（$P < 0.01$）和 46.43±2.85 vs. 99.33±17.11（$P < 0.01$）。CIG 预处理也可明显抑制 OX-LDL 诱导的 DCs 表面分子 CD40、CD1a、HLA-DR 的表达（$P < 0.01$），和 GRb₁ 预处理比较差异无统计学意义（$P > 0.05$）。

2.3　各组 DCs 吞噬功能改变（图 3）

与 PBS 组比较，OX-LDL 组吞噬 Dextran 的

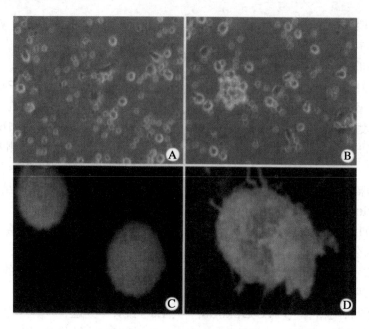

图 1　各组 DCs 的形态学变化

A：GRb$_1$+OX-LDL 组（×200）；B：OX-LDL 组（×200）；C：GRb$_1$+OX-LDL 组（×2000）；D：OX-LDL 组（×2000）；A、B 为 培养第 7 天相差显微镜图像，C、D 为培养第 7 天扫描电镜图像

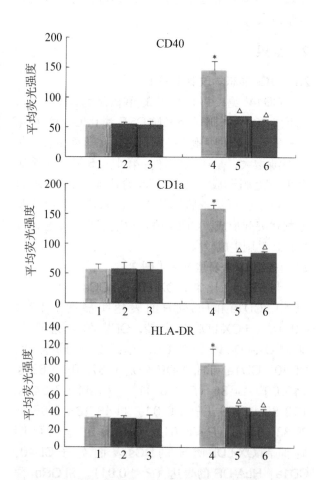

图 2　各组 DCs 表面标志 CD40、CD1a 及 HLA-DR 表达

注：1 为 PBS 组，2 为 GRb$_1$ 组，3 为 CIG 组，4 为 OX-LDL 组，5 为 GRb$_1$+OX-LDL 组，6 为 CIG+OX-LDL 组；与 PBS 组 比 较，*P < 0.01；与 OX-LDL 组比较，△P < 0.01

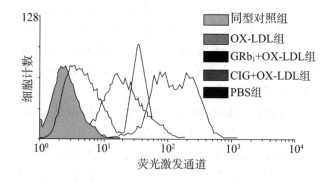

图 3　各组 DCs 吞噬功能的变化

注：GRb$_1$ 组及 CIG 组与 PBS 组 DCs 吞噬功能比较差异 无统计学意义，三者曲线重迭，故 GRb$_1$ 组及 CIG 组曲线 未标识。

DCs 数量明显减少（P < 0.01）；与 OX-LDL 组 比较，GRb$_1$ 预处理明显上调 DCs 的吞噬功能 [吞噬 Dextran 为 （88.13±1.06)% vs. (25.90±5.77)%， P < 0.01]。CIG 预处理也较 OX-LDL 组明显增强 （P < 0.05），但与 GRb$_1$ 预处理组比较差异无统 计学意义（P > 0.05）。

2.4　各组 DCs 培养上清细胞因子浓度改变（表 1）

　　与 PBS 组比较，OX-LDL 干预后 DCs 分泌的 细胞因子 IL-12 和 TNF-α 明显增加（P < 0.01）； GRb$_1$ 预处理明显抑制 OX-LDL 诱导 DCs 分泌 细胞因子 IL-12 和 TNF-α，与 OX-LDL 组比较，

IL-12 和 TNF-α 均明显降低（$P < 0.01$）。CIG 预处理也有抑制 OX-LDL 诱导的 DCs 分泌细胞因子 IL-12 和 TNF-α 的作用（$P < 0.01$），但与 GRb₁ 预处理组比较差异无统计学意义（$P > 0.05$）。

表 1　各组 DCs 培养上清液中细胞因子 IL-12 和 TNF-α 浓度比较（ng/L，$\bar{x} \pm s$）

组别	n	IL-12	TNF-α
PBS	6	53.23± 1.85	93.54± 3.99
GRb₁	6	51.67± 2.89	94.21± 4.16
CIG	6	52.41± 2.57	92.11± 6.42
OX-LDL	6	716.69±36.35[*]	968.11±36.42[*]
GRb₁+OX-LDL	6	88.65± 5.59[△]	133.27±11.98[△]
CIG+OX-LDL	6	90.75± 9.48[△]	97.53± 7.13[△]

注：与 PBS 组比较，[*]$P < 0.01$；与 OX-LDL 组比较，[△]$P < 0.01$

3. 讨论

近年来研究表明，AS 是一种慢性免疫炎症性疾病，体内最强大的专职抗原递呈细胞 DCs 与 AS 发生发展有密切的关系[7]。在正常不易发生 AS 的动脉，DCs 少量散在分布于内膜下层；在承受血流压力较大易于发生 AS 的部位，尤其在人的 AS 斑块中，DCs 的聚集明显增加，而且进展期斑块显著多于起始期斑块，不稳定斑块显著多于稳定斑块，DCs 多簇集在斑块易破裂部位[8-11]。多种 AS 致病因素如 OX-LDL、糖基化终末产物、高糖和热休克蛋白等都可激活动脉内膜中的 DCs，摄取和递呈异物抗原，同时表达黏附分子及 T 淋巴细胞共刺激分子而活化 T 淋巴细胞，损伤血管内皮细胞，激活单核 - 巨噬细胞及血管平滑肌细胞产生炎性细胞因子、炎症趋化因子及基质金属蛋白酶等，启动 AS 免疫炎症反应[12-14]。OX-LDL 还可作为自身抗原刺激局部产生抗 OX-LDL 抗体，促进 DCs 分化成熟。成熟的 DCs 表面高表达两类分子，一类是共刺激分子如 CD1a、CD40、CD86、CD83、CD36 等，其中 CD1a 和 CD40 是其成熟的较特异性标志；另一类是主要组织相容性抗原分子如 HLA-DR。两类刺激分子皆能激活 T 淋巴细胞，其中主要组织相容性抗原分子负责将抗原递呈给 T 淋巴细胞。成熟 DCs 分泌各种细胞因子，如 IL-12、TNF-α、IL-10、IL-19、IL-6 和 INF-γ 等，进一步促进 T 淋巴细胞的免疫应答，其中 IL-12 和 TNF-α 的分泌增加在 DCs 的成熟中具

有重要意义。吞噬作用是 DCs 的主要功能之一，未成熟 DCs 的主要功能是捕获和摄取抗原，而成熟 DCs 在将抗原递呈给 T 淋巴细胞的过程中摄取抗原能力大大降低，吞噬功能明显减弱[15-17]。本研究发现 OX-LDL 能够上调 DCs 表面分子 CD40、CD1a 和 HLA-DR 的表达，增加细胞因子 IL-12 和 TNF-α 的分泌，降低抗原吞噬功能，证实 OX-LDL 能够诱导 DCs 的免疫成熟。

CIG 是过氧化物酶增殖体激活受体 γ 激动剂，可通过影响核转录因子 κB、信号转录子、激活蛋白 -1 介导的信号通路抑制 DCs 的免疫成熟[18-20]。本实验证明，CIG 可抑制 OX-LDL 诱导的 DCs 表面分子 CD40、CD1a、HLA-DR 的表达和 DCs 分泌细胞因子 IL-12 和 TNF-α，表明 CIG 可抑制 DCs 的免疫成熟。

GRb₁ 是五加科植物人参的主要活性成分，具有多种药理学功效，如保护缺血心肌、改善血液循环、调节免疫、调节糖脂代谢等。以 GRb₁ 为主要成分的药物临床广泛用于冠心病、心肌炎、心律失常、糖尿病等的治疗，显示有一定的作用[21,22]。本研究发现，GRb₁ 预处理可明显抑制 OX-LDL 诱导的 DCs 表面分子 CD40、CD1a、HLA-DR 的表达和炎症细胞因子 IL-12、TNF-α 的分泌，增强 DCs 对抗原 Dextran 的吞噬能力，证实 GRb₁ 能够抑制 OX-LDL 诱导的 DCs 免疫成熟。

GRb₁ 可以抑制 OX-LDL 诱导的人单核细胞源 DCs 的免疫成熟，有理由认为 GRb₁ 可通过这一机制调节 AS 发生发展过程中免疫炎症反应，进而具有一定的抗 AS 作用。但是本实验仅为细胞水平的研究，在体是否具有抗 AS 作用，其抑制 OX-LDL 诱导 DCs 成熟的内在机制是什么？皆有待进一步实验研究。

参考文献

[1] Alvarez D, Vollmann EH, von Andrian UH. Mechanisms and consequences of dendritic cells migration. Immunity, 2008，29 (3): 325-342.

[2] Link A, Bohm M. Potential role of dendritic cells in atherogenesis. Cardiovasc Res, 2002，55 (4): 708-709.

[3] Alderman CJ, Bunyard PR, Chain BM, et al. Effects of oxidized low density lipoprotein on dendritic cells: a possible immunoregulatory component of the atherogenic micro-environment. Cardiovasc Res, 2002，55 (4): 806-819.

[4] Flohe SB, Bruggemann J, Lendemans S, et al. Human heat shock protein 60 induces maturation of dendritic cells versus a Th1-promoting phenotype. J Immunol, 2003，170 (5): 2340-2348.

[5] Block KI, Mead MN. Immune system effects of echinacea, ginseng, and astragalus: a review. Integr Cancer Ther, 2003，2 (3): 247-267.

[6] Luo Y, Liang C, Xu C, et al. Ciglitazone Inhibits oxidized-low density lipoprotein induced immune maturation of dendritic cells. J Card iovasc Pharmacol, 2004，44 (3): 3 81-385.

[7] Hansson GK, Libby P. The immune response in atherosclerosis: a double-edged sword. Nat Rev Immunol, 2006，6 (7): 508-519.

[8] Gautier EL, Huby T, Saint-Charles F, et al. Conventional dendritic cells at the crossroads between immunity and cholesterol homeostasis in atherosclerosis. Circulation, 2009，119 (17): 2367-2375.

[9] Hansson GK. Inflammation, atherosclerosis, and coronary artery disease. N Engl J Med, 2005, 352 (16): 1685-1695.

[10] Cao W, Bobryshev YV, Lord RS, et al. Dendritic cells in the arterial wall expresses C1q: potential significance in atherogenesis. Cardiovasc Res, 2003, 60 (1): 175-186.

[11] Bobryshev YV, Lord RS. Mapping of vascular dendritic cells in atherosclerotic arteries suggests their involvement in local immune-inflammatory reactions. Cardiovasc Res, 1998, 37 (3): 799-810.

[12] Ge J, Jia Q, Liang C, et al. Advanced glycosylation end products might promote atherosclerosis through inducing the immune maturation of dendritic cells. Arterioscler Thromb Vasc Biol, 2005, 25 (10): 2157-263.

[13] 姚康，葛均波，孙爱军，等. 高糖对人单核细胞源树突状细胞分化成熟和免疫功能的影响及其机制研究. 中华心血管病杂志，2006，34 (1): 60-64.

[14] 罗育坤，梁春，黄东，等. 氧化修饰低密度脂蛋白促进人单核细胞源树突状细胞的成熟及活化. 复旦学报（医学版），2004，31 (5): 441-444.

[15] Wallet MA, Sen P, Tisch R. Immunoregulation of dendritic cells. Clin Med Res, 2005，3 (3): 166-175.

[16] Guermonprezv P, Valladeau J, Zitvogel L, et al. Antigen presentation and T cell stimulation by dendritic cells. Annu Rev Immunol, 2002，20：621-667.

[17] Tedgui A, Mallat Z. Cytokines in atherosclerosis: pathogenic and regulatory pathways. Physiol Rev, 2006，86 (2): 515-581.

[18] Klotz L, Dani L, Edenhofer F, et al. Peroxisome proliferator-activated receptor gamma control of dendritic cell function contributes to development of CD4$^+$ T cell energy. J Immunol, 2007，178 (4): 2122-2131.

[19] Gosset P, Charbonnier AS, Delerive P, et al. Peroxisome proliferator-activated receptor gamma activators affect the maturation of human monocyte-derived dendritic cells. Eur J Immunol, 2001，31 (10): 2857-2865.

[20] Appel S, Mirakaj V, Bringmann A, et al. PPAR-gamma agonists inhibit toll-like receptor-mediated activation of dendritic cells via the MAP kinase and NF-kappa B pathways. Blood, 2005，106 (12): 3888-3894.

[21] 李利艳，路新国. 人参皂苷的最新研究进展. 四川省卫生管理干部学院学报，2004，23 (4): 293-295.

[22] 王强，莫雪梅，杨小英，等. 人参皂苷治疗心血管疾病的现代研究进展. 心血管病学进展，2006，27 (3): 325-327.

第四章

赤芍川芎有效部位对兔动脉粥样硬化基质金属蛋白酶的影响 *

张　璐　薛　梅　马晓娟　杨　琳　殷惠军

动脉粥样硬化（atherosclerosis，AS）不稳定斑块的破裂是急性卒中事件发生的主要病因之一，对其发生机制的研究及干预具有重要的临床意义 [1]。在 AS 形成过程中，基质金属蛋白酶（matrix metalloproteinases，MMPs）能够降解局部细胞外基质，减少细胞外胶原纤维含量，进而加速斑块破裂 [2]。芎芍胶囊是由赤芍、川芎的有效部位赤芍总苷和川芎总酚组成，实验研究显示其具有消除炎症，稳定 AS 斑块的作用 [3]，那么这种作用是否与 MMPs 有关呢？基于此，我们采用高脂加球囊导管血管损伤术造成 AS 斑块模型，研究赤芍川芎有效部位对 AS 斑块内 MMP-3、MMP-9 和 MMP 组织抑制因子 -1（tissue inhibitor of metalloproteinases-1，TIMP-1）的表达，旨在进一步揭示赤芍川芎有效部位稳定斑块的作用机制。

1.　材料与方法

1.1　实验材料

1.1.1　动物　健康雄性新西兰兔，体重 1.8 ~ 2.2kg，北京维通利华实验动物有限公司提供，动物许可证号：SCXK（京）2005-0002。高脂饲料（基础饲料 +2% 胆固醇 +5% 猪油）由军事医学科学院实验动物中心提供。

1.1.2　药物　辛伐他汀（商品名：舒降之，批号：07432）每片 40mg，杭州默沙东制药有限公司生产；芎芍胶囊（Xiongshao Capsule，XSC）由川芎、赤芍的有效部位川芎总酚和赤芍总苷组成，每粒 0.25g（含芍药苷 ≥ 28mg，总酚酸 ≥ 34mg，阿魏酸 ≥ 3.5mg），中国科学院大连物化所提供，批号：070929。

1.2　实验方法

1.2.1　模型制备　参照相关文献报道 [4] 建立新西兰兔 AS 模型：动物予高脂饲料 100g/d 喂养 2 周后，行腹主动脉球囊导管血管损伤术：3% 戊巴比妥钠（1mL/kg）经耳缘静脉麻醉后，钝性分离出股动脉，插入球囊导管 2.5mm×15mm，深度 15 ~ 17cm，连接压力泵生理盐水充盈球囊，7 ~ 8 个标准大气压，球囊反复牵拉 3 次，退出导管，结扎伤口，逐层缝合伤口。术后肌内注射庆大霉素 8 万单位防治感染。

1.2.2　分组及给药　50 只新西兰兔随机分为 5 组，每组 10 只。正常对照组：给予普通饲料；模型对照组：给予高脂饲料；辛伐他汀组：给予高脂饲料拌入辛伐他汀 2.5mg/(kg·d)；XSC 低剂量组：给予高脂饲料拌入 XSC 0.24g/(kg·d)；XSC 高剂量组：给予高脂饲料拌入 XSC 0.48g/(kg·d)，连续喂养 6 周。

1.3　观察指标和检测方法

1.3.1　血脂检测　分别于造模后第 2 和第 8 周末，耳缘动脉采血（采血前禁食 6h），分离血清，采用生化法（日本 HITACHI 公司 7600-020 型全自动生化分析仪）测定血清总胆固醇（TC）、三酰甘油（TG）、高密度脂蛋白胆固醇（HDL-C）和低密度脂蛋白胆固醇（LDL-C）。

1.3.2　血清 MMPs 检测　第 8 周末取血测定血清 MMP-3、MMP-9 和 TIMP-1，采用酶联免疫吸附测定法（ELISA），按试剂盒（美国 USCNL IFE 公司，MMP-3 批号：080611，MMP-9 批号：081016，TIMP-1 批号：081023）说明进行操作，酶标仪（美国 MULT ISKAN EX PR IMARY EIA V.2.3）在 450nm 处读取各孔吸光度值。以浓度值为横坐标，所测各标准吸光度值为纵坐标，绘制标准曲线。按样本孔测得的吸光度值从标准曲线上查得相应的浓度值，以 μg/L 表示。

1.3.3　斑块组织病理形态学观察　将兔子第 8 周末全部处死，在病变最明显部位（即球囊撕伤内膜处）取下腹主动脉组织，10% 福尔马林固定，常

* 原载于《中国中西医结合杂志》，2009，29（6）：514-518

第四章

规石蜡包埋，间断均匀切片，切片厚度均为 4μm。标本做 HE 染色，在光镜（日本 Olympus BX51 光学显微镜）下观察斑块的基本构成，包括泡沫细胞、脂质沉积和胆固醇结晶等成分。

1.3.4 斑块组织 MMP-3 和 CD40L 蛋白测定

采用免疫组化染色方法检测斑块内 MMP-3 和 CD40L 蛋白表达，免疫组化一抗工作液由北京博奥森生物技术有限公司提供（MMP-3 批号：080501，CD40L 批号：080810），切片在 60℃ 的条件下烘烤 1h，二甲苯和梯度乙醇脱蜡，置 5% 过氧化氢溶液 15min 灭活内源性过氧化物酶；4℃，一抗孵育过夜，二抗结合 30min，DAB 显色，苏木精复染、脱水、中性树胶封片；DAB 显色阳性结果为棕黄色颗粒状。利用美国 Image-Pro Plus Version 4.5.1（IPP）图像分析软件，对阳性区域累积面积进行定量测定，求取斑块内 MMP-3 和 CD40L 阳性区域面积占斑块面积的百分比。

1.4 统计学方法

采用 SPSS 13.0 软件包进行统计学处理，计量用 $\bar{x} \pm s$ 表示，多组两两间比较采用方差分析 LSD 检验。

2. 结果

2.1 一般观察

球囊导管血管损伤术中死亡兔 4 只，术后感染死亡 2 只，4 只未食用完饲料因而退出实验，其余 40 只兔完成实验获得数据。

2.2 各组家兔 AS 斑块病理变化（图 1）

高脂喂养 8 周后，HE 染色显示正常对照组腹

主动脉内膜及中膜均未见泡沫细胞及脂质沉积；模型对照组腹主动脉已形成明显的动脉粥样硬化斑块，内膜明显增厚，内含大量泡沫细胞，内皮下、斑块内有胆固醇结晶，纤维帽形成。各药物干预组内皮细胞肿胀、变性减轻，泡沫细胞及脂质沉积较模型对照组减少。

2.3 各组血脂水平比较（表 1）

高脂饲料喂养 2 周后，模型对照组、辛伐他汀组和 XSC 高、低剂量组血清 TC、TG 和 LDL-C 水平较正常对照组均有显著升高（$P < 0.01$），4 组之间则差异无统计学意义（$P > 0.05$）。药物干预 8 周末，辛伐他汀组、XSC 低剂量组和 XSC 高剂量组血清 TC 与模型对照组均有不同程度降低（$P < 0.05$，$P < 0.01$）；辛伐他汀组还可显著降低血清 TG 和 LDL-C；对 HDL-C，XSC 高剂量组较模型对照组有显著升高（$P < 0.05$），其他各药物组无明显影响。

2.4 各组血清 MMP-3、MMP-9 和 TIMP-1 比较（表 2）

模型对照组和各用药组血清 MMP-3、MMP-9 水平均高于正常对照组（$P < 0.05$，$P < 0.01$）；辛伐他汀组和 XSC 低剂量组 MMP-3 表达降低，与模型对照组比较差异有统计学意义（$P < 0.05$），但辛伐他汀组与 XSC 低剂量组比较，差异无统计学意义（$P > 0.05$）；MMP-9 表达辛伐他汀、XSC 高剂量及 XSC 低剂量组与模型对照组比较，有明显降低（$P < 0.05$），而 3 组之间差异无统计学意义（$P > 0.05$）；TIMP-1 水平模型对照组和各用药组均较正常对照组降低（$P < 0.05$，$P < 0.01$），4 组之间比较差异无统计学

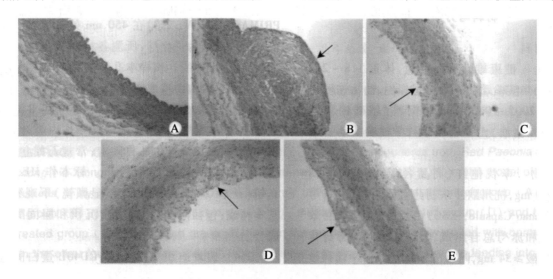

图 1 家兔腹主动脉粥样硬化斑块组织形态变化（HE 染色，×200）
注：A 为正常对照组；B 为模型对照组；C 为辛伐他汀组；D 为 XSC 低剂量组；E 为 XSC 高剂量组

表 1　各组血脂水平比较（mmol/L，$\bar{\chi} \pm s$）

组别	时间	n	TC	TG	HDL-C	LDL-C
正常对照	2 周末	10	1.75±0.81	0.52±0.17	0.37±0.15	0.61±0.39
	8 周末	9	1.75±0.47**	0.51±0.19**	0.43±0.19**	0.91±0.08**
模型对照	2 周末	10	15.77±3.97△	1.92±1.04△	0.78±0.15	7.63±2.41△
	8 周末	7	30.01±3.11	2.79±0.83	0.81±0.21	14.59±2.38
辛伐他汀	2 周末	10	14.65±4.42△	1.75±0.76△	0.88±0.22	7.21±3.62△
	8 周末	8	22.51±2.74**	1.22±0.93**	0.94±0.21	10.41±2.61**
XSC 低剂量	2 周末	10	18.63±6.21△	2.18±0.71△	0.91±0.24	7.46±3.09△
	8 周末	8	26.98±3.09*	2.36±0.64	1.01±0.23	13.14±2.28
XSC 高剂量	2 周末	10	18.91±2.63△	2.20±0.74△	0.95±0.16	6.72±3.43△
	8 周末	8	27.11±3.33*	2.16±0.89	1.05±0.31*	15.10±1.02

注：与模型对照组 8 周末比较，$^*P < 0.05$，$^{**}P < 0.01$；与正常对照组 2 周末比较，$^{\triangle}P < 0.01$

表 2　各组血清 MMP-3、MMP-9 和 TIMP-1 比较（µg/L，$\bar{\chi} \pm s$）

组别	n	MMP-3	MMP-9	TIMP-1
正常对照	9	21.04±2.81**	0.65±0.17**	1.57±0.27
模型对照	7	56.82±18.57△△	1.11±0.07△△	1.20±0.22△
辛伐他汀	8	42.79±13.66*△△	0.90±0.23*△	1.12±0.30△△
XSC 低剂量	8	41.66±10.46*△△	0.89±0.15*△	1.10±0.19△△
XSC 高剂量	8	45.19±13.18△△	0.90±0.13*△	0.95±0.18△△

注：与模型对照组比较，$^*P < 0.05$，$^{**}P < 0.01$；与正常对照组比较，$^{\triangle}P < 0.05$，$^{\triangle\triangle}P < 0.01$

意义（$P > 0.05$）。

2.5　各组斑块内 MMP-3 和 CD40L 阳性面积表达比较

免疫组化和图像分析结果显示，正常对照组腹主动脉内膜光滑，无斑块形成，故阳性面积率无法统计。模型对照组斑块内可见大量棕黄色颗粒，特别是在斑块肩部和基底部明显聚集（图 2，图 3）。与模型对照组比较，辛伐他汀组、XSC 低剂量组和 XSC 高剂量组 MMP-3、CD40L 的阳性染色面积比均显著减少（$P < 0.05$，$P < 0.01$），各用药组间比较差异无统计学意义（$P > 0.05$，表 3）。

表 3　各组斑块组织 MMP-3 和 CD40L 的阳性表达（%，$\bar{\chi} \pm s$）

组别	n	MMP-3	CD40L
正常对照	9	–	–
模型对照	7	18.08±4.71	10.58±2.61
辛伐他汀	8	10.43±2.99**	7.99±1.01*
XSC 低剂量	8	11.15±2.15**	7.40±2.02*
XSC 高剂量	8	9.42±1.79**	7.33±1.99*

注：与模型对照组比较，$^*P < 0.05$，$^{**}P < 0.01$

3. 讨论

AS 形成过程中的血栓形成、血管壁炎症、细胞增生和基质堆积等病理生理改变都与中医的"血瘀证"有内在的联系。活血化瘀中药临床常用于防治 AS 及其相关疾病，并显示有良好的作用[5]。XSC 为我院治疗 AS 和冠心病的有效经验方，是在传统活血化瘀名方血府逐瘀汤的研究基础上，结合现代药理研究，采用其主要药物川芎、赤芍的有效部位川芎总酚、赤芍总苷组成的中药新药复方制剂。以往研究表明，XSC 在降低血脂水平的同时，可通过多种途径直接或间接地发挥抗炎作用，有一定的稳定斑块的作用[3]。关于 XSC 对 AS 斑块 MMPs 及 TIMP-1 表达的影响，尚未见相关研究报道。

MMPs 是一类生物活性依赖于锌离子，降解细胞外基质能力的酶系家族，至今已识别的超过 20 余种。MMPs 按照其底物的特异性可分为 5 个大类别[6]，胶原酶（如 MMP-1）、明胶酶（如 MMP-9）、基质溶解素（如 MMP-3）、膜型基质金属蛋白酶和其他。而 TIMPs 是细胞表达的 MMPs

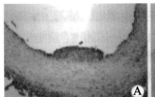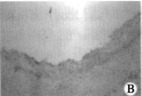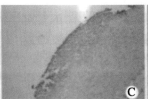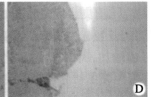

图 2 斑块组织 MMP-3 阳性面积的表达（免疫组化染色，×200）
注：A 为模型对照组；B 为辛伐他汀组；C 为 XSC 低剂量组；D 为 XSC 高剂量组

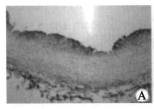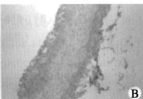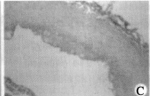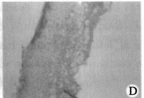

图 3 斑块组织 CD40L 阳性面积的表达（免疫组化染色，×200）
注：A 为模型对照组；B 为辛伐他汀组；C 为 XSC 低剂量组；D 为 XSC 高剂量组

天然抑制物，分 4 个类别，其中 TIMP-1 主要抑制 MMP-1、2、3、9、12。TIMPs 与 MMPs 以 1：1 结合从而抑制其活性，二者互相拮抗，其动态平衡是保持细胞间质稳态的关键。MMPs 参与很多心血管疾病，包括动脉粥样硬化、心室重构、心力衰竭及心房颤动等，其中研究比较深入的是 MMPs 与 AS 斑块破裂、急性冠状动脉综合征（acute coronary syndrome，ACS）的联系。目前已发现多个 MMP 家族成员（MMP-2、3、7、9、13、MT1-MMP）在 AS 斑块中高表达[7,8]。一般认为 MMPs 活性增强可促进 AS 斑块纤维帽中的基质成分的降解，使纤维帽变薄，加速斑块破裂而并发血栓形成，使动脉管腔阻塞程度加重甚至完全阻塞，故认为其与斑块的稳定性密切相关[9]。抑制 MMPs 的表达对于稳定斑块，防治 AS 的发生具有重要意义。

有研究表明，MMP-3 和 MMP-9 都与 AS 斑块的稳定性密切相关[10]，MMP-3 底物较多，并且可以激活许多 MMPs，由于它在 AS 斑块中高表达，被认为对 AS 的进展起了推动作用[6,7]。MMP-9 基因缺失可以减小 AS 斑块面积，降低斑块内巨噬细胞的数量，增加胶原含量，结果较有说服力[11]。本研究中 MMP-3 与 AS 进展相伴随的现象亦支持上述推断，XSC 抑制了血清 MMP-3 和 MMP-9 的表达（同时反映在可以降低斑块内 MMP-3 水平），从而发挥减少斑块局部基质降解的作用，有利于保持斑块的稳定性。XSC 高低剂量组与辛伐他汀组之间差异无统计学意义，提示 XSC 高剂量作用与辛伐他汀相当。本实验中 TIMP-1 各组之间变化不大，XSC 对 TIMP-1 的表达无影响。

CD40L 是肿瘤坏死因子超家族的成员之一，功能性的 CD40L 可表达在 AS 斑块的内皮细胞、巨噬细胞和平滑肌细胞表面，并诱导黏附分子、炎性细胞因子、MMPs、组织因子等明显增加；而且激活的 T 淋巴细胞经 CD40L/CD40 诱导单核 - 巨噬细胞、内皮细胞、血管平滑肌细胞表达 MMPs[12]。本研究结果表明，XSC 高、低剂量组 CD40L 的阳性染色面积与模型对照组比较均有显著减少（$P < 0.05$），同时斑块内 MMP-3 水平亦降低，提示 XSC 可能通过 CD40L 途径发挥调节 MMPs 表达和分泌的作用。

本研究着重观察赤芍川芎有效部位对 AS 斑块 MMPs 的表达，结果表明模型对照组 MMPs 比正常对照组显著提高，提示 AS 时存在着斑块不稳定和细胞外基质降解增加，而 XSC 能显著抑制 MMPs 的表达，显著改善家兔腹主动脉形态学变化，这可能是其稳定粥样斑块、抗动脉粥样硬化的作用机制之一。

参考文献

[1] Arora S, Nicholls SJ. Atherosclerotic plaque reduction: blood pressure, dyslipidemia, atherothrombosis. Drugs Todays (Barc), 2008，44 (9): 711-718.

[2] Ye S. Influence of matrix metalloproteinase genotype on cardiovascular disease susceptibility and outcome. Cardiovasc Res, 2006，69 (3): 636-645.

[3] 徐浩，文川，陈可冀，等. 川芎、赤芍及其有效部位配伍对载脂蛋白E基因缺陷小鼠动脉粥样硬化斑块稳定性影响的研究. 中国中西医结合杂志，2007，27 (6): 513-518.

[4] 韩晓枫，张威，赵益明. 高脂饲料加球囊扩张动脉粥样硬化兔腹主动脉模型的建立. 临床和实验医学杂志，2006，5 (11): 1679-1680.

[5] 蔡春霞，郭玉成. 活血化瘀方药防治动脉粥样硬化的研究近况. 河北医学，2003，9 (8): 760-761.

[6] Visse R, Nagase H. Matrix metalloproteinases and tissue inhibitors of metalloproteinases: structure, function, and biochemistry. Circ Res, 2003, 92 (8): 827-839.

[7] Faia KL, Davis WP, Marone AJ, et al. Matrix metalloproteinases and tissue inhibitors of metallo-proteinases in hamster aortic atherosclerosis: correlation with in-situ zymography. Atherosclerosis, 2002, 160 (2): 325-337.

[8] Carrell TW, Burnand KG, Wells GM, et al. Stromelysin-1 (matrix metalloproteinase-3) and tissue inhibitor of metalloproteinase-3 are overexpressed in the wall of abdominal aortic aneurysms. Circulation, 2002, 105 (4): 477-482.

[9] Abilleira S, Bevan S, Markus HS. The role of genetic variants of matrix metalloproteinases in coronary and carotid atherosclerosis. J Med Genet, 2006, 43 (12): 897-901.

[10] Pollanen PJ, Lehtimaki T, Mikkelsson J, et al. Matrix metalloproteinase-3 and 9 gene promoter polymorphisms: joint action of two loci as a risk factor for coronary artery complicated plaques. Atherosclerosis, 2005, 180 (1): 73-78.

[11] Grav E, Thomas TL, Betmouni S, et al. Elevated matrix metalloproteinase-9 and degradation of perineuronal nets in cerebrocortical multiple sclerosis plaques. J Neuropathol Exp Neuol, 2008, 67 (9): 888-899.

[12] San Miguel Hernndez A, Inglada-Galiana L, Garca Iglesias R, et al. Soluble CD40 ligand: a potential marker of cardiovascular risk. Rev Clin Esp, 2007, 207 (8): 418-421.

辛伐他汀对兔动脉粥样硬化斑块稳定性及斑块内血管新生的影响 *

张 璐 蒋跃绒 薛 梅 吴彩凤 王景尚 殷惠军

动脉粥样硬化（atherosclerosis，AS）斑块的不稳定、破裂，血管收缩和局部血栓形成，导致部分或全部血管阻塞是急性冠状动脉综合征发病的主要机制。研究发现，AS斑块内常出现病理性新生血管，它可能促进粥样硬化病变的发展，甚至诱发斑块内出血和斑块破裂[1]。辛伐他汀（Simvastatin）作为一种降脂药物在临床上已广泛应用。近年来，有研究发现它还具有非特异性抗炎作用，并对斑块能起稳定作用[2]，但辛伐他汀对AS斑块内血管新生的影响仅见个别报道[3]。基于此，我们采用高脂加球囊导管血管损伤术造成动脉粥样硬化斑块模型，研究辛伐他汀对动脉粥样硬化模型斑块稳定性相关指标和斑块内血管新生指标变化，从斑块内血管新生角度探讨辛伐他汀稳定斑块的作用机制。

1. 材料与方法

1.1 材料、试剂与仪器

新西兰兔，雄性，体重 1.8 ~ 2.2kg，北京维通利华实验动物有限公司提供，动物许可证号：SCXK（京）2005-0002。高脂饲料由军事医学科学院实验动物中心生产。辛伐他汀（批号：07432）每片40mg，杭州默沙东制药有限公司生产；酶联免疫吸附测定法（ELISA）试剂盒，美国 Uscnlife 公司提供；免疫组化一抗工作液，由北京博奥森公司提供；日本 HITACHI 公司 7600-020 型全自动生化分析仪；美国 MULTISKAN EX PRIMARY EIA V 2.3 酶标仪；日本 Olympus BX51 光学显微镜；美国 Image-Pro Plus Version4.5.1 (IPP) 图像分析软件。

* 原载于《科学通报》，2009，54（15）：2228-2232

1.2 动物分组及模型制备

30 只健康新西兰兔，随机分为 3 组：正常对照组、模型对照组、辛伐他汀组，每组 10 只。适应性喂养 1 周后，后两组给予高脂饲料（基础饲料 +2% 胆固醇 +5% 猪油），100g/d，测血脂确认已形成高脂血症。喂养高脂 2 周后，行腹主动脉球囊导管血管损伤术，以确保内膜撕伤，3% 戊巴比妥钠（1mL/kg）经耳缘静脉麻醉后，钝性分离出股动脉，插入球囊导管 2.5mm×15mm，深度 15 ~ 17cm，连接压力泵生理盐水充盈球囊，7 ~ 8 个标准大气压（1 个标准大气压 =1.01325×10⁵Pa），球囊反复牵拉 3 次，退出导管，结扎伤口，逐层缝合伤口。术后肌内注射庆大霉素 8 万单位一次防治感染。正常对照组予普通饲料 100g/d；模型对照组予高脂饲料 100g/d；辛伐他汀组予高脂饲料拌入辛伐他汀 2.5mg/(kg·d)，继续喂养 6 周。球囊导管血管损伤术中死亡兔 2 只，术后感染死亡 2 只，2 只未食用完饲料因而退出实验，其余 24 只兔完成实验获得数据。

1.3 取材

分别于第 2 和第 8 周末，即喂养高脂饲料 2 周后及药物干预 6 周后，耳缘动脉采血（采血前禁食 6h），分离血清，–20℃保存备用。第 8 周末将家兔全部处死，在病变最明显部位（即球囊撕伤内膜处）取下腹主动脉组织，10% 福尔马林固定，常规石蜡包埋，间断均匀切片，切片厚度均为 4μm，分别做 HE 染色和免疫组化染色。

1.4 血脂检测

全自动分析仪测定血清总胆固醇（TC）、三酰甘油（TG）、高密度脂蛋白胆固醇（HDL-C）和低密度脂蛋白胆固醇（LDL-C）。

1.5 血清炎症指标及 MMPs 检测

血清 hs-CRP、MMP-3 和 MMP-9 采用酶联免疫法，按试剂盒说明进行操作，最后用酶标仪在 450nm 处读取各孔吸光度值。以浓度值为横坐标，所测各标准吸光度值为纵坐标，绘制标准曲线。按样本孔测得的吸光度值从标准曲线上查得相应的浓度值，以 μg/L 表示。

1.6 斑块组织大体病理形态学观察

HE 染色后在光学显微镜下观察斑块的基本构成，包括泡沫细胞、脂质沉积和胆固醇结晶等成分。利用 IPP 图像分析软件，对各个切面的动脉粥样硬化斑块面积进行分析，测量斑块面积（PA）、血管横截面积（CVA）及计算校正斑块面积（PA/CVA）。

1.7 斑块内血管内皮生长因子 (vascular endothelial growth factor, VEGF)，FⅧRAg, MMP-3 和 CD40L 的蛋白测定

采用免疫组化染色方法检测斑块内 VEGF、FⅧRAg、MMP-3 和 CD40L 抗体的表达，切片在 60℃的条件下烘烤 1h，二甲苯和梯度乙醇脱蜡，置 5% 过氧化氢溶液 15min 灭活内源性过氧化物酶。4℃，一抗孵育过夜，二抗结合 30min，DAB 显色，苏木精复染、脱水、中性树胶封片。DAB 显色阳性结果为棕黄色颗粒状，用 IPP 图像处理软件计数斑块内 VEGF、FⅧRAg、MMP-3 和 CD40L 阳性区域面积占斑块面积的百分比。

1.8 统计学处理

采用 SPSS 13.0 软件包进行统计学处理。计量资料用均数 ± 标准差（$\bar{\chi}$ ±SD）表示。计量资料两组间比较采用配对 t 检验，多组两两间比较采用方差分析 LSD 检验。

2. 结果

2.1 家兔 AS 斑块病理形态学变化

高脂喂养 8 周后，HE 染色显示正常对照组腹主动脉内膜及中膜均未见泡沫细胞及脂质沉积；模型对照组腹主动脉已形成明显的动脉粥样硬化斑块，内膜明显增厚，内含大量泡沫细胞，内皮下、斑块内有胆固醇结晶，纤维帽形成。辛伐他汀组内皮细胞肿胀、变性减轻，泡沫细胞及脂质沉积较模型对照组减少（图 1）。计算机图像分析结果显示各组之间 AS 斑块 PA 和 CAV 差异无显著性，但辛伐他汀可显著降低 PA/CAV，与模型对照组比较差异有显著性（$P < 0.01$）（表 1）。

2.2 血脂水平比较

结果表明，高脂饲料喂养 2 周后模型对照组和辛伐他汀组血清 TC、TG 和 LDL-C 水平较正常对照组均有显著升高（$P < 0.01$）。药物干预 6 周后，辛伐他汀组血清 TC、TG 和 LDL-C 与模型对照组比较均有显著降低（$P < 0.01$）；辛伐他汀组 HDL-C 较模型对照组有升高趋势，但变化无统计学差异（表 2）。

2.3 血清 hs-CRP 水平变化

药物干预 6 周后，各组血清 hs-CRP 浓度明显高于正常对照组，其中模型对照组为（9.80±1.39）μg/mL。辛伐他汀组为（8.65±1.33）μg/mL，与模型对照组比较有显著降低（$P < 0.05$）（表 3）。

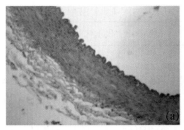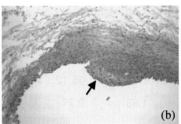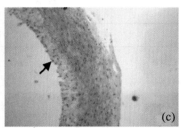

图 1　家兔腹主动脉粥样硬化斑块组织形态变化

（a）正常对照组；（b）模型对照组；（c）辛伐他汀组（HE 染色，×200）

表 1　斑块 PA、CVA 和 PA/CVA 变化比较（$\bar{\chi}$ ±SD）[a]

组别	样本数（n）	PA/mm²	CVA/mm²	PA/CVA（%）
正常对照组	9	–	1.88±0.28	–
模型对照组	7	0.46±0.23	1.90±0.21	28.48±5.47
辛伐他汀组	8	0.29±0.17	1.95±0.17	12.76±3.93**

[a] 与模型对照组比较，**$P < 0.01$

表 2　血脂水平比较（单位：mmol/L，$\bar{\chi}$ ±SD）[a]

组别		样本数（n）	TC	TG	HDL-C	LDL-C
正常对照组	第 2 周	10	1.75±0.81	0.52±0.17	0.37±0.15	0.61±0.39
	第 8 周	9	1.75±0.47**	0.51±0.19**	0.43±0.19**	0.91±0.08**
模型对照组	第 2 周	10	15.77±3.97△△	1.92±1.04△△	0.78±0.15	7.63±2.41△△
	第 8 周	7	30.01±3.11	2.79±0.83	0.81±0.21	14.59±2.38
辛伐他汀组	第 2 周	10	14.65±4.42△△	1.75±0.76△△	0.88±0.22	7.21±3.62△△
	第 8 周	8	22.51±2.74**	1.22±0.93**	0.94±0.21	10.41±2.61**

[a] 与第 8 周末模型对照组比较，* 示 $P < 0.05$；** 示 $P < 0.01$；△△，与第 2 周末正常对照组比较，$P < 0.01$

表 3　血清 hs-CRP 和 MMPs 水平变化（μg/L，$\bar{\chi}$ ±SD）[a]

组别	样本数（n）	hs-CRP	MMP-3	MMP-9
正常对照组	9	7.35±0.44**	21.04±2.81**	0.65±0.17**
模型对照组	7	9.80±1.39△△	56.82±18.57△△	1.11±0.07△△
辛伐他汀组	8	8.65±1.33*△	42.79±13.66*△△	0.90±0.23*△

[a] 与模型对照组比较，* 示 $P < 0.05$，** 示 $P < 0.01$；与正常对照组比较，△示 $P < 0.05$，△△示 $P < 0.01$

2.4　血清 MMP-3 和 MMP-9 水平变化

模型对照组和辛伐他汀组血清 MMP-3、MMP-9 水平明显高于正常对照组（$P < 0.05$，$P < 0.01$）；辛伐他汀组 MMP-3 和 MMP-9 表达与模型对照组比较有明显降低（$P < 0.05$），但两组之间无显著性差异（$P > 0.05$）（表 3）。

2.5　免疫组化定量分析

免疫组化和图像分析结果显示（图 2），正常对照组腹主动脉内膜光滑，无斑块形成，故阳性面积率无法统计；模型对照组斑块内可见大量棕黄色颗粒，特别是在斑块肩部和基底部明显聚集。与模型对照组比较，辛伐他汀组 VEGF、

FⅧ RAg、MMP-3 和 CD40L 的阳性染色面积比均显著减少，组间比较差异具有统计学意义（$P < 0.05$，$P < 0.01$）（表 4）。

3.　讨论

冠心病是目前心血管病致残和死亡的主要原因，也是近年来国际心血管病研究领域的热点，世界上冠心病的发病率呈逐年上升趋势。动脉粥样硬化不稳定斑块是冠心病心肌缺血和各种临床症状的主要原因，且有研究表明冠心病的疾病进程主要由冠状动脉内斑块的生物学性状所决定[4]。因此，稳定斑块、预防斑块破裂和阻止动脉粥样硬化的发

表 4　斑块组织 VEGF、FⅧRAg、MMP-3 和 CD40L 阳性面积表达率（$\bar{\chi} \pm SD$）

组别	样本数（n）	VEGF（%）	FⅧRAg（%）	MMP-3（%）	CD40L（%）
正常对照组	9	–	–	–	–
模型对照组	7	22.65±2.94	15.12±1.45	18.08±4.71	11.08±2.48
辛伐他汀组	8	19.40±1.63	9.77±2.23	10.43±2.99	7.93±0.91
t 值		2.363	4.922	3.467	2.917
P 值		0.046	0.001	0.006	0.015

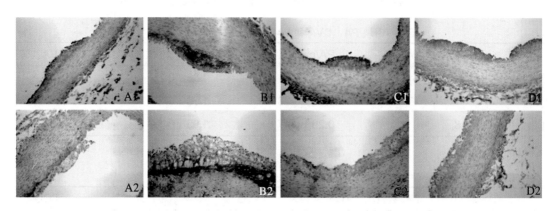

图 2　斑块组织 VEGF、FⅧR Ag、MMP-3 和 CD40L 阳性面积的表达

A，VEGF 阳性面积的表达；B，FⅧR Ag 阳性面积的表达；C，MMP-3 阳性面积的表达；D，CD40L 阳性面积的表达，1，模型对照组；2，辛伐他汀组（免疫组化染色，×200）

展，在一定程度上能改善冠心病病程进展及预后。

近年的研究发现，AS 斑块内常出现病理性新生血管，它们是在 AS 病变基础上发生的，新生血管又促进粥样硬化病变的发展，在 AS 斑块的发生发展中可能是一个核心事件而起着关键性作用[5]。因此，抑制斑块内血管新生可能成为增强斑块稳定性，防治急性冠状动脉综合征的靶点，具有潜在的治疗意义。

他汀类药物能有效减少冠心病的发病率和死亡率，除与其降低低密度脂蛋白胆固醇（LDL-C）有关外，还体现了越来越多的不依赖于降脂作用的心血管保护效应，被称为他汀类药物的多效性，包括改善内皮功能、稳定易损斑块、抗炎、抗氧化、免疫调节、降压、抑制血栓形成等[6]。辛伐他汀为羟甲基戊二酰辅酶 A（HMG CoA）还原酶抑制剂，能抑制内源性胆固醇的合成，进而发挥降低血脂的作用。辛伐他汀在降低血脂水平的同时，还可以抑制内皮细胞的迁移、黏附，降低基质金属蛋白酶的分泌而达到稳定斑块的作用[7]。

动脉粥样硬化是炎症性疾病，炎症反应贯穿于动脉粥样硬化的发展过程，是动脉粥样硬化发生、发展的中心环节，高敏 C 反应蛋白（hs-CRP）是反映动脉粥样硬化炎症过程的敏感指标[8]。本实验结果显示，模型对照组血清 hs-CRP 浓度显著升高，辛伐他汀组比模型组明显降低，表明抑制了 AS 的炎症进程。

MMPs 是一组可消化细胞外基质的重要酶类，它通过降解纤维帽成分，破坏其结构，加速斑块破裂，是造成 AS 斑块不稳定的重要原因[9]。CD40L 可表达在动脉粥样硬化斑块的内皮细胞、巨噬细胞和平滑肌细胞表面，并诱导单核—巨噬细胞、内皮细胞、血管平滑肌细胞表达 MMPs[10]。本实验结果表明，模型对照组血清 MMP-3 和 MMP-9 比正常对照组显著提高，提示 AS 时存在着斑块不稳定和细胞外基质降解增加，而辛伐他汀显著抑制血清 MMP-3 和 MMP-9（同时反映在可以降低斑块内 MMP-3 水平和 CD40L）的表达，从而发挥减少斑块局部的基质降解的作用，有利于保持斑块的稳定性。

VEGF 是迄今发现的具有特异性促进血管内皮细胞有丝分裂的生长因子，已证明在动脉粥样硬化斑块中的表达明显增加，并可能促进斑块的发生与发展[11,12]。FⅧRAg 是广泛存在于内皮细胞表面的一种糖蛋白，是新生血管内皮的特异性标记物，表达于小的毛细血管及毛细血管尚未形成管腔的分支，二者共同参与血管形成过程[13]。本研究结果显示，辛伐他汀可一定程度抑制 VEGF 和 FⅧR Ag 在家兔 AS 斑块模型中的表达。病理学观察结果则显示，在给予高脂饮食的情况下，辛伐他汀组血管形态学指标明显优于单纯高脂饮食组（即模型对照组），也表明辛伐他汀对于改善斑块面积、控制 AS 斑块具有一定作用。

综上所述，辛伐他汀可以抑制炎症反应，并通过降低基质金属蛋白酶的分泌而达到稳定斑块的作用，这和以往的研究结果是一致的[7]。除此之外，辛伐他汀还可抑制在动脉粥样硬化斑块中 VEGF 和 FⅧRAg 的表达，可见抑制斑块内病理性血管新生是其稳定斑块的又一作用机制。

参考文献

[1] Ross J, Staglian N, Donovan M, et al. Atheroselerosis and cancer: common molecular pathways of disease development and progression. Ann N Y Acad Sci, 2001，947：271-292.

[2] Sacco RL, Liao JK. Drug insight, Statins and stroke. Nat Clin Pract Cardiovasc Med, 2005，2：576-584.

[3] Wilson SH, Herrmann J, Lerman LO, et al. Simvastatin preserves the structure of coronary adventitial vasa vasorum in experimental hypercholesterolemia independent of lipid lowering. Circulation, 2002，105：415-418.

[4] Thrall G, Lane D, Carroll D, et al. A systematic review of the effects of acute psychological stress and physical activity on haemorheology, coagulation, fibrinolysis and platelet reactivity: implications for the pathogenesis of acute coronary syndromes. Thromb Res, 2007，120：819-847.

[5] 孙璐，韦立新，石怀银，等. 冠状动脉粥样硬化版块内血管新生与斑块稳定的关系. 中华病理学杂志，2003, 32: 427-431.

[6] 夏城东，殷惠军. 他汀类药物改善内皮功能的多效应研究进展. 心血管进展，2008, 29: 956-960.

[7] Rudd JH, Machac J, Favad ZA. Simvastatin and plaque inflammation. J Am Coll Cardiol, 2007, 48: 1825-1831.

[8] Schlager O, Exner M, Mlekusch W, et al. C-reactive protein predicts future cardiovascular events in patients with carotid stenosis. Stroke, 2007, 38: 1263-1268.

[9] Abilleira S, Bevan S, Markus HS. The role of genetic variants of matrix metalloproteinases in coronary and carotid atherosclerosis. J Med Genet, 2006, 43: 897-901.

[10] San Miguel Hernández A, Inglada-Galiana L, García Iglesias R, et al. Soluble CD40 ligand: a potential marker of cardiovascular risk. Rev Clin Esp, 2007，207: 418-421.

[11] Caldwell RB, Bartoli M, Behzadian MA, et al. Vascular endothelial growth factor and diabetic retinopathy: role of oxidative stress. Curr Drug Targets, 2005, 6: 511-524.

[12] Panutsopulos D, Papalambros E, Sigala F, et al. Protein and mRNA expression levels of VEGF-A and TGF-beta1 in different types of human coronary atherosclerotic lesions. Int J Mol Med, 2005, 15: 603-610.

[13] Galbusera M, Zoja C, Donadelli R, et al. Fluid shear stress modulates von Willebrand factor release from human vascular endothelium. Blood, 1997, 90：1558-1564.

第四章

Panax Quinquefolium Saponins Inhibited Immune Maturation of Human Monocyte-Derived Dendritic Cells via Blocking Nuclear Factor-κB Pathway[*]

LIU Hong-ying   SHI Da-zhuo   WANG Wei   ZHANG Chun-yu   FU Ming-qiang   GE Jun-bo

第四章

1. Introduction

Atherosclerosis (AS) is an inflammatory disease characterized by intense immunological activity and immune responses[1-3]. Dendritic cells (DCs) are the most potent antigen-presenting cells (APC) and are involved in the collaboration between innate and adaptive immunity. In recent years, there are studies revealed that mature DCs could promote the initiation of AS[4,5] and contributed to atherosclerotic plaque destabilization[6]. Panax quinquefolium saponins (PQS) extracted from stems and leaves of *radix panacis quinquefolii* have been regarded as the principal components responsible for various biological activities in anti-atherosclerosis, including anti-inflammation, anti-oxidization, free radical scavenging, lipid metabolic regulation and immune modulation [7-11]. Previous researches showed that PQS could inhibit cytokine release in activated macrophage in vitro[12,13]. However, the effect of PQS on DCs in AS remains unclear.

Given its regulation of proinflammatory genes linked to atherosclerosis, nuclear factor κB (NF–κB) has been regarded as a proatherogenic factor[14,15]. Especially, NF-κB involved in the transcriptional regulation of many genes contributed to the function of DCs[16,17]. Therefore,

we hypothesis that PQS might inhibit the immune maturation of ox-LDL-induced human monocyte-derived DCs via blocking NF-κB signal pathway.

2. Materials and Methods

2.1　Antibodies, Proteins and Reagents

Ox-LDL (AbD serotec Co., UK); fluorescein isothiocyanate (FITC)-labeled or phycoerythrin (PE) -labeled human monoclonal anti-CD1a, anti-CD40，anti-CD86，anti-HLA- DR, anti-CD14 antibodies, IL-12p70，and TNF-αELISA kits, Trizol reagent (Invitrogen, USA); anti-IκBα, anti-phospho-IκBα, anti-Rel A, anti-Rel B, anti-c-Rel, anti-β-actin antibodies (Cell Signaling Technology, USA); human recombinant IL-4 and GM-CSF (R&D Systerm, USA); FITC-labeled dextran of molecular mass 40 kDa, Histopaque-1077 (Sigma Aldrich, USA); human CD14 MicroBeads (Milteny Biotech Co., Germany); RPMI-1640 (Gibco-BRL Life Technologies, UK); FBS (Hyclone Logan, USA); Proteo JET™ cytoplasmic and nuclear protein extraction kit (Fermentas Life Sciences, CA), BCA protein assay kit (Pierce Biotech Co., USA), Annexin V apoptosis detection kit (BD Biosciences, USA), PrimeScript™ RT reagent Kit (Takara Biosciences Inc., Japan), SYBR®

* 原载于 Journal of Ethnopharmacology, 2012, 141（3）：982-988

Premix Ex Taq™ Kit (Takara Biosciences Inc., Japan), TransAM™ NF-κB family kit (Active Motif Inc., USA). PQS was kindly provided by YiSheng Company (Jilin Province, China), and was dissolved into 1 × phosphate-buffered saline (PBS) for the final concentration of 50μg/mL.

2.2 Generation of Human Peripheral Blood Monocyte-derived DCs

Human peripheral blood mononuclear cells (PBMCs) were separated by density gradient centrifugation using Histopaque 1077 according to an established protocol[18]. The monocytes were isolated by positive selection using CD14+ microbeads, then CD14+ cells were seeded into six-well flat-bottom plates with 10^6 cells per well, cultured in 2 mL RPMI-1640 containing 100 ng/mL GM-CSF, 40 ng/mL IL-4，and 10% fetal bovine serum (FBS) for 5 days, then DCs were derived. To investigate the effects of PQS on DCs, 50μg/mL PQS was added to the DCs medium, followed by an addition of PBS, or ox-LDL (50μg/mL) 24 h later, which stayed there for 24 h. Cell viability was over 90% as assessed by Typan blue staining.

2.3 Preparation of PQS

PQS were kindly provided by Jilin Yisheng Pharmaceutic (Jilin, China). The herbal drugs were authenticated and standardized on marker compounds according to the Chinese Pharmacopoeia 2005. PQS were prepared as follows: crude powder of dried stems and leaves of radix panacis quinquefolii (American Ginseng) were dissolved with distilled water, then the aqueous extracts were placed in ethanol after filtration and evaporation, subsequently the ethanol solution were fractionated on a macroporous adsorption resin D 101 column with water and 80% ethanol, PQS were obtained under vacuum drying at 60 ℃. To reduce the dose and purity variability of PQS among different batches, the species, origin, harvest time, medicinal parts, and concocted methods for *radix panacis quinquefolii* were strictly standardized.

2.4 Flow Cytometry Analysis of DCs

The changes in the surface marker expressions of DCs were analyzed by flow cytometry. Briefly, DCs were washed, resuspended in ice-cold 1 × PBS, then incubated with FITC-labeled or PE-labeled monoclonal anti-CD1a, anti-CD40，anti-CD86，anti-HLADR for 30 min at 4 ℃. Cells were washed twice and fixed with 4% paraformaldehyde. Thereafter, the immunofluorescence analysis was performed using a FACS Caliber (BD Biosciences, CA) and analyzed using Cell Quest software.

2.5 Determination of Endocytotic Ability of DCs

Endocytotic ability of DCs was measured as the uptake of FITC-dextran. In medium containing FITC-dextran (1 mg/mL) were incubated 2×10^5 cells per sample at 37℃ for 30 min. After that, the cells were washed twice with cold PBS containing 5% FBS for an analysis with FACS Caliber as described above.

2.6 Measurement of Cytokine Secretion of DCs

The supernatants of cultured DCs were stored at –70 ℃ . The cytokine concentrations of TNF-α, IL-12p70 were analyzed using ELISA kits according to the manufacturer's instructions.

2.7 Preparation of Nuclear and Cytoplasmic Extracts

Nuclear extracts were prepared from DCs using cytoplasmic and nuclear protein extraction kit as described previously[19]. Nuclear and cytoplasmic extracts were stored at –80℃.

2.8 Western Blot Analysis

Nuclear and cytoplasmic cell extracts (20μg per each sample) were subjected to 12% SDS-PAGE (Invitrogen, USA) and proteins were transferred into polyvinylidene fluoride membranes (Millipore, USA). Then, the membranes with blotted protein were blocked, followed by probing with anti-IκBα, anti-phospho-IκBα, anti-Rel A, anti-Rel B, anti-c-Rel, anti-β-actin antibodies at 4℃ overnight. The membranes were washed and incubated at room temperature for 2 h with diluted (1∶5000) secondary HRP-marked antibodies. Immunoreactive proteins were identified using Super Signal West Pico Chemiluminescence Substrate (Thermo, USA). The ChemiDocTM XRS gel documentation system (Bio-Rad, USA) with Quantity One software was used to quantify the immunoreactive proteins. β-actin was used as the loading control.

2.9 Preparation of RNA Extracts and Quantitative Real Time RT-PCR Analysis

Total RNA was extracted from DCs with Trizol reagent according to the manufacturer's instructions. The cDNA was generated by reverse transcriptase from RNA using the PrimeScript™ RT reagent Kit according to the manufacturer's instructions. Then the SYBR® Premix Ex Taq™ Kit was used for real-time PCR reaction according to the manufacturer's instructions. GAPDH, a housweeping gene, was used as an internal control for c-Rel mRNA expression. The sequences for the specific primers used in this study were the following: c-Rel (Gene Bank ID: NM_002908.2) primer sequences were 5′-ttttcctgagagaccaagacct-3′and 5′-gcttgacttgaaacccctgtag-3′, GAPDH (Gene Bank ID: NM 002046.3) primers sequences were 5′-agaaggctggggctcatttg-3′and 5′-aggggccatccacagtcttc-3′. Real-time PCR was performed in an iCycler iQ real-time PCR detection system (Bio-Rad, USA). The c-Rel gene expression in each sample was normalized to GAPDH.

2.10 Analysis of NF-κB Activation

NF-κB activation was measured and quantified by ELISA using a TransAM™ NF-κB family kit as described previously[20]. The absorbance was measured by a spectrophotometer (Eppendorf, Germany) at 450 nm wavelength. The optical density (OD) was normalized to the standard curve.

2.11 Statistical Analyses

Data were expressed as mean ± SD. The comparison between two experimental groups was performed using Student's t test for unpaired data. For multiple comparisons, one-way ANOVA with Bonferroni/Dunn analysis was

used. Statistical analysis was performed with software SPSS 11.5, and a P-value < 0.05 was considered statistically significant.

3. Results

3.1 Exposure to PQS Inhibited the Immune Maturation of ox-LDL-induced DCs

CD14$^+$ microbeads-sorted monocytes were symmetrical, with the purity over 98% (Figure S1). Most of the cells formed different clones 24h later, which grew larger 72 h later, in round shape with needle-like processes. Mature marker expression of co-stimulatory molecules CD1a was examined in 50μg/ml ox-LDL-treated DCs exposed to various concentrations of PQS (0, 25, 50, 100, and 200μg/ml) for 24h. Pilot experiments showed that 50μg/ml PQS could inhibit nearly 60% expression of CD1a (Figure S2). When checking the viability of the cell populations and rate of apoptosis induction by annexin V and propidium iodide double cell staining, we did not detect any increase in the rate of apoptotic and dead cells following exposure to 50μg/ml PQS (Figure S3). This implied that the effect of PQS on CD1a expression was not mediated by induction of apoptosis in DCs. Therefore PQS at a concentration of 50μg/ml was used in the present study.

Next, we explored the effect of PQS on the immune maturation of ox-LDL-induced DCs. Ox-LDL stimulating resulted in an obvious up-regulation of CD1a, CD40, CD86, and HLA-DR expression of DCs, as indicated. Incubation of DCs with PQS reduced up-regulation of expression of these surface markers (Figure 1A). We also investigated the effect of PQS on the antigen-uptake capacity of DCs by FACS. Ox-LDL reduced the antigen-uptake capacity of DCs, which was rescued by PQS pretreatment (Figure 1B). Cytokine secretion by DCs was also compared. Secretion of IL-12 and TNF-α was increased in ox-LDL-treated DCs, but attenuated by the pretreatment with PQS (Figure 1C). These data indicate that PQS can

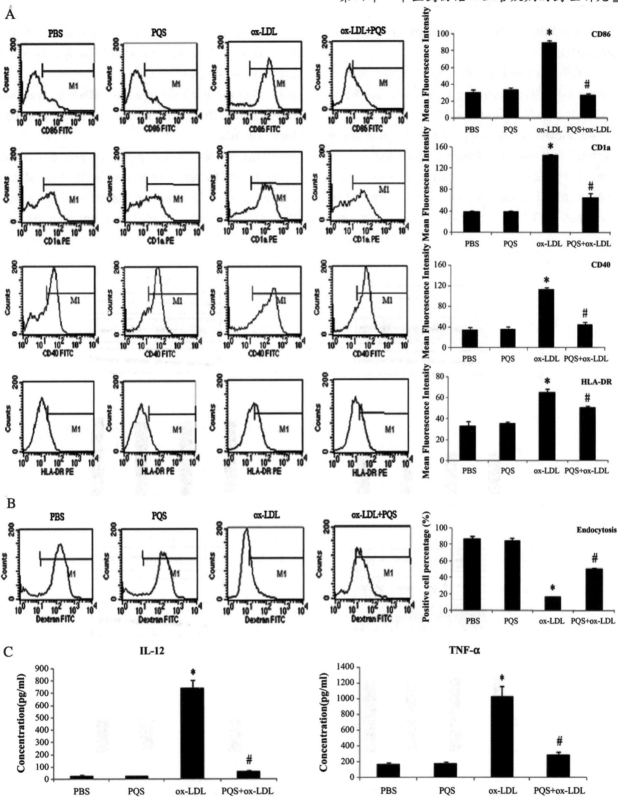

Figure 1　Effects of PQS on Immune Maturation in Human Monocyte-derived DCs. DCs Were Generated as Described above and Stimulated with 50μg/ml ox-LDL or PBS for 24 h in the Absence or Presence of PQS. （A）The expressions of surface molecules （CD40, CD1a, CD86, and HLA-DR）in DCs were analyzed by flow cytometry. The bargraphs represent FITC-labeled or PE-labeled surface markers staining, the black shadows represent loading control, data are from one representative experiment out of three performed. The histograms show mean fluorescence intensity values（mean ± SD）of three independent experiments with similar results in various groups. （B）The endocytic fuction in DCs were analyzed by flow cytometry. The scatter diagrams represent FITC-labeled dextran staining in DCs, data are from one representative experiment out of three performed. The histograms show quantitative results of percentages of positive cells（mean ± SD）of three independent experiments with similar results in various groups. （C）The changes of cytokines secretion in DCs were detected by ELISA. The histograms show the levels of IL-12 and TNF-α（mean ± SD）of three independent experiments with similar results in various groups. *$P < 0.01$ versus PBS and #$P < 0.01$ versus ox-LDL

381

effectively inhibit immune maturation in ox-LDL stimulated DCs.

3.2 PQS Reduced the Protein Expressions of Nuclear c-Rel Transcription Factor but not Rel A and Rel B in ox-LDL-induced DCs

As shown in Figure 2, Western blot analysis revealed that the ctyoplastic protein expression of $pI\kappa B\alpha$ and nuclear-localized c-Rel were significantly increased by ox-LDL stimulation compared with PBS group ($P < 0.01$), but were significantly attenuated with PQS pretreatment ($P < 0.01$). The expressions of Rel A and Rel B proteins were not affected.

3.3 PQS did not Interfere the mRNA Expressions of Nuclear c-Rel Transcription Factor in ox-LDL-Induced DCs

The mRNA expressions of nuclear c-Rel transcription factor were measured by quantitative real time RT-PCR analysis. As shown in Figure3, the mRNA level of c-Rel was not changed by

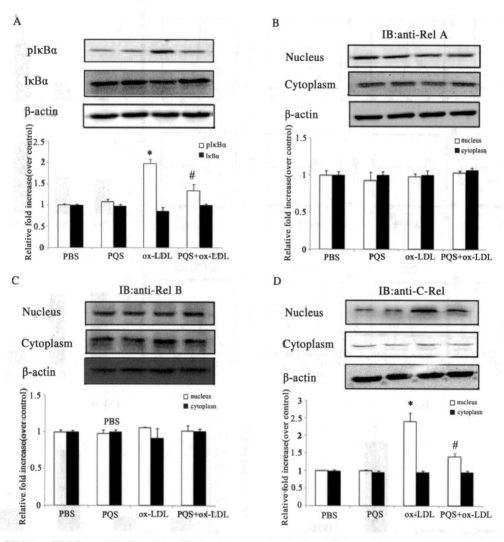

Figure 2　Effects of PQS on NF-κB in Human Monocyte-derived DCs. DCs Were Generated as Described above and Stimulated with 50μg/ml ox-LDL or PBS for 24 h in the Absence or Presence of PQS. Cytoplasmic and nuclear extracts from DCs of various groups were assayed by Western blot analysis. (A) IκBα and pIκBα expressions in cytoplasm. (B) Rel A expression in cytoplasm and nucleus. (C) Rel B expression in cytoplasm and nucleus. (D) c-Rel expression in cytoplasm and nucleus. All experiments were performed in triplicates with similar results. The histograms represent the protein expressions in DCs (mean ± SD), the vertical axis denote fold increase over control (PBS group) after the amount of each protein was normalized to that of β-actin. *$P < 0.01$ versus PBS and #$P < 0.01$ versus ox-LDL

either ox-LDL stimulation or PQS pretreatment in DCs.

3.4 PQS Diminished the Binding Activity of Nuclear c-Rel Transcription Factor in ox-LDL-induced DCs

The binding activity of c-Rel was performed for examining whether PQS-dependent inhibition of ox-LDL-induced DCs maturation associated to down-regulation of c-Rel binding activity. As shown in Figure 4, stimulation with ox-LDL resulted in increased binding activity of c-Rel, while PQS pretreatment diminished binding activity of c-Rel. However, exposure to PQS alone did not affect c-Rel activity without ox-LDL stimulation.

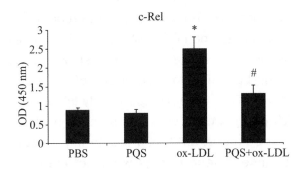

Figure4　Effects of PQS on c-Rel Activation In human Monocyte-derived DCs. DCs Were Generated as Described above and Stimulated with 50μg/ml ox-LDL or PBS for 24 h in the Absence or Presence of PQS. Nuclear extracts from DCs of various groups, and then c-Rel activation was measured and quantified by ELISA using a TransAM™ kit. All experiments were performed in triplicates with similar results. The histograms represent c-Rel activation in DCs (mean ± SD), the vertical axis denote OD at 450 nm detected by spectrophotometer. $^*P < 0.01$ versus PBS and $^\#P < 0.01$ versus ox-LDL

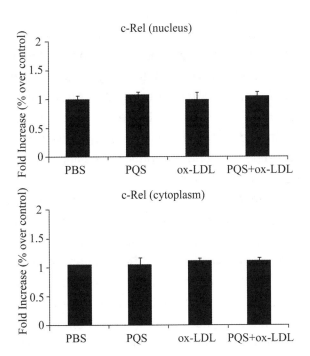

Figure3　Effects of PQS on c-Rel mRNA Expression in Human Monocyte-derived DCs. DCs Were Generated as Described above and Stimulated with 50μg/ml ox-LDL or PBS for 24 h in the Absence Or Presence of PQS. RNA extracts from DCs of various groups were reverse-transcribed, and subsequently assayed by real time PCR analysis. All experiments were performed in triplicates with similar results. The histograms represent the mRNA expressions of c-Rel in DCs (mean ± SD), the vertical axis denote fold increase over control (PBS group) after the amount of each mRNA was normalized to that of GAPDH

4. Discussion

Our study demonstrated that PQS could suppress the immune maturation of DCs induced by ox-LDL partly through inhibiting NF-κB pathway. DCs are professional APCs that are important for the initiation of T cell mediated adaptive immune response[21-23]. DCs maturation is usually accompanied with high expressions of surface marker molecules (e.g., CD40, CD86, CD1a, and HLA-DR) and low endocytosis of antigens, which are necessary for the activation of T lymphocyte. Our study showed that ox-LDL induced up-regulation of CD40, CD1a, CD86, and HLA-DR as well as down-regulation of endocytic function in DCs, and these effects were all significantly attenuated by PQS pretreatment. Both IL-12 and TNF-α are proinflammatory cytokines produced by different APCs, and DCs have emerged as major producers of these cytokines in response to stimuli, such as ox-LDL and LPS[24-27]. IL-12 and TNF-α play a pivotal role in DCs maturation and migration to lymph organs. In addition, they induce the production of other pro-inflammatory cytokines and adhesion molecules, which contribute to the recruitment of monocytes and other cell types, subsequently result in T cell activation[28,29]. Our study showed that ox-LDL-induced secretions of IL-12 and TNF-α in DCs were all significantly inhibited by PQS pretreatment, which might have profound consequences for T cell mediating immune response. These effects were not mediated by induction of apoptosis in DCs, because the analysis of cell viability, which was examined by annexin V and propidium iodide staining, did not reveal a decrease in the apoptosis rate in the presence of PQS. These data suggest that PQS could inhibit phenotypic and functional maturation of DCs induced by ox-LDL.

There are several signaling pathways that contribute to DCs maturation. The most central pathway is mediated by NF-κB as demonstrated in NF-κB knockout mice in previous reports [30,31]. Inhibition of this pathway could block DCs activation, which determined by changed phenotype and function of DCs. In addition, previous studies have shown that ox-LDL could induce maturation in human DCs partly via activation of the NF-κB pathway[27]. Our study identified that PQS pretreatment inhibited the maturation, the transactivation activity and protein expression of NF-κB subunit c-Rel of DC induced by ox-LDL. Therefore, PQS inhibits maturation of ox-LDL stimulated DCs might be related to blocking NF-κB pathway.

NF-κB consists of 5 members, Rel A, Rel B, c-Rel, NF-κB1, and NF-κB2. Rel A, Rel B, and c-Rel are transcriptionally active members, whereas NF-κB1 and NF-κB2 primarily serve as DNA binding subunits. In resting situation, NF-κB dimer is kept inactive in the cytoplasm by an inhibitory protein IκB. Diverse signals induce the nuclear translocation of NF-κB by activating an IκB kinase complex. The complex mediates the phosphorylation of IκB, resulting in its ubiquitination and degradation. Upon translocation to the nucleus, NF-κB regulates gene expression by binding to specific sequences located within the transcriptional regulatory regions of cellular genes. Our study showed that ox-LDL increased the phosphorylation of IκBα, which was significantly repressed by PQS pretreatment. After ox-LDL treatment, the nuclear translocation of c-Rel significantly increased, which was blocked by PQS. These data indicated that PQS inhibited the maturation of DCs induced by ox-LDL through blocking IκBα phosphorylation and subsequently translocation of c-Rel to the nucleus.

DCs development and survival are controlled by different NF-κB subunits[32]. Knockouts of individual NF-κB subunits display distinct phenotypes that likely reflect their ability to regulate different sets of target genes. Our study showed that Rel A and Rel B subunits are not changed upon treatment, while only c-Rel subunit changed significantly following treatment. The underlying mechanism might be different functional subsets of genes are regulated by distinct NF-κB subunits. Evidences accumulated that individual NF-κB subunits show specificity in regulating target gene expression be linked to the sequence of κB sites[33].

Both in vivo and in vitro studies have revealed that c-Rel plays a critical role in the maturation and cytokines induction of DCs[34-38]. We therefore analyzed the expression of c-Rel by quantitative real time RT-PCR and the activity of c-Rel by ELISA. We found the mRNA expressions of c-Rel were not changed in nucleus or in cytoplasm either by ox-LDL stimulation or by PQS pretreatment. This indicated the effect of PQS pretreatment on c-Rel might be at post-transcriptional level. Our study showed here that exposure of ox-LDL-induced DCs to PQS resulted in the binding activity of c-Rel significantly reduced, while PQS alone did not inhibit c-Rel activation. It suggests that PQS could not directly block c-Rel activation. However, the exact mechanisms by which PQS specificity is conferred in regulating NF-κB subunit c-Rel of

DC are presently unknown.

5. Conclusion

In summary, present study demonstrated that PQS could inhibit immune maturation of DCs induced by ox-LDL in vitro, which might be mediated via blocking NF-κB signal pathway. Future studies are warranted to verify whether PQS could attenuate AS in vivo through the above indicating mechanism.

References

[1] Binder CJ, Chang MK, Shaw PX, et al. Innate and acquired immunity in atherogenesis. Nature Medicine, 2002, 8: 1218-1226.

[2] Hansson GK, Libby P. The immune response in atherosclerosis: a double edged sword. Nature Reviews Immunology, 2006, 6: 508-519.

[3] Roberts WC. The cause of atherosclerosis. Nutrition Clinical Practice, 2008, 23: 464-467.

[4] Link A, Bohm M. Potential role of dendritic cells in atherogenesis. Cardiovascular Research, 2008, 55: 708-709.

[5] Ranjit S, Dazhu L. Potential role of dendritic cells for progression of atherosclerotic lesions. Postgraduate Medicine Journal, 2006, 82: 573-575.

[6] Yilmaz A, Lochno M, Traeg F. Emergence of dendritic cells in rupture-prone regions of vulnerable carotid plaques. Atherosclerosis, 2004, 176: 101-110.

[7] Mizuno M, Yamada J, Terai H, et al. Differences in immunomodulating effects between wild and cultured Panax ginseng. Biochemical Biophysical Research Communications, 1994, 200: 1672-1678.

[8] Liu M, Zhang JT. Studies on the mechanisms of immunoregulatory effects of ginsenoside Rg1 in aged rats. Yao Xue Xue Bao, 1996, 31: 95-100.

[9] Kim SH, Park KS. Effects of Panax ginseng extract on lipid metabolism in humans. Pharmacological Research, 2003, 48: 511-513.

[10] Yoon M, Lee H, Jeong S, et al. Peroxisome proliferator-activated receptor alpha is involved in the regulation of lipid metabolism by ginseng. British Journal of Pharmacology, 2003, 138: 1295-1302.

[11] Liao H, Banbury LK, Leach DN. Antioxidant activity of 45 Chinese herbs and the relationship with their TCM characteristics. Evidence Based Complement Alternative Medicine, 2008, 5: 429-434.

[12] Niu YP, Jin JM, Gao RL, et al. Effects of ginsenosides Rg1 and Rb1 on proliferation of human marrow granulocyte-macrophage progenitor cells. Zhongguo Shi Yan Xue Ye Xue Za Zhi, 2001, 9: 178-180.

[13] Haddad PS, Azar GA, Groom S, et al. Natural health products, modulation of immune function and prevention of chronic diseases. Evidence Based Complement Alternative Medicine, 2005, 2: 513-520.

[14] De Winther MP, Kanters E, Kraal G, et al. Nuclear factor kappa B signaling in atherogenesis. Arteriosclerosis Thrombosis Vascular Biology, 2005, 25, 904-914.

[15] Dabŵ J, Kulach A, Gasior Z. Nuclear factor kappa-light-chain-enhancer of activated B cells (NF-kappa B): a new potential therapeutic target in atherosclerosis? Pharmacological Reports, 2010, 62: 778-783.

[16] Tan PH, Sagoo P, Chan C, et al. Inhibition of NF-kappa B and oxidative pathways in human dendritic cells by antioxidative vitamins generates regulatory T cells. Journal of Immunology, 2005, 174: 7633-7644.

[17] Wang J, Wang X, Hussain S, et al. Distinct roles of different NF-kappa B subunits in regulating inflammatory and T cell stimulatory gene expression in dendritic cells. Journal of Immunology, 2007, 178: 6777-6788.

[18] Ge J, Jia Q, Liang C, et al. Advanced glycosylation end products might promote atherosclerosis through inducing the immune maturation of dendritic cells. Arteriosclerosis Thrombosis Vascular Biology, 2005, 25: 2157-2163.

[19] Appel S, BoŴmler AM, Grunebach F, et al. Imatinib mesylate affects the development and function of dendritic cells generated from CD34$^+$ peripheral blood progenitor cells. Blood, 2004, 103: 538-544.

[20] Semnani RT, Venugopal PG, Leifer CA, et al. Inhibition of TLR3 and TLR4 function and expression in human dendritic cells by helminth parasites. Blood, 2008, 112: 1290-1298.

[21] Guermonprez P, Valladeau J, Zitvogel L, et al. Antigen presentation and T cell stimulation by dendritic cells. Annual Review Immunology, 2002, 20: 621-667.

[22] Elbe-Burger A, Stingl G. The role of dendritic cells in immunity. Potential clinical use. Annales de

Dermatologie et de Venereologie, 2004, 131: 93-103.

[23] Wallet MA, Sen P, Tisch R. Immun-oregulation of dendritic cells. Clinical Medicine Research, 2005, 3: 166 -175.

[24] Syme R, Gluck S. Generation of dendritic cells: role of cytokines and potential clinical applications. Transfusion Apheresis Science, 2001, 24: 117-124.

[25] Alderman CJ, Bunyard PR, Chain BM, et al. Effects of oxidised low density lipoprotein on dendritic cells: a possible immunoregulatory component of the atherogenic micro-environment? Cardiovascular Research，2002，55：806-819.

[26] Luo Y, Liang C, Xu C, et al. Ciglitazone inhibits oxidized-low density lipoprotein induced immune maturation of dendritic cells. Journal of Cardiovascular Pharmacology, 2004, 44: 381-385.

[27] Nickel T, Schmauss D, Hanssen H, et al. ox-LDL uptake by dendritic cells induces upregulation of scavenger-receptors, maturation and differentiation. Atherosclerosis, 2009, 205: 442-450.

[28] Correale M, Brunetti ND, Di Biase M. The pro-inflammatory role of cytokines in the mechanism of atherosclerosis. G Italin Cardiology (Rome), 2006, 7: 594-603.

[29] Tedgui A, Mallat Z. Cytokines in atherosclerosis: pathogenic and regulatory pathways. Physiological Reviews, 2006, 86: 515-581.

[30] Dai R, Phillips RA, Ahmed SA. Despite inhibition of nuclear localization of NF-kappa B p65, c-Rel, and RelB, 17-beta estradiol up-regulates NF-kappa B signaling in mouse splenocytes: the potential role of Bcl-3. Journal of Immunology, 2007, 179: 1776-1783.

[31] Wang X, Yu X, Qu S. Protective effect and mechanism of IPQDS on acute myocardial infarction in rats. Zhongguo Zhong Yao Za Zhi, 2009, 34: 3281-3285.

[32] Ouaaz F, Arron J, Zheng Y, et al. Dendritic cell development and survival require distinct NF-κB subunits. Immunity, 2002, 16: 257-270.

[33] Leung TH, Hoffmann A, Baltimore D. One nucleotide in a κB site can determine cofactor specificity for NF-κB dimers. Cell, 2004, 118: 453-464.

[34] Grumont R, Hochrein H, O' keeffe, et al. c-Rel regulates interleukin 12 p70 expression in CD8[+] dendritic cells by specifically inducing p35 gene transcription. Journal of Experimental Medicine, 2001, 194: 1021-1032.

[35] Hsia CY, Cheng S, Owyang AM, et al., c-Rel regulation of the cell cycle in primary mouse B lymphocytes. International Immunology, 2002, 14：905-916.

[36] Mason N, Aliberti J, Caamano JC, et al. Cutting edge: identification of c-Rel-dependent and -independent pathways of IL-12 production during infectious and inflammatory stimuli. Journal of Immunology, 2002, 168: 2590-2594.

[37] Boffa DJ, Feng B, Sharma V, et al. Selective loss of c-Rel compromises dendritic cell activation of T lymphocytes. Cell Immunology, 2003, 222: 105-115.

[38] O' keeffe M, Grumont RJ, Hochrein H, et al. Distinct roles for the NF-kappa B1 and cRel transcription factors in the differentiation and survival of plasmacytoid and conventional dendritic cells activated by TLR-9 signals. Blood, 2005, 106: 3457-3464.

第四章

Effect of Chinese Drugs for Activating Blood Circulation and Detoxifying on Indices of Thrombosis, Inflammatory Reaction, and Tissue Damage in A Rabbit Model of Toxin-Heat and Blood Stasis Syndrome[*]

XUE Mei　YIN Hui-jun　WU Cai-feng　MA Xiao-juan　GUO Chun-yu　HUANG Ye　SHI Da-zhuo　CHEN Ke-ji

Blood stasis is considered as a major contributing factor for the pathogenesis of chronic cardiovascular and cerebrovascular diseases. The pathophysiological basis of blood stasis involves platelet adhesion, aggregation, activation, coagulation, and thrombosis. However, inflammation reaction, oxidative stress injury, tissue necrosis, and other pathological changes during the process of diseases may not be fully explained by blood stasis syndrome. Based on the interpretation of pathogenic roles of toxins in Chinese medicine, it has been believed that "stasis" and "toxin" act together to contribute to the disease etiology. Researches that attempt to elucidate of "toxin" and detoxification have been carried out using modern biology research tools[1-3]. However, the casual relationship and the interaction of "stasis" and "toxin" during pathogenesis are not well understood. Further, there have not been well-established indicators or indices that can be used as sensitive measures for exploring the therapeutic benefit of treatments that are aimed at antagonizing "stasis" and "toxin".

In the current study, utilizing a rabbit compound model of hyperlipidemia, immune injury, and endotoxininduced endothelial injury, we intended to systematically analyze the pathophysiological changes, including tissue damage, inflammation reaction, and thrombosis. At the same time, we planned to evaluate and compare the effect of Chinese medicines with activating blood circulation (ABC) activity and those with activating blood circulation and detoxifying (ABCD) activities on these pathophysiological changes. It was anticipated that the findings in the study would also provide a molecular basis for understanding the interplay of "stasis" and "toxin" in disease pathogenesis.

1. Methods

1.1　Animals and Forage

Fifty-four male purebred New Zealand rabbits, weighting 2.0-2.5 kg, were purchased from Beijing Vital River Experimental Animals Technical Ltd. Co., with a certificate serial number SCXK (Beijing) 2005-0002. Hypercholesterol forage (ordinary forage with 2% cholesterol and 5% lard) was purchased from the Experimental Animal Center of Academy of Military Medical Sciences, China.

1.2　Reagents and Apparatus

Percoll was purchased from Pharmacia (P8370). Rabbit antihuman factor Ⅷ related antigen (CAT: bs-0434R, LOT: 080417) and fluorescein isothiocyanate (FITC) -conjugated

* 原载于 Chinese Journal of Integrative Medicine，2013，19（1）：42-47

polyvalent goat antirabbit IgG (CAT: bsF-0295G, LOT: 080301) were purchased from Beijing Biosynthesis Biotechnology Ltd., Co., China. Bovine serum albumin (A738328) and endotoxin (L2880) were purchased from Roche and Sigma, USA respectively. Enzyme-linked immunoassay (ELISA) kits, which included matrix metalloproteinase-9 (MMP-9) (CAT: E0553Rb, LOT: 090113), tissue inhibitors tometalloproteinase (TIMP-1, CAT: E0128Rb, LOT: 090108), granule membrane protein-140 (GMP-140, CAT: E00602Rb, LOT: 090114), plasminogen activator inhibitor-1 (PAI-1, CAT: E0532Rb, LOT: 090114), highsensitivity C-reactive protein (hs-CRP, CAT: E0821Rb, LOT: 090116), interleukin-6 (IL-6, CAT: E0079Rb, LOT: 090119), and tumor necrosis factor-α (TNF-α, CAT: E0133Rb, LOT: 090114), were all purchased from USCNLIFE Company, China, and a microplate reader (Thermo Multiskan 3, China) was used for the assay.

1.3 Drugs

Simvastatin was purchased from Hangzhou Merck Sharp & Dohme Pharmaceutical Ltd., Co., 40 mg/tablet, batch No. 07432. Simvastatin was grinded into powder form and dissolved in double-distilled water to have a suspension. Xiongshao Capsule (芎芍胶囊, XSC, composed of Rhizoma Chuanxiong and Radix Paeoniae rubra, 0.25 g/capsule, content of drug markers: paeoniflorin $\geqslant$ 28 mg, ferulic acid $\geqslant$ 3.5 mg, and gallic acid $\geqslant$ 34 mg each capsule) was purchased from Dalian Institute of Chemical Physics, China, batch No. 070929. Huanglian Capsule (黄连胶囊), 0.25 g/pill, with ingredient of chinensis Franch, was purchased from Hubei Xianglian Pharmaceutical Ltd., Co., China, with a national medicine permit No. Z19983042. XSC with the ABC activity would be compared with XSC+Huanglian Capsule that possesses ABCD activity.

1.4 Grouping and Model Establishment

After 7 days of acclimation, 10 of 54 rabbits were randomly taken to form the normal control group, which were fed with normal diets. The other 44 rabbits were injected with bovine serum albumin (0.5 g each) and fed with high-fat diet for 6 weŵs. They were then randomly assigned into 1 of 4 treatment groups, namely, the model group (no treatment), simvastatin group, activating blood circulation (ABC) group, and activating blood circulation and detoxifying (ABCD) group, with 11 animals per group. Rabbits with high-fat diet received ear vein injection of endotoxin (1 μg/kg) on the 28th day of highfat diet, and the normal control group received normal saline. The rabbits on high-fat diet continued with the same diet plus treatment of simvastatin[4] (0.93 mg/kg per day), XSC (0.07 g/kg per day), or XSC (0.07 g/kg per day) and Huanglian Capsule (0.14 g/kg per day) administered to the simvastatin group, ABC group, and ABCD group, respectively, for an additional 2 weeks. At the end of the treatment, blood (12 mL) samples from all rabbits were taken from the abdominal aorta. The first 6 mL of the blood was collected into a sodium citrate tube and centrifuged for 15 min at 3 000 r/min. The resulting plasma was stored in a -20 ℃ refrigerator to determine levels of specific serum proteins. The next 3 mL of blood was collected in a siliconized glass tube with 3.8% sodium citrate (0.33 mL) for quantification of circulating endothelial cells [5,6]. The last 3 mL of blood was collected to determine blood lipids.

1.5 Determination of Blood Lipids

Total cholesterol (TC), triglyceride (TG), and low-density and high-density lipoprotein cholesterol (LDL-C and HDL-C) were measured with an automatic biochemical analyzer (Hitachi 7600-020, JAPAN).

1.6 Determination and Quantification of Circulating Endothelial Cells

Circulating endothelia cells (CECs) were separated by Percoll density gradient. Two Percoll suspensions with a specific gravity of 1.060 g/mL and 1.045 g/mL were used. The specific gravity of 1.060 g/mL (100 mL) was obtained by mixing 42.9 mL of stock Percoll suspension, 10 mL of pooled human serum, 37.1 mL of Earle's medium, and 10 mL of 3.8% sodium citrate. The specific gravity of 1.045 g/mL (100 mL) was obtained by mixing 30.3 mL of stock Percoll suspension, 10 mL of pooled human serum, 49.7 mL Earle's medium, and 10 mL of 3.8% sodium citrate. The 3mL of each Percoll suspension was mixed in a centrifuge tube. Anticoagulant blood diluted 1∶1 with Hanks was layered over the mixed Percoll suspension and centrifuged for 20 min at 1 800 r/min at room temperature. The interface containing cells were collected using a capillary pipette and transferred to another a centrifuge tube.

Cells were precipitated by centrifugation and resuspended in 0.5 mL of saline. Cell viability was determined by 0.5% trypan blue staining (viability of > 95% was required). Total cell count was obtained under a light microscope. Indirect immunofluorescence assay was performed to identify the CECs. Cell suspension was spread on a glass slide and fixed with acetone for 30 s at 4℃. Slides were washed with PBS (0.1 mol/L) 3 times, incubated with rabbit anti-human factor Ⅷ related antigen (20 μL) for 30 min at 37℃, washed 3 times with PBS, stained with FITC-conjugated polyvalent goat anti-rabbit IgG (20 μL) 30 min at 37 ℃, washed 3 times with PBS, and embedded in 87% glycerol in PBS (9∶1). CECs were enumerated under a fluorescent microscope (Olympus BX51, JAPAN). Negative controls were processed similarly except the rabbit antihuman factor Ⅷ related antigen was replaced with PBS.

1.7　Pathological Examination of the Atherosclerotic Plaque

At the end of the 2-week treatment, all rabbits were sacrificed and a 1.5-cm-long aortic arch segment was obtained from each rabbit. Samples were rinsed with normal saline, and the section with the most prominent atherosclerotic plaque was dissected. The identical section of the aortic arch was also obtained from the normal control group. Samples were then fixed with 10% formalin, embedded in paraffin, and sliced into 2-μm thickness slices. After HE staining, plaques were examined under the light microscope for foam cells, lipid storage, and cholesterol crystals.

1.8　Determination of Indices of Tissue Damage, Thrombosis and Inflammation Reaction

The indices of tissue damage (serum MMP-9 and TIMP-1), the indices of thrombosis (serum GMP-140 and PAI-1), and the indices of inflammation reaction (serum hs-CRP, IL-6, and TNF-α) were detected by ELISA.

1.9　Statistical Analysis

Statistical analysis was performed with SPSS 11.5 software, and the values of $P < 0.05$ were considered statistically significant. For enumeration data, Chi-square test was used; while for quantitative data, t test was used for comparisons between groups, and one-way ANOVA was applied for significance test in multiple-group comparisons.

2.　Results

2.1　General Observations

After infection of endotoxin, 5 rabbits in the model group, 2 rabbits in Simvastatin group, 5 rabbits in ABC group, and 4 rabbits in ABCD group died of infective fever. Data presented below were taken from the remaining 38 rabbits.

2.2　Comparison of the Levels of Blood Lipids

Compared with the normal control group, the levels of TC, TG, and LDL-C increased in the model group ($P < 0.01$), but there was no change in the level of HDL-C ($P > 0.05$). Compared with the model group, the levels of TC and TG in the simvastatin group and the level of TG in the ABCD group reduced significantly ($P < 0.05$, Table 1).

Table 1   Comparison of the Levels of Blood Lipids（mmol/L, $\bar{\chi} \pm s$）

Group	n	TC	TG	HDL-C	LDL-C
Normal control	10	1.00±0.34	0.72±0.22	1.07±0.43	0.43±0.23
Model	6	29.93±3.10*	4.61±1.29*	0.94±0.29	13.38±3.34*
Simvastatin	9	23.89±3.26△	2.24±0.73△	1.07±0.33	12.21±3.66
ABC	6	28.77±2.86	3.58±1.02	1.17±0.65	13.07±2.74
ABCD	7	27.92±4.38	2.29±0.62△	0.95±0.29	12.31±2.61

Notes：*$P < 0.01$，compared with the normal control group；△$P < 0.05$，compared with the model group

2.3　Pathological Changes in Aortic Arch

Figure 1 shows the HE staining of the aortic arch tissue sections from all groups. There were no foam cells and lipid storage in the aortic media and intima in the normal control group under normal diets. In the model group fed with high-fat diet, the aortic intima was significantly thickened in comparison to the normal control group and contained numerous foam cells. There was a small amount of cholesterol crystals under the endothelium. Compared with the model group, the overall pathological changes in the all drug intervention groups appeared less severe, including thickening of the aortic intima, swelling and degeneration of endothelial cells, and the quantities of foam cells and cholesterol crystals.

2.4　Determination and Quantification of CECs

Endothelial cells after immunofluorescence staining appeared as cells with yellow-green fluorescence under the fluorescence microscope, and none of the cells from the negative control showed any fluorescence, confirming that the fluorescent cells were CECs. Table 2 listed the CECs counts in all groups. Compared with the normal control group, the number of CECs was significantly increased in the model group ($P < 0.01$). In contrast, the number of CECs was significantly reduced after treatment with simvastatin, ABC, or ABCD when compared with the model group ($P < 0.01$). There was no significant difference among the drug intervention groups ($P > 0.05$).

Table 2   Comparison of the Number of CECs in Rabbits among Groups (0.9μL, $\bar{\chi} \pm s$)

Group	n	the number of CECs
Normal control	10	2.00±1.25
Model	6	7.83±1.72*
Simvastatin	9	3.67±1.00△
ABC	6	4.00±0.63△
ABCD	7	4.00±1.41△

Notes: *$P < 0.01$，compared with the normal group; △$P < 0.01$, compared with the model group

2.5　Comparison of Indices of Thrombosis

Compared with the normal control group, serum GMP-140 and PAI-1 were increased significantly in the model group ($P < 0.01$). Compared with the model group, serum GMP-140 and PAI-1 were decreased significantly in the simvastatin group and ABCD group ($P < 0.05$). A decrease in both GMP-140 and PAI-1 was also observed in the ABC group when compared with the model group, but the difference was not statistically significant ($P > 0.05$，Table 3).

Table 3   Comparison of the Levels of GMP-140 and PAI-1 (ng/mL, $\bar{\chi} \pm s$)

Group	n	GMP-140	PAI-1
Normal control	10	0.53±0.12	3.83±0.98
Model	6	1.08±0.31*	7.28±2.01*
Simvastatin	9	0.78±0.33△	5.37±2.26△
ABC	6	0.92±0.20	5.92±1.57
ABCD	7	0.79±0.20△	5.23±1.39△

Notes: *$P < 0.01$，compared with the normal group; △$P < 0.05$, compared with the model group

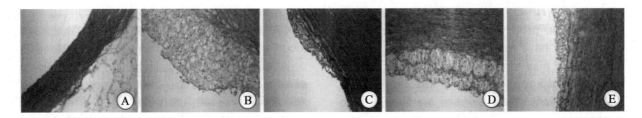

Figure 1　Histomorphologic Changes of Atherosclerosis Plaque in the Aortic Arch（HE staining，×200）

Notes：A：normal control group，B：model group，C：simvastatin group，D：ABC group，E：ABCD group

2.6　Comparison of Indices of Inflammation Reaction

Compared with the normal control group, serum hs-CRP, IL-6, and TNF-α all increased in the model group ($P < 0.01$). Compared with the model group, reductions in levels of all three molecules were evident in all drug intervention groups; however, only reductions in hs-CRP observed in the simvastatin group and IL-6 in the ABCD group were statistically significant *(P < 0.05，Table 4).

Table 4　Comparison of the Levels of Serum hs-CRP, IL-6 and TNF-α ($\bar{\chi} \pm s$)

Group	n	hs-CRP (ng/mL)	IL-6 (pg/mL)	TNF-α (pg/mL)
Normal control	10	5.76±1.61	33.65±7.31	15.24±4.16
	6	11.82±3.52*	54.44±13.56*	31.58±8.39*
Simvastatin	9	8.54±3.76△	44.34±11.32	23.69±9.71
ABC	6	9.53±2.97	44.56±12.26	25.87±7.66
ABCD	7	9.02±2.75	40.64±10.11△	24.14±6.72

Notes: *$P < 0.01$，compared with the normal group; △$P < 0.05$, compared with the model group

2.7　Comparison of Indices of Tissue Damage

Compared with the normal control group, serum MMP-9 was increased in the model group ($P < 0.01$) and serum TIMP-1 was reduced ($P < 0.05$). Compared with the model group, a reduction in MMP-9 and an increase in TIMP-1 were observed for all drug intervention groups, but only the reduction in MMP-9 in the simvastatin group reached statistical significance ($P < 0.05$，Table 5).

Table 5　Comparison of the Levels of Serum MMP-9 and TIMP-1 ($\bar{\chi} \pm s$)

Group	n	MMP-9 (ng/mL)	TIMP-1 (pg/mL)
Normal control	10	0.39±0.11	329.21±91.79
Model	6	0.81±0.24**	195.38±97.34*
Simvastatin	9	0.58±0.26△	239.39±119.18
ABC	6	0.66±0.22	241.66±79.15
ABCD	7	0.63±0.21	290.79±103.89

Notes: *$P < 0.05$，**$P < 0.01$，compared with the normal control group; △$P < 0.05$，compared with the model group

3.　Discussion

With high-fat diets and bovine serum albumin injection, lipid disorders and persistent chronic inflammatory reaction are the main underlying mechanism for plaque formation in the rabbit model of atherosclerosis[7]. Intravenous injection of endotoxin induces systemic inflammatory response, which accelerates the atherogenic process[8]. In the current study, rabbits in the model group, when compared with the normal control group, showed a significant increase in the levels of TC, TG, and LDL-C, atherosclerotic changes in the aortic arch, an increase in CECs, a rapid elevation of serum GMP-140, PAI-1, hs-CRP, IL-6, TNF-α, and MMP-9, and a reduction in TIMP-1. The protein molecules affected in the disease model have been shown in other studies to be markers or play a role in disease pathogenesis. GMP-140 is a known marker of the later stage platelet activation, which is one of the microcosmic dialectical indices of blood stasis[9]；PAI-1 promotes the development of atherosclerosis and thrombosis[10]；hs-CRP, IL-6, and TNF-α are typical inflammatory markers and have a variety of biological effects in body response to infection and tissue damage[11]. The balance between MMP and TIMP plays an important role in the inflammatory response and tissue repair[12].

In the rabbit model, a series of physiological responses and pathological changes occurred, including dyslipidemia, vascular endothelial cells damage, inflammation reaction, platelet activation, thrombosis and tissue damage. Pathological changes, including platelet activation and thrombosis, are always attributed to "blood stasis". Chinese medicine considers "toxin" the etiology of diseases as well as causative agent for pathological changes. Based on this concept, pathological changes, such as tissue necrosis and inflammation reaction, observed in the rabbit model could be attributed to the action of "toxin", the etiologic and pathogenic agent. The overall findings in the model could be attributed to the joint action of "toxin" and "stasis". In this model, injection of bovine serum albumin and endotoxin induced immune damage and fever. These initial responses resemble the diseases caused by pathogenic toxin in humans that are characterized by sudden onset, rapid deterioration, and muscle damage. It appears that the rabbit model used in the current study was established as a result of initial "toxin-heat" attack and subsequent "blood stasis", and both contributed to the eventual changes described above.

Huanglian Capsule is effective in detoxification and heat reduction. XSC was extracted from the traditional activating blood circulation prescription, Xuefu Zhuyu Decoction (血府逐瘀汤), and has been shown to be an effective prescription for the treatment of coronary heart disease. In this study, we used XSC (ABC) and XSC with Huanglian Capsule (ABCD) as two different treatments to assess and compare the effect of the ABC and ABCD activities in the rabbit model of toxic-heat and blood stasis syndrome. Our study results show that the rabbits treated with simvastatin had a decrease in the level of serum TC and TG, a reduction in CECs, and a decrease in the levels of serum GMP-140, PAI-1, hs-CRP, and MMP-9, compared with the rabbits in the model group that received no treatment. The results demonstrated that simvastatin had an anti-inflammatory effect in addition to its lipid lowering function. The results also showed that simvastatin had an anti-atherosclerosis effect as demonstrated by its inhibition in the expression of platelet-activating factor GMP-140, fibrinolytic system PAI-1, and tissue damage factor MMP-9 and by reduction of endothelial injury. Our observation was consistent with the previous findings[13-16]. A similar trend of improvement was also observed in the rabbits treated with the ABCD drug, and this was reflected by the improvement in the serum TG level and in the pathological changes in the aortic arch and a reduction in the number of CECs and in the levels of serum GMP-140, PAI-1, and IL-6.

In contrast, although the rabbits treated with the ABC drug had, to a lesser extent, improvement in the pathological changes in the aortic arch and a reduction in CECs, there was no significant difference in the levels of serum GMP-140, PAI-1, hs-CRP, IL-6, TNF-α, MMP-9, and TIMP-1 when compared with the rabbits in the model group. Previous studies confirmed that some activating blood circulation and detoxifying prescription (extract of *Rhizoma Polygoni Cuspidati* with XSC) and an effective component of activating blood circulation and detoxifying prescription (extrac of *Rhizoma Polygoni Cuspidati* and the alcoholic extract of *Rhubarb*) could reduce the expression of hs-CRP, TNF-α, and MMP-9 in apolipoprotein E gene knockout mice[1-3]. The discrepancy of the findings might be associated with different models utilized and different indices selected in each individual studies.

In our rabbit model of toxin-heat and blood stasis symdrome, a rapid and dramatic rise in the indices selected to represent thrombosis (GMP-140 and PAI-1), inflammation reaction (hs-CRP, IL-6, and TNF-α), and tissue damage (MMP-9 and TIMP-1) was observed in comparison to the normal control group, indicating that these measurements could be used as molecular biomarkers in the diagnosis of toxin-induced stasis and both toxin- and stasis-induced diseases. Further, based on the principle of syndrome differentiation through formula effect assessment, the superior therapeutic benefit of the ABCD drug compared with the ABC drug provided an alternative validation to the rabbit model of toxin-heat and blood stasis. Our study also indicated that serum GMP-140, PAI-1, and IL-6 were sensitive molecular indices for determining the therapeutic effect of drugs with activating blood circulation and detoxifying activities.

References

[1] Zhang JC, Chen KJ, Zheng GJ, et al. Regulatory effect of Chinese herbal compound for detoxifying and activating blood circulation on expression of NF-κB and MMP-9 in aorta of apolipoprotein E gene knocked-out mice. Chin J Integr Tradit West Med, 2007, 27: 40-44.

[2] Zhang JC, Chen KJ, Liu JG, et al. Effect of assorted use of Chinese drugs for detoxifying and activating blood circulation on serum high sensitive C-reactive protein in apolipoprotein E gene knock-out mice. Chin J Integr Tradit West Med, 2008, 28: 330-333.

[3] Zhou MX, Xu H, Chen KJ, et al. Effects of some active ingredients of Chinese drugs for activating blood circulation and detoxicating on blood lipids and atherosclerotic plaque inflammatory reaction in ApoE-gene knockout mice. Chin J Integr Tradit West Med, 2008, 28: 126-130.

[4] Chen Q. Methodological study of Chinese herbs pharmacology. People's Medical Publishing House, 1996, 8: 1103-1105.

[5] Gan WJ, Liu JT, Lin R. The protective effect of quercetin on the vascular endothelial cells injured by homocysteine in rabbits. Chin Pharmacol Bull, 2004, 20 (6): 647-651.

[6] Sbarbati R, D Boer M, Marzilli M, et al. Immunologic detection of endothelial cells in human whole blood. Blood, 1991, 77 (4): 764-769.

[7] Ding J, Chen HY, Kong J, et al. Effect of Rosiglitazone on cardiovascular ultrastructure of atherosclerosis in rabbits. Chin J Gerontology, 2008, 28: 342-344.

[8] Wang KF, Lu FE, Xu LJ, et al. Study on the dynamic changes of body temperature and plasma endotoxin levels in rabbits after infusion with endotoxin. Acta Universitatis Medictnae Tangji, 2001, 30: 129-133.

[9] Chen KJ, Xue M, Yin HJ. The relationship between platelet activation and coronary heart disease and blood-stasis syndrome. Journal of Capital Medical University, 2008, 29: 266-269.

[10] Chen LH, Lu GP, Wu CF, et al. Effect of pravastatin on arterial gene expression of plasminogen activator inhibitor type 1 in atherosclerotic rabbits. Chinese Journal of Cardiology, 2001, 29: 115-117.

[11] Ma XJ, Yin HJ, Chen KJ. Research progress of correlation between blood-stasis syndrome and inflammation. Chin J Integr Med, 2007, 27 (7): 669-672.

[12] Bruno G, Todor R, Lewis I, et al. Vascular extracellular matrix remodeling in cerebral aneurysms. J Neurosurg, 1998, 89: 431-440.

[13] Ji Y, Zhang RY, Lu GP, et al. Effect of simvastatin on the expressions of P-selectin and ICAM-1 in atherosclerotic iliac artery of rabbits. Chin J Geriatrics, 2003, 22 (3): 165-168.

[14] Qin L, Zhu Y, Huang KX. Study on expression of plasminogen activator inhibitor type-1 and its correlation with cholesterolemia in the atherosclerotic rabbits. J Clin Cardiology, 2006, 22 (9): 538-540.

[15] Zhang L, Jiang YR, Xue M, et al. Effect of simvastatin on the atherosclerotic plaque stability and the angiogenesis in atherosclerotic plaque of rabbits. Chinese Sci Bull, 2009, 54 (15): 2228-2232.

[16] Yip HK, Sun CK, Chang LT, et al. Strong suppression of high-sensitivity C-reactive protein level and its mediated pro-atherosclerotic effects with simvastatin: in vivo and in vitro studies. Int J Cardiol, 2007, 121 (3): 253-60.

Correlation between FcγRⅢA and Aortic Atherosclerotic Plaque Destabilization in ApoE Knockout Mice and Intervention Effects of Effective *Components of Chuanxiong Rhizome* and *Red Peony Root**

HUANG Ye   YIN Hui-jun   Ma Xiao-juan   WANG Jing-shang
LIU Qian   WU Cai-feng   CHEN Ke-ji

Coronary heart disease (CHD) is a global cardiovascular disease that remains the principal killer all over the world. Blood stasis syndrome (BSS), a major syndrome type of CHD, is a common Chinese medicine pathological characteristic; its development mechanism and progression are complex and different with a common pathological basement. BSS of CHD is a focus in the field of Chinese medicine and integrative medicine. Our previous study investigated the differential gene expression profiles in peripheral leukocytes of patients with CHD of BSS by oligonucleotide microarray technique. Fc receptor γ ⅢA (FcγRⅢA), one of the differential genes[1], is mainly present on monocytes, which plays a key role in pathological conditions, such as autoimmune diseases and infections [2]. The main pathogenesis of CHD is atherosclerosis. Inflammation and immune response are the key factors of local vulnerable plaques, among which monocytes/macrophages are the main origin of inflammatory factors and plasmas[3]. Atherosclerosis (AS) is a critical and major contributor of CHD and inflammation and immune response play a key role in the pathogenesis of atherosclerosis, while FcγRⅢA contributes to the inflammation and immune response. Thus, we hypothesized that FcγRⅢA, as the target molecule of CHD with BSS, might participate in the occurrence and progression of coronary atherosclerotic plaque destabilization by mediating systemic inflammation.

The apoE knockout (apoE KO) murine model of AS is established, which can mimic the features of fatty streak to plaque formation[4] and the characteristics of stable and unstable atherosclerotic plaque during the progression of AS at different stages[5]. In this study, the AS model by apoE KO mice with 10-week high-fat diet was established and the role of FcγRⅢA in the progression of plaque destabilization and the intervention effects of effective components of Chuanxiong Rhizome and Red Peony Root were analyzed in order to provide a new molecular target for protection and prevention of CHD.

1. Methods

1.1 Drugs and Reagents

Xiongshao Capsule (XSC, 芎芍胶囊) was provided by Beijing International Institute of Biological Products (batch No. 200091), which consists of effective components of Chuanxiong Rhizome and Red Peony Root, 0.25g/capsule. Simvastatin (Sm), 20 mg/tablet, was produced by Hangzhou

* 原载于 Chinese Journal of Integrative Medicine，2011，17（5）：355-360

Moshadong Pharmaceutical Co. Ltd (batch No.100243). Intraperitoneal immunoglobulin (pH 4, IVIG), 5% 50 mL, 2.5 g/bottle, was produced by Chengdu Rongsheng Pharmaceutical Co., Ltd (batch No. 200911B037).

Monoclonal antibody (mAb) against CD14 directly coupled to fluorescein isothiocyanate (FITC) (Clone Sa14-2), mAb against CD16/32 directly coupled to phycoerythrin (PE) (Clone 93), and PE-conjugated anti-mouse IgG2a, κ, the isotypic control mAb, were from BioLegend (USA). OptiLyse C lysing solution (Lot No. 12) was from Beckman Coulter (USA). TRIzol reagent (Lot No. 15596-018) was from Invitrogen (USA). Reverse transcriptase M-MLV kit (Lot No. D2639A) was from Takara (Japan). Real-time PCR amplification kit (Lot No. A4011) was from Bio-Rad (USA). Enzyme-linked immunosorbent assay (ELISA) kit of tumor necrosis factor-α (TNF-α, Lot No. 1011126) was from R&D (USA).

1.2　Animals Grouping and Treatment

Forty 8-week-old male apoE KO mice and eight 18 to 20 g C57BL/6J mice with the same genetic background were obtained from Beijing University Laboratory Animal Center (animal certificate No.SCXK (Jing) 2006-0008). The strain of apoE KO mice was developed in the Jackson Laboratory on a 129/J background. Mice were housed in humidity-controlled 55%±5% rooms at 22±2 ℃ with a 12 h on/12 h off light cycle. After 1 week adaptive fed, mice were switched from normal rodent diet to a high-fat diet[6] that contained 21% fat from lard and supplemented with 0.15% (wt/wt) cholesterol (Experimental Animal Center of the Academy of Military Medical Sciences). Mice were put on a high-fat diet for 10 weeks with different interventions. Eight C57BL/6J mice were selected as the control group and forty apoE KO mice were randomly divided into five groups, model group, IVIG group, Sm group, XSCH group, and XSCL group, 8 mice in each group. Mice in the IVIG group received an intraperitoneal injection of 10 mg IVIG daily over a 5-day period before a high-fat diet. Sm (0.026 g/kg) and XSC (0.39 and 0.195 g/kg) were used in each gavage for 10 weeks in the Sm group, XSCH group, and XSCL group, respectively. Mice in the control group and model group only received the same volume of distilled water per gavage for 10 weeks.

1.3　Sample Preparation

Blood samples from abdominal aorta after anesthesia by intraperitoneal injection of 20% urethane (0.5 mL/100 g) were collected (fasting 24 h before sampling). Monocyte CD16 expression was detected from 0.2 mL ethylenediamine tetraacetate (EDTA) anticoagulant blood by using flow cytometry. Then, the serum was centrifuged 3 000 r/min for 15 min and preserved at −20℃ for TNF-α level analysis. Aorta tissue was taken and preserved at −80℃ for matrix metalloproteinase-9 (MMP-9) mRNA expression analysis.

1.4　Whole-Blood Flow Cytometry Analysis

Monocyte CD16 expression was analyzed by flow cytometry. A total of 200 μL EDTA-anticoagulated whole-blood sample of each group was divided into two tubes, the control tube and the detected tube, and incubated either with anti-CD14 mAb directly coupled to FITC and anti-CD16/32 mAb directly coupled to PE or with the corresponding isotypic control at room temperature in the dark for 20 min. For erythrocyte lysis and fixation of leukocytes, 500 μL OptiLyse C 500 solution was added in each tube. After centrifugation of 1500 r/min for 5 min, cells were washed twice in 3 mL phosphate-buffered saline (PBS) and the final pellet was diluted in 500 μL PBS. EPICS Elite (Beckman Coulter, USA) adjusted by Flow-Chec™ Fluorospheres (Beckman Coulter, USA) was used for flow cytometric analysis. Monocytes were gated in a forward scatter/sideward scatter (FSC/SSC) dotplot. Voltage value of fluorescence channel was determined by analyzing isotypic control and the other tube was measured. EXPO32 software was used to analyze the percentage of CD14$^+$/CD16$^+$ monocytes.

1.5 Real-time Quantitative PCR

Total mRNA was extracted with TRIzol reagent according to the manufacturer's specifications from the aorta. First-strand cDNA was synthesized from 3 μL total RNA samples according to the reverse transcriptase M-MLV manufacturer's specifications. MMP-9 and glyceraldehyde phosphate dehydrogenase (GAPDH) gene sequences from GenBank were synthesized by Shanghai Sangon Biotech Co., Ltd., and were as follows: the primer series for MMP-9: forward 5'-GCGTGTCTGGAGATTCGAC-3' and reverse 5'-CCATGGCAGAAATAGGCTTT-3', length of amplified segment 138 bp; the primer series for GAPDH: 5'-GCACAGTCAAGGCCGAGAA-3' and 5'-CCTCACCCCATTTGATGTTAGTG-3', length of amplified segment 142 bp. PCR amplification of MMP-9 and GAPDH cDNAs was performed according to the real-time PCR amplification kit with 1.5 μL cDNA and same parameters. All reverse transcription-polymerase chain reactions (RT-PCRs) and analysis were performed on the ABI PRISM 7500 sequence detection system (Applied Biosystems). Cycling parameters were both for 94℃ for 15 min; 40 cycles at 94℃ for 15s, 60℃ for 34 s, and 72℃ for 15 s; and 72℃ for 10 min. For each series, the threshold cycle (Ct) value recorded indicates the fractional cycle number at which the amount of amplified target reached a fixed threshold. The housekeeping gene GAPDH was used for internal control. The $2^{-\triangle\triangle Ct}$ method is a convenient way to analyze the relative changes in gene expression from real-time quantitative PCR experiments[7]. The mean Ct value from each sample was normalized to the corresponding GAPDH Ct values, calculated as (Ct$_{experimental\ gene}$-Ct$_{GAPDH}$). The relative gene expression in a particular sample was then given as follows: relative quantification for each gene= $2^{-\triangle\triangle Ct}$ value as mentioned before.

1.6 ELISA Analysis

Serum TNF-α level was determined using a sandwich-type ELISA kit.

1.7 Statistical Analysis

Statistical analysis was performed using SPSS 13.0 for Windows. *P* values less than 0.05 were considered statistically significant. Data were expressed as the mean ± standard deviation. Differences among groups were tested using oneway ANOVA followed by multiple comparisons by LSD test. Spearman's correlation coefficients were calculated to study the relations between monocyte *CD16* expression and aortic MMP-9 mRNA expression or serum TNF-α level.

2. Results

2.1 Comparison of Monocyte CD14$^+$/CD16$^+$ Expression among Groups

Percentage of peripheral monocyte CD14$^+$/CD16$^+$ in the model group was significantly higher than that in the control group and was decreased obviously in IVIG group than that in the model group ($P < 0.01$). After 10-week medication intervention, percentage of CD14$^+$/CD16$^+$ decreased in a different degree in each group compared with that in the model group ($P < 0.01$), but there was no significant statistical difference among these three groups ($P > 0.05$, Table 1, Figure 1).

Table 1 Comparison of Percentage of Peripheral Monocyte CD14$^+$/CD16$^+$ among Groups ($\bar{\chi} \pm s$)

Group	n	Concentration	CD14$^+$/CD16$^+$ (%)
Control	8	0	18.16±4.70
Model	8	0	62.32±11.79*
IVIG	8	10mg	22.28±9.56$^\triangle$
Sm	8	0.026g/kg	32.18±8.38$^\triangle$
XSCH	8	0.390g/kg	35.43±9.83$^\triangle$
XSCL	8	0.195g/kg	38.12±7.35$^\triangle$

Notes: *$P < 0.01$, compared with the control group; $^\triangle P < 0.01$, compared with the model group

2.2 Comparison of Aortic MMP-9 mRNA Expression among Groups

Aortic MMP-9 mRNA expression in the model group was significantly higher than that in the control group and was decreased obviously in the IVIG group compared with the model group ($P < 0.01$). After 10-weŵ medication intervention, aortic MMP-9 mRNA expression decreased in a different degree in each group compared with that in the model group. Aortic MMP-9 mRNA expression in the XSCH group was lowest among these three groups ($P < 0.01$) and this effect was better than that in the Sm group ($P < 0.05$, Table 2).

2.3 Comparison of Serum TNF-α Level among Groups

Serum TNF-α level in the model group was significantly higher than that in the control group ($P < 0.01$) and was decreased in the IVIG group compared with that in the model group ($P < 0.05$). After 10-week medication intervention, TNF-α level decreased in a different degree in each group compared with that in the model group.

The TNF-α level was lowest in the XSCH group ($P < 0.05$) and there was no significant statistical difference between XSCH group and Sm group ($P > 0.05$, Table 2).

2.4 Analyses of Correlation between Monocyte CD16 Expression and Aortic MMP-9 mRNA Expression or Serum TNF-α Level

Correlation analyses showed that monocyte CD16 expression was positively correlated with MMP-9 mRNA expression and serum TNF-α in the IVIG group, XSCH group, and XSCL group (Figure 2).

3. Discussion

FcRs, a group of membrane glycoproteins that belongs to the immunoglobulin superfamily, are the specific receptors for the Fc regions of immunoglobulins that are expressed in almost all leukocytes. FcRs are defined by their specificity for immunoglobulin isotypes. Fcγ receptor (Fcγ R) plays an essential role in the process of immunoinflammatory responses, which is used as an important trigger molecule of inflammation,

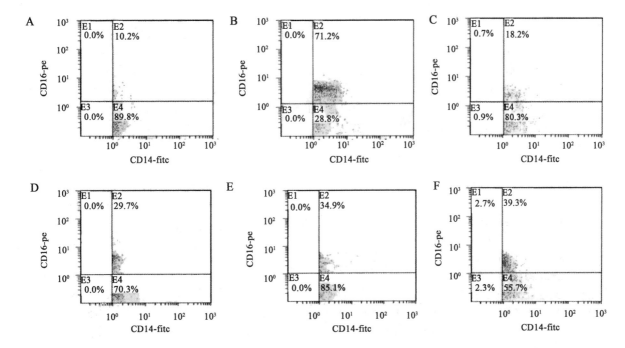

Figure 1　Representative Flow Cytometric Analysis of Monocyte CD16 Expression among Groups

Notes：A：control group；B：model group；C：IVIG group；D：Sm group；E：XSCH group；F：XSCL group

Table 2　Comparisons of Aortic MMP-9 mRNA Expression and Serum TNF-α Level among Groups ($\bar{\chi} \pm s$)

Group	n	Concentration	MMP-9 mRNA （2$^{-\triangle\triangle Ct}$）	TNF-α （pg/mL）
Control	8	0	0.930±0.062	16.193±3.942
Model	8	0	3.968±0.284*	41.758±9.776*
IVIG	8	10mg	2.539±0.359$^{\triangle\triangle}$	26.337±11.855$^{\triangle}$
Sm	8	0.026g/kg	1.991±0.228$^{\triangle\triangle}$	23.768±5.268$^{\triangle}$
XSCH	8	0.390g/kg	1.488±0.123$^{\triangle\triangle}$▲	28.222±8.484$^{\triangle}$
XSCL	8	0.195g/kg	2.330±0.210$^{\triangle\triangle}$	35.596±11.180

Notes：*$P < 0.01$, compared with the control group；$^{\triangle}P < 0.05$, $^{\triangle\triangle}P < 0.01$, compared with the model group；▲$P < 0.05$, compared with the Sm group

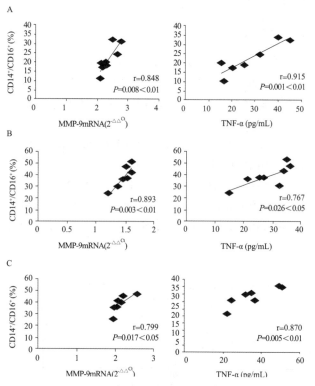

Figure 2　Correlation Analyses between Monocyte CD16 Expression and Aortic MMP-9 mRNA Expression or Serum TNF-α Level

Notes：A：IVIG group；B：XSCH group；C：XSCL group

allergy, and cytophagy. Three different classes of FcγRs have been found on human leukocytes. FcγRⅢ exists in two isoforms, FcγRⅢA and FcγRⅢB. The former is a transmembrane subtype that mainly expresses on monocytes[8]. Researches of FcγRⅢA mainly focus on the relationship between gene polymorphism or expression level and diseases. The FcγRⅢA F158 allele is reported to be a susceptibility

factor for many autoimmune diseases[2], such as rheumatoid arthritis, systemic lupus erythematosus, idiopathic thrombocytic purpura, Wegener's granulomatosis, and CHD[9]. Meanwhile, high levels of FcγRⅢA in a different degree have been observed in patients with coronary bypass operation, Kawasaki disease, and chronic renal failure dialysis[10-12].

AS is a critical and major contributor of CHD. Monocytes play an important role in the early phase of atherogenesis. Recruitment of monocytes from the peripheral blood to the intima of the vessel wall is a primordial event in atherosclerosis[13]. Which role do FcγRⅢA play in the progression of AS? Therefore, we constructed a model by apoE KO mice with high-fat diet to analyze the function of FcγRⅢA in vivo.

IVIG is composed of immunoglobulins, mainly of the IgG isotype. In our study, injections of apoE KO mice with IVIG for 5 days reduced monocyte CD16 expression over the model group. Accordingly, we suggested that IVIG could block FcγRⅢA and suppress its expression and function. This result was consistent with previous study[14].

Inflammation occurs in most vulnerable plaques composed of monocytes, macrophages, and lymphocytes, which is key to plaque rupture[13]. Monocytes themselves produce plenty of MMPs but also release various cytokines, such as TNF-α, which are key players during atherogenesis. MMPs are a family of zinc-dependent enzymes that digest extracellular matrix. Several MMPs are identified in atherosclerotic plaque, playing key roles in vascular remodeling. MMP-9 is essential for plaque destabilization and tissue remodeling and closely related with atherosclerosis[15]. Activation of monocytes and macrophages leads to the release of cytokines, such as TNF-α, which has extensive biological effects. TNF-α, as one of pro-inflammatory cytokines, is also implicated in atherosclerosis[16]. Therefore, we detected MMP-9 and TNF-α as indicators of plaque destabilization and systemic inflammation analyzing by RT-PCR and ELISA, respectively. We found that, after 10-week high-fat diet, these two mediators increased significantly. IVIG and drugs could reduce MMP-9 mRNA expression and serum TNF-α level in order to attenuate atherosclerotic plaque destabilization and suppress systemic inflammation.

Correlation analyses of monocyte CD16 expression, plaque destabilization index, and inflammation factor level in the IVIG group, XSCL group, and XSCH group suggested that IVIG could block FcγR ⅢA and reduce monocyte CD16 expression, MMP-9 mRNA expression, and serum TNF-α level. After 10-week intervention, Sm and XSC could reduce monocyte CD16 expression, MMP-9 mRNA expression, and serum TNF-α level. Moreover, there was significantly positive correlation between monocyte CD16 expression and MMP-9 mRNA expression or serum TNF-α level. Thus, we assume that FcγRⅢA may be involved in the progression of CHD by mediating atherosclerotic plaque destabilization and systemic inflammatory. Researches have proven that XSC is suitable for CHD with BSS by preventing AS, stabilizing plaque, and inhibiting restenosis[17]. In our previous study, we constructed the leukocyte gene expression profile of CHD with BSS using entire genome chip. CHD with BSS was found to be related to

the inflammatory reaction and immune response at molecular level through gene ontology analysis and pathway analysis. Meanwhile, six differential genes of CHD with BSS were screened and identified. FcγRⅢA was one of them[1]. According to the principle of the corresponding formula and syndrome, whether FcγRⅢA is the target of XSC preventing for CHD with BSS, our research proves that FcγRⅢA may participate in atherosclerotic plaque destabilization by mediating systemic inflammation. XSC can stabilize unstable atherosclerotic plaque by attenuating inflammation and its target was relevant to FcγRⅢA.

References

[1] Ma XJ, Yin HJ, Chen KJ. Differential gene expression profiles in coronary heart disease patients of blood stasis syndrome in traditional Chinese medicine and clinical role of target gene. Chin J Integr Med, 2009, 15：101-106.

[2] Ivan E, Colovai AI. Human Fc receptors: critical targets in the treatment of autoimmune diseases and transplant rejections. Hum Immunol, 2006, 67：479-491.

[3] Apple FS, Wu AH, Mair J, et al. Future biomarkers for detection of ischemia and risk stratification in acute coronary syndrome. Clin Chem, 2005, 51：810-824.

[4] Johnson J, Carson K, Williams H, et al. Plaque rupture after short periods of fat feeding in the apolipoprotein E-knockout mouse: model characterization and effects of pravastatin treatment. Circulation, 2005, 111：1422-1430.

[5] van Bochove GS, Straathof R, Krams R, et al. MRI-determined carotid artery flow velocities and wall shear stress in a mouse model of vulnerable and stable atherosclerotic plaque. MAGMA, 2010, 23：77-84.

[6] Johnson J, Carson K, Williams H, et al. Plaque rupture after short periods of fat feeding in the apolipoprotein E-knockout mouse: model characterization and effects of pravastatin treatment. Circulation, 2005, 111：1422-1430.

[7] Livak KJ, Schmittgen TD. Analysis of relative gene expression data using real-time quantitative PCR and the 2-[Delta Delta C (T)] method. Methods, 2001, 25：402-408.

[8] Masuda A, Yoshida M, Shiomi H, et al. Role of Fc

receptors as a therapeutic target. Inflamm Allergy Drug Targets, 2009, 8: 80-86.

[9] Gavasso S, Nygard O, Pedersen ER, et al. Fc gamma receptor Ⅲ A polymorphism as a risk-factor for coronary artery disease. Atherosclerosis, 2005, 180: 277-282.

[10] Stefanou DC, Asimakopoulos G, Yagnik DR, et al. Monocyte Fc gamma receptor expression in patients undergoing coronary artery bypass grafting. Ann Thorac Surg, 2004, 77: 951-955.

[11] Abe J, Jibiki T, Noma S, et al. Gene expression profiling of the effect of high-dose intravenous Ig in patients with Kawasaki disease. J Immunol, 2005, 174: 5837-5845.

[12] Kawanaka N, Nagake Y, Yamamura M, et al. Expression of Fc gamma receptor Ⅲ (CD16) on monocytes during hemodialysis in patients with chronic renal failure. Nephron, 2002, 90: 64-71.

[13] Libby P, Ridker PM, Maseri A. Inflammation and atherosclerosis. Circulation, 2002, 105: 1135-1143.

[14] Samuelsson A, Towers TL, Ravetch JV. Anti-inflammatory activity of IVIG mediated through the inhibitory Fc receptor. Science, 2001, 291: 484-486.

[15] Johnson JL, George SJ, Newby AC, et al. Divergent effects of matrix metalloproteinases 3, 7, 9, and 12 on atherosclerotic plaque stability in mouse brachiocephalic arteries. Proc Natl Acad Sci USA, 2005, 102: 15575-15580.

[16] Stefanadi E, Tousoulis D, Papageorgiou N, et al. Inflammatory biomarkers predicting events in atherosclerosis. Curr Med Chem, 2010, 17: 1690-1707.

[17] Chen KJ, Shi DZ, Xu H, et al. XS0601 reduces the incidence of restenosis: a prospective study of 335 patients undergoing percutaneous coronary intervention in China. Chin Med J, 2006, 119: 6-13.

Effect of Simvastatin on the Atherosclerotic Plaque Stability and the Angiogenesis in the Atherosclerotic Plaque of Rabbits[*]

ZHANG Lu   JIANG Yue-rong   XUE Mei   WU Cai-feng   WANG Jing-shang YIN Hui-jun

Partial or total angiemphraxis resulting from the instability and rupture of atherosclerosis (AS), vasoconstriction and local thrombosis is the main mechanism for the occurrence of acute coronary syndrome. The study found that pathological new vessels often occur in the AS plaque, which may possibly accelerate the progress of the atherosclerotic lesion, and even induce hemorrhage and the rupture of the plaque[1]. Simvastatin, as one kind of lipid lowering agents, has been extensively used clinically. In recent years, it has been found to have non-specific anti-inflammatory actions, and play a plaque stabilization role[2]. However, the effect of simvastatin on the angiogenesis in the AS plaque was rarely reported[3]. On the basis of these reports, effects of simvastatin on related indices of the plaque stability in the AS model and changes of angiogenetic indices in the plaque were studied using high fat forage and balloon injury induced AS plaque models, hoping to explore the roles of simvastatin in stabilizing the plaque from the angiogenesis in the plaque.

---

* 原载于 Chinese Science Bulletin, 2009, 54 (17): 3061-3066

1. Materials and Methods

1.1 Experimental Materials

New Zealand male rabbits, 1.8-2.2 kg, were provided by Beijing Vital River Lab Animal Technology Co., Ltd. (the animal certificate No.: SCXK (Jing) 2005-0002). The high fat forage was produced by the Experimental Animal Center of the Academy of Military Medical Sciences. Simvastatin (the batch No.: 07432), 40 mg per tablet, was produced by Hangzhou Moshadong Pharmaceutical Co., Ltd.

Enzyme-linked immunosorbent assay (ELISA) kit was provided by the American Uscnlife Company. The immunochemical primary working solution was provided by Beijing Biosynthesis Biotechnology Co., Ltd.; Automatic Biochemical Analyzer type 7600-020 provided by HITACHI, Japan. V 2.3 enzyme-labeled instrument by MULTISKAN EX PRIMARY EIA, USA; Japan Olympus BX51 light microscope and the American Image-Pro Plus Version 4.5.1 (IPP) Software were also used.

1.2 Animal Grouping and Model Preparation

Thirty healthy New Zealand rabbits were randomly divided into the normal control group, the model control group and the simvastatin group, 10 in each group. After one week of adaptive feeding, high fat forage (consisting of basic forage, 2% cholesterol, and 5% lard) was administered to rabbits at the daily dose of 100 g in the latter two groups. The established hyperlipemia model was confirmed using blood lipids determination. After feeding the high fat forage for two weeks, the balloon injury via the abdominal aorta was conducted to guarantee the intima tear. The femoral artery was bluntly dissected after anesthesia through the ear edge vein using 3% sodium pentobarbital (1 mL/kg). The Foley's tube, 2.5 mm × 15 mm, was inserted to the depth of 15-17 cm to connect the booster pump, using normal saline to engorge the balloon under 7-8 standard atmosphere pressure. The balloon was repeatedly dragged for 3 times, and then the Foley's tube was withdrawn. The wound was ligated and sutured layer-by-layer. 80 000 IU gentamycin was once intramuscularly injected to prevent the infection. The common forage was fed to rabbits in the normal control group at the daily dose of 100 g; high fat forage fed to those in the model control group at the daily dose of 100 g; high fat forage mixed with 2.5 mg/kg body weight to those in the simvastatin group. All were fed for 6 successive weeks. Two rabbits died during the balloon injury surgery, 2 died due to post-surgical infection, 2 were dropped out of the experiment since they had not eaten the forage. Data were obtained from the rest 24 rabbits that completed the experiment.

1.3 Sampling

Blood sampling from the ear edge artery was collected (fasting 6 h before sampling) at the end of the 2nd and the 8th week respectively, i.e., 2 weeks after high fat forage feeding and 6 weeks after medication intervention. Then the serum was centrifuged and preserved at $-20\ ^\circ\text{C}$ for later use. All rabbits were sacrificed at the end of the 8th week. The lower abdominal aorta tissue was taken from the site with the most obvious lesion (i.e., the balloon intima tear), and fixed in 10% formalin, embedded with routine paraffin, sectioned evenly at the width of 4 μm. Then HE staining and immunochemical staining were respectively performed.

1.4 Detection of Blood Lipids

Serum total cholesterol (TC), triglyceride, high-density lipoprotein (HDL-C) and low-density lipoprotein (LDL-C) were determined using an autoanalyzer.

1.5 Serum Inflammatory Indices and MMPs Detection

Serum levels of hs-CRP, MMP-3 and MMP-9 were detected using enzyme-linked immunosorbent assay (ELISA) and operated according to the instruction of the kit. Finally the absorbance value of each pore was read at 450 nm using an enzyme-labeled instrument. The concentration value was taken as the X-axis, and each standard absorbance value measured as the Y-axis, thus drawing a standard curve. The corresponding concentration value was checked from the standard curve referring to the absorbance value measured at the sample pore and expressed as μg/L.

1.6 Macroscopically Pathomorphological Observation of the Plaque Tissue

The basic structure of the plaque observed under a light microscope after HE staining included foam cells, lipidoses, and cholesterol crystal, etc. compositions. Using IPP imaging analytic software, the area of the AS plaque of each section was analyzed. The plaque area (PA) and the cross-sectional vascular area (CVA) were measured, and the correcting plaque area (PA/CVA) calculated.

1.7 The Protein Expressions of the Vascular Endothelial Growth Factor (VEGF), Factor VIII related antigen (FVIII RAg), MMP-3 and Cluster of Differentiation Antigen 40 Ligand (CD40L) in the Plaque

The expressions of the VEGF, FVIII RAg, MMP-3, and CD40L in the plaque were detected using the immunohistochemical method. The sections were baked at 60 ℃ for 1 h, and deparaffined with dimethyl benzene and gradient alcohol. They were put in 5% dioxogen for 15 min to deactivate endogenous peroxydase. They were incubated with the primary antibody at 4 ℃ overnight, and conjugated with the secondary antibody for 30 min, colorated with DAB, after being stained with hematine, dehydrated, and mounted with neutral gum. The positive findings of the DAB coloration showed brownish yellow granule. The percentages of the positive area of VEGF, FVIII RAg, MMP-3 and CD40L to the plaque area were calculated using IPP imaging management software.

1.8 Statistical Analysis

Statistical analysis was conducted using SPSS 13.0 software package. The measurement data were expressed as mean ± standard deviation ($\bar{\chi} \pm s$). t-test was used for comparison of the measurement data, and LSD test used for intra-group comparison.

2. Results

2.1 The Pathomorphological Changes of the AS Plaque in Rabbits

After 8-week high fat forage feeding, HE stain results showed no foam cells or lipidoses in the abdominal aortic tunica intima and media of the normal control group. In the model control group, obvious AS plaque had formed in the abdominal aorta, with obviously thickened intima. It was full of foam cells. There was cholesterol crystal under the intima and in the plaque, with the fiber cap formation. In the simvastatin group, the swelling and degeneration of endothelial cells were attenuated, with lesser foam cells and lipidoses when compared with those of the model control group (Figure 1). Results of the computer imaging analysis showed no significance in the PA and CAV among the 3 groups. But simvastatin could significantly lower the PA/CAV, showing significant difference to that of the model control group ($P < 0.01$) (Table 1).

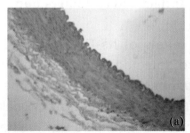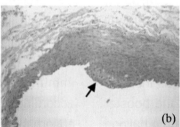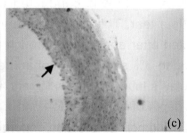

Figure 1　The Morphological Changes in the Rabbit Abdominal Aortal AS Plaque. (a) The normal control group; (b) the model control group; (c) the simvastatin group. HE staining, ×200

Table 1　Comparison of Changes in the PA，CVA，and PA/CVA（$\bar{\chi} \pm s$）[a]

Group	n	PA（mm^2）	CVA（mm^2）	PA/CVA（%）
The normal control group	9	–	1.88 ± 0.28	–
The model control group	7	0.46 ± 0.23	1.90 ± 0.21	28.48 ± 5.47
The simvastatin group	8	0.29 ± 0.17	1.95 ± 0.17	$12.76 \pm 3.93^{**}$

[a] **，$P < 0.01$，compared with the model control group

Table 2　Comparison of Blood Lipids（mmol/L，$\bar{\chi} \pm s$）[a]

Group	Time	n	TC	TG	HDL-C	LDL-C
The normal control group	2nd week	10	1.75 ± 0.81	0.52 ± 0.17	0.37 ± 0.15	0.61 ± 0.39
	8th week	9	$1.75 \pm 0.47^{**}$	$0.51 \pm 0.19^{**}$	$0.43 \pm 0.19^{**}$	$0.91 \pm 0.08^{**}$
The model control group	2nd week	10	$15.77 \pm 3.97^{\triangle\triangle}$	$1.92 \pm 1.04^{\triangle\triangle}$	0.78 ± 0.15	$7.63 \pm 2.41^{\triangle\triangle}$
	8th week	7	30.01 ± 3.11	2.79 ± 0.83	0.81 ± 0.21	14.59 ± 2.38
The simvastatin group	2nd week	10	$14.65 \pm 4.42^{\triangle\triangle}$	$1.75 \pm 0.76^{\triangle\triangle}$	0.88 ± 0.22	$7.21 \pm 3.62^{\triangle\triangle}$
	8th week	8	$22.51 \pm 2.74^{**}$	$1.22 \pm 0.93^{**}$	0.94 ± 0.21	$10.41 \pm 2.61^{**}$

[a] **，$P < 0.01$，compared with the model control group at the end of the 8th week. $\triangle\triangle$，$P < 0.01$，compared with the normal control group at the end of the 2nd week

2.2　Comparison of Blood Lipids

Results showed that serum levels of TC, TG and LDL-C were significantly elevated after 2-week high fat forage feeding in the model control group and the simvastatin group when compared with the normal control group ($P < 0.01$). After 6-week medication intervention, serum levels of TC, TG and LDL-C were significantly lowered in the simvastatin group when compared with the model control group ($P < 0.01$). The serum level of HDL-C in the simvastatin group had an increasing tendency when compared with the model control group, but with insignificantly statistical difference (Table 2).

2.3　Changes in the Serum hs-CRP Level

After 6-week medication intervention, serum hs-CRP concentration in each group was obviously higher than that of the normal control group. Of them, it was (9.80 ± 1.39) μg/mL in the model control group. It was (8.65 ± 1.33) μg/mL in the simvastatin group, showing a significantly lower level when compared with the model control group ($P < 0.05$) (Table 3).

2.4　Changes in Serum MMP-3 and MMP-9 Levels

The serum MMP-3 and MMP-9 levels in the model control group and the simvastatin group were obviously higher than those of the normal control group ($P < 0.05$, $P < 0.01$). The expressions of MMP-3 and MMP-9 in the simvastatin group were obviously lower when compared with those of the model control group ($P < 0.05$), but with insignificant difference ($P > 0.05$) (Table 3).

Table 3　Changes in Serum hs-CRP and MMPs（μg/L，$\bar{\chi} \pm s$）[a]

Group	n	hs-CRP	MMP-3	MMP-9
The normal control group	9	$7.35 \pm 0.44^{**}$	$21.04 \pm 2.81^{**}$	$0.65 \pm 0.17^{**}$
The model control group	7	$9.80 \pm 1.39^{\triangle\triangle}$	$56.82 \pm 18.57^{\triangle\triangle}$	$1.11 \pm 0.07^{\triangle\triangle}$
The simvastatin group	8	$8.65 \pm 1.33^{*\triangle}$	$42.79 \pm 13.66^{*\triangle\triangle}$	$0.90 \pm 0.23^{*\triangle}$

[a] *，$P < 0.05$；**，$P < 0.01$，compared with the model control group. $\triangle$，$P < 0.05$；$\triangle\triangle$；$P < 0.01$，compared with the normal control group

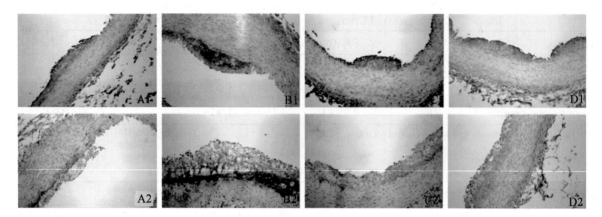

Figure 2 Expressions of VEGF, FVⅢRAg, MMP-3 and CD40L Positive Areas in the Plaque Tissue. A, Expression of the VEGF positive area; B, Expression of the FVⅢRAg positive area; C, Expression of the MMP-3 positive area; D, Expression of the CD40L positive area. 1, The model control group; 2, the simvastatin group. Immunohistochemical staining, ×200

Table 4   The Expression Percentage of VEGF, FVⅢRAg, MMP-3 and CD40L Positive Areas in the Plaque Tissue ($\bar{x} \pm s$)

Group	n	VEGF（%）	FVIII RAg（%）	MMP-3（%）	CD40L（%）
The normal control group	9	–	–	–	–
The model control group	7	22.65±2.94	15.12±1.45	18.08±4.71	11.08±2.48
The simvastatin group	8	19.40±1.63	9.77±2.23	10.43±2.99	7.93±0.91
t value		2.363	4.922	3.467	2.917
P value		0.046	0.001	0.006	0.015

2.5 Quantitatively Immunohistochemical Analysis

The immunohistochemical and imaging analyses showed (Figure 2) that the abdominal aortic intima was smooth in the normal control group, with no plaque formation. Therefore, it was impossible to calculate the positive area. A great deal of brownish yellow granules could be seen in the plaque of the model control group, which was obviously aggregated at the shoulder and basilar part of the plaque. Compared with the model control group, the positively stained area percentages of VEGF, FVⅢRAg, MMP-3 and CD40L in the simvastatin group were significantly reduced, showing statistical significance in inter-group comparisons ($P < 0.05$, $P < 0.01$) (Table 4).

3. Discussion

Coronary heart disease (CHD) is the main cause for the disability and death of cardiovascular diseases. It has also become a highlight in the international field of cardiovascular diseases. The incidence of CHD shows a year-on-year increasing tendency worldwide. The atherosclerotic unstable plaque is the main reason for the myocardial ischemia of CHD and various clinical symptoms. Besides, one study shows that the progression of CHD is determined mainly by biological features of the plaque in the coronary artery[4]. Therefore, the plaque stabilization, the prevention of the plaque rupture, and the prohibition of the development of atherosclerosis can improve the progress and prognosis of CHD to a certain extent.

A recent study[5] found that pathological new vessels often occur in the AS plaque. They occur on the basis of AS lesion, whilst new vessels also accelerate the progress of the atherosclerotic

第四章

lesion. It may possibly be one core event in the occurrence and development of the AS plaque and plays a critical role. Therefore, inhibition of angiogenesis in the plaque may possibly become the target to enhance the plaque stability and prevent acute coronary syndrome with potential therapeutic significance.

Statins can effectively reduce the incidence and mortality of CHD. In addition to its LDL-C lowering effect, it shows its cardiovascular protective effect independent of blood lipids lowering. This is called as pleiotropic effects of statins, including improvement of endothelial functions, stabilization of vulnerable plaques, anti-inflammation, anti-oxidation, immunoregulation, blood pressure lowering, and inhibition of thrombopoiesis, and so on[6]. Simvastatin, as one hydroxyl-methyle-glutaryl coenzyme A (HMG-CoA) reductase inhibitor, can inhibit the synthesis of endogenous cholesterols, thus further playing a role in lowering blood lipids. While lowering blood lipids levels, simvastatin may also inhibit the migration and adhesion of endothelial cells, and lower the secretion of MMPs, thus arriving at the effect on the plaque stabilization[7].

AS is an inflammatory disease. The inflammatory reaction runs through the developing process of AS, being the central link of the occurrence and development of AS. hs-CRP is a sensitive marker to reflect the atherosclerotic inflammatory process[8]. Results of this experiment showed that serum hs-CRP concentration was significantly increased in the model group. It was obviously decreased in the simvastatin group when compared with the model control group, showing the atherosclerotic inflammatory process was inhibited.

MMPs are one important enzyme group capable of digesting the extracellular matrix. It may accelerate the plaque rupture through degrading compositions of fiber caps and destroying their structures, which is an important reason for unstable atherosclerotic plaques[9].

CD40L may be expressed on the surface of endothelial cells, macrophages, and smooth muscle cells in the atherosclerotic plaque, and induce monocytes/macrophages, endothelial cells, vascular smooth muscle cells to express MMPs[10]. Results of this experiment showed that serum MMP-3 and MMP-9 levels were more significantly elevated in the model control group than in the normal control group, indicating the existence of unstable plaques and increased degradation of extracellular matrix in AS. However, simvastatin significantly inhibited serum expressions of MMP-3 and MMP-9 (Similarly this may be reflected by lowering serum MMP-3 level and CD40L in the plaque), thus playing a certain role of reducing local matrix degradation in the plaque. It is conducive to the maintenance of the plaque stability.

VEGF, one growth factor with the specificity to promote the mitosis of vascular endothelial cells, has been proved to be express obviously in the atherosclerotic plaque, and possibly accelerate the occurrence and development of the plaque[11,12]. FVIIIRAg, one glycoprotein extensively existing on the surface of endothelial cells, is a specific marker for the neogenetic vascular endothelium. It is expressed at the small blood capillaries and the branch of capillaries without forming the lumens. VEGF and FVIIIRAg both participate in the angiogenesis[13]. Results of this study showed simvastatin may prohibit expressions of VEGF and FVIIIRAg in the rabbit AS plaque model to some extent. Results of pathological observation showed that under the condition of high fat forage feeding, the vascular morphological indices in the simvastatin group were superior to those in the model control group (fed with high fat forage alone). It also indicated simvastatin played a role in improving PA and controlling the AS plaque.

To sum up, simvastatin may inhibit the inflammatory reaction, and reach the plaque stabilization through lowering the secretion of

MMPs, which is in line with previous results[7]. Besides, simvastatin may also inhibit expressions of VEGF and FⅧRAg in the atherosclerotic plaque. We may infer that inhibition of pathological angiogenesis in the plaque is its another mechanism of action on stabilizing the plaque.

References

[1] Ross J, Staglian N, Donovan M, et al. Atheroselerosis and cancer: common molecular pathways of disease development and progression. Ann N Y Acad Sci, 2001, 947: 271-292.

[2] Sacco RL, Liao J K. Drug Insight: statins and stroke. Nat Clin Pract Cardiovasc Med, 2005, 2: 576-584.

[3] Wilson S H, Herrmann J, Lerman LO, et al. Simvastatin preserves the structure of coronary adventitial vasa vasorum in experimental hypercholesterolemia independent of lipid lowering. Circulation, 2002, 105: 415-418.

[4] Thrall G, Lane D, Carroll D, et al. A systematic review of the effects of acute psychological stress and physical activity on haemorheology, coagulation, fibrinolysis and platelet reactivity: implications for the pathogenesis of acute coronary syndromes. Thromb Res, 2007, 120: 819-847.

[5] Sun L, Wei LX, Shi HY, et al. The relation between angiogenesis and the plaque stability in the atherosclerotic plaque. Chin J Pathol, 2003, 32: 427-431.

[6] Xia CD, Yin HJ. Progress of researches on pleiotropic effects of statins in improving endothelial functions. Adv Cardiovasc Dis, 2008, 29: 956-960.

[7] Rudd JH, Machac J, Favad ZA. Simvastatin and plaque inflammation. J Am Coll Cardiol, 2007, 48: 1825-1831.

[8] Schlager O, Exner M, Mlekusch W, et al. C-reactive protein predicts future cardiovascular events in patients with carotid stenosis. Stroke, 2007, 38: 1263-1268.

[9] Abilleira S, Bevan S, Markus HS. The role of genetic variants of matrix metalloproteinases in coronary and carotid atherosclerosis. J Med Genet, 2006, 43: 897-901.

[10] San Miguel Hernández A, Inglada-Galiana L, García Iglesias R, et al. Soluble CD40 ligand: a potential marker of cardiovascular risk. Rev Clin Esp, 2007, 207: 418-421.

[11] Caldwell RB, Bartoli M, BŴzadian MA, et al. Vascular endothelial growth factor and diabetic retinopathy: role of oxidative stress. Curr Drug Targets, 2005, 6: 511-524.

[12] Panutsopulos D, Papalambros E, Sigala F, et al. Protein and mRNA expression levels of VEGF-A and TGF-beta1 in different types of human coronary atherosclerotic lesions. Int J Mol Med, 2005, 15: 603-610.

[13] Galbusera M, Zoja C, Donadelli R, et al. Fluid shear stress modulates von Willebrand factor release from human vascular endothelium. Blood, 1997, 90: 1558-1564.

第五节　中医药抗血小板、抑制血栓形成的研究

Correlation between Platelet Gelsolin and Platelet Activation Level in Acute Myocardial Infarction Rats and Intervention Effect of Effective Components of Chuanxiong Rhizome and Red Peony Root[*]

LIU Yue　YIN Hui-jun　JIANG Yue-rong　XUE Mei　GUO Chun-yu
SHI Da-zhuo　CHEN Ke-ji

1. Introduction

Despite recent medical advances, cardiovascular diseases remain the predominant cause of morbidity and mortality all over the world [1,2]. Rupture of atherosclerotic plaque and the ensuing thrombotic changes are the triggers for acute coronary event. Platelet activation and aggregation play crucial roles in this process of atherothrombosis. The emergence of antiplatelet drug is the milestone of prevention and therapy of cardiovascular disease and provides the primary therapeutic strategy to combat cardiovascular diseases. The proper application of antiplatelet drug in reducing the mortality and morbidity of acute myocardial infarction successfully has been verified by a large number of large-scale clinical trials [3]. Antiplatelet drug, such as aspirin, now is recommended for the secondary prevention of cardiovascular disease (CVD) in patients with CVD because it decreases the risk of CVD events and mortality in clinical trials of men and women with CVD [4]. But many clinical problems arose along with the wide range of application of antiplatelet drugs (such as aspirin and clopidogrel, etc.) during the past 10 years [5,6]. Despite their proven benefits, recurrent cardiovascular events still occur in those taking antiplatelet drugs. This has led to the concept of "antiplatelet drug resistance", most commonly aspirin or clopidogrel resistance. The latest research shows that aspirin prophylaxis in people without prior CVD does not lead to reductions in cardiovascular death, for the benefits are further offset by clinically important bleeding events [7], which limit the clinical practice of antiplatelet drugs widely. These phenomena suggest that other pathways capable of stimulating platelet activation may exist and provide an impetus for developing new antiplatelet drugs which possess higher efficacy and fewer adverse effects.

Proteomics technology has been successfully applied to platelet research during the past 5 years, contributing to the emerging

* 原载于 Evidence-Based Complementary and Alternative Medicine，2013，Article ID：985746

field of platelet proteomics which led to the identification of a considerable amount of novel platelet proteins, many of which have been further studied at their functional level [8]. Our previous work [9] indicated that platelet gelsolin is the main platelet differential functional protein between patients of coronary heart disease and healthy people by platelet proteomics. Studies have also shown that platelet gelsolin is highly expressed in patients with acute coronary syndrome (ACS) and the blood-stasis syndrome (BSS) of traditional Chinese medicine (TCM) [10,11]. Gelsolin is known to have one of the key roles in extracellular actin-scavenger system (EASS) [12], but the biological role of platelet gelsolin in platelet activation of acute myocardial infarction (AMI) is unclear. On the prevention of atherosclerosis or vulnerable plaque, Chinese medicine and Western medicine agree on stabling plaque and promoting blood circulation. Based on the agreed thoughts of the Eastern and Western worlds, the application of Chinese herbs for activating blood circulation (ABC herbs) has valuable significance in the exploration of reducing the risk of cardiovascular event [13,14]. Chuanxiong rhizome and Red peony root are the two classical ABC herbs in China and have been used for thousands of years in the prevention and treatment of CVD. Xiongshao capsule (XSC) is a patent drug in China and is composed of effective components of Chuanxiong rhizome and Red peony root. Our previous studies have showed that paeoniflorin, ferulic acid and total phenolic acid are the major active principles of the water extract from Xiongshao capsule [15,16]. Clinical studies indicated that XSC can effectively prevent restenosis after percutaneous coronary intervention (PCI) [17], but the antiplatelet target of XSC is not defined.

In the present study, we used AMI as a disease model to investigate the correlation between platelet gelsolin and platelet activation level in rat model of AMI and the prophylaxis mechanism of XSC *in vivo*.

2. Materials and Methods

2.1 Drug and Reagents

Xiongshao Capsule (XSC), which contained paeoniflorin (more than or equal to 28 mg each capsule), ferulate (more than or equal to 3.5 mg each capsule), and total phenolic acid (more than or equal to 34 mg each capsule), 0.25 g per capsule, were provided by Beijing International Institute of Biological Products (batch no. 200091, Beijing, China); aspirin, 0.1 g per capsule, was purchased from Bayer Health Care Manufacturing (batch no. BJ01653, Beijing, China); verapamil, 0.04 g per tablet, was purchased from the Central Pharmaceutical Co., Ltd (batch no. 100402, Tianjing, China). All the drugs were dissolved in pure water before use.

Fluo-3AM was purchased from Sigma (St Louis, MO, USA); rabbit anti-gelsolin polyclonal antibody was purchased from Abcam (San Francisco, USA); mouse anti-β-actin monoclonal antibody was purchased from Sigma (St Louis, MO, USA); FITC-Phalloidin was purchased from Sigma (St Louis, MO, USA); enzyme-linked immunosorbent assay (ELISA) kit of P-selectin, gelsolin, F-actin, vitamin D binding protein (VDBP), CK-MB, cTnI, TXB_2, and COX-1 were purchased from Huamei Biological Technology Company (Wuhan, Hubei province, China).

2.2 Animal Grouping and Treatment

Sprague Dawley (SD) rats (male, weight 220-250 g, *n*=90) were obtained from Beijing University Laboratory Animal Center (the animal certificate No: SCXK (Jing) 2006-0009). The rats were housed in humidity-controlled $(55 \pm 5)\%$ rooms at (22 ± 2) ℃ with a 12 h on/12 h off light cycle. The animals were maintained with free access to standard diet and tap water.

After one week of adaptive feeding, we randomly allocated the SD rats into six groups of 15 rats each as follows: Model group, Sham group, Aspirin group, Xscd group (the high dose group), Xscx group (the low doses group), and Verapamil group. Aspirin 40 mg/ (kg·day), verapamil 4mg/ (kg·day), and XSC 390 mg/ (kg·day), 195 mg/ (kg·day) per gavage for 3 consecutive weeks were administrated to the aspirin, verapamil, Xscd and Xscx groups respectively. Rats in the Sham and Model groups received the same volume of distilled water, per gavage for 3 weeks. After 3 weeks, myocardial infarction (MI) model was created in rats by ligating the left anterior descending coronary artery (LAD) as described before [18]. The Animal Care and Use Committee of Xiyuan Hospital approved the experimental protocol.

2.3　Sample Preparation

After 3 hours of ligation, all the rats were killed after anesthesia by intraperitoneal injection of 20% urethane (0.5 mL/100 g). Fresh blood (10 mL) was drawn from the abdominal aorta and collected into vacutainer tubes containing acid citrate dextrose (ACD) 9% v/v (trisodium citrate 22.0 g/L, citric acid 8.0 g/L, dextrose 24.5 g/L) as anticoagulant. The initial 2 mL of blood was discarded to avoid spontaneous platelet activation. The blood was centrifuged for 10 min at $150 \times g$ at room temperature to obtain plateletrich plasma (PRP) and the remaining blood centrifuged for 20 min at $800 \times g$ to obtain platelet poor plasma (PPP).

Ischemic heart tissue was taken after blood collection and preserved at -80℃ for detection of gelsolin expression by western blotting.

2.4　Enzyme-linked Immunosorbent Assay Analysis

The concentration of PRP and PPP of gelsolin, plasma F-actin, VDBP, CK-MB, cTnl, TXB_2, COX-1 were determined by enzyme-linked immunoadsorbent assay (ELISA), as per the manufacturer's instructions. The absorbance was measured at 450 nm in an ELISA reader.

2.5　Western Blotting Analysis

The level of gelsolin in ischemic heart tissues was determined by Western blot analysis according to the standard procedure as described previously[19]. β-actin was used as a loading control.

2.6　Detection of MFI of Platelet Calcium Ion

Platelet-rich plasma was prepared and incubated with 4μmol/L Fluo-3-AM (Sigma, Saint Louis, MO, USA) at 37℃ for 40min. The calcium concentration of platelets was determined using flow cytometry to measure the mean fluorescence intensity (MFI), as previously described [20].

2.7　Statistical Analysis

Data are presented as mean $\pm$ SD. The SPSS Statistics 11.0 package was utilized to analyze the data. Differences among groups were analyzed using the one-way analysis of variance (ANOVA), followed by multiple comparisons by Least-Significant Difference (LSD) test. Spearman's correlation coefficients were calculated to study the relations between gelsolin concentration in PRP and plasma P-selectin level. Differences between groups were at $P < 0.05$.

3.　Results

3.1　General Condition

All the rats in the different groups survived and exhibited normal physical appearance and behavior during the gavage period of different drugs. The outcome among the different groups after ligation of LAD is presented in Table 1.

Table 1　The Outcome among the Different Groups after Ligation of LAD

Group	N	Dead rats (n)	Surviving rats (n)
Sham	15	6	9
Model	15	6	9
Aspirin	15	5	10
Xscd	15	6	9
Xscx	15	7	8
Verapamil	15	7	8

3.2　XSC Reduces the Concentration of Myocardial Injury Markers

We chose CK-MB and cTnl as the myocardial injury markers in rats with acute myocardial infarction (AMI). Compared with the Sham group, the concentration of CK-MB and cTnl of Model group increased significantly after ligation of LAD for 3 hours ($P < 0.01$). The high dose of XSC (390 mg/(kg·day)) can reduce the concentration of CK-MB and cTnI markedly ($P < 0.05$); this has similar effect with aspirin in vivo (see Table 2).

Table 2　Effect of Xiongshao Capsule (XSC) on the Concentration of Myocardial Injury Markers of AMI Rats

Group	N	CK-MB (ng/mL)	cTnI (pg/mL)
Sham	9	0.279±0.074	9.81±2.62
Model	9	0.386±0.043**	15.18±4.3**
Aspirin	10	0.340±0.024†	12.04±1.19†
Xscd	9	0.336±0.027†	12.23±1.41†
Xscx	8	0.351±0.013	13.85±3.02
Verapamil	8	0.358±0.017	14.43±2.98

**P < 0.01 compared to Sham group and †P < 0.05 compared to Model group

3.3　XSC Inhibits the Platelet Activation Level

We choose the plasma P-selectin as the marker of platelet activation level. Compared with Sham group, the plasma P-selectin concentration of the Model group increased significantly after ligation of LAD for 3 hours ($P < 0.01$). The high dose of XSC can inhibit P-selection level markedly ($P < 0.05$), this has similar effect with the Aspirin group (see Figure 1).

3.4　XSC Reduces the Platelet Gelsolin Level and Enhances the Activity of Extracellular Actin-Scavenger System (EASS)

Plasma gelsolin and VDBP are the main components of the EASS which undertake the responsibility as scavenger of the abnormal increased extracellular filament actin (Factin). Compared with the Sham group, the plasma gelsolin and VDBP of the Model group was reduced significantly ($P < 0.05$) and F-actin increased markedly ($P < 0.01$), while platelet gelsolin it increased markedly ($P < 0.01$). High dose of XSC can reduce platelet gelsolin and F-actin level ($P < 0.05$), while it increased plasma gelsolin and VDBP significantly ($P < 0.05$) (see Figures 2, 3, and 4).

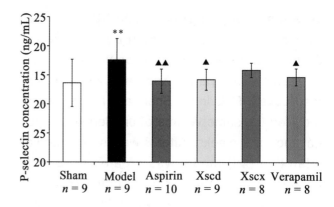

Figure 1　Effect of Xiongshao Capsule (XSC) on P-selectin Concentration of AMI Rats. **$P < 0.01$ compared to Sham group, and ▲$P < 0.05$ or ▲▲$P < 0.01$ compared to Model group

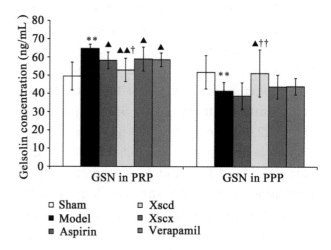

Figure 2　Effect of Xiongshao Capsule (XSC) on Gelsolin Concentration among PRP and PPP of AMI Rats. **$P < 0.01$ compared to Sham group, ▲$P < 0.05$ or ▲▲$P < 0.01$ compared to Model group, and †$P < 0.05$ or ††$P < 0.01$ compared to Aspirin group

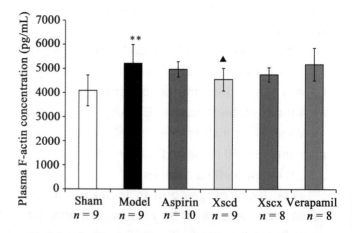

Figure 3　Effect of Xiongshao Capsule (XSC) on Plasma F-actin Concentration of AMI Rats. **$P < 0.01$ compared to Sham group, and ▲$P < 0.05$ compared to Model group

3.5　XSC Inhibits the Activation of TXB₂ and COX-1

Compared with Sham group, the concentration of TXB_2 and COX-1 of Model group increased significantly after ligation of LAD for 3 hours $(P < 0.01)$. High dose of XSC can reduce COX-1 and TXB_2 level significantly $(P < 0.05)$; this has similar effect with the Aspirin group (see Figure 5).

3.6　XSC Inhibits the MFI of Calcium

Compared with Sham group, the MFI of calcium of the Model group increased markedly $(P < 0.01)$. High dose of XSC can inhibit platelet calcium increase $(P < 0.05)$. This has similar effect to the Verapamil group $(P < 0.05)$ (see Figure 6).

3.7　XSC Attenuates the Expression of Gelsolin in Infarcted Myocardium

Compared with Sham group, the gelsolin expression of infarcted myocardium of Model group increased markedly, and XSC can inhibit gelsolin expression of infarcted myocardium, but

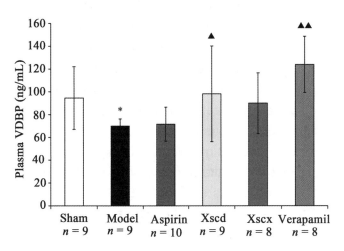

Figure 4　Effect of Xiongshao Capsule（XSC）on Plasma VDBP Concentration of AMI Rats. *$P < 0.05$ compared to Sham group, and ▲$P < 0.05$ or ▲▲$P < 0.01$ compared to Model group

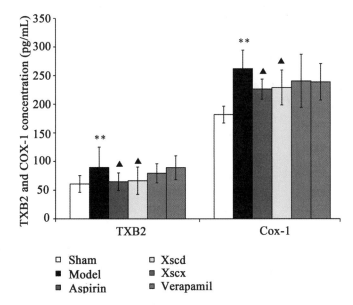

Figure 5　Effect of Xiongshao Capsule（XSC）on Plasma TXB₂ and COX-1 Concentration of AMI Rats. **$P < 0.01$ compared to Sham group, and ▲$P < 0.05$ compared to Model group

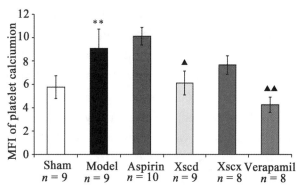

Figure 6　Effect of Xiongshao Capsule（XSC）on MFI of Platelet Calciumion Concentration of AMI Rats. **$P < 0.01$ compared to Sham group, and ▲$P < 0.05$ or ▲▲$P < 0.01$ compared to Model group

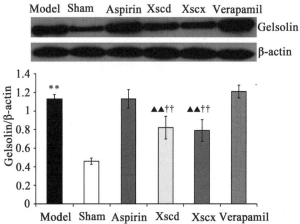

Figure 7　Effect of Xiongshao Capsule（XSC）on Protein Level of Gelsolin in Ischemic Heart Tissue of AMI Rats. **$P < 0.01$ compared to Sham group, and ▲▲$P < 0.01$ compared to Model group, ††$P < 0.01$ compared to Aspirin group

411

verapamil has no such effect (see Figure 7).

3.8 Analyses of Correlation between Platelet Gelsolin Concentration and Plasma P-Selectin Level

Next we investigated any potential correlation between the platelet gelsolin concentration and plasma P-selectin levels that may exist in the Model group and Xscd group. Correlation analysis showed that platelet gelsolin concentrations were high positively correlated with plasma P-selectin levels in the Model group (see Figure 8 (a)) and Xscd group (see Figure 8(b)).

4. Discussion

Gelsolin is a calcium-regulated actin filament (F-actin) severing and capping protein, which is expressed as both cytoplasmic and plasma isoforms. The functions of extracellular gelsolin are less well defined. Gelsolin is also an important cytoskeletal protein, which is a key actin binding protein (ABPs) as well. Increasingly evidence has shown that gelsolin has close relationship with many diseases and pathological processes, such as cancer, apoptosis, infection and inflammation, pulmonary diseases, and aging [21]. During the past 5 years, many scholars began to focus on gelsolin's possible role in the development of

cardiovascular diseases [22]. Activated platelets play a pivotal role in the formation of arterial thrombi, and antiplatelet drugs become the core in the prevention and treatment of CVD. Platelet activation not only causes the changes of membrane protein, but also a series of morphological changes, from inviscid, discotic circulating platelets to a paste-like, protruding platelet jelly, that affects the regulation of platelet cytoskeletal proteins.

Using differential proteomics of platelet, our previous study [9] indicated that platelet gelsolin was the main platelet differential functional proteins between patients with coronary heart disease and healthy people. In addition, data from our previous clinical studies demonstrated that [10,11] platelet gelsolin was highly expressed in patients with acute coronary syndrome (ACS) and the blood stasis syndrome (BSS) of traditional Chinese medicine. Meanwhile, based on the Chinese medicine principle of "prescription to syndrome". Platelet gelsolin may be viewed as a new target for ABC herbs. In this study, we evaluated the biological role of platelet gelsolin in the development of platelet activation in a rat model of AMI and the potential contribution of XSC prophylaxis in this progress *in vivo*.

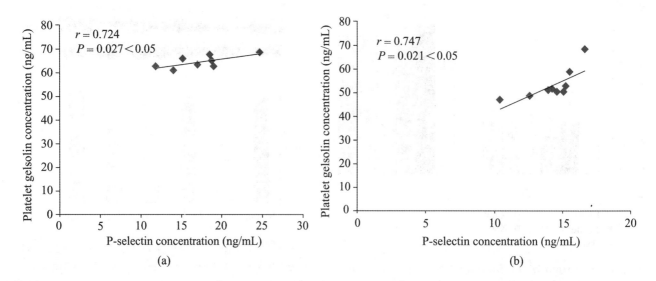

(a)

(b)

Figure 8　Correlation between Gelsolin Concentration in PRP and Plasma P-selectin Level of Model Group and Xscd Group. (a) Model group and (b) Xscd group

As we know, P-selectin is a 140 kD glycoprotein that is presented in the granules of platelets and translocates rapidly to the cell surface after platelet activation; it is generally considered as the gold marker of platelet activation[23]. In this study, after ligation of LAD for 3 hours, the concentration of CK-MB and cTnI and the P-selectin level of the Model rats increased significantly compared with Sham rats, which indicated that the Model rats had myocardial injury and platelet activation.

The actin cytoskeleton plays a central role in many fundamental cellular processes involving the generation of force and facilitation of movement, which are enabled by the assembly of actin monomers into filaments and cooperation with a wide variety of ABPs [21], including gelsolin. Actin monomers (G-actin) spontaneously associates to form F-actin under physiological conditions and vice versa. This dynamic progress keeps in balance all the time. In the presence of tissue injury or cell death, G-actin is released into the circulation where it can interact with components of the haemostatic and fibrinolytic systems, or polymerize and form F-actin excessively. Studies [24] have suggested that F-actin can lead to platelet aggregation directly *in vitro*, and the presence of excessive F-actin in blood vessels, which can plug smaller vessels and decrease blood flow to promote the formation of blood clots, can be fatal. Infusion of high doses of G-actin in rabbits caused the rapid and fatal formation of massive F-actin-containing thrombi in arterioles and capillaries of pulmonary veins [25]. An extracellular actinscavenger system (EASS) [12] was therefore likely to exist. Plasma gelsolin, together with vitamin D binding protein (VDBP), another extracellular ABPs, were regarded as potentially important components of this system. They are capable of removing F-actin from the circulation and inhibiting F-actin elongation to alleviate the vascular toxicity of excessive F-actin. In this study, the concentration of gelsolin in PRP of AMI rats increased accompanied by the high platelet activation and increased level of F-actin while gelsolin in PPP decreased which indicates the EASS of AMI rats was suppressed. Correlation analysis showed that platelet gelsolin concentrations were high, positively correlated with plasma P-selectin levels in the Model group.

Xiongshao capsule (XSC) is a patent drug developed from Xue Fu Zhu Yu Decoction. It is the classic formula used for activating blood circulation (ABC) in China for hundreds of years. Clinical studies have shown that XSC can effectively prevent restenosis after percutaneous coronary intervention (PCI) [17]. XSC was shown to enhance the protective effect of ischemic postconditioning on rat with myocardial ischemic reperfusion injury [26]. It was also shown to stabilize atherosclerotic plaque by suppressing inflammation and the expression of FcγR ⅢA [27]. But the potential antiplatelet mechanism of XSC prophylaxis is unclear. In this study, we found that high dose of XSC prophylaxis could decrease the concentration of myocardial injury markers, CK-MB and cTnI, and reduce the plasma P-selectin level of AMI rats as well. The antiplatelet mechanism of aspirin involves the inhibition of COX-1 and TXA_2, our study shows that high dosage of XSC can inhibit the activation of TXB_2 and COX-1 *in vivo*, which has similar cardioprotection effect with aspirin *in vivo*. Meanwhile, high dosage of XSC prophylaxis inhibited the expression of platelet gelsolin in AMI rats by inhibiting the platelet calcium influx, but increased the concentration of plasma gelsolin and plasma VDBP simultaneously, so the EASS was activated, and the concentration of F-actin in AMI rats decreased which indicated that the F-actin was being removed from the circulation. Calcium ions not only promote gelsolin secretion but also play a vital role in the development of platelet activation. Studies have shown increased platelet $[Ca^{2+}]_i$ in patients with CVD [28], and that calcium channel blocker (CCB) could reduce platelet $[Ca^{2+}]_i$ and inhibit platelet aggregation [29]. Verapamil is a classic CCB agent and a previous

413

study *in vivo* [30] shows that verapamil exhibits a dose-dependent inhibitory effect on platelet aggregation and thrombus formation in rats. In this study, our results show that high dosage of XSC can mimic the calcium channel antagonist effect.

We have also investigated the expression of the gelsolin in infarcted myocardium of AMI rats. The results indicate that the gelsolin expression of infarcted myocardium of the Model group increased markedly; while XSC can inhibit gelsolin expression of infarcted myocardium significantly, verapamil or aspirin has no such effect, holding that other pathway existed in the regulation of gelsolin as well. Heart failure (HF) is the end stage of CVD (including after AMI). It is of great importance to know the effects and mechanism of XSC on cardioprotection at earlier stages of CVD. Ventricular remodeling after AMI is the main pathological change of HF. A previous study[31] has showed that gelsolin is an important contributor to heart failure progression through novel mechanisms of HIF-1α and DNase I activation and downregulation of antiapoptotic survival factors. Based on these results and our study, we propose that gelsolin inhibition is a promising target for CVD therapy besides antiplatelet agent.

5. Conclusion

We have provided experimental evidence supporting our conclusion that high correlation between platelet gelsolin and platelet activation level in AMI rats, the aspirin-like cardioprotection, and antiplatelet effects of XSC are related to its inhibition on platelet gelsolin, platelet calcium influx and activate d the EASS. Taken together, our results suggest that platelet gelsolin is a potential antiplatelet target and XSC is a promising lead compound for antiplatelet and cardiovascular therapy.

References

[1] Choi J, Kermode JC. New therapeutic approaches to combat arterial thrombosis. Molecular Interventions, 2011, 11 (2): 111-123.

[2] Tseeng S, Arora R. Reviews: aspirin resistance: biological and clinical implications. Journal of Cardiovascular Pharmacology and Therapeutics, 2008, 13 (1): 5-12.

[3] Michelson AD. Antiplatelet therapies for the treatment of cardiovascular disease. Nature Reviews Drug Discovery, 2010, 9, (2): 154-169.

[4] Baigent C, Blackwell L, Collins R, et al. Aspirin in the primary and secondary prevention of vascular disease: collaborative meta-analysis of individual participant data from randomized trials. The Lancet, 2009, 373 (9678): 1849-1860.

[5] Juurlink DN, Gomes T, Ko DT, et al. A population-based study of the drug interaction between proton pump inhibitors and clopidogrel. Canadian Medical Association Journal, 2009, 180 (7): 713-718.

[6] Mega JL, Close SL, Wiviott SD, et al. Cytochrome P-450 polymorphisms and response to clopidogrel. New England Journal of Medicine, 2009, 360 (4): 354-362.

[7] Seshasai SR, Wijesuriya S, Sivakumaran R, et al. Effect of aspirin on vascular and nonvascular outcomes: meta-analysis of randomized controlled trials. Archives of Internal Medicine, 2012, 172, (3): 209-216.

[8] Garca A. Clinical proteomics in platelet research: challenges ahead. Journal of Thrombosis and Haemostasis, 2010, 8 (8): 1784-1785.

[9] Li XF, Jiang YR, Wu CF, et al. Study on the correlation between platelet function proteins and symptom complex in coronary heart disease. Zhongguo Fen Zi Xin Zang Bing Xue Za Zhi, 2009, 9 (6): 326-331.

[10] Liu Y, Yin HJ, Chen KJ. Research on the correlation between platelet gelsolin and blood-stasis syndrome of coronary heart disease. Chinese Journal of Integrative Medicine, 2011, 17 (8): 587-592.

[11] Liu Y, Yin HY, Jiang YR, et al. Correlation between platelet gelsolin level and different types of coronary heart disease. Chinese Science Bulletin, 2012, 57 (6): 631-638.

[12] Lee WM, Galbraith RM. The extracellular actin-scavenger systemand actin toxicity. New England

Journal of Medicine, 1992, 326 (20): 1335-1341.

[13] Chen KJ. Explore the possibilities of Chinese herb and formulas for promoting blood circulation and removing blood stasis on reducing the cardiovascular risk. Zhongguo Zhong Xi Yi Jie He Za Zhi, 2008, 28 (5): 389.

[14] Liu Y, Yin HJ, Shi DZ, et al. Chinese herb and formulas for promoting blood circulation and removing blood stasis and antiplatelet therapies. Evidence-Based Complementary and Alternative Medicine, 2012, Article ID 184503.

[15] Zhang Z, Qing LM, Chen KJ. Study on the pharmacokinetics of paeoniflorin contained in Xiongshao capsule in canine. Zhongguo Shi Yan Fang Ji Xue Za Zhi, 2000, 6 (6): 21-24.

[16] Zhang Z, Yan YF, Chen KJ. Study on the pharmacokinetics of ferulic acid in canine serum after giving an intragastrical single dose of Xiongshao capsules to a dog. Beijing Zhong Yi Yao Da Xue Xue Bao, 2001, 24 (1): 25-28.

[17] Chen KJ, Shi DZ, Xu H, et al. XS0601 reduces the incidence of restenosis: a prospective study of 335 patients undergoing percutaneous coronary intervention in China. Chinese Medical Journal, 2006, 119 (1): 6-13.

[18] Sun M, Dawood F, Wen WH, et al. Excessive tumor necrosis factor activation after infarction contributes to susceptibility of myocardial rupture and left ventricular dysfunction. Circulation, 2004, 110 (20): 3221-3228.

[19] Li GH, Shi Y, Chenet Y, et al. Gelsolin regulates cardiac remodeling after myocardial infarction through DNase I-mediated apoptosis. Circulation Research, 2009, 104 (7): 896-904.

[20] Zhuang MM, Wen YX, Liu SL, et al. Determination of the level of cytopplasmic free calcium in human platelets with flow cytometry. Xi An Jiao Tong Da Xue Xue Bao, 2005, 26 (5): 508-510.

[21] Li GH, Arora PD, Chen Y, et al. Multifunctional roles of gelsolin in health and diseases. Medicinal Research Reviews, 2012, 32 (5): 999-1025.

[22] Liu Y, Jiang YR, Yin HJ, et al. Gelsolin and cardiovascular diseases. Zhongguo Fen Zi Xin Zang Bing Xue Za Zhi, 2011, 11 (1): 50-53.

[23] Michelson AD, Furman MI. Laboratory markers of platelet activation and their clinical significance. Current Opinion in Hematology, 1999, 6 (5): 342-348.

[24] Vasconcellos CA, Lind SE. Coordinated inhibition of actin-induced platelet aggregation by plasma gelsolin and vitamin D-binding protein. Blood, 1993, 82 (12): 3648-3657.

[25] Haddad JG, Harper KD, Guoth M, et al. Angiopathic consequences of saturating the plasma scavenger system for actin. Proceedings of the National Academy of Sciences of the United States of America, 1990, 87 (4): 1381-1385.

[26] Zhang DW, Zhang L, Liu JG, et al. Effects of Xiongshao capsule combined with ischemic postconditioning on monocyte chemoattractant protein-1 and tumor necrosis factor-α in rat myocardium with ischemic reperfusion injury. Zhongguo Zhong Xi Yi Jie He Za Zhi, 2010, 30 (12): 1279-1283.

[27] Huang Y, Yin HJ, Ma XJ, et al. Correlation between FcγR III A and aortic atherosclerotic plaque destabilization in ApoE knockout mice and intervention effects of effective components of Chuanxiong Rhizome and Red Peony Root. Chinese Journal of Integrative Medicine, 2011, 17 (5): 355-360.

[28] Yoshimura M, Oshima T, Hiraga H, et al. Increased cytosolic free Mg^{2+} and Ca^{2+} in platelets of patients with vasospastic angina. American Journal of Physiology, 1998, 274 (2): R548-R554.

[29] Fujinishi A, Takahara K, Ohba C, et al. Effects of nisoldipine on cytosolic calcium, platelet aggregation, and coagulation/fibrinolysis in patients with coronary artery disease. Angiology, 1997, 48 (6): 515-521.

[30] Li M, Liu Y, Huang Y, et al. Effect of verapamil on the thrombogenesis and nitric oxide level in the serum of rats. Nanjing Yi Ke Da Xue Xue Bao, 2007, 27 (10): 1080-1083.

[31] Li GH, Shi Y, Chenet Y, et al. Gelsolin regulates cardiac remodeling after myocardial infarction through DNase I-mediated apoptosis. Circulation Research, 2009, 104 (7): 896-904.

Effect of Chinese Herbal Medicine for Activating Blood Circulation and Detoxifying on Expression of Inflammatory Reaction and Tissue Damage Related Factors in Experimental Carotid Artery Thrombosis Rats*

XUE Mei ZHANG Lu YANG Lin JIANG Yue-rong GUO Chun-yu YIN Hui-jun CHEN Ke-ji

The lesion of thrombosis in cardio-/cerebrovascular diseases is based on atherosclerosis, and many clinical and lab researches have confirmed that thrombosis due to atherosclerosis is closely related to inflammation[1-3]. The etiology and pathogenesis of platelet activation and thrombosis in the process of cardiac and cerebral thrombotic diseases are considered as "blood stasis" in Chinese medicine (CM). A series of therapeutic principles and methods of promoting blood circulation and removing blood stasis was formed under the guidance of this theory, which showed a positive therapeutic effect on the prevention and treatment of cardio-/cerebrovascular diseases. However, the pathological changes such as tissue necrosis and inflammation cannot be considered only as CM blood stasis[4]. Based on the combination of the basic theory of blood stasis and pathogenic toxins of CM, experimental carotid artery thrombosis rats model were used in this study. The pathophysiological changes were reflected in thrombosis, inflammatory reaction and tissue damage in three aspects, and the difference of the therapeutic effects of Chinese drugs for activating blood circulation to that of activating blood circulation and detoxifying were compared as well. We then tried to determine the micro-pathological basis of the relationship between blood stasis and the pathogenic toxin, and provide an objective experimental basis for the CM treatment of cardiac and cerebral thrombotic diseases.

1. Methods

1.1 Animals

Fifty SPF Wistar rats, half male and half female, weighing 190 ± 10 g, were provided by Experimental Institute of Chinese Academy of Medical Sciences [Certificate No. SCXK (Beijing) 2005-0013].

1.2 Main Reagents and Instruments

Enzyme-linked immunosorbent assay (ELISA) kit, matrix metalloproteinases (MMP-9, batch number: 20080413), tissue inhibitors to metalloproteinase (TIMP-1, batch number: 20080617), granule membrane protein-140 (GMP-140, batch number: 20080621), tissue-type plasminogen activator (t-PA, batch number: 080523), high-sensitivity C-reactive protein (hs-CRP, batch number: 20080617), interleukin-6 (IL-6, batch number: 20080524), were provided by R&D Systems Inc, USA and were sub-packaged by Shanghai Boatman Biotech Inc., which were detected by micro-plate reader (Thermo MK3, USA).

* 原载于 Chinese Journal of Integrative Medicine，2010，16（3）：247-251

1.3 Medication

Simvastatin (Hangzhou MSD Pharmaceutical Co. Ltd., batch number: 07432), 40 mg each tablet, was made into powder in mortar and dissolved into suspension with double-distilled water. Xiongshao Capsule (芎芍胶囊, XSC, Dalian Institute of Chemical Physics, batch number: 070929), 0.25 g each capsule, contained paeoniflorin (more than or equal to 28 mg each capsule), ferulate (more than or equal to 3.5 mg each capsule) and total phenolic acid (more than or equal to 34mg each capsule). Huanglian Capsule (黄连胶囊, HLC, Hubei XiangLian Pharmaceutical Co. Ltd.), each Capsule contained 0.25g Coptis *Chinensis Franch*.

1.4 Grouping and Methods of Model Establishment

Fifty Wistar rats were randomly divided into the sham operation group, the model group, the Simvastatin group, the activating blood circulation (ABC) group and the activating blood circulation and detoxifying (ABCD) group, with 10 in each group. The dose was determined by equivalent conversion method according to the animals' body surface area ratio[5]. Simvastatin (1.8 mg/kg), XSC (0.135g/kg) and Xiongshao Capsule and Huanglian Capsule (XSHLC, 0.135g/kg) were administered to the simvastain group, ABC group and ABCD group by gastrogavage, respectively, once every 24 h for two weeks, and an equal volume of normal saline was given to the sham operation group and the model group. One hour after the last administration, the anesthetized rats (20% urethane solution 0.6mL/100g, intraperitoneal injection) were set on the operating table in supine position with head fixed, stretched limbs lashed and neck fully exposed.

The right side of the neck was shaved, with local skin sterilized with 75% alcohol and incised. According to Kurz's method[6], the right common carotid artery was separated about 2 cm, a small piece of plastic film was put (4 cm × 1.8 cm) under

it to protect surrounding tissues, and then filter paper (1cm × 1cm) soaked in 20 μL FeCl$_3$ (70%) was used, which was placed on the vessel to induce the injury. Filter paper soaked in an equal volume of normal saline was used in the sham operation group. Thirty minutes later the filter paper was removed, local tissue was flushed with normal saline and sutured and the rats were put back to the feeding room. After 24 h, the blood samples were collected from the abdominal aorta of rats and kept in a red biochemical procoagulant tube at room temperature for 30 min. The serum was separated by low-speed centrifugation (2 000r/min for 15 min) and then was stored at −20℃ for use. Two rats in each group were randomly selected randomly, and about 1.5 cm of the right common carotid artery was cut down and fixed with 10% formaldŴyde for the follow-up biopsy.

1.5 Items of Observation and Methods

The serum level of MMP-9, TIMP-1, GMP-140, t-PA, hs-CRP and IL-6 were detected with enzyme-linked immunosorbent assay. The thrombosis from the common carotid artery was observed by HE staining with an optical microscope (Olympus BX51, Japan).

1.6 Statistical Analysis

All statistical analyses were performed with SPSS 11.5, and $P < 0.05$ was considered as statistically significant. The analysis of variance (ANOVA) were applied in the intergroup comparison of measurement data, and the χ^2 test was used in the comparison of enumeration data.

2. Results

2.1 Pathological Changes of Common Carotid Artery

The histophysiological structure of the sham operation group was clear and complete, arranged in neat rows. The structures of the tunica media and tunica externa were normal, and the tunica intima was smooth and complete without foreign bodies. In the other groups, the vessel wall was thin and a cord-like mixed thrombus was formed, which had a homogeneous red staining region (mainly composed of platelets and fibrin) and a small amount of plasma with some cracks. There were also large stained areas (mainly composed by cracked red blood cells and white blood cells) in the vessel. The tunica intima was damaged, covered with hemosiderin and cracked macrophages, and the basic structure of the tunica media and tunica externa maintained integrity while the elastic layer was thinner. See Figure 1.

2.2 Comparison of Thrombosis-related Indicators among Groups

Compared with the sham operation group, the serum level of GMP-140 was significantly increased and the serum level of t-PA was significantly decreased in the model group ($P < 0.01$, $P < 0.05$). The serum level of GMP-140 was significantly decreased and the serum level of t-PA was significantly increased in the Simvastatin, ABC and ABCD groups compared with those in the model group ($P < 0.05$, Table 1).

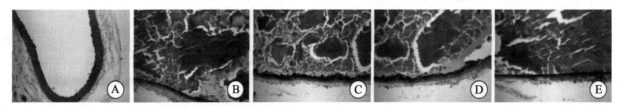

Figure 1 Pathological Changes of Common Carotid Artery in Each Group（HE Staining，×200）

Notes：A：Sham operation group；B：Model group；C：Simvastatin group；D：ABC group；E：ABCD group

Table 1 Comparison of the Serum Levels of GMP-140 and t-PA among Groups（pg/mL, $\bar{\chi} \pm s$）

Group	n	GMP-140	t-PA
Sham operation	10	657.18±247.75**	1089.14±299.19*
Model	10	1319.37±403.94	689.90±292.63
Simvastatin	10	946.95±404.67*	1095.38±451.44*
ABC	10	956.64±366.72*	1055.29±377.24*
ABCD	10	967.77±432.22*	1130.23±505.08*

Notes：*$P < 0.05$, **$P < 0.01$, compared with the model group

2.3 Comparison of Inflammation-related Indicators among Groups

Compared with the sham operation group, the serum levels of hs-CRP and IL-6 were significantly increased in the model group ($P < 0.01$). The serum levels of hs-CRP and t-PA were significantly decreased in the simvastatin group, ABC group and ABCD group compared with those in the model group ($P < 0.05$, $P < 0.01$). The level of serum hs-CRP in ABCD decreased significantly compared with that in ABC ($P < 0.05$, Table 2).

Table 2 Comparison of the Serum Levels of hs-CRP and IL-6 among Groups（$\bar{\chi} \pm s$）

Group	n	hs-CRP (ng/mL)	IL-6 (pg/mL)
Sham operation	10	6.29±2.64**	234.07±99.22**
Model	10	13.55±3.56	433.55±224.34
Simvastatin	10	8.96±4.28**	246.23±147.07*
ABC	10	10.14±3.07*	277.67±152.56*
ABCD	10	7.17±2.50**△	246.40±161.76*

Notes：*$P < 0.05$, **$P < 0.01$, compared with the model group；△$P < 0.05$, compared with the ABC group

2.4　Comparison of Tissue Damage-related Indicators among Groups

Compared with the sham operation group, the serum level of MMP-9 was significantly increased in the model group ($P < 0.01$). The serum levels of MMP-9 were significantly decreased in simvastatin group, ABC group and ABCD group compared with the model group ($P < 0.05$). There was no significant difference in the serum levels of TIMP-1 among the different groups ($P > 0.05$, Table 3).

Table 3　Comparison of the Serum Levels of MMP-9 and TIMP-1 among Groups (pg/mL, $\bar{\chi} \pm s$)

Group	n	MMP-9	TIMP-1
Sham operation	10	228.12±74.51**	272.83±55.11
Model	10	466.05±173.15	284.25±78.27
Simvastatin	10	341.17±123.71*	305.94±75.20
ABC	10	336.84±88.34*	328.79±107.78
ABCD	10	334.47±110.16*	298.07±101.75

Notes: $^*P < 0.05$, $^{**}P < 0.01$, compared with the model group

3.　Discussion

Blood stasis syndrome and its treatment by promoting blood circulation is one of the most active fields in CM research, which has made remarkable progress on the pathogenic characteristics, determination of standards, scoring and pathologic changes. This has significantly improved the clinical diagnosis and treatment efficacy towards cardiac and cerebral thrombotic diseases. Although there were many discourses about the status of the pathogenic toxin in the pathogenesis of cardio-/cerebrovascular diseases, no common understanding with regards to its pathogenic characteristics, whole- and micro-pathological changes, and syndrome differentiation and disease identification has been up to standard. Especially, there has been inadequate understanding of whether the toxin or the combination and transformation of the toxin and blood stasis of CM are involved in the pathogenesis of cardio-/cerebrovascular diseases. This limited the in-depth study and improvement of clinical efficacy of CM in the treatment and prevention of cardio-/cerebrovascular diseases.

Modern research has confirmed that modern physiochemistry-related indicators of cardio-/cerebrovascular thrombosis diseases considered to be CM blood stasis syndrome are involved in platelet activation, adhesion, congregation and thrombosis, etc. However, some scholars have made modern biological indices and connotation on the toxin and the therapeutic method of detoxifying. The combined use of Chinese herbal medicine for detoxifying and activating blood circulation (*Polygonum Cuspidatum Sieb. et Zucc.*, XSC) could reduce the expression of nuclear factor-κB and MMP-9 in the aorta of ApoE (-/) mice, and the effect of the combination is superior to that of use of either of them alone[7], which could also reduce the serum hs-CRP level[8]. Active ingredients from Chinese drugs for activating blood circulation and detoxifying, including *Panax notoginseng saponins*, *Rhizoma Coptidis*, *Polygonum Cuspidatum Sieb. et Zucc* could lower the blood lipid levels in ApoE knockout mice, and a significant difference was still seen between *Polygonum Cuspidatum Sieb. et Lucc* and the others. However, a significant decrease in the level of tumor necrosis factor-α was seen only in the rhubarb treated group[9]. But whether toxin and blood stasis are the reciprocal causations involved in the disease process, or which modern pathological and biochemical indicators may be involved, or whether the therapeutic method of activating blood circulation and detoxifying is superior to that of activating blood circulation, or which indices are sensitive indicators, remain unanswered and there are still no systematic researches about these.

Atherosclerosis (AS) is a common basis for thrombosis in cardio-/cerebrovascular diseases. According to CM theory, the pathogenetic factors involved in the formation of AS such as platelet aggregation, thrombosis, and vascular endothelial proliferation have an intrinsic relationship with blood stasis, and Chinese drugs for activating blood circulation have shown better efficacy in clinics in the prevention and treatment of AS and its related diseases [10]. Meanwhile, the pathological changes such as inflammatory cell infiltration and increased levels of inflammation markers in the AS process have similar presentations with toxin and blood stasis. According to the CM theory of blood stasis and pathogenic toxins, we made the experimental carotid artery thrombosis rat model using Kurz's method, tried to imitate the pathological process of disease due to blood stasis combined with under standing of the etiology and pathogenesis of blood stasis and the pathogenic toxin of CM, and compared the therapeutic effects of Chinese drugs for activating blood circulation to that for activating blood circulation and detoxifying. The results showed that the serum levels of GMP-140，hs-CRP, IL-6，and MMP-9 increased and the serum level of t-PA decreased in the model group compared with those in the sham operation group.

XSC is, based on experience, an effective prescription for the treatment of coronary heart disease in our hospital, whose composition is based on the classic prescription of Xuefu Zhuyu Decoction (血府逐瘀汤) and its modern pharmacological study. The capsule is composed of the effective part of Chuanxiong total phenols and red peony glycoside. HLC is a heat-clearing and detoxifying herb, so we used XSC as the therapeutic drug of ABC and used XSC and HLC as the therapeutic drugs of ABCD. Compared with the model group, the levels of serum GMP-140，hs-CRP, IL-6 and MMP-9 in ABC group and ABCD group were significantly reduced ($P < 0.05$), while the level serum of hs-CRP in ABCD group decreased more significantly compared with that in ABC group ($P < 0.05$).

GMP-140，a member of the selectin family,

can be only expressed on the surface of the platelet after degranulation, which is the specific marker for late stage platelet activation and one of the micro-cosmic indicators for blood stasis syndrome[11]. t-PA is mainly secreted by vascular endothelial cells, which can reflect the state of fibrinolysis and coagulation. AS is a chronic inflammation of the endarterium, and CRP is closely related with cardiovascular diseases such as acute coronary syndrome, while hs-CRP may be a predictor for the risk of cardiovascular disease. IL-6 has extensive biological activities, and plays many biological roles in inflammatory reaction, infection and injury[12]. In our study, the results showed that platelets and the coagulation system could be activated after $FeCl_3$ injured the tunica intima, increased the expression of GMP-140 and formed the obstructive thrombus in the injured local tissue. Thus, the content of t-PA in the blood decreased and the thrombosis model of "blood stasis" was formed. The increase of serum hs-CRP and IL-6 levels compared with that in the sham operation group just confirmed an inflammatory response.

XSC used alone or combined with HLC can reduce the serum levels of GMP-140，hs-CRP, IL-6 and MMP-9 and increase the serum level of t-PA, so as to inhibit platelet activation and relieve inflammation. XSC combined with HLC could decrease the serum level of hs-CRP than either used alone, which showed that hs-CRP might be one of the sensitive indicators for evaluation of the therapeutic effect of ABCD drugs. The relative balance between MMP and TIMP plays an important role in many physiological and pathological conditions, such as infection, autoimmune reactions and hypoxia/ischemia etc[13]. In this study, the serum level of MMP-9 could be decreased in the simvastatin, ABC and ABCD groups compared with that in the model group, but the level of serum TIMP-1 showed no significant difference among the groups, which may be related to blood samples drawing time after modeling, and should be explored in our future study.

References

[1] Paoletti R, Gotto AM Jr, Hajjar DP. Inflammation in atherosclerosis and implications for therapy. Circulation, 2004, 109 (23 Suppl 1): III 20-26.

[2] Zouridakis E, Avanzas P, Arroyo-Espliguero R, et al. Markers of inflammation and rapid coronary artery disease progression in patients with stable angina pectoris. Circulation, 2004, 110: 1747-1753.

[3] Nijm J, Wikby A, Tompa A, et al. Circulating levels of proinflammatory cytokines and neutrophil-platelet aggregates in patients with coronary artery disease. Am J Cardiol, 2005, 95：452-456.

[4] Shi DZ, Xu H, Yin HJ. Combination and transformation of toxin and blood stasis in etiopathogenesis of thrombotic cerebrocardiovascular diseases. Chin J Integr Med, 2008, 6: 1105-1108.

[5] Chen Q, ed. Methodology of research on pharmacology of traditional Chinese medicine. Beijing: People's Medical Publishing House, 1996：1103-1105.

[6] Kurz KD, Main BW, Sandusky GE. Rat model of arterial thrombosis induced by ferric chloride. Thromb Res, 1990, 60: 269-280.

[7] Zhang JC, Chen KJ, Zheng GJ, et al. Regulatory effect of Chinese herbal compound for detoxifying and activating blood circulation on expression of NF-κB and MMP-9 in aorta of apolipoprotein E gene knocked-out mice. Chin J Integr Tradit West Med, 2007, 27: 40-44.

[8] Zhang JC, Chen KJ, Liu JG, et al. Effect of assorted use of Chinese drugs for detoxifying and activating blood circulation on serum high sensitive C-reactive protein in apolipoprotein E gene knock-out mice. Chin J Integr Tradit West Med, 2008, 28：330-333.

[9] Zhou MX, Xu H, Chen KJ, et al. Effects of some active ingredients of Chinese drugs for activating blood circulation and detoxicating on blood lipids and atherosclerotic plaque inflammatory reaction in ApoE-gene knockout mice. Chin J Integr Tradit West Med, 2008, 28: 126-130.

[10] Shi DZ, Ma XC, Gao XA. Research overview of the prevention and treatment of atherosclerosis by prescriptions for activating blood circulation. Journal of Traditional Chinese Medicine, 1995, 36: 433-435.

[11] Chen KJ, Xue M, Yin HJ. The relationship between platelet activation and coronary heart disease and blood-stasis syndrome. Journal of Capital Medical University, 2008, 29：266-269.

[12] Ma XJ, Yin HJ, Chen KJ. Research progress of correlation between blood-stasis syndrome and inflammation. Chin J Integr Tradit West Med, 2007, 27: 669-672.

[13] Candelario-Jalil E, Yang Y, Rosenberg GA. Diverse roles of matrix metalloproteinases and tissue inhibitors of metalloproteinases in neuroinflammation and cerebral ischemia. Neuroscience, 2009, 158：983-994.

第四章

第六节 中医药保护血管内皮细胞、抑制血管平滑肌细胞增殖的研究

活血解毒中药含药血清对氧化低密度脂蛋白诱导的内皮细胞损伤和凋亡的影响 *

缪 宇 蒋跃绒 杨 琳 夏城东 张 璐 吴彩凤 史大卓 殷惠军 陈可冀

心脑血管血栓性疾病是严重危害人类健康的常见疾病，动脉粥样硬化（atherosclerosis, AS）作为心脑血管疾病的主要病理基础受到人们的高度关注。大量研究认为血管内皮细胞损伤及其功能异常是 AS 形成的始动环节[1]。本研究根据血栓性疾病内皮损伤的机制，利用氧化低密度脂蛋白（oxidized low-density lipoprotein, ox-LDL）为刺激物诱导内皮细胞损伤模型，从氧化损伤和凋亡方面观察内皮细胞损伤后病理生理改变，比较活血化瘀和活血解毒治法作用环节和靶点的差异，从细胞损伤角度阐释"瘀毒"病因相互联系的科学内涵。

1. 材料与方法

1.1 实验材料

1.1.1 实验动物 Wistar 大鼠 32 只，体重 (200±20) g, SPF 级，雌雄各半，由中国医学科学院医学实验动物研究所提供，动物质量合格证明号为 SCXK（京）2005-0013。大鼠自由饮水，在室温 23～25℃、湿度 50%～70% 的环境饲养，光照 12h，黑暗 12h。

1.1.2 药物与试剂 芎芍胶囊由川芎、赤芍的有效部位川芎总酚和赤芍总苷组成，每粒 0.25g，每克提取物分别含芍药苷≥112mg, 阿魏酸≥14mg, 总酚酸≥136mg, 由大连化学物理研究所提供，批号为 070929；黄连胶囊每粒 0.25g，由湖北香连药

业有限责任公司生产，批号为 070502，批准文号为国药准字 Z19983042；辛伐他汀，每片 40mg，杭州默沙东制药有限公司生产，批号为 07432。

达尔伯克改良伊格尔培养基 (Dulbecco's modified Eagle's medium, DMEM)（低糖型）和优级胎牛血清购自美国 HyClone 公司；表皮细胞生长因子 (epidermal growth factor, EGF)、胰酶、胶原酶I和四氮唑蓝 (methyl thiazolyl tetrazolium, MTT) 均购自美国 Sigma 公司；ox-LDL 购自中国医学科学院基础医学研究所生化室，浓度 1.5mg/mL，以硫代巴比妥酸反应法测定丙二醛 (malondialdehyde, MDA) 含量来确定其氧化修饰程度，MDA 值 24.9nmol/L；超氧化物歧化酶 (superoxide dismutase, SOD) 测试盒和 MDA 测定试剂盒均购自南京建成生物工程研究所；乳酸脱氢酶 (lactate dehydrogenase, LDH) 试剂盒购自北京北化康泰临床试剂有限公司；Annexin V 异硫氰酸荧光素 (fluorescein isothiocyanate, FITC) / 碘化丙啶 (propidium iodide, PI) 凋亡检测试剂盒购自美国 BD-Pharmingen 公司，健康产妇脐带取自北京海淀区妇幼保健医院。

1.2 实验方法

1.2.1 含药血清的制备 取正常大鼠 32 只，随机分为空白对照组、阳性对照（辛伐他汀）组、活血（芎芍胶囊）组和活血解毒（芎芍胶囊加黄连胶囊）组，每组 8 只。根据临床成人剂量，按

* 原载于《中西医结合学报》，2011, 9 (5)：539-545

体表面积比等效剂量法折算大鼠用量，阳性对照组、活血组和活血解毒组大鼠分别按辛伐他汀 1.8mg/kg、芎芍胶囊 0.135g/kg、芎芍胶囊和黄连胶囊各 0.135g/kg 的剂量给药，药物均用蒸馏水稀释后，按 10mL/kg 体质量灌胃，每日 1 次，连续 7d。空白对照组予等体积蒸馏水作对照。末次给药后 1h，无菌条件下经腹主动脉取血，4℃ 静置 1h，900×g 离心 15min，分离含药血清。将同组大鼠含药血清混匀，56℃ 水浴 30min 灭活血清，微孔滤膜过滤除菌，冻存管分装，–70℃ 保存备用。

1.2.2　人脐静脉内皮细胞的分离、培养与鉴定　人脐静脉内皮细胞 (human umbilical vein endothelial cell, HUVEC) 的分离与培养参照文献方法 [2]。无菌条件下收集健康产妇正常分娩的新生儿脐带，胶原酶消化法收集细胞，5% CO_2、37℃ 条件下用含 20% 胎牛血清、10ng/mL EGF、40μU/mL 胰岛素，40U/mL 肝素，2mmol/L 谷氨酰胺，50U/mL 青霉素，50μg/mL 链霉素，1mmol/L 丙酮酸钠的全 DMEM 培养。实验用第 3 代细胞。倒置相差显微镜下观察细胞形态，并采用免疫组织化学法进行Ⅷ因子表达鉴定。

1.2.3　实验分组　将人脐静脉内皮细胞随机分为 5 组：空白对照组、ox-LDL 对照组、辛伐他汀含药血清组、活血药含药血清组和活血解毒药含药血清组。Ox-LDL 对照组加入刺激剂 ox-LDL（终浓度 100μg/L）和 10% 空白大鼠血清，活血药物血清组、活血解毒药物血清组和辛伐他汀含药血清组分别加入相应的 10% 含药血清，并同时加入 ox-LDL（终浓度 100μg/L），空白对照组仅加入等量的空白大鼠血清，共孵育 24h。

1.2.4　MTT 法检测细胞增殖　将对数生长期的细胞以 $1×10^4$ 个 /mL 的密度接种于 96 孔板，继续培养至细胞基本融合后，按上述分组方法加入相应试剂，每组 4 个复孔，继续孵育 24h。每孔加入 5mg/mL MTT 10μL, 37℃、5% CO_2 孵育 4h；弃上清，每孔加入 150μL 二甲基亚砜；震荡摇匀 10min; 用 Tecan Sunrise 酶联免疫检测仪（奥地利）在波长 492nm 处测定吸光度值。

1.2.5　LDH 释放测定　取细胞培养上清液及细胞冻融裂解液（–20℃ /37℃ 反复冻融 3 次）分别测定乳酸脱氢酶活性，按试剂盒说明书进行操作。LDH 漏出率 =[细胞培养上清液 LDH 活性 /（细胞培养上清液 LDH 活性 + 细胞裂解液 LDH 活性）]×100%。每组 4 个复孔。

1.2.6　细胞 SOD 活性和 MDA 含量测定　细胞于 –20℃ /37℃ 反复冻融 3 次，取冻融细胞裂解液，按照试剂盒说明书测定细胞内 SOD 活性，按照 MDA 试剂盒说明书，硫代巴比妥酸法测定细胞 MDA 含量，细胞蛋白质定量采用 Lowry 法。每组 8 个复孔。

1.2.7　内皮细胞凋亡检测　采用 Annexin VFITC/PI 双染试剂盒进行凋亡检测。

收集脱落和仍贴壁的细胞，用冰磷酸盐缓冲液 (phosphate-buffered saline, PBS) 洗 2 次，100μL 结合缓冲液 (10mmol/L Hepes pH 7.4, 140mmol/L NaCl, 2.5mmol/L $CaCl_2$) 重悬细胞，加入 Annexin V-FITC 和 PI 室温下避光 15min，最后用 400μL 结合缓冲液终止反应，进行流式细胞仪分析。凋亡时细胞膜磷脂的不对称性丧失，原位于质膜内侧的磷脂酰丝氨酸暴露于外侧，与 Annexin V 结合呈绿色荧光（FITC 呈绿色），而 PI 则能使坏死细胞标记上红色荧光。因此，将细胞用两种染料同时染色后，可以检测出非凋亡的活细胞（Annexin V 阴性 /PI 阴性）、早期凋亡细胞（Annexin V 阳性 /PI 阴性）及晚期凋亡和坏死细胞（Annexin V 阳性 /PI 阳性），计算凋亡细胞比率。每组 5 复孔。

1.3　统计学方法

所得实验数据以 $\overline{\chi} \pm s$ 表示，采用 SPSS for Windows 11.0 统计软件包进行统计学处理。计量资料多组间比较采用单因素方差分析，多组间两两比较采用 LSD-t 检验。

2. 结果

2.1　对 HUVEC 形态的影响

在倒置相差显微镜下观察到空白对照组内皮细胞呈梭形或多角形，细胞形态饱满，数目较多，排列密集；ox-LDL 对照组细胞数目显著减少，排列疏松，胞内颗粒物质增多；各药血清组细胞状态介于空白对照组和 ox-LDL 对照组之间，以辛伐他汀含药血清组最为接近空白对照组。见图 1。

2.2　对 HUVEC 活力的影响

与空白对照组相比，ox-LDL 对照组 HUVEC 吸光度值明显减少 ($P < 0.05$); 与 ox-LDL 对照组比较，活血药物血清、活血解毒药物血清及辛伐他汀含药血清组吸光度值明显增加 ($P < 0.05$, $P < 0.01$)；各用药组间比较，差异无统计学意义。见表 1。

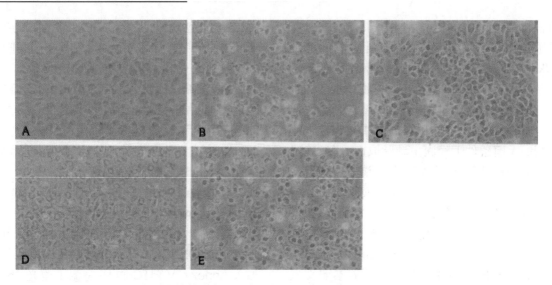

图1 各组人脐静脉内皮细胞形态特征（倒置相差显微镜，×100）

A：Blank control group；B：Ox-LDL group；C：10% simvastatin-containing serum group；D：10% Xiongshao capsule-containing serum group；E：10% Xiongshao capsule plus Huanglian capsule-containing serum group

2.3 对 HUVEC LDH 释放的影响

与空白对照组相比，ox-LDL 对照组 HUVEC 上清液中 LDH 活性明显增加（$P < 0.05$）；与 ox-LDL 对照组比较，活血药物血清组、活血解毒药物血清组及辛伐他汀药物血清组细胞上清液中 LDH 活性下降，但差异无统计学意义。各组 LDH 漏出率比较，差异无统计学意义。见表 2。

表1 各组人脐静脉内皮细胞活力（$\bar{\chi} \pm s$）

Group	n	Optical density value
Blank control	4	0.21 ± 0.04
Ox-LDL	4	$0.17 \pm 0.02^*$
10% simvastatin-containing serum	4	$0.25 \pm 0.04^{\triangle\triangle}$
10% XS-containing serum	4	$0.22 \pm 0.03^{\triangle}$
10% XSHL-containing serum	4	$0.26 \pm 0.03^{*\triangle\triangle}$

$^*P < 0.05$, vs blank control group; $^\triangle P < 0.05$, $^{\triangle\triangle}P < 0.01$, vs ox-LDL group. XS: Xiongshao capsule; XSHL: Xiongshao capsule plus Huanglian capsule

2.4 对细胞 SOD 活性和 MDA 含量的影响

与空白对照组相比，ox-LDL 对照组 HUVEC 细胞裂解液 SOD 活性下降（$P < 0.01$），MDA 含量明显升高（$P < 0.01$）；活血中药和辛伐他汀药物血清均可逆转 ox-LDL 诱导的 HUVECSOD 活性下降和 MDA 含量增多（$P < 0.01$，$P < 0.05$），活血解毒中药含药血清作用不明显。活血解毒药物血清组 SOD 活性和 MDA 含量与活血药物血清组比较差异无统计学意义。见表 3。

2.5 对 ox-LDL 刺激的 HUVEC 凋亡的影响

与空白对照组相比，ox-LDL 对照组 HUVEC 早期凋亡细胞（Annexin V 阳性 /PI 阴性）及晚期凋亡和坏死细胞（Annexin V 阳性 /PI 阳性）比率明显增加（$P < 0.01$，$P < 0.05$）；活血、活血解毒中药血清及辛伐他汀含药血清孵育 24h 后，ox-LDL 诱导的 HUVEC 早期凋亡率明显下降（$P < 0.05$），各药物血清治疗组晚期凋亡率变化不明显。见表 4。

3. 讨论

血管内皮细胞极易受到血液及其周围有害因素的影响而发生结构和功能的改变，引起内皮细胞损伤。Ox-LDL 作为最重要的致粥样硬化因子，具有细胞毒性作用，与血凝素样氧化低密度脂蛋白受体 1（lectin-like oxidized LDL receptor, LOX-1）特异性结合后，可激活内皮细胞合成和分泌大量黏附分子，加速单核细胞与活化的内皮细胞间的黏附、聚集，并迁移至内皮下形成泡沫细胞，是 AS 的早期主要事件[3]。

本研究结果显示，与空白对照组比较，100μg/L ox-LDL 刺激 24h 后，HUVEC 活力下降，细胞上清液中 LDH 生成增加，细胞内 SOD 活性下降，而细胞 MDA 含量明显增加，提示该实验条件下 ox-LDL 对 HUVEC 产生了氧化损伤。MDA 是脂质过氧化的代谢产物，其水平的高低可反映脂质过氧

表2 各组人脐静脉内皮细胞 LDH 释放（$\bar{\chi} \pm s$）

Group	n	Intracellular LDH（U/mL）	Supernatant LDH（U/mL）	LDH leakage（%）
Blank control	4	2.32±0.80	16.05±6.09	87±1
Ox-LDL	4	3.51±0.77	24.40±3.58*	87±3
10% simvastatin-containing serum	4	2.37±0.87	18.16±6.12	88±2
10% XS-containing serum	4	2.53±1.07	20.17±6.14	89±16
10% XSHL-containing serum	4	2.48±0.29	18.00±2.57	88±1

*$P < 0.05$, vs blank control group. XS：Xiongshao capsule；XSHL：Xiongshao capsule plus Huanglian capsule；LDH：lactate dẆydrogenase

表3 各组人脐静脉内皮细胞 SOD 活性和 MDA 含量（$\bar{\chi} \pm s$）

Group	n	SOD（U/mg）	MDA（nmol/mg）
Blank control	8	45.99±5.66	21.16±6.84
Ox-LDL	8	21.59±6.10**	35.05±4.89**
10% simvastatin-containing serum	8	48.22±6.53△△	24.39±8.89△△
10% XS-containing serum	8	34.64±11.53*△	28.19±8.02△*
10% XSHL-containing serum	8	29.19±6.25**	30.50±3.48**

*$P < 0.05$, **$P < 0.01$, vs blank control group；△△$P < 0.05$, △△$P < 0.01$, vs ox-LDL group. XS：Xiongshao capsule；XSHL：Xiongshao capsule plus Huanglian capsule；SOD：superoxide dismutase；MDA：malondial dẆyde

表4 各组人脐静脉内皮细胞凋亡情况（$\bar{\chi} \pm s$，%）

Group	n	Annex in V+/PI-	Annexin V+/PI+
Blank control	5	1.86±1.82	1.04±1.60
Ox-LDL	5	7.60±1.93**	4.46±2.54*
10% simvastatin-containing serum	5	4.22±1.32△	3.60±2.78
10% XS-containing serum	5	4.88±1.17*△	3.94±2.15
10% XSHL-containing serum	5	4.90±0.53*△	4.26±2.02*

*$P < 0.05$, **$P < 0.01$, vs blank control group；△$P < 0.05$, vs ox-LDL group. XS：Xiongshao capsule；XSHL：Xiongshao capsule plus Huanglian capsule

化损伤的程度。SOD 作为自由基清除剂，广泛地存在于生物体组织内，能催化超氧阴离子等自由基，发生歧化反应，阻止自由基的连锁反应。LDH 是一种细胞内的糖酵解酶，广泛存在于细胞浆内。当细胞破坏或细胞膜通透性增加时，LDH 水平明显增高，可反映细胞或细胞膜损伤的程度。培养液中 LDH 的活力明显增强，意味着 LDH 从细胞中漏出增多。

细胞凋亡也参与了动脉粥样硬化的进程[3]。作为氧自由基的携带者，ox-LDL 是否诱导血管内皮细胞的凋亡依赖于氧化的程度[4]。Ox-LDL 诱发的内皮细胞凋亡与其降低线粒体呼吸链多种酶活性和增加活性氧生成有关，这些效应促进了高胆固醇和氧化应激状态下的血管损伤和动脉硬化，LOX-1 介导了 ox-LDL 诱发的细胞凋亡[5]。本研究也发现，ox-LDL 孵育 24h 可使 HUVEC Annexin V+/PI-、AnnexinV+/PI+ 比率均明显增加。Annexin V+/PI- 反映早期凋亡，细胞包膜完整；AnnexinV+/PI+ 反映细胞晚期凋亡和坏死。但本方法不能区分经凋亡途径死亡的细胞和经坏死途径死亡的细胞，两者均表现为 Annexin V+/PI+[6]。本研究结果表明，ox-LDL 刺激 24h 后，细胞早期凋亡、晚期凋亡和坏死细胞均明显增加。

传统中医认为 AS 为本虚标实之证，本虚多为气虚，标实则以血瘀、痰浊、气滞多见。现代中医理论多从痰、瘀、毒来解释其病机。AS 过程中的一系列炎症变化如淋巴细胞、巨噬细胞等炎症细胞浸润，炎症反应标志物、炎症介质水平增高等与毒邪致病学说有关。毒邪致病后，脏腑气机失调，津凝为痰，血聚为瘀。痰、瘀、毒三者相互促生，导致 AS 的发生[7]。因此，本研究采用 ox-LDL 诱导的内皮细胞损伤模型，模拟血栓性疾病"瘀毒互结"的病理基础，并比较传统活血化瘀中药和活血化瘀解毒中药治疗作用的差异。

芎芍胶囊是在传统活血化瘀名方血府逐瘀汤基础上，反复精简、提取有效部位、优化配比而成的有效组分配伍制剂，由川芎总酚和赤芍总苷配伍而成，是我院治疗冠心病的有效经验方。黄连味苦性寒，归心、脾、胃、肝、胆、大肠经，具有清热燥湿、泻火解毒的功效，始载于《神农本草经》，列为上品。黄连胶囊由黄连加工而成，具有解毒清热的作用。与直接采用中药粗制剂进行体外实验相比，以相应的含药血清为研究对象，不仅可有效克服制剂理化性质对实验结果产生的干扰，且其实验条件更接近于药物在体内产生效应的内环境，得到的结果也更加可信[8]。本研究分别使用芎芍胶囊、芎芍胶囊联用黄连胶囊的含药血清作为干预药物，结果显示，单纯活血药物血清和活血解毒药物血清均可改善 ox-LDL 诱导的 HUVEC 活力下降和早期凋亡增加。活血中药含药血清可明显逆转 ox-LDL 诱导的 HUVECSOD 活性下降和 MDA 含量增多，活血解毒与活血中药药物血清比较，差异无统计学意义。说明在抗内皮细胞氧化损伤和早期凋亡方面，活血解毒中药配伍与单纯活血中药作用相似，也提示早期细胞凋亡可能不是中药解毒作用的敏感指标。

References

[1] Sima AV, Stancu CS, Simionescu M. Vascular endothelium in atherosclerosis. Cell Tissue Res, 2009；335 (1): 191-203.

[2] Jiang YR, Chen KJ, Xu YG, et al. Effects of propyl gallate on adhesion of polymorphonu clear leukocytes to human endothelial cells induced by tumor necrosis factor alpha. Chin J Integr Med, 2009, 15 (1): 47-53.

[3] Vannini N, Pfeffer U, Lorusso G, et al. Endothelial cell aging and apoptosis in prevention and disease: E-selectin expression and modulation as a model. Curr Pharm Des, 2008, 14 (3): 221-225.

[4] Roy Chowdhury SK, Sangle GV, Xie X, et al. Effects of extensively oxidized low-density lipoprotein on mitochondrial function and reactive oxygen species in porcine aortic endothelial cells. Am J Physiol Endocrinol Metab, 2010, 298 (1): e89-e98.

[5] Lu J, Yang JH, Burns AR, et al. Mediation of electronegative low-density lipoprotein signaling by LOX-1: a possible mechanism of endothelial apoptosis. Circ Res, 2009, 104 (5): 619-627.

[6] Homburg CH, de Haas M, von dem Borne AE, et al. Human neutrophils lose their surface Fc gamma RⅢ and acquire Annexin V binding sites during apoptosis in vitro. Blood, 1995, 85 (2): 532-540.

[7] 范砚超, 张国平, 唐明, 等. 从毒论治动脉粥样硬化初探. 山东中医杂志, 2004, 23 (5): 261-263.

[8] 徐海波, 吴清和. 中药血清药理学研究进展. 湖南中医药导报, 1999, 5 (8): 11-14.

人参三七组方对人脐静脉内皮细胞血管内皮生长因子分泌及其受体 2 表达的影响 *

雷　燕　田　伟　朱陵群　杨　静　陈可冀

血管生成在缺血性疾病发病机制和治疗方面的研究已成为目前医学研究的热点课题。在血管生成的过程中，内皮细胞不仅参与整个过程，而且也是重要的靶细胞。近年的研究表明，血管内皮生长因子 (vascular endothelial growth factor, VEGF) 直接作用于血管内皮细胞，具有促使内皮细胞分裂、增殖、诱导新生血管形成的作用，在组织缺血性疾病，尤其是难治性冠心病的治疗中展现出良好的前景 [1]。VEGF 的这些生物效应是通过其特异受体——血管内皮细胞生长因子受体 2 (vascular endothelial growth factor receptor-2，VEGFR-2) 介导的。本实验通过体外培养内皮细胞，观察人参三七组方对人脐静脉内皮细胞 (human umbilical vein endothelial cell, HUVEC) 分泌 VEGF 以及对 VEGFR-2 表达的影响，旨在探讨人参三七组方对血管生成的作用，从而为临床上治疗缺血性疾病提供可靠的实验依据。

1.　材料与方法

1.1　实验材料

1.1.1　细胞株　人脐静脉内皮细胞 (HUVEC-2C, cat No. C-023-5C, Lot No. 4C0218), 购自 Cascade Biologics 公司。

1.1.2　实验药物　外用重组牛碱性成纤维细胞生长因子 (bovine basic fibroblast growth factor, bFGF), 珠海亿胜生物制药有限公司生产，批准文号为国药准字 S10980075，产品批号为 20070301；人参颗粒剂（批号：0609089）和三七颗粒剂（批号：0612051），购自广东一方制药有限公司，均经水提后精制而成，按 2∶1（人参∶三七）配比，用时用完全培养基（Medium 200+ 低血清生长因子补充物）配成所需浓度，经 0.22μm 微孔滤膜过滤除菌，分装，4℃保存。

1.1.3　试剂与仪器　完全培养基 (Cascade Biologics 公司)，多聚赖氨酸溶液、VEGFR-2 免疫细胞化学试剂盒、VEGF 酶联免疫吸附测定 (enzyme-linked immunosorbent assay, ELISA) 试剂盒 (武汉博士德生物技术有限公司)，四甲基偶氮唑蓝 (Amresco 公司)，VEGFR-2 兔抗人单克隆抗体 (美国 Epitomics 公司)。酶标仪 (芬兰 Labsystems 公司)，倒置相差显微镜 CK2 型 (日本 Olympus 公司)，彩色图像分析仪 MIS-2000SP (美国 3Y 公司)。

1.2　实验方法

1.2.1　ELISA 法检测 VEGF 含量　消化培养至第 4 代的 HUVEC，终浓度调至 3×10^4 个 /mL, 以 100μL/ 孔接种于 96 孔培养板，共 5 组，每组设 8 个复孔，置于 37℃，5% CO_2 饱和湿度培养箱中培养。24h 后吸出无血清培养基，加入 100μL 不同质量浓度的人参三七组方，使其终浓度分别为 0.4mg/mL（高剂量组），0.2mg/mL（中剂量组），0.1mg/mL（低剂量组，相当于生药人参 0.67mg/mL，生药三七 0.33 mg/mL，其配比及浓度是根据四甲基偶氮唑盐法实验所筛选出的最佳有效作用浓度）。另设加入 bFGF (320 U/mL) [1] 的细胞悬液对照组和只加培养液的空白对照组。置于 37℃，5% CO_2 饱和湿度培养箱中培养。24 h 后取上清液低温离心备用。ELISA 检测方法参考试剂盒说明书进行。酶标仪检测波长为 450 nm 时的吸光度值，再将吸光度换算为 VEGF 含量（ng/L）。

1.2.2　免疫细胞化学法检测 VEGFR-2 蛋白表达　用多聚赖氨酸包被载玻片，分别放入 24 孔培养板中，调整 HUVEC 浓度为 2×10^4 个 /mL, 以 1 mL/ 孔接种于载玻片上。每个药物浓度设 6 个复孔。按照试剂盒说明书检测 VEGFR-2 表达，一抗为 VEGFR-2 兔抗人血清，二抗为羊抗兔 IgG，

* 原载于《中西医结合学报》，2010，8（4）：368-372

427

二氨基联苯胺室温显色。镜下控制反应时间，以 PBS 代替一抗作阴性对照。光学显微镜下（×200 倍）观察细胞胞浆中呈现棕褐黄色颗粒者为阳性细胞。采用 3Y 图像分析仪 counter/size 程序，分析载玻片上 VEGFR-2 阳性表达产物的光密度（optical density，OD）值并计数阳性细胞。每张载玻片取 4 个视野，将所得细胞数及 OD 的均值作为该样本的平均细胞数和 OD 值。

1.2.3　蛋白印迹法检测 VEGFR-2 蛋白表达　分别收集细胞，加入蛋白提取液并用细针头反复吹打，置冰上 15 min, 4℃、11 500×g 离心 10 min, 转移上清液至新的 EP 管中。二喹林甲酸法测定蛋白浓度。取各蛋白样品 20μg，加入蛋白样品缓冲液变性后将蛋白样品加入 12% 十二烷基硫酸钠 - 聚丙烯酰胺凝胶中电泳，直至蓝色条带泳出分离胶底部。采用电转移法将蛋白质从十二烷基硫酸钠 - 聚丙烯酰胺凝胶转移至硝酸纤维素膜，转膜成功后，以 5% 脱脂牛奶 TBS-T 液体封闭硝酸纤维素膜上的非特异蛋白位点，按 1：1 000 比例加入 VEGFR-2 兔源性单克隆抗体或加入抗 β-actin 抗体，4℃过夜。次日经过洗膜，加入 1：3 000 稀释的羊抗兔辣根过氧化物酶标记二抗，再洗膜后，杂交膜显色反应按照电化学发光试剂盒的说明进行。采用数字扫描成像系统分析特异条带的强度。每组重复 3 次扫描，并将所得数据进行分析。

1.3　统计学方法

计量资料数据用 $\bar{\chi} \pm s$ 表示，采用 SPSS 13.0 统计软件进行统计分析，均数间经方差齐性检验后，进行单因素方差分析，组间两两比较采用 q 检验。

2. 结果

2.1　各组 HUVEC 上清液中 VEGF 含量

与空白对照组相比，bFGF 组和高剂量中药组 HUVEC 上清液中 VEGF 含量增加（$P < 0.05$）；中、低剂量中药组上清液中 VEGF 含量与空白组相比有升高趋势，但差异无统计学意义（$P > 0.05$）。中、低剂量中药组上清液中 VEGF 含量与 bFGF 组比较，差异有统计学意义 ($P < 0.05$)。见表 1。

2.2　蛋白印迹法检测各组 HUVEC VEGFR-2 蛋白表达

各组细胞均有不同程度的 VEGFR-2 蛋白表达，其中 bFGF 组与高剂量中药组表达最为明显，与空白对照组相比差异有统计学意义 ($P < 0.05$),而中、低剂量中药组表达较弱。见表 1 和图 1。

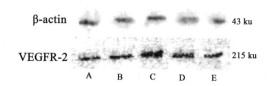

图 1　蛋白印迹法检测各组细胞 VEGFR-2 蛋白表达

A：Blank control group；B：bFGF group；C：High-dose formula group；D：Medium-dose formula group；E：Low-dose formula group

2.3　免疫细胞化学法检测各组 HUVEC VEGFR-2 蛋白表达

倒置相差显微镜下可见细胞呈梭形或多边形。边界清楚，胞浆丰富，胞浆内有棕黄色沉淀，胞核

表 1　各组 VEGF 含量、VEGFR-2 阳性细胞数量和 VEGFR-2 蛋白表达（$\bar{\chi} \pm s$）

Group	VEGF（ng/L，$n=8$）	Number of VEGFR-2-positive HUVECs（$n=6$）	OD value of VEGFR-2-positive HUVECs（$n=6$）	VEGFR-2/β-actin（$n=3$）
Blank control	67.61±8.54	13.18±5.79	0.149±0.002	1.583 9±0.102 8
BFGF	93.68±11.35*	18.08±6.06**	0.183±0.002*	2.113 9±0.211 5*
High-dose formula	89.24±12.16*	18.29±4.98**	0.171±0.003*	2.074 5±0.189 8*
Medium-dose formula	74.57±8.90△	13.81±4.31△△□□	0.168±0.003*	1.482 2±0.173 0
Low-dose formula	72.81±9.26△	12.79±4.10△△□□	0.147±0.003△▲□	1.388 8±0.262 0

*$P < 0.05$, **$P < 0.01$, *vs* blank control group；△$P < 0.05$, △△$P < 0.01$, *vs* bFGF group；▲$P < 0.05$, *vs* medium-dose formula group；□$P < 0.05$, □□$P < 0.01$, *vs* high-dose formula group

椭圆居中，核仁不清。给药后 24 h 检测，各组细胞均有 VEGFR-2 表达。bFGF 组和高剂量中药组阳性细胞数最多，与空白对照组、中剂量和低剂量中药组比较，差异有统计学意义（$P < 0.01$）；bFGF 组，高、中剂量中药组阳性细胞 OD 值高于空白对照组和低剂量中药组，差异有统计学意义（$P < 0.05$）。空白对照组 VEGFR-2 蛋白表达物呈淡褐色；而 bFGF 组和高、中剂量中药组 VEGFR-2 蛋白表达明显上调，VEGFR-2 蛋白被染成深褐色。见表 1 和图 2。

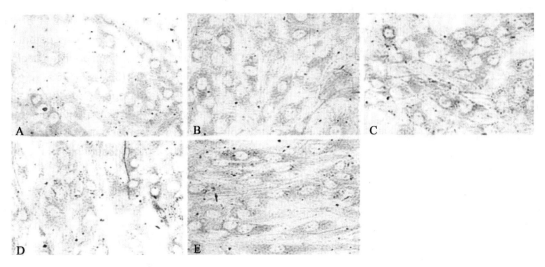

图 2 免疫细胞化学法检测各组 VEGFR-2 阳性细胞表达（光学显微镜，×200）

A：Blank control group；B：bFGF group；C：High-dose formula group；D：Medium-dose formula group；E：Low-dose formula group

3. 讨论

益气活血中药治疗冠心病的机制可能在于其具有促进血管生成的作用，从而有利于冠心病患者心脏侧支循环的形成，减轻心肌缺血缺氧危害[2-4]。本研究重在探索人参三七组方对 HUVEC 分泌 VEGF 的影响以及对 VEGFR-2 的表达的影响，旨在为人参三七组方促血管生成的研究奠定基础。

大量研究表明，人参具有增强机体免疫功能、抗缺氧、扩张冠状动脉、促进微循环、改善心肌缺血、减轻心肌损伤等作用；三七具有良好的养血止血功效，能改善心脏微循环，扩张血管[5,6]。二药配伍，具有益气活血、化瘀生新的作用。

VEGF[7] 是一类多功能生长因子，由多种细胞分泌，并通过旁分泌机制作用于受体而发挥作用。VEGF 和其受体结合后最明显的生物学效应是促使内皮细胞有丝分裂，诱导血管内皮细胞增殖和迁徙。增殖和迁徙的内皮细胞又分泌其他生长因子，一方面作用于非内皮细胞促进它们的有丝分裂，以此和内皮细胞形成新生血管；另一方面还可以使非内皮细胞分泌 VEGF，再通过旁分泌机制作用于内皮细胞。它与细胞表面的 VEGFR 结合，通过激活酪氨酸激酶信号转导途径发挥功能。VEGF 的生物学活性主要是通过两个酪氨酸受体所介导的[8,9]，即 VEGFR-1 (fms-like tyrosine kinase, Flt-1) 和 VEGFR-2 (kinase insert domain-containing receptor/fetal liver kinase, KDR/Flk-1)。VEGFR-1 是内皮细胞特异性生长因子受体，其表达主要与鼠胚胎时期血管形成和伤口愈合有关，较少涉及内皮细胞增殖。VEGFR-2 是 VEGF 的主要功能受体，主要分布于内皮细胞表面，VEGF 对内皮细胞的存活、增殖、分化等起着关键性的作用，其主要生物学功能都是通过 VEGFR-2 实现的。Brekken 等[10] 研究发现，VEGFR-2 在 VEGF 所诱导的血管生成中起主要作用，单独使用 KDR 的抑制剂，就能阻断 VEGF 和 bFGF 所诱导的血管生成。VEGFR-2 和 VEGF 结合后发生二聚体化，并且胞内的酪氨酸残基自身发生磷酸化，引发胞内信号向下游传递。VEGFR-2-/- 型小鼠在胚胎期的 8.5 ～ 9.5 d 因血管缺陷死亡，说明 VEGFR-2 在血管发育过程中发挥关键作用[1]。这也是实验选用 VEGFR-2 为切入点的原因。

本研究结果表明，各组细胞培养的上清液中 VEGF 的含量不同，且人参三七组方各组

第四章

VEGFR-2 阳性细胞数以及阳性细胞的 OD 值都有不同程度的改变，说明药物干预后，通过某种途径使 HUVEC 的 VEGFR-2 表达有所增加。这样的结果在蛋白印迹法的实验中得到进一步的证明。有意义的是，上清液中 VEGF 含量增加的一组正好与其受体 VEGFR-2 蛋白表达增加的一组相吻合。因此，可以得出人参三七组方促进 HUVEC 增殖可能是通过促进 HUVEC 分泌 VEGF，同时促进其受体 VEGFR-2 的表达来完成这一生物学过程的。

References

[1] Lazarous DF, Shou M, Stiber JA, et al. Adenoviral-mediated gene transfer induces sustained pericardial VEGF expression in dogs: effect on myocardial angiogenesis. Cardiovasc Res, 1999, 44 (2): 294-302.

[2] Lei Y, Gao Q, Chen KJ. Effects of extracts from Panax Notoginseng and Panax Ginseng fruit on vascular endothelial cell proliferation and migration in vitro. Chin J Integr Med, 2008, 14 (1): 37-41.

[3] 田伟，雷燕. 中医药在治疗性血管生成中的研究进展. 中国中医基础医学杂志，2008, 14 (4): 319-321.

[4] 雷燕，王培利，林燕林，等. 当归补血汤煎剂对实验性心肌梗死衰老大鼠缺血心肌的促血管生成作用. 中国中医基础医学杂志，2005, 11 (12): 892-894.

[5] 刘郁，刘连新. 人参功效再认识. 时珍国医国药，

2006，17 (2): 289.

[6] 张喜平，齐丽丽，刘达人. 三七及其有效成分的药理作用研究现状. 医学研究杂志，2007, 36 (4): 96-98.

[7] Ferrara N, Gerber HP, LeCouter J. The biology of VEGF and its receptors. Nat Med, 2003, 9 (6): 669-676.

[8] La DS, Belzile J, Bready JV, et al. Novel 2, 3-dihydro-1, 4-benzoxazines as potent and orally bioavailable inhibitors of tumor-driven angiogenesis. J Med Chem, 2008, 51 (6): 1695-1705.

[9] Weiss MM, Harmange JC, Polverino AJ, et al. Evaluation of a series of naphthamides as potent, orally active vascular endothelial growth factor receptor-2 tyrosine kinase inhibitors. J Med Chem, 2008, 51 (6): 1668-1680.

[10] Brekken RA, Overholser JP, Stasmy VA, et al. Selective inhibition of vascular endothelial growth factor (VEGF) receptor 2 (KDR/Flk 1) activity by a monoclonal anti-VEGF antibody blocks tumor growth in mice. Cancer Research, 2000, 60 (18): 5117-5124.

[11] Marioni G, Giacomelli L, D'Alessandro E, et al. Laryngeal carcinoma recurrence rate and disease-free interval are related to CDI05 expression but not to vascular endothelial growth factor 2 (Flk-1/Kdr) expression. Anticancer Res, 2008, 28 (1B): 551-557.

人参三七川芎提取物延缓血管紧张素 II 诱导内皮细胞衰老机制的研究 *

杨 静 雷 燕 方素萍 崔 巍 陈可冀

随着老龄化社会的到来，研究和防治与增龄有关的疾病，有效延缓衰老的进程已成为社会需要。高血压、冠心病、心功能不全等心血管疾病发生率随增龄急剧上升[1]，这些疾病中存在明显的心血管老化的表现。近来研究发现，血管内皮细胞衰老与存在血管老化的心血管疾病有许多联系，因此从内皮细胞衰老入手研究血管老化值得关注。本实验以 Ang II 诱导内皮细胞衰老，观察中药人参三七川芎提取物能否延缓 Ang II 诱导的内皮细胞衰老，初步探讨益气活血中药延缓血管老化的机制。

1. 材料与方法

1.1 材料

1.1.1 药物制备 人参三七川芎提取物为醇提物，

* 原载于《中西医结合学报》，2009, 29 (6): 524-528

第四章

三者之比为 3：2：4（含 3.164g 生药 /g 浸膏），由中国中医科学院中药所提供；缬沙坦（valsartan）购自 Novartis 公司（批号 H20040217）。

1.1.2　试剂　脐静脉内皮细胞（HUVEC-2C，美国 Cascade Biologics 公司，cat No：C-023-5C，Lot No：4C0218）；培养基 Medium 200（美国 Cascade Biologics 公司，cat No：M-200PRF-500；Lot No：061115-902）；低血清生长因子补充物（美国 Cascade Biologics 公司，cat No：S-003-10，Lot No：061121-901）；Ang II、荧光探针 2′,7′-Dichloro fluorescin diacetate DCFDA（美国 Sigma 公司）；细胞衰老测定试剂盒（上海杰美基因医药科技有限公司，Cat No：GMS 10012.1，Lot No：11-52818-12）；NO 试剂盒、抗超氧阴离子自由基及产生超氧阴离子自由基测试盒（南京建成生物工程研究所）；AT_1R、AT_2R 多克隆抗体（武汉博士德公司）；p47phox 多克隆抗体（美国 Santa cruz 公司）。

1.1.3　仪器　TCS-SP2 激光扫描共聚焦显微镜（Leica，德国）；恒温 CO_2 培养箱（Sanyo，日本）；倒置显微镜（OLYMPUS，日本）；流式细胞仪（BD，美国）；酶标仪（BIO-TEK，美国）。

1.2　实验方法

1.2.1　分组　实验用细胞分为 5 组：(1) 空白对照组（完全培养基 M200+LSGS）；(2) Ang II 衰老模型组（10^{-6}mol/L Ang II）；(3) 人参三七川芎高剂量组（10^{-6}mol/L Ang II +50mg/L 人参三七川芎提取物）；(4) 人参三七川芎低剂量组（10^{-6}mol/L Ang II +20mg/L 人参三七川芎提取物）；(5) valsartan 组（10^{-6}mol/L Ang II +10^{-6}mol/L valsartan）。人参三七川芎提取物所采用的浓度是根据噻唑蓝 (MTT) 法[2] 实验筛选出的最佳有效作用浓度。

1.2.2　细胞培养　按照内皮细胞培养方法[3]，将细胞传至 5 代，待细胞贴壁后，人参三七川芎提取物高剂量组、低剂量组培养液中分别加入 50mg/L、20mg/L 人参三七川芎提取物，随每次换液各加入相应浓度药物。各组细胞铺至瓶底 80% 左右后，无血清同步 6h。除空白对照组外，Ang II 组、人参三七川芎高剂量组、低剂量组分别加入终浓度为 10^{-6}mol/L 的 Ang II，持续刺激 48h，第 12 和 24h 各补充 Ang II 1 次；Valsartan 组加入 valsartan 后 1h 加入 Ang II，valsartan 及 Ang II 的终浓度均

为 10^{-6}mol/L，第 12h 和 24h 各补充 Ang II 1 次，第 23h 补充 valsartan1 次，持续刺激 48h。细胞用 0.25% 的胰酶消化，4℃，1500r/min 离心收集。

1.2.3　衰老细胞鉴定　SA-β-gal 是一种可鉴定衰老细胞的生物学标志物[4]，按照细胞衰老测定试剂盒说明检测，观察并计数显微镜下胞浆内有蓝色细胞的百分数，判断细胞衰老的情况。

1.2.4　细胞周期分析　每组细胞以 0.25% 胰蛋白酶消化、收集细胞，用预冷的 PBS 洗涤 2 次，调整细胞数至 $1×10^6$ 个 /mL，逐滴加入预冷的 70% 乙醇固定，4℃过夜。次日，离心，PBS 洗涤，用含有终浓度为 20mg/mL RN aseA 酶的 50mg/L 的碘化丙啶（PI）染液避光染 30min，300 目筛网过滤细胞后，流式细胞仪检测。应用 Cell QuestPro 软件获取至少 20 000 个细胞的荧光 2 (FL-2A) 直方图，通过 ModiFit 软件分析细胞周期分布。

1.2.5　ROS 含量　以 $5×10^4$/孔细胞接种于 6 孔培养板中，加入 1mL 预温至 37℃ 的 10μmol/L DCFDA 工作液，轻轻混匀。37℃ 孵育 30min，无血清培养基清洗 2 次，激光共聚焦显微镜下观察结果。ROS 特异性荧光探针 DCFDA 储存液（10mmol/L，0.1mL）临用前按 1：1000 用无血清培养液稀释为工作浓度 10μmol/L。由蓝光激发，发绿色荧光，激发波长 488nm，发射波长 525nm。

1.2.6　抗超氧阴离子自由基含量测定　检测细胞培养液内抗超氧阴离子自由基活力的含量，间接反映细胞内 O_2^- 的情况，操作依据试剂盒说明进行。

1.2.7　NO 含量测定　内皮损伤时 NO 其合成减少或生物活性降低[5]，O_2^- 的产生导致 NO 的耗竭，通过检测细胞培养液中 NO 含量，可间接反映内皮细胞的衰老情况。采用硝酸还原酶法，按照 NO 试剂盒说明操作。

1.2.8　细胞 AT_1R、AT_2R、NAD (P) H 氧化酶 p47phox 蛋白表达　采用 Western blot 检测方法[6]。RIPA buffer 裂解液提取总蛋白，考马斯亮蓝法测蛋白含量，调整蛋白浓度，煮沸变性 5min，12.5% SDS-PAGE 电泳后半干转印仪转膜，5% 脱脂奶粉的 TBST（0.05% 的 Tween-20）封闭 1h，1：300 稀释的一抗 4℃ 孵育过夜，辣根过氧化物酶标记的二抗孵育 1.5h，Odyssey 荧光扫描，β-actin 为内对照。

1.3 统计学方法

采用 SPSS 13.0 软件进行统计处理，观察指标以均数 ± 标准差 ($\bar{\chi} \pm s$) 表示，采用单因素方差分析。

2. 结果

2.1 β-gal 细胞衰老测定

衰老细胞在酸性条件下 β- 半乳糖苷酶活性增加，催化生成深蓝色的沉积产物，观察蓝色表达的细胞作为细胞衰老的分子特征来识别和探测衰老细胞。β-gal 染色显示，空白对照组几乎不表达 β-gal 蓝染阳性细胞；Ang II 诱导衰老模型组蓝染阳性细胞数明显增加，约 78.33%；余用药组阳性细胞数较 Ang II 衰老模型组明显减少，中药高剂量组约 65.00%，低剂量组约 55.33%；valsartan 组约 50.33%。

2.2 各组细胞周期变化比较（表 1）

通过细胞 DNA 含量来判断细胞周期时相。流式细胞仪分析表明与空白对照组比较，Ang II 模型衰老组细胞周期向 G_0-G_1 期明显停顿；与 Ang II 模型衰老组相比，人参三七川芎高、低剂量组及 valsartan 组，G_0-G_1 期细胞明显减少，处于 G_2-M 期的细胞明显增多，差异有统计学意义（$P < 0.05$），表明人参三七川芎高、低剂量组在一定程度上可延缓 Ang II 诱导的细胞衰老，促进细胞增殖。

表 1 各组细胞周期变化比较 (%, $\bar{\chi} \pm s$)

组别	n	G_0-G_1 期	G_2-M 期	S 期
空白对照	3	40.45±0.88	55.21±1.14	4.34±0.49
Ang II 衰老模型	3	60.77±2.64*	38.74±5.56*	5.16±1.59
人参三七川芎高剂量	3	45.93±3.50△	49.25±3.90△	4.83±1.69
人参三七川芎低剂量	3	44.59±1.28△	50.72±0.57△	4.69±0.79
Valsartan	3	42.12±2.35△	54.08±2.01△	3.79±0.59

注：与空白对照组比较，*$P < 0.05$；与 Ang II 衰老模型组比较，△$P < 0.05$

2.3 各组 ROS 含量比较（表 2，图 1）

DCFDA 是 ROS 特异性荧光探针，通过激光共聚焦显微镜发射发射光和激发光，使 ROS 呈现绿色荧光。与空白对照组比较，Ang II 衰老模型组、人参三七川芎高、低剂量组细胞内 ROS 所发荧光强度明显增强（$P < 0.05$）；与 Ang II 衰老模型组比较，人参三七川芎高、低剂量组、valsartan 组的荧光强度明显减弱，差异均有统计学意义（$P < 0.05$）。

表 2 人参三七川芎提取物对细胞内 ROS 含量的影响 ($\bar{\chi} \pm s$, n=4)

组别	n	ROS 含量（荧光像素数）
空白对照	3	125.77±3.53△
Ang II 衰老模型	3	285.43±5.25*
人参三七川芎高剂量	3	231.52±2.51*△
人参三七川芎低剂量	3	221.67±3.84*△
Valsartan	3	218.37±4.13*△

注：与空白对照组比较，*$P < 0.05$；与 Ang II 衰老模型组比较，△$P < 0.05$

2.4 各组抗超氧阴离子与 NO 含量比较（表 3）

与空白对照组比较，Ang II 衰老模型组培养液内的抗超氧阴离子和 NO 含量明显减少（$P < 0.05$），说明 Ang II 诱导后衰老的内皮细胞功能异常，产生 O_2^- 增多；与 Ang II 衰老模型组比较，人参三七川芎高、低剂量组及 valsartan 组培养液内的抗超氧阴离子和 NO 含量明显增加，差异有统计学意义（$P < 0.05$）。

表 3 人参三七川芎提取物对细胞培养液抗超氧阴离子与 NO 含量的影响 ($\bar{\chi} \pm s$)

组别	n	抗超氧阴离子（U/L）	NO (μmol/L)
空白对照	4	99.67±0.38	26.51±0.19
Ang II 衰老模型	4	80.70±0.30*	11.90±0.67*
人参三七川芎高剂量	4	87.45±0.58△	17.35±0.70△
人参三七川芎低剂量	4	88.47±0.54△	17.67±0.51△
Valsartan	4	93.69±0.79△	18.85±0.66△

注：与空白对照组比较，*$P < 0.05$；与 Ang II 衰老模型组比较，△$P < 0.05$

2.5 各组细胞 p47phox、AT_1R、AT_2R 蛋白表达比较（表 4，图 2）

与空白对照组比较，Ang II 模型衰老组

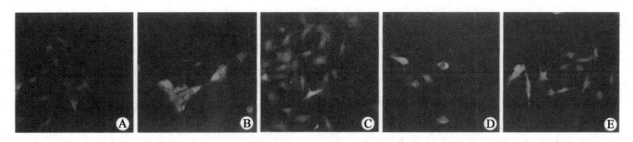

图1　人参三七川芎提取物对细胞内 ROS 含量影响（×400）

注：A 为空白对照组；B 为 AngⅡ 衰老模型组；C 为人参三七川芎高剂量组；D 为人参三七川芎低剂量组；E 为 Valsartan 组

p47phox、AT_2R 蛋白表达上调，AT_1R 表达下调；与 AngⅡ模型衰老组比较，人参三七川芎低剂量组 p47phox、AT_2R 蛋白表达下调，AT_1R 表达则上调；Valsartan 组与人参三七川芎高剂量组 p47phox 下调，AT_1R 表达上调，AT_2R 表达无改变。

表4　各组细胞 p47phox、AT_1R、AT_2R 蛋白表达比较（$\bar{\chi} \pm s$）

组别	n	p47phox	AT_1R	AT_2R
空白对照	3	0.401± 0.001△	0.436± 0.006△	0.337± 0.002△
AngⅡ 衰老模型	3	0.539± 0.001*	0.292± 0.003*	0.423± 0.002*
人参三七川芎高剂量	3	0.484± 0.003△	0.316± 0.004△	0.416± 0.001
人参三七川芎低剂量	3	0.474± 0.003△	0.317± 0.004△	0.409± 0.002△
Valsartan	3	0.444± 0.002△	0.372± 0.001△	0.415± 0.005

注：与空白对照组比较，*$P < 0.05$；与 AngⅡ 衰老模型组比较，△$P < 0.05$

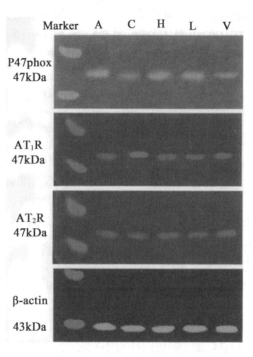

图2　各组细胞 p47phox、AT_1R、AT_2R 蛋白表达比较

注：A 为 AngⅡ模型组；C 为空白对照组；H 为人参三七川芎高剂量组；L 为人参三七川芎低剂量组；V 为 Valsartan 组

3. 讨论

人参、三七、川芎属于中药益气活血药范畴，中医学认为其有"延年不老"的功效。现代药理学研究显示，三种药物的有效成分与抗衰老作用密切相关。本实验通过观察人参三七川芎提取物对内皮细胞衰老的影响，研究益气活血中药是否具有延缓血管老化的作用。

活性氧 (ROS) 学说是目前较公认的衰老假说。随增龄活性氧产生增加，氧化损伤产物在细胞内积聚，最终导致细胞功能失调和衰老[7]。研究表明，老年内皮功能紊乱是由于 ROS 与内生保护抗氧化剂之间的失衡造成的，而 NAD (P) H 氧化酶是血管壁内皮细胞 ROS 的主要来源[8]。Ang Ⅱ 在调节

血管老化的刺激和信号中有关键作用，可导致血管内皮细胞衰老[9]。NAD (P) H 氧化酶可由 AngⅡ 激活[10]，导致 ROS 的产生[11]，ROS 作为 AngⅡ 信号级联中的第二信使，参与血管损伤过程许多细胞信号转导，可引起内皮细胞衰老，其中 p47phox 是 NAD (P) H 氧化酶活性必需的亚单位。Ang Ⅱ 通过对血管的病理生理作用引起血管的损伤，促进其衰老，出现各种衰老表现。本研究以 AngⅡ 诱导的内皮细胞衰老为模型，观察中药提取物能否从 Ang Ⅱ 致衰途径延缓内皮细胞衰老。

实验中首先观察到，在 AngⅡ 诱导下，β-gal 染色阳性细胞显著增加，应用高、低剂量中药处理后，衰老细胞数明显减少；激光共聚焦显微镜观察发现，中药高、低剂量组的细胞 ROS 所发荧光强

度明显低于衰老模型组，提示中药提取物能降低内皮细胞 ROS 的合成。在细胞周期研究中发现，应用中药干预后的细胞，G_0-G_1 期细胞显著降低，G_2-M 期的细胞明显增加，表明中药能够使处于休眠静止期的细胞重新活跃，进入增殖期，在一定程度上延缓了细胞的衰老。NO 能抑制炎细胞的浸润，减少氧自由基生成，加速氧自由基灭活[5]，Ang II 致衰的细胞应用中药培养后培养液中 NO 含量和抗超氧阴离子活力显著上升，间接证明了给予中药后的细胞氧自由基生成减少，扩血管物质生成增加，减少了内皮的损伤，延缓了细胞衰老。

本研究进一步观察益气活血中药对 Ang II 刺激后衰老内皮细胞 AT_1R、AT_2R、p47phox 的表达，结果表明，高、低剂量中药可降低衰老细胞中 p47phox 的表达，进而减少活性氧生成；现有研究发现 AT_1R 介导大多数已知的 Ang II 的生物学效应，如促进血管收缩、细胞增生、刺激活性氧生成等[12,13]。实验结果中 AT_1R 在致衰各组细胞中表达下降可能是 Ang II 刺激后受体代偿性表达下调的结果，衰老模型组下调最明显；致衰各组 AT_2R 在 Ang II 刺激后与空白对照组比较仍表现为上调，可能是衰老细胞对 AT_1R 所致的不良效应产生的保护性反应。现有的研究支持 AT_2R 可拮抗 AT_1R 的效应，但 AT_2R 具有抑制细胞生长、促进凋亡等作用[13]，而内皮细胞凋亡是血管衰老的表现之一，AT_2R 过度表达同样有不利之处，人参三七川芎低剂量组能下调 AT_2R 表达，而高剂量组表达无改变，说明人参三七川芎可能对 AT_2R 途径也有影响。高、低剂量人参三七川芎干预后，内皮细胞培养液 O_2^- 生成减少，细胞 p47phox 蛋白表达下降，支持中药提取物可能经由 AT_1R 途径下调 p47phox 表达，减少活性氧生成，延缓内皮细胞衰老。

综上所述，益气活血中药人参三七川芎提取物可能经由 AT_1R 从蛋白水平下调 NADPH 氧化酶 p47phox 的表达，使 HUVECs 产生活性氧减少，从而延缓 Ang II 诱导的内皮细胞的衰老，对 AT_2R 途径的影响还需进一步研究证实。

参考文献

[1] Lakatta EG, Levy D. Arterial and cardiac aging: major shareholders in cardiovascular disease enterprises part I：aging arteries: a "set up" for vascular disease. Circulation, 2003, 107 (1): 139-146.

[2] Mosmann T. Rapid colormietric assay for cellular growth and surviva: application to proliferation in cytotoxicity assay. J Immunol Methods, 1983, 65 (1-2): 55-65.

[3] 薛俊丽，冯波. 人脐静脉内皮细胞培养方法. 同济大学学报，2007, 28 (5): 110-113.

[4] Dmiri GP, Lee X, Basile G, et al. A biomarker that identifies senescent human cells in culture and in aging skin in vivo. Proc Natl Acad Sci USA, 1995, 92 (20): 9363-9367.

[5] 王玉筵. 血管内皮功能紊乱与血管老化. 岭南心血管病杂志，2006, 12 (6): 452-453.

[6] 汪家政，范明. 蛋白质技术手册. 北京：科学出版社，2001：77-100.

[7] Shringarpure R, Davies KJ. Protein turnover by the proteasome in aging and disease. Free Radic Bio-Med, 2002，32 (2): 1084-1089.

[8] Griendling KK, Sorescu D, Ushio-Fukai M. NAD(P)H Oxidase role in cardiovascular biology and disease. Circ Res, 2000，86 (5): 494-501.

[9] Shan HY, Bai XJ, Chen XM. Angiotensin II induces endothelial cell senescence via the activation of mitogen-activated protein kinases. Cell Biochem Function, 2008, 26 (4): 459-466.

[10] Berry C, Hamilton CA, Brosnan MJ, et al. Superoxide excess in hypertension and aging: a common cause of endothelial dysfunction. Hypertension, 2001, 37 (2): 529-534.

[11] Dandona P, Kumar V, Aljada A, et al. Angiotensin II receptor blocker valsartan suppresses reactive oxygen species generation in leukocytes, nuclear factor-kappa B, in mononuclear cells of normal subjects: evidence of an anti inflammatory action. J Clin Endocrinol Metab, 2003, 88 (9): 4496-4501.

[12] Carey, Robert M. Update on the role of the AT2 receptor. Curr Opin Nephrol Hypertens, 2005, 14 (1): 67-71.

[13] 肖梅. 肾素 - 血管紧张素系统在心血管疾病进展中的作用. 心血管病学进展，2005, 26 (2): 137-140.

人参三七川芎提取物延缓内皮细胞复制性衰老的机制研究 *

杨　静　雷　燕　崔　巍　方素萍　陈可冀

我国已进入老龄化社会，因而研究和防治与增龄有关的疾病，有效延缓衰老的进程已成为社会需求。研究发现，衰老是造成心血管疾病相关发病率和死亡率增高的主要独立危险因素之一[1]，并且心血管疾病中存在明显的血管老化表现，如内皮细胞功能的紊乱和衰老。人参三七川芎属于中药益气活血药范畴，中医学认为其有"延年不老"的功效。现代药理学研究显示，这三种药物的有效成分与抗衰老作用密切相关[2-4]。因此，本实验以内皮细胞复制性衰老为衰老模型，观察人参三七川芎提取物能否延缓内皮细胞的复制性衰老，为研究益气活血中药延缓血管老化作用做初步探讨。

1. 材料

1.1　药物制备

人参（*Panax ginseng*），产自吉林抚松镇；三七（*Panax notoginseng*），产自云南；川芎（*Ligusticum chuanxiong*），产自四川，经中国中医科学院中药研究所黄璐琦研究员鉴定均符合《中国药典》2005 年版标准。人参三七川芎提取物为醇提物，由中国中医科学院中药研究所提供（实验用药加入 3 倍 70% 乙醇提取 3 次，每次 2h，滤过，弃药渣，将醇提取液进行乙醇回收，浓缩至无醇味，制成中药浸膏），生药含量 3.164g/g 浸膏；VitE 购自 Sigma 公司，批号 085K1584。

1.2　细胞及试剂

脐静脉内皮细胞（HUVEC-2C, 美国 Cascade Biologics 公司, cat No: C-023-5C, Lot No: 4C0218）；培养基 Medium 200（美国 Cascade Biologics 公司, cat M-200PRF-500；Lot 061115-902）；低血清生长因子补充物（美国 Cascade Biologics 公司, cat S-003-10, Lot 061121-901）；荧光探针 7′-Dichlorofluorescin diacetate DCFDA（美国 Sigma 公司，批号 077K4037）；细胞衰老测定试剂盒（上海杰美基因医药科技有限公司，cat No: GMS10012.1，Lot No: 11-52818-12）；二甲基亚砜（DMSO，批号 T20080814，上海诺泰化工有限公司）；NO 试剂盒（南京建成生物工程研究所，批号 20071117）、抗超氧阴离子自由基及产生超氧阴离子自由基测试盒（南京建成生物工程研究所，批号 20071218）；AT$_1$R 多克隆抗体（武汉博士德公司，货号 BA0582）、AT$_2$R 多克隆抗体（武汉博士德公司，货号 BA0583）；p47phox 多克隆抗体（美国 Santa cruz 公司，货号 sc-17844）。

1.3　器材

TCS-SP2 激光扫描共聚焦显微镜（Leica, 德国）；MCO-20AIC 型恒温 CO_2 培养箱（Sanyo, 日本）；CK2 型倒置相差显微镜（OLY-MPUS, 日本）；FACS Calibur 型流式细胞仪,（BD, 美国）；SIAFRT SYNERGYHT 型酶标仪（BIO-TEK, 美国）。

2. 方法

2.1　分组

细胞分为 4 组：8 代衰老模型组（完全培养基 M200+LSGS）；人参三七川芎高、低剂量组 (50, 20mg／L)；VitE 组 (50mg/L)。人参三七川芎提取物所采用的剂量是根据噻唑蓝 (MTT) 法实验筛选出的最佳有效作用浓度；VitE 组将 VitE 中加入体积分数为 2‰ DMSO 助溶，其余各组加入相同剂量 DMSO，达到同期对照的目的。

2.2　细胞培养

参照内皮细胞培养方法[5]进行细胞传代，5 代始细胞贴壁后，各用药组随每次换液加入相应药物浓度，2d 换液 1 次，持续刺激，传至第 8 代，待各组细胞铺满瓶底 80% 左右，用质量分数 0.25% 的胰酶消化，4℃，1500r／min 离心收集。

* 原载于《中国中药杂志》，2009，34（12）：1544-1548

2.3 8 代复制性衰老内皮细胞的判定

将 2 代 HUVEC-2C 和 8 代 HUVEC-2C 从细胞形态学、SA-β-gal 染色和细胞周期三方面进行比较，判断 8 代内皮细胞衰老状况。

2.4 衰老细胞鉴定

衰老相关 β- 半乳糖苷酶 (SA–β-gal) 是一种可鉴定衰老细胞的生物学标志物 [6]，按照细胞衰老测定试剂盒说明检测，观察并计数显微镜下胞浆内有蓝色细胞的百分数，判断细胞衰老的情况。

2.5 细胞周期分析

每组细胞以 0.25% 胰蛋白酶消化、收集细胞，用预冷的 PBS 洗涤 2 次，调整细胞数至 1×10^6 个 /mL，逐滴加入预冷的 70% 乙醇固定，4℃过夜。次日，离心，PBS 洗涤，用含有 20g / L RNaseA 酶的 50mg / L 的碘化丙啶 (PI) 染液避光染 30min，300 目筛网过滤细胞后，流式细胞仪检测。应用 CellQuestPro 软件获取至少 2 万个细胞的荧光 2 (FL-2A) 直方图，通过 ModiFit 软件分析细胞周期分布。

2.6 细胞内 ROS 含量

以 5×10^4 个 / 孔细胞接种于 6 孔培养板，加入 1mL 预温至 37℃ 的 10μmol / L DCFDA 工作液，轻轻混匀。37℃孵育 30min，无血清培养基清洗 2 次，激光共聚焦显微镜观察结果。ROS 特异性荧光探针 DCFDA 临用前用无血清培养基稀释成 10μmol / L 的溶液。蓝光激发，激发波长 488nm，发射波长为 525nm。

2.7 抗超氧阴离子自由基含量测定

检测细胞培养液内抗超氧阴离子自由基活力的含量，间接反映细胞内 O^{2-} 的情况，操作依据试剂盒说明进行。

2.8 NO 含量测定

内皮损伤时 NO 合成减少或生物活性降低 [7]，通过检测细胞培养液中 NO 含量，可间接反映内皮细胞的衰老情况。采用硝酸还原酶法，按照 NO 试剂盒说明操作。

2.9 细胞 NAD (P) H 氧 化 酶 p47phox、AT_1R、AT_2R 蛋白表达采用 Western blot 检测方法

用 RIPA buffer 裂解液提取总蛋白，通过考马斯亮蓝法测蛋白含量，调整蛋白浓度，煮沸变性 5min，12.5% SDS-PAGE 电泳后半干转印仪转膜，5% 脱脂奶粉的 TBST（0.05% 的聚氧乙烯脱水山梨醇单油酸酯）封闭 1h，1：300 稀释的一抗 4℃ 孵育过夜，辣根过氧化物酶标记的二抗孵育 1.5h，

Odyssey 荧光扫描，β-actin 为内对照。

2.10 统计学方法

采用 SPSS 13.0 软件进行统计处理，观察指标以 $\bar{\chi} \pm s$ 表示，采用单因素方差分析，$P < 0.05$ 为差异有显著性。

3. 结果

3.1 8 代复制性衰老内皮细胞的判定

预实验中通过细胞形态学观察到，2 代内皮细胞体呈多角形，相互嵌合，胞浆清澈透明，细胞轮廓不清晰，呈单层铺路石状排列；8 代内皮细胞大小不均，形状混浊，胞体轮廓变清晰，体积增大，生长缓慢，排列稀疏，难于形成单层细胞。SA-β-gal 染色显示，2 代内皮细胞基本不表达蓝染细胞，8 代内皮细胞组表达 β-gal 蓝染细胞较多 ($P < 0.05$)，约 78.33%。细胞周期研究显示，2 代内皮细胞 S 期细胞比例较高，G_0/G_1 期细胞比例较低，G_2/M 期细胞活跃；8 代内皮细胞与 2 代细胞相比，G_1 期进入 S 期的细胞比例明显降低，G_2/M 期细胞明显减少，差异有统计学意义 ($P < 0.05$)。表明 8 代内皮细胞已属于复制性衰老细胞，可用于细胞衰老的相关实验研究。

3.2 SA-β-gal 细胞衰老测定

β-gal 染色显示，VitE 组蓝染阳性细胞数约为 39.00%；8 代衰老模型组表达 β-gal 蓝染细胞较多 ($P < 0.05$)，约为 78.33%；中药高、低剂量组阳性细胞数分别为 49.33%、44.67%，较 8 代衰老模型组明显减少，差异有统计学意义 （均 $P < 0.05$)。

3.3 细胞周期分析

流式细胞仪分析表明，与 Vit E 组比较，8 代衰老模型组细胞周期向 G_0/G_1 期明显停顿，G_2/M 期细胞明显减少；与 8 代衰老模型组比较，中药高、低剂量组及 VitE 组 G_0/G_1 期细胞明显减少，处于 G_2/M 期的细胞明显增多，差异有统计学意义 ($P < 0.05$)；但与 VitE 组比较，中药高、低剂量组 G_0/G_1 期细胞增多，G_2/M 期细胞减少 ($P < 0.05$)。这表明随传代进行，人参三七川芎提取物高、低剂量组在一定程度上能够延缓细胞的衰老（表1）。

3.4 细胞内 ROS 含量测定

DCFDA 是 ROS 特异性荧光探针，通过激光共聚焦显微镜发射发射光和激发光，使细胞内活性氧呈现绿色荧光。8 代衰老模型组细胞所发荧光强

度强，与 8 代衰老模型组比较，中药高、低剂量组和 VitE 组的荧光强度明显减弱，差异有统计学意义（$P < 0.05$），但中药 2 个剂量组荧光强度比 VitE 组稍强（图 1）。

3.5　抗超氧阴离子与 NO 含量测定

与各用药组比较，8 代衰老模型组培养液内的抗超氧阴离子和 NO 含量明显减少（$P < 0.05$）；中药高、低剂量组培养液内的抗超氧阴离子和 NO 含量比衰老组明显增加，但较 VitE 组含量降低，差异有统计学意义（均 $P < 0.05$）。提示 8 代衰老内皮细胞产生的超氧阴离子（O_2^-）相对增多，而人参三七川芎提取物高、低剂量组能在一定程度上改善内皮的功能，增强抗氧化能力，从而延缓细胞衰老（表 2）。

3.6　Western blot 结果

与 8 代衰老模型组比较，中药高、低剂量组与 VitE 组 p47phox、AT_1R、AT_2R 表达明显下调，差异有统计学意义（均 $P < 0.05$）；与 Vit E 组比较，中药高、低剂量组 p47phox 和 AT_2R 表达上调（$P < 0.05$），AT_1R 表达仅有上调趋势，差异无统计学意义（表 3）。

4.　讨论

本实验在人参三七川芎提取物延缓小鼠血管老化整体实验进行的基础上，通过观察人参三七川芎提取物对内皮细胞衰老的影响，进一步研究益气活血中药是否具有延缓血管老化的作用。

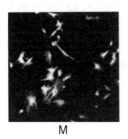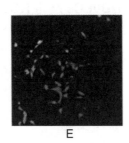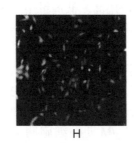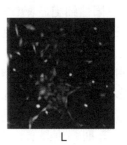

M　　　　　　　E　　　　　　　H　　　　　　　L

图 1　人参三七川芎提取物对细胞内 ROS 含量影响（×100）

M. 8 代衰老模型组；E. Vit E / 50mg / L 组；H. 中药 50mg / L；L. 中药 20mg / L 组

表 1　人参三七川芎提取物对各组细胞周期影响分析（$\bar{\chi} \pm s$, n=3）

分组	剂量（mg / L）	G_0/G_1（%）	G_2/M（%）	S（%）
衰老模型	–	54.16±0.23[1]	35.97±1.18[1]	9.86±0.96
中药提取物	50	33.97±0.13[1,2]	59.83±0.82[1,2]	6.19±0.70
	20	29.64±1.04[1,2]	64.25±0.22[1,2]	6.11±0.86
Vit E	50	16.62±0.34[2]	78.88±0.12[2]	4.50±0.34

注：与 VitE 组相比 [1] $P < 0.05$；与衰老模型组相比 [2] $P < 0.05$（表 2，3 同）。

表 2　人参三七川芎提取物对细胞培养液抗超氧阴离子与 NO 含量的影响（$\bar{\chi} \pm s$, n=4）

分组	剂量（mg / L）	抗超氧阴离子（U / L）	NO（μmol / L）
衰老模型	–	80.71±0.31[1]	8.14±0.44[1]
中药提取物	50	88.73±0.33[1,2]	12.19±0.35[1,2]
	20	91.00±0.37[1,2]	13.62±1.17[1,2]
Vit E	50	96.53±1.09[2]	18.12±0.37[2]

表 3　人参三七川芎提取物对细胞 p47 phox、AT_1R、AT_2R 蛋白表达的影响（$\bar{\chi} \pm s$, n=3）

分组	剂量（mg / L）	P47phox	AT_1R	AT_2R
衰老模型	–	0.498±0.006[1]	0.461±0.007[1]	0.566±0.001[1]
中药提取物	50	0.482±0.004[1,2]	0.350±0.016[2]	0.467±0.005[1,2]
	20	0.462±0.001[1,2]	0.324±0.005[2]	0.460±0.004[1,2]
Vit E	50	0.387±0.006[2]	0.303±0.003[2]	0.392±0.002[2]

第四章

ROS 学说是目前较公认的衰老假说。随增龄活性氧产生增加，氧化损伤产物在细胞内积聚，最终导致细胞功能失调和衰老[8]。研究表明，老年内皮功能紊乱是由于 ROS 与内生保护抗氧化剂之间的失衡造成的，而 NAD (P) H 氧化酶是血管壁内皮细胞 ROS 的主要来源[9]，其中 p47phox 是 NAD (P) H 氧化酶活性必需的亚单位。ROS 参与血管损伤过程中许多细胞信号转导，可引起内皮细胞衰老。本研究在前期预实验的基础上，结合相关文献的研究方法[10]，从细胞形态学、β- 半乳糖染色和细胞周期三方面进行分析，确定以 8 代 HUVEC-2C 为复制性衰老细胞模型，观察中药提取物能否从活性氧途径延缓内皮细胞衰老。

实验中首先观察到，8 代衰老内皮细胞 β- 半乳糖染色阳性细胞显著增加，应用高、低剂量中药和 Vit E 处理后，阳性细胞数明显减少。观察细胞内活性氧发现，中药高、低剂量组细胞 ROS 所发荧光强度明显低于 8 代衰老模型组，比 Vit E 组稍强，提示中药提取物能降低衰老内皮细胞 ROS 的合成。细胞周期研究中发现，应用中药干预后的细胞，G_0/G_1 期细胞显著降低，G_2/M 期的细胞明显增加，表明中药能够使处于休眠静止期的细胞重新活跃，进入增殖期，在一定程度上延缓了细胞的衰老。NO 能抑制炎细胞的浸润，减少氧自由基生成，加速氧自由基灭活[7]。对细胞培养液 NO 和抗超氧阴离子的检测发现，8 代衰老模型组 NO 含量、抗超氧阴离子活力降低，在应用中药培养后 NO 含量和抗超氧阴离子活力显著上升，间接证明了给予中药后的细胞氧自由基生成减少，扩血管物质生成增加，减少了内皮的损伤，延缓细胞的衰老。

进一步观察益气活血中药对衰老细胞 p47phox，AT_1R、AT_2R 显示，8 代衰老内皮细胞 p47phox 的蛋白表达上调，中药高、低剂量组降低衰老细胞 p47phox 的表达，低剂量组比高剂量组下调更明显。内皮细胞可释放内皮源性收缩因子如 Ang Ⅱ，当内皮功能受损时，Ang Ⅱ 合成和释放增加，可引起血管紧张度增加、血小板聚集、白细胞黏附和血栓形成等[11-12]。本实验通过观察 Ang Ⅱ 受体 AT_1R 和 AT_2R 发现，8 代衰老内皮细胞 AT_1R、AT_2R 含量明显增高，表明衰老内皮细胞 AT_1R、AT_2R 表达相对较多。各用药组与衰老组比较，AT_1R、AT_2R 表达均显著减少，提示益气活血中药与 Vit E 可能影响内皮源性收缩因子 Ang Ⅱ 的释放，改

善内皮功能。研究报道，AT_2R 具有促凋亡、抑增殖的作用[13]，而外源性 Ang Ⅱ 可通过 AT_1R 途径经由 NADPH 氧化酶刺激活性氧增加，引起内皮细胞衰老[14]，对于本实验中用药后内皮细胞释放的 Ang Ⅱ 引起的 AT_1R 的改变是否与 NADPH 氧化酶亚单位 p47phox 的降低存在直接关系，还需进一步研究。以上结果分析表明，中药高、低剂量组干预后，内皮细胞培养液 O^{2-} 生成减少，细胞 p47phox 蛋白表达下降，支持中药提取物通过活性氧途径下调 NADPH 氧化酶亚单位 p47phox 表达，减少活性氧生成，延缓内皮细胞衰老。

综上，益气活血中药人参三七川芎提取物可延缓内皮细胞复制性衰老，可能经由活性氧途径通过下调 NADPH 氧化酶 p47phox 的表达，使 HUVECs 产生 ROS 减少，从而延缓细胞的衰老。研究中发现，中药提取物能降低衰老内皮细胞 AT_1R、AT_2R 的表达，但是否通过细胞产生的 Ang Ⅱ 引起的相关途径使 p47phox 下调，导致内皮细胞的复制性衰老，有待进一步研究。

参考文献

[1] Susic D, Frohlich ED. The aging hypertensive heart: a brief update. Nat Clin Pract Cardiovasc Med, 2008, 5 (2): 104.

[2] 符路娣, 田丙坤, 蔡海云, 等. 中医药抗衰老的试验研究述评. 四川实验动物, 2006, 6: 20.

[3] 周晓慧, 周晓霞, 杨鹤梅. 三七总皂甙防治动脉粥样硬化的研究进展. 承德医学院学报, 2003, 20 (4): 350.

[4] 周江. 川芎有效成分及其药理作用研究. 浙江中医杂志, 2007, 42 (10): 615.

[5] 薛俊丽, 冯波. 人脐静脉内皮细胞培养方法. 同济大学学报, 2007, 28 (5): 110.

[6] Dimri GP, Lee X, Basile G, et al. A biomarker that identifies senescent human cells in culture and in aging skin in vivo. Proc Natl Acad Sci USA, 1995, 92: 9363.

[7] 王玉筵. 血管内皮功能紊乱与血管老化. 岭南心血管病杂志, 2006, 12 (6): 452.

[8] Shringarpure R, Davies KJ. Protein turnover by the proteasome in aging and disease. Free Radic Biol Med, 2002, 32: 1084.

[9] Griendling KK, Sorescu D, Ushio-Fukai M. NAD(P) H oxidase role in cardiovascular biology and disease. Circ Res, 2000, 86: 494.

[10] 赵海梅, 杨彬, 成蓓. 血管内皮细胞生长过程中与衰老相关的细胞生物学特征的变化. 中国微循环, 2006,

10 (2): 130.

[11] Horning, Drexler H. Reversal of endothelial in humans. Coron Artery Dis, 2001，12：463.

[12] Kharbanda RK, Deanfield. Function softhehealthy endothelium. Coron Artery Dise, 2001，12：485.

[13] 肖梅 . 肾素 - 血管紧张素系统在心血管疾病进展中的作用 . 心血管病学进展，2005，26 (2): 137.

[14] 李虹，白小涓，刘强，等 . 血管紧张素体外诱导内皮细胞衰老的机制研究 . 中国现代医学杂志，2007，17 (1): 51.

Effect of Chinese Herbal Drug-Containing Serum for Activating-Blood and Dispelling-Toxin on Ox-LDL-Induced Inflammatory Factors' Expression in Endothelial Cells[*]

JIANG Yue-rong　MIAO Yu　YANG Lin　XUE Mei　GUO Chun-yu

MA Xiao-juan　YIN Hui-jun　SHI Da-zhuo　CHEN Ke-ji

Atherosclerosis (AS) is a kind of inflammation injured disease. It has been shown by many researches that the oxidized low-density lipoprotein (ox-LDL) plays an important role in the pathologic process of AS and could activate the vascular endothelial cells to enhance expressions of multiple adhesive factors and cytokines in cells. Our research group has worked in recent years to recognize AS from pathogenetic angle of "stasis-toxin" and discovered that Chinese drugs for activating blood and dispelling toxin are more effective than those for activating-blood to resolve stasis singly in attenuating and stabilizing AS plaque[1-3]. This study was designed to explain the relationship of the two pathogens (stasis and toxin) from cell injury and inflammation response aspects by comparing the difference of acting links and targets between the two kinds of Chinese drugs in ox-LDL injured endothelial model cells through observing the physio-pathologic changes that occurred after endothelial injury in expressions and releasing of factors related to tissue damage and inflammation response.

1. Methods

1.1 Experimental Animal

Wistar rats, weighing 200 ± 20 g, SPF grade, supplied by the Institute of Experimental Animal, Chinese Academy of Medical Sciences, certification No. SCXK (Jing) 20050013.

1.2 Testing Drugs

Xiongshao Capsule (芎芍胶囊，XS), 0.25 g/capsule, containing drug's markers of paeoniflorin 28 mg, ferulic acid 3.5 mg, and total phenolic acid 34 mg, was provided by Dalian Institute of Physics and Chemistry, China, batch No. 070929.

Huanglian Capsule (黄连胶囊，HL), 0.25 g/capsule, product of Hubei Xianglian Pharmaceutical Co., Ltd., China, batch No. 070502，certification No. Z19983042.

2. Reagents

DMEM culture medium (high-sugar type) and top-grade fetal bovine serum were purchased from Hyclone Co. Epidermal growth factor

* 原载于 Chinese Journal of Integrative Medicine，2012，18（1）：30-33

(EGF), pancreatin, collagenase I, L-glutamine, gelatin, HEPES, EDTA, and sodium pyruvate were products of Sigma Co., USA. Penicillin, streptomycin, heparin, and short-acting insulin injection were made in China, analytic pure. Ox-LDL was purchased from the Biochemical Department of Basic Medical Institute, Chinese Academy of Medical Sciences, which showed single protein strip in agarose gel electrophoresis. Kits for enzyme immunoassay testing human interleukin-6 (IL-6), tumor necrosis factor-α (TNF-α), and soluble intercellular adhesion molecule-1 (sICAM-1) were products of R&D Co., sub-packed in China. Healthy human umbilical cord was from Hospital for Mother and Child Health Care of Haidian District, Beijing, China. CD54-FITC antibodies (IgG 2α, κ, MEM-111), CD62E-PE antibodies (mouse IgG 2α, κ, Clone HCD62E), and their homotype controls were purchased from BioLegend Co., USA.

2.1 Experimental Instruments

Flow cytometer, EPICS Elite, product of Beckman Coulter Co., USA; automatic enzyme-labeled detector, Wellscan type MK3, product of Labsystems Dragon Co., Finland.

2.2 Drug-Containing Serum Preparation

Thirty-two Wistar rats were divided into four groups equally: the blank group treated with distilled water, the positive control group treated with simvastatin (1.8 mg/kg), the test group I treated with Chinese herbal compound for activating blood (XS 0.135 g/kg), and the test group II treated with Chinese herbal compound for both activating blood and dispelling toxin (XS 0.135 g/kg and HL 0.135 g/kg). All treatments were administered once a day for 7 successive days by gastric infusion. Blood of rats was collected 1 h after final administration from abdominal aorta under sterilization, kept unchanged for 1 h, and centrifuged at 3 000 r/min for 15 min to separate the drug-serum. The drug-sera from rats of the same groups were mixed, subjected to 56 ℃ water bath for 30 min to inactivate, filtrated with microporous membrane to eliminate germs, sub-packaged in

tubes, and preserved under −70 ℃ until ready for testing.

2.3 Isolation, Cultivation, and Identification of Human Umbilical Vein Endothelial Cells

Referring to Jaffe's method[4] with a little modification, human umbilical cords of newborn collected in aseptic condition from healthy puerperal were processed by collagenase digestive method to separate cells. Human umbilical vein endothelial cells (HUVECs) were cultured with DMEM culture medium containing 20% fetal bovine serum, 10 ng/mL EGF, 40μU/mL insulin, 40 U/mL heparin, 2 mmol/L glutamine, 50 U/mL penicillin, 50μg/mL streptomycin, and 1 mmol/L sodium pyruvate. Cells of the third generation were taken for experiment after identification by factor VIII immunochemical test and morphological observation with an inverted phase-contrast microscopy.

2.4 Cell Grouping and Treatment

HUVECs were divided into five groups: the blank control group, the model group, the positive control group, the test group I, and the test group II. Cells of each group (1×10^8/L) were inoculated in 30 mm culture disc separately, and when grown to confluence condition, they were treated as follows: except those in the blank control group, HUVECs were made into injured model cells by adding ox-LDL of inducing dosage (final concentration of 100 5 μg/mL, which had been determined in advance) to culture medium. At the same time, 10% drug-serum from corresponding groups of rats was added to the medium of the latter three groups, respectively, while serum from rats of the blank control group was added in medium of the first two groups. Cells were then incubated in an incubator for 24 h.

2.5 Items and Methods of Detection

Levels of IL-6, TNF-a, and sICAM in the supernatant from centrifugation were detected by enzyme-linked immunosorbent assay (ELISA).

The expressions of ICAM-1 and E-selectin on HUVECs' surface were detected using flow cytometry adopting the following procedures:

cells were collected, digested with pancreatin, and washed with PBS to prepare single-cell suspension of 1×10^6/mL in concentration. Each sample was divided into two tubes. The corresponding monoclonal antibodies of CD54-FITC and CD62E-PE were added into the first tube, while the corresponding isotype control of mouse IgG2α-FITC and mouse IgG2α-PE were added in the second tube and then were mixed sufficiently, incubated for 30 min at room temperature light protectively, and washed with PBS. The supernatant was discarded, and cells were put in a flow cytometer to detect the respective index by multi-color analysis, adopting FS/SS gate method to sort cells, and the percentage of positive expressed cells was calculated by EXPO32 software.

2.6　Statistical Analysis

Data were expressed by mean $\pm$ standard deviation ($\overline{\chi} \pm s$), managed by software SPSS 13.0. The comparison among multiple groups was managed by single-factor variance analysis, and the paired comparison between groups was managed by LSD test.

3.　Results

3.1　Effects on Levels of IL-6, TNF-α, and sICAM-1 in the Supernatant

Compared with the blank control group, levels of IL-6, TNF-α, and sICAM-1 in the supernatant of the model group were significantly higher ($P < 0.01$), while these abnormal changes, except sICAM level in test group I, could be reversed in the three treated groups (positive control, test I, and test II) significantly, showing statistical differences ($P < 0.01$ or $P < 0.05$). As for comparisons of effects between the two test groups, no significant difference on IL-6 and TNF-α was found, although the decrease in the test group II seemed more significant (Table 1).

Table 1　Effects on Levels of IL-6, TNF-α, and sICAM-1 in the Supernatant of HUVEC Culture (pg/mL, $\overline{\chi} \pm s$, n=8)

Group	IL-6	TNF-α	sICAM-1
Blank	63.38$\pm$1970	82.70$\pm$27.14	819.60$\pm$75.45
Model	128.18$\pm$14.01**	168.83$\pm$18.68**	1323.75$\pm$286.12**
Test I	93.06$\pm$28.93**$^{\triangle\triangle}$	121.13$\pm$38.63**$^{\triangle\triangle}$	1144.13$\pm$252.65**
Test II	89.80$\pm$9.71$^{\triangle\triangle}$	116.67$\pm$12.89*$^{\triangle\triangle}$	1003.64$\pm$180.37$^{\triangle\triangle}$
Positive control	88.48$\pm$24.97$^{\triangle\triangle}$	115.67$\pm$33.77*$^{\triangle\triangle}$	1023.23$\pm$175.39$^{\triangle}$

Notes：*$P < 0.05$, **$P < 0.01$, compared with the blank control group；$^{\triangle}P < 0.05$, $^{\triangle\triangle}P < 0.01$, compared with the model group

3.2　Effect on the Cell Surface Positive Expression Rates of ICAM-1 and E-selectin

Compared with the blank control group, levels of cell surface ICAM-1 (CD54) and E-selectin (CD62E) expression increased significantly in the model group ($P < 0.01$) and were lower in the three treated groups than those in the model group, respectively, showing significant differences ($P < 0.05$). However, insignificant differences among the three groups were found (Table 2).

Table 2　Effects on Cell Surface Positive Rate of CD54 and CD62E (%, $\overline{\chi} \pm s$, n=3)

Group	CD54 positive rate	CD62E positive rate
Blank	56.27$\pm$20.43	18.70$\pm$13.66
Model	96.13$\pm$1.34**	43.97$\pm$12.33**
Test I	79.00$\pm$8.88*$^{\triangle}$	25.73$\pm$9.37$^{\triangle}$
Test II	76.37$\pm$10.30$^{\triangle}$	21.93$\pm$3.12$^{\triangle}$
Positive control	74.73$\pm$10.31$^{\triangle}$	25.93$\pm$4.79$^{\triangle}$

Notes: *$P < 0.05$, **$P < 0.01$, compared with the blank control group; $^{\triangle}P < 0.05$, compared with the model group

4. Discussion

AS is a disease manifested mainly by vascular inflammation response, and its pathogenesis involves many factors. Abnormal blood lipid metabolism-induced hyperlipidemia and lipo-peroxidation are the crucial factors for AS genesis and development process. Among them, the effect of ox-LDL in promoting the inflammation response of AS has been assured by many researchers[5]) ; it could injure vascular endothelium through multiple paths, including advancing the production of inflammation factors and adhesive molecules. The pathogenetic initiating step of AS is the adhesion of monocytes on vascular endothelium, which could be promoted by the adhesive molecules, such as ICAM-1 (CD54), VCAM-1, and E-selectin.

Being a cellular constituent-type expressed adhesive molecule, ICAM-1 plays central actions in the process of leukocyte recruitment to endothelium[6], and it could mediate adherence and spillage of various types of leukocyte toward endothelium[7]. E-selectin (CD62E) is a functional cell membranous adhesive molecule that belongs to the selectin family, and it is expressed in the very early stage of inflammation course but is limited in the vascular endothelium only.

The adhesive molecules-mediated leukocyte adhesion could enhance the instability of AS plaques and attenuate their fibrous cap, thus accelerate the breakage of plaque and the formation of thrombus, which is manifested in clinics as instable angina and myocardial infarction [8,9].

Considering the Chinese medicine (CM) recognition of "stasis and toxin" and combining with the relevant modern medical ideals, our research group suggested that most of the pathologic damages, such as tissue-injured necrosis caused by breakage of AS plaque and thrombosis obstruction, inflammatory cascade reaction, oxidized lipid deposition, calcium overload, and cell apoptosis, are similar to that of CM evil pathogens (stasis and toxin) in specialties such as acute initiation, rapid transmitting and changing, direct attack to internal organs, and great damage to tissues[1,8]. Therefore, a full-scale Chinese medical explanation on genetic specialty and pathogenesis of vascular thrombotic cardio-cerebral diseases could be made by combining the two pathogens. Many small-sample clinical observations have illustrated the reliable clinical effectiveness of Chinese drugs for clearing heat and dispelling-toxin in preventing and treating instable angina and apoplexy[9], and a study regarding the intervening effect of Chinese drugs on AS instable plaque in apolipoprotein E gene defect mice has proven that the effect of drugs for activating blood and dispelling toxin is superior to those simply for activating blood to remove stasis[2], which indicated from an experimental aspect the important role of "toxin" in the pathogenesis of arterial thrombotic diseases.

XS is composed of the effective ingredients of Chinese herbal medicines, total phenols of *Radix Paeoniae rubra*, and total glycosides of *Radix Chuanxiong*. It was shown by a previous study as being effective as anti-AS. This study was designed to compare the effectiveness of drug-serum of XS+HL (drugs for both activating blood and dispelling toxin) to that of XS alone (drugs for activating blood only) on ox-LDL-stimulated HUVECs. The results showed that ox-LDL stimulation could significantly raise the levels of IL-6, TNF-α, and sICAM in the culture supernatant as well as the expressions of ICAM-1 and E-selectin in cell surface, and these abnormally heightened indices, except sICAM level in the test group I, could be reduced to some extent by the test drug-sera, with the effect similar to that of simvastatin (the positive control), suggesting that the combination of XS+HL has definite inhibitory actions on the vascular endothelial inflammation response injured by ox-LDL. However, its concrete mechanism awaits further studies.

References

[1] Shi DZ, Xu H, Yin HJ, et al. Combination and transformation of toxin and blood stasis in etiopathogenesis of thrombotic cerebrocardiovascular diseases. J Chin Integr Med, 2008, 6：1105-1108.

[2] Wen C, Xu H, Huang OF, et al. Effect of drugs for promoting blood circulation on blood lipids and inflammatory reaction of atherosclerotic plaques in apoE gene deficiency mice. Chin J Integr Tradit West Med, 2005, 25：345.

[3] Zhang JC, Chen KJ, Zheng GJ, et al. Regulatory effect of Chinese herbal compound for detoxifying and activating blood circulation on expression of NF-κB and MMP-9 in aorta of apolipoprotein E gene knocked-out mice. Chin J Integr Tradit West Med, 2007, 27：40-44.

[4] Jiang YR, Chen KJ, Xu YG, et al. Effects of Propyl Gallate on adhesion of polymorphonuclear leukocytes to human endothelial cells induced by tumor necrosis factor alpha. Chin J Integr Med, 2009, 15：47-53.

[5] Ou HC, Lee WJ, Lee IT, et al. Ginkgo biloba extract attenuates ox-LDL-induced oxidative functional damages in endothelial cells. J Appl Physiol, 2009, 106：1674-1685.

[6] Landsberger M, Wolff B, Jantzen F, et al. Cerivastatin reduces cytokine-induced surface expression of ICAM-1 via increased shedding in human endothelial cells. Atherosclerosis, 2007, 190：43-52.

[7] Xenos ES, Stevens SL, Freeman MB. Nitric oxide mediates the effect of fluvastatin on intercellular adhesion molecule-1 and platelet endothelial cell adhesion molecule-1 expression on human endothelial cells. Ann Vasc Surg, 2005, 19：386-392.

[8] Hopkins AM, Baird AW, Nusrat A. ICAM-1：targeted docking for exogenous as well as endogenous ligands. Adv Drug Deliv Rev, 2004, 56：763-778.

[9] Kaski JC, Fernández-Bergés DJ, Consuegra-Sánchez L, et al. A comparative study of biomarkers for risk prediction in acute coronary syndrome-results of the SIESTA (Systemic Inflammation Evaluation in non-ST-elevation Acute coronary syndrome) study. Atherosclerosis, 2010, 212：636-643.

[10] Zhang JC, Chen KJ. Theoretical thinking on relationship between toxic-stasis pathogenicity and atherosclerotic vulnerable plaque. Chin J Integr Tradit Westn Med, 2008, 28：366-368.

[11] Lu XH, Ding SW. Clinical effect and mechanism on treating unstable angina pectoris by Huanglian Jiedu Capsule. J Shandong Univ Tradit Chin Med, 2005, 29：457-460.

Effects of Propyl Gallate on Adhesion of Polymorpho-nuclear Leukocytes to Human Endothelial Cells Induced by Tumor Necrosis Factor Alpha[*]

JIANG Yue-rong   CHEN Ke-ji   XU Yong-gang   YANG Xiao-hong   YIN Hui-jun

Leukocyte adhesion to the vascular endothelium is a critical initiating step in inflammation and atherosclerosis[1]. Upon exposure to pro-inflammatory cytokines, such as tumor necrosis factor alpha (TNF-α) or interleukin -1β (IL-1β), endothelial cells (Ecs) synthesize and express on their surface numerous adhesion molecules and other molecules such as intercellular adhesion molecule-1 (ICAM-1 or CD54), vascular cell adhesion molecule-1 (VCAM-1) and E-selectin (CD62E)[2], which participate in leukocyte and platelet recruitment,

* 原载于 Chinese Journal of Integrative Medicine，2009，15（1）：47-53

coagulation and inflammation. Various drugs, including statins, non-steroidal anti-inflammatory drugs (NSAIDs) and antioxidants, were reported to have the effects of regulating adhesion molecule expression and inhibiting the adhesion of leukocytes to ECs[3].

Propyl Gallate (PrG, molecular formula: $C_{10}H_{12}O_5$, structure formula: see Figure 1), also named as Radix Paeoniae 801, is an alkyl ester derivative of gallic acid, one of the active ingredients of radix Paeonia rubra. PrG is a strong antioxidant and has various effects such as blocking lipooxygenase and cyclooxygenase activities, scavenging free radicals, inhibiting arachidonic acid-induced platelet aggregation, and anti-inflammation[4-6]. It is clinically used for the treatment of coronary heart disease, cerebral thrombosis, thrombotic phlebitis, dysmenorrhea and so on in China.

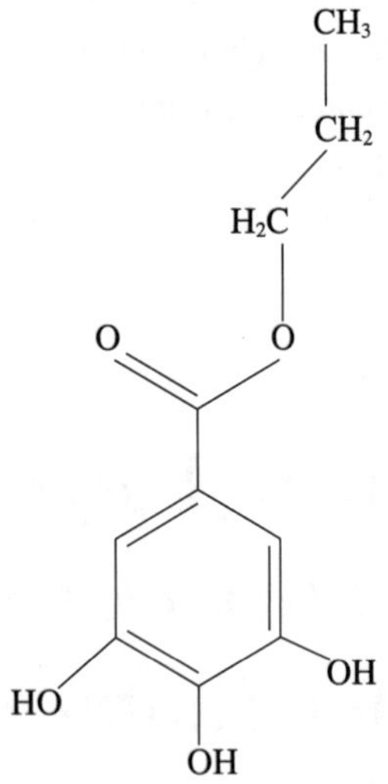

Figure 1　Chemical Structure of Propyl Gallate

Several anti-inflammatory effects of PrG have been reported including its inhibitory action on acute inflammatory reactions induced by carragheenin, bradykinin or 5-hydroxytryptamine (5-HT) [7]. However, the effects of PrG on vascular inflammatory responses and underlying cellular mechanisms are still not known. In the present study, we tested the hypothesis that PrG, an inhibitor of lipooxygenase and cyclooxygenase-2[8] with potent antioxidant property, could inhibit

TNF-α-induced endothelial adhesion to human polymorphonuclear cells (PMNs), an early sign of vascular inflammatory reaction.

1.　Methods

1.1　Reagents

Monoclonal antibody against CD54 directly coupled to FITC (mouse IgG_1 κ, Clone 84H10) and FITC-conjugated anti-mouse IgG, the isotypic control monoclonal antibody, were from Beckman Coulter (Immunonotech, Mareille, France). The monoclonal antibody against CD62E directly coupled to PE (mouse IgG_1, Clone 68-5H11) and PE-conjugated anti-mouse IgG the isotypic control monoclonal antibody, were from Pharmingen (Becton Dickinson, USA). PrG was provided by Fujian Mindong Rejuvenation Pharmaceutical Co., Ltd., China (batch No.030505). Acetylsalicylic acid (ASA) was from Sigma (Lot No. 033K0026). Stock solutions (0.1 mol/L) of PrG and ASA were made in dimethylsulfoxide (DMSO) and then diluted to proper concentrations just before application. Dulbecco's modified Eagle medium (DMEM, with D-glucose at 4500 mg/L, Lot No.1136551) was from GIBCO. Fetal calf serum (FCS, Lot No. ALA 12918) was from Hyclone (USA). Epidermal growth factor (Lot No. 060305H253) and TNF-α (Lot No. 22CY25) were from Perprotech (USA). Human lymphocyte isolation medium was from Tianjin Haoyang Biological Manufacture Co., Ltd., China (Lot No. 060305H253). Collagenase I, trypsin, HEPES, L-glutamine, gelatin and sodium pyruvate were from Sigma (USA).

1.2　Culture of Endothelial Cells and Experimental Conditions

Human umbilical vein endothelial cells (HUVECs) were obtained from newborn infant umbilical cord veins by digestion with 0.1% collagenase according to the method described by Jaffe[9] with some modifications. The resulting cells were cultivated on gelatin and grown to subconfluence in DMEM culture medium containing 20% FCS and supplemented with 40 U/mL heparin,

40μ U/mL insulin, 10 ng/ mL EGF, 2 mmol/L glutamine, 50 U/mL penicillin, 50μg/mL streptomycin and 1 mmol/L sodium pyruvate at 37 ℃ under 5%CO_2. Cells were judged to be more than 99% endothelial cells by their characteristic cobblestone morphology in an inverted microscope (Leica DMIRB, Germany) and by immunocytochemical demonstration of factor Ⅷ staining. HUVECs were used for experiments at the third to fourth passages of individual preparations. They were seeded in either 96-well plates (0.5 mL/well) for adhesion experiments, or in 30 mm culture dishes for cytometry analysis.

1.3 Preparation of Peripheral Blood PMN

Whole blood from normal healthy donors was collected in syringes containing 3.8% sodium citrate (9 : 1 v/v). PMNs were isolated by lymphocyte isolation medium gradient centrifugation (20℃, $500 \times g$ for 30 min). Mononuclear cells banded on the surface of the upper layer. PMNs banded at the interface of the two density concentrations and erythrocytes banded at the bottom. PMNs were obtained from the interface after gradient centrifugation and erythrocytes were removed from this fraction with hypotonic lysis. PMNs were then washed three times with phosphate-buffered saline (PBS) and placed in DMEM medium with 10% FCS at the concentration of 1×10^6/mL.

1.4 Analysis of Surface Levels of Adhesion Molecules

Surface adhesion molecules in HUVECs were analyzed by flow cytometry. When HUVECs at the third passage grew to confluence, ECs were pre-incubated with various concentrations of PrG (0.001, 0.01, 0.1, 1, 2, and 5 mmol/L) or 1‰ DMSO (v : v) or 10 mmol/L ASA for 1 h, and then were stimulated with 10 ng/mL TNF-α for 6 h; 1‰ DMSO served as the negative control. The HUVEC monolayer was then washed twice with PBS, detached by trypsin and neutralized by the addition of medium with 10% FBS. Cells were then transferred to flow cytometry tubes, washed three times with PBS and adjusted to be at the

concentration of 1×10^6/mL. Each specimen was divided into two tubes and incubated either with anti-CD54 monoclonal antibody (mAb) directly coupled to FITC and anti-CD62E mAb directly coupled to PE or with the corresponding isotypic control at 4℃ in the dark for 30 min and then washed twice. EPICS Elite (Beckman Coulter, USA) was used for flow cytometric analysis. Forward light scatter was measured as an index of cell size and fluorescence. The calibration of fluorescence positivity was performed as follows. The negative control was cells incubated with an FITC-labeled mouse IgG and a PE-labeled mouse IgG, and this was set so that the fluorescence-positive rate was infinitely close to 1%. All cells above this setting were regarded as positive. EXPO32 software was used to analyze the percentage of cells staining positive above the gate and mean fluorescence intensity (MFI) of all cells.

1.5 PMN Adherence Assays

Rose bengal vital staining was performed to measure PMN adherence to HUVECs according to Gamble[10]. HUVEC cells were plated in DMEM culture medium containing 20% FCS into 96-well plates at approximately 1×10^5/mL and grown to confluence. ECs were pre-incubated with various concentrations of PrG (0.001, 0.01, 0.1, 1, 5 mmol) L) or 1‰ DMSO (v : v) or 10 mmol/L ASA for 1 h, and then were stimulated with 10 ng/mL TNF-α for 6 h. Prior to assay, the medium was removed and the HUVEC monolayer washed once by PBS. PMNs were then added to the HUVEC monolayer in a volume of 200 μL per well at 37℃ for 30 min. The non-adherent cells were removed by aspiration and each well washed twice. All medium was removed by aspiration and 100 μL of a 0.25% solution of Rose Bengal in PBS was added to each well for 5 min at room temperature. The stain was then aspirated off, and each well washed twice by PBS. Then 200 μL of a solution of ethanol : PBS (1 : 1) was added. After approximately 30 min, when total release of stain from the cells had occurred, the optical density (OD) at wavelength 570 nm was determined for each well using an ELISA reader (Wellscan MK3, Labsystems Dragon, Finland). The OD value of each well was proportional to the number of adherent PMNs.

1.6 Statistics

Five different preparations of HUVECs were tested. Results were expressed as mean ± standard deviation. Differences among groups were tested using One-Way ANOVA, followed by multiple comparisons by LSD test using SPSS 11.0 for Windows and significance was calculated at $P < 0.05$.

2. Results

2.1 Effects on Fluorescence-Positive Rate and MFI of FITC-CD54

As shown in Table 1, CD54 was constitutively expressed in $32.53 \pm 1.98\%$ of HUVECs and the corresponding MFI of CD54 was 2.36 ± 0.72. After 6 h of incubation with 10 ng/mL TNF-α, CD54 was expressed in $95.70 \pm 2.52\%$ of HUVECs, while the corresponding MFI was 10.37 ± 3.30 ($P < 0.01$). Compared with basal levels, the percentage of fluorescence-positive cells and MFI of surface FITC-CD54 increased significantly after stimulation by TNF-α for 6 h ($P < 0.01$). PrG at doses ranging from 1 mmol/L to 5 mmol/

L decreased CD54 surface expression in a dose-dependent way. PrG at doses ranging from 0.001 mmol/L to 0.1 mmol/L did not alter the TNF-α-mediated increase in CD54 surface expression. ASA at dose of 10 mmol/L could significantly decrease the MFI of CD54 ($P < 0.05$, Figure 2).

2.2 Effects on Fluorescence-Positive Rate and MFI of PE-CD62E

Without stimulation, about $9.16 \pm 3.43\%$ of HUVECs constitutively expressed CD62E and the corresponding MFI was 1.53 ± 0.58. After 6 h of incubation with 10 ng/mL TNF-α, CD62E was expressed in $42.58 \pm 5.91\%$ of HUVECs, while the corresponding MFI was 5.68 ± 1.46. Compared with basal levels, CD62E surface expression increased significantly after stimulation by TNF-α (10 ng/mL) for 6 h ($P < 0.01$). PrG at doses ranging from 1 mmol/L to 5 mmol/L dose-dependently decreased CD62E surface expression ($P < 0.01$). PrG at doses ranging from 0.001 mmol/L to 0.1 mmol/L did not alter the TNF-α-mediated increase in CD62E surface expression. However, PrG at doses lower than 0.1 mmol/L showed a trend of slight increase in CD62E ($P > 0.05$). ASA did not alter the MFI and positive rate of CD62E ($P > 0.05$, Table 2 and Figure 2).

Table 1　Effects on Fluorescence-Positive Rate and MFI of FITC-CD54 in HUVEC ($\bar{\chi} \pm s$)

Group	n	Concentration	CD54 positive rate（%）	CD54 MFI
Control	5	0	32.53 ± 1.98	2.36 ± 0.72
TNF-α	5	10ng/mL	95.70 ± 2.52**	10.37 ± 3.30**
TNF-α+ASA	5	10mmol/L	86.40 ± 2.46	6.27 ± 1.70*
TNF-α+PrG	5	5 mmol/L	16.87 ± 3.77 $^{\triangle\triangle}$	2.03 ± 0.41 $^{\triangle\triangle}$
TNF-α+PrG	5	2 mmol/L	52.20 ± 20.09 $^{\triangle\triangle}$	2.46 ± 0.81 $^{\triangle\triangle}$
TNF-α+PrG	5	1 mmol/L	84.30 ± 9.90 $^{\triangle}$	3.67 ± 1.26 $^{\triangle\triangle}$
TNF-α+PrG	5	0.1 mmol/L	95.10 ± 3.58	9.48 ± 2.75
TNF-α+PrG	5	0.01 mmol/L	96.00 ± 1.01	10.80 ± 1.15
TNF-α+PrG	5	0.001 mmol/L	98.10 ± 0.97	10.26 ± 2.85

Notes：$^{*}P < 0.05$, $^{**}P < 0.01$, compared with the control; $^{\triangle}0P < 0.05$, $^{\triangle\triangle}P < 0.01$, compared with the TNF-$\alpha$ control

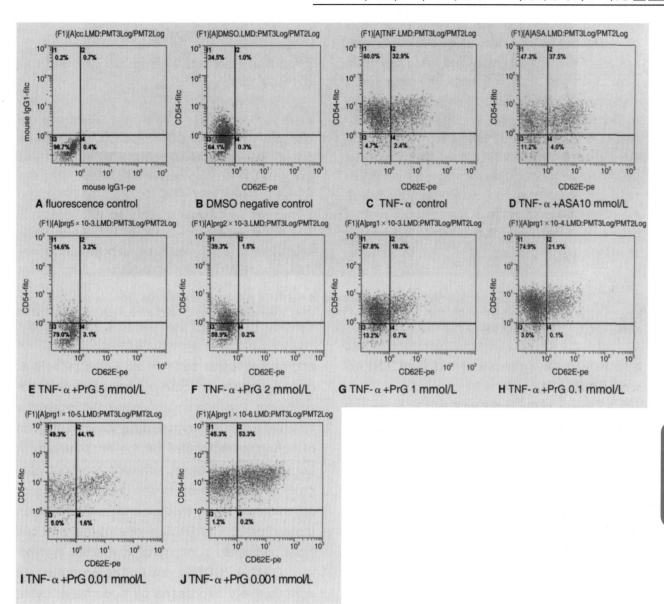

Figure 2 Representative Flow Cytometric Analysis from One of Three Separate Experiments of CD54 and CD62E Surface Expression in TNF-α-activated HUVEC. The Number of Positive Cells（%）Is Indicated in the Different Panels. A：Fluorescence control，B：DMSO negative control，C：TNF-α control，D：TNF-α+ASA10mmol/L，E：TNF-α+PrG 5mmol/L；F：TNF-α+PrG 2mmol/L，G：TNF-α+PrG 1mmol/L，H：TNF-α+PrG 0.1mmol/L；I：TNF-α+PrG 0.01mmol/L，J：TNF-α+PrG 0.001mmol/L

Table 2 Effects on Fluorescence-Positive Rate and MFI of PE-CD62E in HUVEC（$\bar{\chi} \pm s$）

Group	n	Concentration	CD62E positive rate（%）	CD62E MFI
Control	5	0	9.16±3.43	1.53±0.58
TNF-α	5	10ng/mL	42.58±5.91*	5.68±1.46*
TNF-α+ASA	5	10mmol/L	47.25±4.25	4.35±1.85
TNF-α+PrG	5	5 mmol/L	8.99±2.30△	1.53±0.21△
TNF-α+PrG	5	2 mmol/L	13.83±2.23△	1.63±0.06△
TNF-α+PrG	5	1 mmol/L	30.32±5.08	2.67±0.76△
TNF-α+PrG	5	0.1 mmol/L	43.66±9.55	4.82±1.16
TNF-α+PrG	5	0.01 mmol/L	45.20±6.04	5.93±0.47
TNF-α+PrG	5	0.001 mmol/L	50.96±9.77	7.46±0.92

Notes：*$P < 0.01$, compared with the control；△$P < 0.01$, compared with the TNF-α control

447

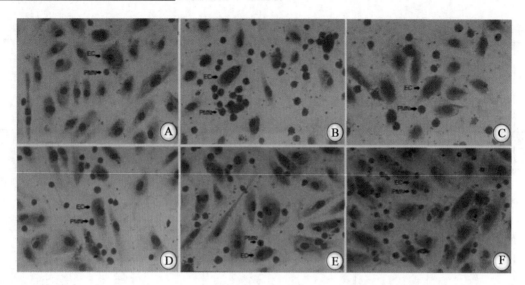

Figure 3 Rose Bengal Staining of PMNs Adhered to HUVECs with Inverted Microscope（× 400）
Notes：A：DMSO negative control; B：TNF- α control; C：TNF-α+PrG 1 mmol/L; D：TNF-α+PrG 0.1 mmol/L; E：TNF-α+PrG 0.01mmol/L; F：TNF-α+ASA 10 mmol/L

2.3 Effects on Adhesion of PMNs to TNF-α-activated HUVECs

As shown in Figure 3 and Table 3, compared with non stimulated HUVECs, TNF-α enhanced the ability of HUVECs to attach PMN cells (OD values from 0.276 ± 0.023 to 0.357 ± 0.071). At doses ranging from 0.1 mmol/L to 5 mmol/L, PrG significantly reduced the adhesion of PMN induced by TNF-α ($P < 0.01$). ASA did not alter the adhesion of PMN to HUVECs.

Table 3 Effect of PrG on Adhesion of PMNs to TNF-α-Activated HUVECs ($\bar{\chi} \pm s$)

Group	n	Concentration	OD value
Control	5	0	0.276±0.023
TNF-α	5	10ng/mL	0.357±0.071*
TNF-α+ASA	5	10mmol/L	0.361±0.043
TNF-α+PrG	5	5 mmol/L	0.300±0.065 △
TNF-α+PrG	5	1 mmol/L	0.282±0.033 △△
TNF-α+PrG	5	0.1 mmol/L	0.296±0.050 △
TNF-α+PrG	5	0.01 mmol/L	0.307±0.023
TNF-α+PrG	5	0.001 mmol/L	0.317±0.029

Notes: *$P < 0.01$, compared with the control; △$P < 0.05$, △△$P < 0.01$, compared with the TNF-α control

3. Discussion

Endothelial cells provide a non-thrombogenic and non-adhesive surface, but under pathologic conditions they become pro-adhesive and pro-coagulant. Pro-inflammatory cytokines initiate the vascular inflammatory response via up-regulation of adhesion molecules on the endothelium[11]. Leukocyte and platelet adhesion to endothelial cells, an early step in the pathogenesis of atherosclerosis, is mediated through adhesion molecules[12]. The PMN is one of the vital cell types participate in inflammatory reaction *in vivo*.

ICAM-1 (CD54), an adhesion molecule constitutively expressed by endothelial cells, is an important member of the immunoglobulin superfamily (IgSF) that is centrally involved in trafficking of leukocytes to endothelial and epithelial barriers[13]. Upon stimulation by cytokines or bacterial lipopolysaccharides (LPS), the increased ICAM-1 expression contributes to the initiation and continuation of the inflammatory reaction. CD54 mediates adhesion and extravasation of all classes of leukocytes to and through the endothelium[14]. The predominant function of CD54 and related cell adhesion molecules, such as VCAM-1 and E-selectin (CD62E), is related to the recruitment and trafficking of leukocytes via interactions with leukocyte-expressed integrins[15]. The leukocyte adhesion mediated by adhesion molecules may promote the instability of atheromatous plaques, and the consequent fissuring or rupture of these plaques and the formation of thrombus, which may play a key role in the pathogenesis of unstable angina and myocardial infarction[16].

The basal expression of CD54 and CD62E, as well as the expression after incubation with TNF-α, are an indication that the cells are in a good condition[17]. In the present study, CD54 and CD62E were constitutively expressed in 32.53 ± 1.98% and 9.16 ±3.43% of HUVECs, respectively. The corresponding MFIs of CD54 and CD62E were 2.36 ± 0.72 and 1.53 ±0.58, respectively. After 6 h of incubation with 10 ng/mL TNF-α, CD54 and CD62E were expressed in 95.70 ± 2.52% and 42.58 ± 5.91 % of HUVECs respectively, while the corresponding MFIs of CD54 and CD62E were 10.37 ± 3.30 and 5.68 ± 1.46 respectively. These expression levels were in agreement with levels found in other published studies[17], indicating that the cells were in a good condition.

According to Kapiotis[18], ASA at high doses (i.e., 10 mmol/L), by inhibition of NF-κB mobilization, inhibited VCAM-1, but not CD54 expression and adhesion of U937 monocytic cells in HUVECs. The NSAID Ibuprofen was identified as a potent inhibitor of IL-1α and TNFα-induced surface expression of VCAM-1 and a less potent inhibitor of pyrogen-induced expression of ICAM-1, whereas no effect on CD62E was found. Ibuprofen caused a significant ($P < 0.01$ at 2 mmol/L) dose-dependent inhibition of pyrogen-induced expression of VCAM-1 and CD54 on HUVECs (IC$_{50}$ 0.1-0.3 mmol/L). Ibuprofen (at 2 mmol/L) did not affect PMN-adherence to HUVECs.

In the present study, pre-treatment with PrG suppressed TNFα-induced surface expression of CD54 and CD62E ($P < 0.05$ at 1-5 mmol/L). PrG also reduced the adherence of PMNs to TNFα-treated HUVECs at doses ranging from 0.1 mmol/L to 5 mmol/L. Hence, PrG showed the effect of inhibiting TNFα-induced up-regulation of these adhesion molecules, similar to non-selective cyclooxygenase inhibitors ASA and Ibuprofen. With the dose of ASA tested in our study (10 mmol/L), we did not detect a significant inhibitory effect on the expression of CD54 or CD62E. Thus the concentrations of ASA needed to affect CD54 expression seem to be higher than those of PrG in the presence of TNF-α. PrG inhibited CD54 and CD62E in endothelial cells, which may indicate an additional anti-inflammatory property of this drug.

On the other hand, PrG at doses lower than 0.1 mmol/L showed a trend of slight increase in CD62E ($P > 0.05$), which was similar to the effect of atorvastatin on potentiating TNF-α-mediated CD62E induction according to Denis Bernot's report, in which atorvastatin (1.0 μmol/L) up-regulated the TNF-α-induced expression of VCAM-1, ICAM-1 and E-selectin at the endothelial cell surface, and also altered the surface distribution of adhesion molecules, which may account for its reduced binding of monocytes[19].

In conclusion, our results show that PrG (0.1-5 mmol/L) decreased adhesion of PMNs to human endothelial cells by regulating the surface expression of adhesion molecules. Although our in vitro results cannot be directly extrapolated to the in vivo situation, they suggest a potential therapeutic mechanism of PrG for its intervention in cytokine-mediated vascular inflammatory processes at the endothelial cell level.

References

[1] Nomura S. Tandon NN, Nakamura T, et al. High-shear-stress-induced activation of platelets and microparticles enhances expression of cell adhesion molecules in THP-1 and endothelial cells. Atherosclerosis, 2001, 158: 277-287.

[2] Landsberger M, Wolff B, Jantzen F, et al. Cerivastatin reduces cytokine-induced surface expression of ICAM-1 via increased shedding in human endothelial cells. Atherosclerosis, 2007, 190: 43-52.

[3] Desideri G, Croce G, Tucci M, et al. Effects of bezafibrate and simvastatin on endothelial activation and lipid peroxidation in hypercholesterolemia:

evidence of different vascular protection by different lipid-lowering treatments. J Clin Endocrinol Metab, 2003, 88: 5341-5347.

[4] Reddan JR, Giblin FJ, Sevilla M, et al. Propyl gallate is a superoxide dismutase mimic and protects cultured lens epithelial cells from H2O2 insult. Exp Eye Res, 2003, 76: 49-59.

[5] Huang JD, Song Z, Li J, et al. Study on the therapeutic mechanism of the active principle of the Chinese drug Paeoniae Radix 801 through affinity biosensors IAsys plus quartz crystal microbalance. Chin J Integr Med, 2005, 11: 37-40.

[6] Franzone JS, Natale T, Cirillo R, et al. Influence of propyl-gallate and 2-mercaptopropionylglycine on the development of acute inflammatory reactions and on biosynthesis of PGE_2. Boll Soc Ital Biol Sper, 1980, 56: 2539-2545.

[7] Soares DG, Andreazza AC, Salvador M. Sequestering ability of butylated hydroxytoluene, propyl gallate, resveratrol, and vitamins C and E against ABTS, DPPH, and hydroxyl free radicals in chemical and biological systems. J Agric Food Chem, 2003, 51: 1077-1080.

[8] Yin HJ, Jiang YR, Wu XH, et al. Effect of propyl gallate on activity of cyclooxygenase 1 and 2 in mice's peritoneal macrophages. Chin J Integr Med, 2004, 10: 213-217.

[9] Jaffe EA. Culture of human endothelial cells derived from umbilical veins. Identification by morphologic and immunologic criteria. J Clin Invest, 1973, 52: 2745-2754.

[10] Gamble JR, Vadas MA. A new assay for the measurement of the attachment of neutrophils and other cell types to endothelial cells. J Immunol Methods, 1988, 109: 175-184.

[11] Jiang MZ, Tsukahara H, Hayakawa K, et al. Effects of antioxidants and NO on TNF-alpha-induced adhesion molecule expression in human pulmonary microvascular endothelial cells. Respir Med, 2005, 99: 580-591.

[12] Xenos ES, Stevens SL, Freeman MB, et al. Nitric oxide mediates the effect of fluvastatin on intercellular adhesion molecule-1 and platelet endothelial cell adhesion molecule-1 expression on human endothelial cells. Ann Vasc Surg, 2005, 19: 386-392.

[13] Hopkins AM, Baird, AW, Nusrat A. ICAM-1: targeted docking for exogenous as well as endogenous ligands. Adv Drug Deliv Rev, 2004, 56: 763-778.

[14] Carlos TM, Harlan JM. Leukocyte-endothelial adhesion molecules. Blood, 1994, 84: 2068-2101.

[15] Springer TA. Adhesion receptors of the immune system. Nature, 1990, 346: 425-434.

[16] Crea F, Biasucci LM, Buffon A, et al. Role of inflammation in the pathogenesis of unstable coronary artery disease. Am J Cardiol, 1997, 80 (5A): 10E-16E.

[17] Lanbeck P, Odenholt I, Riesbeck K. Dicloxacillin and erythromycin at high concentrations increase ICAM-1 expression by endothelial cells: a possible factor in the pathogenesis of infusion phlebitis. J Antimicrob Chemother, 2004, 53: 174-179.

[18] Kapiotis S, Sengoelge G, Sperr WR, et al. Ibuprofen inhibits pyrogen-dependent expression of VCAM-1 and ICAM-1 on human endotheial cells. Life Sci, 1996, 58: 2167-2181.

[19] Bernot D, Benoliel AM, Peiretti FP, et al. Effect of atorvastatin on adhesive phenotype of human endothelial cells activated by tumor necrosis factor alpha. J Cardiovasc Pharmac, 2003, 41: 316-324.

第四章

第五章

糖、脂代谢异常的相关研究及其他

西洋参茎叶总皂苷对脂肪细胞糖脂代谢及胰岛素抵抗信号转导的影响 *

张颖　陈可冀　杨领海　白桂荣　殷惠军

胰岛素抵抗（insulin resistance，IR）是指胰岛素分泌量在正常水平时刺激靶细胞（肝细胞、骨骼肌细胞、脂肪细胞等）摄取和利用葡萄糖的生理效应显著减弱，或者是靶细胞维持摄取、利用葡萄糖的正常生理效应需要超常量的胰岛素。IR 是联系多种代谢相关疾病（如冠心病、糖尿病、高血压、血脂异常、肥胖等）的共同病理生理基础。其生理效应的发挥是通过与靶细胞膜表面的胰岛素受体结合，启动受体后信号转导，调节代谢及基因表达而实现的。胰岛素信号转导异常是导致机体 IR 和糖脂代谢异常的重要环节之一。

西洋参茎叶总皂苷（*Panax quinquefolius saponin*，PQS）是从国产西洋参茎叶中提取的活性成分。研究表明 PQS 确实同时具有调整脂质代谢、降低血糖和改善心肌缺血的作用。那么，该药调脂降糖的机制是什么？是否是通过改善胰岛素抵抗而实现的？其改善 IR 的机制又是什么？本研究以 3T3-L1 脂肪细胞 IR 为对象，观察药物 PQS 对脂肪细胞糖脂代谢及胰岛素抵抗信号转导的影响。

1. 材料与方法

1.1 细胞系

小鼠 3T3-LI 前脂肪细胞株来源于 American Type Culture Collection（ATCC），由中国医学科学院协和医科大学细胞中心购得。细胞用含 10% 优级胎牛血清及青链霉素的高糖（25mmol/L glucose）IMDM 培养液（GIBCO 公司）传代培养，培养条件为 37℃，5% CO_2。

1.2 药物

PQS 由我院制剂室外购干燥的西洋参茎叶，水煎、醇提、回收乙醇，每克生药可提取 40mg 皂苷，用蒸馏水配液，过滤灭菌后用于细胞培养，实验时终浓度分别为 0.02、0.04、0.08mg/mL。二甲双胍的实验时终浓度为 1mmol/L。

1.3 试剂与仪器

磷酸化的胰岛素受体抗体（Lot No.4，CELL SIGNALING）、磷酸化的蛋白激酶 B 抗体（Lot No.27730，UPSTATE）、山羊抗兔 IgG 抗体（Lot No.23795A、UPSTATE）、山羊抗鼠 IgG 抗体（Lot No.23796A，UPSTATE）、兔抗绵羊 IgG 抗体（Lot No.23650A，UPSTATE）、抗胰岛素受体 β 亚单位抗体（Lot No.C2905，SANTA CRUZ）、磷酸化的胰岛素受体底物 1 抗体（Lot No.D0104，SANTA CRUZ）、肿瘤坏死因子 α（TNF-α，Sigma 公司 Lot No.302CY25）、蛋白浓度测定试剂盒（CALBIOCHEM 公司）、游离脂肪酸测定试剂盒（南京建成生物工程研究所）、电泳仪（BIO-RAD 公司，型号 DYY-Ⅲ 12 型）、转印仪（美国伯乐公司，型号 TRANS-BIOT）、酶标仪（TECAN 公司，型号 SUN-RISE A-5082）。

1.4 实验方法

1.4.1 分组　参考 Ross SA[1] 等的方法将 3T3-L1 前脂肪细胞诱导分化为成熟脂肪细胞后，传于 6 孔板，分为 6 组：空白对照组（对照组）、模型组、二甲双胍组以及 PQS 大、中、小剂量组。

1.4.2 造模方法[2]　模型组与各药物治疗组细胞均先用含 0.65mmol/L 棕榈酸、1%BSA、10nmol/L 葡萄糖的 KRP 缓冲液（131.2mmol/L NaCl，4.71mmol/L KC1，2.48mmol/L $Na_3PO_4 \cdot 12H_2O$，1.24mmol/L $MgSO_4$，2.47mmol/L $CaCl_2$，10mmol/L HEPES，pH 7.2 ~ 7.4）孵育 12h，每 2h 换液 1 次。对照组用不含棕榈酸的上液做同样处理。12h 后，均用含 1mmol/L 丙酮酸钠、1%BSA 的 KRP 缓冲液孵育 1h。再用含 1%BSA 的 KRP 缓冲液孵育 1h。然后全部换用全 IMDM 孵育。至此，模型成功，可用于实验。

1.4.3 观察项目及方法

1.4.3.1 PQS 对葡萄糖消耗作用研究　诱导分化成熟的脂肪细胞造模成功后予相应药物 [二甲双胍

---

* 原载于《中国中西医结合杂志》，2010，30（7）：748-751

1mmol/L、PQS 大（0.08mg/mL）、PQS 中（0.04mg/mL）、PQS 小（0.02mg/mL）] 剂量培养 24h。取培养液，用葡萄糖氧化酶法测培养液中葡萄糖残存量，以未接种细胞空白复孔的糖含量均值为基础值，计算出各孔细胞葡萄糖消耗量。

1.4.3.2 脂肪分解的检测 诱导分化成熟的细胞，于 6 孔培养板中生长融合，分别设对照组、TNF-α 组及各药物治疗组。除对照组外，均用 TNF-α 诱导脂解，培养液中终浓度为 1.5nmol/L。各药物治疗组在培养液中，除加 TNF-α 外，还分别加入相应药物培养 48h。48h 后，吸取培养液，用试剂盒检测培养液中游离脂肪酸（free fatty acid，FFA）的浓度。以 0.1mol/L NaOH 液裂解细胞，用 MERCK 蛋白浓度检测试剂盒测定蛋白浓度，以校正 FFA 浓度。

1.4.3.3 PQS 对胰岛素抵抗状态下信号蛋白磷酸化水平的影响 将诱导分化成熟的脂肪细胞传于 100mm 的培养皿，分 6 组，每组 6 孔，造模成功后予相应药物培养 48h。48h 后，制备细胞蛋白样品，步骤如下：（1）用 Human insulin 150nmol/L 刺激细胞；（2）30min 后用冰冷的 PBS 洗细胞 1 次；（3）消化：加胰酶消化液，收集细胞悬液，离心；（4）洗涤：用冰冷 PBS 吹洗 2 次，离心；（5）裂解：加 50μL modified RIPA buffer/ 支（modified RIPA buffer 成分：Tris-HCl 50mmol/L，pH 7.4；NP40 2%；TritonX-100 1%；sodium deoxycholate 0.5%；NaCl 150mmol/L；EDTA 1mmol/L；PMSF 1mmol/L；Na$_3$VO$_4$ 1mmol/L；NaF 1mmol/L）；（6）分装入 2 个 0.5mL EP 管，1 支用于测定蛋白浓度（Bradford Coomassie dye-binding assay），另 1 支用于 Western-blot，–80℃ 保存。用 Western-blot 法检测磷酸化蛋白水平，步骤如下：（1）将蛋白样品用上样缓冲液稀释，95～100℃ 煮 5min；（2）SDS-PAGE 蛋白电泳，3% 的浓缩胶，10% 的分离胶，上样量 20μL/ 孔；（3）转膜：硝酸纤维素膜用含 20% 甲醇的转膜液浸泡 5min，半干法转膜，恒定电流 0.8mA/cm²，时间 1h；（4）封闭及抗体孵育：封闭液：TBS/T+5%（w/v）脱脂奶粉。室温，摇动 1h，用 TBS/T 洗膜，杂交袋中与一抗（以封闭液 1：100 稀释）孵育，4℃ 过夜，TBS/T 洗膜；杂交袋中与二抗（以封闭液 1：1000 稀释）孵育，室温 1.5h；TBS/T 洗膜；（5）显色：化学增强发光法 (ECL)，曝光时间为 2min。

1.5 统计学方法

所得数据用 $\bar{\chi}\pm s$ 表示，采用 SPSS 13.0 统计软件包进行统计学处理，对各组数据进行正态性检验和方差齐性检验，Levene 方差齐性检验示方差齐，计量资料组间比较采用单因素方差分析，多组间两两比较采用 LSD-t 检验。

2. 结果

2.1 PQS 对葡萄糖消耗量的影响（表 1）

模型组葡萄糖消耗量低于对照组（$P < 0.01$）；与模型组比较，各用药组葡萄糖糖消耗量显著增加（$P < 0.01$），且随着 PQS 用药剂量的增加，葡萄糖消耗量也有逐渐增加的趋势。

表 1 各组葡萄糖消耗量比较（$\bar{\chi}\pm s$）

组别	n	葡萄糖消耗量（mmol/L）
对照	6	14.133±1.305
模型	6	5.250±2.671*
二甲双胍	6	11.807±1.358△
PQS 大剂量	6	10.784±2.373△
PQS 中剂量	6	10.217±1.237△
PQS 小剂量	6	9.984±2.006△

注：与对照组比较，*$P < 0.01$，与模型组比较，△$P < 0.01$

2.2 PQS 对脂肪分解的影响（表 2）

TNF-α 组培养液中 FFA 浓度显著高于对照组（$P < 0.01$）。各用药组培养液中 FFA 浓度均显著低于 TNF-α 组（$P < 0.01$），且随着 PQS 用药剂量的加大，培养液中 FFA 浓度有逐渐减少的趋势。

表 2 各组 TNF-α 的脂解作用比较（$\bar{\chi}\pm s$）

组别	n	FFA 浓度（nmol/μg）
对照	6	1.320±0.538
TNF-α	6	2.479±0.597*
二甲双胍	6	1.210±0.566△
PQS 大剂量	6	1.105±0.631△
PQS 中剂量	6	1.108±0.260△
PQS 小剂量	6	1.201±0.593△

注：与对照组比较，*$P < 0.01$；与 TNF-α 组比较，△$P < 0.01$

453

2.3 PQS 对胰岛素抵抗时胰岛素信号转导途径中信号蛋白磷酸化的影响（图 1）

Western blot 结果发现，胰岛素刺激 30min 后，胰岛素抵抗模型组胰岛素受体 β 亚单位酪氨酸磷酸化水平（phospho-insulin receptor）、IRS-1 酪氨酸磷酸化水平（phospho-IRS1）、PKB 的 Ser473 磷酸化水平（phospho-PKB）均较对照组减低；与模型组比较，PQS 中、大剂量和二甲双胍组信号蛋白磷酸化水平均有不同程度增高的趋势。

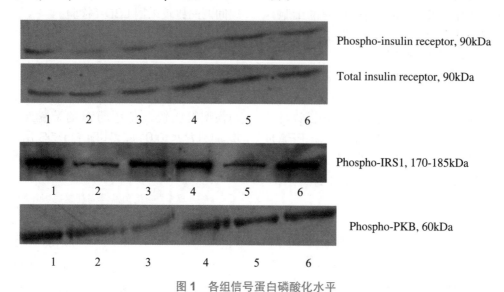

图 1　各组信号蛋白磷酸化水平

注：1 为对照组；2 为模型组；3 为 PQS 小剂量组；4 为 PQS 中剂量组；5 为 PQS 大剂量组；6 为二甲双胍组

3. 讨论

胰岛素生理效应的发挥是通过与靶细胞膜表面的胰岛素受体 α 亚基结合，解除其对 β 亚基的抑制，受体酪氨酸蛋白激酶活化，酪氨酸发生自身磷酸化引起构象改变，从而能与三磷腺苷（ATP）及胰岛素受体底物接触，将受体底物蛋白的酪氨酸残基磷酸化。胰岛素受体底物（insulin receptor substrates，IRSs）包括 IRS-1、IRS-2、IRS-3、IRS-4、SHC、CBL、APS、SH2B、GAB-1、GAB-2、DOCK-1、DOCK-2。转基因小鼠的研究提示，胰岛素的效应大部分由 IRS-1 和 IRS-2 介导。IRS-1 主要调控外周胰岛素效应（脂肪、骨骼肌）和身体生长，其酪氨酸磷酸化后，可与效应蛋白（如 P13-K、酪氨酸磷酸酶 SHP2、酪氨酸激酶 fyn）和接头蛋白结合，使胰岛素信号向下传递。活化的胰岛素受体可经以下途径进行信号转导：（1）磷脂酰肌醇 3 激酶（PI3-K）信号转导途径：活化的 IRSs 与 PI3-K 调节亚基 p85 结合，使催化亚基 p110 活化。PI3-K 活化后，催化细胞浆膜侧的 4、5- 二磷酸磷脂酰肌醇 PI（4，5）P2 转变成三磷酸磷脂酰肌醇（PIP3）。PIP3 可将 PKB、PIP3 依赖的蛋白激酶 -1（PDK-1）和非典型蛋白激酶 C（aPKC）募集至细胞浆膜侧附近，在那里 PDK-1 使 PKB 的 Ser473 磷酸化，进而产生多种生物学效应（如促进葡萄糖转运，抗脂肪分解，促进糖原、蛋白及脂肪合成，抑制细胞凋亡，促进内皮细胞产生一氧化氮，促进特定基因表达等[3-5]）。（2）活化的胰岛素受体可通过 CAP/Cbl 途径，与 PI3-K 途径协同，促进 GLUT4 转位和葡萄糖转运。（3）Ras 信号转导途径[6]：IRSs 与生长因子受体结合蛋白 2（Grb-2）结合，后者与鸟苷酸交换因子结合进而激活 Ras，通过 MAP 激酶级联系统调节基因表达。胰岛素信号转导异常是导致机体 IR 和糖脂代谢异常的重要环节之一，促进胰岛素信号转导是改善胰岛素抵抗的有效途径之一。

本研究表明：模型组葡萄糖糖消耗量显著低于对照组（P < 0.01），提示 FFA 可以减少脂肪细胞对葡萄糖的消耗，诱导 IR 的发生，而二甲双胍和 PQS 3 个剂量组葡萄糖糖消耗量均较模型组显著增加（P < 0.01），且随着 PQS 用药剂量的增加，葡萄糖消耗量也逐渐增加。同时，TNF-α 还可诱导脂肪分解，使细胞培养液中 FFA 浓度显著升高（P < 0.01），而二甲双胍和 PQS 3 个剂量组培养液中 FFA 浓度均较 TNF-α 组显著下降（P < 0.01），且随着 PQS 用药剂量的加大，其抗脂解作用有逐渐增强的趋势。以上结果提示：PQS 能够促进脂

第五章

肪细胞利用葡萄糖，并抑制 TNF-α 的促脂解作用，从而调节糖脂代谢。

其次，胰岛素信号转导的研究结果显示：FFA 诱导脂肪细胞发生胰岛素抵抗时，胰岛素刺激下的胰岛素受体 β 亚单位和 IRS-1 的酪氨酸磷酸化水平降低，PKB 的 Ser473 磷酸化水平下降、活性下降，胰岛素信号转导通路受阻，终至葡萄糖转运障碍，脂肪细胞摄取利用葡萄糖下降，葡萄糖消耗量减少。而 PQS 同二甲双胍均有不同程度的促进胰岛素受体 β 亚单位、IRS-1 酪氨酸磷酸化及 PKB 第 473 位丝氨酸磷酸化的趋势，从而促进脂肪细胞摄取利用葡萄糖，改善胰岛素抵抗。

结合本研究室其他研究结果：PQS 可促进胰岛素刺激下的 GLUT-4 转位、葡萄糖转运、CAP 基因转录[7]。我们可以得出如下结论：PQS 可调节脂肪细胞糖脂代谢，这可能与其促进胰岛素信号转导、改善机体胰岛素抵抗状态有关。但 FFA 可诱导脂肪细胞发生胰岛素抵抗，FFA 和葡萄糖二者之间供能的竞争可能是 FFA 引发血糖升高及 IR 的重要原因，故 PQS 所致胰岛素受体后信号转导的改善是药物的直接效应还是通过"影响脂肪细胞脂肪代谢使脂肪分解减少、FFA 释放减少"而发挥的间接效应尚待进一步的研究来证实。

参考文献

[1] Ross SA，Chen XL，Hope H，et al. Development and comparison of two 3T3-LI adipocyte models of insulin resistance：increased glucose flux vs glucosamine treatment. Biochem Biophys Res Commun，2000，273（3）：1033-1041.

[2] Van Epps-Fung M，Williford J，Wells A，et al. Fatty acid-induced insulin resistance in adipocytes. Endocrinology，1997，138（10）：4338-4345.

[3] Nesto RW. The relation of insulin resistance syndromes to risk of cardiovascular disease. Rev Cardiovas Med，2003，4（Suppl 6）：S1-S18.

[4] Woodgett JR. Recent advances in the protein kinase B signaling pathway. Cell Biol，2005，17（2）：150-157.

[5] Feuvray D，Darmellah A. Diabetes-related metabolic perturbations in cardiac myocyte. Diabetes Metab，2008，34：S3-S9.

[6] Halevy O，Cantley LC. Differential regulation of the phos-phoinositide 3-kinase and MAP kinase pathways by hepatocyte growth factor vs insulin-like growth factor-I in myogenic cells. Exp Cell Res，2004，297（1）：224-234.

[7] 殷惠军，张颖，杨领海，等. 西洋参茎叶总皂苷对胰岛素抵抗脂肪细胞葡萄糖转运、GLUT-4 转位和 CAP 基因表达的影响. 中国药理学通报，2007，23（10）：421-426.

脂康颗粒与辛伐他汀降脂治疗随机对照研究 *

赵福海　刘国兵　吕树铮　卢燕玲

血脂异常是心脑血管疾患重要的危险因素，中国人群血脂流行病学数据显示，我国血脂异常人群总数达到 1.6 亿，其中胆固醇起了不容忽视的作用，而胆固醇水平升高是导致心脑血管死亡的主要原因[1]。有研究证实：他汀类药物不但可以减慢甚至逆转动脉粥样硬化斑块的进展，而且可以降低低密度脂蛋白水平，对于冠心病的一级和二级预防有明显作用[2-4]。本研究观察了中药脂康颗粒的降血脂作用，并与辛伐他汀比较，现报告于下。

1. 临床资料

1.1　诊断标准

血脂异常诊断参照 2006 中国成人血脂异常防治指南[1]。正常饮食情况下，2 周内非同日两次禁食 12 ~ 14h 后的血脂水平，符合以下任意一条者即可诊断为血脂异常：（1）总胆固醇（TC）≥ 6.24mmol/L；或合并低密度脂蛋白胆固醇（LDL-C）≥ 4.16mmol/L；（2）三酰甘油（TG）≥ 2.27mmol/L；或合并 LDL-C ≥ 4.16mmol/L；（3）TC ≥ 6.24mmol/L，并

* 原载于《中国中西医结合杂志》，2010，30（10）：1052-1055

TG ≥ 2.27mmol/L；或合并 LDL-C ≥ 4.16mmol/L；
（4）高密度脂蛋白胆固醇（HDL-C）< 1.04mmol/L；
或合并 LDL-C ≥ 4.16mmol/L。

1.2 临床资料

门诊筛选符合诊断标准的原发性血脂异常的
患者，按照 2：1 的比例随机分为两组，脂康颗粒
组 30 例，男 16 例，女 14 例；年龄 45 ～ 72 岁，
平均（58.9±10.1）岁；既往病史：糖尿病史 5 例
（17.3%），高血压病史 18 例（60.6%），冠心病
史 17 例（58.4%）。辛伐他汀组 15 例，男 7 例，
女 8 例；年龄 45 ～ 73 岁，平均（59.4±10.3）岁；
既往病史：糖尿病史 3 例（19.5%），高血压病史
9 例（57.8%），冠心病史 9 例（62.6%）。两组资
料比较，差异无统计学意义（P > 0.05）。所有患
者均签署书面知情同意书。筛选期内采用低脂肪、
低胆固醇膳食。

2. 方法

2.1 给药方案

脂康颗粒由天大药业（珠海）有限公司提供，
由决明子、山楂、红花、桑葚、枸杞子组成，批
号：960108。脂康颗粒组采用脂康颗粒 8.0g，每
天 2 次冲服，共 24 周；12 周治疗结束后进行疗
效评定为无效者，采用脂康颗粒 8.0g，每天 3 次
冲服，至 24 周治疗结束。辛伐他汀组采用辛伐他
汀，每天 40mg 口服，共 24 周。

2.2 检测指标及方法

分别在治疗前，治疗 4、8、12 和 24 周检测
所有研究对象空腹血 TC、LDL-C、HDL-C、TG、
丙氨酸氨基转移酶（ALT）、天冬氨酸氨基转移酶
（AST）、高敏 C 反应蛋白（hs-CRP）、空腹血糖
（FBG）、血肌酐（Cr）和血尿酸（UA）水平；采
用 Roehe Modullr P800 型全自动生化检测仪。

2.3 疗效评定标准

根据 2001 美国国家胆固醇教育计划 ATP Ⅲ
标准[5]：LDL-C ≤ 2.59mmol/L 定为理想，即
达标，2.60 ～ 3.34mmol/L 为高于理想水平，
≥ 3.35mmol/L 为边缘性升高；TC ≤ 5.17mmol/L
定为理想，即达标，5.18 ～ 6.19mmol/L 为高于理想
水平，≥ 6.20mmol/L 为边缘性升高。治疗无效：
经 12 周治疗后如果 TC、LDL-C、TG 任一指标下
降 < 10%，或 HDL-C 上升 < 0.104mmol/L 者判定

为治疗无效。

2.4 统计学方法

计量数据用 $\bar{x}±s$，组内比较采用重复测量数
据的方差分析，组间比较采用独立样本的 t 检验分
析；分类资料用卡方检验，Fisher 确切概率法分析，
P < 0.05 为差异有统计学显著性。用 SPSS 13.0
软件进行统计学处理。

3. 结果

3.1 两组治疗前后 TC、TG、HDL-C 及 LDL-C 比较（表 1）

脂康颗粒组：治疗 4、8、12、24 周与治疗
前 TC、LDL-C 水平比较，差异有统计学意义（P
< 0.01）；TG、HDL-C 水平比较，差异均无统计
学意义（P > 0.05）；辛伐他汀组：治疗 4、8、
12、24 周与治疗前 TC、LDL-C 水平比较，差异
有统计学意义（P < 0.01）；TG 水平差异无统计
学意义（P > 0.05）。治疗 4、8、12、24 周 TC、
LDL-C、HDL-C 和 TG 水平两组间比较，差异均
无统计学意义（P > 0.05）。

3.2 两组 4、8、12 及 24 周 LDL-C、TC 达标比较（表 2、3）

治疗 12 周时，LDL-C 达标：脂康颗粒组
与辛伐他汀组分别为 11 例（36.7%）和 9 例
（60.0%），差异有统计学意义（P < 0.05）；
TC 达标脂康颗粒组与辛伐他汀组分别为 26 例
（86.7%）和 15 例（100.0%），差异无统计学意
义（P > 0.05）。治疗 24 周时，LDL-C 达标率脂
康颗粒组与辛伐他汀组分别为 16 例（53.3%）和
9 例（60.0%），差异无统计学意义（P > 0.05）；
TC 达标率脂康颗粒组与辛伐他汀组分别为 27 例
（90.0%）和 14 例（93.3%），差异无统计学意义
（P > 0.05）。治疗 12 周时脂康颗粒组有 3 例患
者因无效而加药，辛伐他汀组治疗无效者例数为
0；24 周时两组治疗无效患者均为 0。

3.3 两组治疗前后血生化指标比较（表 4）

两组治疗前 ALT、AST、Cr、UA、FBG 及
hs-CRP 比较，差异无统计学意义（P > 0.05）；
治疗 12、24 周随访，组内、组间比较，差异均无
统计学意义（P > 0.05）。

表1　两组治疗前后 TC、TG、HDL-C 及 LDL-C 比较（mmol/L, $\bar{\chi} \pm s$）

组别	例数	时间	TC	TG	HDL-C	LDL-C
脂康颗粒	30	治疗前	6.06±0.61	1.67±0.65	1.00±0.21	3.01±0.96
		治疗4周	4.49±0.98*	1.75±0.57	1.05±0.22	3.01±0.96*
		8周	4.31±1.02*	1.59±0.55	1.03±0.27	2.86±1.01*
		12周	4.19±0.83*	1.48±0.98	0.95±0.20	2.85±0.75*
		24周	4.28±0.86*	1.63±0.60	0.99±0.21	2.55±0.85*
辛伐他汀	15	治疗前	6.05±0.59	1.50±0.60	0.99±0.27	4.61±0.57
		治疗4周	4.28±0.35*	1.68±0.38	1.19±0.28	2.58±0.40*
		8周	3.85±0.56*	1.63±0.54	1.05±0.38	2.51±0.45*
		12周	3.82±0.82*	1.47±1.08	0.85±0.14	2.54±0.87*
		24周	4.08±0.83*	1.58±0.72	0.96±0.23	2.45±0.60*

注：与本组治疗前比较，*$P < 0.01$

表2　两组4、8、12及24周 LDL-C 达标比较［例（%）］

组别	例数	时间	LDL		
			< 2.59mmol/L	2.60 ~ 3.34 mmol/L	≥ 3.35 mmol/L
脂康颗粒	30	4周	26（86.7）	2（6.7）	2（6.7）
		8周	30（100.0）	0（0）	0（0）
		12周	11（36.7）*	13（43.3）*	6（20.0）
		24周	16（53.3）	9（30.0）	5（16.7%）
辛伐他汀	15	4周	15（100.0）	0（0）	0（0）
		8周	15（100.0）	0（0）	0（0）
		12周	9（60.0）	4（26.7）	2（13.3）
		24周	9（60.0）	5（33.3）	1（6.7）

注：与辛伐他汀组同一时间点比较，*$P < 0.05$

表3　两组4、8、12及24周 TC 达标比较［例（%）］

组别	例数	时间	TC		
			< 5.17mmol/L	5.18 ~ 6.19 mmol/L	≥ 6.20 mmol/L
脂康颗粒	30	4周	24（80.0）*	5（16.7）*	1（3.3）
		8周	25（83.3）*	3（10.0）*	2（6.7）
		12周	26（86.7）	4（13.3）*	0（0）
		24周	27（90.0）	2（6.7）	1（3.3）
辛伐他汀	15	4周	15（100.0）	0（0）	0（0）
		8周	15（100.0）	0（0）	0（0）
		12周	15（100.0）	0（0）	0（0）
		24周	14（93.3）	1（6.7）	0（0）

注：与辛伐他汀组同一时间点比较，*$P < 0.05$

第五章

表4 两组治疗前后血生化指标比较（$\bar{x} \pm s$）

组别	例数	时间	ALT	AST	Cr	UA	FBG	hs-CRP
			(u/L)		(μmol/L)		(mmol/L)	(mg/L)
脂康颗粒	30	治疗前	25.5±15.6	21.5±8.7	72.9±17.9	306.9±81.4	6.5±2.3	3.9±4.3
		治疗12周	21.8±8.3	20.7±5.5	71.7±17.8	306.8±88.9	5.5±1.4	2.8±3.5
		治疗24周	23.8±14.5	22.1±12.3	85.4±25.2	346.7±95.6	5.8±1.6	3.9±5.5
辛伐他汀	15	治疗前	24.4±10.5	21.1±3.9	73.7±14.5	302.9±106.6	5.1±0.6	3.8±7.1
		治疗12周	26.2±19.3	21.3±10.4	81.3±29.4	314.9±94.2	6.4±2.5	4.5±5.1
		治疗24周	23.1±14.0	21.5±8.3	68.5±25.6	336.3±78.7	5.3±1.4	4.9±6.4

4. 讨论

本研究表明脂康颗粒具有明确降脂作用，其疗效并不次于他汀类降脂药物辛伐他汀。脂康颗粒是临床长期治疗血脂异常的经验方，由决明子、山楂、红花、桑葚、枸杞子组成，其中决明子是君药；桑葚、枸杞子为臣药；山楂、红花为佐药；全方具有滋阴清肝，活血通络功效，用于肝肾阴虚挟瘀之高脂血症。其调脂作用主要通过以下4个途径实现：（1）抑制肠道吸收；（2）抑制内源性TC、TG合成；（3）影响体内脂类代谢；（4）促进体内胆固醇排泄[6]。我们研究发现，治疗期间两组血脂水平均有明显降低，脂康颗粒组主要以TC、LDL-C水平降低为主，而降低TG和升高HDL-C的作用则相对较弱。随访期间，脂康颗粒组和辛伐他汀组LDL-C达标率治疗12周分别为36.7%和60%（$P < 0.05$），治疗24周时分别为53.3%和60%（$P > 0.05$）；TC达标率治疗12周分别为86.7%和100.0%（$P > 0.05$），治疗24周分别为90.0%和93.3%（$P > 0.05$）。说明脂康颗粒具有明确的降脂治疗作用，其具体作用机制有待深入研究。

研究表明：他汀类药物具有独立于降低LDL-C水平之外的抗炎活性，他汀类药物具有明显的抑制CRP的表达及其相关的促炎效应[7]。研究中我们观察到无论是脂康颗粒组还是辛伐他汀组，其治疗前后hs-CRP水平变化不明显（$P > 0.05$）。推测与入选人群均为病情相对稳定的患者，且排除急性冠脉综合征等炎症反应水平较高人群有关。

安全性是药物评价的一项重要指标，本研究发现长期应用脂康颗粒安全性高，6个月的观察期间未发现其对肝功能、肌酶有明显影响，安全性较高。且未发现如他汀类药物应用中所见的肝功能损害（转氨酶升高）、白细胞异常、肌痛及横纹肌溶解的不良反应[8]。对血糖代谢、血尿酸水平无影响，提示脂康颗粒作为纯中药制剂临床效果肯定，而且长期应用安全可靠。

本研究表明：脂康颗粒具有肯定的降低血TC及LDL-C的作用，而且其安全性高。但作为小样本随机对照研究，其结果仍有一定的局限性，有待进一步大样本随机对照临床试验证实。

参考文献

[1] 中国胆固醇教育计划教材编写委员会编. 中国胆固醇教育计划全国培训教材. 上海：同济大学出版社，2006：8-19.

[2] Tani S, Nagao K, Anazawa T, et al. Coronary plaque regression and lifestyle modification in patients treated with pravastatin. Assessment mainly by daily aerobic exercise and an increase in the serum level of high-density lipoprotein cholesterol. Circ J, 2010, 74 (5): 954-9611.

[3] Takayama T, Hiro T, Yamagishi M, et al. Effect of rosuvastatin on coronary atheroma in stable coronary artery disease：multicenter coronary atherosclerosis study measuring effects of rosuvastatin using intravascular ultrasound in Japanese subjects (COSMOS). Circ J, 2009，73 (11): 2110-2117.

[4] Nasu K, Tsuchikane E, Katoh O, et al. Effect of fluvastatin on progression of coronary atherosclerotic plaque evaluated by virtual histology intravascular ultrasound. JACC Cardiovasc Interv, 2009,2 (7): 689-696.

[5] Expert Panel on Detection, Evaluation, and Treatment of High Blood Cholesterol in Adults. Evaluation and treatment of high blood cholesterol in adults：executive summary of the third report of the national cholesterol education program (NCEP) expert panel

on detection, evaluation and treatment of high blood cholesterol in adults (Adults Treatment Panel Ⅲ). J AMA, 2001, 285 (19): 2486-2497.

[6] 田相同，姜良花. 脂康颗粒调节血脂异常临床研究. 中西医结合心脑血管病杂志，2006，4（2）：121-122.

[7] Ridker PM, Rifai N, Lowenthal SP. Rapid reduction in

creative protein with cerivastatin among 785 patients with primary hypercholesterolemia. Circulation, 2001, 103 (9): 1191-1193.

[8] Dale KM, White CM, Henyan NN, et al. Impact of statin dosing intensity on transominase and creatine kinase. Am JM ed, 2007, 120 (8): 706-712.

LC-ESI-MS^n 法鉴定心悦胶囊中西洋参皂苷类成分 *

杨琳　缪宇　殷惠军　史大卓　陈可冀

心悦胶囊是以西洋参茎叶总皂苷（*Panax quinquefolius* saponin，PQS）为原料药的上市中药制剂，具有益气养阴、和血之功效，临床用于气阴两虚冠心病心绞痛患者的治疗，具有较好的疗效[1]。PQS 是从五加科植物西洋参的茎和叶中提取得到的皂苷成分，主要为人参皂苷类物质，包括达玛烷型（dammarane）[又分为原人参二醇型（protopanaxadiol）和原人参三醇型（protopanaxatriol）]、齐墩果烷型（oleanane）和奥克梯隆型（ocotillol）3 种类型的皂苷[2]。虽然已往对西洋参茎叶中提取的皂苷类成分进行了研究[3]，但临床常用药心悦胶囊的具体组成成分和药效物质目前并不清楚。为了深入探讨心悦胶囊的作用机制，有必要对其成分进行系统的研究。

目前关于人参皂苷类成分的分析方法主要有 HPLC-DAD[4]、HPLC-ELSD[5] 和 LC-MS[6] 等，其中 LC-MS 技术集液相的高效分离和质谱的高灵敏度、定性专属性强的特点，在该领域中尤为多用。在人参皂苷的 LC-MS 分析测定中，APCI 源[7] 和 ESI 源[3,6,8] 是两种常见的离子源，而以 LC-ESI-MS 正离子检测模式的报道最多。人参皂苷类尤其是原人参二醇型和原人参三醇型皂苷在 ESI-MS 正离子检测模式下易同时形成 [M+H]$^+$ 和 [M+Na]$^+$ 峰，这就降低了二级质谱分析时母离子的浓度，在一定程度上降低分析的灵敏度。本实验采用 LC-ESI-MS^n 负离子检测模式，对中成药心悦胶囊中的人参皂苷类成分进行了系统的分析，流动相采用乙腈 - 水系统，获得了较好的分析效果。

1. 材料与方法

1.1 仪器和材料

Finnigan LCQ Classic 离子阱液相色谱 - 质谱联用仪（美国 Thermo-Finnigan 公司），包括 Finnigan SpectraSystem P4000 泵；Xcalibre 2.0 数据处理系统；Millipore-Biocel 超纯水处理系统。

甲醇、乙腈为色谱纯（美国 Fisher 公司）；水为自制超纯水（18.2MΩ）。心悦胶囊由吉林益盛药业股份有限公司提供；人参皂苷 Rg$_1$、Re 和拟人参皂苷 F$_{11}$（pseudoginsenoside F$_{11}$）对照品购自中国药品生物制品检定所，人参皂苷 Rb$_2$、Rb$_3$、Rc、Rd、Rg$_3$、Rg$_2$、F$_2$ 购自天津一方科技有限公司，质量分数均大于 98%。

1.2 样品制备

1.2.1 供试品溶液的制备：取心悦胶囊 3 粒，取内容物混匀。精密称取内容物 300.0mg（相当于 1 粒胶囊内容物的量），加甲醇 15mL，密封，室温浸泡 15min，超声提取 30min 后，离心（10000r/min）6min，分取上清液。精密吸取该上清液 10μL，置 10mL 量瓶中，加甲醇至刻度，摇匀，取适量，离心（10000r/min）6min，上清液作为供试品溶液。

1.2.2 空白对照溶液的制备：精密称取心悦胶囊辅料 241.2mg（相当于 1 粒胶囊的辅料量），加甲醇 15mL，按"1.2.1"项下方法操作，得空白对照溶液。

1.2.3 人参皂苷混合对照品溶液的制备：分别精密称取人参皂苷 Rb$_2$、Rb$_3$、Rc、Rd、Re、Rg$_1$、

---

* 原载于《中草药》，2010，41（12）：1942—1947

Rg$_2$、Rg$_3$、F$_2$和拟人参皂苷 F$_{11}$ 适量，加甲醇制成 200μg/mL 的对照品溶液，分别精密吸取各对照品溶液 25μL，置 10mL 量瓶中，加甲醇至刻度，摇匀，取适量，离心（10 000r/min）6min，上清液作为人参皂苷混合对照品溶液（相当于各对照品的质量浓度为 500ng/mL）。

1.3 色谱与质谱条件

1.3.1 液相色谱条件：色谱柱为 Waters symmetry C$_{18}$（100mm×2.1mm，3.5μm）；流动相为 A：乙腈，B：20% 乙腈 - 水，梯度洗脱程序：0 ～ 4min，0 ～ 13% A；3 ～ 14min，13% ～ 15% A；14 ～ 24min，15% ～ 30%A；24 ～ 27min，30% ～ 31% A；27 ～ 37min，31% ～ 42% A；37 ～ 50min，42% ～ 88% A；50 ～ 60min，88% A。体积流量：0.3mL/min；柱温：室温；进样量：10μL。

1.3.2 质谱条件：ESI 源，负离子检测模式。扫描范围：m/z 300 ～ 2000。离子阱条件为喷雾电压：3.5kV；壳气（N$_2$）：4.137×10^5 Pa；辅助气（He）：6.895×10^4 Pa；离子传输管温度：250℃；离子传输管电压：–35V；套管镜头电压：–15V。

2. 结果

电喷雾电离（ESI）属于软电离，人参皂苷类成分在 ESI 源作用下，不发生结构裂解而给出准分子离子峰，从而得到化合物相应的相对分子质量信息。ESI-MS^n 能够得到化合物的多级裂解质谱，为化合物的结构解析提供丰富的信息。人参皂苷类成分的多级质谱裂解规律表明，在碰撞能的作用下，人参皂苷主要发生糖苷键的断裂，质谱给出失去一个或多个糖的次级苷和苷元的碎片离子。西洋参中的皂苷类成分依据其母核的不同，裂解形成的皂苷元主要为原人参二醇、原人参三醇和奥克梯隆醇，在 ESI（负离子）检测模式下分别给出 m/z 459、475 和 491 的特征苷元碎片离子，这些离子可以作为皂苷类型鉴定的有利证据。图 1 分别给出了人参皂苷 Rd（原人参二醇型）、Re（原人参三醇型）和拟人参皂苷 F$_{11}$（奥克梯隆型）的 MS 谱图。

2.1 样品的 LC-MS 分析

取"1.2 样品制备"项下的空白、供试品及对照品溶液，按照上述液相和质谱条件分别进行 LC-MS 分析，得到各样品的总离子流色谱图

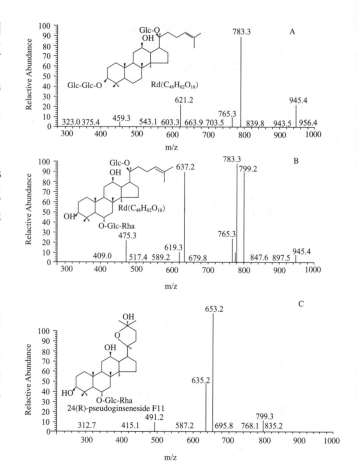

图 1 人参皂苷 Rd（A），人参皂苷 Re（B）和拟人参皂苷 F$_{11}$（C）的负离子质谱

（TIC），见图 2。与空白对照溶液相比，心悦胶囊供试品溶液的 TIC 谱图中出现了 16 个明显的色谱峰，按照出峰的先后顺序将其标示为 1 ～ 16，保留时间见表 1。在 TIC 中，谱峰 1 给出 m/z 945 和 799 的 [M-H]$^-$ 准分子离子峰，谱峰 12 给出 m/z 765、783 的 [M-H]$^-$ 准分子离子峰，谱峰 2 ～ 11 和 13 ～ 16 依次给出 m/z 799、783、783、1077、1077、1077、945、915、915、765、783、783、765 和 765 的 [M-H]$^-$ 准分子离子峰。初步推断心悦胶囊中含有 18 个主要单体成分。

2.2 样品的 LC-MS^2 及 LC-MS^3 分析

为了确定各化合物的结构，对各准分子离子进行了 MS^2，甚至 MS^3 裂解分析，表 1 中列出了各化合物 MS^2 碎片离子。

保留时间为 5.27min 的谱峰 1，给出 [M-H]$^-$ 为 m/z 945 和 799 的准分子离子峰，表明谱峰 1 可能包含 2 个化合物。对 m/z 945 的 [M-H]$^-$ 准分子离子进行 MS 裂解分析，质谱给出了 m/z 799、783、765、637、619、475 的碎片离子；m/z

第五章

799 为母离子 *m/z* 945 失去 1 个脱水的鼠李糖基产生的碎片离子 [M-(Rha-H$_2$O)-H]$^-$，*m/z* 783 为 *m/z* 945 失去 1 个脱水的葡萄糖基得到的碎片离子 [M-(Glc-H$_2$O)-H]$^-$，*m/z* 765 为母离子失去 1 个脱水的葡萄糖基后再失去 1 个水得到的碎片离子 [M-(Glc-H$_2$O)-H$_2$O-H]$^-$，*m/z* 637 为母离子失去 1 个脱水的鼠李糖基和 1 个脱水的葡萄糖基产生的碎片离子 [M-(Rha-H$_2$O)-(Glc-H$_2$O)-H]$^-$，*m/z* 619 对应于母离子失去 1 个脱水的鼠李糖基和 1 个脱水的葡萄糖基后再失去 1 个水产生的碎片离子 [M-(Rha-H$_2$O)-(Glc-H$_2$O)-H$_2$O-H]$^-$，*m/z* 475 对应于 *m/z* 945 失去 1 个脱水的鼠李糖基和 2 个脱水的葡萄糖基后生成的碎片离子 [M-(Rha-H$_2$O)-2(Glc-H$_2$O)-H]$^-$，*m/z* 475 碎片离子的产生说明该人参皂苷为原人参三醇型皂苷。综合上述分析，*m/z* 945 的 [M-H]$^-$ 峰代表相对分子质量为 946、结构中含有 1 个鼠李糖和 2 个葡萄糖的原人参三醇型皂苷，这与文献报道的人参皂苷 Re 的质

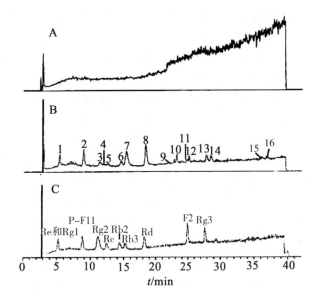

图 2　空白（A），心悦胶囊（B）和人参皂苷对照品混合物（C）在负离子模式下的总离子流色谱图

表 1　化合物 1 ~ 16 在 ESI 负离子检测模式中的 MS 光谱数据

编号	t_R/min	化合物	[M-H]$^-$（*m/z*）	MS^2（*m/z*）（%）
1	5.27	人参皂苷 Re	945	945（8），799（96），783（100），765（32），637（94），619（20），475（38）
		人参皂苷 Rg1	799	799（28），637（100），475（18）
2	8.74	拟人参皂苷 F11	799	799（18），653（100），635（38），491（22）
3	11.21	G-Rg2	783	783（18），637（100），619（34），475（70）
4	11.81	G-Rg2 异构体	783	783（28），637（100），619（28），475（64）
5	12.37	G-Rc	1077	945（100），915（70）
6	14.38	Rb2	1077	1077（60），945（100），915（96），783（68），765（20）
7	15.20	Rb3	1077	1077（22），945（100），915（32），783（66），765（14），621（6），603（4），459（6）
8	18.23	G-Rd	945	945（14），783（100），765（6），621（20），459（6）
9	22.61	gypenoside IX	915	915（22），783（100），765（4），753（8），621（24），603（2），459（4）
10	23.02	gypenoside IX isomer	915	915（2），783（100），765（2），753（2），621（32），459（4）
11	24.62	G-Rg6	765	765（10），619（100），601（32），457（2）
12	24.99	G-Rg6 异构体	765	765（6），619（100），601（24）
		G-F2	783	783（10），621（100），459（26）
13	27.73	G-Rg3	783	783（24），621（100），459（38）
14	28.36	G-Rg3 异构体	783	783（24），621（100），459（44）
15	35.88	Rk1	765	765（22），603（100）
16	36.61	Rg5	765	765（22），603（100）

谱数据相同[7-8]。经与人参皂苷 Re 对照品质谱图（图 1-B）及 LC 保留时间（图 2-C）比较，确定该化合物为人参皂苷 Re（G-Re）。

对谱峰 1 中 [M-H]⁻ 为 m/z 799 的准分子离子进行 MS² 裂解分析，质谱给出了 m/z 637、475 的碎片离子峰，分别对应于 [M-（Glc-H₂O）-H]⁻ 和 [M-2（Glc-H₂O）-H]⁻，说明该化合物为原人参三醇型皂苷，结构中含有 2 个葡萄糖，这与人参皂苷 Rg1 的结构相符[7-8]。采用人参皂苷 Rg1 对照品在相同条件下进行分析，结果与该化合物的 LC 保留时间及质谱数据一致，故鉴定该化合物为人参皂苷 Rg₁（G-Rg₁）。

保留时间为 8.74min，[M-H]⁻ 准分子离子为 m/z 799 的谱峰 2，MS 谱图给出 m/z 653、635、491 的碎片离子，分别对应于 [M-（Rha-H₂O）-H]⁻、[M-（Rha-H₂O）-H₂O-H]⁻ 和 [M-（Rha-H₂O）-（Glc-H₂O）-H]⁻，说明化合物结构中含有 1 个鼠李糖和 1 个葡萄糖，而 m/z 491 碎片的生成说明该化合物为奥克梯隆醇型皂苷。经与拟人参皂苷 F₁₁ 对照品质谱图（图 2-C）及 LC 保留时间比较，确定该化合物为拟人参皂苷 F₁₁（P-F₁₁）。

保留时间为 11.21 和 11.81min 的谱峰 3 和 4 均给出 m/z 783 的 [M-H]⁻ 峰，MS 谱图也均给出 m/z 637、619 和 475 的碎片离子，见表 1，说明谱峰 3 和 4 代表的化合物互为同分异构体。m/z 637 的碎片离子为母离子 m/z 783 失去 1 个脱水的鼠李糖基产生的碎片离子，该离子进一步脱去 1 个 H₂O 后产生 m/z 619 的碎片离子。m/z 475 的碎片离子为母离子 m/z 783 失去 1 个脱水的鼠李糖基和 1 个脱水的葡萄糖基产生的碎片离子，该离子的产生说明谱峰 3 和 4 代表的化合物均为原人参三醇型皂苷。综上所述，谱峰 3 和 4 代表相对分子质量为 784、结构中含有 1 个鼠李糖和 1 个葡萄糖的原人参三醇型皂苷。查阅相关文献，迄今为止，从西洋参（包含根、茎、叶、花、果实）中发现的人参皂苷类化合物相对分子质量为 784 的仅有 4 种，分别为人参皂苷 Rg₂、G-F₂、20（S）-Rg₃ 和 20（R）-Rg₃[9-10]，后 3 者均属于原人参二醇型皂苷，仅有人参皂苷 Rg₂ 属于原人参三醇型皂苷，且结构中含有 1 个葡萄糖和 1 个鼠李糖。采用人参皂苷 Rg₂ 对照品进行分析比较，结果 G-Rg₂ 的 LC 保留时间及质谱数据与谱峰 3 一致，故鉴定谱峰 3 为人参皂苷 Rg₂（G-Rg₂）。谱峰 4 与谱峰 3 的 MS 谱图极为相似，且 LC 保留时间非常接近，

无法完全分离，与文献[11]比较，初步推测谱峰 4 为人参皂苷 Rg₂ 的异构体 20（R）-ginsenoside Rg₂（G-Rg₂ isomer），结构有待于进一步确证。

保留时间为 12.37、14.38 和 15.20min 的谱峰 5、6 和 7，均给出 m/z 1077 的 [M-H]⁻ 峰，是互为同分异构体的 3 个化合物。谱峰 5 的 MS 谱图中碎片离子信号强度非常低，仅给出 m/z 945 和 915 的碎片离子，未能得到苷元的离子信息。m/z 945 为母离子失去 1 个脱水的五碳糖基（Ara 或 Xyl）后生成的碎片离子，m/z 915 为母离子失去 1 个脱水的葡萄糖基所得到的碎片离子，数据说明该化合物分子中至少含有 1 个五碳糖和 1 个葡萄糖。谱峰 6 的 MS² 谱图给出 m/z 945、915、783 和 765，分别对应于碎片离子 [M-（Ara/Xyl-H₂O）-H]⁻、[M-（Glc-H₂O）-H]⁻、[M-（Ara/Xyl-H₂O）-（Glc-H₂O）-H]⁻ 和 [M-（Ara/Xyl-H₂O）-（Glc-H₂O）-H₂O-H]⁻，说明该化合物是相对分子质量为 1078，结构中含有 1 个五碳糖和至少 1 个葡萄糖的皂苷，但 MS 谱图未能得到苷元信息。谱峰 7 的 MS² 谱图给出 m/z 945、915、783、765、621、603 和 459，分别对应于碎片离子 [M-（Ara/Xyl-H₂O）-H]⁻、[M-（Glc-H₂O）-H]⁻、[M-（Ara/Xyl-H₂O）-（Glc-H₂O）-H]⁻、[M-（Ara/Xyl-H₂O）-（Glc-H₂O）-H₂O-H]⁻、[M-（Ara/Xyl-H₂O）-2（Glc-H₂O）-H]⁻、[M-（Ara/Xyl-H₂O）-2（Glc-H₂O）-H₂O-H]⁻ 和 [M-（Ara/Xyl-H₂O）-3（Glc-H₂O）-H]⁻，m/z 459 的苷元离子碎片的生成，说明该化合物为原人参二醇型皂苷，谱峰 7 代表相对分子质量为 1078、结构中含有 1 个五碳糖和 3 个葡萄糖的原人参二醇型皂苷。虽然谱峰 5、6 和 7 的质谱数据相似，但由于它们的 LC 保留时间不同，它们的极性不同。与文献比较[3,7]，推测谱峰 5、6 和 7 分别为人参皂苷 Rc、Rb₂ 和 Rb₃。采用人参皂苷 Rc、Rb₂ 和 Rb₃ 对照品在相同条件下进行分析（见图 2-C），数据与推测结果一致。谱峰 5、6 和 7 分别为人参皂苷 Rc（G-Rc）、Rb₂（G-Rb₂）和 Rb₃（G-Rb₃）。

保留时间为 18.23min 的谱峰 8，准分子离子峰 [M-H]⁻ 为 m/z 945，MS 谱图给出 m/z 783、765、621 和 459 的碎片离子，分别对应于碎片离子 [M-（Glc-H₂O）-H]⁻、[M-（Glc-H₂O）-H₂O-H]⁻、[M-2（Glc-H₂O）-H]⁻ 和 [M-3（Glc-H₂O）-H]⁻，说明该化合物为相对分子质量为 946，结构中含有 3 个葡萄糖的原人参二醇型皂苷。经与文献比较[7]，推测其为人参皂苷 Rd。采用 Rd 对照品对照，质谱数据

第五章

及 LC 保留时间与该化合物一致，鉴定谱峰 8 为人参皂苷 Rd（ginsenoside Rd）。

保留时间为 22.61 和 23.02min 的谱峰 9 和 10，LC-MS 谱图给出 m/z 915 的 [M-H]⁻ 峰，MS 谱图均给出 m/z 783、765、753、621、603 和 459 的碎片离子，分别对应于母离子失去 1 个脱水的五碳糖基、失去 1 个脱水的五碳糖基和 1 个水、失去 1 个脱水的葡萄糖、失去 1 个脱水的五碳糖和 1 个脱水的葡萄糖、失去 1 个脱水的五碳糖和 1 个脱水的葡萄糖后再失去 1 个水、失去 1 个脱水的五碳糖和 2 个脱水的葡萄糖基产生的碎片离子，说明它们均为结构中含有 1 个五碳糖和 2 个葡萄糖的原人参二醇型皂苷。经与文献对照[12]，推测谱峰 9 和 10 为 gypenoside IX 和 gypenoside IX 的异构体。

保留时间为 24.62min 的谱峰 11，LC-MS 谱图给出 m/z 765 的 [M-H]⁻ 峰。谱峰 11 的 MS 谱图给出 m/z 619、601 和 457 的碎片离子，分别对应于碎片离子 [M-(Rha-H₂O)-H]⁻、[M-(Rha-H₂O)-H₂O-H]⁻、[M-(Rha-H₂O)-(Glc-H₂O)-H]⁻，说明化合物结构中含有 1 个鼠李糖和 1 个葡萄糖，m/z 457 的碎片离子的产生，说明该化合物的母核比原人参二醇多 1 个不饱和度。为了进一步确证母核的碎片离子，对二级质谱中产生的 m/z 619[M-(Rha-H₂O)-H]⁻ 进行了 MS³ 裂解分析，并证实 m/z 619 进一步裂解后的子离子为 m/z 457。综合目前关于西洋参的化学成分研究结果，推测该化合物为人参皂苷 Rg₆（G-Rg₆）[8,13]。

保留时间为 24.99min 的谱峰 12，LC-MS 谱图给出 m/z 765 和 783 的 [M-H]⁻ 峰，该谱峰中包含 2 个未分开的化合物。对 m/z 765 的准分子离子进行二级 MS 分析，结果 MS 谱图给出 m/z 619 和 601 的碎片离子，质谱数据与 G-Rg₆ 相似，以 m/z 619 为二级母离子对其进行 MS³ 裂解分析，但未得到满意的子离子碎片。与文献对照[11]，推测谱峰 12 为 GRg₆ 的同分异构体（G-Rg₆ isomer），结构有待于进一步确定。

对谱峰 12 中 [M-H]⁻ 为 m/z 783 的化合物进行 MS² 分析，在碰撞能的作用下，m/z 783 给出了 m/z 621[M-(Glc-H₂O)-H]⁻ 和 m/z 459[M-2(Glc-H₂O)-H]⁻ 碎片离子，说明该化合物为结构中含有 2 个葡萄糖的原人参二醇型皂苷。目前关于西洋参化学成分的研究表明[8-9]，符合该质谱裂解规律的人参皂苷有 20（S）-Rg₃、20（R）-Rg₃ 和 G-F₂ 3 种，

但这 3 种成分的极性不同，人参皂苷 F₂ 的极性较小[9]，通过分析比较，初步推测谱峰 12 中 m/z 783 的化合物可能为人参皂苷 F₂。采用人参皂苷 F₂ 对照品在相同条件下进行分析，结果表明 G-F₂ 与该化合物的 LC 保留时间及质谱数据一致，鉴定该化合物为人参皂苷 F₂（G-F₂）。

保留时间为 27.73 和 28.36min 的谱峰 13 和 14，准分子离子 [M-H]⁻ 均为 m/z 783，相应的 MS 谱图均给出 m/z 621[M-(Glc-H₂O)-H]⁻ 和 459[M-2(Glc-H₂O)-H]⁻ 碎片离子，质谱裂解规律均与 G-F₂ 相同，经与文献比较[7,8,14]，推测这两个化合物分别为 20（S）-G-Rg₃ 和 20（R）-G-Rg₃。采用 20（S）-G-Rg₃ 对照品进行比较，20（S）-G-Rg₃ 与谱峰 13 代表的化合物的 LC 保留时间及 MS 谱图数据一致，故鉴定 13 为 20（S）-G-Rg₃。谱峰 14 为其异构体 20（R）-G-Rg₃。

保留时间为 35.88 和 36.61min 的谱峰 15 和 16 均给出 m/z 765 的 [M-H]⁻ 准分子离子，它们的 MS² 谱图均仅给出 m/z 603[M-(Glc-H₂O)-H]⁻ 碎片离子，说明化合物结构中均含有 1 个葡萄糖，与文献[11]对照，初步推测其分别为人参皂苷 Rk₁（G-Rk₁）和 Rg₅（G-Rg₅）。由于化合物在样品中的量较低，未能得到满意的 MS³ 谱图数据，这两个化合物的结构有待于进一步的确定。

3. 讨论

本实验首次采用 LC-MSⁿ 联用技术分析了中成药心悦胶囊中主要的皂苷类成分。通过与胶囊辅料提取物的总离子流谱图比较，发现了胶囊提取物中的 18 个主要的皂苷类成分，与文献报道的质谱数据和液相保留时间比较，将其依次鉴定为 G-Re、GRg₁、P-F₁₁、G-Rg₂、G-Rg₂ isomer、G-Rc、G-Rb₂、G-Rb₃、G-Rd、gypenoside IX、gypenoside IX isomer、G-Rg₆、G-Rg₆ isomer、G-F₂、20（S）-G-Rg₃、20（R）-G-Rg₃、G-Rk₁ 和 G-Rg₅，并采用 G-Re、G-Rg₁、P-F₁₁ 等 10 个对照品对相应的成分进行了确证。本实验发现的这 18 个皂苷类成分为心悦胶囊的主要组成成分。

心悦胶囊中的皂苷类成分以原人参二醇型皂苷居多，包括 G-Rd、G-Rb₂、G-Rb₃、G-Rg₃、G-Rg₃ isomer、G-F₂、gypenoside IX 和 gypenoside IX isomer，而 G-Rd、G-Rb₃、G-Rb₂ 和奥克梯隆醇型皂苷 P-F₁₁ 在胶囊中的量相对较高，推测它们为心悦胶囊的主要药效物质。人参皂苷 Rb₁ 在胶囊

中的量相对较少，未能给出理想的 LC-MS 及 MS^2 谱图，这与文献报道的"G-Rb$_1$ 在西洋参茎、叶中的含量低"的结果一致 [4]。

本研究建立了心悦胶囊中主要皂苷类成分的快速、准确的 LC-MS^n 分析方法，首次阐明了胶囊中的主要皂苷类成分的结构，为心悦胶囊的药效物质基础研究提供了科学依据。

参考文献

[1] 王苏平. 二类新药产自废弃西洋参茎叶. 中国社区医师，2005，7（21）：83.

[2] 梦祥颖，任跃英，李向高，等. 西洋参中皂苷类成分的研究综述. 特产研究，2001，(3)：43-47.

[3] Ligor T, Ludwiczuk A, Wolski T, et al. Isolation and determination of ginsenosides in American Ginseng Leaves and root extracts by LC-MS. Anal Bioanal Chem, 2005, 383: 1098 -1105.

[4] 许传莲，郑毅男，崔淑玉，等. RP-HPLC 法测定西洋参茎叶中 6 种人参皂苷的含量. 吉林农业大学学报，2002，24（3）：50-52.

[5] 赵岩，刘金平，卢丹，等. 反相高效液相色谱-蒸发光散射检测法测定西洋参和西洋红参中人参皂苷的含量. 时珍国医国药，2006，17（10）：1956-1958.

[6] Wan XM, Sakuma T, Asafu-Adjaye E, et al. Determination ofginsenosides in plant extracts from panax ginseng and Panax quinquefolius L. by LC/MS/MS. Analy Chem, 1999, 71 (8): 1579-1584.

[7] Ma XQ, Xiao HB, Liang XM. Identification of ginsenosides in Panax quinquefolium by LC-MS. Chromatographia, 2006, 64 (1-2): 31-36.

[8] 张海江，蔡小军，程翼宇. 高效液相色谱-电喷雾质谱法鉴别人参、西洋参和三七的皂苷提取物. 中国药学杂志，2006，41（5）：391-394.

[9] Besso H, Kasai R, Wei JX, et al. Further studies on dammarane-saponins of American ginseng, roots of Panax quinquef olium L. Chem Pharm Bull, 1982, 30 (12): 4534-4538.

[10] 李亚萍，郝秀华，李铣. 西洋参果中配糖体成分的研究. 中草药，1999，30（8）：563-565.

[11] 王占良，王弘，陈世忠. 高效液相色谱-二极管阵列检测/质谱法分析生脉饮煎剂中的人参皂苷类成分. 色谱，2006，24（4）：325-330.

[12] 王金辉，李铣. 加拿大产西洋参茎叶的化学研究（I）十一种三萜皂苷的分离和鉴定. 中国药物化学杂志，1997，7（2）：130-132.

[13] Dou DQ, Li W, Guo N, et al. Ginsenoside Rg$_8$, a new dammarane-type triterpen oid saponin from roots of Panax quinquef olium. Chem Pharm Bull, 2006, 54 (5): 751-753.

[14] 苏健，李海舟，杨崇仁. 吉林产西洋参的皂苷成分研究. 中国中药杂志，2003，28（9）：830-833.

Influence of High Blood Glucose Fluctuation on Endothelial Function of Type 2 Diabetes Mellitus Rats and Effects of *Panax Quinquefolius* Saponin of Stem and Leaf *

WANG Jing-shang   YIN Hui-jun   GUO Chun-Yu
HUANG Ye   XIA Cheng-dong   LIU Qian

The outcomes of cardiovascular events in diabetics are equal to those found in patients with coronary artery diseases (CAD) not associated with type 2 diabetes mellitus (T2DM). T2DM is hence upgraded from "risk factor" to "equivalent" of CAD[1]. Vascular endothelial dysfunction plays a critical role in the occurrence and development of diabetic cardiovascular complications, which is also termed as one of the most important pathophysiologic basis of these diseases[2]. The key feature of diabetes is hyperglycemia, which accounts for the long-term complications[3].

---

* 原载于 Chinese Journal of Integrative Medicine, 2013，19（3）：217-222

Good blood glucose control is an effective way to prevent or delay the complications of diabetes[4]. There are two kinds of behaving form of hyperglycemia. One is steady high blood glucose, and the other is fluctuant high blood glucose. Normally, the level of blood glucose changes within a limited range. However, the inter-and intra-day glucose fluctuations are relatively high in diabetic patients[5]. Several epidemiological investigations have confirmed that glucose fluctuations is an independent risk factor for diabetic cardiovascular complications as well as an independent predictor of high mortality rate[6]. For the fluctuant, high blood glucose may have more deleterious influences than constant high glucose on endothelial function and diabetes chronic cardiovascular complications; study on glucose fluctuations has recently become a research focus in the field of diabetic cardiovascular disease.[7,8]

Panax Quinquefolius Saponin (PQS) of stem and leaf are the active parts of American ginseng, which can regulate lipid metabolism, lower the blood glucose, improve insulin resistance and myocardial ischemia, and so on simultaneously[9-12]. In this study, we aimed to observe the influence of high blood glucose fluctuations on endothelial function in T2DM rats and the effects of PQS.

1. Methods

1.1 Drugs and Reagents

PQS was provided by Jilin Ji'an Yisheng Pharmaceutical, Co., Ltd. (batch No. 081002), China. Metformin hydrochloride (batch No. 1005052) was produced by Sino-American Shanghai Squibb Pharmaceuticals, Co., Ltd. (0.5g per tablet) . Streptozotocin (STZ batch No. AB0162-050121) was produced by Sigma, USA. Insulin radioimmunoassary kit was from Science and Technology Development Center of general Hospital of PLA (batch No. 20100908), China. Nitric oxide (NO) kit was from Nanjing Jiancheng Bioengineering Institute, China. Enzyme-linked immunosorbent assay (ELISA) kit of Endothelin-1 (ET-1), soluble intercellular adhesion molecule 1 (sICAM-1), tumor necrosis factor α (TNF-α), and hepatocyte growth factor (HGF) were all from R&D (USA, batch No. 20100927，20101015，20100921，20100916).

1.2 Animals

There were 80 male rats, 180-220g, obtained from Beijing University Laboratory Animal Center [certificate No：SCXK (Jing) 2006-0008]. Animal feeds were provided by the Experimental Animal Center of the Academy of Military Medical Sciences. High fat laboratory chow contains 10% lard (wt/wt), 10% sucrose (wt/wt), 2.5% cholesterol, and 0.25% cholate (wt/wt).

1.3 Establishment of Animal Model and Grouping

After two weeks of adaptive feeding, 10 rats were randomly chosen as the normal control (NOR) group. Feed of the other 70 rats were switched from normal rodent diet to a high fat and high caloric laboratory chow. After 6-week high fat and high caloric diet, rats received only one intraperitoneal injection of a small dose of STZ (35 mg/kg) and then were fed with normal rodent diet for 2 weeks. During the 10th week, fasting blood glucose levels of rats were measured every morning by collecting blood samples from their caudal veins；meanwhile, fasting blood glucose coefficient of variation (FBG-CV= interday blood glucose means/standard deviation) was calculated. Rats, in which the blood glucose levels were higher than 16.7 mmol/L, were regarded to be successful models of T2DM diabetes, which finally were 50. Same processes were performed to the normal controls at the same time, and FBG-CV was calculated as well. Rats with higher FBG-CV values of diabetes were divided into fluctuant high blood glucose (FHG) group, and the others were in steady high blood glucose (SHG) group. There were 40 rats in FHG group and 10 in SHG group for the study. FHG rats were then divided into 4 groups according to the level of FBG-CV and fasting blood glucose, 10 rats in each group：PQS 30 mg/ (kg·d) (PQSL) group, PQS 60 mg/

(kg·d) (PQSH) group, metformin hydrochloride control (MHC) group, and FHG control (FHGC) group. All rats were fed with high caloric laboratory chow except normal control rats.

1.4 Specimen Collection

At the 17th week, all rats were executed after anesthesia with intraperitoneal injection of 20% urethane (0.6 mL/100g, fasting 12 h before sampling). Blood samples were collected from abdominal aorta. The serum was centrifuged 3,000 r/min for 15 min and preserved at -20℃ for biochemistry analysis. The top 2 cm of thoracic aorta tissue was removed and fixed with 20% formaldehyde as soon as possible.

1.5 Biochemical Assays

Serum fasting blood-glucose (FBS), total cholesterol (TC), and triglyceride (TG) were determined by enzymic technique. High-density lipoprotein cholesterin (HDL-C) and low-density lipoprotein cholesterin (LDL-C) were analyzed by immunoturbidimetry. All kits used were purchased from BioSino Bio-technology and Science Inc., China. Fasting plasma insulin (FINS) was measured using radioimmunoassay by Beijing PaTeLaiLi Biomedical Technology, Co., Ltd., China.

1.6 Pathological Morphologic Analysis

Thoracic aorta, fixed in 20% formaldehyde, was imbedded with paraffin, sectioned, and stained with hemotoxylin and eosin (HE). Then, the pathomorphological changes of aorta were observed under light microscopes.

1.7 Index of Endothelial Injury and Inflammatory Factors

Serum NO level was determined with

biochemical technology. Serum ET-1, TNF-α, sICAM-1, and plasma HGF levels were analyzed with ELISA. Operation tests were all carried out according to the kit instructions strictly.

1.8 Statistical Analysis

Data were expressed as the mean ±standard deviation. Differences among groups were tested using One-way ANOVA, followed by multiple comparisons by LSD test. Statistical analysis was performed using SPSS 13.0 for Windows and P values less than 0.05 were considered statistically significant.

2. Results

2.1 Comparison of Rat Weight and Serum Biochemical Indices among Groups

Compared with the NOR group, weights of rats with T2DM and plasma FINS in the SHG group and the FHGC group decreased obviously $(P < 0.01)$, and serum FBG, TC, and TG increased significantly $(P < 0.01)$. However, there was no significant difference between the SHG and FHGC groups. It suggested that the fluctuations of high blood glucose and high blood lipid in rats with T2DM might not be accordant. Compared with the FHGC group, serum FBG, TC, and TG in the PQSL, PQSH, and MHC groups decreased significantly $(P < 0.05$ or $P < 0.01)$, while plasma FINS increased obviously $(P < 0.05$ or $P < 0.01)$. It suggested that PQS and MHC could ameliorate the state of high blood glucose and high blood lipid and increase plasma insulin level. In this study, PQS and MHC did not change the weight of rats with T2DM (Table 1).

Table 1 Comparison of Biochemical Indices among Groups ($\bar{\chi} \pm s$)

Group	n	Weight (g)	FBG (mmol/L)	FINS (mIU/L)	TC (mmol/L)	TG (mmol/L)
NOR	10	577.83±40.10	5.97±1.02	35.45±5.92	1.10±0.23	0.66±0.23
SHG	10	306.00±40.06*	26.88±4.14*	24.48±5.01*	8.93±1.41*	4.83±0.46*
FHGC	10	308.25±39.46*	26.09±2.50*	22.19±5.64*	8.67±0.88*	4.80±0.41*
PQSL	10	312.13±66.36*	23.00±2.83*△	25.14±6.47*	5.80±1.43*△△	2.10±0.39*△△
PQSH	10	341.78±43.76*	22.70±3.06*△	30.59±8.54△△	5.48±1.05*△△	2.08±0.43*△△
MHC	10	362.13±65.85*	20.39±3.01*△△	27.76±6.10*△	4.25±1.43*△△	2.09±0.44*△△

Notes：*$P < 0.01$, compared with the NOR group；△$P < 0.05$, △△$P < 0.01$, compared with the FHGC group

2.2　Aortic HE Staining

After 10 weeks, compared with the NOR group, the aortic endothelium of rats with T2DM appeared of disorder and damage to a certain degree. However, there was no difference between the SHG and FHGC groups. Structure of aortic endothelium in rat of the PQS and MHC groups improved. This result might be related to shortage of model number and drugs intervene.

2.3　Comparison of Serum NO and ET-1 among Groups

As compared with the NOR group, serum NO and ET-1 in the SHG and FHGC groups increased obviously ($P < 0.01$). Compared with the SHG group, serum NO and ET-1 in the FHGC group increased obviously ($P < 0.05$). Compared with the FHGC group, serum NO, and ET-1 of PQSL, PQSH and MHC groups were reversed ($P < 0.01$, Table 2).

2.4　Comparison of Serum TNF-α and sICAM-1 among Groups

Compared with the NOR group, serum TNF-α and sICAM-1 in the SHG and FHGC groups increased significantly ($P < 0.01$). Compared with the SHG group, serum TNF-α and sICAM-1 in FHGC group increased obviously ($P < 0.01$). Compared with FHGC group, serum TNF-α and sICAM-1 in the PQSL, PQSH, and MHC groups decreased obviously ($P < 0.01$, Table 3).

Table 2　Comparison of Serum NO and ET-1 in T2DM Rats among Groups ($\bar{\chi} \pm s$)

Group	n	NO (μmol/L)	ET-1 (pg/mL)
NOR	10	34.80 ± 9.02	33.50 ± 6.18
SHG	10	$65.25 \pm 10.33^{*}$	$49.66 \pm 6.04^{*}$
FHGC	10	$74.60 \pm 9.56^{* \triangle}$	$57.13 \pm 7.86^{* \triangle}$
PQSL	10	$54.59 \pm 9.33^{\blacktriangle}$	$44.01 \pm 6.45^{\blacktriangle}$
PQSH	10	$47.49 \pm 8.816^{\blacktriangle}$	$37.53 \pm 8.56^{\blacktriangle}$
MHC	10	$49.92 \pm 10.41^{\blacktriangle}$	$40.83 \pm 8.39^{\blacktriangle}$

Notes：$^{*}P < 0.01$，compared with the NOR group；$^{\triangle}P < 0.05$，compared with the SHG group；$^{\blacktriangle}P < 0.01$，compared with the FHGC group

2.5　Comparison of Serum HGF

Plasma HGF, as a protective mechanism of vascular endothelial injury, which will be significantly increased along with the aggravation of injury, plays an important role in forecasting vascular endothelial injury. Compared with the NOR group, plasma HGF in SHG group and FHGC groups increased obviously ($P < 0.01$). Compared

Table 3　Comparison of Serum TNF-α and sICAM-1 in T2DM Rats among Groups ($\bar{\chi} \pm s$)

Group	n	TNF-α (pg/mL)	sICAM-1 (ng/mL)
NOR	10	26.19 ± 6.22	1.06 ± 0.16
SHG	10	$50.79 \pm 7.91^{*}$	$1.54 \pm 0.26^{*}$
FHGC	10	$59.08 \pm 6.98^{* \triangle}$	$1.82 \pm 0.20^{* \triangle}$
PQSL	10	$45.03 \pm 5.72^{\blacktriangle}$	$1.47 \pm 0.18^{\blacktriangle}$
PQSH	10	$38.40 \pm 7.47^{\blacktriangle}$	$1.23 \pm 0.17^{\blacktriangle}$
MHC	10	$40.68 \pm 6.44^{\blacktriangle}$	$1.35 \pm 0.24^{\blacktriangle}$

Notes：$^{*}P < 0.01$，compared with the NOR group；$^{\triangle}P < 0.01$，compared with the SHG group；$^{\blacktriangle}P < 0.01$，compared with the FHGC group

with SHG group, plasma HGF in FHGC group increased significantly ($P < 0.01$). Compared with FHGC group, serum HGF in PQSL group, PQSH group, and MHC group decreased obviously ($P < 0.01$, Table 4).

Table 4　Comparison of serum HGF in T2DM Rats among Groups ($\bar{\chi} \pm s$)

Group	n	HGF (pg/mL)
NOR	10	259.36 ± 41.27
SHG	10	460.42 ± 79.80*
FHGC	10	528.29 ± 74.58*△
PQSL	10	374.58 ± 54.72▲
PQSH	10	336.99 ± 92.06▲
MHC	10	355.37 ± 59.91▲

Notes: *$P < 0.01$, compared with the NOR group; △$P < 0.01$, compared with the SHG group; ▲$P < 0.01$; compared with FHGC group

3. Discussion

The occurrence and development of diabetes complications is relevant not only to the general blood sugar level but also the glucose fluctuations[13-16]. Endothelial dysfunction is the initial factor and pathophysiologic basis of diabetic cardiovascular diseases. In recent decades, a large number of in vitro experiments have showed that FHG have more deleterious influences on endothelial function than SHG and induce human umbilical vein endothelial cells more vulnerable to apoptosis[17,18]. However, there is few experiments in vivo. The existing glucose fluctuation animal models were usually established using artificial intervention, such as poorly maintained insulin-control, feeding maltose, glucose injections, et al[19-21]. However, these models all increase the confounding factors during the experiments in varying degrees. Meanwhile, it is hard for them to meet the requirements of clinical practice. In this study, the T2DM rats were divided into SHG group and FHG group using FBG-CV. FBG-CV can decrease the confounding factors and meet the requirements of the clinical practice better. After eight weeks drugs treatment, compared

with SHG group, serious endothelial dysfunction appeared in the FHG group obviously. With this method, the rat model is reliable for use. In addition, it proved that high glucose fluctuation could accelerate the injury and dysfunction of vascular endothelium.

As well-known, high glucose fluctuation induces endothelial dysfunction more obviously than uncontrolled hyper glycemia. However, the exact mechanisms involved are still unclear. In vitro experiments showed that high glucose fluctuation could easily promote nitrotyrosine and 8-hydroxydeoxyguanosine (8-OHdG) production by poly ADP-ribose polymerase (PARP) pathway, promote ROS synthesis by mitochondrial respiratory chain, enhance oxidative stress, induce endothelial cell apotosis, and simultaneously increase the expression levels of cell-adhesion molecule ICAM-1, VCAM-1, and E-selectin, while PKC inhibitor bisindolylmaleimide-I (BIMI-I) and PKCβ specific inhibitor LY379196 could decrease their expression[18,22-25]. Ceriello A, et al[22] reported that, for patients with diabetes mellitus, acute glucose fluctuation induced more serious oxidative stress and endothelial dysfunction than steady high glucose. The findings in this study were consistent with the previous results. Plasma HGF in 10-week diabetes rats increased significantly in FHGC group compared with SHG group and NOR group. Plasma HGF, a protective mechanism of vascular endothelial injury, which will be significantly increased along with the aggravation of injury, is an important parameter forecasting vascular endothelial injury. It indicated that there might be obvious vascular endothelial injury in diabetes model rats. Glucose fluctuation could aggravate the endothelial injury further.

Serum TNF-α and sICAM-1 in diabetes rats were increased dramatically compared with NOR group and were further increased in FHGC group compared with SHG group. The results indicated that there was obvious vascular endothelial dysfunction and white blood cells activation in diabetes rats；glucose fluctuation could aggravate the endothelial injury further. The expression serum vasoconstrictor ET-1 and vasorelaxant substance NO in FHGC group also significantly increased as compared with SHG group, which indicated that the endothelial vasomotor dysfunction in early diabetes rats might be related to increasing vessel stress, ET-1 production, and compensating the increase of NO.

American ginseng typically grows on the east coast of Canada and the U.S. According to Chinese medicine (CM) theories, American ginseng is cold in property, bitter, and sweet in taste. It mainly distributes to Lung (Fei), Liver (Gan), and Kidney (Shen) meridians, with the effects of supplementing qi, nourishing yin, promoting body fluid and eliminating restlessness, which can be used for qi and yin deficiency. The PQS of stem and leaf are the active parts of American ginseng, which have been shown to regulate lipid metabolism, lower the blood glucose, improve insulin resistance and myocardial ischemia, reduce myocardium oxygen consumption, ameliorate myocardial remodeling, inhibit platelet aggregation, etc[9-12]. A multicenter double-blind randomized control clinical trial organized by the Ministry of Public Health of the Peoples Republic of China proved the above effects of PQS[26]. In this study, the administration of PQS showed similar effects with metformin hydrochloride on lowering blood glucose and adjusting glycolipid metabolism. Also, PQS and metformin hydrochloride both have the effect of alleviating vascular endothelial injury on T2DM rats with high glucose fluctuations, which may be related to its effects of relieving vessel stress, decreasing vasoconstrictor ET-1 production, preventing compensated increase of NO, and reducing inflammatory reaction. However, it is very hard to say whether adjusting glycolipid metabolism or the above effects plays a more important role in its protective effects on endothelial function. In comparison with steady high glucose, does PQS have better effects on fluctuation high glucose condition? This is still not clear at present.

For now, metformin has been recommended as the first-line treatment and essential drug of combination therapy in international guidelines and many national guidelines for the type 2 diabetic patients[27]. This study showed that PQS had similar effects with metformin. The results in this study indicated that Chinese herbs would be promising to play a stronger role in treating and preventing diabetic cardiovascular complications in the future.

References

[1] Expert Panel on Detection, Evaluation, and Treatment of High Blood Cholesterol in Adults. Executive Summary of the Third Report of the National Cholesterol Education Program (NCEP) Expert Panel on Detection, Evaluation, and Treatment of High Blood Cholesterol in Adults (Adult Treatment Panel Ⅲ). JAMA, 2001, 285：2486-2497.

[2] Guerci B, Kearney-Schwartz A, Böhme P, et al. Endothelial dysfunction and type 2 diabetes. Part 1：physiology and methods for exploring the endothelial function. Diabetes Metab, 2001, 27：425-434.

[3] Mazzone T, Chait A, Plutzky J. Cardiovascular disease risk in type 2 diabetes mellitus：insights from mechanistic studies. Lancet, 2008, 371：1800-1809.

[4] Nordwall M, Arnqvist HJ, Bojestig M, et al. Good glycemic control remains crucial in prevention of late diabetic complications—the Linkoping Diabetes Complications Study. Pediatr Diabetes, 2009, 10：168-176.

[5] Bonora E, Muggeo M. Postprandial blood glucose as a risk factor for cardiovascular disease in type Ⅱ diabetes：the epidemiological evidence. Diabetologia, 2001, 44：2107-2114.

[6] Hirsch IB, Brownlee M. Should minimal blood-variability become the gold standard of glycemic control? J Diabetes Complic, 2005, 19：178-181.

[7] Monnier L, Colette C. Glycemic variability：should we and can we prevent it? Diabetes Care, 2008, 31 (Suppl2)：S150-S154.

[8] O'Sullivan EP, Dinneen SF. Benefits of early intensive glucose control to prevent diabetes complications were sustained for up to 10 years. Evid Based Med, 2009, 14：9-10.

第五章

[9] Yin HJ, Zhang Y, Jiang YR, et al. Effects of *panax quinquefolium* saponin (PQS) on blood lipid metabolism of alloxan diabetic rats. Chin J Integr Med Cardio/Cerebrovasc Dis, 2004, 2: 647-648.

[10] Yin HJ, Zhang Y, Shi DZ, et al. Effects of *panax quinquefolium* saponin (PQS) onglucose transportation, GLUT-4 translocation and CAP mRNA expression of insulin resistance adipocytes. Chin Pharmacol Bull, 2007, 23: 1332-1337.

[11] Zhang Y, Chen KJ, Yang LH, et al. Effects of *panax quinquefolius* saponin of stem and leaf on glucose-lipid metabolism and insulin signal transduction in insulin resistant model adipocytes. Chin J Integr Med, 2010, 30: 748-751.

[12] Fan BJ, Fei F, Zhao XZ. Effects of *panax quinquefolium* saponin (PQS) on the vascular endothelial function of the myocardial hypertrophied rats. Chin Jgerontol, 2009, 29: 811-812.

[13] Muggeo M, Zoppinig, Bonora E, Brun E, et al. Fasting plasma glucose variability predicts 10-year survival of type 2 diabetes patients: the Verona Diabetes Study. Diabetes Care, 2000, 23: 45-50.

[14] Piconi L, Quagliaro L, Assaloni R, et al. Constant and intermittent high glucose enhances endothelial cell apoptosis through mitochondrial superoxide overproduction. Diabetes Metab Res Rev, 2006, 22: 198-203.

[15] Azuma K, Kawamori R, Toyofuku Y, et al. Repetitive fluctuations in blood glucose enhance monocyte adhesion to the endothelium of rat thoracic aorta. Arterioscler Thromb Vasc Biol, 2006, 26: 2275-2280.

[16] Kilpatrick ES. Arguments for and against the role of glucose variability in the development of diabetes complications. J Diabetes Sci Technol, 2009, 3: 649-655.

[17] Risso A, Mercuri F, Quagliaro L, et al. Intermittent high glucose enhances apoptosis in human umbilical vein endothelial cells in culture. Am J Physio, 2001, 281: E924-E930.

[18] Piconi L, Quagliaro L, Assaloni R, et al. Constant and intermittent high glucose enhances endothelial cell apoptosis through mitochondrial superoxide overproduction. Diabetes Metab Res Rev, 2006, 22: 198-203.

[19] Horvath EM, Benko R, Kiss L, et al. Rapid "glycaemic swings" induce nitrosative stress, activate poly (ADP-ribose) polymerase and impair endothelial function in a rat model of diabetes mellitus. Diabetologia, 2009, 52: 952-961.

[20] Mita T, Otsuka A, Azuma K, et al. Swings in blood glucose levels accelerate atherogenesis in apolipoprotein E-deficient mice. Biochem Biophys Res Commun, 2007, 358: 679-985.

[21] Tu Q, Weng YJ, Tong Z, et al. Establishment of blood glucose fluctuation model on diabetes mice and its damage to viscera. J Fudan Univ, 2008, 47: 647-651.

[22] Ceriello A, Esposito K, Piconi L, et al. Oscillating glucose is more deleterious to endothelial function and oxidative stress than mean glucose in normal and type 2 diabetic patients. Diabetes, 2008, 57: 1349-1354.

[23] Quagliaro L, Piconi L, Assaloni R, et al. Intermittent high glucose enhances ICAM-1, VCAM-1 and E-selectin expression in human umbilical vein endothelial cells in culture: the distinct role of protein kinase C and mitochondrial superoxide production. Atherosclerosis, 2005, 183: 259-267.

[24] Piconi L, Quagliaro L, Da Ros R, et al. Intermittent high glucose enhances ICAM-1, VCAM-1, E-selectin and interleukin-6 expression in human umbilical endothelial cells in culture: the role of poly (ADPribose) polymerase. J Thromb Haemost, 2004, 2: 1453-1459.

[25] Piconi L, Corgnali M, Da Ros R. The protective effect of rosuvastatin in human umbilical endothelial cells exposed to constant or intermittent high glucose. J Diabetes Complic, 2008, 22: 38-45.

[26] Zhang Y, ed. Effect of *Panax Quinquefolius* saponin on insulin sensitivity in patients of coronary heart disease and its mechanism. Beijing: China Academy of Chinese Medical Sciences, 2006.

[27] Chinese Diabetes Society. The 2007 guideline of Chinese type 2 diabetes prevents and controls. Nat Med J China, 2008, 88: 1227-1245.

第五章

Panax Quinquefolius Saponin of Stem and Leaf Attenuates Intermittent High Glucose-Induced Oxidative Stress Injury in Cultured Human Umbilical Vein Endothelial Cells via PI3K/Akt/GSK-3β Pathway[*]

WANG Jing-shang　YIN Hui-jun　HUANG Ye　GUO Chun-yu　XIA Cheng-dong
LIU Qian　ZHANG Lu

1. Introduction

Vascular disorders, especially cardiovascular disorders, are major causes of morbidity and mortality in diabetic patients [1]. Intermittent high glucose (IHG) and constant high glucose are two general phenomena in diabetes. Recent studies have shown that IHG may be more dangerous for the development of diabetes-related complications including cardiovascular disorders, and thus for diabetic patients [2].

Although the precise mechanism underlying the action of IHG remains unclear, significant progress has been made. Recent studies have shown that IHG could induce an increased rate of apoptosis, protein kinase C activation, nicotinamide adenine dinucleotide phosphate oxidase activation in cultured endothelial cells, and monocytes adhesion to endothelial cells in diabetic rats. These effects are even more pronounced than those of constant high glucose [3-7]. Moreover, there is growing evidence that an acute increase of glycemia is accompanied by oxidative stress that may contribute to the generation of vascular endothelial dysfunction [8]. Meanwhile, clinical evidence suggests that *in vivo* glucose fluctuations may be damaged for endothelial cells, which could be mediated by oxidative stress [9,10]. And enhanced oxidative damage after diverse stimuli has been confirmed to be an initial event in the development of cardiovascular diseases [11,12]. It is, therefore, thought that prevention of intermittent high glucose-induced oxidative damage on endothelial cells may have important implications for pharmacologic attempts to prevent these complications.

PQS is the effective parts of American ginseng, a herb widely used in clinical Chinese medicine for diabetes and cardiovascular diseases treatment. In fact, there is growing evidence demonstrating the significant beneficial effects of PQS consumption on diabetic patients, including lowering blood sugar, keeping blood sugar stable, improving insulin resistance, regulating lipid metabolism, and cardio protective effects such as antimyocardial ischemia, reducing myocardium oxygen consumption, ameliorating myocardial remodeling, and inhibiting platelet aggregation [13-16]. A multicenter, double-blind, randomized control clinical trial organized by Ministry of Public Health of the People's Republic of China showed the similar results [17]. Our previous study had demonstrated that PQS could improve endothelial function in diabetes mellitus in experimental rats with high glucose fluctuation [18]. However, as far as we know, little evidence exists concerning the effect of PQS on oxidative damage in endothelial cells induced by intermittent high glucose.

---

* 原载于 Evidence-Based Complementary and Alternative Medicine，2013，Article ID：196283

PI3K and Akt are downstream effectors of insulin signaling [19], as well as important signaling molecules in the regulation of glycogen metabolism in myocytes, lipocytes, and hepatocytes [20,21]. Uncoupling of insulin signaling at PI3K-Akt in response to high glucose concentrations in these cell types has been implicated in the pathogenesis of insulin resistance and T2DM [22]. By regulating angiogenesis, proliferation, microvascular permeability, survival, cellular transformation, and embryonic differentiation, PI3K-Akt also plays an important role in regulation of endothelial cell (EC) function [23,24]. Cells respond via PI3K-Akt signaling to a variety of cytokines, G protein-coupled receptor ligands, and growth factors as well as to cellular stresses, including heat shock, hypoxia, and oxidative stress [25]. It has been reported that prolonged exposure of ECs to high glucose concentrations would result in reduced proliferation and survival through altered PI3K-Akt signaling[26]. The nitric oxide production, followed by Akt activation, had been confirmed to prevent steady high blood glucose-induced endothelial cell injury [27]. Our previous study had observed that PQS could improve insulin sensitivity by increasing the tyrosine phosphorylation of insulin receptor and IRS1 and the Ser473 phosphorylation of Akt [15]. A potential target of PQS may also be the serine/threonine kinase Akt.

Therefore, the aims of our present study were to (1) determine whether treatment with PQS attenuates intermittent high glucose-induced stress injury in HUVECs and, if so, (2) investigate the signaling pathway involved.

2. Materials and Methods

2.1　Chemicals and Reagents

PQS was provided by Jilin Jian Yisheng Pharmaceutical Co. Ltd. Dulbecco's-Modified Eagle's Medium (DMEM) was purchased from Gibco (Grand Island, NY, USA). Fetal bovine serum (FBS) was obtained from HyClone. The antibodies against Akt, phosphorylated-Akt (Ser473), GSK3β, GSK3β, phosphorylated-GSK3β (Ser9) and β-Actin were purchased from Cell Signaling Technology (USA). The LY294002 and 3- (4，5-dimethylthiazol-2-yl) 2，5-diphenyltetrazolium bromide (MTT) were purchased from Sigma-Aldrich (St. Louis, USA). Malonyldialdehyde (MDA) and superoxide dismutase (SOD) assay kits were obtained from Jian Cheng Biological Engineering Institute (Nanjing, China). All other biochemicals used were of the highest purity available.

2.2　Isolation and Culture of Human Umbilical Vein Endothelial Cells (HUVECs)

HUVECs were isolated and pooled from umbilical cords obtained from normal vaginal deliveries by the procedure described by Jaffe et al. [28] The cells were cultured ingelatin-coated 60 mm Petri dishes (Corning) and grown in DMEM, supplemented with 20% heat-inactivated fetal bovine serum, 20 mM glutamine (Sigma-Aldrich), 10 ng/mL endothelial cell growth supplement (Sigma-Aldrich), 40 U/mL heparin (Gibco), 50 U/mL penicillin, 50μg/mL streptomycin (Gibco), 20 mM Hepes (Sigma-Aldrich), and 0.11 mg/mL sodium pyruvate (Sigma-Aldrich). The Petri dishes were incubated at 37 ℃, in 5% CO_2-95% air gas mixture. Primary cultures were fluid-changed 24 h after seeding and were subcultured on reaching confluence by the use of 0.25% Trypsin-EDTA, inactivated by dilution. More than 99% HUVECs were identified to be endothelial cells by their characteristic cobblestone morphology (Figure 1A) under an inverted microscope (Leica DMIRB, Germany) and characterized by brown granules in cytoplasm using immunocytochemical staining of factor Ⅷ (Figure 1B). Only HUVECs of the second passage were used in the study to avoid age-dependent cellular modification. HUVECs were seeded at equal density ingelatin-coated 60 mm Petri dishes or plates, allowed to attach overnight, and then exposed to the following experimental conditions for 8 days：(1) continuous DMEM

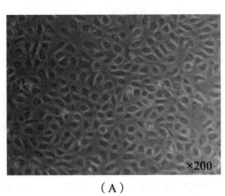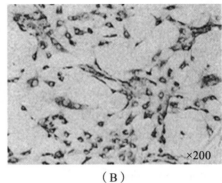

×200   ×200

（A）   （B）

Figure 1   Morphology and Immunocytochemical Staining of HUVEC. （A）Characteristic cobblestone morphology of HUVEC under an inverted microscope. （B）Immunocytochemical staining of HUVEC

containing normal (5.56 mmol/L) glucose (NG), (2) continuous DMEM containing high (25 mmol/L) glucose (HG), (3) alternating normal and high-glucose media every 24 h (IHG), (4) as (3), with the addition of 0.05 mg/mL PQS, and (5) as (3), with the addition of 0.1 mg/mL PQS. To further examine the role of the PI3K/Akt/GSK3 β pathway on the effect of PQS, another two groups of HUVECs were pretreated with the specific PI3K inhibitor LY294002 (20μmol/L；Sigma) for 30 min before PQS was added.

2.3   Cell Viability Measurement (MTT Assay)

Cell viability was determined by MTT assay. HUVECs were seeded in 96-well culture plates at a density of 1×10^5 cells with 200μL culture medium per well. Four hour before the culture was terminated, 10μL assay medium containing 5 mg/mL MTT was added to each well. After 4 h of incubation at 37℃, the medium was removed and the cells lysed by addition of 150μL DMSO. The optical density of each sample was measured in an ELISA microplate reader using test and reference wavelengths of 490 nm.

2.4   Preparation of Cell Lysates

The cells were seeded at a density of 1×10^5 cells/mL in 24-well plates and were allowed to attach for 24 h before treatment. Upon completion of the incubation studies, the cells were scraped from the plates into ice-cold RIPA lysis buffer (50 mM Tris with pH 7.4, 150 mM NaCl, 1% Triton X-100, 1% sodium deoxycholate, 0.1% SDS, and 0.05 mM EDTA), and protein concentration

was determined by the bicinchoninic acid method, using BSA as a reference standard. Aliquots were stored at −80℃ until detection for MDA and SOD activity.

2.5   Assay for Intracellular Contents of SOD and MDA

The activities of SOD and the concentration of MDA were both determined by using commercially available kits. All procedures completely complied with the manufacturer's instructions. The activities of SOD were expressed as units per milligram protein. MDA was measured at a wavelength of 532 nm by reacting with thiobarbituric acid to form a stable chromophoric production. Values of MDA level were expressed as nanomoles per milligram protein.

2.6   Western Blot Analysis

Cells were lysed in iced lysis buffer. Total protein (50 mg/lane) was separated by SDS-PAGE and transferred to a polyvinylidene fluoride membrane. After incubation in blocking solution (5% nonfat milk) (Sigma), membranes were incubated with primary antibodies for Akt, phosphorylated-Akt, GSK3β, phosphorylated-GSK3β, or β-Actin for overnight at 4℃. Membranes were washed and then incubated with 1：2000 dilution horseradish peroxidase-conjugated secondary antibody (ZSGB-BIO, Beijing, China). The relative density of each protein band was normalized to that of β-Actin. All results were representative of at least 3 independent

2.7 Statistical Analysis

All data were expressed as mean ± SD. The SPSS Statistics 15.0 package was utilized to analyze the data. Differences among groups were analyzed using the one-way analysis of variance (ANOVA), followed by multiple comparisons by LSD test. The $P < 0.05$ was considered statistically significant.

3. Results

3.1 Effects of PQS on Intermittent High Glucose-Induced Loss of HUVEC Viability

After 8 days of experiment, we observed that the cell viability in HG (0.8 ± 0.12) decreased significantly in comparison with NG, and this decrease was even more marked in IHG (0.61 ± 0.08). Two different concentrations (0.05 or 0.1 mg/mL) of PQS improved cell viability significantly (0.9 ± 0.11 or 0.89 ± 0.15). However, pretreatment with LY294002 (PI3K inhibitor) abolished PQS's effect on cell viability in cultured endothelial cells exposed to intermittent high glucose (0.63 ± 0.07 or 0.65 ± 0.13) (Figure 2).

3.2 Effects of PQS on SOD and MDA Levels

As shown in Table1 and Figure 3 A, after 8 days of experiment, the SOD level significantly decreased in IHG compared with either NG or HG. Pretreatment HUVECs with PQS (0.05 mg/mL or 0.1 mg/mL) inhibited the decreased SOD level induced by intermittent high glucose, which was abrogated by LY294002.

The content of MDA in the medium was increased significantly after treatment with intermittent high glucose for 48 h, compared with either normal or stable high glucose condition. Pretreatment HUVECs with PQS (0.05 mg/mL or 0.1 mg/mL) inhibited the elevation of MDA concentration elicited by intermittent high glucose significantly, which was abolished by LY294002 (Table 1 and Figure 3 (B)).

Together, these results showed that blood glucose fluctuation produced higher

suppression of antioxidant capacity and more oxidative damage than stable high glucose alone. However, pretreated with PQS, all these were reversed.

3.3 Effects of PQS on Decreased Akt and GSK3β Phosphorylation Levels Induced by Intermittent High Glucose

To investigate the underlying mechanism for protective effects of PQS, we examined the effect of PQS (0.1 mg/mL) on Akt and GSK3β level in intermittent high glucose-treated HUVECs. As shown in Figure 4 (A), HG significantly reduced the phosphorylation of Akt without alteration of total Akt expression in comparison with conditioning, and this decrease was even more marked in IHG. Pretreatment of HUVECs with PQS led to a significant increase in the phosphorylation of Akt in endothelial cells exposed to intermittent high glucose. And PQS had no effect on the Akt protein level. The specific PI3K inhibitor LY294002 markedly suppressed the effects of PQS on Akt activity.

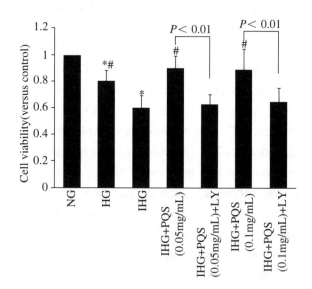

Figure 2 Effects of PQS on Intermittent High Glucose-Induced Loss of HUVEC Viability. Cell viability was determined by MTT assay. Cell viability was expressed as a percentage of cytoprotection vs. control group set at 100%. Data were presented as means ± SD. (n = 5) . *P < 0.01 vs. NG; #s < 0.01 vs. IHG

Table 1　Effects of PQS on SOD and MDA levels（*n*=5）

Group	SOD U/mg protein	MDA nmol/mg protein
NG	53.8 ± 7.62	24 ± 2.41
HG	30.81 ± 6.97*#	39.9 ± 7.18*#
IHG	20.73 ± 3.75*	47.16 ± 7.77*
IHG + PQS（0.05 mg/mL）	32.69 ± 2.66#	39.15 ± 6.86#
IHG +PQS（0.05 mg/mL）+ LY	21.41 ± 2.05▲	52 ± 4.72▲
IHG + PQS（0.1 mg/mL）	35.9 ± 3.37#	33.11 ± 3.07#
IHG +PQS（0.1 mg/mL）+ LY	17.66 ± 5.93▲	44.2 ± 3.66▲

Note：*$P < 0.01$ *vs* NG；#$P < 0.01$ *vs* IHG. ▲$P < 0.01$ *vs* IHG + PQS（0.05 mg/mL or 0.1 mg/mL）

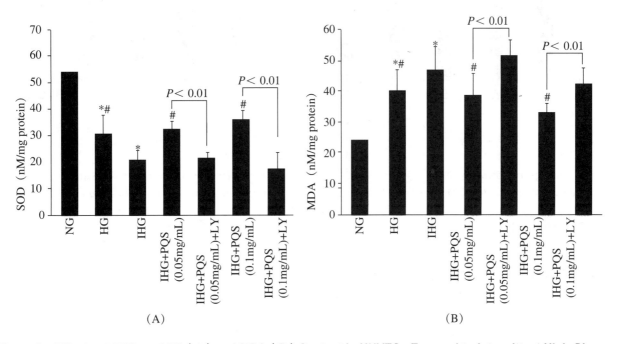

Figure 3　Effects of PQS on SOD（A）and MDA（B）Content in HUVECs Exposed to Intermittent High Glucose. Data were presented as means ± SD（*n*=5）. *$P < 0.01$ *vs* NG, #$P < 0.01$ *vs* IHG

Furthermore, similar to the effects of HG/IHG and PQS on Akt phosphorylation, IHG inhibited GSK3β phosphorylation without alteration of total GSK3β expression, compared with NG or HG. PQS treatment significantly attenuated the decreased phosphorylation of GSK3β induced by intermittent high glucose, which was abolished by LY294002 (Figure 4 (B)).

4.　Discussion

There are two novel observations in our present experiment. Firstly, we have provided direct *in vitro* evidence that treatment with PQS attenuates intermittent high glucose-induced oxidative stress injury in HUVECs. Secondly, we have demonstrated that the protective effect of PQS on HUVECs was PI3K/Akt/GSK3β-dependent.

Hyperglycemia is generally regarded as one of the major causes of pathological consequences of both type I and type II diabetes [29]. Much of this damage is thought to be a consequence of elevated production of ROS and oxidative stress has recently been proposed as the unifying

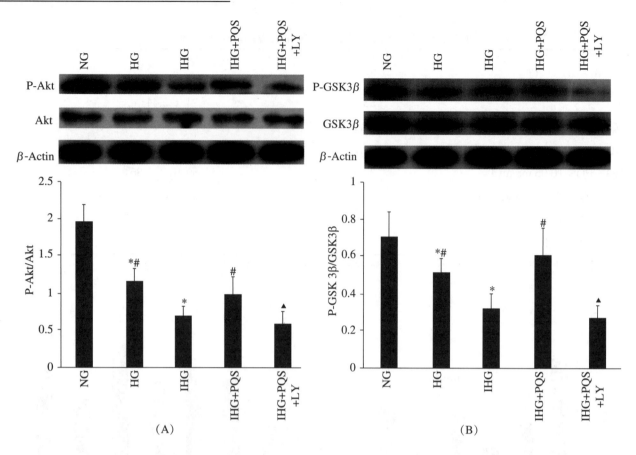

Figure 4   Phosphorylation of Akt（A）and GSK3 β（B）in Cultured Human Umbilical Vein Endothelial Cells Determined by Western Blot. Data obtained from quantitative densitometry were presented as mean ± SD（*n*=3）. Before PQS was added，HUVECs were pretreated with LY294002 for 30 min. $^*P < 0.01$ *vs.* NG，$^\#P < 0.01$ *vs.* IHG；$^\blacktriangle P < 0.01$ *vs.* IHG + PQS. PQS，panax quinquefolius saponin of stem and leaf（0.1 mg/mL）

explanation of the hyper glycemia-related diabetic complications [30,31]. In normal subjects, blood glucose is strictly controlled within a narrow range, while blood glucose in diabetic patients often changes obviously within a single day. Though there is still an extensive debate about glucose variability as a risk factor for complications independent of HbA1c in diabetes [32,33], more and more lines of evidence have found that glucose fluctuations may play a significant role in the pathogenesis of diabetic complications. According to *in vitro* experimental settings and animal studies, fluctuating glucose levels display a more deleterious effect on endothelial cells than constantly high glucose exposure and that this effect should be mediated by an oxidative stress [3-7]. Moreover, human studies have shown that acute and chronic blood glucose fluctuations in T2DM levels could increase oxidative stress significantly [9,10], although short-term glucose variability is not associated with raised oxidative stress markers in healthy volunteers [34].

In this study, we employed a cellular experimental model in which primary cultures of human endothelial cells were exposed to intermittent high glucose, a condition that partly mimics glucose excursions occurring in diabetes *in vivo*. As known to all, MDA is a by-product of lipid peroxidation induced by excessive ROS and widely used as a biomarker of oxidative stress [35]. On the other hand, SOD, as an endogenous antioxidant, plays a pivotal role in preventing cellular damage caused by ROS [36]. Enhanced oxidative damage after diverse stimuli has been confirmed to be an initial event in the development of cardiovascular diseases. In agreement with previous studies [6,7], we confirmed that intermittent high glucose, as seen in diabetic patients, was more deleterious than those of stable high glucose and that oxidative stress was convincingly involved. In our present study, a more obvious decrease of cell viability was observed in HUVECs exposed to intermittent high glucose for 8 days, which was associated with an elevation of MDA production and a significant decrease in SOD. Nonetheless, when HUVECs were preincubated with PQS, these intermittent high glucose-induced cellular events were blocked to agreat extent. These results together suggested that enhancement of endogenous antioxidant preservation and attenuation of lipid peroxidation may represent a major mechanism of cellular protection by PQS.

The underlying mechanism by which PQS protects HUVECs from intermittent high glucose-induced oxidative damage is an important question raised by the results presented in this study.

Akt, downstream of PI3K, is thought to be one of the important factors in cell survival. In endothelial cells, Akt activation has been reported to promote cell survival [37,38]. And evidence has shown that the PI3K/Akt pathway plays an important role in preventing endothelial cell injury induced by high glucose. Our previous study had confirmed that PQS could increase insulin sensitivity by increasing the tyrosine phosphorylation of insulin receptor and IRS1 and the Ser473 phosphorylation of Akt. Based on these observations, we examined the contribution of the PI3K/Akt pathway to the protective effect of PQS. In the present study, we confirmed the inhibitory effect of high glucose on Akt activation as previous report [39] and meanwhile observed a more obvious inhibitory effect in intermittent high glucose condition. We also demonstrated that PQS treatment attenuated the decrease in Akt phosphorylation induced by intermittent high glucose, which was abolished by PI3K inhibitor. Furthermore, LY294002 significantly abolished

the protective effect of PQS on oxidative damage induced by intermittent high glucose, which indicated that PQS exerted its protective effect through PI3K/Akt pathway.

Among the various intracellular downstream effectors of Akt, GSK3β phosphorylation and inactivation are considered important mechanisms of cell survival [40]. In the present study, we confirmed for the first time that decreased GSK3β phosphorylation level was involved in high glucose-induced oxidative damage. And the decrease was even more obvious in intermittent high glucose condition. Pretreatment with PQS significantly improved the decreased GSK3β phosphorylation levels induced by intermittent high glucose, which was also blocked by LY294002, indicating that PQS-promoted GSK3β phosphorylation depends on PI3K-Akt activation. Taken together, these results provide strong evidence that the PI3K/Akt/GSK3β pathway is involved in the antioxidative damage effect of PQS.

In summary, the present study shows that PQS inhibits intermittent high glucose-induced oxidative damage in cultured HUVECs through the PI3K/Akt/GSK3β pathway. It provides further strong evidence that PQS, as well as traditional Chinese herb, might offer an alternative strategy for diabetic cardiovascular complications prevention.

References

[1] Ali MK, Narayan KMV, Tandon N. Diabetes & coronary heart disease：current perspectives. Indian Journal of edical Research, 2010, 132 (11)：584-597.

[2] Brownlee M, Hirsch IB. Glycemic variability：a hemoglobin A1c-independent risk factor for diabetic complications. Journal of the American Medical Association, 2006,295 (14)：1707-1708.

[3] Watada H, Azuma K, Kawamori R. Glucose fluctuation on the progression of diabetic macroangiopathy-new findings frommonocyte adhesion to endothelial cells. Diabetes Research and Clinical Practice, 2007, 77 (3) supplement：S58-S61.

[4] Mita T, Otsuka A, Azuma K, et al. Swings in

477

blood glucose levels accelerate atherogenesis in apolipoprotein E-deficient mice. Biochemical and Biophysical Research Communications, 2007, 358 (3): 679-685.

[5] Piconi L, Quagliaro L, Da Ros R, et al. Intermittent high glucose enhances ICAM-1, VCAM-1, E-selectin and interleukin-6 expression in human umbilical endothelial cells in culture: the role of poly (ADP-ribose) polymerase. Journal of Thrombosis and Haemostasis, 2004, 2 (8): 1453-1459.

[6] Piconi L, Quagliaro L, Assaloni R, et al. Constant and intermittent high glucose enhances endothelial cell apoptosis through mitochondrial superoxide overproduction. Diabetes/Metabolism Research and Reviews, 2006, 22 (3): 198-203.

[7] Horvàth EM, BenkoR, Kiss L, et al. Rapid "glycaemi-cswings" induce nitrosative stress, activate poly (ADP-ribose) polymerase and impair endothelial function in a rat model ofdiabetes mellitus. Diabetologia, 2009, 52 (5): 952-961.

[8] Giacco F, Brownlee M. Oxidative stress and diabetic complications. Circulation Research, 2010,107 (9): 1058-1070.

[9] Chang CM, Hsieh CJ, Huang JC, et al. Acute and chronic fluctuations in blood glucose levels can increase oxidative stress in type 2 diabetes mellitus. Acta Diabetologica, 2012, 49 (supplement 1): S171-S177.

[10] Monnier L, Mas E, Ginet C, et al. Activation of oxidative stress by acute glucose fluctuations compared with sustained chronic hyperglycemia in patients with type 2 diabetes. Journal of the American Medical Association, 2006, 295 (14): 1681-1687.

[11] Lakshmi SVV, Padmaja G, Kuppusamy P, et al. Oxidative stress in cardiovascular disease. Indian Journal of Biochemistry and Biophysics, 2009, 46 (6): 421-440.

[12] Elahi MM, Kong YX, Matata BM. Oxidative stress as a mediator of cardiovascular disease. Oxidative Medicine and Cellular Longevity, 2009, 2 (5): 259-269.

[13] Yin HJ, Zhang Y, Jiang YR, et al. The effect of panax quinquefolium saponins on blood lipid level in Alloxan-Induced hyperglycemia rat model. Chinese Journal of Integrative Medicine on Cardio/Cerebrovascular Disease, 2004, 2 (11): 647-648.

[14] Yin HJ, Zhang Y, Yang LH, et al. The effects of PQS on glucose transport, GLUT4 translocation

and CAP mRNA expression of adipocytes. Chinese Pharmacological Bulletin, 2007, 23 (10): 1332-1337.

[15] Zhang Y, Chen KJ, Yang LH, et al. Effects of panax quinquefolius saponin of stem and leaf on glucose-lipid metabolism and insulin signal transduction in insulin resistant model dipocytes. Zhong guo Zhong Xi Yi Jie He Za Zhi, 2010, 7: 748-751.

[16] Fan BJ, Fei F, Zhao XZ. Effects of panax quinquefolium saponin (PQS) on the vascular endothelial function of the myocardial hypertrophied rats. Chinese Journal of Gerontology, 2009, 29 (7): 811-812.

[17] Zhang Y. Effect of panax quinquefolius saponin on insulin sensitivity in patients of coronary heart disease and its mechanism. China Academy of Chinese Medical Sciences, 2006.

[18] Wang JS, Yin HJ, Guo CY, et al. Influence of high blood glucose fluctuation on the endothelial function of type 2-evidence-based complementary and alternative medicine 7 diabetes mellitus rats and the effects of panax quinquefolius saponin of stem and leaf. Chinese Journal of Integrative Medicine, 2013, 19 (3): 217-222.

[19] Galetic I, Andjelkovic M, Meier R, et al. Mechanism of protein Kinase B activation by insulin/insulin-like growth factor-1 revealed by specific inhibitors of phosphoinositide 3-kinase-significance for diabetes and cancer. Pharmacology and Therapeutics, 1999, 82 (2-3): 409-425.

[20] Hernandez R, Teruel T, Lorenzo M. Akt mediates insulin induction of glucose uptake and up-regulation of GLUT4 gene expression in brown adipocytes. FEBS Letters, 2001, 494 (3): 225-231.

[21] Tremblay F, Lavigne C, Jacques H, et al. Defective insulin-induced GLUT4 translocation in skeletalmuscle of high fat-fed rats is associated with alterations in both Akt/protein kinase B and atypical protein kinase C (zeta/lambda) activities. Diabetes, 2001, 50 (8): 1901-1910.

[22] Vosseller K, Wells L, Lane MD, et al. Elevated nucleocytoplasmic glycosylation by O-GlcNAc results in insulin resistance associated with defects in Akt activation in 3T3-L1 adipocytes. Proceedings of the National Academy of Sciences of the United States of America, 2002, 99 (8): 5313-5318.

[23] Gousseva N, Kugathasan K, Chesterman CN, et al. Early growth response factor-1 mediates insulin-inducible vascular endothelial cell proliferation and regrowth after injury. Journal of Cellular Biochemistry,

2001, 81 (3)：523-534.

[24] Shioi T, McMullen JR, Kang PM, et al. Akt/protein kinase B promotes organ growth in transgenic mice. Molecular and Cellular Biology, 2002, 22 (8)：2799-2809.

[25] De Luca A, Maiello MR, D'Alessio A, et al. The RAS/RAF/MEK/ERK and the PI3K/AKT signaling pathways：role in cancer pathogenesis and implications for therapeutic approaches. Expert Opinion on Therapeutic Targets, 2012, 16 (supplement 2)：S17-S27.

[26] Varma S, Lal BK, Zheng R, et al. Hyperglycemia alters PI3k and Akt signaling and leads to endothelial cell proliferative dysfunction. American Journal of Physiology, 2005, 289 (4)：H1744-H1751.

[27] Zhang W, Wang R, Han SF, et al. α-Linolenic acid attenuates high glucose-induced apoptosis in cultured human umbilical vein endothelial cells via PI3K/Akt/eNOS pathway. Utrition, 2007, 23 (10)：762-770.

[28] Jaffe EA, Nachman RL, Becker CG, et al. Culture of human endothelial cells derived from umbilical veins. Identification by morphologic and immunologic criteria. The Journal of Clinical Investigation, 1973, 52 (11)：2745-2756.

[29] Shamoon H, Duffy H, Fleischer N, et al. The effect of intensive treatment of diabetes on the development and progression of long-term complications in insulin-dependent diabetes mellitus. The New England Journal of Medicine, 1993, 329 (14)：977-986.

[30] Ceriello A, Esposito K, Piconi L, et al. Oscillating glucose is more deleterious to endothelial function and oxidative stress than mean glucose in normal and type 2 diabetic patients. Diabetes, 2008, 57 (5)：1349-1354.

[31] Brownlee M. The pathobiology of diabetic complications：a unifying mechanism. Diabetes, 2005, 54 (6)：1615-1625.

[32] Siegelaar SE, Holleman F, Hoekstra JBL, et al.

Glucose variability: does it matter? Endocrine Reviews, 2010, 31 (2)：171-182.

[33] Kilpatrick ES, Rigby AS, Atkin SL. Glucose variability and diabetes complication risk：we need to know the answer. Diabetic Medicine, 2010，27 (8)：868-871.

[34] Wakil A, Smith KA, Atkin SL, et al. Short term glucose variability in healthy volunteers is not associated with raised oxidative stress markers. Diabetes, Obesity & Metabolism, 2012, 14 (11)：1047-1049.

[35] Cini M, Fariello RG, Bianchetti A, et al. Studies on lipid peroxidation in the rat brain. Neurochemical Research, 1994, 19 (3)：283-288.

[36] Luo T, Xia Z. A small dose of hydrogen peroxide enhances tumor necrosis factor-alpha toxicity in inducing human vascular endothelial cell apoptosis：reversal with propofol. Anesthesia and Analgesia, 2006, 103 (1)：110-116.

[37] Kim I, Kim HG, So JN, et al. Angiopoietin-1 regulates endothelial cell survival through the phosphatidylinositol 3'-kinase/Akt signal transduction pathway. Circulation Research, 2000, 86 (1)：24-29.

[38] Fulton D, Gratton JP, McCabe TG, et al. Regulation of endothelium-derived nitric oxide production by the protein kinase Akt. Nature, 1999, 399 (6376): 597-601.

[39] Ho FM, Lin WW, Chen BC, et al. High glucose-induced apoptosis in human vascular endothelial cells is mediated through NF-κB and c-Jun NH2-terminal kinase pathway and prevented by I3K/Akt/eNOS pathway. Cellular Signalling, 2006, 18 (3)：391-399.

[40] Park KW, Yang HM，Youn SW, et al. Constitutively active glycogen synthase kinase-3β gene transfer sustains apoptosis, inhibits proliferation of vascular smooth muscle cells, and reduces neointima formation after balloon injury in rats. Arteriosclerosis, Thrombosis, and Vascular Biology, 2003, 23(8): 1364-1369.

第
五
章

Effect of Puerarin on the PI3K Pathway for Glucose Transportation and Insulin Signal Transduction in Adipocytes[*]

ZHAO Ying   ZHOU You   YIN Hui-jun   ZHANG Ying

Puerarin, one of the active ingredients of kudzuvine root, has extensive bioactivity, especially its effects in treating diabetes mellitus and in alleviating insulin resistance had been proved by lots of researches and received universal attention in present years[1-3]. But there is no report yet regarding its effect on insulin resistance signal transduction so far. In this article, the effects of puerar in on glucose metabolism and the molecular mechanism of its improvement on insulin resistance were explored by using insulin resistance adipocytes model induced by free fatty acid, and the insulin receptor (IR), insulin receptor substrate-1 (IRS-1) and protein expression of protein kinase B (PKB) as the indexes were investigated.

1. Materials

1.1　Cell Line, Testing Drug and Reagents

The 3T 3-L1 cell line comes from American Type Culture Collection (ATCC) was purchased from the Center of Cells, Peking Union Medical College, Chinese Academy of Medical Sciences.

Puerarin injection was the product of Yantai Luyin Pharmaceutical Group, batch No.0310211.

The biosynthetic insulin injection was purchased from Nuohenuode Co., Danmark, batch No. PW52526；cetylic acid from Beijing Company of Chemical Reagents, batch No.940902；C salt from Celite Co. and Serva Co.；Cytochalasin B from Sigm a Co.；2-deoxy-d-glucose from Beijing Co. Ltd. of Atomic Nuclear Tech.；rabbit multi-clonal phosphorylated insulin receptor antibody (Lot3021) from Cell Signaling Co.；mouse multi-clonal PKB antibody (Lot 27730) from Upstate Co. and goat multi-clonal phosphory lated IRS-1 antibody (Lot D0104) from Saanta Cruz Co.

1.2　Chief Instruments

Thermostatic CO_2 incubator was product of REVCO, USA；liquid-scintillator, product of Perkin Elmer Co.；centrifuge type 3K30，product of Sigma Co.；enzyme labeling apparatus, product of TECAN Co.，and the Sartorius analytical balance type BP211D, product of Gilson SAS Co.

2. Methods

2.1　Lypocyt Differentiation

After the 3T 3-L1 preadipocytes being cultured in the protoculture fluid to form cellular fusion, they were cultured for 48h, referring to Ross's method[4]，with the Iscove's modified Dulbecco's medium (IMDM), containing 10% fetal bovine serum (FBS), 1μM dexam ethasone, 10μg/mL insulin and 0.5mM of isobutyl methyl xanthine, and then the cells were continuously cultured in IMDM containing 10μg/mL insulin and 10% FBS (changed every 2-3 days), until the 9th day, when over 90% cells was differentiated to mature adipocytes.

2.2　Establishment of Insulin Resistance Model

* 原载于 Journal of Harbin Institute of Technology (New Series), 2009，16 (1)：47-50

and Grouping

The mature adipocytes were seeded in six-well culture dishes and divided into 6 groups,. ie. the model group, the control group, and the drug administrating groups treated respectively with dimethyl biguanide (DMBG 1mM), high (1.5mg/mL) and low (0.75mg/mL) concentration of puerarin (Group Pue H and Pue L) and propyleneglycol (1.5mg/mL, Group PG).

Cells in the model group and the 4 treated groups were incubated firstly for 12h with Krebs-Ringer phosphate (KRP) buffer (131.2 mmol/L NaCl, 4.71mmol/L KCl, 2.48mmol/L Na$_3$PO$_4$· 12H$_2$O, 1.24mmol/L MgSO$_4$, 2.47mmol/ L CaCl$_2$, and 10mmol/L hydroxyethyl piperazine ethanesulfonic acid, pH=7.2-7.4) containing 0.65 mmol/L cetylic acid, 1% benzenesulfonic acid (BSA) and 10nmol/L glucose, 2mL in each well. The solution was renewed every 4h. For the cells in the control group, they were incubated in the same way but without cetylic acid in buffer. Then they were washed twice with KRP buffer containing 1 mmol/L sodium pyruvate and 1% BSA, and then incubated with same solution for 1h, washed with D-Hank's solution for two times, incubated again with whole IMDM, to establish the model successfully. The model cells in the drug treated groups were continuously incubated with corresponding testing drugs. Ready for following experiments.

2.3 Determination of Glucose Consumption in Insulin Resistant Adipocytes

After 24 h incubation the culture was taken to determine the residue volume of glucose by glucose oxidase method. The glucose consumption was calculated based on the glucose content in the culture without cell incubated.

2.4 Determination of Glucose Transportation after Insulin Stimulation

The model cells after being reacted with corresponding testing drugs for 48 h were washed three times with D-Hank's solution; added in IMDM with 100nmol/L of rapidly effective insulin to incubate 30min under 37℃; added 20μL of 2-Deoxy-d-1-3H glucose mother fluid to make the final concentration 50μmoL/L and the radio-activity 1μCi/mL, incubated 10min; washed with ice PBS twice; cracked by 0.1mol/L NaOH, 1mL for each well. Then the fluid with cracked cells was divided into two portions and placed in two 1.5mL EP tubes, preserved under −20 ℃. One portion is for determining the radio-activity with liquid-scintillator by adding 200 μL scintillation solution into 100μL of the fluid. The other is for measuring the protein concentration for correcting the intake of 3H-glucose. Besides, two pore cells incubated with medium containing Cytochalas in B was treated in the same way as mentioned above, and the data was taken as the non-specific intake of 3H-glucose, then, the specific intake after insulin stimulation could be obtained by subtract it from the amount of scintillate counting.

2.5 Analysis of IR, IRS-1 and PKB Protein Expressions

2.5.1 Preparation of Cellular Protein Sample

Cellular protein sample was prepared along the following procedures. Cells were stimulated with 150nmol of human insulin; washed once with 6mL of ice PBS for each plate; digested with 6mL of pancreatin digestion solution for each plate; collect the supernate into a 15mL centrifuge tube and then centrifuged at 1000r/m in for 5min; blowing washed twice with 2mL of ice PBS; centrifuged at 1000r/m in for 5min; cracked with 50μL of modified RIPA buffer (consisted of Tris-HCl 50mM, pH 7.4; NP 40.2%; Triton X-100 1%; Sodium deoxycholate 0.5%; NaCl 150mM; EDTA 1mM; PMSF 1mM; Na$_3$VO$_4$ 1mM; NaF 1mM); separated into two 0.5mL EP tubes, one for determining protein concentration using Bradford Coomassie dyebinding assay, the other for being preserved under −80℃ for Western blot.

2.5.2 Western Blot Test The Western blot test was conducted as follows: the sample was diluted with buffer, $20\mu L$ for every $10\mu L$ of cell cracked solution; boiled at 95-100 ℃ for 5min; carried out SDS-PAGE protein electrophoresis with 3% concentrated latex and 10% separating latex for every $20\mu L$ of sample in each well; wiped nitro-cellulose film by soaking the sample in the film wipping solution (containing 20% methanol being double diluted with electrode buffer solution) for 5min, semidry processed, $0.8mA/cm^2$, 1h. Then the blocking and antibody incubation was conducted: blocked with TBS/T plus 5% (W/V) skim milk powder, room temperature, shook for 1h; washed three times with TBS/T, 5min each time; incubated in a hybrid bag with prim aryantibody (diluted to 1:100 with blocking fluid, 4 ℃, overnight); washed three times with TBS/T, 5min each time; incubated in a hybrid bag with secondary antibody (diluted to 1:100 with blocking fluid, room temperature, 1.5h); washed three times with TBS/T, 5min each time. And finally, the sample was colorated with enhanced chemical luminescent method with 2 min of exposure.

2.6 Data Management and Statistical Analysis

All the data obtained were expressed by mean±standard deviation and analyzed using the software SPSS 8.0. The comparison among multiple groups was conducted adopting single variance analysis, $P < 0.05$ was regarded as having statistical significance, and $P < 0.01$ as having very significant difference.

3. Results

3.1 Effect of Puerarin on the Glucose Consumption

The experiment data listed in Tab 1, showed that the glucose consumption in the model group was lower than that in the control group ($P < 0.01$), indicating that the free fatty acid could reduce the glucose consumption, and induce insulin resistance, which was identical with the outcome reported. Compared with the model

group, the glucose consumption in group DMBG, Pue H and Pue L significantly increased, but not changed in group PG, indicating that both DMBG and puerarin, either high or low dose, could promote the glucose utilization of adipocytes, while propylene, as a solvent, couldn't influence it at all.

Table 1 Effects of Puerarin on the Glucose Consumption ($n=6$, $\bar{\chi} \pm s$)

Group	Consumption of glucose/ (mmol/L)
Control	3.45 ± 0.09
Model	2.68 ± 0.19**
DMBG	3.33 ± 0.09▲▲
Pue H	3.12 ± 0.08▲▲#
Pue L	2.89 ± 0.10▲
PG	2.71 ± 0.22*

Notes: *$P < 0.05$, **$P < 0.01$, compared with control group; ▲$P < 0.05$, ▲▲$P < 0.01$, compared with model group; #$P < 0.01$, compared with the PG

3.2 Effect of Puerarin on Insulin Stimulated Glucose Transportation

Data in the Tab. 2 showed that the radio activity, indicating the glucose transportation was significantly lower in model group than that in control group, suggesting that free fatty acid could reduce the intake of glucose in adipocytes, which indicated the success of model establishing. As compared with that in model group, the radio activity was significantly higher in group DMBG, Pue H and Pue L, which illustrated that both DMBG and puerarin could enhance the sensitivity of adipocytes to insulin and thus to alleviate the insulin resistance.

Table 2 Effects of Puerarin on Glucose Transportation ($n=6$, $\bar{\chi} \pm s$)

Group	Glucose transportation/ (pmol/μg)
Control	5.05 ± 0.66
Model	2.23 ± 0.63*
DMBG	4.29 ± 0.70▲
Pue H	3.92 ± 0.55▲#
Pue L	4.09 ± 0.29▲#
PG	2.70 ± 0.45

Notes: *$P < 0.01$, compared with the control group; ▲$P < 0.01$, compared with the model group; #$P < 0.01$, compared with the PG

3.3 Effect of Puerarin on IR, IR-1 and PKB Expression

As shown in Figures 1-3, the levels of tyrosine phosphory lation of IR subunitβ, IRS-1 and PKB Ser473 were lower in model group than that in control group respectively. As compared with the model group, the level of tyrosine phosphorylation of IR was significantly higher in groups of Pue H, Pue L and DMBG, and puerarin showed the effect superior to that of BMDG. Besides, low dose of puerar in showed a significant effecting increasing tyrosine phosphorylation of IRS-1 level, but all the testing drugs showed insignificant effect on that of PKB Ser473.

4. Discussions

Fat tissue could secrete several active substances to influence the insulin sensitivity and metabolic balance in organism, besides, the adipocytes themselves are the target tissue of insulin action, involved in metabolic diseases. Adipocytes has been regarded as the best cell model for studying them echanism of insulin in promoting glucose transportation signal.

The insulin resistance, in previous studies, are mostly induced by high insulin or high glucose[5,6]. But since the recognition on pathogenesis of insulin resistance is turned from glucose metabolism centered to lipid-toxic theory, which holds that it could be directly induced by the elevation of blood plasm a free fatty acid[7], therefore, the author considered that an insulin resistance adipocytes model induced by free fatty acid used in this study was more suitable than others for its higher conformity to the nature developing process of insulin resistance.

It is well-known in current studies that the paths of insulin stimulating glucose transportation are mainly the phosphatidylinosito-l3-kinase pathway (PI3K pathway) and the Cb1/CAP pathway. The PI3K mediated path is the principal one for insulin signal transduction, which initiated from the phosphorylation of IR, with the IRS-1 and

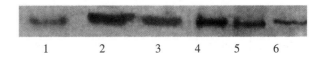

Figure 1   Result of Western Blot on Phosphorylation of IR Protein Expression

1.Model；2.Control；3.DMBG；4.Pue H；5.Pue L；6.PG

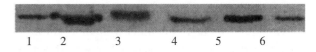

Figure 2   Result of Western Blot on Phosphorylation of IRS-1 Protein Expression

1.Model；2.Control；3.DMBG；4.Pue H；5.Pue L；6.PG

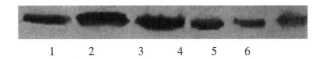

Figure 3   Result of Western Blot on PPK-B Protein Expression

1.Model；2.Control；3.DMBG；4.Pue H；5.Pue L；6.PG

PKB as the key proteins for signal transmission[7]. Results of this study showed that after insulin resistance being induced in adipocytes by free fatty acid, the insulin stimulated tyrosine phosphorylation level of IR and IRS-1, as well as the phosphorylation level and activity of PKB Ser473 reduced significantly, which lead to the blocking of insulin signal transduction, and finally the obstacle of glucose transportation, lowering of glucose intake and utilization in adipocytes and decrease of glucose consumption. The results also showed that both puerarin and DMBG could increase the tyrosine phosphorylation level of IR subunit β；low dose of puerarin could also obviously raise the tyrosine phosphorylation level of IRS-1 level, suggesting that the mechanism of puerarin on promoting glucose transportation and consumption in adipocytes to alleviate insulin resistance might be related with its effects in enhancing the tyrosine phosphorylation of IR and IRS-1.

References

[1] Zhang L, Chen L, Ni HX, et al. Effect of puerarin on glucose transportation protein 4 expression of fatty

cells in rats diabetic model induced by streptozotocin. Chinese Journal of Clinical Rehabilitation, 2006, 10 (39)：135-138.

[2] Cao L, GU ZL, Mao CP. Effect of puerarin on insulin resistance in diabetic mice. Chinese Traditional and Herbal Drugs, 2006, 37 (6)：901-904.

[3] Han HM, Wang SHG. Study on the treatment of insulin resistance with puerarin in patients with non-insulin dependent diabetes mellitus. Chinese Journal of Integrated Traditional Chinese and Western Medicine in Intensive and Critical Care, 2006, 13 (2)：117-119.

[4] Ross SA, Chen XL, Hope H, et al. Development and comparison of two 3T3-L1 adipocyte models of insulin

resistance：increased glucose flux vs glucosamine treatment. Biochem Biophys Res Commun, 2000, 273 (3)：1033-1041.

[5] LI CHG, Ningguang, Chen JL. Establishment and certification of Hep G2 cell model of insulin resistance. Chinese Journal of Diabetes, 1999, 7：198-200.

[6] Wu Hr, Xiang GSH, LU HL, et al. Insulin resistance of fat cell induced by high concentrated glucose. Journal of Hua Zhong University of Sciences and Technology (Medica ledition), 2006, 35 (1)：66-78.

[7] Chen JI, Jia WP, Li Q, et al. Relationship between the serum free fatty acid and insulin secretory function in early stage sugar regulation impaired patients. Shanghai Medicine, 2004, 27：470-472.

Expression Changes of Akt and GSK-3β during Vascular Inflammatory Response and Oxidative Stress Induced by High-fat Diet in Rats[*]

WANG Jing-shang   YIN Hui-jun   HUANG Ye   GUO Chun-yu   XIA Cheng-dong   ZHANG Lu

1. Introduction

Atherosclerosis is the pathological basis of cardiovascular diseases which represent the leading cause of death worldwide；and recent epidemiological data have strongly suggested that hyperlipidemia, characterized by elevated serum total cholesterol and low density and very low density lipoprotein cholesterol and decreased high density lipoprotein, is an important risk factor for coronary heart disease and this increased risk appears to be independent of other known risk factors [1,2]. Recent research has shown that inflammation plays a key role in coronary artery disease and atherosclerosis development [3,4]. It also has become clear that oxidative stress represents a common pathogenic mechanism

for atherosclerosis, from lipid streaks formation to plaque rupture and thrombosis. A particularly important mechanism for ROS-mediated atherosclerosis appears to be through stimulation of proinflammatory events [5]. Among all confirmed mechanisms, vascular endothelium injury is claimed to an important initial event at the onset of atherosclerosis [6].

Phosphatidylinositol-3-kinase (PI3K) and Akt are downstream effectors of insulin signaling as well as important signaling molecules in the regulation of glycogen metabolism in myocytes, lipocytes, and hepatocyte. By regulating angiogenesis, proliferation, microvascular permeability, survival, cellular transformation, and embryonic differentiation, PI3K/Akt also

* 原载于 Journal of Biomedical Science and Engineering, 2013，6：1-5

plays an important role in the regulation of endothelial cell functions [7]. Among the various intracellular downstream effectors of Akt, GSK-3β phosphorylation and inactivation are considered important mechanisms of cell survival [8]. However, as yet, little is known about the role of Akt and GSK-3β expressions in the vascular endothelium inflammation and oxidative stress induced by hyperlipidemia.

Therefore, in the current study, we aimed to determine the influence of high-fat diet feeding on endothelial inflammation and oxidative stress in rats and thus to investigate the possible role of PI3K/Akt/GSK-3β pathway involved.

2. Materials and Methods

2.1 Drugs and Reagents

Superoxide dismutase (SOD) and malondialdehyde (MDA) assay kits were obtained from Nanjing Jiancheng Bioengineering Institute, China. Enzyme-linked immunosorbent assay (ELISA) kitsof soluble intercellular adhesion molecule 1 (sICAM-1), tumor necrosis factor α (TNF-α), hepatocytegrowth factor (HGF) and Lectin-like oxidized cellulose low density lipoprotein receptor-1 (LOX-1) were all purchased from R&D (USA). The antibodies against Akt, phosphorylated-Akt (Ser473), GSK-3β, phosphorylated-GSK3β (Ser9) and β-actin were purchased from Cell Signaling Technology (USA). All other biochemicals used were of the highest purity available.

2.2 Establishment of Hyperlipidmia Model and Groupsing

20 male Sprague-Dawley rats, 180-220g, were obtained from Vital River Laboratory Animal Technology Co. Ltd. Beijing. Rats were housed in the facility at Xiyuan hospital, China Academy of Chinese Medical Sciences according to the guidelines for laboratory animals approved by Beijing Experimental Animal Management Center. After 1 week of adaption, 10 rats were selected randomly to switch from normal diet (control group, CON) to high fat diet (hyperlipidmia group,

HLP) which contained 10% fat (wt/wt), 10% sugar (wt/wt), 2.5% cholesterol (wt/wt) and cholate 0.25%(wt/wt) for 18 weeks.

The establishment of the hyperlipidmic rats was evaluated by analyzing blood lipid levels including TC, TG, LDL-C and HDL-C.

2.3 Specimen Collection

At the 20th week, all rats were executed after anesthesia with intraperitoneal injection of 20% urethane (0.6 mL/ 100g, fasting 12 h before sampling). Blood samples were collected from abdominal aorta. The aorta was removed for Westen-blot analysis.

2.4 Assay for Lipid Parameter, MDA and SOD

TC and TG were determined by enzymic technique. HDL-C and LDL-C were analyzed by immunoturbidimetry. The activities of SOD and the concentration of MDA were both determined by using commercially available kits.

2.5 ELISA Assay

Serum TNF-α, soluble ICAM-1 (sICAM-1) levels and plasma HGF and LOX-1 from rats were measured by ELISA according to the instructions from R&D Systems (USA).

2.6 Western Blot Analysis

Total protein (50 mg/lane) from aorta was separated by SDS-PAGE and transferred to a polyvinylidene fluoride membrane. After incubation in blocking solution (5% nonfat milk) (Sigma), membranes were incubated with primary antibodies for Akt, phosphorylated Akt, GSK3β, phosphorylated-GSK-3β or β-actin for overnight at 4°C. Membranes were washed and then incubated with 1 : 2000 dilution horseradish peroxidase-conjugated secondary antibody (ZSGB-BIO, Beijing, China). The relative density of each protein band was normalized to that of β-actin. All results were representative of at least 3 independent experiments.

2.7 Statistical Analysis

The results were presented as means ± SD. The SPSS statistics 15.0 package was utilized to analyze the data. Differences between these two groups were analyzed using t test. The $P < 0.05$

was considered statistically significant.

3. Results

3.1 Effect of High-Fat Diet on Body Weight and Serum Lipid Parameters

As shown in Table 1, compared to the control, the body weight and the serum levels of TC, TG, LDL-C increased after high-fat diet for 18 weeks ($P < 0.05$ or $P < 0.01$), whereas the HDL-C level in sera decreased significantly ($P < 0.01$).

3.2 Effect of High-Fat Diet on Plasma HGF and LOX-1 Levels

As shown in Figure 1, plasma HGF and LOX-1 levels showed a significant in crease in rats with high-fat diet compared with the control ($P < 0.01$).

3.3 Effect of High-Fat Diet on Serum SOD and MDA Levels

As shown in Table 2, after high-fat diet for 18 weeks, the serum level of SOD decreased significantly ($P < 0.01$), whereas MDA level increased obviously compared with the control ($P < 0.01$).

3.4 Effect of High-Fat Diet on Serum TNF-α and sICAM-1 Levels

As shown in Figure 2, compared with the control, serum levels of TNF-α and sICAM-1 increased significantly ($P < 0.01$), which indicated that inflammation activated and

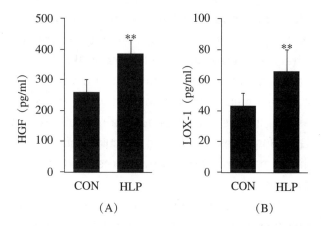

Figure 1 Changes in Plasma Hepatocyte Growth Factor（HGF, pg/mL）（A）and Lectin-Like Oxidized Cellulose Low Density Lipoprotein Receptor-1（LOX-1, pg/ml）（B）Levels after High-fat Diet for 18 Weeks. Data are presented as the means ± SD.（n= 10）. **$P < 0.01$, Compared with the control group

increased cell adhesion ability in rats with high-fat diet for 18 weeks.

3.5 Effect of High-Fat Diet on Akt and GSK-3β Phosphorylation Levels

To investigate the underlining mechanism of high fat diet induced endothelial injury accompanied by obvious inflammation and oxidative stress, we examined the expression changes of Akt and GSK-3β in rat aorta. As shown in Figure 3, in comparison with the control, the protein phosphorylation of Akt and GSK-3β decreased obviously in rats with high-fat diet.

Table 1 Changes of Body Weight and Serum Lipid Parameters

Group	Body weight（g）	TC（mmol/L）	TG（mmol/L）	HDL-C（mmol/L）	LDL-C（mmol/L）
NOR	577.83 ± 40.10	1.10 ± 0.23	0.66 ± 0.23	0.48 ± 0.05	0.34 ± 0.07
HLP	646.00 ± 52.78*	3.78 ± 0.16**	1.58 ± 0.16**	0.28 ± 0.06**	0.63 ± 0.09**

Data are presented as the means ± SD（$n = 10$）. *$P < 0.05$, **$P < 0.01$, compared with the control group

Table 2 Effect of High-fat Diet on Serum SOD and MDA Levels

Group	SOD（U/mg protein）	MDA（nmmol/mg protein）
NOR	43.79 ± 11.48	2.93 ± 0.70
HLP	27.50 ± 2.52**	5.15 ± 0.63**

Data are presented as the means ± SD（$n = 10$）. **$P < 0.01$, compared with the control group

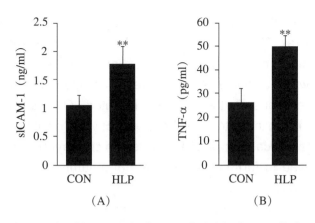

Figure 2　Changes in Serum Soluble Intercellular Adhesion Molecule 1（sICAM-1，ng/mL）（A）and Tumor Necrosis Factor α（TNF-α，pg/ml）（B）Levels After High-fat Diet for 18 Weeks. Data are presented as the means ±SD（n = 10）.P < 0.01, compared with the control group**

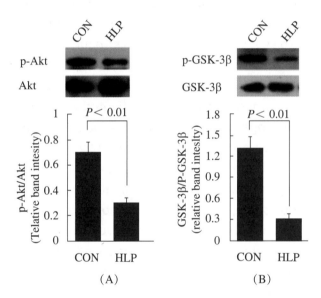

Figure 3　Phosphorylation of Akt（a）and GSK-3β（b）in Rat Aorta was Determined by Western Blot. Data obtained from quantitative densitometry were presented as mean ±SD of 3 independent experiments

4. Discussion

Hyperlipidemia is an independent risk factor of atherosclerosis [1]. Epidemiological investigations so far have shown that the plasma cholesterol levels are increased in most patients with atherosclerosis and the severity of atherosclerosis is positively correlated with the increase of plasma low density lipoprotein and total cholesterol levels [2]. Animals fed a fatty diet with long term showed marked atherosclerosis [9,10], further proof showed that hyperlipidemia played an important role in the atherosclerosis development. In recent years, it has become apparent that atherosclerosis is a chronic inflammatory process affecting large- and medium-sized arteries throughout the cardiovascular system. And inflammation has been recognized as an important initial event at the onset of atherosclerosis, meanwhile involved in the development of atherosclerosis [11]. Besides, some experts have pointed out that abnormal lipid metabolism and inflammation are the most promising targets for the atherosclerosis intervention. Therefore, it will give us more effective means for atherosclerosis intervention by exploring the explicit pro-inflammatory effects of hyperlipidemia and its detailed mechanism.

In our study, animal model of hyperlipidemia was verified by measurement of body weight and blood lipid levels. After high-fat diet for 18 weeks, we observed the obvious increase in body weight, TC, TG, and LDL-c levels and decreased HDL-c level in SD rats. Plasma HGF, which increases significantly along with the aggravation of injury, has been identified as a protective factor of vascular endothelial injury. So, herein HGF was used to evaluate the extent of vascular injury [12]. Our study showed that the plasma HGF level was increased obviously in rats with high-fat diet compared with the control, which indicated that a short-term high-fat diet can lead to obvious vascular endothelial injury.

Oxidative stress and inflammation are the main mechanisms of vascular endothelial injury, which has been thought as the initial step of atherosclerosis [13]. As known, MDA is a by-product of lipid peroxidation induced by excessive ROS and widely used as a biomarker of oxidative stress [14]. On the other hand, SOD, as an endogenous antioxidant, plays a pivotal role in preventing cellular damage caused by ROS and indicates antioxidant capacity of the body [14,15]. In our present study, marked MDA content increase

第五章

and SOD activity decrease were found in rats with high-fat diet, which indicated that 18 weeks-high-fat diet can induce obvious oxidative stress in rats accompanied by significant antioxidant capacity decrease.

Previous experiments have shown that the elevated blood lipids can increase the phosphoinositide hydrolysis, synthesis and release of endothelin in endothelial cells, then activate the endothelial adhesion molecules secretion and promote the circulating monocytes adhesion to vascular well. Tumor necrosis factor α (TNF-α), as an important medium in inflammation and multiple pathophysiological processes, can lead to a series of inflammatory damage and mediate the adhesion of leukocytes to vascular endothelial cells [16]. Intercellular adhesion molecules (ICAMs), as one part of the immunoglobulin superfamily, play important role in inflammation, immune responses and in intracellular signalling events [17]. Animal experiments confirmed that the degree of atherosclerosis decreased significantly in Apolipoprotein E-deficient (ApoE$^{-/-}$) mice with ICAM-1 knockout [18]. In clinical studies, the serum level of ICAM-1 in patients with atherosclerosis is higher than that in the healthy control, which decreased gradually when patients getting better. Therefore, adhesion molecules have been regarded as a key factor in the pathogenesis of atherosclerosis. Oxidized low density lipoprotein (ox-LDL) plays a critical role in the development of atherosclerosis [19]. Recent studies show that ox-LDL may be the main factor inducing endothelial cells and smooth muscle cells injury [20]. Lectin-like oxidized low-density lipoprotein (ox-LDL) receptor-1 (LOX-1) is the primary endothelial receptor for ox-LDL, and both its expression and function are associated with vascular inflammation. And ox-LDL has been shown to upregulate expression of LOX-1 [19]. Meanwhile LOX-1 can upregulate the expressions of VCAM-1, ICAM-1, E-selectin and MCP-1 and can lead to the aggregation of monocytes to

endothelial cells [21]. In this study, we observed that TNF-α and ICAM-1 levels increased significantly after high-fat diet for 18 weeks, which indicating obvious vascular inflammatory reactions. Furthermore, the elevated LOX-1 level in sera indicated that there were obvious oxidative modifications of LDL in rats, which may in turn lead to further development of inflammatory in artery.

Phosphatidylinositol-3-kinase/protein kinase B (PI3K/Akt) signaling pathway is an important cell signaling pathways in vivo, which plays an important role in the cell mobilization, migration, differentiation and apoptosis [7]. Meanwhile, PI3K/Akt signaling pathway, as one of the insulin signaling pathways, plays an important role in the glucose transport, glycogen synthesis, glycolysis and gluconeogenesis regulation, and the protein synthesis and lipolysis process [22]. Akt is the most important signaling molecule of the downstream in PI3K. Activated Akt has a wide range of biological effects including anti-apoptosis and prosurvival functions by promoting the glycogen synthase kinase-3β (GSK-3β) phosphorylation, a downstream effector of Akt [8]. In our study, decreased phosphorylation levels of Akt and GSK-3β were observed in rat aorta after 18 weeks' high-fat diet, which indicated that elevated blood lipids might inhibit the activity of PI3K/Akt obviously.

Collectively, our study confirmed that short-term high-fat diet can damage the function of endothelium, and the main mechanism may be the inflammatory response induced by oxidative stress, meanwhile PI3K/Akt/GSK-3β pathway plays an important role in the process.

References

[1] Malloy MJ, Kane JP. Hyperlipidemia and cardiovascular disease. Current Opinion in Lipidology, 2012, 23: 591-592.

[2] Ingelsson E, Massaro JM, Sutherland P, et al. Contemporary trends in dyslipidemia in the Framingham Heart Study. Archives of Internal Medicine, 2009, 169: 279-286.

[3] Ross R. Atherosclerosis—an inflammatory disease. The New England Journal of Medicine, 1999, 340：115-126.

[4] Hansson GK. Inflammation, atherosclerosis, and coronary artery disease. The New England Journal of Medicine, 2005, 352：1685-1695.

[5] Stocker, R, Keaney Jr, JF. Role of oxidative modifications in atherosclerosis. Physiological Reviews, 2004, 84：1381-1478.

[6] Vanhoutte PM. Endothelial dysfunction：the first step toward coronary arteriosclerosis. Circulation Journal, 2009, 73：595-601.

[7] Franke TF. PI3K/Akt：getting it right matters. Oncogene, 2008, 27：6473-6488.

[8] Park KW Yang, HM, Youn SW, et al. Constitutively active glycogen synthase kinase-3beta gene transfer sustains apoptosis, inhibits proliferation of vascular smooth muscle cells, and reduces neointima formation after balloon injury in rats. Arteriosclerosis, Thrombosis, and Vascular Biology, 2003, 23: 1364-1369.

[9] Jenner A, Ren M, Rajendran R, et al. Zinc supplementation inhibits lipid peroxidation and the development of atherosclerosis in rabbits fed a high cholesterol diet. Free Radical Biology & Medicine, 2006, 42：559-566.

[10] Ma KL, Ruan XZ, Powis, SH, et al. Inflammatory stress exacerbates lipid accumulation in hepatic cells and fatty livers of apolipoprotein e knockout mice. Hepatology, 2008, 48：770-781.

[11] Davis NE. Atherosclerosis—an inflammatory process. Journal of Insurance Medicine, 2005, 37：72-75.

[12] Jiang, WG, Hiscox S. Hepatocyte growth factor/scatter factor, a cytokine playing multiple and converse roles. Histology and Histopathology, 1997, 12：537-555.

[13] Bonomini F, Tengattini S, Fabiano A, et al. Atherosclerosis and oxidative stress. Histology and Histopathology, 2008, 23：381-390.

[14] Del Rio D, Stewart AJ, Pellegrini N. A review of studies on malondialdehyde as toxic molecule and biological marker of oxidative stress. Nutrition, Metabolism & Cardiovascular Diseases, 2005, 15，316-328.

[15] Luo T, Xia Z. A small dose of hydrogen peroxide enhances tumor necrosis factor alpha toxicity in inducing human vascular endothelial cell apoptosis：reversal with propofol. Anesthesia & Analgesia, 2006, 103: 110-116.

[16] Kleinbongard P, Heusch G, Schulz, R. TNF-alpha in atherosclerosis, myocardial ischemia/reperfusion and heart failure. Pharmacology & Therapeutics, 2010, 127：295-314.

[17] Frank PG, Lisanti MP. ICAM-1：role in inflammation and in the regulation of vascular permeability. American Journal of Physiology—Heart and Circulatory Physiology, 2008, 295: H926-H927.

[18] Bourdillon MC, Poston RN, Covacho C, et al. ICAM-1 deficiency reduces atherosclerotic lesions in double-knockout mice (ApoE（-/-）/ICAM-1 (-/-)）fed a fat or a chow diet. Arteriosclerosis, Thrombosis, and Vascular Biology, 2000, 20: 2630-2635.

[19] Mitra S, Goyal T, Mehta JL. Oxidized LDL, LOX-1 and atherosclerosis. Cardiovascular Drugs and Therapy, 2011, 25: 419-429.

[20] Girona J, Manzanares JM, Marimón F, et al. Oxidized to non-oxidized lipoprotein ratios are associated with arteriosclerosis and the metabolic syndrome in diabetic patients. Nutrition, Metabolism &Cardiovascular Diseases, 2008, 18: 380-387.

[21] Chen M, Masaki T, Sawamura T. LOX-1，the receptor for oxidized low-density lipoprotein identified from endothelial cells：implications in endothelial dysfunction and atherosclerosis. Pharmacology & Therapeutics, 2002, 95: 89-100.

[22] Riley JK, Carayannopoulos MO, Wyman AH, et al. Phosphatidylinositol 3-kinase activity is critical for glucose metabolism and embryo survival in murine blastocysts. The Journal of Biological Chemistry, 2006, 281：6010-6019.

第
五
章

第六章

名老中医经验继承

陈可冀院士冠心病病证结合治疗方法学的创新和发展 *

史大卓

病证结合是传统中医学临床诊治疾病的一种重要方法,早在 2000 年前的中医经典《黄帝内经》中就已初具雏形;东汉张仲景在《黄帝内经》的基础上,建立了在辨病论治体系下辨证论治的模式;唐代孙思邈《千金方》中既有辨病论治,按病列方,也有在辨病基础上辨证论治,按证列方。清代徐灵胎《兰台规范》指出:"欲治病者,必先识病之名,能识病名,而后求其病之所由生,知其所由生,又当辨其生之因各不同,而病状所由异,然后考其治之法。"陈可冀院士在前人基础上,倡导并践行病证结合方法治疗疾病,尤其在冠心病治疗方面,病证结合应用活血化瘀法,显著提高了临床疗效。

1. 活血化瘀法治疗冠心病心绞痛

冠心病是危害人类健康的重大疾病,我国目前冠心病死亡率约为 86.9/10 万,而且呈逐年上升趋势 [1]。冠心病心绞痛是由于冠状动脉供血不足,心肌急剧、暂时缺血与缺氧引起的临床综合征,以阵发性胸前压榨性疼痛为主要特点,属中医学"胸痹"、"心痛"的范畴。汉代张仲景将胸痹心痛的病机概括为"阳微阴弦",指出"阳微阴弦,即胸痹而痛,所以然者,责其极虚故也。今阳虚知其在上焦,所以胸痹、心痛者,以其阴弦故也",并创立了栝蒌薤白白酒汤、栝蒌薤白半夏汤、枳实薤白桂枝汤等系列宣痹通阳方剂。宋代伊始,活血化瘀法被应用于治疗胸痹心痛,《太平圣惠方》《圣济总录》等书中均载有不少以活血化瘀立法治疗胸痹心痛的方剂。明清时期,某些医家开始重视行气开郁法,如王肯堂强调"凡治诸般心痛,必以开郁行气为主,此其要法也"。

在继承传统学术思想的基础上,陈可冀院士认为冠心病心绞痛患者血小板黏附、聚集,血栓形成,微循环障碍,动脉内膜增厚,脂质沉积,血管狭窄等病理改变,皆可影响血液的正常运行,导致血行不畅,滞而不行,因此可将其归属于中医"血瘀"的范畴 [2];冠心病患者胸痛、舌色紫暗、瘀点

瘀斑、舌下脉曲张、口唇发绀等,皆为瘀血的临床表征。陈院士将宏观表征与微观病理改变有机结合,认为冠心病心绞痛主要中医病机为"血脉瘀滞",活血化瘀治法可作为中医治疗冠心病的基本治法。根据血瘀兼证虚实的不同,相继研制了冠心 II 号方、抗心梗合剂、愈梗通瘀汤、愈心痛方、川芎嗪、元胡索素、赤芍 801、芎芍胶囊等 10 余种活血化瘀方药治疗冠心病,并首先在国内采用随机、双盲、双模拟方法进行临床试验评价活血化瘀中药治疗冠心病的效果,证实活血化瘀法治疗冠心病心绞痛,具有改善心绞痛症状、抗心肌缺血的作用,开辟了中医药及中西医结合临床双盲随机对照试验的先河 [3]。

陈可冀院士不仅倡导活血化瘀治疗冠心病心绞痛,而且临证诊病时十分注重气血相关、病邪相兼及脏腑气机生化,在活血化瘀治法的基础上衍化出理气活血、化痰活血、益气活血、温阳活血等多种治法,丰富和完善了活血化瘀治法的内容。在以活血化瘀为主辨证治疗冠心病心绞痛方面,陈院士对各种不同虚实证候的主症、次症、治法、方药等进行了规范,主持建立了冠心病辨证标准、冠心病疗效评价标准,这些皆成为国家的行业标准和新药疗效评价标准,得到了国内外的普遍认可。

2. 益气活血、化浊通腑法治疗急性心肌梗死

急性心肌梗死 (acute myocardial infarction, AMI) 是在冠状动脉粥样硬化基础上,伴有斑块破裂、出血、血栓形成或冠状动脉持续痉挛等引起冠状动脉急性闭塞,导致冠状动脉血流中断或急剧减少,导致心肌缺血性坏死的一种急性冠状动脉综合征。AMI 后,由于梗死区心肌收缩功能丧失,左室心肌节段性收缩运动异常,可导致左室整体收缩功能降低,甚至心脏泵功能衰竭。AMI 患者临床多有剧烈胸痛、大汗淋漓、呼吸困难、喘憋、面色苍白、四肢逆冷等表现。20 世纪 70—80 年代,陈院士等认为,患者胸闷、呼吸困难、面色苍白、多汗、脉微欲绝,属中医学"气虚"、"阳虚"甚

* 原载于《中国中西医结合杂志》,2011,31 (8):1017-1020

第六章

至"阳脱"的表现；患者冠状动脉管腔狭窄和闭塞，属于中医学"血瘀"的范畴。由此提出气虚、心脉瘀阻是 AMI 的主要病机，主张益气活血法治疗 AMI，并研制了抗心梗合剂，方由黄芪、丹参各30g，党参、黄精、郁金、赤芍各15g组成，用于治疗 AMI。临床研究表明，可明显改善患者的临床症状，降低 AMI 的住院并发症和病死率[4]。

在临床实践中，陈院士发现 AMI 急性期患者多有大便秘结、口气臭秽、舌苔黄腻或厚腻、脉弦滑或滑数等症状和体征，认为其病机在气虚血瘀基础上，应兼有瘀血、痰浊胶结，秽浊蕴积。患者动脉粥样硬化 (atherosclerosis, AS) 斑块破裂、溃疡、出血、脂质成分外溢、血栓形成等病理改变，可归于中医学"痰瘀互结"的范畴，提出痰瘀互结、秽浊蕴积是 AMI 病机的一个重要方面。在以往益气活血基础上，主张结合化浊通腑法治疗AMI，并研制出益气活血、化浊通腑的愈梗通瘀汤。本方由生晒人参 10～15g、生黄芪 15g、紫丹参15g、全当归 10g、延胡索 10g、川芎 10g、广藿香 12g、佩兰 10g、陈皮 10g、半夏 10g、生大黄6～10g组成。方中人参、黄芪并用，心气、宗气、元气并补；黄芪具有益气托腐生肌之效，人参以生晒参或红参为好，津液亏虚者可用西洋参，党参虽也可用，但作用平补和缓，似不能与生晒参等温补益气之效同日而语；方中当归、丹参并用，调气养血活血，使气血各有所归；当归的有效成分阿魏酸钠有改善红细胞变形能力及清除超氧自由基的功用[5]。"损其心者调其营卫"，血虚当得补，血滞当能通；丹参补血之力虽逊于当归，但通瘀之力强于后者，前者宜于偏热，后者宜于偏寒，而相配伍，可得通治；延胡索、川芎并用，可增强理气定痛、化瘀通脉之功；延胡索苦辛，性温无毒，入肝经，兼入心包、肾、脾、肺四经，《雷公炮炙论》有"心痛欲死，速觅延胡"之论，李时珍也有"止痛妙不可言"之喻；川芎为血中气药，理气定痛而活血通瘀，抗血小板黏聚功能尤好[6]。AMI 患者临床常见苔腻脉滑、纳呆呕恶、大便干结等症状，本方大黄之用，可以通瘀、化浊而推陈致新；藿香辛微温无毒，通常认为系清暑药，实际上醒脾和胃、辟恶止吐，四时皆可应用；佩兰苦辛温无毒，化湿浊而定痛。至于方中半夏，张仲景早有"呕加半夏"之训，配以陈皮理气和中，治疗浊阻；《本草纲目》对陈皮本有可治"途中心痛"之语。诸药合用，通补兼施，共奏益气生肌、行气活血定痛、化

瘀通脉、通腑化浊之功。药理研究证实，该方能增加冠状动脉血流量、改善心肌供血、修复损伤心肌，缩小梗死面积；小样本临床观察证实，在西医常规治疗基础上，采用此方治疗 AMI 患者，可降低 AMI 住院患者的病死率，减少早期并发症，改善心功能[7,8]。

3. 活血化瘀方药干预冠心病介入治疗后再狭窄

20 世纪 80 年代开始，冠心病的治疗进入了冠状动脉介入治疗时代，但介入治疗后再狭窄的问题一直未能理想解决。2000 年以前，冠心病介入治疗后再狭窄发生率约为 30% 左右；随着药物涂层支架的广泛应用，支架置入术后再狭窄率降低到5% ～ 10%[9]，但再狭窄的防治仍是目前心血管病研究领域普遍关注的一个焦点和难点问题。

经皮冠状动脉介入治疗 (percutaneous coronary intervention, PCI) 术后，由于血管内皮细胞损伤、内膜撕裂、基底膜暴露等因素，发生局部炎症和血栓形成。血栓中的血小板释放出大量生长因子、细胞因子和血管活性物质，促进血管平滑肌细胞增殖、迁移，使管腔再次狭窄[10]。陈院士认为血小板活化、血管内膜损伤、平滑肌细胞增殖、胶原沉积、血栓形成等病理改变属于中医学"血脉瘀滞"的病理改变，倡导活血化瘀制剂防治冠心病介入治疗后再狭窄。在国家"八五""九五""十五"攻关期间，首先对经典活血化瘀方血府逐瘀汤制剂进行研究，证实其在预防介入治疗后再狭窄方面确有疗效。然后对方药进行简化和精制，提取方中的有效部位，选川芎、赤芍有效部位最佳剂量配比制成芎芍胶囊。通过大规模、多中心、随机、双盲、安慰剂对照的临床试验进一步评价活血化瘀中药预防 PCI 后再狭窄的效果，证实芎芍胶囊能降低介入后再狭窄发生率，减少复合终点事件的发生，预防心绞痛的复发[11]，为活血化瘀中药制剂预防冠心病介入治疗后再狭窄形成和心绞痛复发，改善患者长期预后提供了一个有效的中药治疗途径。

4. 活血解毒法稳定 AS 斑块

AS 斑块的稳定与否取决于斑块内脂质池的大小和纤维帽的厚度。脂质核心随着泡沫细胞的死亡和血浆脂类的沉积而不断增大，纤维帽因为巨噬细胞浸润释放大量的水解酶降解胶原纤维而逐渐变

薄，斑块的稳定性下降[12]。在 AS 急性心血管事件中，血小板活化、黏附、聚集和血栓形成等病理改变以及胸痛、舌暗、瘀斑、舌下静脉曲张等宏观体征，中医学多将其归于"血脉瘀阻"的范畴，但血栓闭塞引发的炎症瀑布反应、氧化脂质沉积、细胞凋亡和组织损伤坏死等病理损害，以及病情凶险、疼痛剧烈、舌苔垢浊、舌质紫绛、口气秽臭的临床特点，却似非单一"血瘀"病因所能概括。陈院士采用病证结合方法，把心血管血栓性疾病发病的病理改变及临床特点与中医"毒"邪致病起病急骤、传变迅速、直中脏腑和腐肌伤肉等特点相结合，提出心血管血栓性疾病"瘀毒"病因学说，认为"瘀"、"毒"从化联合致病是冠心病的主要病因，"毒瘀"互结，坏血损脉，贯穿心血管血栓性疾病的整个过程，并据此提出了采用活血解毒治法稳定 AS 斑块的思路。实验研究采用不同活血化瘀中药配伍干预 ApoE 基因缺陷小鼠 AS 不稳定斑块，结果证实活血药和解毒药皆有一定的稳定 AS 斑块的作用，但具有活血解毒作用的中药作用优于单纯活血药或解毒药，活血和解毒配伍可提高稳定斑块的效果，从实验角度验证了瘀毒病因认识的正确性[13]；临床通过 1500 余例的前瞻性队列研究，规范了瘀毒互结的临床表征和微观病理改变，并证明瘀毒互结表征重者和心血管血栓性临床事件有一定的关联。

陈院士长期致力于病证结合治疗心血管疾病的研究：一方面，他强调把中医整体辨证和疾病病理生理变化辨识相结合，在传统中医宏观辨证的基础上，运用现代科学技术方法对各证候内在的生理、病理变化进行研究，为临床提供可量化辨证的依据；另一方面，他强调现代医学病理生理变化和中医的辨证理论认识有机结合，把西医理化诊断纳入到中医辨证的体系，借助现代科学技术延展中医四诊的视野。陈院士指出：中医病证结合论治的产生和发展，是中医临床医学发展的一个重要模式。每一个疾病发生、发展及转化，皆具有"病"与"证"在疾病不同阶段的相互融合和演变。着眼于贯穿疾病基本病理改变的辨病论治和整体认识指导

下辨证论治的结合，会对疾病病理生理变化有更清晰的认识，由此而进行的治疗也会获得更理想的效果。

参考文献

[1] 陈娜萦. 冠心病的发病形势与预防. 中华慢病杂志，2005，4（2）：41-44.

[2] 陈可冀，李连达，翁维良，等. 血瘀证与活血化瘀研究. 中西医结合心脑血管病杂志，2005，3（1）：1-2.

[3] 陈可冀，钱振淮，张问渠，等. 精制冠心片对冠心病心绞痛双盲法治疗 112 例疗效分析. 中华心血管病杂志，1982，10（2）：85-89.

[4] 中医研究院西苑医院内科，东直门医院内科，广安门医院内科，等. 以"抗心梗合剂"为主治疗急性心肌梗塞 118 例疗效分析. 中华内科杂志，1976，1（4）：212-215.

[5] 杨慧，吴宏. 当归多糖对脐血造血细胞冷冻损伤的可恢复性研究. 中草药，2008，9（11）：1684-1688.

[6] 王欢，唐于平，郭建明，等. 当归 - 川芎药对不同配比组方对家兔血小板聚集和凝血功能的影响. 中国实验方剂学杂志，2010，16（2）：73-77.

[7] 廖欣，罗陆一. 愈梗通瘀汤治疗冠心病心绞痛的临床观察. 中国中西医结合杂志，1998，18（10）：594-597.

[8] Schapiro-Dufour E, Cucherat M, Velzenberger E. et al. Drug-eluting stents in patients at high risk of restenosis：assessment for France. Int J Technol Assess Health Care, 2011, 27 (2)：108-117.

[9] McDowell G, Slevin M, Krupinski J. Nanotechnology for the treatment of coronary in-stent restenosis：a clinical perspective. Vasc Cell, 2011, 3 (1)：8.

[10] Chen KJ, Shi DZ, Xu H, et al. XS0601 reduces the incidence of restenosis：a prospective study of 335 patients undergoing percutaneous coronary intervention in China. Chin Med J, 2006, 119 (1)：6-13.

[11] Magnani G, Demola MA, Fava C, et al. From vulnerable plaque to vulnerable patient. Cardiology, 2010, 11 (12)：6-9.

[12] 史大卓，徐浩，殷惠军，等. "瘀"、"毒"从化——心脑血管血栓性疾病病因病机. 中西医结合学报，2008，6（11）：1105-1108.

传承岳美中教授崇高的人文精神遗产 *

陈可冀

岳美中教授是我国中医药学界的一代宗师，并且是1981年成立的中国中西医结合研究会（现中国中西医结合学会）第一届顾问。我有幸从学和从业岳老二十余年，感到他对中华民族传统文化的情商、智商均至为高洁，实令人有明月不染之感。他嗜书如命，终生浸润于我国传统文史典籍之中，不仅精读经史子集，警句佳作背诵如流，一部《二十四史》亦时常反复研读，求知欲极强；对于声韵、训诂、诗词之类，情趣尤浓；其诗作《锄云诗集》载诗一千余首，不仅涉及时政兴废、世事沧桑、奇山异水、梅菊芭蕉、医事经历，乃至亲友师生离合之情，常感而发之，亲自工整笔录，今日审读，犹若岳老本人私事之记事本云。他在诊疗之余，亦常乐于与我等师生对谈所感，例如司马迁之逆境奋发，苏东坡之达观豪放，孟轲之"吾善养浩然之气"，张衡之热爱真理，傅山之工诗画，孔学之"仁者爱人"等，盖实际上无不属于从善抑或从恶之教。岳老常常幽默与学问熔于一炉，师生对坐，其乐融融焉，以至于我等师生"文革"期间曾被张贴大字报列为一项"不务正业"之罪状而被"揭发"。岳老认为学习中国传统文化知识是我们后人继承前人历史观、道德观、哲学思想、意识形态，以及怎样做人等的重要内容，我们大家不可以数典忘祖。他认为在传承学习中国文化和中医药学术时，对所提倡的"取其精华，去其糟粕"的理解，也应在学习理解实践的基础上有所作为，不可以自掘坟墓，不可与先贤古典绝了缘分。他常说："覆巢之下，无复完卵"，他更不赞成"五四"时期有人说的"汉字不灭，中国必完"（鲁迅《病中答情报访员》）的言论。今天看来，岳老的教导对年轻一代的中医药从业人员，实有甚大的教育意义；我所接触到的他们之中，虽不少毕业于高等中医药院校，但大多与古典医籍并不直接谋面，实有中医药"文化赤字"或蜻蜓点水之嫌，足资师道者戒。

对于数千年以来的中医药学术文明史，岳老属于经方派专家，认为"法从仲景思常沛，医学长沙自有真"，但他认为经方应用实应重视学习其辨证论治与专病、专方、专药相结合辨证思维精神或理念。《伤寒论》及《金匮要略》中之此类遣方用药实例在在可见，1961年我随他与梁漱溟到福建，岳老曾为福建中医学界专家做了有关这一方面的专题报告。他也十分欣赏李杲和叶桂的理论和临床经验，主张应结合临床实际，各取其长，而不应偏执一己之见，他告诫我们不可以自傲，所谓"桃子万家宗一脉，纷纷井底各言天"，进而不免贻误病家。

岳老在从事日常医疗业务中，以"治心何日能忘我，操术随时可误人"为座右铭，主张"治急性病要有胆有识，治慢性病要有方有守"。根据国家指派，岳老先后为多个国家元首治病，获得了周恩来总理、吴阶平教授等的赞扬。岳老闲章有"北国青囊，南洋丹鼎，东瀛鸿爪，西土萍踪"之中医药扬威海外之感怀之刻，是为旁箴。尽管"文革"期间岳老被勒令作为"反动学术权威"扫厕所、挖粪石之类劳动，他也是默默地做得尽善尽美。我当年时常偷偷去看他低头弯腰俯地劳动的情景，深深为之同情。我理解他老人家，所以整个"文革"期间，我没有贴过他的任何一张大字报，没有说过他任何一句不好的话。他的解放，是周总理在人民大会堂立等他去给越南胡志明治疗心肌梗死而实现的。当时因被抄家，岳老走时只好穿了周总理的鞋，以及吴阶平教授的袜子登上了前去急救的飞机。

"文革"后，他前后身为全国政协四届医卫副组长，全国五届人大常委，身负重任。鉴于中医人才匮乏，岳老上书中央，倡议并获批创办我国首批高级中医研究班、高级研究生班，为我国改革开放培养了一大批中医精英，可谓功德无量。

《左传》称"太上有立德，其次有立功，其次有立言，虽久不废，此之谓不朽"，岳老应是三者俱全。岳老为人很低调，但他有爱国主义精神，有事业心，有激情，有勇气，有中华儿女的人文情

* 原载于《中国中西医结合杂志》，2012，32 (6)：725

怀，憧憬着中医药的未来。他不封闭、不固执，坚韧而和谐，支持我从事中西医结合事业。他眼睛不好，多半低着头走路，但内心锐气十足。我和维养每次见到他往颐和园方向走去，背地里就相互地

说：此乃"韬光养晦，浅水卧龙"也。是的，他是中医药学历史上永远值得我们感念的巨人，伟大的中医药学者。伟大的时代造就了岳老的传奇人生。

岳美中教授病证结合治疗常见病的临证经验 *

张京春

岳美中，当代著名中医学家，一生从事中医医疗和教学工作，临证时重视平衡阴阳、调理脾胃，较早地提出了专病、专方、专药与辨证论治相结合的原则，促进了病证结合这一中西医结合治疗观的发展。作为经方派大师，岳老善用经方治大病，学宗张仲景、李东垣和叶天士三家，而《伤寒论》和《金匮要略》更为他所推崇，故有"法崇仲圣思常沛，医学长沙自有真"之警句。他倡办了全国中医研究班和研究生班，培养了一大批中医高级人才，并多次出国从事重要医事活动，在国内外享有盛誉。今借助北京市中医局立项的岳美中名家研究室支持，在室站负责人岳老亲传优秀弟子陈可冀老师指导下总结岳老的学术经验，概览岳老著作及其传人的相关文章，特别将岳老善治的肾病、肝病及心系疾病分述如下，以期对后人有所借鉴。

1. 肾炎

1.1 病因病机

岳老综合《内经》《丹溪心法》及《中藏经》等古籍中有关肾的病理生理的描述，形成了自己的肾病发病观，认为肾病的形成，肾虚是关键。一是肾本虚，导致开合失司，膀胱气化不利，影响水液代谢，形成肾病；二是因肾虚，导致脾、肺、三焦功能失调，形成肾病。肾阳不足，不能温煦脾阳，脾失健运，水湿内停，溢于肌肤而为水肿。或因脾气不足，清气不升，浊阴不降，小便因而不利，形成肾病。肾阴不足，不能上滋肺，肺气不利，不能通调水道，亦可形成水肿。肾虚不能行水，水液内停，致三焦气机不畅，又可引起气滞水停，形成本病。

岳老不仅认识到肾虚是导致脏腑功能失调、水液代谢障碍引起水肿的重要因素，而且还认识

到，外感所致的风水证，也是先有"肾先亏损"，后感外邪所致。慢性肾盂肾炎在中医学中大部分属于"劳淋"范畴，一部分则属于"血淋"或"膏淋"。这些患者多表现为易疲倦、面色不华、肌肤不润、腰酸腰痛、夜尿频繁等虚弱症状，呈慢性疾患，多属气血不足之证。有些患者有不同程度的蛋白尿或间歇脓尿，甚至合并慢性膀胱炎而有尿血，排尿不适，脉滑数，舌淡，则为水道有瘀血或湿热之证。

1.2 治则治法

岳老认为，肾炎多虚，治以扶正为主，水肿轻者，缓则治其本，宜补肾制水为主；重者，急则治其标，以利水攻水为先；体质极虚者攻补兼施。岳老治肾炎虽始终体现了同病异治的辨证论治思想，及权衡标本缓急的具体治疗法则，但还是能体会他治肾病重在扶正的原则。其中或补肾阳为主，或补肾阴为主，或补肾气为主，或补脾胃为主，或补肺肾，或补脾肾等。

岳老长于治疗肾炎。他认为成年人之慢性肾炎多由急性转来。急性肾炎时，多取发汗或峻下的方法，如越婢加术汤和浚川散。刚从急性转为慢性之初，以利水为主，用胃苓汤加枳壳、党参；中期者，宜扶正利水，用苓桂术甘汤等；肾变性期，水肿显著，蛋白尿亦重，可用防己黄芪汤，此期"收效关键，仍在守方，守方之中须注意观察病之动向，以消息方药"；末期者，阳虚证用罗止园治肿胀方，阴虚证用加味知柏地黄汤，肾阴阳两虚兼脾肺不足采用自制芡实合剂（芡实30g、白术12g、茯苓12g、怀山药15g、菟丝子24g、金樱子24g、黄精24g、百合18g、枇杷叶9g、党参9g），脾胃不和、脾湿不化用自制调和脾胃之肾炎

* 原载于《中国中西医结合杂志》，2012，32（7）：879-881

方（云茯苓 9g、泽泻 6g、猪苓 6g、白芍药 4.5g、川厚朴 4.5g、川枳壳 4.5g、陈皮 1g、甘草 1g）。善后办法，可投黄芪粥等，以消除蛋白尿。对于黄芪，岳老认为适用于慢性虚弱病症，必须久服多服才能收效，而不似附子干姜下咽即效。诚如《本经疏证》"大气一转，其气乃散"，营卫畅达，则水祛湿蠲。

2. 泌尿系统结石

泌尿系统结石又称为尿石症，包括肾结石、输尿管结石、膀胱和尿道的结石。由于肾和输尿管的结石与膀胱和尿道的结石，在发病年龄、性别、病因及结石成分上有差别，而在临床表现上又各有偏重，因此，将肾和输尿管结石合称为上尿路结石，膀胱和尿道结石称为下尿路结石，其中上尿路结石发病率较高。岳老曾治疗印尼苏加诺总统的左肾结石肾功能消失症，取得了溶化结石恢复肾功能的效果。

2.1　病因病机

泌尿系统结石多属于中医学"石淋"范畴。岳老认为，其形成机理，在于"阴阳偏盛"、"气血乖和"与"湿热交蒸"，同时又存在地方水土因素。

2.2　治则治法

岳老认为，使用中药治疗结石的治则是利水通淋，古人多用八正散、石韦散二方及单味药金钱草等。岳老在治疗结石症时除继承传统治法外，常选用强肾之药如杜仲、续断、苁蓉、桑寄生等以图"扶正祛邪"。此外，在结石进入输尿管后，则加重利水通淋之力，以图"因势利导"。

岳老指出要根据患者具体情况进行辨治，形体壮实者以排石为主；形体虚衰者须同时辅以扶正药物，攻补兼施。另外，按结石部位所在为治，如肾内结石，以补肾为主；输尿管结石，以下行加分利为主。

岳老对本病临症，每用金钱草为主药，剂量轻者 30g，重者 210g，以 90～150g 居多数。在药物的选择和组合方面，岳老亦指出应当"专方专药"与"辨证论治"相结合。如八正散、猪苓汤、金钱草、石韦、海金沙等，均为有效之方药，并自制排尿路结石方（金钱草、海金砂、草梢、冬葵子、牛膝、大生地、当归、琥珀末、王不留行）治疗实型结石。岳老还根据自己的临床实践，提出了 15 类治疗尿路结石的药物，其中如降下排石药、溶解结石药、防止结石复发药等，以及对孤立的鹿角状结石用药、解除痉挛药等。岳老指出，凡一般

输尿管和膀胱结石，其体积在尿道中有通过之可能者，均有可能予服中药以排出。至于服中药是否能把结石破碎或化解，在临床上尚须累积经验。

值得提出的是，岳老在阐述尿路结石用药谱时已明确指出，木通"此味有影响肾功能的不良反应，在肾虚者勿用"。

3. 肝炎

3.1　病因病机

岳老认为，"伤寒发黄"包括黄疸型传染性肝炎。发黄的病机主要是湿热郁蒸。在急性阶段有热重、湿重、湿热并重三种不同类型，且多数是热重于湿。

慢性肝炎常反复发作，患者症状不一，或胁痛，或腹胀、食欲不振、或恶心欲吐，或腹泻肠鸣等胃肠症状；触诊多有肝、脾肿大。化验检查可表现为长期肝功能异常。多属中医学"胁痛""积聚"等病范畴。其病因病机较复杂，或湿热留恋不去，或湿阻气滞，或气滞血瘀，或日久正气亏损等导致脾胃升降失调、肝胆疏泄失职，出现上述诸症。

3.2　治则治法

岳老认为，治疗肝病应本着肝病病程中主症出现的先后、轻重、缓急，择以效方。简而言之，初期邪盛而正不虚，祛邪即扶正；中期邪正交争，邪尚盛而正将不支，则祛邪兼以扶正；末期正衰不能敌邪，则扶正即祛邪。至于救逆，亦宜遵从这些普遍规律。但也有寒热夹杂、阴阳错综、虚实混淆之非单纯症象者，则方药亦宜错综变化，随机制宜。

岳老在治疗慢性肝炎时，采用了"清化开泄"兼"扶正"之法。"清化"有清热化瘀和清化痰浊之意；"开泄"是指通过辛苦之品，辛开兼具清化痰浊之效。其方有半夏泻心汤、小陷胸汤、柴胡疏肝散、大柴胡汤等。较普遍用到了半夏泻心汤、小陷胸汤，方中均具有辛温之半夏，苦寒之黄连，黄连配半夏既辛开苦降，又寒热平调，配伍其他药物，使脾胃升降有序，运化有常，对改善胃肠道症状有立竿见影之效，亦起到恢复肝功能的作用。慢性肝炎病的治法一般多采取清热利湿化瘀为主，在初、中期是有效的，若病程过长，甚至 3～5 年不愈，并有肝硬化倾向者，则应考虑是否久服攻利克伐之剂而有伤气血、损及阴阳的不良反应。在脘闷胁痛（多刺痛）等瘀滞症状与肝功能不正常时，亦应顾及是无力康复，或正虚似邪，宜慎重投药。若果有虚象，则用四物养血，相应加入他药，可以消除症状，恢复肝功能。慢性肝炎由于经年不愈，

病邪久积，或治疗不当，日久必伤及气血，损及阴阳。因此，岳老治慢性肝炎时，除了考虑"久病入络"，以治疗方中适当加入活血化瘀通络之品外，常常注重扶正的治疗。

岳老在治疗急性肝炎中还体现了"不胶执在肝炎患者的肝功能某一项指标上"的辨证思想。

4. 冠心病

4.1 病因病机

冠心病中医常以胸痹心痛论治。岳老根据《黄帝内经》总结胸痹心痛的病因分为内因和外因，内因则为机体阳气素虚，卫阳力量不够，时有厥气上逆，寒气聚于清阳之府胸中，久留而不去，导致胸阳亦微。外因寒气侵袭胸阳，内外相和导致脉管蜷缩而绌急，故心绞痛发作。依中医学理论，胸阳衰弱，浊阴干犯清阳之府，乃是该病之基本病机。当胸阳衰弱之时，血行则缓慢，瘀即随之而成，甚至造成阴血凝固。此乃胸痹形成血瘀之病理。在治法上活血化瘀，兼以宣痹行气，当以切合病机。因气为血帅，气行则血行，宣痹须行气，宣痹行气即可收化瘀之效。

4.2 治则治法

岳老认为胸为清阳之府，心体阴而用阳，一有浊阴，则发生胸痹之证，必须采用阳药及通药以廓清阴邪，不可掺杂阴柔滋敛之品以助长阴邪。胸痹证舌苔多为白苔坐底，上罩一层薄黄苔，且多滋润，不可误认为热像，一为阴邪踞阳位，不免表面阳化，二因阴邪逼胸阳上腾，也可使表面阳化，所以上罩薄黄滋润之苔，是基于阳化而又无力祛除阴邪以廓清阳位，切不可从阳论治。

胸痹夜间发作者多为心阳虚微，轻则用干姜、桂枝、薤白温通心阳，重则用附子、肉桂回阳救逆。岳老常以宣痹通阳法治之，方选栝蒌薤白白酒汤、栝蒌薤白半夏汤、枳实薤白桂枝汤及薏苡附子散等。

岳老认为心痛多相当于现代医学的心肌梗死。常以如下分型辨证: (1) 芳香开窍：心肌梗死发生猝心痛，在病理上中医学认为是气滞血瘀，经脉不通，不通则痛引起的急证，岳老认为此等紧急情况下须采用芳香开窍以通之治法，有一定的疗效。《太平惠民和剂局方》苏合香丸主之。西苑医院宽胸丸（荜茇 900g，良姜、延胡索、檀香各 450g，细辛 150g，冰片 30g）亦可用之。另对心绞痛发作，也有温通解痛的作用。 (2) 活血化瘀：冠心病临床所见的心绞痛、胸闷、心律失常、心肌梗死、

舌质紫黯，原于心阳式微，或心气不足，而导致心脉痹阻，气滞血瘀，更所谓不通则痛，是冠心病的共性。中医学多用活血化瘀法治之。用化"死血"方（当归尾 15g、川芎 9g、丹皮 9g、苏木 9g、红花 9g、延胡索 9g、桂枝 9g、桃仁 9g、赤曲 9g、降香 3g、通草 3g、大麦芽 6g、穿山甲 9g）。水煎成，入童便、酒、韭汁，饮之。若瘀血严重者，用变通血府逐瘀汤（当归尾 9g、川芎 9g、桂心 9g、栝蒌 18g、薤白 12g、桔梗 6g、枳壳 6g、红花 9g、桃仁 9g、怀牛膝 18g、柴胡 9g），本方是治心肌梗死比较全面的一个方剂。此方曾在临床上进行疗效验证，证实该方对改善症状、心功能的恢复有较好的效果。对血瘀痰阻之胸痹心痛见胸闷气短，天阴更觉胸膺发憋，性情急躁等用加味冠通汤（党参 12g、当归 12g、薤白 18g、红花 9g、延胡索 12g、广郁金 9g、丹参 12g、糖栝蒌 24g、鸡血藤 24g）。(3) 回阳救逆：急性心肌梗死猝心痛时，患者面色苍白，心悸气短，恶寒冷汗，四肢厥逆或疼痛，或下利清谷，甚则指端青紫，唇青面黑，舌质紫黯，大小便不禁，脉微欲绝或见结代。用回阳救逆急救，张仲景四逆汤主之。

另有临床实验证实采用岳老的经验方人参三七琥珀以 1:1:1 比例治疗冠心病心绞痛或 2:2:1 比例治疗充血性心力衰竭，均取得了较好的疗效。

5. 高血压

岳老对高血压的治疗提倡专病专方治疗，尤其对于舒张压较高的患者，经验更为独到。

5.1 气虚证

岳老认为此类患者之气虚，可有肾气虚及中气虚之不同。用苦寒泻肝或二仙汤之类不起效用，用大量黄芪有时可有一定作用。一般黄芪用 1 两以上，配陈皮 1 钱。王清任《医林改错》中的补阳还五汤也有一定效果，但有"火热"者不宜用。还可以用李东垣的升阳益胃汤，原是治疗"肺与脾胃虚"的方剂。岳老常用此方治高血压，气短倦怠，左脉弦滑，右脉虚大，兼见湿热偏盛症状为标者。方中君药是黄芪，臣药是人参、炙甘草、半夏，其他如白芍、羌活、防风等皆为佐使之品。

5.2 阴虚阳亢证

岳老认为张锡纯《医学衷中参西录》镇肝熄风汤（淮牛膝 30g、代赭石 30g[先煎]、生龙骨 10g[先煎]、生牡蛎 15g[先煎]、生龟版 15g[先煎]、生白芍 15g、元

参 15g、天冬 15g、川楝子 6g、生麦芽 6g、茵陈 6g、甘草 5g）。功用：镇肝熄风。主治：阴虚阳亢，肝风内动之证或建瓴汤（怀山药 30g、怀牛膝 30g、生赭石 24g、生地黄 18g、生龙骨 18g、生牡蛎 18g、生杭芍 12g、柏子仁 12g）。功用：镇肝熄风，滋阴安神；主治：肝阳上亢之证。

5.3 痰浊上扰证

以加味半夏白术天麻汤每能见功。岳老认为本方对于湿痰中停，胃气不降，症见眩晕较甚，如坐舟车，血压高低波动颇大，舌苔白腻，脉弦滑者较好。其不仅是治太阴痰气上逆之方，更是一个双向调节人体机能的重要方剂，尤其是对血压波动者

有良效。不但对发作性头痛食后嗜睡之低血压有效，对由于肠胃虚弱、头痛体倦之高血压也有效。其施于虚证高血压，偏于实证者则不宜。

岳老除对上述疾病有丰富经验，还善治咳喘、脾胃病、老年病、热性病及妇科病等诸多疾病。常以外感内伤辨治咳喘病，并创制许多有效方剂，在肺痈、肺痨的治疗中，岳老继续发扬其倡导的"专病专方"思想，方选千金苇茎汤治肺痈、黄连方治肺痨。由陈可冀院士整理、记录补益六法的《岳美中老中医治疗老年病的经验》一书，是新中国成立后国内最早介绍老年病证治的中医著作，曾被日本医学刊物全书译载。

基于关联规则的清宫胸痹医案用药规律研究 *

张京春　陈可冀　刘玥

胸痹是指以胸部闷痛、甚则胸痛彻背、气短喘息不得卧为主症的一种疾病，其病因多与寒邪内侵、饮食不当、情志波动、年老体虚等有关。中医药有着丰富的胸痹诊疗经验，本文采用关联规则的数据挖掘方法，对清代宫廷治疗胸痹的用药经验进行挖掘、分析，以期对现今临床诊治胸痹疾病提供参考。

1. 资料

1.1 医案来源

医案来源于《清宫医案集成》[1]，其中汇集了上启顺治、下至光绪年间清代宫廷的诊疗医案。

1.2 医案纳入及排除标准

纳入以"胸闷""胸膈满闷""胸隔堵满"或"胸中刺疼"为主症，并具有完整的症状、证候、治疗方药的胸痹医案（当同一医案中有多个主症时，结合该患者诊疗连续性的侧重点确定病名诊断，每一个医案只确定一个病名诊断）。排除病名判别有歧义的医案及只有外治方法或内服丸药（只有方剂名称无组成药物）而无内服药物治疗的医案。

2. 方法

2.1 资料处理

采集医案的基本信息，包括：诊治时间、患者、医家、症状、证候、治法、方剂名称、药物组

成、特殊煎服法、用药剂量共 10 项，其中症状、证候、治法、药物组成为必备项，将以上医案信息点录入由中国科学院计算技术研究所协助设计的清宫医案分析系统中，所有数据由 2 人 2 机分别录入，最后经审核校对所有信息点与原始医案一致，形成可分析的结构化文本。

2.2 数据的规范化处理

数据录入完成后，形成清宫胸痹医案数据库，将医案中出现的中药处方名、俗称等统一规范成标准的药名，将《中华本草》[2]中药物的正名作为标准药名，对中药名进行统一规范，制定标准化文本，同时参照《中药学》[3]将中药按照功效进行分类，建立中药功效分类标准化文本。

2.3 数据挖掘方法

运用频数统计方法对胸痹医案的总体用药情况进行分析，统计每味药物的使用频数，找出用药频率较高者进行分析，寻找清宫胸痹医案用药的核心药物；通过关联规则以及频繁项集找出一些已知和未知的药对，同时对清宫胸痹医案治疗方剂的组成药物类别进行分析，以发现其基本组方结构。

3. 结果

3.1 清宫胸痹医案常用药物频数统计

共纳入清宫胸痹医案 81 例。

---

* 原载于《中医杂志》，2013，54（9）：789-791

表1 清宫胸痹医案主要用药频数统计

序号	药物	频次	频率 (%)	序号	药物	频次	频率 (%)
1	青皮	57	70	14	橘红	21	26
2	枳壳	56	69	15	木香	20	25
3	瓜蒌	52	64	16	茯苓	19	23
4	香附	46	57	17	沉香	17	21
5	厚朴	35	43	18	生地黄	15	19
6	栀子	35	43	19	当归	15	19
7	大黄	33	41	20	牡丹皮	15	19
8	黄连	31	38	21	薄荷	13	16
9	延胡索	27	33	22	赤芍	13	16
10	龙胆草	26	32	23	陈皮	13	16
11	半夏	25	31	24	腹皮子	12	15
12	黄芩	24	30	25	焦山楂	12	15
13	白芍	23	28	26	白术	10	12

清宫胸痹医案常用药物频数具体见表1，其中最常用的5味药依次为青皮、枳壳、瓜蒌、香附、厚朴，说明清宫治疗胸痹病主用理气之品，疏肝破气的青皮、理气宽中的枳壳、利气宽胸的瓜蒌、理气解郁的香附使用频率都在50%以上。针对胸痹病常见兼夹的胃蓄湿饮证，青皮还可行滞消胀，枳壳兼能消积化滞；针对肝热证，瓜蒌同时可以清热化痰，香附疏肝调经止痛。

3.2 清宫胸痹医案常用药物关联规则分析

3.2.1 常用药物二项关联分析 表2示，清宫胸痹医案中最常用的10个药对依次为大黄-枳壳、龙胆草-青皮、沉香-青皮、当归-香附、赤芍-香附、香附-青皮、半夏-瓜蒌、枳壳-青皮、枳壳-瓜蒌及青皮-瓜蒌，体现清宫胸痹医案治疗中常用行气、活血、化痰治法。

3.2.2 常用药物三项关联分析 表3示清宫胸痹医案中出现最多的三项药物组合均是理气药＋当归或半夏或栀子、龙胆草、延胡索。值得注意的是厚朴、枳壳、大黄这三味药物是小承气汤的组成，半夏、瓜蒌、黄连是小陷胸汤的组成，两个经方加起来至少使用了31次，可见清宫胸痹医案证候多为气滞、痰热互结所致，其中胸痹病的清热之品多用栀子、大黄、龙胆草三者在一起使用的机会也很高，特别是当大黄、栀子一起用时，有80%的可能也会用龙胆草，而龙胆草具有清热泻肝之功效，更进一步说明了清宫胸痹病治疗中多用理气、清热、清肝、化痰、活血之法。

3.2.3 常用方剂三类药组方结构关联分析 表4示，清宫胸痹医案中常用方剂的三类药组方结构中，关联度最高的前10位组合依次为理气药＋芳香化湿药＋清化热痰药、理气药＋芳香化湿药＋清热燥湿药理气药＋清化热痰药＋清热燥湿药、理气药＋芳香化湿药＋温化寒痰药、理气药＋清化热痰药＋温化寒痰药、理气药＋芳香化湿药＋消食药、理气药＋活血止痛药＋清热凉血药、理气药＋活血止痛药＋发散风热药、理气药＋补气药＋利水消肿药、理气药＋清热凉血药＋清热泻火药。

表2 清宫胸痹医案常用药物二项关联分析（支持度≥10）

序号	二项关联药物	支持度	置信度 (%)
1	大黄⇒枳壳	29	90
2	龙胆草⇒青皮	24	90
3	沉香⇒青皮	16	90
4	当归⇒香附	14	90
5	赤芍⇒香附	12	90
6	香附⇒青皮	35	80
7	半夏⇒瓜蒌	19	80
8	枳壳⇒青皮	41	70
9	枳壳⇒瓜蒌	38	70
10	青皮⇒瓜蒌	37	70
11	枳壳⇒香附	32	60
12	栀子⇒龙胆草	19	50
13	延胡索⇒沉香	11	40

表 3　清宫胸痹医案常用药物三项关联分析（支持度 ≥ 10）

序号	三项关联药物	支持度	置信度 (%)
1	当归,枳壳⇒香附	10	100
2	龙胆草,栀子⇒青皮	18	90
3	半夏,青皮⇒瓜蒌	12	90
4	沉香,延胡索⇒青皮	10	90
5	半夏,瓜蒌⇒黄连	15	80
6	大黄,栀子⇒龙胆草	11	80
7	枳壳,青皮⇒瓜蒌	28	70
8	枳壳,青皮⇒大黄	25	60
9	瓜蒌,枳壳⇒大黄	23	60
10	瓜蒌,青皮⇒大黄	21	60
11	厚朴,枳壳⇒大黄	16	60
12	枳壳,青皮⇒厚朴	21	50
13	半夏,瓜蒌⇒香附	10	50
14	栀子,瓜蒌⇒生地黄	11	40

表 4　清宫胸痹医案三类药组方结构关联分析（支持度 ≥ 10）

序号	关联药物类别	支持度	置信度 (%)
1	理气药、芳香化湿药⇒清化热痰药	21	33.87
2	理气药、芳香化湿药⇒清热燥湿药	18	29.03
3	理气药、清化热痰药⇒清热燥湿药	18	29.03
4	理气药、芳香化湿药⇒温化寒痰药	15	24.19
5	理气药、清化热痰药⇒温化寒痰药	15	24.19
6	理气药、芳香化湿药⇒消食药	13	20.97
7	理气药、活血止痛药⇒清热凉血药	12	19.35
8	理气药、活血止痛药⇒发散风热药	12	19.35
9	理气药、补气药⇒利水消肿药	11	17.74
10	理气药、清热凉血药⇒清热泻火药	10	16.13

4. 讨论

数据挖掘分析主要采用频繁项集、关联规则和聚类分析等方法，关联规则是寻找同一事件中不同项的相关性，运用关联分析可以挖掘隐藏在数据间的相互关系，探测以前未发现的隐藏着的模式，当其满足一定的可信度时就具有一定的普遍性规则[4]。通常采用支持度和置信度两个术语来表示规则的兴趣度，如药物 A⇒药物 B，其中支持度为同时包含 A 和 B 的事物数，在本研究中即清宫胸痹医案数据库中 A 和 B 两味药物同时出现在一个医案中的次数；置信度为包含 A 和 B 的事物占只包含 A 的事物的百分比，或者说是在 A 给定情况下关于 B 的条件概率，即 A、B 两味药物同时出现的频数占药物 A 出现的总频数的比例。药物频数越高，则支持度越高；置信度越高，则反映关联分析可信度越高，意义越大。本研究采用频数分析和关联规则方法分析清宫胸痹病的治疗经验，从配伍层次分析清宫胸痹医案的用药规律。

本研究结果发现，清宫胸痹医案中主用理气之品，如青皮、枳壳、香附等，配伍清肝、化痰、清热、活血止痛之品。值得注意的是胸痹医案中多用于活血止痛的延胡索，其性温，味辛苦，入心、脾、肝、肺，是活血化瘀、行气止痛之妙品，尤以止痛之功效而著称。李时珍在《本草纲目》中归纳延胡索有"活血，利气，止痛，通小便"功效，并推崇其"能行血中气滞，气中血滞，故专治一身上下诸痛"，可以看出延胡索在胸痹胸痛症状的缓解上亦有重要作用。

方剂或中药复方是中医临床治疗的主要手段，而配伍组方是中医处方的核心，也是反映临床医生学术思想的精华所在，清宫胸痹医案中常见的中药配伍模式是理气药＋芳香化湿药的同时配伍清化热痰药或清热燥湿药，同时胸痹医案中经常使用的方剂有小陷胸汤和小承气汤，以方测证表明清宫胸痹病多由气滞肝郁、痰热互结所致。通过对清宫医案

中方剂配伍规律的挖掘、分析，可以深刻领会清宫太医对于疾病的治疗经验，把握用药规律，对于进一步指导目前中医临床处方用药具有一定的参考价值。

参考文献

[1] 陈可冀. 清宫医案集成. 北京：科学出版社，2009.
[2] 国家中医药管理局《中华本草》编委会. 中华本草. 上海：上海科学技术出版社，1999.
[3] 高学敏. 中药学. 北京：人民卫生出版社，2004.
[4] 张云涛，龚玲. 数据挖掘原理与技术. 北京：电子工业出版社，2004：70-75.

从治法入手探讨名老中医临床经验应用研究的思路和方法*

高铸烨　付长庚　张京春

名老中医是将中医药学基本理论、前人经验与当今实际相结合，解决临床疑难问题的典范，是中医药学术的带头人，他们的临床经验是在长期的实践中与中医学理论结合、突破、创新的结果，是中医行业的宝贵财富。十一五国家科技支撑计划所立项的名老中医临床经验应用研究，是在对名老中医诊疗经验分析整理的基础上，重点研究其有独特疗效的诊疗方法，并在临床中应用、发展、创新[1]。文章从治法入手探讨了名老中医临床经验应用研究的思路和方法，兹述如下。

1. 理法方药相一致是名老中医临床经验应用研究的前提

中医药学是一门实践性、经验性很强的学科，理法方药的紧密结合是中医药学的基本特点，理法方药理论体系是随着临床实践和理论认识的不断加深而不断发展和完善的[2]。中医在临证诊察疾病时主张四诊合参、谨守病机，进而确立治则治法、组方用药，整个过程体现了理法方药相一致的临床思维特点。纵观中医药学发展的历史，杰出的医学大师无一不是贯穿着理法方药思维的一致性、整体

性，尤其是有创见发明、贡献较大的医家，大都是理论上有所突破，随之深化和扩大了某些治法的应用，或创制了一些新的治则，并根据临床的不同表现，研制和阐述体现自己学术思想的方剂和药物，使之形成一个完整的体系。金元四大家就是典型的例子，如刘河间在《素问》病机十九条的启示下，提出"六气皆能化火"之说，改变了当时喜用温燥药的习惯，根据祛风泻火、清热燥湿等治则，创用天水散、凉膈散等以寒凉为主的方剂，形成寒凉学派。张从正根据"先论攻邪，邪去而元气自复"提出"汗、吐、下"祛邪三法，开拓了临床思路，丰富了有关方药的临床应用。李东垣以升降为枢纽，进一步发展了脾胃学说，并创制了补中益气汤、升阳散火汤等与其理论相一体的方剂，丰富了黄芪、升麻、柴胡、葛根等药物的临床应用。朱丹溪以"阳常有余，阴常不足"立论，以滋阴降火为原则，加深了后世对黄柏、知母、山栀子等药的认识，被称为"滋阴派"。从他们的成功之路不难看出他们所取得的成就得益于他们广博的学识和深邃的思辨，得益于将中医理法方药的完美结合和创新发展[3]。中医临床关键在于辨证施治，辨证的关键

---

* 原载于《中华中医药杂志》，2010，25（12）：2043-2045

第六章

是辨析病因病机，施治的关键是因证选方、因方遣药，即坚持理法方药相一致的原则。当然，名老中医临床经验应用研究更不能脱离或忽视理法方药的一致性。

2. 以治法为切入点是名老中医临床经验应用研究的突破口

治法是中医根据病证的病因病机设立的治疗方法，是多种因素集约的合理运用。治法具有针对性（法随证立）、层次性（如虚者补之→补气→补脾气）、广泛性、兼容性（诸法联用）、可创性（不断发展创新）、抽象性和灵活性（法随证变）等特点[4]。在辨证论治体系中，治法作为病证和方药的中介，使中医辨证论治的药物治疗学内容构成密切联系的整体。治法一方面蕴含病证、病因、病机和组方配伍规律的内容，包涵着方-证相关的内在逻辑性；另一方面治法对证、方、药具有提纲挈领和逻辑分类的重要作用。

治法可以指导组方用药，处方药物可以体现"治法"，但二者并不相等。一个治法可以根据具有相同功效药物组成不同的方剂，同一"治法"指导下所组成的不同方剂虽然有其相同的功效，但由于所组成药物的不同、剂量的差异、煎煮方法的区别而又表现出每个具体方剂的特有功效。因此，治法作为理论（理）联系实际（方药）的纽带和桥梁，针对具体病症确立相应的治法是提高中医临床疗效的关键，也是名老中医临床经验继承、发展、创新的突破口。尤其在当前证候的标准化、客观化研究难以取得明确结论之时，以相对固定的证型来描述证候时容易出现表述不统一，造成辨证的牵强附会。而以治法为核心，进行名老中医临床经验应用研究，能够体现病情的复杂多样性、个体性和辨证的灵活性，以免陷于僵化的固定分型，或可解决名老中医学术经验继承与临床应用脱节的问题，从而保持中医理论的特色和优势，促进名老中医学术思想的发展和创新。通过对不同治法的横向比较和纵向分析，不仅可以证实方药在某些功效方面程度上的差别，还有望发现不同治法的某些特殊功效。如陈可冀教授提出的"三通两补法"治疗冠心病的学术经验，就是在病证结合理论指导下，对冠心病病因病机深刻认识的基础上，结合自身多年临床经验的高度概括和总结，并被临床广泛应用[5-6]。

3. 病证结合是名老中医临床经验应用研究的重要途径

病证结合，即辨病与辨证相结合，是一种既重视对病的诊断、又注重辨证论治的临床诊疗体系[7]。辨病是辨西医之病，寻找病源，明确诊断，对疾病的病因、病机、病情的发展、转归、预后等从整体上进行把握；辨证是辨中医之证，根据疾病某一发展阶段的病理特点而做出阶段性判断。病主要反映机体整个生理病理系统的基本矛盾，而证则反映疾病当前阶段的主要矛盾；病决定证的基本特征与发展方向，证体现疾病不同阶段的病机特点；两者结合既掌握了疾病的基本矛盾，又能解决证候的主要矛盾。病证结合的临床实践是在确定疾病的情况下，结合辨证论治，综合考虑疾病因人、因地、因时等因素所表现出的不同证候来确立治则治法，从而实现个体化治疗。病证结合的临床研究是用中医辨证论治理论来重新认识、解释现代医学所诊之疾病，是中西医结合研究的重要模式。从某种意义上来说，病证结合是对中医辨证论治体系的补充与完善，有利于加深对疾病性质的认识，有助于掌握不同疾病的特殊性及发展、转归规律，弥补了中医学在诊断、疗效评判标准方面缺乏统一性的缺点。病证结合诊疗模式有助于我们准确理解治则治法在辨证施治过程中的重要性，突出了中医理法方药一致性的特色和优势，是实现证候疗效评价价值的可行途径[8]，也是从治法入手进行名老中医临床经验应用研究的重要途径。

4. 展望

名老中医代表着当前中医学术和临床发展的最高水平，发展和创新名老中医临床经验和学术思想对中医学的发展具有举足轻重的作用，基于此进行的理论提炼将是未来中医药学发展的核心驱动力量[9]。就名老中医临床经验应用研究而言，若仅从病证结合角度来选药组方治疗疾病显然有悖于中医的理论体系，若只凭中医理法方药体系来辨证组方治病似也较难尽快推动中医向较深层次发展。只有西医的辨病与中医的辨证相结合，并根据辨证施治的原则，遵循理法方药一致性，依据君臣佐使的规律和中药的性味归经、药效特点来配伍组方；再结合现代医学认识，把握不同疾病的病变规律和临床特点，方可彰显名老中医学术思想和临床经验的特色和优势，进而便于推广应用、创新发展。总之，坚持病证结合、理法方药相一致的原则，以临床诊疗实践进行效果的衡量和评价，从治法方面入手进行名老中医临床经验应用研究，将达到治法各异的殊途同归之妙，进而使名老中医临床经验在继承中应用，在应用中不断发展和创新。

参考文献

[1] 薛钧，贺兴东，翁维良，等．名老中医学术经验"研究型继承"的实践．世界中医药，2008，3 (1)：46-47.

[2] 任秀玲．论中医学的理论医学特征．中华中医药杂志，2006，21 (6)：4-6.

[3] 任秀玲．中医学本质论．中华中医药杂志，2009，24 (6)：693-696.

[4] 李姿慧，胡建鹏，王健．中医治则治法研究与探讨．安徽中医学院学报，2007，26 (6)：1-4.

[5] 张京春．陈可冀院士治疗冠心病心绞痛学术思想与经验．中西医结合心脑血管病杂志，2008，3 (7)：634-636.

[6] 张京春．陈可冀院士治疗冠心病心绞痛学术思想与经验（续完）．中西医结合心脑血管病杂志，2008，3 (8)：712-713.

[7] 谢元华，张京春，陈可冀．病证方药相应及其意义．中西医结合心脑血管病杂志，2008，6 (1)：1-2.

[8] 李建生，余学庆，李素云．病证结合诊疗模式下实现证候疗效评价价值的可行途径．中华中医药杂志，2009 (3)：261-264.

[9] 周学平，叶放，周仲瑛．中医理论传承与创新研究的思路和方法．中医杂志，2009，50 (2)：101-103.

郭士魁活血化瘀学术经验初探 *

张东　李秋艳

活血化瘀作为一种有效的治疗方法早在《内经》中就已经提出来了，并为历代医家所推崇。如清代医家王清任把活血化瘀应用于多种疾病的治疗当中，并总结了益气活血、通窍活血、通下活血等多种治疗方法，扩大了活血化瘀治法的应用范围。

在现代，医家中倡导活血化瘀治疗方法的不乏其人，中国中医研究院西苑医院的郭士魁先生 (1915—1981) 就是其中较为著名的一位。20 世纪六七十年代，大多数医家主要应用以栝楼薤白半夏汤为代表的通阳宣痹的方法治疗冠心病，那时郭士魁先生就较早地提出了活血化瘀治疗冠心病的思路，并不断应用于临床实践，总结了丰富的临床经验，到今天活血化瘀已经成为治疗冠心病最重要的方法之一。本文兹就郭士魁先生关于活血化瘀方面的思路和方法做一介绍。

1. "冠心 2 号"的创立

郭士魁先生在 20 世纪 70 年代研制出了"冠心 2 号"，并广泛应用于临床。"冠心 2 号"由红花、赤芍、丹参、降香、川芎组成，红花"破血、和血、调血"、"通利血脉"；丹参"功同四物"，"破宿血，补生新血"，与红花并入心经，"补心定志、安神宁心"，二者一温一凉，相得益彰。川芎为血中气药，辛燥温散；赤芍柔肝活血，与川芎相配一刚一柔，刚柔相济。而此方尤妙在降香，降香不但"行血破滞，宣五脏郁气"，而且芳香温通，此处用降香配伍活血药，蕴含了王清任通窍活血汤活血通窍之意。用降香有麝香芳香通窍之意，但避免了麝香的耗散峻烈之缺点，而且降香兼有行气活血，又蕴含了血府逐瘀汤行气活血、"气为血之帅"的制方原理。一药兼有两方之长，使"冠心 2 号"集理气活血芳香温通于一体，成为冠心病治疗的一个经典方剂。

病案 1 李某，男，48 岁，1976 年 1 月 20 日初诊因情绪不好或劳累后胸闷，伴头晕、恶心、耳鸣，某医院诊断冠心病 1 年，平时心电图示 T 波改变（Ⅱ、Ⅲ、AVF 倒置，TV4 ~ 5 低平）。检查：舌质暗苔白，脉沉弦。郭老会诊后辨证为胸痹眩晕（气滞血瘀兼有痰浊）。立法：活血理气化痰。方用：川芎 12g、红花 12g、赤芍 12g、丹参 24g、降香 9g、郁金 18g、鸡血藤 18g、葛根 24g、泽泻 15g、白术 12g、栝楼 18g。

* 原载于《中国中医基础医学杂志》，2010，16 (12)：1189-1190

1976年1月27日二诊：服药后头晕、恶心、耳鸣缓解，劳累后仍有胸闷。舌质暗苔白，脉沉弦。上方加薤白、桃仁各9g继服。1976年2月3日三诊：服上方6剂，近来无胸闷及心痛，舌质暗苔薄白，脉弦细。又服上方18剂，心电图T波倒置有改善。再未发生胸闷及耳鸣、头晕。

按：本例患者辨证为胸痹、眩晕（气滞血瘀兼痰浊），方选冠心2号之红花、川芎、赤芍、丹参、降香理气活血、芳香通窍；辅以郁金、葛根、鸡血藤加强活血通络之力，栝楼、薤白、白术、泽泻宽胸化痰浊。

2. 芳香温通活血

郭士魁先生借用治疗牙痛的民间验方哭来笑去散，创立了以芳香温通为主的宽胸丸，方选荜拨、良姜、细辛、檀香、元胡等药物温通活血，能迅速缓解冠心病心绞痛的发作。对于冠心病心绞痛的长期治疗或配合活血化瘀的方药，或在活血化瘀药物中根据病情的轻重缓急灵活选用荜拨、良姜、细辛、檀香中的几味加于处方之中，共奏温通活血之功。

案例2 田某，男，62岁，病历号210457。1975年10月16日会诊：患者因急性心肌梗死，在外院治疗4d后，现仍有轻度胸痛、胸闷、发憋、腹胀，大便隔日一行，四肢冷，出汗。查：舌暗紫舌体胖，中心苔黄腻，脉沉细左细弱。辨证：气虚血瘀兼痰浊。立法：益气温阳，活血化浊。方用：生黄芪18g、当归15g、丹参18g、红花9g、川芎18g、赤芍15g、栝楼30g、薤白15g、桂枝15g、良姜9g、荜拨9g、木香9g、香附15g、干晒参9g（另煎兑服）、元胡粉0.9g、冰片粉0.6g（后2味冲服）。1975年10月23日二诊：服药后胸痛、胸闷完全缓解，出汗减少，大便通畅，腹胀缓解，舌质暗紫苔白，脉沉细左细弱，上方继服。

1975年10月30日三诊：一般状况好，无胸闷、胸痛，睡眠可，已下地活动，无其他不适；舌暗苔薄白，脉沉细，继予益气温阳，活血化瘀。方用：党参15g、黄芪15g、当归9g、丹参18g、川芎18g、红花9g、赤芍15g、栝楼30g、薤白12g、香附12g、木香9g。

按：患者真心痛，心阳、心气受损，心脉瘀阻致胸闷、胸痛，四肢冷为阳气虚。汗出、腹胀、大便不畅为气虚。郭老给予益气活血、开窍化痰之剂。黄芪、人参益气，当归养血，荜拨、良姜、元胡、冰片为宽胸丸加减，芳香温通止痛；丹参、川芎、红花、赤芍为冠心2号加减，活血化瘀；桂枝温通心阳；栝楼、薤白化痰宽胸；香附、木香理气止痛。

3. 安神养心活血

郭老对于心血管疾病的治疗非常重视"心主血，心藏神"这一中医传统理论。在临床应用活血化瘀或益气活血药物的同时，非常注重养心血、养心阴。如临床多用当归、生地、玉竹等药物，在活血化瘀的基础上，灵活配伍益气、化痰、清热等药物。郭老非常重视心藏神，无论是对于冠心病、心律失常的治疗，还是对于心力衰竭、高血压病的治疗，经常加用养心安神的药物，如酸枣仁、五味子、柏子仁、首乌藤、珍珠母等。郭老认为，血脉瘀阻则心神不藏，反之心神不藏则心血易阻，因此郭老多在益气活血、理气活血、开窍活血等诸多方法中又增加了安神活血一法。

案例3 郭某，女47岁，工人，1976年1月20日初诊：半年来心悸、烦躁、出汗、眠差，月经3个月未至。心电图为窦性心动过速、房性期前收缩。近来诸症加重，心慌、心烦不安。舌质略暗，边尖赤中心有裂，苔薄白，脉沉弦细数有促象，可闻期前收缩10～15次/分，未闻病理性杂音，心率：94次/分，血压130/86mmHg。心电图：窦性心律，频发性房性期前收缩，T波改变。郭老诊后辨证为胸痹（气虚、气滞血瘀）。辨证：心阴虚损，心神不宁。立法：育阴养心，镇静安神。方用：百合15g、生地15g、珍珠母24g、柏子仁9g、菖蒲16g、远志9g、川芎16g、鸡血藤18g、麦冬9g、元参16g、乌梅16g、炙甘草6g。

1976年2月3日二诊：进上方14剂。心悸、心慌完全缓解，睡眠进步，心烦减轻。舌质略暗边尖赤，中心裂，苔薄白，脉沉弦细，心律齐，心率86次/分，血压120/85mmHg，上方继服。

1976年2月17日三诊：服上药，精神好转，心烦减轻，无心悸、心慌，睡眠进步，复查心电图正常。继服上方6～12剂。

按：本例患者心阴不足，见舌红有裂，心神不宁、心烦不安，心悸脉结。治疗选用育阴养心、镇静安神之剂。百合、生地为《金匮要略》中的百合地黄汤，有养阴安神之功，再配伍元参、麦冬、乌梅养阴；柏子仁、菖蒲、远志、珍珠母镇静宁心安神；炙甘草养心调和诸药，共奏育阴养心、镇静安神之功。

4. 疑难杂病诸法并用

心血管疾病病程长，病变复杂，单纯用一种方法很难取得长期满意的疗效，因此郭老经常会诸法并用。郭老认为，对于心脏，心气、心血、心阴、心阳、心神往往相互影响、互为因果，不能截然分开。因此，郭老常常融益心气、养心阴、活心血、温心阳、安心神、宽胸化痰等诸法于一方或交替使用，治法虽多，但井然有序，针对病情，丝丝入扣。

案例4 李某，女，79岁，病历号15506。1977年12月2日郭老会诊：患者原有高血压病，冠心病3年。近1年来经常胸闷、胸痛，并向左肩放射，含硝酸甘油可缓解。头晕、心慌、经常昏厥，曾到某医院看急诊2次，诊断为冠心病、高血压病、阵发性心房颤动、心动过缓（窦房结功能低下）。曾用地高辛、阿托品等药物治疗未愈。昨日来院急诊，监测心律为：阵发性心房颤动，心室率100～110次/分，阵发性完全性房室传导阻滞，交结性逸搏，偶见窦性停搏，心房颤动转复时，窦停较长，起搏较晚，致昏厥。舌质红中心龟裂少津，苔少，脉缓结代，心律不整，心率40～44次/分。血压：140/80mmHg。郭老诊后辨证为气阴两虚，心脉瘀阻。立法：益气育阴，养心活血。

方用党参18g，黄芪18g，丹参24g，红花9g，川芎16g，五味子15g，麦冬16g，生地18g，浮小麦30g，炙甘草18g，全栝楼18g，薤白16g，生龙牡各18g。

1977年12月16日二诊：服药后，胸闷、憋气好转，心悸仍有发生，每在心房颤动转复时头晕、乏力但无昏厥。舌质红龟裂，苔薄白，脉沉细缓，心律整，心率46次/分，血压140/80mmHg。方用党参18g、葛根18g、生地18g、柏子仁16g、生黄芪18g、干姜16g、丹参24g、川芎15g、红花9g、桂枝16g、炙甘草18g、珍珠母30g。

1977年12月23日三诊：服药后，2d未发生心房颤动，昨日发作1次，心率120次/分，转

复时有轻度头晕。近来无胸闷及心绞痛，舌质红，中心裂，苔薄白。脉沉细缓，心律整，心率46次/分。方用：党参24g、黄芪15g、当归16g、白术16g、茯苓18g、陈皮9g、升麻6g、葛根18g、丹参30g、川芎16g、桂枝9g、柏子仁9g、五味子16g、炙甘草16g。

1978年1月11日四诊：服药后，心悸减少，有3d未发生心房颤动，但有轻度胸闷，无心绞痛，睡眠可。舌质红中心裂，苔薄白，脉弦细迟偶有代象，心律偶有不整，心率42～48次/分，血压140/80mmHg。方用：党参18g、生地18g、麦冬16g、五味子9g、桂枝9g、葛根18g、桃仁9g、川芎16g、当归16g、黄芪18g、细辛3g、丹参18g、补骨脂15g、炙甘草16g。

1978年1月25日五诊：服药后，无胸闷及心绞痛，心悸很少发生，近2周发生1次心房颤动，约30min自动转复，无明显头晕，睡眠好，舌质略红中心裂，苔薄白，脉细缓，心律整，心率48～50次/分，血压130/70mmHg，继服上方。

按：本例患者病变复杂，有冠心病、高血压、阵发性心房颤动、心动过缓、阵发性完全性房室传导阻滞、交结性逸搏、窦性停搏，心率快至120次/分，慢至心率40次/分，伴胸闷、胸痛、心悸、头晕甚至昏厥。辨证为气阴两虚、心脉血瘀，以党参、黄芪补心气；生地、麦冬养心阴；浮小麦、炙甘草、五味子、柏子仁、生龙牡宁心神；川芎、丹参、红花活心血；栝楼、薤白化痰宽胸，后又以桂枝、干姜、细辛温通心阳。对于复杂之病变，集补心气、温心阳、养心阴、安心神、活心血，诸法并用，可谓面面俱到，如此才能取得较好的疗效。

参考文献

[1] 翁维良，于英奇整理.郭士魁临床经验选集——杂病证治.北京：人民卫生出版社，2005：53-94.

[2] 翁维良.中国百年百名中医临床家丛书—郭士魁.北京：中国中医药出版社，2001：101-202.

[3] 翁维良.翁维良临床经验辑要.北京：中国医药科技出版社，2001，82-110.

[4] 钱超尘，温长路.王清任研究集成.北京：中医古籍出版社，2006，272.

翁维良应用活血化瘀法的学术经验 *

张东 李秋艳

中国中医科学院西苑医院翁维良教授是中国中医科学院首席研究员，博士生导师，博士后导师，全国老中医药专家学术经验继承导师，科学技术委员会委员，第七、八届国家药典委员会委员，科学技术部中医 (973 计划) 专家组成员，国家食品药品监督管理局新药审评专家，中华中医药学会临床药理学会副主任委员。翁老行医 50 余年，擅于应用活血化瘀的方法治疗心血管疾病以及各种疑难病，用药精炼，疗效显著。笔者有幸师从翁老，侍诊左右，觅得一鳞半爪，兹介绍如下。

1. "冠心 3 号" 的创立

"冠心 3 号" 由红花、赤芍、丹参、郁金、川芎组成，其中红花 "破血、和血、调血" "通利血脉"，丹参 "功同四物" "破宿血，补生新血"，与红花并入心经，并有 "补心定志、安神宁心" 之功，二者一温一凉，相得益彰。川芎，血中气药，辛燥温散；赤芍柔肝活血，与川芎相配一刚一柔，刚柔相济。郁金，行气、解郁、凉血、破瘀。此方是由已故名老中医郭士魁先生创立的冠心 2 号变化而来，两方仅有一味之差即冠心 2 号用降香，而冠心 3 号用郁金。冠心 2 号用降香是取其芳香温通、行血破滞之功，降香配伍活血药，蕴含了王清任通窍活血汤活血通窍之意。用降香有麝香芳香通窍之意，但避免了麝香的耗散峻烈之缺点，而且降香兼能行气活血，又蕴含了血府逐瘀汤行气活血、"气为血之帅" 的制方原理。一药兼有两方之长，使 "冠心 2 号" 集理气活血、芳香温通于一体，成为冠心病治疗的一个经典方剂。

翁维良教授在临床中应用 "冠心 2 号" 得心应手。但在不断的临床实践中翁老发现由于冠心病是一个慢性疾病，往往需要长期服药，翁老有一些较重的患者服药三五年的很常见，因此临床上就需要一个适合长期服用的方剂。"冠心 2 号" 的药性虽然已近平和，但降香一味长期服用毕竟芳香耗散，用于冠心病急性期有较好的缓解心绞痛的作用，但若长期服仍嫌其有伤正之弊，因此翁老从临床出发，改降香为郁金，用郁金既保留了降香活血、行气、通窍的长处，又较为温和，避免了降香久服耗散气血的弊端，因此郁金、红花、川芎、丹参、赤芍成为了翁老临床常用的固定方剂，翁老称为 "冠心 3 号"。翁老应用此方非常灵活，郁金通散活血，但性味寒凉，改降香为郁金，是变 "温通" 为 "凉通"，为血瘀有热不适合温通的冠心病患者提供了一个新的方法。而对于血瘀有寒又要长期服药的病人，翁老则又巧妙地改郁金为姜黄，姜黄性味辛、苦、温，与郁金是同一植物的不同部位，但性味变温，换郁金为姜黄，"凉通" 又变为 "温通"，但不伤正气，一药之换，颇具巧思。即使对于同一个患者，翁老也常常根据其寒热变化，甚至季节的改变，交替应用郁金和姜黄，以应对病情的需要，翁老的灵活辨证由此可见一斑。

病例 1 患者，女，59 岁，2008 年 11 月 6 日就诊。阵发胸痛 6～7 年，每次疼痛 5～10 min，自服硝酸甘油 3 min 可缓解，走路快或上楼时发作，尤其着急时胸痛发作明显，秋冬重，春夏较轻，眠差，脉细，舌质紫暗，苔薄白。辨证：胸痹，气滞血瘀，心脉瘀阻。治则治法：活血理气。处方：柴胡 10g、郁金 12g、红花 12g、赤芍 12g、川芎 12g、丹参 15g、元胡 12g、川牛膝 15g、珍珠母 20g、夜交藤 20g、五味子 10g、枣仁 12g、路路通 15g、决明子 12g、水煎服，7 剂。2008 年 11 月 14 日复诊：走路、上楼胸痛减轻，睡眠好转，脉细，舌质紫暗，苔薄白。辨证：气滞血瘀，心脉瘀阻。治则治法：活血理气，上方去夜交藤、路路通，继服 14 剂。

按：患者着急时胸痛发作明显，舌质紫暗，为气滞血瘀之证，翁老应用冠心 3 号为主，红花、赤芍、丹参、郁金、川芎活血，又加柴胡、元胡、川牛膝、路路通理气活血通络，珍珠母、夜交藤、酸枣仁安神养心，使胸痛得以明显缓解。

* 原载于《北京中医药》，2010，29 (11)：823-825

2. 芳香开窍温通活血

宽胸丸是西苑医院治疗冠心病不稳定型心绞痛的一个经典方剂，以芳香温通活血化瘀的荜拨、良姜、细辛、檀香、元胡等药物为主。荜拨，辛热，"破滞气，开郁结"；高良姜，"辛热纯阳，除一切陈寒痼冷"；细辛，"芳香最烈，故善开结气，宣泄郁滞"，有"开通诸窍之功"；檀香，"芳香辛行，温散寒邪"；元胡，"能行血中气滞，气中血滞，里一身内外上下诸痛"。诸药合用，芳香开窍，温通活血。翁老在临床常常应用此方。或用成方，或是根据病情的轻重缓急选用其中的一两味药物，配伍其他活血药灵活选用。然此方温散，临床多用于气虚、阳虚有寒的患者。而翁老对于血瘀有热的患者亦敢于应用此法，通过配伍清热的凉药如黄芩、黄连等，既避免了温热药物性温助热之过，又保留了荜拨、檀香等药物芳香通窍之长。对于阴虚有热的患者则配伍生地、麦冬、玄参等滋阴清热但不滋腻的药物，避免了温散之品助热伤阴的弊端，同时又加强了通窍活血的力量，这种不拘一格灵活变通的思想在翁老的临床治疗中颇为多见。

病例 2 患者，男，79 岁，2008 年 11 月 6 日就诊。患者 20 年前开始间断胸痛，1990 年因心肌梗死入院行冠状动脉造影，前降支植入 2 个支架，1991 年因心前区不适再次行冠状动脉造影，回旋支植入 2 个支架。平时规律服用拜阿司匹林 100 mg 每晚 1 次，硫酸氢氯吡格雷（波立维）75 mg 每日 1 次，单硝酸异山梨酯 20 mg 每日 2 次，此后多次因胸痛住院。高血压病史 38 年，最高血压 180/100 mmHg，糖尿病病史 2 年，肾功能不全病史 1 年，脑梗死病史 3 年，脂代谢异常病史年份不详，吸烟史 20 年，平均每日 5 ~ 10 支，已戒 10 年。饮酒史 30 年，白酒多少不等，已戒 10 年。近两个月来频发心前区疼痛，每日发作 1 ~ 2 次，活动后加重，自服硝酸甘油可以好转，每日吸氧 2 次，伴心慌、乏力、头晕、大便秘结，2 日 1 次。舌黯红苔薄黄，脉弦。心电图示：窦性心律，Ⅰ、Ⅱ、aVF 导联 P 波低平，Ⅰ、V6 导联 T 波倒置，Ⅱ导 T 波消失，V5 导联 T 波撤向，V6 ST 段压低 0.1 mV。中医诊断：胸痹（气虚血瘀）。西医诊断：(1) 冠状动脉粥样硬化性心脏病（不稳定型心绞痛 PCI 支架术后）；(2) 高血压 3 级（极高危）；(3) 2 型糖尿病；(4) 高脂血症；(5) 肾功能不全；(6) 陈旧脑梗死；(7) 多发动脉粥样硬化并狭窄。

治法：益气活血，温通心脉。处方：葛根 15g、生黄芪 15g、太子参 15g、川芎 12g、红花 12g、郁金 12g、丹参 15g、赤芍 12g、当归 12g、良姜 10g、姜黄 12g。宽胸丸 1 丸，日 3 次。2009 年 1 月 19 日二诊：白天心绞痛明显好转，但夜间心绞痛发作 1 ~ 2 次，服硝酸甘油可缓解，纳差，大便干，舌黯苔薄黄，脉弦。治法：益气养阴活血，处方：葛根 15g、生黄芪 15g、太子参 15g、黄精 15g、玉竹 12g、五味子 12g、川芎 12g、红花 12g、郁金 12g、丹参 15g、姜黄 12g。2009 年 2 月 1 日三诊：心绞痛好转，大便仍干，纳差，眠可，原方去姜黄加麻仁 12g、决明子 15g 润肠通便。

按：患者心绞痛频繁发作，随时有发生心肌梗死的可能，因此要迅速有效地控制心绞痛的发作。翁老在益气活血的基础上汤药加良姜 10g、姜黄 12g，再加宽胸丸芳香通络，温通血脉，心绞痛得以迅速控制；二诊患者夜间心绞痛发作频繁，因此加用养阴之黄精、玉竹，但仍用姜黄温通血脉，使心绞痛进一步得到控制。可见温通心阳对于缓急止痛、迅速缓解心绞痛取得了较好的疗效。

3. 注重益气养阴活血

翁老治疗心血管疾病时非常重视心气、心阴与心血之间的关系，翁老认为气为血之帅，气虚则行血不利则产生瘀血，但阴为血之源，心阴不足、血干而枯同样会导致瘀血，反之血瘀又会耗气伤阴，加重气血之虚。对于不同的疾病，气虚、血虚以及血瘀的原因和轻重缓急的比例也不同，如心肌炎多是热毒内侵，大多先伤阴，进一步耗气，气阴两虚使一部分患者最后会导致血瘀，所以对于心肌炎的患者则大多以益气养阴、清热解毒为主，辅以活血化瘀。对于心力衰竭的患者则大多是先有心气耗损，气虚导致血瘀，进一步气不生血，瘀血耗阴导致心阴虚，所以心力衰竭以气虚血瘀为主，后期则兼有阴虚。冠心病的患者则大多数是先有瘀血阻于心络，瘀血既生，长期则耗气伤阴，导致气阴两虚。而心律失常则较为复杂，气虚、阴虚、瘀血可以互为因果，或为气虚进一步导致气阴两虚兼有血瘀，或先为气滞血瘀，继而耗伤气阴，则要根据患者的病情灵活应用。选用益气养阴的药物，翁老常用黄芪、党参、沙参、麦冬、五味子、玉竹、生地等配伍活血化瘀的药物，但翁老认为黄芪补脾肺之气，偏于走表；党参既补脾气，同时也补心气，偏于走里；而太子参，不但补心气，而且气阴双补，所以对于典型的气阴两虚的患者，翁老更多地选用太子参。

病例3 患者，男，65岁，2008年6月30日就诊。患者2005年9月因心力衰竭、心房颤动在某院诊断为扩张型心肌病，左室内径74 mm，射血分数39%，2007年进一步加重，喘憋不能平卧，经治疗好转。近日时有喘憋，但可平卧，活动后加重，出汗多，烦躁，心悸，咳嗽，咳痰，耳鸣，脉结代，舌质暗，苔中部黄。辨证：喘证，气阴两虚，瘀血内阻。治则治法：益气养阴，兼以活血，处方：生黄芪15g、黄精15g、玉竹12g、丹参15g、红花12g、赤芍12g、葛根15g、杏仁10g、桔梗15g、远志10g、茯苓15g、泽泻15g。7剂。2008年7月14日复诊，喘憋减轻，活动量增加，仍汗出，但较前稍好，早上痰多，乏力较重，辨证：喘证，气阴两虚，瘀血内阻。治则治法：益气养阴，兼以活血，处方：生黄芪15g、黄精15g、白术12g、防风12g、玉竹12g、丹参15g、红花12g、赤芍12g、桔梗15g、土茯苓15g、车前草15g。14剂，以后以此方出入加减。至2009年4月30日就诊，患者活动量较大，可上五层楼，每天可去集贸市场购物，出汗减少，少量咳痰，脉细弦，苔干而黄，辨证：喘证，气阴两虚，瘀血内阻。治则治法：益气养阴，兼以活血，处方：太子参15g、北沙参15g、麦冬15g、五味子10g、玉竹12g、黄芪20g、山萸肉10g、赤芍12g、红花12g、川芎12g、银杏10g、茯苓15g。14剂。患者一直以益气养阴活血之法出入加减，于2009年10月复查超声左室内径60 mm，射血分数45%。

按：患者诊断为扩张型心肌病，心衰较重，翁老辨证为气虚血瘀，以生黄芪、太子参、白术益气，黄芪、白术、防风又为玉屏风散之意；黄精、玉竹、北沙参、麦冬、五味子、山萸肉养阴，太子参、麦冬、五味子又为生脉饮，为益气养阴之代表方；赤芍、红花、川芎活血，桔梗、杏仁等止咳化痰，茯苓、泽泻利水。翁老以此方出入加减，患者坚持服用，终使活动耐量明显增加，左室内径减小，射血分数增加，取得了较好的疗效。

4. 心主血，心藏神的应用

翁老非常重视"心主血，心藏神"这一中医理论在心血管疾病的治疗当中的应用，认为心神不藏则心神不宁，心神不宁则气血不能平和，气血不能平和则易致气滞血瘀，血脉易阻，因此心神不宁是导致瘀血的原因之一；而瘀血阻滞又可以导致或加重心神不宁，因此心神安定平和，血脉才能顺畅，反之亦然，因此心主血、心藏神二者相互影响、密切相关。翁老在治疗上把"心主血，心藏神"二者有机地结合起来，在益气活血、养阴活血、开窍活血等诸法中加用安神养心，无论是对于冠心病、心律失常还是对于心力衰竭、高血压病的治疗，都明显增强了疗效。翁老经常选用养心安神的药物如酸枣仁、五味子、柏子仁、首乌藤、珍珠母等。

病例4 患者，女，57岁，2008年5月26日就诊，患者阵发心前区疼痛3年，3年前诊断冠心病，近1个月时有胸痛、胸闷，走路时发作较明显，伴乏力、气短，睡眠可，大便日2次，不溏，脉细，舌质暗，苔薄白，辨证：胸痹，气虚血瘀，治则治法：益气活血，佐以安神。处方：生黄芪15g、黄精12g、葛根15g、珍珠母20g、枣仁15g、夜交藤15g、菊花12g、荷叶15g、丹参15g、赤芍12g、郁金12g、红花12g、川芎12g。14剂。2008年6月26日复诊：胸痛减轻，但仍与劳累有关，胸闷亦减轻，但天气闷热时会偶有加重，脉细，舌质暗，苔薄黄，辨证：胸痹，气虚血瘀。治则治法：益气活血，佐以安神。处方：原方去菊花、珍珠母、夜交藤，加神曲12g、路路通15g、藿香12g，14剂继服。

按：患者胸痛、胸闷、乏力、气短、舌质暗，翁老辨证为气虚血瘀，以生黄芪、黄精益气养阴，丹参、赤芍、郁金、红花、川芎活血，患者虽然睡眠可，但翁老仍用了珍珠母、枣仁、夜交藤安神养心，意在心神安定才能使血脉条畅，使瘀血去而胸痛止。

5. 藤类通络

王清任创立通经逐瘀汤，以皂角刺、穿山甲、麝香等药物走窜入于经络，配伍地龙、桃仁、红花等活血药共奏通经逐瘀之功。翁老认为通经逐瘀汤攻逐之力较猛，长期服用未免伤正，且麝香价格昂贵，亦不适合多服，因此翁老借鉴中医"藤类入络"的理论，应用藤类药物配伍活血化瘀药物治疗心脑血管病。此法既有通散活血之功，又有引药入络之意，为冠心病、高血压、脑血管病等慢性病的长期治疗找到了一个较好的方法。翁老在临床上常用络石藤、路路通2味为对药，络石藤祛风湿，

第六章

通经络；路路通，通经利水，二者均可治疗跌打损伤、经行不畅，故又均有活血化瘀之效，既加强了活血化瘀的作用，又避免了损伤正气，尤其适合慢性患者长期服用。

病例5 患者，男，51岁，2008年8月21日就诊。患者患高血压病一年余，血压波动在(90～200)/(50～100)mmHg，去年在某院诊断为肾动脉狭窄，置入2枚支架，后又因为急性左心衰、阵发心房颤动、慢性肾衰竭多次住院，目前血压仍波动较大，目前血压170/100mmHg，头晕，头发麻，头胀，视物不清，睡眠差，偶有胸闷，脉弦细，舌质暗红，舌苔薄黄。辨证：眩晕，气虚血瘀，络脉瘀阻。治则治法：益气活血通络，处方：生黄芪15g、北沙参12g、路路通15g、络石藤15g、川牛膝12g、丹参12g、赤芍12g、红花12g、姜黄12g、川芎12g、当归12g、天麻

12g、钩藤15g、薏米15g。7剂。2008年9月4日复诊：血压波动减轻，波动在（150～90）/（60～80）mmHg，头发麻，头胀，视物不清等症状减轻，脉弦细，舌质暗红，舌苔黄。辨证：肝阳上亢，络脉瘀阻，治则治法：平肝通络，处方：葛根15g、天麻12g、钩藤15g、杜仲12g、丹参15g、红花12g、赤芍12g、川芎12g、路路通15g、络石藤15g、珍珠母20g、土茯苓15g、黄芩15g、泽泻12g。7剂继服。

按：患者患肾动脉狭窄，继发性高血压，头晕，脉弦细，舌质暗红。翁老辨证气虚血瘀，络脉瘀阻，以生黄芪、北沙参益气养阴，路路通、络石藤祛风湿，通经络，配伍丹参、红花、赤芍、川芎共奏化瘀通络之功，兼天麻、钩藤平肝，土茯苓、泽泻、黄芩、薏米化湿清热，全方益气活血通络祛湿，扶正祛邪兼顾，相得益彰。

病证结合治疗观与临床实践[*]

陈可冀

科学技术进步总是继承与创新互动，保持永恒和与时俱进互动，中医药临床实践中的病证结合治疗观的演变和进步，很能说明这个问题。

1. 当代中医临床诊疗的几种模式

当代中医临床诊疗的模式主要有以下几种：(1)经典（传统）模式：中医辨病论治与辨证论治的结合；(2)中医辨证论治模式：证因脉治、方证相应；(3)中医辨症与专方专药的应用模式；(4)西医辨病与中医辨证论治结合模式：即现代病证结合模式；(5)西医辨病与专方的应用模式；(6)无病从证、无证从病模式。在这些代表性模式中，当代中医药界及中西医结合界最为普遍应用的是西医辨病与中医辨证论治相结合的现代病证结合模式，这也是中西医结合的重要成果，更是中医现代临床实际的需求。新中国成立以来我国国家食品药品监督管理局先后批准的中成药新药近万种，其中95%以上既有西医适应证病种，又有中医的证候适应证标

准。中医药界大多数临床医生也普遍要求应用病证结合、方证对应的原则进行处方遣药。当然，在一部分高水平的中医老专家以及基层中医师中，还是有很多医生特别只注重临床中医辨证论治的模式，体现中医传统的治疗特色。在很多综合性医院里，很多西医则采用西医辨病与专方应用的模式，简单易行，也有一定成效。几种模式各有优越性和局限性，理当互为补充，才能更好地满足临床诊疗的需求。

2. 现代病证结合模式的医学科学与文化意义

西医辨病与中医辨证论治结合治疗的模式之所以推广较好，应用面较广泛，是因为它有如下优点：(1)体现了东西方医学科学与文化的优势互补大趋势（辨识疾病本质并全面了解症象表现）；(2)体现了经典理论与经验的传承；(3)体现了临床服务能力与临床水平的提高；(4)体现了科学认识

* 原载于《中国中西医结合杂志》，2011，31 (8)：1016-1017

和治疗疾病及疗效评价；(5) 体现了有利于治疗和诊断上的原始性创新；(6) 有利于国际交流、沟通。当然，从不同角度思考，现代病证结合模式也必然会对中医自身以病机（风、寒、暑、湿、燥、火、热、瘀、水、饮、痰、毒等）为核心的辨证思维体系的发展存在一定程度的冲击。

3. 病证结合治疗观的历史沿革

辨证论治是中医药学的主要学术特色和价值表现。不过，数千年来，实际上中医药学在临床实践中也还是注重辨病论治与辨证论治相结合的，其文献依据可见于《五十二病方》《黄帝内经》《伤寒论》《金匮要略》《肘后备急方》等著作。中医辨病论治中所列的很多病名不少现代还在广泛应用，如卒中与中风、胬肉攀睛、疔疮、感冒、缠腰火丹、历节风、乳岩、天行赤眼、鼻渊、牛皮癣、痔、痈、子痫、麻疹、水肿、消渴、淋病、黄疸、宿食、心痛等，只不过现代医学的进步丰富了这些疾病的内涵。中医证候的名称也是有很多切合实际应用的，如郁证、痹证、虚劳、痰饮等。这些都值得在实际工作中很好地加以更好地继承和发扬。

《金匮要略》是最典型、的最有实用价值的辨病论治与辨证论治相结合的专著。各篇均题揭为"辨病脉证治"，所载病种达 60 余种，计 262 方。宋、金、元及明清时代在辨证论治学术方面陆续有很大的进步，学派蜂起，在一定程度上倾向于在临床中更多地注重辨证论治，辨病论治也相应深入。对后世以及今天都有深远的影响。清徐灵胎在《兰台轨范·序》中说："欲治病者，必先识病之名。能识病名，而后求其病之所由生。知其所有生，又当辨其生之各不同，而病状所由异，然后考其治之法。一病必有主方，一方必有主药"，其论点很有代表性。温病学派在卫气营血辨证、三焦辨证、湿热病辨证等方面都有很多创新性的见解。王清任主张"治病之要诀，在明白气血"；程钟龄在《医学心悟·医门八法》中也是强调八纲辨证论治的。我在临床中也常加上气血两纲以成十纲辨证，加以应用，感觉很能够得心应手。

近现代汇通医派如张锡纯首开西法断病结合中医辨证的先河，最引起现代医学界广为注意的代表性方剂是石膏阿司匹林汤。现代名医陆渊雷、施今墨、金寿山、岳美中、姜春华、朱良春、祝谌予等也都倡导病证结合的临床实践，他们的论点和临床案例都有文献可查，证明他们都是讲究实际的优秀的临床家。

4. 病证结合临床研究的病种选择和方法学思考

病证结合临床治疗可以针对目标疾病、目标证候（证与候）、目标症状或四者兼顾（病、证、症、候取向，或症、候、证、病取向），或从整体调节入手，或从局部问题入手，能解决其中某一环节就是了不起的成果。其病种选择应侧重在：(1) 适应当代国家/社会的需求，严重危害人民健康严重的常见病、多发病，如肿瘤、心脑血管病糖尿病等；(2) 凸显中医药疗效优势的病种，如功能性疾病、免疫性疾病、过敏性疾病、病毒性疾病、皮肤病、消化及泌尿系统病、情志病、骨关节病、小儿及老年性疾病、更年期综合征等。如我们针对冠心病介入治疗后再狭窄这一心血管领域的难题，在西医常规治疗基础上加用活血化瘀中药芎芍胶囊等调节气血方药，按照循证医学原则采用多中心、随机、双盲、安慰剂对照方法证实加用中药组可以明显降低介入治疗术后再狭窄的发生率，为在我国国情下再狭窄的预防干预提供了一种有效的手段。

在病证结合临床研究方面，随机化和对照观察是很重要的原则。应进一步重视循证医学和转化医学的引入。在当前条件下，可提倡多元模式临床医疗的研究设计和疗效评价，包括双重的目标病种选择（社会需求＋中医优势），双重的研究方法思考（疾病＋证候、症状），双重的评价标准的整体复合（定量＋定性），以及进一步的循证医学引入，建立增强式的病证结合、宏微观和整体局部统一的循证医学模式，解决可重复性的病证结合临床实用的标准化范式或框架，传承发展，提高自主创新的能力，以期进一步提高疗效，促进中医药的学术及产业化发展，走向世界。当然，药品临床试验管理规范 (Good Clinical Practice, GCP) 的规范化要求及有关随机临床试验报告的声明 (CONSORT 声明) 等，都应考虑结合实际采用。

《论语》有"温故而知新"之说，我们要尊古出新，要温故知新，不可以温故而不出新、温故而不去知新。有的科学家强调，高科技价值链依次应为：信息 (information)、知识 (knowledge)、创意 (ideas)、创新 (innovation)、创业 (therapeutic approach/product developments/marketing) 等多个环节，思路和方法学先行，不断攀升，这些来自实际的经验概括，很值得临床家们思考。

稳步促进中西医结合临床路径的实施 *

陈可冀

我国正在逐步推进有关各临床学科和有关各病种的临床路径的制定、实施和管理的工作。中医/中西医结合临床路径的构建和实施也应当切实稳步做好。吴大嵘、吕玉波教授等对中医/中西医结合临床路径研发的关键问题做了较系统的分析，简要回顾了临床路径的发展史，并指出了中医/中西医结合临床路径研发应注意的一些基本原则和策略[1]。本期又发表了王磊博士、张敏州教授等关于急性心肌梗死中西医结合临床路径的构建及初步评价研究，其结果认为该病治疗中如能以益气活血法为基础的急性心肌梗死中西医结合临床路径进行处理，临床上可以降低患者的住院时间，控制直接经皮冠状动脉介入治疗 (percutaneous coronary intervention, PCI) 的住院费用和缩短该病患者入院时的时间，提高医疗质量[2]，认为临床路径的构建是十分必要和可行的。本期刘建平教授等[3]也对临床路径的制定与实施作出具体讨论。

其实，临床路径 (clinical path 或 clinical pathway)，说到底也就是相当于做好单病种的管理，有一个医疗机构和医疗人员共同照顾好患者的医疗及护理规范或标准遵循，控制和改进医疗质量，并实现合理而有效的跨学科服务，降低相应的医院及患者的费用开支。如果已有相应比较成熟的临床诊疗指南、建议或共识，更可以作为临床路径制定的参照，可以更切合实际，提高科学技术水平。

实事求是的临床路径可以为大多数患者提供最有序、最有效的整体医疗管理步骤或模式。但是由于中医/中西医结合的医疗措施强调个体化差异较西医要突出得多，在诊疗过程中，有"同病异治""异病同治"等辨证思维及处理范例，要求医生要特别注意这一点差异性的处理，体现中医/中西医结合的临床诊疗技术特色，既要重视路径、标准或规范，又不为其所束缚，提高疗效，减少不良反应，并减少不必要的开支，医患应该合作调整并克服这一屏障，以提高有效性、满意度和时

效性；要有质量第一的认识 (quality-first attitude)。据一般估计，实际上大约 80% 的患者可比较正常应用所制定的临床路径实施，但还可能有 20% 左右的患者需另按中医传统思维作个例处理 (case management)。

为了制定和实施好各有关病种的临床路径，以医院或科室为单位成立临床路径发展或管理小组 (clinical path development team) 是必要的，这种跨学科或不同职责人员的多元化组织，定期进行研讨，会更有利于发现和解决问题，可以及时处理好各类差异，检查实施情况，不断提高整体服务质量，改善医患关系。

临床路径的制定、实施及管理，也是一个系统工程，涉及医生、护理人员、信息沟通、管理得力、各自的责任心以及仪器设备条件等诸多层面的种种问题；从多个方面看，有时会认为做好临床路径的实施难度较大；但是为了患者的健康，应该不断改进质量。如能如上所述，认真参考各有关病种的临床循证指南和转化医学成就，以之作为桥梁，尊重中医/中医结合传统思维，可能有助于进一步克服障碍，合理医疗支出费用，往前走去[4-5]。

参考文献

[1] 吴大嵘，周罗晶，张军，等．中医、中西医结合临床路径研发的关键问题．中国中西医结合杂志，2010，30 (11)：1206-1208.

[2] 王磊，张敏州，张军，等．急性心肌梗死中西医结合临床路径的构建及初步评价研究．中国中西医结合杂志，2011，31 (1)：7-10.

[3] 刘建平，王思成，吴大嵘，等．循证中医临床路径的制定与实施．中国中西医结合杂志，2011，31 (1)：115-119.

[4] Haynes B, Haines A. Barriers and bridges to evidence based clinical practice. BM J, 1998, 25 (7153)：273-276.

[5] Zerhouni E. Medicine. The NIH Roadmap. Science, 2003, 302 (5642)：63-72.

* 原载于《中国中西医结合杂志》，2011，31 (1)：6

第六章

高敏心肌肌钙蛋白的临床应用：优势与挑战 *

陈可冀 刘 玥

2012 年公布的《中国心血管病报告 2011》中指出目前我国心血管病死亡率仍然高居不下，其中 2010 年心血管病死亡率高居首位，明显高于肿瘤及其他疾病。急性心肌梗死 (AMI) 因其发病急骤、致死率高而在心血管病的防治中占有极其重要的地位，因此在一级预防的基础上，急性胸痛的患者得到尽早明确诊断、及时再灌注治疗对于降低其死亡率意义重大。

1. 高敏心肌肌钙蛋白临床应用的优势

心肌肌钙蛋白 (cardiac troponin，cTn) 因具有高度的心肌特异性和敏感性而成为诊断 AMI 的"金指标"。欧洲心脏病学会 (European Society of Cardiology, ESC)、美国心脏病学会基金会 (American College of Cardiology Foundation, ACCF)、美国心脏学会 (American Heart Association, AHA) 和世界心脏联盟 (World Heart Federation, WHF) 自 2000 年以来先后发布的 3 个版本"心肌梗死统一定义"中均推荐将 cTn 作为临床诊断 AMI 的首选血清生物标志物，而该定义历次版本的修订基本也围绕 cTn 检测技术的不断更新发展而做出。cTn 的正常值被定义为应低于正常健康人群参考范围上限 (upper reference limit, URL) 的第 99 百分位值，若高于这一正常值（变异系数 ≤ 10%），同时具备相应的临床症状和（或）心电图或影像学特征性改变就应该考虑 AMI 的诊断。但以往由于 cTn 检测技术的限制，许多临床实验室往往在表面正常的人群中都检测不到 cTn，就更加难以确认其正常上限的第 99 百分位值，部分人群其 cTn 的值即使超过正常值上限的第 99 百分位值仍未能检测出，同时检测精确度也难以达到其对变异系数 ≤ 10% 的要求。

近年来，心肌肌钙蛋白检测技术的不断发展，新一代高敏肌钙蛋白 (highly sensitive cardiac troponin, hs-cTn) 检测试剂盒的出现基本解决了上述问题，从其问世之日起就引起了全球心血管病研究者的极大关注，围绕 hs-cTn 在 AMI 的诊断、预后中的作用等方面做了许多研究，取得了一系列成果。目前多项大型临床研究结果发现，hs-cTn 在诊断 AMI 的准确率方面显著高于传统的 cTnT，同时其在早期诊断 AMI 方面的表现也同样引人注目 [1-3]。有学者单独分析胸痛发生在 3h 之内的患者，发现 hs-cTn 诊断 AMI 的准确性亦大大优于传统的 cTn 检测 [4]。新近研究还发现，对于急性胸痛的患者，应用 hs-cTn 检测还可以快速鉴别出胸痛是由 AMI 引起还是由其他心脏疾病（如心律失常、心力衰竭及心肌炎）引起，具有指导临床治疗的重要价值 [5]。在对 AMI 预后的危险分层方面，hs-cTn 在预测不良的心血管事件的发生上也有重要作用 [6]。不仅如此，其在对稳定型冠心病、心力衰竭、表面健康人群中的预后判断也有一定的参考价值 [7-9]。

2. 高敏心肌肌钙蛋白给临床应用带来的挑战

值得注意的是，任何事物都有双面性，hs-cTn 的出现给 AMI 的临床诊断及预后评估带来了诸多优势，但同时也对临床实际应用带来了诸多挑战 [10,11]。

首先，hs-cTn 目前尚缺乏明确的定义及参考范围。有学者把 CV 等于 10% 时的最小检测值很接近第 99 百分位值的 cTn 检测方法称为 hs-cTn，也有学者认为，能在部分或全部表面健康人群中检测到 cTn、同时第 99 百分位值的检测不精密度的 CV ≤ 10% 才是 hs-cTn [12]。而对检测性能进行恰当评估是合理选择 cTn 检测方法的重要环节，早在 2009 年，美国著名心血管病专家 Apple 博士就提出一个评价方案，表面健康人群中的 cTn 检出率 > 50% 即被认定为高敏检测方法，而将 CV ≤ 10% 定义为"指南可接受"，CV > 10% 但 ≤ 20% 定义为"临床可接受"，而 CV > 20% 定义为"不可接受" [13]。一般认为，一定时间内观察到 cTn 增高或降低的变化是提高 AMI 诊断特异性的关键之一，但是升高的幅度目前也缺乏共识，有专家将此幅度定为 20%，有的定为 30%，还有定

* 原载于《医学研究杂志》，2013，42 (2)：1-3

第六章

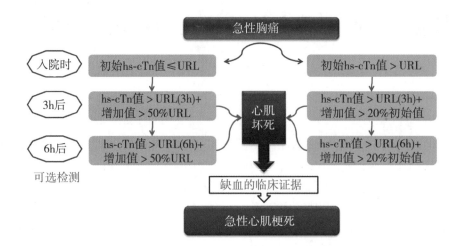

图 1　一种利用 hs-cTn 检测 3h 内快速诊断 AMI 的模式流程图（译自文献 [14] 中图 1）

为 50% 者，不一而同。除此之外，对 hs-cTn 的正常参考范围也缺乏统一标准，hs-cTn 在表面健康人群中存在因年龄、性别以及种族之间的变异，如欧美学者研究发现男性的检测值普遍高于女性（1.2 ～ 2.4 倍）；黑色人种检测值普遍高于高加索人种（1.2 ～ 2.6 倍）等，同时发现临床研究试验所建立的参考范围与试剂盒生产厂商所提供的标准资料也存在较大的差异 [14]。不仅如此，2012 版心肌梗死统一定义一发布，其中对于"操作相关性心肌梗死（PCI 相关性心肌梗死与 CABG 相关性心肌梗死）"的诊断标准引起了学者的许多争议，特别是对于其中 hs-cTn 标准的部分。这些都提示目前对于 hs-cTn 的相关标准的建立还缺乏系统共识，因此目前阶段各国各地建立适合本实验室条件的 hs-cTn 参考范围是非常必要的，目前针对亚洲人的 hs-cTn 的参考范围及相关影响因素的大型临床研究尚不多，因此在中国 hs-cTn 临床应用时更加不能简单地照搬国外生产厂商提供的源自国外人群研究结果的数据。值得高兴的是，2012 年 10 月《中华心血管病杂志》上发布了"高敏心肌肌钙蛋白在急性冠状动脉综合征中的应用中国专家共识"以及"hs-cTn 在中国人群中的部分应用经验"，相信未来随着基于中国人群的 hs-cTn 临床研究资料的不断丰富，必将为 hs-cTn 在中国的临床推广应用带来更加详实的循证依据 [15,16]。

其次，临床如何快速排除 hs-cTn 升高是 AMI 还是其他疾病尚缺乏统一规范。以往心血管病医师看到 cTn 阳性结果就等同于诊断 AMI，并随之开展一系列治疗，包括抗血小板治疗及介入治疗等，但随着高敏感检测技术的应用，极低浓度的 cTn 也能被检测出来，但许多都不是由 AMI 引起的，但

是近 10 年来 AMI 被诊断人数逐年增加，是我们过去漏诊了太多的 AMI 还是现在误诊了太多的 AMI？2012 版"心肌梗死统一定义"专门辟出一章讨论由 hs-cTn 升高导致的"心肌损伤"的范畴，并详细列出了多种可能引起 cTn 升高的非 AMI 原因 [17]。有多项临床研究发现使用非高敏检测 cTn 阴性而高敏检测 cTn 阳性的 70% ～ 90% 的患者都不是 ACS，这就需要临床大夫在实际工作中快速排除 AMI，以避免对其进行不恰当的治疗。值得高兴的是，目前已有许多学者对此做出了探索性的研究，如有学者开发出了 1h 内快速排除 AMI 的新算法 [18]，而又有学者提出另一种 3h 快速诊断 AMI 的算法模式 [14]（图 1）。当然这些都需要结合临床症状和心电图的动态变化做出综合评估，虽然这些算法还需要大量的临床实践的验证，但毕竟为 hs-cTn 的广泛临床应用提供了有益的借鉴。

3. 展望

随着 hs-cTn 检测未来在临床的广泛使用，普通病房和急诊室中的 hs-cTn 阳性患者较之以往必然会大量增多，伴随的后续多次 hs-cTn 复测、心血管系统的检查、住院日期及急诊留观日期的延长等，这些都会给医院以及急诊医师、心血管医师以及普通内科医师带来极大的挑战，可能会带来医疗资源的紧张以及医疗费用的增高，还可能对医保政策产生一定影响 [10]。另一方面，对于不典型的胸痛患者，特别是非高敏检测 cTn 阴性而高敏检测 cTn 阳性的患者，应该如何进行早期管理尚缺乏循证依据，值得开展进一步研究，以期建立成熟的"高 hs-cTn"早期诊断管理方案，为 AMI 的早期诊断、早期干预，降低病死率做出贡献。

参考文献

[1] Reiter M, Twerenbold R, Reichlin T, et al. Early diagnosis of acute myocardial infarction in patients with pre-existing coronary artery disease using more sensitive cardiac troponin assays. Eur Heart J, 2012, 33 (8)：988-997.

[2] Apple FS, Pearce LA, Smith SW, et al. Role of monitoring changes in sensitive cardiac troponin T assay results for early diagnosis of myocardial infarction and prediction of risk of adverse events. Clin Chem, 2009, 55 (5)：930-937.

[3] Potocki M, Reichlin T, Thalmann S, et al. Diagnostic and prognostic impact of copeptin and high-sensitivity cardiac troponin T in patients with pre-existing coronary artery disease and suspected acute myocardial infarction. Heart, 2012, 98 (7)：558-565.

[4] Reichlin T, Hochholzer W, Bassetti S, et al. Early diagnosis of myocardial infarction with sensitive cardiac troponin assays. N Engl J Med, 2009, 361 (9)：858-867.

[5] Haaf P, Drexler B, Reichlin T, et al. High-sensitivity cardiac troponin in the distinction of acute myocardial infarction from acute cardiac noncoronary artery disease. Circulation, 2012, 126 (1)：31-40.

[6] Ndrepepag, Braun S, Schulz S, et al. Comparison of prognostic value of high-sensitivity and conventional troponin T in patients with non-ST-segment elevation acute coronary syndromes. Clin Chim Acta, 2011, 412 (15-16)：1350-1356.

[7] Koenig W, Breitling LP, Hahmann H, et al. Cardiac troponin T measured by a high-sensitivity assay predicts recurrent cardiovascular events in stable coronary heart disease patients with 8-year follow-up. Clin Chem, 2012, 58 (8)：1215-1224.

[8] Sato Y, Fujiwara H, Takatsu Y. Cardiac troponin and heart failure in the era of high-sensitivity assays. J Cardiol, 2012, 60 (3)：160-167.

[9] deFilippi CR, de Lemos JA, Christenson RH, et al. Association of serial measures of cardiac troponin T using a sensitive assay with incident heart failure and cardiovascular mortality in older adults. JAMA, 2010, 304 (22)：2494-2502.

[10] Scott IA, Cullen L, Tate JR, et al. Highly sensitive troponin assays—a two-edged sword? Med J Aust, 2012；197 (6)：320-323.

[11] Giannitsis E, Katus HA. Pros and cons of high-sensitivity assays for cardiac troponin. Nat Rev Cardiol, 2012, 9 (11)：616-618.

[12] 潘柏申. 迎接高敏感方法检测心肌肌钙蛋白时代的到来. 中华心血管病杂志, 2011, 39 (8)：689-692.

[13] Apple FS. A new season for cardiac troponin assays：its time to keep a scorecard. Clin Chem, 2009, 55：1303-1306.

[14] Thygesen K, Mair J, Giannitsis E, et al. How to use high-sensitivity cardiac troponins in acute cardiac care. Eur Heart J, 2012, 33 (18)：2252-2257.

[15] 中华医学会心血管病分会. 高敏心肌肌钙蛋白在急性冠状动脉综合征中的应用中国专家共识. 中华心血管病杂志, 2012, 40 (10)：809-812.

[16] 叶平, 王凡. 高敏心肌肌钙蛋白在心血管事件风险预测中的价值. 中华心血管病杂志, 2012, 40 (10)：889-891.

[17] Thygesen K, Alpert JS, Jaffe AS, et al. Third universal definition of myocardial infarction. Eur Heart J, 2012, 33 (20)：2551-2567.

[18] Reichlin T, Schindler C, Drexler B, et al. One-hour rule-out and rule-in of acute myocardial infarction using high-sensitivity cardiac Troponin T. Arch Intern Med, 2012, 13 (8)：1-8.

2013年中美国家心血管病报告要点对比解读及其启示[*]

陈可冀　刘玥

心血管疾病的发生和流行与社会经济水平、生活方式以及生态环境等因素密切相关，并伴随国家工业化、城镇化及老龄化进程而加快[1]。近年来，随着生活水平的不断提高以及不健康生活方式

* 原载于《中国中西医结合杂志》, 2013, 33 (3)：293-297

515

的持续蔓延，中国已成为全球心血管疾病的高发区，因此及时制定符合中国国情的合理防治策略至关重要。2012年8月和2013年1月，中国和美国相继正式公布了各自最新的国家心血管病报告[2,3]，两国报告中的统计数据均更新至2010—2011年，具有良好的对比度。对中、美两国最新心血管病统计报告要点进行对比解读，有利于深入分析和探究中国心血管病的流行现状、原因及发展趋势，且可为其防治策略的制定提供一定的参考。

1. 概况

《中国心血管病报告2011》中指出，我国总体人群的心血管疾病（包括心脏病和脑卒中）患病率仍在持续上升，估计全国心血管病患者有2.3亿，即每5个成人中有1人患病，其中高血压2亿人，脑卒中至少700万人，心肌梗死200万人，心力衰竭420万人，肺心病500万人。中国每年约有350万人死于心血管疾病，每死亡5人中就有2人是心血管疾病，约占全因死亡的41%，居各死亡原因首位，每天有9590人死于心血管疾病，大约每10秒就有1人死亡，其中农村居民心血管病死亡率增速高于城市居民。此外，高血压、吸烟、血脂异常、肥胖/超重、体力活动不足、不合理膳食等主要心血管危险因素仍呈进行性增长态势，防控形势严峻[2]。

美国大约有8360万成年人患有一种或多种心血管疾病，其中年龄在60岁以上的患者约占一半以上。冠心病患者大约有1540万人，心力衰竭患者510万人，脑卒中患者680万人。1999—2009年，美国总体人群因心血管病死亡人数下降了32.7%，但仍占死亡总人数的1/3左右。2009年美国心血管病死亡率约为236.1/10万人，其中白人男性、黑人男性、白人女性、黑人女性的死亡率（每10万人）分别为281.4、387.0、190.4及267.9人。每天有超过2000人死于心血管疾病，大约每40秒就有1人死亡，每25秒就会发生1次冠状动脉事件；每死亡6个人中就有1人是冠心病，每死亡19人中就有1人是脑卒中。对于心血管病主要危险因素的统计数据表明，有3190万美国成人（≥20岁）血清TC水平超过240 mg/dL；约有7800万成人有高血压（约占美国总人口的1/3）；有1970万被诊断患有糖尿病（约占美国总人口的8.3%），且糖尿病前期人口约占总人口的38.2%[3]。

2. 心血管疾病危险因素

2.1 高血压

《中国心血管病报告2011》中指出，新中国成立后中国进行过4次大规模的高血压患病率调查，历年的调查结果表明我国高血压患病率呈明显上升趋势。估计全国高血压患病人数为2亿，每5个成年人中就有1个是高血压。其中，2002年的成人高血压患病率为18.8%，男性患病率高于女性，患病率随年龄的增加而呈上升趋势，近年来部分区域性调查显示成人高血压患病率达25.0%左右。根据2002年的全国性调查结果，我国人群高血压的知晓率为30.6%，治疗率为24.7%，控制率为6.1%，对于接受治疗的患者，控制率可达到25.0%。随着年龄的增加，知晓率、治疗率和控制率都在升高，且城市高于农村。1991—2004年，我国6～17岁儿童青少年血压水平显著上升，采用"中国儿童高血压参照标准"诊断，儿童高血压患病率从1991年的7.1%上升到2004年的14.6%，年平均上升速度为0.58%[2]。

美国目前约有7800万成人高血压患者，约占美国总人口的1/3左右，每3个成年人中就有1个是高血压。2007年美国成人高血压患病率平均为29.0%左右，预测2030年美国成人高血压患病率较2013年增长约7.2%。2007—2010年美国人群高血压的知晓率为81.5%，治疗率为74.9%，控制率为52.5%，2003—2008年的研究数据显示成人高血压患者中约有8.9%为难治性（或顽固性）高血压患者。一项研究表明1999—2006年间美国青少年高血压患病率约为3.6%[3]。

2.2 血脂异常

《中国心血管病报告2011》中指出，近20年来我国居民血脂水平呈持续上升的趋势，特别是青少年的血脂水平。2002年全国调查，成人血脂异常患病率为18.6%，其中高胆固醇血症（TC ≥ 5.72 mmol/L）患病率为2.9%，高甘油三脂血症（TG ≥ 1.70 mmol/L）患病率为11.9%，低高密度脂蛋白胆固醇血症（HDL-C < 1.04 mmol/L）患病率为7.4%。儿童青少年（3～17.9岁）胆固醇升高（TC ≥ 5.72 mmol/L）患病率为0.8%，甘油三酯升高（TG ≥ 1.70 mmol/L）患病率2.8%。成人血脂异常知晓率3.2%，检测率6.4%，估计目前血脂异常者至少有2亿人。2003—2007年，北京、上海、南京等大城市对不同类型人群抽

样调查结果之间显示血脂异常患病率均较高，在35.4% ～ 59.6%[2]。

2007—2010年美国大约有3190万成人（≥ 20岁）血清TC水平超过240 mg/dL，总体患病率为13.8%。近20年来，美国成人的血清TC水平从206 mg/dL（1988—1994年）降低到203 mg/dL（1999—2002年），血清LDL-C水平从129 mg/dL（1988—1994年）降低到123 mg/dL（1999—2002年）。1999—2006年，美国成人高低密度脂蛋白胆固醇血症患病人数降低了33.0%左右。美国成人血脂异常知晓率从42.0%（1999—2000年）增长到50.4%（2005—2006年），治疗率从28.4%（1999—2002年）增长到48.1%（2005—2008年）。2007—2010年美国青少年（12 ～ 19岁）血脂异常比例约为20.3%，约7.8%的青少年血清TC水平≥ 200 mg/dL[3]。

2.3 代谢综合征

《中国心血管病报告2011》中指出，2002年中国居民营养与健康状况调查数据证实18岁以上代谢综合征的患病率粗率平均为10.2%。北京地区2005年的统计数据表明，16442名调查对象，依据国际糖尿病联盟（International Diabetes Federation, IDF）代谢综合征诊断标准，患病率为27.9%，依据美国国家胆固醇教育计划（National Cholesterol Education Project, NCEP）成人治疗专家组Ⅲ（ATP Ⅲ）代谢综合征诊断标准，患病率为19.5%。2010年新疆分层抽样抽取30 ～ 70岁维吾尔族居民1379人，哈萨克族居民1123人，采用ATP Ⅲ代谢综合征诊断标准，经年龄调整的代谢综合征患病率分别为10.3%和3.3%。2010年中国7城市的心脏研究纳入心内科住院患者3465例，依据IDF标准定义代谢综合征，调整性别、年龄、吸烟、BMI、是否诊断心血管疾病等因素的影响，代谢综合征患者发生慢性肾病的危险性是无代谢综合征的1.27倍[2]。

基于2003—2006年美国健康与营养调查统计数据（National Health and Nutrition Examination Surveys, NHANES），大约有34.0%的美国成人符合代谢综合征诊断标准，其中男性约为35.1%，女性约为32.6%。怀孕女性代谢综合征患病率从17.8%（1988—1994年）增长到26.5%（1999—2004年）。美国民众对于代谢综合征的知晓率还很有限[3]。

3. 心血管疾病不良生活方式

3.1 吸烟

《中国心血管病报告2011》中指出，我国男性吸烟率一直是世界上最高的几个国家之一。2010年全球成人烟草调查（Global Adult Tobacco Survey, GATS）—中国项目（覆盖中国28个省的人群）调查显示，我国15岁及以上男性总吸烟率为62.8%，现在吸烟率为52.9%，男性吸烟者总数达3.4亿，现在吸烟者2.9亿；女性总吸烟率为3.1%，现在吸烟率为2.4%，女性吸烟者总数为1639万人，现在吸烟者1046万。我国男性吸烟率处于平台期，而女性吸烟人群不断增加。1996年和2002年中国男性医师和教师的吸烟率均超过50.0%。2010年GATS调查表明，男性医师和教师的现在吸烟率分别为40.0%和36.5%，下降幅度较为明显，但仍是世界上男性医师吸烟率最高的国家之一。2005年的全国调查发现，11 ～ 23岁的大中学生中，男女生现在吸烟率分别为22.4%和3.9%，我国青少年吸烟低龄化倾向特别明显。2010年GATS调查数据表明20 ～ 34岁的现在吸烟者中，52.7%在20岁以前就成为每日吸烟者。2002年中国非吸烟者被动吸烟的比例高达51.9%，被动吸烟者5.4亿。中国多省市心血管病危险因素队列研究入选了30000例年龄在35 ～ 64岁的观察对象进行的10年随访结果证实吸烟是急性冠心病事件和急性缺血性卒中的独立危险因素之一。多因素分析显示，吸烟者的急性冠心病事件、缺血性脑卒中事件和出血性脑卒中事件的发病危险分别是不吸烟者的1.75倍、1.37倍和1.21倍[2]。

美国每5个成人就有1人吸烟。2010年大约有6960万大于12岁的美国居民是现在吸烟者，比例约为27.4%，较2007年的28.6%有所下降。2011年美国成人现在吸烟率男女性分别为21.3%和16.7%，平均为19.0%左右，较1998年的24.1%明显下降，美国44个州及哥伦比亚地区成人吸烟率明显下降。美国非吸烟人群血清尼古丁代谢产物coninine的检测阳性率由52.5%（1999—2000年）降低到40.1%（2007—2008年），其中在儿童少年人群（3 ～ 19岁）较成年人（≥ 20岁）下降较为明显。美国学生（9 ～ 12年级）大约有23.4%有吸烟史，其中男学生居多，12 ～ 17岁青少年吸烟率由2002年的13.0%下降至2010

年的 8.3%。2005 年，由吸烟导致的死亡约占美国成人死亡原因的 19.1%，其中大约有 1/3 的死亡与心血管疾病相关。2000—2004 年，吸烟导致每年约有 443 595 个美国人死亡，其中男性 269 655 人，女性 173 940 人；吸烟相关性死亡人群中约有 49 000 例死亡病例 (11.0%) 与吸食"二手烟"相关；每年怀孕妇女吸烟可导致 776 例婴儿死亡。据统计，美国男性吸烟人群较非吸烟人群寿命缩短约 13.2 年，女性吸烟人群寿命缩短约 14.5 年 [3]。

3.2 缺乏体力活动

《中国心血管病报告 2011》中指出，我国居民体力活动水平呈明显下降趋势，18 ~ 55 岁居民体力活动主要来源于职业活动和家务活动，除休闲时的体力活动稍有增加外，其他形式的体力活动均呈下降趋势，与 1997 年相比，2006 年男性总体力活动量减少了 27.8%，女性减少了 36.9% [2]。

2011 年的统计数据表明，约有 2/3 的美国成人休闲时缺乏身体活动，其中女性 (33.2%) 明显高于男性 (29.9%)，且随着年龄的增大这个比例显著上升。小于 18 岁的年轻人群中不参加规律体力活动者比例很高，且其比例随年龄增长而不断升高。17.7% 的女孩和 10.0% 的男孩均有连续七天内没有参加过 60 min 左右的中等至高强度身体活动的情况 [3]。

3.3 超重和肥胖

《中国心血管病报告 2011》中指出，基于 2002 年的调查数据，我国居民中超重者 (BMI 24.0 ~ 27.9 kg/m²) 约 2.0 亿人，肥胖者 (BMI ≥ 28 kg/m²) 约 6000 万人。如按 2006 年我国人口估计，18 岁以上超重者和肥胖者分别达到 2.4 亿和 7000 万，呈明显增加趋势 [2]。

2010 年，美国成人超重或肥胖人口约有 1.5 亿，约占 68.2%；约有 34.6% 的美国成人达到肥胖的标准 (BMI 30 kg/m²)。31.8% 的儿童或青少年人群超重或肥胖（约 2390 万人）[3]。

3.4 不健康膳食

《中国心血管病报告 2011》中指出，自 2002 年以来，我国居民膳食整体结构已发生明显变化，但一些膳食特点明显不利于心血管疾病的预防，如谷类食物摄入量下降，脂肪摄入增加，水果、蔬菜摄入量较低，食盐摄入量大大超过膳食指南推荐每天小于 6g 的标准 [2]。

在美国，情况与中国类似，谷物、水果及蔬菜摄入量明显不足，而脂肪和甜食的摄入量明显过

量。此外，只有 8% ~ 11% 的白人，9% ~ 11% 的黑人以及 13% ~ 19% 的墨西哥人每日钠的摄入量小于 2.3g。2005 年，美国推荐高血压人群、中老年人群以及黑人每日钠的摄入量应该少于 1.5g [3]。

4. 心血管疾病防治

4.1 冠心病

《中国心血管病报告 2011》中指出，2008 年中国城市缺血性心脏病的患病率为 15.9‰，农村地区为 4.8‰，城乡合计为 7.7‰，与 2003 年调查数据相比明显上升。2009 年中国城市居民冠心病死亡粗率为 94.96/10 万，农村居民冠心病死亡粗率为 71.27/10 万，与 2008 年的数据相比有所上升。总体来看，城市地区冠心病死亡粗率高于农村地区，男性高于女性。在冠心病介入治疗方面，近三年我国冠状动脉介入数量有了大幅度的增长，同时开展了一系列的支架介入治疗安全性与有效性的循证评价研究。冠心病药物治疗及二级预防方面，2008 年的研究表明，中国内地慢性稳定性心绞痛的治疗大体上遵循指南，但与指南要求和优化治疗相比仍存在差距，β 受体阻滞剂和他汀类药物的应用明显不足。老年冠心病患者的血压、血脂和血糖达标率均较低，尤其血压、血脂达标率亟待提高 [2]。

2010 年美国成人冠心病患病率约为 6.4%，男、女性患病率分别为 7.9% 和 5.1%。心肌梗死的患病率约为 2.9%，男、女性分别为 4.2% 和 1.7%。每 34 秒就有 1 个美国人发生心肌梗死。2011 年美国约有 63.5 万人初发冠状动脉事件（首次入院的心肌梗死或冠心病死亡），约 28 万人再发冠状动脉事件。首次心肌梗死的发病年龄男性平均为 64.7 岁，女性为 72.2 岁。2009 年美国因冠心病死亡人数为 386 324 人，平均每 6 个死亡患者中就有 1 人是冠心病。1999—2009 年，美国因冠心病年死亡率降低 40.3%，实际死亡人数降低约 27.1%。2010 年美国共有 95.4 万住院患者行冠状动脉介入术 (PCI)，39.7 万人行冠状动脉旁路移植术 (CABG) [3]。

4.2 脑卒中

《中国心血管病报告 2011》中指出，2008 年我国城市居民脑血管疾病患病率为 13.6‰，农村居民为 8.3‰。2009 年的城市居民脑血管疾病死亡粗率为 126.27/10 万，农村为 152.09/10 万。近年来，脑血管疾病死亡率不断增加，男性高于女

性，农村地区高于城市地区。在中国局部地区的研究表明，拉萨和香港的脑卒中患病率与死亡率均高于中国其他地区，且明显高于欧美等发达国家。在缺血性脑卒中治疗方面的研究表明，随着年龄增长，溶栓、华法林、糖皮质激素及降脂药的使用率下降，残疾和并发症发生率升高[2]。

美国每年大约有 79.5 万人新发或复发脑卒中，其中大约有 61 万人为首次脑卒中患者。87% 为缺血性脑卒中，每 40 秒就会发生 1 例脑卒中。2007—2010 年的研究数据表明，约有 680 万成人（≥ 20 岁）有脑卒中史，这 4 年间脑卒中的患病率约为 2.8%，老年人、黑人、受教育不足人群以及美国东南部居民脑卒中发病率较高。2009 年的数据表明，美国每 19 例死亡患者中就有 1 例脑卒中患者。2009 年美国脑卒中死亡率约为 38.9/10 万人。1999—2009 年，美国脑卒中年死亡率下降了 36.9%，实际死亡率下降了 22.9%。2010 年，美国约有 10 万人接受了动脉内膜切除术 (endarterectomy)，颈动脉内膜切除术是预防脑卒中最常用的外科治疗。1998—2004 年美国医保人群接受颈动脉内膜切除术的人数略有下降，但行颈动脉支架手术人群大幅度上升。1998 年行颈动脉支架术的比例还不足 3%，而 2008 年已经增至 13% 左右[3]。

5. 心血管疾病负担

《中国心血管病报告 2011》中指出，世界银行预测，2010—2030 年中国心肌梗死、脑卒中、糖尿病和慢性阻塞性肺病负担（生命年损失）增幅将超过 50%，其中心肌梗死和脑卒中的比重将过半。中国的心血管病死亡率明显高于日本和欧美等发达国家，如不采取积极应对措施，2005—2015 年，心血管病、脑卒中和糖尿病将给中国造成约 5500 亿美元的经济损失[2]。

美国每年直接或间接因心血管疾病造成的医疗费用约为 3126 亿美元，明显高于因肿瘤引起的医疗费用的增加（2280 亿美金）。据预测，至 2030 年，约有 40.8% 的美国人患有心血管疾病，2013—2030 年因心血管疾病带来的直接医疗费用将由目前的 3200 亿美金增至 8180 亿美金，非直接损失会由 2013 年的 2030 亿美金增至 2030 年的 3080 亿美金，增幅将高达 52% 左右[3]。

6. 思考及展望

2012 年国际著名医学期刊《The Lancet》杂志刊登研究指出，至 2010 年，男性出生时的预期寿命与 1970 年相比已上升了 11.1 年，女性上升了 12.1 年。但尽管寿命延长，人类却更多地受到疾病的侵扰，罹患如心血管疾病和癌症等非传染性疾病 (non-communicable diseases, NCD) 的患者越来越多，真正与贫困相关的疾病风险在全球层面上转变为与一系列 NCD 和人类生活方式更密切相关的风险[4]。心血管疾病是一种最常见的 NCD，已成为全球范围内危害人民健康、妨碍社会和经济发展的严重公共卫生和社会问题[5]。根据中国冠心病政策模型预测[6]，2010—2030 年若仅考虑人口老龄化和人口增加的因素，中国 35～84 岁人群心血管疾病（心绞痛、心肌梗死、冠心病猝死和脑卒中）事件发生数增加将超过 50%；若考虑血压（收缩压年上升 0.17～0.21 mmHg）、TC（TC 上升至 5.4 mmol/L）、糖尿病（糖尿病患病率上升 15%）、吸烟（下降）的因素，心血管病事件数将额外增加 23% 左右。2010—2030 年中国心血管病事件数将增加约 2130 万，死亡人数增加约 770 万左右。由上可知，目前我国心血管疾病的患病率及死亡率均处于持续上升阶段，而美国近十年来的统计数据表明其心血管疾病的患病率及死亡率均呈现明显下降趋势（图 1），但其比例较其他疾病为多，美国亦承受心血管疾病重荷。

心血管疾病具有可防、可治的特点，自美国 Framingham 心脏病研究 1961 年首次提出"危险因素"的概念以来，积极控制危险因素成为近半个

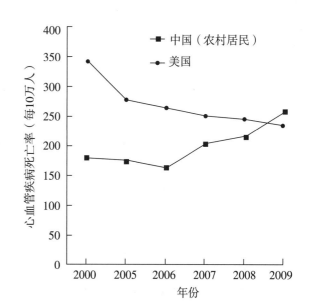

图 1 2000—2009 年中美两国心血管疾病死亡率趋势图比较
注：本图根据文献 [2，3] 中的相关统计数据重新制图而成

世纪全球心血管病防治的重心。美国曾经也是心血管疾病的高发国，然而近年来其发病率及死亡率却大幅度降低，其心血管一级预防功不可没，其他国家的实践经验也表明，控制危险因素能够大幅度降低心血管疾病的患病率和死亡率。中国学者通过研究证实，高血压、吸烟、超重或肥胖、高胆固醇血症是我国成年男性心血管疾病发病的主要危险因素。心血管疾病的这 4 个主要危险因素的人群归因危险度合计超过 70%。高血压和吸烟是中国成年男性心血管疾病的最重要的危险因素。血压在中国人群对心血管疾病发病风险的强度比在西方人群大。继续加强对这些危险因素的预防和干预，特别是控制血压和戒烟是减少我国男性人群心血管疾病发病最有效的途径[7]。从以上数据对比可以看出，无论是对危险因素的防控、主要心血管疾病的防治及健康教育方面，我国与美国均存在巨大落差。美国居民对至少 1 种脑卒中危险因素的知晓率已由 1995 年的 59% 增长到 2000 年的 71%，对 3 种脑卒中危险因素的知晓率虽较低但仍逐年增长（1995 年为 5.4%，2000 年为 12.0%，2005 年为 15.7%）[3]。而中国居民对于心脑血管危险因素的知晓率还很低，因此需要积极加强对于心血管危险因素的控制，应由政府主导，医疗机构及医务人员积极配合开展健康教育，向患者、公众及媒体普及正确的心血管危险因素及不良生活方式的防治常识。中国男性医师的吸烟率与其他国家相比仍处在较高水平，医务人员需要身体力行，起示范作用，如积极戒烟、减肥、合理膳食、积极运动等，用自己的健康行为去影响周围更多的人[5]。

另一方面，需要向社会大众普及心血管急救常识及常用急救方法。调查表明 79% 的美国民众知晓如何进行医学急救，98% 会使用自动体外除颤器（automated external defibrillator, AED）对突发心室纤颤患者进行体外除颤以恢复正常心律，60% 熟悉心肺复苏术的操作[3]，这些都为美国心血管疾病死亡率的降低做出了积极贡献。

值得关注的是，从统计报告可以看出，无论是中国还是美国，儿童青少年超重或肥胖的比例都在不断上升，研究表明肥胖带来的高血压、高血脂等健康风险在青少年身上已有明显体现，肥胖青少年在多项健康风险指标上都超过体重正常的青少年，如血压平均高出 7.49 mmHg，此外血脂、血糖水平也更高，这都为未来心血管疾病的发生留下了隐患[8]。人们要重视让青少年养成健康饮食和定期锻炼的习惯，不要让他们带着潜在的心血管健康风险长大。

随着我国中医药学与西医药学的发展以及两种医药学在真实医疗环境中的相互交叉、渗透，中西医结合医学应运而生，成为我国独具特色的医疗体系之一。我国政府也依据科学发展规律及中国国情制定了坚持中西医结合和促进中西医结合的科技政策和方针[9]。中医药学是世界传统医学的杰出代表，而中西医结合体现了不同文化包容发展的精神，是传统与现代相结合的整合医学的典范[10]。调查表明，中国超过 71.2% 的患者会选择中西医结合的治疗方法，结合医学在我国医疗卫生体系中发挥了不可替代的作用[11]。我国已制定了中国慢性病防治工作规划（2012—2015 年），其中对于心血管疾病的防治占据了很重要的位置，我们应该充分发挥中西医结合医学的优势与潜力，在心血管疾病一级预防和二级预防方面做到有所为有所不为、扬长避短，为降低我国心血管疾病的患病率与死亡率做出贡献。

参考文献

[1] 王文，刘明波，隋辉，等．中国心血管病的流行状况与防治对策．中国心血管病杂志，2012，17 (5)：321-323.

[2] 卫生部心血管病防治研究中心中国心血管病报告 2011．北京：中国大百科全书出版社，2012.

[3] Go AS, Mozaffarian D, Roger VL, et al. Heart disease and stroke statistics—2013 update：a report from the American Heart Association. Circulation, 2013, 127 (1)：e6-e245.

[4] Salomon JA, Vos T, Hogan DR, et al. Common values in assessing health outcomes from disease and injury：disability weights measurement study for the Global Burden of Disease Study 2010. Lancet, 2012, 380 (9859)：2129-2143.

[5] 高润霖．行动起来，积极应对非传染性疾病的挑战．中华医学杂志，2012，92 (1)：1-2.

[6] Moran A, Gu D, Zhao D, et al. Future cardiovascular disease in China：markov model and risk factor scenario projections from the coronary heart disease policy model in China. Circ Cardiovasc Qual Outcomes, 2010, 3 (3)：243-252.

[7] Ji JF, Pan EC, Li JX, et al. Classical risk factors of cardiovascular disease among Chinese male steel workers：a prospective cohort study for 20 years. BMC Public Health, 2011, 11：497.

第六章

[8] Friedemann C, Heneghan C, Mahtani K, et al. Cardiovascular disease risk in healthy children and its association with body mass index: systematic review and meta-analysis. BMJ, 2012, 345: e4759.

[9] 毛平，孔令青，刘岩，等.中西医结合人才社会需求调研报告.中国中西医结合杂志，2012，32 (12)：1684-

1686.

[10] 王文健.关于发展中西医结合医学的共识.中国中西医结合杂志，2011，31 (6)：837-838.

[11] 陈可冀，吕爱平，陈士奎，等.中国中西医结合医学发展状况调查报告.中国中西医结合杂志，2006，26 (6)：485-488.

稳定性冠心病：PCI 还是药物治疗的选择——一项新的 Meta 分析结果的启示 *

陈可冀　刘　玥

为了评价比较经皮冠状动脉介入治疗 (percutaneous coronary intervention, PCI) 和药物治疗对稳定性冠心病患者的临床疗效，美国纽约州立大学石溪分校医疗中心的 Kathleen Stergiopoulos 博士和 David L.Brown 博士进行了临床随机对照试验的 Meta 分析，该项最新研究结果发表于 2012 年 2 月 27 日的国际著名医学期刊《Archives of Internal Medicine》（《内科学文献》）上 [1]。文章选取的前瞻性随机对照临床试验均来源于 MEDLINE 数据库中 1970 年至 2011 年 9 月间的检索结果，并且排除了接受 PCI 治疗不足 50% 的临床试验，通过随机效应模型得出相应的 OR 值。8 项临床随机对照试验共纳入 7229 例患者，其中，3 项试验的研究对象为心肌梗死后病情稳定的患者，而 5 项试验的研究对象为稳定性心绞痛患者和（或）压力测试显示心肌缺血的患者，加权平均随访时间为 4.3 年（表 1）。临床以死亡、非致命性心肌梗死、计划外的血运重建以及持续性心绞痛作为观察终点。结果表明，PCI 和药物治疗的不良事件发生率分别为：死亡：8.9% vs 9.1% (OR, 0.98；95%CI, 0.84 ~ 1.16)；非致命性心肌梗死：8.9% vs 8.1% (OR, 1.12；95% CI, 0.93 ~ 1.34)；计划外血运重建：21.4% vs 30.7% (OR, 0.78；95% CI, 0.57 ~ 1.06)；持续性心绞痛：29% vs 33% (OR, 0.80；95% CI, 0.60 ~ 1.05)。因此，研究人员得出结论，在预防死亡、非致命性心肌梗死、计划外血运重建或持续性心绞痛方面，与药物治疗相比，稳定性冠心病患者行 PCI 并未额外获益。

值得注意的是，这篇最新的 Meta 分析所得出的结论其实并不新颖，早在 2007 年发表的 COURAGE 研究（Clinical Outcomes Utilizing Revascularization and Aggressive Drug Evaluation, 血运重建和优化药物治疗的临床转归）结果即表明对于稳定性冠心病患者，与单纯药物优化治疗 (optimal medical treatment, OMT) 相比，PCI 治疗在降低全因死亡率及非致命性心肌梗死发生率方面并不具明显优势 [2]。并且当时我们也对 COURAGE 研究做出了自己的思考 [3]，那么，这项最新的 Meta 分析的结果又有什么新的特点，给我们带来了哪些新的启示呢？我们认为可能有以下几个方面。

1. 纳入的随机对照试验更加全面，结论更为可信

COURAGE 研究，包括以往的临床研究所报告的结果都为欧美人群的资料，对亚裔人群的研究很少，并且很少关注合并冠心病等危症时的情况，因此所得出的结论可能存在一定的局限性。而最新的 Meta 分析纳入的 8 项随机对照试验，其中 2008 年发表的 JASP 研究 [4]（Japanese Stable Angina Pectoris Study, 日本稳定性心绞痛研究）是一项多中心的随机对照试验，所纳入的病例均为亚裔人群；而 2009 年发表在《新英格兰杂志》上的 BARI-2D 研究 [5]（Bypass Angioplasty Revascularization Investigation 2 Diabetes, 2 型糖尿病患者冠状动脉旁路移植血运重建研究），首次同时关注了冠心病和 2 型糖尿病并存状态时的

---

* 原载于《中国中西医结合杂志》，2012，32 (5)：583-584

表 1   稳定性冠心病 PCI *vs* 药物治疗纳入的随机对照研究

研究名称	病例数	研究期限	随访年限	纳入标准
TOAT, 2002	66	1997—1999	1	前壁 Q 波型心肌梗死，LAD 闭塞，无胸痛
Hambrecht et al, 2004	101	1997—2001	1	稳定型心绞痛，有缺血证据
DECOPI, 2004	212	1998—2001	3	Q 波型心肌梗死 15 天，无缺血证据，梗死相关动脉完全闭塞，稳定期患者
OAT, 2006	2166	2000—2005	4	心肌梗死后 3 ~ 28 天，梗死相关动脉完全闭塞，稳定期患者
MASS Ⅱ, 2007	408	1995—2000	5	稳定型心绞痛或压力测试心肌缺血患者
COURAGE, 2007	2287	1999—2004	4.6	稳定型心绞痛；稳定的不稳定型心绞痛患者；心肌缺血或狭窄 > 80%
JSAP, 2008	384	2002—2004	3.3	劳累性心绞痛或可诱导的心肌缺血；狭窄 ≥ 75%
BARI 2D, 2009	1605	2001—2005	5	糖尿病患者同时有可诱导的心肌缺血或心绞痛

注：本表译自文献 [1] 中的表 2

治疗策略，结果表明对稳定性冠心病患者血运重建治疗并不优于积极的药物治疗，即使对高危的 2 型糖尿病人群也同样如此。由此可以看出本次 Meta 分析在种群以及临床试验覆盖面上更为全面，因此得出的结论应该更为可信。

2. 合理选择 PCI，做到有所为有所不为

最新 Meta 分析的结果进一步证实，与单纯药物治疗比较，稳定型冠心病患者行 PCI 治疗对终点事件无额外益处。稳定性冠心病治疗的主要目的是改善预后和缓解症状，因此治疗策略的选择是整个治疗过程中的关键环节，具体来说就是"药物治疗优先"还是"血运重建治疗优先 [包括 PCI 和冠状动脉旁路移植术 (CABG)]"，要结合临床症状、客观的心肌缺血证据、危险因素的综合考虑等[6]。毋庸置疑，PCI 的临床应用为缺血性心脏病的治疗提供了又一利器，但其主要应用领域在于对急性冠状动脉综合征 (acute coronary syndrome, ACS)，特别是 ST 段抬高的急性心肌梗死的早期干预，及时再通血管，挽救缺血心肌，拯救生命；而对稳定性冠心病患者，若在改善生活方式和合理用药的基础上仍不能控制心绞痛的发作，PCI 治疗可能有助于缓解症状。但是，任何治疗手段都有一定的适用范围，不应过度应用，做到有所为有所不为。在当今冠心病治疗学领域，改善生活方式和合理药物治疗的基石地位不可动摇，不能滥用 PCI，让支架乱飞[7]，要做到有理、有据、有节。

3. 落实证据比获得证据更加重要

正如《Archives of Internal Medicine》编辑部为该文配发的特邀评论[8]中指出，COURAGE 研究、BARI-2D 研究以及许多其他临床研究的结果并未得到重视，即并未将其落实到临床实践当中去，临床医师表面上以循证医学的研究结果为圣经，但临床实践中却在有选择地利用循证医学的结论，即选择那些貌似支持现存治疗理念的研究结果为我所用，而摒弃那些不受欢迎的、看似与现存治疗理念相违背或相冲突的研究结果。COURAGE 研究结论发布近 5 年，但目前仍有不少医院遇到稳定性冠心病患者还是采取"PCI 优先"的治疗策略，这其中或许有利益的驱动，但是临床循证研究的目的就在于客观评价目前治疗策略的优劣，进而选择更加合适的临床治疗策略，因此落实临床证据之路任重道远，正如评论的标题中呼吁的"再要怎么做才能完全扭转目前的治疗策略？"(What More Will It Take to Turn the Tide of Treatment?)

4. 中西医结合在冠心病防治中大有可为

最新的 Meta 分析以及之前的 COURAGE 等研究结果表明，对于稳定性冠心病，优化药物治疗加 PCI 并未表现出相对于单纯优化药物治疗的优越性。原因在于，虽然 PCI 能较快地改善缺血区的血运，但其并没有完全阻断动脉粥样硬化的发展。因此 PCI 治疗后仍会发生再狭窄及血栓形成，

即冠状动脉粥样硬化的病理改变仍在继续，其终点事件发生率与单纯优化药物治疗的终点事件发生率差异无统计学意义。因此单纯优化药物治疗在冠心病治疗中举足轻重。而中西医结合疗法在其中大有可为。中西医学在对冠心病动脉粥样硬化防治方面有着稳定病变、"通其血脉"的共同看法，东西方这种理念上的一致性，使得应用传统活血化瘀方药在降低心血管风险可能性的探索上具有一定的实际意义[9]。目前活血化瘀中药在防治 PCI 术后再狭窄、抗血小板治疗、内皮保护、梗死后血管新生等方面都有较好的疗效，未来可以进一步深入研究，为其扩大临床应用提供扎实的循证依据。

参考文献

[1] Stergiopoulos K, Brown DL. Initial coronary stent implantation with medical therapy *vs* medical therapy alone for stable coronary artery disease. Arch Intern Med, 2012, 172 (4)：312-319.

[2] Boden WE, O' Rourke RA, Teo KK, et al. COURAGE Trial Research Group. Optimal medical therapy with or without PCI for stable coronary disease. N Engl J Med, 2007, 356 (15)：1503-1516.

[3] 陈可冀. COURAGE 临床研究对中西医结合治疗冠心病的启示. 中国中西医结合杂志，2007, 27 (8)：677.

[4] Nishigaki K, Yamazaki T, Kitabatake A, et al. Japanese Stable Angina Pectoris Study investigators. Percutaneous coronary intervention plus medical therapy reduces the incidence of acute coronary syndrome more effectively than initial medical therapy only among patients with low-risk coronary artery disease：a randomized, comparative, multicenter study. JACCC ardiovasc Interv, 2008, 1 (5)：469-479.

[5] BARI 2D Study Group, Frye RL, August P, et al. A randomized trial of therapies for type 2 diabetes and coronary artery disease. N Engl J Med, 2009, 360 (24)：2503-2515.

[6] 陈可冀，赵福海，蒋跃绒. 慢性稳定型心绞痛的中西医结合治疗进展. 中国实用内科杂志，2011，31 (7)：481-482.

[7] 赵福海，陈可冀. 审慎对待合理应用冠心病介入治疗手段. 中国中西医结合杂志，2011，31 (3)：295-296.

[8] Boden WE. Mounting evidence for lack of PCI benefit in stable ischemic heart disease—what more will it take to turn the tide of treatment. Arch Intern Med, 2012, 172 (4)：319-321.

[9] 陈可冀. 活血化瘀方药降低心血管风险可能性的探索. 中国中西医结合杂志，2008，28 (5)：389.

2012 年全球心肌梗死统一定义亮点解读 *

陈可冀　刘　玥

心肌梗死是危害全球人类健康的重要杀手，同时也是全球心血管病医师一直以来关注的热点领域。"心肌梗死统一定义 (universal definition of myocardial infarction)" 是一个全球化的文件，由欧洲心脏病学会 (ESC)、美国心脏病学会基金会 (ACCF)、美国心脏学会 (AHA) 和世界心脏联盟 (WHF) 领衔全球心血管病医师共同制定统一发布，并推荐在全世界范围内应用，目前我国的心血管病诊疗指南中亦推荐使用该定义。继 2000 年、2007 年发布的第 1 版[1]和第 2 版[2]统一定义之后，2012 年 8 月 ESC/ACCF/AHA/WHF 工作联盟又发布了修订后的第 3 版心肌梗死全球统一定义[3]。每次定义的修订都有一些亮点所在，或是理念的与时俱进、或是概念的逐步明晰，早在 2007 年统一定义的第 2 版发布时我们就对此做过相关解读[4]，并推荐中医界及中西医结合界同仁们也使用这个全球心肌梗死新定义。时隔 5 年，该定义又更新推出了现在的新版本，又有哪些亮点值得我们关注呢？

2012 年新定义的亮点之一是更新了血运重建治疗 [包括经皮冠状动脉介入治疗 (PCI) 和冠状动脉旁路移植术 (CABG)] 相关性心肌梗死的诊断标

* 原载于《中国中西医结合杂志》，2012，32 (11)：1445-1447

准，特别是重新设定了对心脏肌钙蛋白（cTnI 或 cTnT）水平的要求。众所周知，血运重建治疗已在全世界范围内普遍开展，已成为冠心病治疗中的主要手段，而血运重建治疗相关性心肌梗死的出现亦成为其术后影响患者预后的重要因素，但多年来对其诊断标准尚不明晰，很多急性心肌梗死患者接受血运重建治疗后 cTn 出现增高并伴有缺血症状，无法明确是由之前心肌梗死过程产生还是血运重建治疗操作所致？如果有证据表明血运重建治疗后 cTn 的提高所致随后事件（诸如死亡）发生风险增高，那么明确诊断血运重建治疗相关性急性心肌梗死是至关重要的。

2012 版定义中仍首选心肌 cTn（I 或 T）水平作为检测心肌梗死最为敏感的生化标志物，同时沿用上一版定义中心肌梗死的分型标准[2,4]，不同的是在对操作相关性心肌梗死的诊断中更新了对 cTn 水平的要求（表 1）。其中 4 型 a PCI 相关性心肌梗死被定义如下：基线 cTn 水平正常的患者，在接受 PCI 治疗后 48h 内 cTn 水平升高至超过参考值上限 (URL) 第 99 百分位的 5 倍者；或者基线水平升高的患者，cTn 水平上升超过 20%，且保持稳定或逐渐下降者。同时需要至少具备以下诸项中的 1 项：心肌缺血症状，新出现的缺血性心电图改变或新出现的左束支传导阻滞 (left bundle branch block, LBBB)，血管造影结果与 PCI 并发症相一致，或有存活心肌新损失或新出现局部心壁运动异常的影像学证据。而在 2007 版定义中，cTn 阈值为超过 URL 第 99 百分位的 3 倍，本次提高 cTn 阈值的依据是对接受 PCI 治疗者的长期随访的结果。

2012 版定义同时也提高了 5 型 CABG 相关性心肌梗死的 cTn 阈值，对于 cTn 基线水平正常的患者，在接受 CABG 术后的第一个 48h 内，cTn 阈值从 2007 版定义中的 URL 第 99 百分位的 5 倍增至 10 倍。同时也需至少具备以下诸项中的 1 项：新出现病理性 Q 波或新出现的 LBBB，或血管造影显示移植物或原有冠状动脉新出现闭塞，或有存活心肌新损失或新出现局部心壁运动异常的影像学证据。

2012 年新定义的亮点之二是系统阐释了对"心肌损伤"概念的理解及范围的界定。众所周知，所有医生（不仅是心脏科医生）都会在临床实践中遇到 cTn 水平升高超过阈值的问题，有太多的重症患者存在心肌损伤，但这些心肌损伤并不是心肌梗死（无其他心肌缺血的临床证据）。因此在本版定义中新增了一部分——"心肌损伤伴坏死生物标志物的测定"，首次对可能引起 cTn 水平升高的所有心肌损伤的原因（包括心肌缺血和非心肌缺血）做了详细的列表分类和阐述（表 2），尤其详细列出了由非缺血因素导致心肌损伤的可能的各类疾病（包括心力衰竭）。新版定义中还指出某些诸如经导管主动脉瓣置换术 (transcatheter aortic valve implantaion, TAVI) 或二尖瓣钳夹等新术式可能也会导致心肌损伤伴坏死，且其可能与 CABG 相似的是，生物标志物水平升高越明显，预后就越差，但目前尚缺乏相关的临床研究证据。

同时，新版定义中把那些基线 cTn 水平正常，在接受 PCI 治疗后 48h 内 cTn 水平升高但不超过 URL 第 99 百分位的 5 倍或即使超过 5 倍但无临床影像学证据的患者诊断为"心肌损伤"而不是 PCI 相关性心肌梗死。由此看出，界定 cTn 水平升高属于"心肌梗死"还是"心肌损伤"，其关键是看是否具备临床或影像学证据。正因如此，2012 版定义还包含了用于鉴别和确诊心肌梗死的各类影像学检查，详细阐释了超声心动图、核素扫描、磁共振和计算机断层扫描在诊断急性心肌梗死时的作用。近年来影像学检查在急性心肌梗死的诊断上发挥着越来越重要的作用，尤其在缺乏典型临床表现或心电图表现不明确时，通过辅助检查尤其是影像学检查来帮助确诊心肌梗死尤为重要。

从以上对亮点的解读可以看出，2012 版新定义的修订主要是围绕对高敏 cTn (hs-cTn) 检测技术的发展做出的。cTn 对心肌组织具有高度特异性和临床敏感性，可直接反映心肌坏死的程度。研究表明，cTnI 水平是心血管疾病预后的独立预测因

表 1　心肌梗死统一临床分型

1 型		自发型心肌梗死
2 型		缺血心肌氧供失衡型心肌梗死
3 型		突发意外型心脏性猝死（猝死前无血样采集）
4 型	4 型 a	PCI 相关性心肌梗死（2012 版定义更新见文内）
	4 型 b	支架血栓所致的心肌梗死（冠状动脉造影或尸检证实）
5 型		CABG 相关性心肌梗死（2012 版定义更新见文内）

注：本表译自文献 [3] 中的表 2，有删减和调整

第六章

表2 引起 cTn 水平升高的各种原因所致的心肌损伤

心肌缺血性心肌损伤

斑块破裂

冠状动脉管腔内血栓形成

心肌缺血氧供失衡性心肌损伤

快速性 / 缓慢性心律失常

主动脉夹层或严重主动脉瓣疾病

肥厚性心肌病

心源性 / 低血容量性 / 感染性休克

严重的呼吸衰竭、严重贫血

高血压病（伴或不伴左心室肥大）

冠状动脉痉挛、冠状动脉栓塞或血管炎

冠状动脉内皮功能障碍（无实质性冠心病）

非心肌缺血性心肌损伤

心脏挫伤、外科手术、消融、除颤等

横纹肌溶解（心脏相关）

心肌炎、心脏毒性药物所致

其他原因所致的心肌损伤

心力衰竭应激性心肌病

严重的肺栓塞或肺动脉高压

败血症和危重病患者、肾衰竭

严重的神经系统疾病，如脑卒中、蛛网膜下腔出血

浸润性疾病，如淀粉样变、肉状瘤病

剧烈运动

注：本表译自文献 [3] 中的表 1，有调整

子，hs-cTn 检测可以在极早期诊断心肌梗死，同时可以预测稳定性高危人群心肌梗死和心血管死亡的风险[5]，虽然降低其检测阈值可更早发现心肌梗死且对改善预后具有重要意义，但是检测阈值的降低会导致许多非心肌梗死患者出现 hs-cTn 水平升高的可能性增加[6]，因此动态监测 hs-cTn 的变化可以增加诊断的特异性[7]。已有学者[8]提出一种采用 hs-cTnT 测定值的简单算法——即使用 hs-cTnT 的初始值以及其在第 1h 内的变化绝对值来快速鉴别胸痛患者是否为急性心肌梗死，当然这种新算法实际应用于临床诊断还需要经过大规模的临床验证和对比研究。

2012 版心肌梗死全球新定义的发布对于心血管病的临床研究会带来极大的益处，即全球可以用一个标准的方法来解释和对比不同的临床试验。近年来，随着临床循证指南的广泛应用和中医药规范化工作的开展，中医及中西医结合心血管病临床指南的制定也正在进行当中[9]，而临床指南的制定需要基于大量的临床研究的结果，为了便于国际交流和与世界接轨，我们在此同样推荐中医界和中医结合界也应采用 2012 版全球心肌梗死的统一定义来进行和开展临床研究。

参考文献

[1] The Joint European Society of Cardiology / American College of Cardiology Committee. Myocardial infarction redefineda consensus document of the Joint European Society of Cardiology / American College of Cardiology Committee for the redefinition of myocardial infarction. Eur Heart J, 2000, 21 (18)：1502-1513.

[2] Thygesen K, Alpert JS, White HD. Joint ESC/ACCF/AHA/WHF task force for the redefinition of myocardial infarction. Universal definition of myocardial infarction. Eur Heart J, 2007, 28 (20)：2525-2538.

[3] Thygesen K, Alpert JS, Jaffe AS, et al. The writing group on behalf of the Joint ESC/ACCF/AHA/WHF task force for the universal definitionof myocardial infarction. Third universal definition of myocardial infarction. Eur Heart J, 2012, doi：10. 1093/eurheartj/ehs184.

[4] 陈可冀, 蒋跃绒. 推荐应用全球性心肌梗死新定义. 中国中西医结合杂志, 2009, 29 (7)：581-582.

[5] Kavsak PA, Xu L, Yusuf S, et al. High-sensitivity cardiac troponin I measurement for risk stratification in a stable high-risk population. Clin Chem, 2011, 57 (8)：1146-1153.

[6] Agewall S, Giannitsis E, Jernberg T, et al. Troponin elevation in coronary vs non-coronary disease. Eur Heart J, 2011, 32 (4)：404-411.

[7] Mueller M, Biener M, Vafaie M, et al. Absolute and relative kinetic changes of high-sensitivity cardiac troponin T in acute coronary syndrome and in patients with increased troponin in the absence of acute coronary syndrome. Clin Chem, 2012, 58 (1)：209-218.

[8] Reichlin T, Schindler C, Drexler B, et al. One-hour rule-out and rule-in of acute myocardial infarction using high sensitivity cardiac troponin T. Arch Intern Med, 2012, 13 (8)：1-8.

[9] 陈可冀, 蒋跃绒. 中医和中西医结合临床指南制定的现状与问题. 中西医结合学报, 2009, 7 (4)：301-305.

第六章

开拓心血管病领域中西医结合研究 *

陈可冀

1. 世界医学史上经病理证实的年代最早的冠心病患者

1972 年长沙马王堆汉墓出土一具女尸，我院耿鉴庭教授参与鉴定。不久，我也到现场考察。病理证实该女尸左冠状动脉粥样硬化，斑块及血栓阻塞管腔，超过 3/4，病变达到四级；左前降支上 1/3 接近完全闭塞；左室前壁近心尖部的瘢痕灶示生前有心肌梗死。随墓出土的有不少芳香温通药物，包括藿香、辛夷、高良姜、花椒、肉桂等。经查医学史文献，意大利解剖学家 Manin Lancisi (1654—1720)、苏格兰解剖学家 John Hunter (1728—1792) 最早报告冠状动脉病变尸检病例，古病理学家 Shattock (1909) 和 Ruffer (1911) 分别报告埃及"法老"尸解所见，但缺乏冠状动脉标本，因制作木乃伊时已将内脏挖空。上述随墓中草药，都是现今芳香定痛的常用药。

2. 美国著名心脏病学家怀特 (Paul White) 教授关于中医药治疗冠心病可能性的观点

十年动乱后期，国门初开。20 世纪 70 年代初期，美国著名心脏病学家怀特教授率美国心脏病学家代表团访华。在北京时，吴阶平院士、吴英恺院士为主的十多人在北京饭店与之座谈，我和著名中医学家郭士魁教授也参加了。我和郭老的任务是介绍 10 分钟关于中医药对冠心病的认识和治疗。我们很认真和紧张地作了哪怕是很短发言的准备。郭老发言讲到《黄帝内经》和《金匮要略》中关于心绞痛有关经典描述和我们自己的治疗经验。怀特说："中国医学历史悠久，我相信中医药里面可以找到治疗冠心病的有效方法。"我对怀特教授的这一段话，这样理解和认识，印象深刻。当时黄宛教授和方圻教授也在座。

3. 活血化瘀方药治疗心血管病的开发并辐射全国，感到所谓"活血化瘀现象"

20 世纪 50 年代中后期，我和郭士魁教授对活血化瘀方药应用于心血管病已有初步重视。1958 年后，中国中医研究院与中国医学科学院阜外医院（现为阜外心血管病医院）开始了长达数年的关于冠心病和高血压病的协作研究，这方面的理解有了进一步加深。20 世纪 70 年代初，周恩来总理指示要加强对冠心病的研究，于是由吴英恺院士（当年阜外医院院长）为组长，西苑医院和中国人民解放军总医院为副组长单位的北京 16 家医院组成的北京地区防治冠心病协作组应运而生。经大家充分讨论，提出以冠心 II 号复方（由丹参、川芎、赤芍、红花、降香组成）为切入点，进行对冠心病心绞痛的防治临床及基础研究。黄宛、陈在嘉、金荫昌、邵耕、顾复生、崔吉君、寇文熔、石湘芸、陈文为等教授都积极投入，最初总结 600 例临床经验，证明有一定疗效。随后又改进为精制冠心片进行阜外医院、西苑医院、同仁医院三家医院多中心 RCT 研究，其结果"精制冠心片双盲法治疗冠心病心绞痛 112 例疗效临床分析"论文发表于 1982 年第 2 期《中华心血管病杂志》，这是我国中医药及中西医结合领域第一篇多中心 RCT 临床论著。在此前后，活血化瘀方药的研究进一步成为全国最活跃的中西医结合领域之一，被称为"活血化瘀现象"。此后，我们还首先应用川芎嗪治疗缺血性中风，现尚在城乡推广应用。基础实验工作也很系统。

4. 中西医结合防治 PCI 后再狭窄的探索

1981 年《中华医学杂志》英文版编委会在南京召开，我和刚从美国回归的北医三院院长、心血管专家陈明哲教授会议期间同住一室，他精于冠状动脉介入治疗。我提到因为尚有若干病例介入后冠状动脉再狭窄，这个问题值得关注，可否我们合作进行中医药防治再狭窄的探索研究，他很赞成。不久，我们就制订计划由北医三院和西苑医院合作进行基础和临床试验。我和博士研究生史大卓、马晓昌医师、李立志医师、徐凤芹医师等参加了相关的临床和实验研究工作，证明了血府逐瘀汤及其精简

* 原载于高润霖、胡大一主编：《中国心血管病学 30 年回顾》，人民卫生出版社，2009，120-122

方有抑制内皮细胞、平滑肌细胞增殖的效果，临床也看到作用；史大卓的博士课题也是在陈明哲教授、韩启德院士和我共同指导下完成的。近年，我们又与北京安贞医院吕树铮教授、中日友好医院柯元南教授、广东省中医院等合作，研究了由该方有效部位川芎酚及赤芍苷组成的芎芍胶囊的冠状动脉介入后多中心 RCT 临床研究，共 335 例，证实中西医结合治疗较单用西药的再狭窄率减少，论文发表于《Chinese Medicine Journal》2006 年第 1 期，并进行了其作用的分子机制研究，算是引领了这一领域的中西医结合的探索研究。

5. 冠心病血瘀证实质及有关抗血小板中药研究

我们在多年的工作中注意到不少活血化瘀方药具有抗血小板功能。2004 年起，在国家自然基金重大研究计划重点项目的支持下，开展了冠心病血瘀证血小板活化相关因子基因组学研究。采用病例对照研究设计，以血小板 GPⅢa、GPⅡb、GPⅠb 的 HPA-1、HPA-3、HPA-2 基因多态性为切入点，分析其多态性与冠心病血瘀证的相关性，并研究了 GPⅠb、GPⅡb-Ⅲa、GMP-40 活性与冠心病血瘀证的相关性。结果显示 HPA-1、HPA-2 多态位点不是汉族人冠心病和冠心病血瘀证的独立危险因素，HPA-3 多态位点是汉族人冠心病发病的独立危险因素，但它不是冠心病血瘀证的危险因素。在冠心病和冠心病血瘀证的发生发展过程中，GPⅡb-Ⅲa、GMP-140 活性明显增强，可作为血瘀证微观辨证的客观指标之一，而 GPⅠb 活性不是冠心病血瘀证的敏感指标。通过对冠心病血瘀证、冠心病非血瘀证、非冠心病血瘀证患者和健康对照者的全基因组芯片筛查研究，构建了冠心病血瘀证差异基因表达者。基于芯片数据挖掘和相关差异基因的分子功能及生物学通路的分析，从核酸水平提示了冠心病血瘀证发生发展与炎症免疫反应的相关性，并运用定量 RT-PCR 对所筛选的目标基因进行鉴定，进一步通过临床血清学实验验证目标基因白介素 -8 与疾病的相关性。白介素 -8 功能分析显示 IL-8 可能通过影响血小板活化程度而介导了冠心病血瘀证的客观化诊断奠定了一定基础，同时为冠心病发病机制的进一步深入研究和血瘀证证候实质的探讨提供了新的研究方向。上述研究分别发表于《Chinese Journal of Integrative Medicine》2008 年第 4 期，《Chinese Science Bulletin》2009 年第 5 期，及《Tohoku J Exp Med》2008 年第 1 期等杂志上，我们希望为抗血栓形成提供一些线索。

病证结合治疗观的过去与现在 *

陈可冀　蒋跃绒　谢元华

辨证论治是中医临床的特色和优势，也是中医药学诊治疾病的主要原则和方法。但是，纵观中医学的发展，实际上"辨证论治"与"辨病论治"一直是两种主要的思维模式，且"辨病"早于"辨证"。早在《内经》《伤寒论》《金匮要略》中，已确定了观察和处理疾病时，证和病必须结合的原则，对后世医学发展产生了极大的影响[1]。因"病"的含义不同，病证结合可分为古典（或传统）病证结合与现代病证结合。前者指中医辨病与中医辨证相结合，后者指西医辨病（西医疾病诊断）与中医辨证相结合。

1. 传统的病证结合治疗观

1.1 传统病证结合治疗观的历代发展

先秦时期《五十二病方》《黄帝内经》等贯穿了辨病论治的原则，并初具病证结合的雏形；东汉张仲景奠定了辨病基础上辨证论治的基础；隋唐时期在辨病论治、专病专方上进一步发展；宋金元及以后的明清时期，逐步形成以辨证论治为主的病证结合论治模式。

1.1.1　先秦时期　以辨病论治为主，初具病证结合的雏形。现存最古老的医方书《五十二病方》中载有癫疾、疣、马不痫、蛊、疽病等 52 种病名，

* 原载于《中国中西医结合杂志》，2011，31（4）：437-443

均以疾病作为篇目标题，如《疽病》方："治白蔹、黄芪、芍药、桂、姜、椒、茱萸，凡七物。骨疽倍白蔹，肉疽倍黄芪，肾疽倍芍药。"既列出了疽病通用之方，又因骨疽、肉疽、肾疽的不同，治疗也有倍白蔹、黄芪、芍药之别，为后世提供了中医药学早期辨病和辨证论治的思想依据。《黄帝内经》也以辨病论治为主要治疗形式。其中载有十二方，如《素问·腹中论》以鸡矢醴治臌胀，《素问·病能论》生铁落饮治怒狂、泽泻饮治酒风等，以辨病用方为主，初具运用专病专方的规模[2]。《黄帝内经》涉及的病名达100余种，其中有许多专"病"的论述，如《疟论》《咳论》《痹论》《痿论》"寒热病""癫狂病"等，对疾病的病因病机、鉴别诊断、治疗及预后等均作了详细阐述。《黄帝内经》当时已认识到临床上同病异证的问题，如将疟病分为寒疟、热疟、风疟、瘅疟等。《素问·至真要大论》并指出："谨守病机，各司其属"，其实质即强调在临证中当周密地进行辨证论治之意[2]。所论病机十九条，既有对"掉眩""收引""肿满""鼓栗""呕"等"症"的辨识，也有"疮""痿""痉"等"病"的诊断。这种简练的辨证、辨病方式，可看作是后世辨证与辨病相结合的思想雏形。

1.1.2 汉晋时期 首倡"辨病脉证并治"，奠定了病证结合的基础。东汉末年，张仲景继承与发展了《黄帝内经》的辨病、辨证论治的思想，重视在辨病的基础上辨证论治，奠定了病证结合论治的基础[3]。《伤寒论》和《金匮要略》大多篇名冠以"辨某病脉证并治"，重视在辨病的基础上辨证论治。其中《伤寒论》倡"六经辨证"，提及病名约40种，先按六经病分类，再分析脉证，多为辨证论治，如桂枝汤证、大承气汤证、陷胸汤证等。《金匮要略》倡"脏腑经络先后病脉证治"，提出病名约160种，遵循着以病为纲、按病论述、据病立法、病分各类、逐类设证、因证制方、按方用药这样一种较为成熟的理法方药俱备的体例模式[4]。均先讲辨病，后讲辨证，如百合病、疟病、肺痿、胸痹等，并重视疾病鉴别。

专病专证专方或疾病通治方与辨证论治相结合的方法，在汉晋时期也多有体现。如《伤寒论》在具体治疗中，某病以某方"主之"，即为专病专证专方[3]，某病证"可与"或"宜"某方，体现了辨证与辨病结合，随宜治之的思想。《金匮要略》多以专病专证成篇。如百合病责之"心肺阴虚"，

主以百合剂，又因见证不同，而有百合地黄汤、百合知母汤、百合鸡子汤、滑石代赭汤、百合滑石散之异。晋代葛洪指出，临床应"分别病名，以类相续，不先错杂"，其《肘后备急方》对卒心痛、伤寒、痢疾、天行疫疠、疟病等的治疗，基本上不以分型论治，而是以通治方，加减施治。

1.1.3 隋唐时期 辨病结合辨证论治进一步发展，专病专方专药得到丰富。隋唐时期是我国医学发展承前启后的重要时期，病证结合论治得以继承和发展。唐代孙思邈《备急千金要方·论诊候第四》："夫欲理病，先察其源，候其病机"，主张积极辨识疾病及其证候产生的机制。

《备急千金要方》《千金翼方》中既有辨病论治，按病列方，也有辨病基础上辨证，按证列方。如《千金要方·消渴淋闭方》中载消渴方五十三首，其中既有消渴通治方，即辨病用方，如黄连丸猪肚丸；也有分证列方，如茯神汤，治胃腑实热，引饮常渴。王焘《外台秘要》也是依此体例。唐代《新修本草·诸病通用药》即按病列药，如瘿瘤所列海藻、昆布、文蛤、半夏、贝母等，寸白所列槟榔、芜荑、贯众、狼牙、雷丸等。说明隋唐时期，辨病基础上结合辨证论治有了进一步的发展。《千金方》和《外台秘要》在专病专方专药方面进一步发挥，如治疟用常山，治瘿用羊靥、海藻、昆布方，治消渴用地黄剂、黄连剂，治痢用苦参，治夜盲用羊肝等，极大地丰富了专病专方专药的内容。

1.1.4 宋金元时期 以辨证论治为主的病证结合模式初步形成。宋金元时期，一方面由于受理学的影响，思辨、感悟、取类比象的思维方式占一定的主导地位，辨证论治也相应取得了显著进展。另一方面，由于当时科学技术条件的限制，原有的辨病方式没有得到较大的发展，逐渐形成了以辨证论治为主的病证结合模式。南宋陈无择首倡"三因论"，主张"断其所因为病源，然后配合诸证，随因施治"，与后世"审因论治"相吻合。金元四大家则从不同角度丰富了辨证论治，刘完素主"火"论，倡"六气皆从火化"；张从正力主"邪去则正安"，倡汗、吐、下三法；李杲辨内伤外感，倡"人以胃气为本"，"内伤脾胃，百病由生"之说；朱震亨主相火，谓"阳常有余，阴常不足"，并提出"百病多因痰作祟"的观点，因时代环境之不同，对证候辨识各有所见。辨病论治渐被忽视。

宋代陈无择《三因极一病证方论·五科凡例》："故因脉以识病，因病以辨证，随证以施治"。

朱肱《类证活人书》:"庶几因名识病,因病识证,如暗得明,胸中晓然,而处病不瘳矣"。皆主张先识病,因病辨证,随证施治,初步形成了以辨证论治为主的治疗模式。

1.1.5 明清时期 以辨证论治为核心,辨病论治在某些方面得到深入。明清时期,辨证论治思想得到迅速发展,辨病论治或病证结合论治在某些方面也有了进一步深入,但仍以辨证论治为核心。八纲辨证、卫气营血辨证、三焦辨证等从不同角度扩展了辨证论治的范畴。

明代张景岳集宋金元辨证思想之大成,力主八纲辨证。赵献可辨证重命门;缪希雍倡甘凉滋润、酸甘化阴为治疗脾阴虚之大法;明末清初喻昌论大气与秋燥,更强调八纲辨证施治;清代王清任主张"治病之要诀,在明白气血"等,从不同角度丰富了中医辨证方法学。程钟龄《医学心悟·医门八法》指出:"论病之情,则以寒热虚实表里阴阳八字统之。而论治病之方,则又以汗和下消吐清温补八法尽之",也强调辨证论治。明清时期的温病学家,如叶桂辨卫气营血,吴瑭倡三焦辨证,薛雪论湿热病证,对外感热病的辨证论治分别做出了重要贡献。

辨病论治在某些方面有了深入发展,如明代医家孙志宏所著《简明医彀》,对每一病证均列主方,并附加减法;清代王清任治疗中风病半身偏瘫,专立补阳还五汤,以应常达变。徐灵胎《兰台轨范·序》中指出:"欲治病者,必先识病之名。能识病名,而后求其病之所由生。知其所由生,又当辨其生之因各不同,而病状所由异,然后考其治之之法。一病必有主方,一方必有主药"。说明了病证结合论治的重要性以及先识病后辨证的诊治步骤。

1.2 传统病证结合治疗观的主要形式

历代医家在长期的医疗实践中,逐渐形成以辨证为主结合辨病和以辨病为主结合辨证的两种治疗形式。

1.2.1 辨病为主,结合辨证 "辨病为主,结合辨证"是着眼于病的共性,在解决疾病基本矛盾的基础上,结合辨证论治。如《金匮要略》对胸痹之病,责之于"阳微阴弦",主以栝蒌薤白剂。又因邪气轻重、病情缓急而有实证之枳实薤白桂枝汤、虚证之人参汤,痰滞重症之栝蒌薤白半夏汤,轻证之茯苓杏仁甘草汤、橘枳姜汤等的不同。《简明医彀》:"医有成法、有活法,成法师古不可悖,活法

因时不可拘"。对每一病证皆列主方,随证加减。如治疗怔忡,主方以"当归、人参、黄连、远志、炙草、茯神、石菖蒲(炒,各一钱)加竹叶、龙眼、灯心煎成,调朱砂(飞一钱,临睡服)。心虚加柏子仁,麦冬;有汗,黄芪、枣仁;痰加半夏、胆星、橘红,痰多,在膈上稀涎散吐之,膈下滚痰丸利之……"皆为在辨病的基础上随证治之。

1.2.2 辨证为主,结合辨病 辨证论治在病证结合治疗中占有重要地位。辨病是对疾病整个过程变化规律的认识和概括,辨证是对疾病某一阶段病因、病位、病性、病势等方面的辨析和综合。"辨证为主、结合辨病"是着眼于证的共性,在解决机体某一阶段或某一状态下特殊矛盾的基础上,结合辨病论治。如治疗肾阳虚的肾气丸,明《奇效良方》载其"治肾气虚乏,下元冷惫,心火炎上,渴欲饮水。或肾水不能摄养,多吐痰唾,及脾虚不能克制肾水,亦吐痰唾,而不咳者,脐腹疼痛,夜多漩溺,尺脉缓弱,肢体倦怠,面色痿黄或黧黑,及虚劳不足,渴欲饮水,腰重疼痛,小便不利,脚气上攻,小腹不仁,男子消渴,小便反多,妇人转胞,小便不通,并皆治之。"水肿、咳喘、消渴、妇人转胞、癃闭及虚劳诸病在一定阶段均可出现肾阳虚证者,同证异病,皆可用肾气丸,此为辨证为主结合辨病的形式。

2. 近代汇通医派的病证结合治疗观

近代汇通医派首开西法断病结合中医辨证的先河,成为后世中西医病证结合诊疗模式的先导。19世纪中叶以后,西医大量传入中国,出现了汇通学派。早期汇通医家朱沛文认为中医"精于穷理,而拙于格物",但"信理太过,而或涉于虚";西医"专于格物,而短于穷理",但又"逐物太过,而或涉于固",主张汇通中西,以临床验证为标准求同存异。陆渊雷《伤寒论今释》卷一:"余以为理论当从西医之病名,治疗当宗仲景致审证为宜也[5]。"提出中医辨证当与西医辨病相结合。

张锡纯《医学衷中参西录》一书,既采用西医辨病,专病专方专药论治,又以衷中为主,体现辨证论治精神。如其"医方"篇中治肺病方、治癫狂方、治霍乱方、治痢方、治消渴方、治黄疸方等,皆为辨病基础上辨证论治。张锡纯善于汇通西医理论,针对病原、病因或病机的侧重点,选用专病专药,并结合辨证论治。如治毒淋,必用鸦胆子于诸辨证方中,认为"鸦胆子味至苦,而又善化瘀

解毒清热凉血，其能消毒菌之力，全在于此"。又如他在实践中发现"水蛭破瘀血，而不伤新血"，"其破瘀血者，乃此物之良能"，而妇女月闭癥瘕以瘀为主者，单用水蛭辨病论治。此外，他在实践中尝试运用西法诊病，中医治病。如张锡纯认为西人所谓"脑充血"，"实为类中风之证"，《内经》名之为煎厥、大厥、薄厥。《素问·调经论》曰："血之与气，并走于上，此为大厥，厥则暴死。气反则生，气不反则死。"并于经文之中悟得此证治法，以镇肝熄风汤主之，多有效验。而西人所谓"脑贫血"，即《灵枢·口问》谓："上气不足，脑为之不满……"脑为之不满，其脑中贫血可知[6]，用加味补血汤治疗。治疗中他常中西药物并用。他认为西医用药在局部，其重在治标，中医用药求其因，重在治本，二者结合，必获良效。

由于历史和时代的局限性，"衷中参西"不可避免地存在着中西医简单对应，甚至牵强附会之处，但"中体西用"顺应了当时中医发展的历史性与特殊性，对后世中西医病证结合起到了承前启后的作用。

3. 现代的病证结合治疗观

随着现代疾病谱的改变和中医临床实践经验的不断积累，辨病的含义发生了变化。现代医学辨病基础上的病证结合是传统病证结合的进一步发展。

著名中医施今墨先生强调辨证论治，但诊病时也重视参照西医医疗检查结果，并注意采用西医病名。金寿山先生《金匮诠释·自序》中提出应辨病与辨证相结合、辨脉与辨因相结合、通治方与专治方相结合的观点，强调"病"是纲，"证"是目，纲举则目张[7]。著名中医岳美中先生也指出："若能不停留于辨认证候，还进而辨病、辨病名（包括中医病名与西医病名），论治时注意古今专方专药的结合运用，一定效果更好；同时，也只是在此情况下，因人、因时、因地制方的作用才更有治疗价值[2]。"

3.1 现代病证结合治疗观的主要模式

3.1.1 西医诊病，中医辨证模式 西医诊病、中医辨证的病证结合临床模式源于近半个世纪的中西医结合临床诊疗实践，目前，已被广大中西医结合工作者广泛地应用于临床实践中。病证结合临床诊疗和研究模式是中西医结合的重要模式[8]。西医疾病诊断与中医辨证相结合的病证结合在临床中的

广泛应用，充分体现了中西医两种医学的优势互补[9]。中医学强调宏观和整体，西医则比较注重微观和局部，病证结合是两种医学最好的结合模式，只有两者的有机结合才能准确反映疾病及患者的状态，才能更有针对性地治疗患者，以达到最好的治疗目的。病证结合的临床诊疗和研究思想体现了疾病共性规律与患病个体个性特征的有机结合，为在科学层面开展中医药学的研究提供了可能。

3.1.2 辨证论治与专病专方专药论治结合模式 著名中医学家岳美中先生较早提出专病专方专药与辨证论治相结合的主张[2]，曾列举治黄疸之用茵陈剂、硝石矾石剂，治下利脓血之用白头翁汤、马齿苋、鸦胆子、大蒜等，麻风病之用毒蛇剂、大枫子剂等专方专药。姜春华先生认为"既要为病寻药，又不废辨证论治，为医者须识病辨证，才能做到辨病与辨证相结合"，并就如何从《外台秘要》寻找特异方药介绍了经验，认为若能寻找到专病专方专药，治病常有特效[10]。近年来，随着对辨病论治的重视，通过大量的临床实践及药理研究，发掘出许多专病专药，如蒲黄、红曲治血脂异常，五味子降转氨酶，靛玉红治慢性粒细胞白血病，雷公藤治结缔组织病，水蛭用于脑卒中，青皮升压等。专病专方专药治病主要是针对疾病的基本病机，属辨病论治范畴。由于疾病的基本矛盾和各个阶段的主要矛盾有时是不一致的，如果一味固守专方，就会陷入机械化，影响疗效。在专病专方基础上结合辨证论治，就会弥补这一不足。运用专病专方专药结合辨证论治已成为病证结合论治的重要模式之一。

3.1.3 疾病分期分阶段论治模式 疾病分期分阶段论治是指在掌握疾病基本病机和演变规律，确立治疗大法的基础上，根据疾病不同阶段、不同分期的主要矛盾进行辨证论治。著名中医朱良春先生在1962年即提出辨病与辨证相结合的主张[11]，强调谨守病机，分期论治。如治疗泌尿系统结石，认为其病机演变规律为下焦湿热，气滞血瘀，湿热久留，每致耗伤肾阴或肾阳。据此确立治疗大法为新病应清利湿热，通淋化石，以通淋化石汤；久病则需侧重补肾或攻补兼施，以增液益气排石汤、济生肾气加三金汤，分别针对久病肾阴虚或肾阳虚证。三方均重用鸡内金化石、金钱草排石，并酌用海金沙、石韦、冬葵子等以通淋，为辨病论治，至于实证清利，虚证补养，则为辨证论治[12]。

3.1.4 辨中医基本病机结合辨证论治模式 辨中

医基本病机结合辨证论治，即在中医理论指导下，辨识疾病的基本病机，因机立法，在此基础上结合辨证，随证施治。如糖尿病的中医基本病机是阴虚燥热，临床以气阴两虚较为常见，著名中医祝谌予先生自创"降糖对药方"针对这一基本病机[13]，临床多数情况下以此方随证加减，每获良效，但若消渴日久，脾虚生湿化热，湿热蕴结脾胃而出现脘腹痞闷、舌苔黄腻、脉濡缓等证，则应改投清热化湿之剂，如黄芩滑石汤。

3.1.5 无病从证，无证从病模式 一般情况下，西医辨病与中医辨证各有所据，辨病与辨证结合治疗，可相互补充，相济为用。但随着现代医学的发展，出现了很多传统中医四诊"无证可辨"或因信息量少"难以辨证"，而实验室检查或影像学诊断发现的疾病，如无症状性心肌缺血、隐匿性肾炎、隐性糖尿病等；或者某些疾病经过治疗，"证"消失，而现代医学检查显示疾病未愈的情况。此时，应无证从病，辨病论治为主。对一些西医无法明确诊断的疾病、病因未明的疾病、功能性疾病等，可无病从证，辨证论治为主。

3.2 现代病证结合治疗观的不同层次

3.2.1 理论层次 (1) 以中医理论辨识现代疾病。在中医理论指导下，通过对发病特点、病变部位、疾病表现于外的临床症状、体征等的辨识，并吸收现代医学先进的检测手段，延长和拓宽传统望、闻、问、切四诊的诊断视野，分析、总结疾病的病因、病机和内在规律。如再生障碍性贫血，其病变在骨髓造血干细胞，根据中医"肾主骨生髓"的理论，采用补肾生血法治疗，确有疗效。又如对冠心病介入术后再狭窄，其形成过程中的血栓形成、血管壁炎症、细胞增生等病理改变与中医学"心脉痹阻"、"心脉不通"有类似之处，从"血瘀证"论治，采用血府逐瘀制剂、芎芍胶囊等治疗[14]，经大样本、多中心 RCT 试验证实疗效可信。(2) 中西医理论合参，病证结合优势互补。中医学强调宏观和整体，重哲学思辩，重经验与观察，重表征和过程，动态、个体化辨证论治是其优势。西医学重视定量科学，注重微观和局部，重证据分析，强调结构，重视还原论，应用化学药物及侵入性方法治疗方面有显著优势。根据中西医理论各自优势和不足，中西医病证结合优势互补，发挥协同作用有助于提高临床疗效。如肿瘤的治疗，常于西医手术、放疗或化疗针对局部肿瘤病灶的同时，结合中医辨证论治、扶正固本祛邪法调节机体免疫功能，减轻

不良反应，提高生命质量。(3) 中西医结合基础研究成果的临床转化应用。中医学具有数千年的临床经验积累和浩瀚的古典文献记载，这些宝贵经验经过现代研究技术和方法明确其药效物质基础、作用靶标和机制、循证疗效证据等，可收到更大的获益。如从传统抗疟草药黄花蒿中分离出来的抗疟新药青蒿素及其衍生物和复方的研发，从治疗慢性白血病经验方当归芦荟丸中所含的有效中药青黛中分离提取的有效成分靛玉红用于慢性粒细胞白血病，从通过诱导细胞凋亡和分化治疗急性早幼粒细胞白血病的砷制剂的研究，临床转化应用均起到了很好的疗效。

3.2.2 诊断层次 现代病证结合治疗观在诊断层次的体现，即中西医辨病和辨证双重诊断，要求对同一患者既作出中医疾病和辨证诊断，又作出西医疾病诊断，这也是目前中医临床诊治疾病应用最广泛的模式。(1) 西医疾病诊断与中医病证诊断相结合。同一现代医学的疾病可涵盖多种中医学的疾病，如现代医学的充血性心力衰竭，可对应中医学的"喘证""水肿""胸痹"等多种病名，辨证可以完全相同，也可能完全不同。而同一中医病名，也可对应多种西医学的疾病，如中医学的头痛，可见于现代医学的高血压病、脑血管病、脑膜炎、血管性头痛、神经衰弱、鼻窦炎等多种疾病，其预后各异，中医辨证也可能完全不同。这就要求中西医双重诊断，辨病与辨证相结合，才能更准确地把握病情。(2) 结合疾病病理生理变化分期分阶段辨证。一方面，疾病基本的病理生理变化和演变规律决定了证的特点和转归；另一方面，证又有一定的独立性和自身的发展规律。将疾病病理生理变化和证候演变规律相结合，建立病证结合的分期分阶段辨证体系，有助于更好地处理诊断过程中个体化和共性的问题。(3) 宏观辨证与微观辨证相结合，功能辨证与形态辨证相结合。传统中医辨证论治为宏观辨证，其特点是具有动态性、整体性和灵活性，重功能、轻形态，通过对四诊收集到的各种症状和体征加以分析、综合，判断为某种"证"。其局限性在于带有一定的主观臆测性和不确定性，缺乏定量和客观化。近年来，在传统中医宏观辨证和功能辨证的基础上，提出"微观辨证""形态辨证"的概念[15,16]。微观辨证是在中医学理论指导下，采用现代先进的检测手段，从器官、组织、细胞、分子、基因等水平辨识证候。形态辨证是以现代解剖和病理形态学为依据辨识证候。前者如将唾液淀粉

酶活性下降，尿中 D- 木糖排泄率降低，作为脾虚证辨证诊断的微观参考指标，后者如以胃镜征象与辨证分型相结合治疗浅表性胃炎。在中医学理论指导下，将现代实验室检查、影像学检查、组织病理学检查等先进技术作为中医传统四诊的延伸，宏观辨证与微观辨证相结合、功能辨证与形态辨证相结合，是病证结合诊疗的重要发展方向之一。

3.2.3　治疗层次　(1)"同病异治"、"异病同治"与"同证异治"、"异证同治"　病与证的关系具体可表现为同病同证、同病异证、异病同证、异病异证等几种形式。从辨证的角度出发，同病异治和异病同治是中医的重要治则，体现了中医整体观和辨证论治的特点。然而从中医辨病的角度出发，中医治则也应有"同证异治"和"异证同治"。一方面，不同疾病虽可表现为相同的"证"，但其治疗也会有较大的差异。如冠心病、脑梗死、慢性肾炎、肝纤维化、痛经、肿瘤等多系统疾病皆可出现"血瘀证"，反映了这些疾病在某一阶段的共性，但因为病位、病性等的不同，其治疗各有其特点。另一方面，就某病而言，临床虽可表现为诸多不同的证，但因受疾病本身病理生理改变影响，治疗上也会存在类似性。如消渴病，虽有上、中、下三消之分，以及兼气虚血瘀之别，但始终贯穿着阴虚燥热这一基本病机，治疗也终不离滋阴润燥清热之法。(2) 辨病论治与辨证论治的有机结合。现代病证结合治疗观，并不是西医辨病与中医辨证治疗的简单相加，而在于用中医理论认识现代疾病，"以人为本"，实现二者的有机结合、优势互补。对西医辨病与中医辨证均很明确的情况，可以辨病论治与辨证论治相结合或择优治疗；对西医辨病明确，而中医无证可辨的"潜证"、"隐证"，可以辨病治疗为主，处以专病专方或经验方；对中医辨证明确，而西医病因不明或缺乏特异性疗法的情况，可以中医辨证论治为主。

4. 辨病、辨证、传统与现代病证结合各自的优势与局限

在现代医学迅猛发展的今天，中医执业者所面对的不仅是一些内涵和外延较为模糊的古代病名，如咳嗽、眩晕、痰饮病等，更多的是诊断明确的现代医学疾病。应注意在中医理论指导下，实现辨证与辨病的有机结合，中西互参，优势互补。

4.1　辨病与辨证各自的优势与局限

辨病有助于掌握疾病整个病理过程的基本矛盾，弥补单纯辨证的不足，解决某些疾病潜伏期、初期或无症状期无证可辨的问题。如无症状性心肌缺血，临床可无任何症状，而核素心肌扫描冠状动脉造影可发现冠状动脉病变。结合中医对这些病理改变的认识，辨病论治，采用益气活血法治疗，多可延缓或改善病情。如不采用辨病的方法，就无法对这些"隐证"、"潜证"做出早期诊断和治疗。辨病是针对疾病病理生理改变的认识，其局限性在于尚未能从动态的个体化和整体的角度去把握病情，重视社会环境精神体质等对疾病的影响。只注重辨病，强调对疾病病理改变治疗的针对性，忽视对患者疾病的动态变化个体化及整体状态的调节，对一些西医无法明确诊断的疾病（无病可辨）、功能性疾病、甚至复杂的器质性疾病的治疗，就可能无所适从。

中医辨证的局限性在于偏重对疾病外在症状表现的分析、综合，具有一定程度的主观性、经验性、模糊性和不确定性，对疾病内在病理生理改变的重视不足。有时经辨证治疗，症状虽可减轻或消失，但疾病却不一定真正根除。如不与辨病结合，仅满足于症状的改善，则难以获得疾病的真正治愈。只注重辨证，强调整体调节，治疗就会缺乏针对性。对许多无证可辨的情况，如仅有实验室指标的异常，而无明显临床症状（包括舌、脉异常）者，还会增加辨证的困难。

4.2　传统病证结合治疗观与现代病证结合治疗观各自的优势与局限

传统以中医辨病与中医辨证相结合为特点的治疗观，其局限性在于病证诊断和疗效判定多由主观经验判断，缺乏客观指标和可靠的定量标准。许多中医病名和证候诊断与预后并无直接关系。如中医学的胃痛，可能包括现代医学的急慢性胃炎、胃痉挛、消化道溃疡、消化道肿瘤、冠心病等疾病，其预后是完全不同的。现代以西医辨病与中医辨证相结合为特点的病证结合治疗观以病统证，可提高中医辨证的确定性，弥补单纯中医辨证缺乏标准化、规范化、客观化和不确定性的不足，使治疗更具针对性，避免只注重症状的改善和功能状态的调整而忽视对疾病病理改变的针对性治疗。其缺陷在于不利于中医辨病体系的自身发展，易导致单纯西医辨病、中医辨证的机械化倾向。对西医无法诊断的疾病，传统中医辨病和辨证则可弥补现代医学的不足。

5. 中西医统一的病证结合治疗观

病证结合治疗观在理论上涵盖了传统中医药学与现代医学诊疗实践的原则。由于中西医学对"病"的认识不尽相同，"证"又处于动态的变化中，因此"病证结合"在疾病的发生发展过程中应分不同层次与多个阶段予以处置，其统一性存在于整个诊疗过程当中，与患者的需求相一致。当症状或体征出现时，患者有了就医的诉求。医生根据症状、体征及实验室指标进行病证归纳与判别，依照病证相关的诊断处以方药或其他治疗。临床既要重视病证关联，也重视方证关联、药证关联等[17]，实现"法随证立，方从法出，方以药成"的思路，实现病、证、方相应的诊疗原则，解决病与证在具体实际中表现出纷繁复杂的多样性与不确定性问题[18]。也就是说，临床上为了实现医疗目标，需要贯彻病证结合的治疗观，明确与结合病、证的诊断，给予最有效的治疗，即如《伤寒论》所说"病皆与方相应者，乃服之"，"观其脉证，知犯何逆，随证治之"，同时也将现代医学所重视的对因、对症治疗统一贯穿起来，体现了灵活性与针对性的高度结合。

日本自江户时代汉方古方派医家提出方证相对的概念，方证相对便成为汉方诊疗体系的指导思想，对现代汉方医学的临床和科研产生了巨大的影响，如将《伤寒论》的古方大量成品化，提取其有效部位或单体制剂作为临床用药，方便使用，对汉方医疗的普及与推广意义重大；但同时也可能由于定证定方僵化的医疗模式，为汉方医学的衰落埋下了伏笔[17]。统一的病证结合治疗观真实地反映了临床实际的诊疗过程，同时也反映了中国中西医并存并重的医疗现实，或可为中西两种医学融会贯通奠定相关的理论基础，对临床产生与发挥重要的指导意义，推进我国医疗体制改革与卫生事业。

参考文献

[1] 欧阳锜. 证病结合用药式. 长沙：湖南科学技术出版社，1993：2.

[2] 岳美中教授原著，陈可冀等合编. 岳美中医学文集. 北京：中国中医药出版社，2000：3-12.

[3] 童舜华，童瑶，段逸山. 张仲景病证结合论治思想探析. 江西中医药，2003，34 (8)：10-11.

[4] 蒋明. 论以辨病为前提之《金匮要略》病证结合模式. 南京中医药大学学报，2003，19 (2)：65-68.

[5] 陆渊雷. 伤寒论今释. 北京：人民卫生出版社，1956：1-55.

[6] 张锡纯. 医学衷中参西录. 石家庄：河北人民出版社，1980：111-175.

[7] 金寿山. 金匮诠释. 上海：上海中医学院出版社，1986：1-6.

[8] 陈可冀，宋军. 病证结合的临床研究是中西医结合研究的重要模式. 世界科学技术-中医药现代化，2006，8 (2)：1-5.

[9] 张京春，陈可冀. 病证结合是中西医结合临床的最佳模式. 世界中医药，2006，1 (1)：14-15.

[10] 单书健，陈子华. 古今名医临证金鉴：外感热病（上）. 北京：中国中医药出版社，1999：166.

[11] 朱良春. 辨证与辨病相结合的重要性及其关系的探讨. 中医杂志，1962，4 (4)：16.

[12] 朱建平，邱志济. 朱良春治疗泌尿系统结石"对药"特色. 辽宁中医杂志，2000，27 (12)：532-533.

[13] 董振华，季元. 祝谌予治疗糖尿病慢性并发症的经验. 中医杂志，1997，38 (1)：12-14.

[14] Chen KJ, Shi DZ, Xu H, et al. XS0601 reduces the incidence of restenosis：a prospective study of 335 patients undergoing percutaneous coronary intervention in China. Chin Med J, 2006, 119 (1)：6-13.

[15] 蔡定芳. 论机能辨证与形态辨证相结合. 中国中西医结合杂志，1999，19 (4)：241-243.

[16] 沈自尹. 微观辨证和辨证微观化. 中医杂志，1986，27 (2)：55-57.

[17] 谢元华，张京春，陈可冀. 病证方药相应及其意义. 中西医结合心脑血管病杂志，2008，6 (1)：1-2.

[18] 秋叶哲生. 證の歴史と現代的課題. 漢方の臨床，2010，57 (12)：2017-2024.

审慎对待合理应用冠心病介入治疗手段 *

陈可冀　赵福海

冠心病介入技术的诞生，毋庸置疑对缓解心绞痛症状、挽救急性心肌梗死患者的生命、降低病死率起到举足轻重的作用，它代替了部分冠状动脉旁路移植术，减少了患者的创伤和痛苦。可是任何医学技术都是有界限的，一旦超越界限，就会走向反面，因此应该合理地把握其适应证，规范其应用范围。

1. 把握介入治疗的适应证

2010 年 11 月，美国心脏病学会杂志 (Journal of the American College of Cardiology, JACC) 杂志报道[1]一个 56 岁的男性冠心病患者，在过去的 10 年间接受了 28 次冠状动脉造影检查，共植入 67 个支架。我们并不清楚该患者的具体病情，但作为心内科介入医生，不应只见病变，而忽视患者的整体情况。刘茜倩[2] 和胡大一[3] 医师分别以"让支架飞"和"关于让支架飞和让 CT 飞"在《医师报》做过评论，很实际。确实，对造影发现的病变应具体分析，是否所有病变都应支架置入？对单支血管多处病变、多支血管病变、临界病变或者侧支循环丰富的慢性闭塞病变，应该进行血流贮备分数测定，寻找"罪犯病变或罪犯血管"，而不应千篇一律，以支架简单覆盖。

因此遵循指南，应将合理把握指征时刻牢记在胸。欧洲心脏病学会 (ECS) 2010 心肌血运重建指南指出：稳定性心绞痛患者如药物治疗能很好地控制症状，无明确的大面积心肌缺血证据；非 ST 段抬高急性冠状动脉综合征危险分层中低危者；ST 段抬高心肌梗死患者发病 3 ~ 28 天的患者均不建议介入治疗[2]。

2. 合理应用辅助检查诊断冠状动脉疾病与心肌缺血

眼下不少心内科医生离开辅助检查寸步难行，以至于不问病史、不进行体格检查便开出一大堆检查单。其实典型冠心病常常通过简单的病史和心电图即可做出诊断。

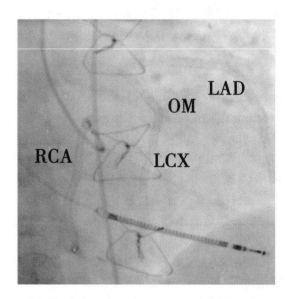

图 1　在过去的 10 余年间，这位 56 岁的患者，共接受 28 次冠状动脉造影，置入了 67 个支架（转引自 JACC, 2010, 56:1605）

NCDR 研究表明：在 398 978 例进行冠状动脉造影的患者中，仅 37.6% 的患者显示有临床意义的狭窄，其中 39.2% 的患者狭窄小于 20%[3]。试想通过简单仔细的询问病史、危险因素评价、必要的无创检查便可排除冠心病的诊断，为何要用昂贵的有创手段，换来如此高的阴性结果呢？

如果临床医生能更多地发挥自己的主观能动性，而不是被检查束缚住手脚，采用定势思维，下面的"医源性"悲剧就不会发生。2010 年 12 月，《Archives of Internal Medicine》报道 1 位不伴危险因素的女性患者，因不典型胸痛行冠状动脉 CT 造影，发现钙化和动脉硬化斑块，行有创冠状动脉造影检查时发生严重并发症——左主干夹层，不得已行紧急冠状动脉旁路移植术，6 个月后因移植血管退化，于移植血管植入了药物洗脱支架，术后不到 8 周又因支架内血栓而发生 ST 段抬高的心肌梗死并难治性心源性休克，最终接受了心脏移植手术[4]。多排螺旋 CT (MDCT) 诊断冠状动脉疾病的阴性预测值为 83% ~ 89%[5]，而阳性患者中

* 原载于《中国中西医结合杂志》，2011，31 (3)：295-296

第六章

仅 50% 为有血流动力学意义的狭窄，因此它并不能准确评价冠状脉狭窄病变，且有高估阻塞性冠状动脉疾病严重程度的可能[6]。鉴于此，对胸痛患者应依其疼痛特征，合理应用负荷心电图 / 超声 / 核素心肌扫描判断是否有心肌缺血，再应用 MDCT/MRI 判断是否存在冠状动脉疾病，结合病情及以上检查决定是否有行有创冠状动脉介入检查的必要。

3. 重视中西医结合在冠心病治疗中的价值

现在业界相当多的人对介入治疗顶礼膜拜，忽视了药物在冠心病治疗中的基础作用。COURAGE 研究表明：对有客观心肌缺血证据的稳定性心绞痛患者，无论接受强化的药物治疗还是在药物基础上联合介入治疗，长期随访两组在死亡、心肌梗死、卒中、因不稳定性心绞痛而住院方面并无差异[7]；OAT 研究表明：急性 ST 段抬高心肌梗死发病 3～28 天的患者，如果没有胸痛或可诱发的心肌缺血，尽管开通闭塞的梗死相关动脉，患者并不能从介入治疗中获益[8]。因此笔者体会强化冠心病二级预防策略，包括介入后的并发症等问题，结合活血化瘀等相关方药的合理使用，可使相当部分患者从药物治疗中获益[9]，当然，也需要在这方面做更科学的探讨和研究。

4. 在获益与风险之间探寻适合的治疗策略

冠心病治疗要考虑患者的全身情况，例如有出血风险的肿瘤患者、近期需要行外科手术的患者、因经济原因无力支付双重抗血小板治疗或对抗血小板药物抵抗的患者，选择金属裸支架可在最大程度上降低支架内血栓的风险；而多支血管病变、左主干分叉等病变，如采用介入治疗，则支架内血栓风险明显增高，而外科旁路移植可明显降低再次血运重建的比例，最大程度使患者获益；药物治疗可有效地稳定心绞痛患者，则既不需介入，也不需旁路移植。

切记介入治疗仅仅是冠心病的一种治疗手段，至少我们不要对患者造成伤害！

参考文献

[1] Khouzam RN, Dahiya R, Schwartz R. A heart with 67 stents. J Am Coll Cardiol, 2010, 56 (19)：1605.

[2] 刘茜倩 . 让支架飞 . 医师报 .2011-01-06：20.

[3] 胡大一 . 关于让支架飞和让 CT 飞 . 医师报 .2011-01-13：06.

[4] Guidelines on myocardial revascularization：The Task Force on Myocardial Revascularization of the European Society of Cardiology (ESC) and the European Association for Cardio-Thoracic Surgery (EACTS). Eur Heart J, 2010, 31 (20)：2501-2555.

[5] Patel MR, Peterson ED, Dai D, et al. Low diagnostic yield of elective coronary angiography. N Engl J Med, 2010, 362 (10)：886-895.

[6] Becker MC, Galla JM, Nissen SE. Left main trunk coronary artery dissection as a consequence of inaccurate coronary computed tomographic angiography. Arch Intern Med. Published online 2010, December13.

[7] Miller JM, Rochitte CE, Dewey M, et al. Diagnostic performance of coronary angiography by 64-row CT. N Engl J Med, 2008, 359 (22)：2324-2336.

[8] Sarno G, Decraemer I, Vanhoenacker PK, et al. On the inappropriateness of noninvasive multidetector computed tomography coronary angiography to trigger coronary revascularization：a comparison with invasive angiography. JACC Cardiovasc Interv, 2009, 2 (6)：550-557.

[9] Boden WE, O'Rourke RA, Teo KK, et al. Optimalmedical therapy with or without PCI for stable coronary disease. N Engl J Med, 2007, 356 (15)：1503-1516.

[10] Hochman JS, Lamas GA, Buller CE, et al. Coronary intervention for persistent occlusion after myocardial infarction. N Engl J Med, 2006, 355 (23)：2395-2407.

[11] Chen KJ, Shi DZ, Xu Hao, et al. XS0601 reduces the incidence of restenosis：a prospective study of 335 patients undergoing PCI in China. Chin Med J, 2006, 119 (1)：6-13.

第六章

中西医优势互补治疗冠心病心绞痛 *

史大卓

冠心病是在冠状动脉粥样硬化 (atherosclerosis, AS) 斑块的基础上形成血管狭窄、痉挛或血栓形成，导致心肌供血不足，临床出现一系列心肌缺血症状的一类疾病，为导致人类死亡和致残的一个主要原因。冠心病尽管有许多分类方法，但目前一般分为稳定型心绞痛 (stable angina, SA) 和急性冠状动脉综合征 (acute coronary syndrome, ACS)。其中ACS 又可分为不稳定型心绞痛 (unstable angina, UA)、非 ST 段抬高心肌梗死 (non-ST-segment elevation myocardial infarction, NSTEMI) 和 ST 段抬高心肌梗死 (ST-segment elevation myocardial infarction, STEMI)。ACS 共同的病理基础包括如下几个方面：(1) 不稳定粥样斑块内出血，斑块迅速增大；(2) 斑块破裂或表面破损，局部血小板聚集继而血栓形成；(3) 血管痉挛等。心绞痛和心肌梗死的主要区别在于是否发生心肌坏死。尽管 UA 和心肌梗死有相似的病理基础，但因心肌损伤的程度不同，治疗和预后方面也存在差异。本文主要讨论冠心病心绞痛包括 SA 和 UA 的治疗。

冠心病心绞痛是因心肌暂时缺血、缺氧引起的以发作性心前区不适为主要表现的一组临床综合征，通常见于冠状动脉至少 1 支或主要分支管腔直径狭窄 ≥ 50% 的患者。当体力活动或精神应激时，冠状动脉血流不能满足心肌代谢的需要，导致心肌缺血，诱发心绞痛。中医对本病的临床症状早在《内经》中即描述，如"胸痹"、"心痛"等，症状严重者则描述为"真心痛"、"厥心痛"。

1. 冠心病心绞痛的现代西医治疗

自 1977 年首例开展经皮冠状动脉腔内球囊扩张成形术 (PTCA) 治疗冠心病以来，从 PTCA 到金属裸支架、药物洗脱支架，以及新近尝试用于临床的药物洗脱球囊，经皮冠状动脉介入治疗 (percutaneous coronary intervention, PCI) 已成为冠心病治疗的一个主要有效方法。对于有较大范围心肌缺血证据的 SA 患者，PCI 疗效较为肯定；对于危险分层（TIMI 评分或 Grace 评分）为极高危的非 ST 段抬高的 ACS 患者应进行紧急PCI (< 2h)，中高危非 ST 段抬高的 ACS 患者应进行早期 PCI (< 72h) [1]。但是，包括介入治疗和旁路移植术的血运重建术仅是心血管疾病治疗手段之一，药物的二级预防仍是冠心病治疗的基础。COURAGE 研究提示，对于稳定型心绞痛患者，介入治疗的优势可能仅限于改善心绞痛症状，并不能显著改善患者预后 [2]，与药物治疗相比不能降低病死率及心肌梗死发生率 [1]。

冠心病的药物治疗的目的在于预防心肌梗死和猝死的发生，改善生存率和生活质量。目前临床用于治疗冠心病心绞痛的药物主要有如下几类：

1.1 抗血小板药物

包括阿司匹林、噻吩吡啶、血小板糖蛋白(GP) Ⅱb/ Ⅲa 受体拮抗剂等。阿司匹林可抑制环氧化酶和血栓烷 (thromboxane, TXA_2) 的合成，抗血小板聚集，只要没有禁忌证，仍为首选抗血小板药物。噻吩吡啶类药物氯吡格雷可选择性不可逆地抑制血小板 ADP 受体，阻断 ADP 依赖激活的GPⅡb / Ⅲa 复合物，减少 ADP 介导的血小板激活和聚集。主要用于急性冠状动脉综合征、支架植入后及有阿司匹林禁忌证者；普拉格雷属于第三代噻吩吡啶类抗血小板药物，可直接阻断 P2Y12 受体，抗血小板活性是氯吡格雷的 10 ~ 100 倍，且受代谢影响较小，但其出血事件明显高于氯吡格雷，特别是老年、低体重和既往缺血性脑血管发作的患者 [3,4]；替卡格雷是一种环戊三唑吡啶类药物，能直接作用于 ADP 受体，不需经过肝代谢，不受体内代谢影响，疗效优于氯吡格雷，而且对 ADP 受体的拮抗为可逆性，故不增加出血风险 [5,6]。GPⅡb / Ⅲa 受体拮抗剂包括阿昔单抗、依替巴肽、替罗非班等，对行 PCI 的 UA 患者可能明显受益，而对不拟行 PCI 的低危患者获益不明显。

---

* 原载于《中国中西医结合杂志》，2011, 31 (6)：732-735

1.2　抗凝血酶类药物

包括肝素和低分子肝素，多用于 UA 患者，可降低患者心肌梗死和心肌缺血的发生率，联合使用阿司匹林获益更大。介入治疗手术前或手术期间，建议优先选普通肝素，且可与 GP Ⅱ b / Ⅲ a 受体拮抗剂合用；手术后或接受早期保守治疗和延迟 PCI 者，建议使用低分子肝素。

1.3　他汀类药物

他汀类药物能有效降低血清总胆固醇 (TC) 和低密度脂蛋白胆固醇 (LDL-C)，因此可降低心血管事件。他汀类药物还有延缓 AS 斑块进展、稳定斑块和抗炎等作用。冠心病患者 LDL-C 的目标值为 < 2.60mmol/L，极高危患者的目标值为 LDL-C < 2.07 mmol/L，高危或中危者 LDL-C 应至少降低 30% ~ 40%。同时存在高甘油三酯 (TG) 或低高密度脂蛋白 (HDL-C) 的高危患者，可考虑联合使用他汀类药物和贝特类药物（非诺贝特）或烟酸。PROSPER 研究表明，他汀类药物能显著减少老年人心肌梗死风险，直到 80 岁以上患者，均可从他汀类药物中获益[7]。

1.4　β- 受体阻滞剂

β- 受体阻滞剂同时兼有改善预后及减轻症状两方面的作用，只要无禁忌证，应作为稳定型心绞痛的初始治疗药物。有心肌梗死、左室收缩功能异常或心力衰竭病史的心绞痛患者更应长期甚至终身服用 β- 受体阻滞剂。β- 受体阻滞剂能降低心肌梗死后 SA 患者死亡和再梗死的风险。具有内在拟交感活性的 β- 受体阻滞剂，心脏保护作用较差，推荐使用无内在拟交感活性的 β- 受体阻滞剂。临床应用应从小剂量开始，逐级增加剂量，以静息心率不低于 50 次 / 分为宜。

1.5　血管紧张素转换酶抑制剂 (ACEI)

所有合并糖尿病、心力衰竭、左室收缩功能异常、高血压病或慢性肾病的冠心病心绞痛患者，均应使用 ACEI，其他冠心病患者也建议长期服用 ACEI，但低危患者获益可能较小。一项包括 33960 例冠心病患者的荟萃分析表明，ACEI 可减少冠心病患者（包括无左室功能障碍或心力衰竭患者）的病死率和主要心血管事件[8]。不能耐受 ACEI 的慢性心绞痛患者，可改用血管紧张素受体拮抗剂 (ARB) 作为替代治疗[9]。

1.6　硝酸酯类

硝酸酯类药物为内皮依赖性血管扩张剂，能扩张冠状动脉，改善心肌组织灌注，从而改善心绞痛症状。硝酸酯类药物可反射性增加交感神经张力，使心率加快，因此临床常联合 β- 受体阻滞剂应用。

1.7　其他

二氢吡啶类和非二氢吡啶类钙拮抗剂均有抗心绞痛作用，长效钙拮抗剂可作为抗心绞痛的初始治疗药物，不一定在其他药物无效后才使用或加用，其有效性和安全性已在 ACTION、CAMELOT、ALLHAT 及 ASCOT 研究中得到证实[10-13]。非二氢吡啶类钙拮抗剂地尔硫䓬或维拉帕米可作为对 β 受体阻滞剂有禁忌证患者的替代治疗。改善代谢性药物曲美他嗪和钾通道开放剂尼可地尔、If 通道阻滞剂伊伐布雷定等，由于应用时间短，相关研究证据较少，目前多被用于冠心病的辅助治疗。

2. 冠心病心绞痛的中医药治疗

《素问·痹论》指出："胸痹者，脉不通"。概括了胸痹的基本病机为"脉不通"，不通则痛。《金匮要略·胸痹心痛短气病脉证治》将"胸痹"主要表现总结为胸中气塞、胸痛彻背、背痛彻心、短气等，认为其病理关键为"阳微阴弦"，即胸部"阳气"亏虚，阴寒痰浊上乘阳位，痹阻心脉，不通则痛，为本虚标实证，并创制系列栝蒌薤白剂用于临床，至今仍为治疗冠心病心绞痛的一个主要治疗方法。后世医家对胸痹的认识皆不断有所发展，如明代虞抟《医学正传》指出，本病与"污血冲心"有关；清代叶天士强调久病入络，主张用活血通络法治疗胸痹心痛；王清任则创制血府逐瘀汤治疗胸痹心痛。陈可冀院士集前人经验，病证结合，认为"脉不通"的基本病机在于血脉瘀滞，倡导活血化瘀治疗冠心病，并研制冠心Ⅱ号、愈心痛胶囊、芎芍胶囊等活血化瘀制剂用于临床，较以往单纯应用宣痹通阳法治疗冠心病明显提高了疗效。在此基础上，陈可冀院士根据冠心病心绞痛本虚标实的病机和疾病不同阶段的轻重缓急，将冠心病心绞痛的治法概括为三通两补，即"芳香温通"、"宣痹通阳"、"活血化瘀"之三通和"补肾"、"补气血"之两补，对指导中医临床治疗冠心病心绞痛起到了执简驭繁的作用。

2.1　心绞痛发作期治疗

心绞痛是心肌缺血缺氧的信号，改善心肌缺血缺氧是缓解疼痛的关键。疼痛发作时中医的基本病机为心脉闭阻、不通则痛，以标实为主，可有气滞、血瘀、寒凝、热结、痰阻等不同，治疗当急治其标，予以温阳散寒、行气活血、通阳泄浊、豁痰开窍为法，以达通则不痛的目的。温散通脉多选用芳香温通之品，其气味芳香，性温善行，既有通脉宣痹之力，又有较快缓解疼痛之用。现代许多芳香温通的中成药如苏合香丸、苏冰滴丸、冠心苏合丸、速效救心丸、宽胸丸、宽胸气雾剂等，皆可在心绞痛发作时含服、喷雾或吞服，可迅速缓解血管痉挛，增加冠状动脉血流量，改善心肌血供。但芳香温通药多辛散走窜，不宜过用久服，以免散气耗阴，必要时可配伍补心气、养心阴药物，以取通脉而不伤正之效。此外，在芳香温通的基础上，可适当配伍疏肝理气之品，如苏梗、柴胡、香附等调理气机，以使气行血行。

2.2 心绞痛缓解期治疗

冠心病缓解期病机多为本虚标实：虚者，心之气血阴阳不足或兼肝、脾、肾脏腑亏损；实者则如上述。冠心病缓解期的治疗不外乎补虚与通痹两法：补虚应在补元气、补心气和滋补阴血的同时，辨气血阴阳以定性，分肝、脾、肾脏腑以定位；通痹则当芳香温通、宣痹通阳、活血化瘀，辨其寒热属性、瘀滞轻重和病位的深浅，或活血、或化瘀、或通络、或宣痹化痰，目的在于使心气、宗气以运血脉，宣通血脉痹阻。由于本病为终身疾病，病程日久，常存在阳损及阴、阴损及阳、寒热错杂为患的病理过程，既可因虚致心脉痹阻，也可因血瘀、气滞、痰阻、寒凝、热结等而致心脉痹阻、损伤正气，最终导致虚实并存。因此，临床遣方用药当标本兼治，通中寓补，补中有通。陈可冀院士总结的三通两补治法具有提纲挈领作用，值得领会应用。临床常见中医证型有血脉瘀滞、气虚血瘀、痰浊痹阻以及久病耗气伤阴导致的气阴两虚、心肾阴虚等，可作为稳定型心绞痛辨证施治参考。

2.3 UA

UA是介于SA与急性心肌梗死之间的一种病情较为严重的临床状态，和SA相比，UA具有疼痛程度重、持续时间长、硝酸酯类药物疗效差、易发展为急性心肌梗死或发生猝死的特点。结合UA的临床表现及病理变化，中医学认为UA多有瘀血凝结、久病入络、心脉瘀阻的病机，其血瘀程度多较SA严重。由于患者素体禀赋差异，UA患者临床可表现出气滞血瘀、气虚血瘀、阳虚血瘀及痰瘀互阻等不同的病机。因此，临床治疗UA，除注意一般心绞痛治疗的规律外，还要注意以下几方面：(1) 温阳重在心肾，活血不忘祛瘀：UA的病机

特点是阳虚与血瘀程度都较严重，中医治疗应注重温阳以通血脉。疼痛发作时治以芳香温通，使阴寒散，阳气复，心脉调畅，心痛缓解。UA的活血化瘀治疗，一要偏于辛温柔润，二要破瘀散结；(2) 病证结合，谨察虚实：不同类型的UA患者有各不相同的病机。如初发劳累型心绞痛以标实为主，应重用活血化瘀药，适当应用破血逐瘀药可提高疗效；恶化劳累型心绞痛因患病时间较长，往往由稳定劳累型心绞痛发展演变而来，与中医"久心痛"类似，应攻补兼施，采用益心气、补宗气、生肾元、活血祛瘀为法；自发型心绞痛与活动无明显的关系，以夜间及凌晨发作多见，应重在温阳散寒，兼用活血祛瘀之法；卧位型心绞痛多属于严重的劳累型心绞痛，其治疗应重用益气，兼以活血化瘀。对于伴有心功能不全的患者，在益气扶正的基础上，佐以活血利水，可望收到较好的疗效。

2.4 介入治疗后冠心病心绞痛

近年来，对介入治疗后冠心病的中西医综合干预研究，取得一定进展。陈可冀等[14]采用多中心、随机双盲对照研究方法，临床观察活血化瘀中药制剂联合西医常规治疗PCI后冠心病患者的疗效，证明在西医常规治疗的基础上加用活血化瘀制剂，可明显降低PCI后患者半年内的心绞痛发生率、减少再狭窄形成和降低终点事件的发生，表明活血化瘀中药制剂可进一步提高介入治疗后冠心病患者的疗效。有研究观察发现，PCI对于血瘀证有一定的改善作用，但对气虚证无改善作用。相反，PCI在一定程度上加重了气虚证，因而对于冠心病介入术后的患者，中医辨证治疗应以益气为主，活血通脉为辅[15]。研究证明，中医药干预冠心病介入术后冠心病，有抑制血管平滑肌细胞增生、保护血管内皮细胞、纠正血脂紊乱、抗血小板聚集等作用[16]，显示有良好的临床应用前景，值得进一步验证，为扩大临床应用提供可靠的证据。

尽管近年来在系列临床研究和系统评价的基础上，国内外皆建立了指导临床实践的冠心病心绞痛诊疗指南，但其疗效仍存在个体差异，个体化治疗仍为治疗冠心病心绞痛获得理想疗效的主要途径。其他如阿司匹林抵抗、血运重建后心肌组织无灌注和缓慢灌注、心肌缺血后系统炎症反应、内皮功能障碍等，现代医学尚无理想的干预措施。现代药理研究表明，中医药具有广泛的药理效应，如抗血小板黏附聚集、抑制血栓形成、扩张血管、改善血管内皮功能、调节炎症反应、促进心肌毛细血管

再生和增加心肌组织灌注等，可作用于冠心病心绞痛的许多病理环节。利用现代西医学的微观形态学和分子生物学的病理生理观察，提高中医药治疗的靶向性；利用中医整体辨证、个体化诊疗的理念，综合西医靶向治疗产生更佳的整体综合效应，需要药理、药学、毒理、临床和生物信息学等多学科结合，进而促进研究成果转化为临床应用，为提供临床疗效做出新的贡献。

参考文献

[1] 中华医学会心血管病学分会，中华心血管病杂志编辑委员会. 经皮冠状动脉介入治疗指南. 中华心血管病杂志，2009，37 (1)：4-25.

[2] Boden WE, O'Rourke RA, Teo KK, et al. Optimal medical therapy with or without PCI for stable coronary disease. N Engl J Med, 2007，356 (15)：1503-1516.

[3] O'Donoghue M, Antman EM, Braunwald E, et al. The efficacy and safety of prasugrel with and without a glycoprotein Ⅱb / Ⅲa inhibitor in patients with acute corohary syndromes undergoing percutaneous intervention：a TRITONTIM I 38 (Trial to assess improvement in therapeutic outcomes by optimizing platelet inhibition with prasugrel-thrombolysis in myocardial infarction 38) analysis. J Am Coll Candiol, 2009，54 (8)：678-685.

[4] Seidel H, Rahman MM, Scharf RE. Monitoring of antiplatelet therapy: Current limitations, challenges, and perspectives. Hamostaseologie, 2011，31 (1)：41-51.

[5] White HD. Oral antiplatelet therapy for atherothrombotic disease：current evidence and new directions. Am Heart J, 2011，161 (3)：450-461.

[6] Nawarskas JJ, Clark SM. Ticagrelor：A novel reversible oral antiplatelet agent. Cardiol Rev, 2011，19 (2)：95-100.

[7] Sattar N, Murray HM, McConnachie A, et al. C-reactive protein and prediction of coronary heart disease and global vascular events in the Prospective Study of Pravastatin in the Elderly at Risk. Circulation, 2007，115 (8)：981-989.

[8] Danchin N, Cucherat M, Thuillez C, et al. Angio tensin-converting enzyme inhibitors in patients with coronary artery disease and absence of heart failure or left ventricular systolic dysfunction：an overview of long-term randomized controlled trials. Arch Intern Med, 2006, 166 (7)：787-796.

[9] Fraker TD, Finn SD, Gibbons RJ, et al. 2007 chronic angina focused update of the ACC / AHA 2002 guidelines for the management of patients with chronic stable angina：a report of the American College of Cardiology / American Heart Association Task Force on Practice Guidelines Writing group to develop the focused update of the 2002 guidelines for the management of patients with chronic stable angina. J Am Coll Cardiol, 2007, 50 (23)：2264-2274.

[10] Poole-Wilson PA, Lubsen J, Kirwan BA, et al. Effect of long-acting nifedipine on mortality and cardiovascular morbidity in patients with stable angina requiring treatment (ACTION trial)：randomized controlled trial. Lancet, 2004，364 (9437)：849-857.

[11] Nissen SE, Tuzcu EM, Liby P, et al. Effect of antihypertensive agents on cardiovascular events inpatients with coronary disease and normal blood pressure：the CAMELOT study：a randomized controlled trial. JAMA, 2004，292 (18)：2217-2225.

[12] Allhat Collaborative Reseach Group. Major cardiovascular events in hypertensive patients randomized to doxazos in vs chlorthalidone：the antihypertensive and lipid-lowering treatment to prevent heart attack trial. JAMA, 2000, 283 (15)：1967-1975.

[13] Dahl-fB, Sever PS, Poulter NR, et al. Prevention of cardiovascular events with an antihypertensive regimen of amlodipine adding perindoprilas required versus atenolol adding bendroflum ethiazide as required, in the Anglo-Scandinavian Cardiac Outcomes Trial-Blood Pressure Lowering Arm：amulticentre randomized controlled trial. Lancet, 2005, 366 (9489)：895-906.

[14] Chen KJ, Shi DZ, Xu H, et al. XS0601 reduces the incidence of restenosis：a prospective study of 335 patients undergoing percutaneous coronary intervention in China. Chin Med J, 2006, 119 (1)：3-7.

[15] 陈伯钧，潘宗奇，苏学旭，等. 冠心病介入治疗前后中医证型变化的研究. 中国中西医结合杂志，2007，27 (8)：689-691.

[16] 张翔炜，张敏州，李松，等. 通冠胶囊对冠心病经皮冠脉介入术后患者凝血纤溶系统的影响. 中国中西医结合杂志，2004，24 (12)：1065-1068.

病因病机研究与提高中西医结合临床水平 *

史大卓　高铸烨

病因病机研究是提高中医药临床水平的重要方面。早在两千多年前的《黄帝内经》中即有"夫百病之所生者，必起于燥湿、寒暑、风雨、阴阳、喜怒、饮食、居处"的病因认识，强调辨证治疗过程中应"审察病机，无失气宜"；并将特定病因致病的病理变化归纳为"病机十九条"，以执简驭繁，指导临床。金元四大家之一刘河间对"六气皆从火化"和"五志过极，皆为热甚"病因病机的阐释；李东垣对"内伤脾胃，百病由生"和"火与元气不两立"病因病机的论述；朱丹溪对"阳有余而阴不足"和"湿热相火"等病因病机的认识；吴又可对温疫病疫疠时气病因的发现；清代叶天士对卫气营血、久病入络病因病机的阐发以及王清任瘀血病因病机的认识等，都推动了中医病因病机学的发展和临床实践的进步。综观传统中医学的发展历史，应当说临床诊疗模式的每一次发展，无不以病因病机认识的发展和创新为前提。

病因病机是对机体疾病产生的原因和疾病发生、发展、变化机制的阐释。现代医学多从致病微生物（细菌、病毒）及器官、细胞、基因、蛋白质等方面的生理病理改变，以求其病因；传统中医学则多从审症求因、辨证求因或以效析因的角度，采用取类比象、演绎推理方法，阐释整体和相关脏腑"有诸形于内，必形于外"的病因。尽管两者认识病因的方法不同，但对象皆是患病机体，目的皆为求患病之因。在中医学现代病因病机研究方面，两者相互补充，宏观和微观结合，辨病和辨证结合，可以提高认识水平，并加以深化：例如再生障碍性贫血的中医病因病机认识从脾肾亏虚到肾亏精竭、痰瘀互结；类风湿性关节炎的病因病机认识从"风寒湿三气杂至合而为痹"发展到现代的"肝肾亏虚、邪毒深伏经筋骨骱"；中风的病因病机认识，唐宋以前多以外风立论，其后逐渐认识到"内风"为患，至清·王清任则强调半身元气亏虚，血脉瘀滞不利，再到当代风、火、痰、毒、瘀、虚的认识等。这些对传统病因病机认识的发展和突破皆导致

了临床治疗方法学的转变，显著提高了临床疗效。

冠心病的中医治疗，上世纪60—70年代以前多遵循汉·张仲景提出的"阳微阴弦"病因病机，采用宣痹通阳的栝蒌薤白类方剂进行治疗。近年来，陈可冀等根据冠心病血小板黏附聚集、血管管腔狭窄、血栓形成等病理改变和中医"血脉不通则痛"的认识，倡导冠心病血脉瘀滞的病因病机，主张应用活血化瘀为主进行治疗，辐射全国，显著提高了临床疗效。随着现代医学有关冠心病病理生理研究的深入，多将冠心病发病过程中的临床表征如胸痛、舌质暗及血小板活化、黏附聚集和血栓形成等微观病理变化的病因病机概括为"血瘀"；但其发病急骤、传变迅速、腐肌伤肉的致病特点及组织坏死、过氧化应激损伤、炎症反应等病理改变，似非单一"血瘀"病因病机所能全面概括，而这些致病特点与传统中医因毒致病特点颇为相似。有关因毒致病的病因病机，自古就有阐述：如清·尤在泾 [1] 认为系因"邪气蕴结不解"；王冰 [2] 认为"夫毒者，皆五行标盛暴烈之气所为也"。现代学者多认为毒为病因之甚，提出了内毒 [3]、热毒、寒毒、浊毒、瘀毒等因毒致病的病因病机认识 [4]。近年来，围绕因毒致病进行了不少研究，但是关于冠心病有关因毒致病作用的认识尚不统一，且未建立冠心病因毒致病辨证的标准，成为因毒致病理论转化为临床应用的瓶颈，限制了冠心病中医治疗方法学的创新和疗效的提高。

陈可冀院士等在以往冠心病血脉瘀滞的病因病机基础上，结合传统中医有关因毒致病的认识及冠心病中医临床表征和微观变化特点，提出毒瘀互结、因毒致变是其主要病因病机。围绕这一认识 [5-7]，在国家重点基础研究发展计划（973计划）资助下，进行了有关"毒"病因病机的文献研究、实验研究、临床随机对照研究和前瞻性大样本队列研究，同时结合现代信息生物学分析，从宏观临床表征和微观理化指标变化两方面，建立了冠心病稳定期因毒致病的辨证标准，进行了量化诊断规范，

* 原载于《中国中西医结合杂志》，2011，31 (3)：293-294

并分析了毒作为病因致病的归因危险度，结果表明 84.35% 的冠心病心血管事件归因于"毒邪"病因致病。说明此标准可用于冠心病稳定期高危患者的辨识和毒邪病因致病的诊断，为冠心病"毒"作为病因病机认识转为指导临床应用提供了依据。

中医病因病机学的发展和创新，是一个不断临床实践、反复检验和逐渐凝练升华的过程。本刊本期发表了陈可冀等[8]制定的冠心病稳定期因毒致病的辨证诊断量化标准，建立在文献研究、专家临床经验和现代前瞻性大样本队列研究的基础上，既体现了传统中医关于因毒致病认识的特点，又涵盖了临床可操作性强的微观指标，符合循证医学理念，为现代中医病因病机学的研究提供一个范例。难能可贵的是，该研究在病因学分析的基础上，通过大样本队列研究的数据进行反向验证，表明冠心病因毒致病的标准有较高归因度。该标准的建立，对促进中医在冠心病防治领域发挥既病防变相关干预措施的优势、提高临床疗效，将产生积极的规范和指导作用。

参考文献

[1] 孙中堂. 尤在泾医学全书. 北京：中国中医药出版社，1999：109.

[2] 张登本，孙理军. 王冰医学全书. 北京：中国中医药出版社，2006：233.

[3] 徐中环，王承平. 中医"内毒"论. 中国中医基础医学杂志，2002，8 (5)：7-9.

[4] 张艳，杨关林，于睿，等. 动脉粥样硬化中医虚瘀痰毒病因病机实质研究探讨. 时珍国医国药，2007，18 (6)：1513-1514.

[5] 徐浩，陈可冀. 从对动脉粥样硬化认识转变看中西医结合的优势与切入点. 中国中西医结合杂志，2007，27 (1)：5-7.

[6] 徐浩，史大卓，殷惠军，等. "瘀毒致变"与急性心血管事件：假说的提出与临床意义. 中国中西医结合杂志，2008，28 (10)：934-938.

[7] 史大卓，徐浩，殷惠军，等. "瘀"、"毒" 从化——心脑血管血栓性疾病病因病机. 中西医结合学报，2008，6 (11)：1105-1108.

[8] 陈可冀，史大卓，徐浩，等. 冠心病稳定期因毒致病的辨证诊断量化标准. 中国中西医结合杂志，2011，31 (3)：313-314.

以临床实践数据为导向构建中西医结合临床指南的设想 *

徐 浩 史大卓 刘保延 陈可冀

临床指南 (clinical guideline)，又称临床实践指南 (clinical practice guideline)，是按照循证医学原则，以当前最佳证据为依据，按照系统和规范方法，在多学科人员合作下制定的有关陈述和建议，旨在供医务工作者为患者制定最恰当的医疗卫生服务方案。

最近几十年来，临床各科出现了大量的循证临床指南，对于规范临床实践起到了重要的作用。中医药诊治疾病有其自身的理论体系，中西医结合更是以复杂干预为特点，按照现代医学研究证据制定临床指南的方法，对中医药及中西医结合指南的制定存在不完全适用的具体情况。本文即提出以临床实践数据为导向构建中西医结合临床指南，与循证临床指南互为补充，并结合初步的临床实践加以探讨，以期为中西医结合临床指南的构建提供新的思路。

1. 循证临床指南——证据的分级与评价

既往多数指南都是基于当地或国内专家的意见、教科书、标准治疗或传统医疗制定。但现在对指南的认识已经发生了根本变化。随着科学证据的逐渐增多，个体观察、病理生理推理和专家观点虽仍很需要，但已不足以为患者提供最好的医疗护理，临床医学界急切需要平衡成本、效益、风险的最佳决策依据。20 世纪 90 年代初英国 James Petrier 教授首次提出临床实践指南的概念[1]。现

* 原载于《中国中西医结合杂志》，2009，29 (6)：544-547

在，撰写循证临床实践指南的过程与以往有很大不同，它包括提出相关临床问题，系统检索文献和使用正确的方法对证据级别进行评分，再根据证据的级别和强度提出推荐意见。证据质量存在等级差别，分级依赖于不同研究的设计强度，如随机对照试验（RCT）、队列研究和病例对照研究等[2]。还包括以下内容：单盲或双盲的应用、是否采用意向治疗分析及其结果、随访时间与失访率、基线情况、对照的可比性、研究结果的类型及范围、95%可信区间等。作为评价临床试验的质量，上述分级标准毋庸置疑，但作为形成临床实践指南的证据，其过多地强调研究的方法学，而对该证据在临床应用的可重复性、灵活性和临床实用性、患者的个体差异和偏好以及来自临床实践的数据则缺乏足够的重视[3,4]。

2. 中医药临床指南——如何认识和合理应用 RCT

中医药学虽历经数千年的发展，积累了丰富的临床实践经验，以辨证论治、个体化治疗为其一大特色。但是按循证医学的相关标准，其证据级别相对较低，主要为 2 级，甚至 3 级以下的证据。中医药浩如烟海的古籍文献中的记载，仅能归属于专家经验，而被列为 3 级以下证据。而对于证据级别较高的 RCT，尤其是设计规范、科学性强的 RCT 研究还较少。因此，近年来中医药领域的 RCT 研究明显增加。但需要指出的是，我们要避免一提"循证"就"必做 RCT"的盲动倾向，甚至没有太多工作基础就去做多中心、大样本RCT，其结果可能适得其反，劳民伤财。RCT 也有其适用范围，要根据需要解决的临床问题（如病因、诊断、治疗、预后等）去选择合适的研究方法。我们鼓励有长期临床基础、效果可靠的中成药制剂或者较成熟的治疗方案进行多中心 RCT加以验证，哪怕在疾病某一环节被证明有价值也是非常有意义的。

另外，中医药临床指南的难点在于辨证论治的疗效评价问题。以 RCT 为主的临床研究方法多基于群体性特征，强调基线均衡、控制混杂因素（其实这正是患者和疾病的个体化特征因素和医生个体化辨证施治的关键），要求避免"干扰"和"沾染"（但实际上因涉及国情、经费、伦理学及患者依从性问题等很难避免），难以满足中医临床辨证论治个体化诊疗模式中以多维时空、诸多因

素、非线性、复杂性为主要特征临床研究的需要。因此以个体化诊疗为特点的中医药临床指南期望以RCT 等研究为主要证据显然有一定局限性。如何解决这一瓶颈问题，成为制定中医药临床指南的关键。以临床实践数据为基础，前瞻性设计观察指标（证型宜粗不宜细），在积累足够样本量基础上，充分利用临床终点事件、生活质量、卫生经济学等现代医学公认的指标，基于数据二次分组进行疗效评价，寻找个体化特征与临床疗效的相关性，无疑是可采取的方法之一，这对于基于群体特征的循证临床实践指南必将是有益的补充。

3. 中西医结合临床指南——治疗方案优化是前提和基础

中西医结合医学以其疗效突出、优势互补等特点越来越多地被医生和广大患者所接受，成为我国医疗实践的三大医学体系之一[5]。与中医药临床指南相比，中西医结合临床指南既有与其相似之处，也有其自身的特点。例如在诊断学方面，采用病证结合的方法已基本上成为共识，既有国际通用的疾病诊断标准，如 ICD 10（国际疾病分类），又有反映中医学特点的"证"，突出中医辨证论治的优势。但在治疗方面，西医指南、中医药临床指南的制定，虽然对于中西医结合临床指南的制定具有重要参考价值，但决不是前两者的简单相加。这是因为两种指南的制定，均是着眼于该医学体系本身在临床实践中如何更好地应用，如同样是高血压病患者，西医指南有规范的降压治疗方案，中医药指南也可以分出若干证型，给出代表方剂或中成药。但如果以患者为中心去考虑，是不是把两种方案加在一起就是最佳的方案呢？答案显然是不确定的。这其中除牵涉到中西药物的相互作用（协同作用？相互牵制？减少不良反应？增加不良反应？）对疗效和安全性的影响外，卫生经济学同样是需要考虑的问题。理想的治疗方案应该是在循证医学理念指导下各种治疗方法的有机结合，并以进一步提高临床疗效、减少不良反应和降低（或不明显增加）医疗开支为目的。中西医各有所长，应优势互补、有机结合，在疾病的哪些环节中西医结合疗效高于单纯中医或单纯西医？以谁为主？怎么结合？最佳剂量多少？疗程多长？有哪些潜在的相互作用？……这些不能凭空臆测或从理论上推断，也不能仅凭个人经验，均需要有证据的支持。因此，中西医结合临床指南面临的最大挑战就是中西医指南的整合，

也即治疗方案的优化问题。

4. 以临床实践数据为导向优化中西医结合治疗方案的思路与体会

基于此，我们提出在"临床科研一体化"思想指导下，通过建立结构化临床信息采集系统，按照循证医学理念，前瞻性科研设计，动态采集临床信息，构建中西医结合诊疗数据仓库，借助现代数据挖掘及统计分析方法，以临床实践数据为导向两次分组评价临床疗效，优化中西医结合治疗方案的新思路。该系统和方法具有以下优点：(1) 数据来源于临床实践，更符合临床个体化诊疗及复杂性干预的原貌 (real world)；(2) 通过标准化术语的应用和高度结构化的设计，信息采集更加规范，有别于一般的临床记录和以文本内容为主的电子病历，数据质量高，可利用性强，便于分析总结；(3) 将临床数据采集与临床业务工作一体化，寓科学研究于临床实践当中，不仅可通过模板设计、优化界面等方便临床业务流程，提高临床医生的积极性，而且由于记录内容同时将作为医疗档案保存，也确保了数据的准确性和可靠性；(4) 与 RCT 不同，不干预临床医生的诊疗行为，可操作性强；(5) 前瞻性设计记录内容、随访内容和观察指标，如症状程度、量表计分、住院费用、终点事件等，便于可以基于不同指标和结局（症状、理化检查指标、生活质量、卫生经济学、终点事件等）进行疗效的评价；(6) 是观察和研究中西药物相互作用的最佳方法；(7) 可以很好地监测现有指南的执行情况，发现潜在问题，有利于在现有指南基础上方案的进一步优化。其缺点在于临床干预措施复杂，混杂因素较多，要想得出某一方面结果，可能需要极大的样本量。

2002—2006 年，我们依托北京市科委重大项目"中医药防治重大疾病个体诊疗评价体系的研究"及子课题"冠心病诊治规律及综合治疗方案的研究"，在"临床科研一体化"思想指导下，以冠心病为切入点，对基于数据的临床研究模式进行了探索性研究，搭建了高度结构化的冠心病临床个体化诊疗信息采集平台，并在京津地区 9 家医院应用，建立了 5284 例冠心病患者临床诊疗信息存储、挖掘为一体的数据仓库；制定了冠心病中医临床信息基本术语及采集规范，对随机行走模型、关联规则、支持向量机、Bayes 网络等数据挖掘方法进行了研究，人机结合，以人为主，探索了符合冠心病个体化诊疗临床主题需求的挖掘分析方法；并将数据挖掘和统计分析方法相结合，分析了冠心病中医证候特点和用药规律，探索了基于临床实践数据的复杂干预疗效评价方法 [6-9]。针对中西医结合治疗方案的优化，我们建立了基于治疗有效患者，疾病、证候、中药、西药多因素结合关联规则挖掘分析，根据支持度、置信度大小，优化中西医结合治疗方案的新方法。如分析结果显示，在心肌梗死合并心功能不全，同时中医证型是阴虚、痰浊、血瘀时，常用的药物组合是抗凝类、生脉注射液、硝酸酯类、抗血小板类、果糖针、利尿剂、调脂药、麦冬、太子参、半夏、栝蒌。根据所支持数据的多少，可以得出相应的治疗组合，这种病证互参、中西医结合的治疗方案对临床具有一定参考价值。需要说明的是，这些治疗方案是在现有数据基础上产生的，因此还是很初步的。但我们有理由相信，随着数据的积累和挖掘分析方法的改进，治疗方案将得到不断优化，方案中各种治疗方法的主次地位、疗程与剂量、疾病不同发展阶段的治疗差别等也可以得到进一步细化和完善。

5. 从临床实践数据转化为临床实践指南证据的可行性

临床实践数据，就是对临床实践过程的真实记录，与作为指南证据"金标准"的 RCT 研究结果有着很大的区别。RCT 为临床研究，科学性强，但不一定符合临床原貌，适用范围有限，数据的可靠性和患者依从性受多种因素影响，对复杂干预方案研究不太适合，耗资巨大。而且，研究结论可能受潜在的经济利益影响。在 2003 年 5 月出版的一期《英国医学杂志》中就同时刊登有两篇有关分析"厂家赞助与研究结果和可靠性"方面的文章 [10,11]。结果均提示：厂家的资助研究常常会得出有利于资助厂家的文章。作者甚至以"Evidence b (i) ased medicine"作为标题。这正是我们都不愿看到、希望回避却又不得不面对的现实。而临床实践数据由于来源于临床实践，具有真实、可靠的特点，可以客观反映没有"人为因素干扰"情况下的临床原貌。更为重要的是，它可以回答 RCT 排除在外的部分患者（如肾衰竭、妊娠、高龄患者等）的临床治疗问题，从而适用于更大范围的患者群，因此实际上更具备形成临床实践指南的前提和基础。

证据水平的分级来自于对某个临床问题的论

证强度，RCT 由于按照现代临床流行病学方法进行了严谨的科研设计，最大程度地减少了研究结果的偏差，因此被认为证据力度较强。有人认为，临床实践数据只能算观察性研究，科学性较差。需指出的是，验证性研究（如 RCT）固然重要，但基于临床实践数据的观察性研究同样不可或缺，它可以发现临床中潜在的问题，为下一步验证性研究提供线索，而且对于复杂性干预难以直接进行验证，在干预因素明确之前观察性研究必不可少；此外，虽然一般的观察性研究样本量小，连续性差，临床意义有限，但通过我们的实践看出，如果建立结构化的临床信息采集系统，对临床实践数据进行动态、连续的记录，同时前瞻性设计记录内容和观察指标，实际上也蕴含了现代临床流行病学科研设计思路，体现了循证医学理念。临床流行病学方法中的"随机抽样"，最根本的目的是能反映和代表总体疗效，而基于临床实践数据的研究模式样本可以积累到接近无限大，基本可以反映总体疗效；循证医学方法重视临床终点硬指标和动态长期观察，而海量临床信息采集形成的数据库也具有可长期保存、无限扩展、便于动态监测的特点；临床流行病学的"对照"原则亦可以采用基于临床实践数据的二次分组临床研究模式，利用大样本的优势，采用分层分析或多元回归分析等方法控制混杂因素影响，平衡组间基线水平。而对于 RCT 所难以完成的复杂治疗方案优化问题，也有可能通过现代数据挖掘和统计分析方法加以解决。因此，从理论上讲，前瞻性设计、观察的临床实践数据也是基于循证医学原则的高水平证据（相当于临床流行病学的队列研究、非随机对照研究），与回顾性总结、个人经验、专家共识等截然不同，因此临床实践数据转化为临床实践指南的证据，在方法学和技术层面上具有可行性。

6. 前景展望

随着循证医学理念的深入人心，构建循证临床实践指南已逐渐成为制定指南的趋势，它强调证据的分级与评价，更重视来自于临床试验（如RCT），而非临床实践的证据。然而，近年来循证临床实践指南制定的方法学、对个体化临床实践的指导作用也受到一定的质疑 [3,4,12,13]，使其在贯彻执行过程中受到了极大的挑战 [14,15]。随着现代信息技术和数据挖掘技术的飞速发展，为以临床实践数据为导向构建临床指南，尤其是以个体化诊疗和复杂干预为特点的中西医结合临床指南提供了有力的技术支撑。相信将临床实践数据与循证医学证据有机结合的临床实践指南已经为期不远，也必将因其科学性、实用性、灵活性、开放性、动态更新等特点为临床实践提供更大的指导作用。

参考文献

[1] Handley MR, Stuart ME. An evidence-based approach to evaluating and improving clinical practice：guideline development. HMO Pract, 1994, 8 (1)：10-19.

[2] Harbour R, Miller JA. A new system for grading. recommendations in evidence based guidelines. BM J, 2001, 323 (7308)：334-336.

[3] Doherty S. Evidence-based medicine：arguments for and against. Emerg Med Australas, 2005, 17 (4)：307-313.

[4] Latov N. Evidence-based guidelines：not recommended. J Am Phys Surg, 2005, 10 (1)：18-19.

[5] 陈可冀，吕爱平，陈士奎，等. 中国中西医结合医学发展状况调查报告. 中国中西医结合杂志，2006，26 (6)：485-488.

[6] 高铸烨，徐浩，史大卓，等. 急性心肌梗死中医辨证分型的聚类研究. 中国中医急症，2007，16 (4)：432-434.

[7] 高铸烨，徐浩，史大卓，等. 基于关联规则挖掘对急性冠脉综合征遣药组方规律的分析. 辽宁中医杂志，2007，34 (3)：284-285.

[8] 高铸烨，徐浩，陈可冀，等. 用随机行走模型评价生脉注射液治疗冠心病的临床疗效. 中西医结合学报，2008，6 (9)：902-906.

[9] 徐浩，高铸烨，陈可冀. 1864 例老年冠心病患者诊疗状况及其预后的前瞻性研究. 中华老年医学杂志，2008，27 (8)：617-622.

[10] Lexchin J, Bero LA, Djulbegovic B, et al. Pharmaceutical industry sponsorship and research outcome and quality：systematic review. BMJ, 2003, 326 (7400)：1167-1170.

[11] Melander H, AhlqvistRastad J, Meijerg, et al. Evidence b (i) ased medicine-selective reporting from studies sponsored by pharmaceutical industry：review of studies in new drug applications. BMJ, 2003, 326 (7400)：1171-1173.

[12] Caplan LR. Evidence based medicine：concerns of a clinical neurologist. J Neurol Neurosurg Psychiatry, 2001, 71 (5)：569-574.

[13] Woolf SH, Grol R, Hutchinson A, et al. Clinical guidelines：potential benefits, limitations, and harms

第六章

of clinical guidelines. BMJ, 1999, 318 (7182)：527-530.

[14] O'Connor PJ, Amundsong, Christianson J. Performance failure of an evidence-based upper respiratory infection clinical guideline. J Fam Pract, 1999, 48 (9)：

690-697.

[15] Gaziano TA. The South African Hypertension guideline 2006 is evidence-based but not cost-effective. S Afr Med J, 2006, 96 (11)：1170-1173.

病证结合治疗快速性心律失常经验举隅[*]

蒋跃绒

陈可冀老师临证倡导中西医病证结合，优势互补。每以辨证论治兼顾疾病特点，辨病用方贯穿辨证论治之精神，重视辨证论治与专病专方专药结合。快速性心律失常包括期前收缩、阵发性心动过速（室上性、室性）、扑动与颤动（房性、室性）、预激综合征等，属中医学"心悸"、"怔忡"的范畴。本文所论陈可冀老师治疗的快速性心律失常主要包括期前收缩、阵发性心房颤动、短阵室上性心动过速，其他类型未包括在内。

1. 辨病辨证要点：多从虚、瘀、痰、火论治

陈可冀老师临诊快速性心律失常多从虚、瘀、痰、火论治，重视详辨阴阳、气血、虚实，因证施治。《千金要方·心脏脉论》有"因虚致悸"的论述。《丹溪心法·惊悸怔忡》指出心悸"当责之虚与痰"。清代王清任《医林改错》首倡活血化瘀治疗用归脾安神等方不效的心悸。陈可冀老师则认为本病主要责之于虚瘀痰火，病位在心、脾、肝、肾，以虚者居多，常见虚实夹杂，以虚为本，以实为标。虚者以气虚和阴虚多见，实者有瘀血、痰火的不同。

2. 遣方用药规律：疾病通治方与辨证用方相结合

陈可冀老师曾自创新补心丹，以西洋参、黄芪、麦冬、元参、生地，益气养阴清热为主，佐以丹参活血，柏子仁、酸枣仁宁心安神，鹅不食草清热解毒，用于病毒性心肌炎、甲状腺功能亢进、高血压病等病见心悸，证属气阴两虚、阴虚内热者。此为常法或通治之法。临证还需变通应用，如气阴

两虚者也常以生脉散、黄芪生脉散加味；阴虚内热者常以天王补心丹、新补心丹、知柏地黄汤；血虚肝旺者以四物安神汤加减；气虚血少、脉结代者，以炙甘草汤加减；瘀血内阻者，以冠心Ⅱ号方、血府逐瘀汤加减；痰火内扰者以黄连温胆汤、小陷胸汤加减；兼痰浊者，以栝蒌薤白半夏汤、茯苓杏仁甘草汤、桔枳姜汤加减，水饮内停者，以防己茯苓汤、猪苓汤、五皮饮等；阴阳两虚、心肾不交者以桂枝加龙骨牡蛎汤加减；伴头昏脉弦阴虚阳浮者，选加天麻钩藤饮、杞菊地黄丸。对一组陈可冀老师治疗快速性心律失常患者的处方用药分析发现，其用药主要为以下几组：滋阴养血药：麦门冬、干地黄、玄参、五味子、当归；益气药：黄芪、太子参、甘草、党参；活血药：延胡索、赤芍、干地黄、川芎、丹参、红花、桃仁、丹皮；清热药：苦参、黄连、黄芩、丹皮、竹茹；化痰祛湿药：茯苓、半夏、佩兰、薤白、藿香、车前草、泽泻、栝蒌、竹茹；安神药：酸枣仁、柏子仁、珍珠母。频数分析发现，其中用药频次排在前5位的依次为麦冬(46.15%)、甘草(43.59%)、五味子、延胡索(41.02%)、黄芪、太子参(33.33%)、赤芍(28.21%)、苦参、干地黄、半夏(25.64%)。以上体现了陈可冀老师治疗本病，重视益气养阴法的应用，根据挟瘀、痰、火的不同，随证施治的特点。

3. 诊治特色：辨证基础上结合辨病用药、重视宁心安神

陈可冀老师在辨证论治的基础上，注意结合使用延胡索、郁金、苦参等经临床筛选及现代研究证实具有抗心律失常的药物。如曾用苦参片

* 原载于《中国中西医结合杂志》，2012，32 (8)：1136-1137

第六章

7.5g/d 治疗用普鲁卡因胺不能完全控制的频发室性期前收缩。对快速性心律失常证属气滞血瘀者，常选延胡索、郁金。延胡索生物碱有抗实验性家兔氯化钡和大鼠乌头碱诱发的心律失常及抗缺血再灌注心律失常的作用。对阵发性心房颤动可选延胡索末分次温水冲服，剂量以每日＜9g为宜，个别患者剂量＞12g 时可能出现药物热。陈可冀老师治疗本病还常加用宁心安神药物，实证者多选珍珠母、石决明重镇安神，虚证者多选酸枣仁、柏子仁滋阴养血安神，使心神得宁，惊悸自止。

4. 医案举隅

患者，男，58 岁，主因反复心悸 10 年，加重半个月于 2006 年 2 月 8 日来诊。患者于 1996 年无诱因出现发作性心悸，心电图示阵发性心房颤动。2003 年因发作频繁，于安贞医院、阜外医院等就诊，口服普罗帕酮（心律平）后未再发作。2005 年 3 月于北京市第六医院行冠状动脉造影，诊断为"X 综合征"，后停用心律平，改用胺碘酮。2006 年春节前后至今房颤反复发作，每次 2 ～ 4h，2 ～ 3 天发作 1 次。现时常感觉心悸。既往患 2 型糖尿病史 10 年，对四环素过敏。嗜烟 30 年，饮酒 30 年，已戒酒。其母患有房颤。舌质暗红，苔黄腻，脉弦细，口气浊臭。血压：150/70mmHg，心率：68 次 / 分。实验室检查：C 反应蛋白 6.8mg/L。超声心动图（2005 年 7 月 26 日，北京市第六医院）：心内结构大致正常，左室舒张功能减退。西医诊断：阵发心房纤颤；中医诊断：心悸，

痰热内扰。予黄连温胆汤加减：川黄连 12g、法半夏 10g、陈皮 10g、云茯苓 10g、麸枳壳 10g、青竹茹 10g、生甘草 12g、珍珠母 20g、生石决明 20g。嘱忌食辛香温燥之品。西医治疗不变：曲美他嗪 20mg 每天 1 次，厄贝沙坦（安博维）0.075g 每天 1 次，胺碘酮 0.2g 每天 1 次。二诊：2 月 23 日。诉近 2 周房颤发作次数减少，每周 1 ～ 2 次，每次 1 ～ 2min，睡眠好转。舌暗，苔黄厚腻，脉沉弦。心率 64 次 /min。前方珍珠母、生石决明均增至 30g。三诊：3 月 16 日。房颤由原来 2 ～ 3 天 1 次减为 2 周 1 次。舌暗，苔黄腻，脉沉弦。血压 140/80mmHg，心率 60 次 /min。前方加栝蒌 30g，元胡 12g，黄连增至 15g。生甘草易为炙甘草。四诊：3 月 23 日。患者近 12 日未发作房颤，纳眠可，二便调。血压 140/80mmHg，心率 78 次 / 分。舌稍暗，苔黄腻，脉沉弦。前方黄连增至 20g，法半夏增至 15g。五诊：3 月 30 日。患者 7 天前房颤发作 1 次，持续 6h，纳眠可。舌苔黄腻，脉沉弦。心率 64 次 / 分。前方加藿香、佩兰各 15g，赤芍、郁金各 20g。六诊：4 月 13 日。服前方后近 20 日未发作心房颤动，纳眠可，余无不适。舌质偏暗，苔腻微黄，脉沉弦。心率 56 次 / 分，律齐。效不更方，前方继服。

按：本案主要从痰火论治，兼顾血瘀，以黄连温胆汤为主方，先后加用珍珠母、生石决明重镇安神，元胡、郁金理气活血且具有抗心律失常作用的药物，反映了陈可冀老师以辨证论治为主，兼顾辨病的临证特色。

病证结合临床研究的关键问题 *

徐 浩

病证结合模式为中医临床的重要诊疗模式，陈可冀院士不仅在应用病证结合方法治疗心血管病、老年病方面具有丰富的临床经验，而且对于如何开展病证结合临床研究有独到的见解。他认为，病证结合是中西医结合研究的最佳切入点之一，"病"与"证"在研究中的碰撞，不仅为进一步优

化疾病辨识方法、提高临床疗效奠定了基础，对中西两种医学的互补融合、乃至新医学体系的创建也具有重要意义。

病证结合临床研究涉及范围广泛，包括疾病证候分布特点研究、疾病证候演变规律研究、疾病证候客观化研究、疾病证候分类及诊断标准研究、

* 原载于《中国中西医结合杂志》，2011，31 (8)：1020-1021

病证结合干预性治疗研究等。陈可冀院士认为，病证结合临床研究的最终目的是进一步凸显中医药治疗的优势和特色，以提高疗效、应用推广为目标，力争所研究的治疗方案或中药制剂为中医、中西医结合界普遍认可。因此，基于病证结合的干预性治疗临床研究应当作为研究重点，当然，也应鼓励进一步进行证候分类、诊断标准和流行病学调查等研究，为病证结合干预性治疗研究奠定基础。

作为补充替代医学的重要组成部分，中医药到底对哪些疾病有优势？病证结合临床研究应选择哪些病种？陈可冀院士认为，病证结合临床研究的病种选择应以国际上关注的现代医学疗效欠佳的中医药优势病种[1]及重大疾病为主，二者都不可或缺。结合临床实际，中医优势病种可选择风湿免疫疾病如类风湿关节炎、过敏性疾病如哮喘、病毒感染性疾病、炎症性肠病、功能性胃肠病、妇科疾病、皮肤病如湿疹和银屑病、心身疾病等；重大疾病尽管西医可能有疗效确切的治疗方法（如冠心病的介入治疗），但由于此类疾病危害巨大，单纯西医治疗难以满足临床，社会需求广泛，而且在疾病的某个点、某个环节或某个阶段中医药仍有一定优势（如冠心病介入治疗后的无复流），以此为切入点，中西医优势互补将可望进一步提高重大疾病的临床疗效，为人类健康事业做出贡献。

陈可冀院士认为，病证结合临床研究的干预方法可以为治疗方案，也可以为专方专药，应结合具体疾病而定，但必须体现中医药的特点和疗效优势，才有进一步临床推广的价值。治疗方案可以是多种方法的综合应用，能充分体现中医药个体化、动态诊疗的优势，但要注意规范性、可操作性及可推广性，尤其推荐专科学会在临床实践文献分析及广泛征求专家意见基础上推出的治疗方案（而不是一家之言或一地之经验），因为其验证后更便于临床推广，这方面政府相关部门的参与和推动也非常重要。专方专药则要求有较好的前期工作或临床应用基础，疗效确切，质量可控，安全性好。干预方法不同，病证结合临床研究的设计方案也会有所差异，但都应遵循临床流行病学方法和原则，注意研究方法的适宜性，干预方法为一种治疗方案时，可考虑采用实用性随机对照试验、队列研究等临床设计；专方专药研究推荐随机对照试验设计，条件许可的情况下建议应用双盲、安慰剂对照设计，尤其是疗效评价以主观指标为主的临床研究。在不能使用双盲观察时，需注意终点指标评价及数据分析时

的盲法原则。

关于病证结合临床研究中评价指标的选择，目前是中医界讨论的焦点。有人认为，证候改善是中医的优势，应将其作为主要指标，而不必考虑西医的理化指标。然而，西医不懂中医证候，因此仅把这种证候的改善作为疾病疗效评价指标很难获得西医界的认可。陈可冀院士指出，病证结合临床研究中的评价指标包括终点指标、替代指标、症状体征、证候计分、生活质量和患者报告的结局指标等，应根据研究目标选择应用，而不能有所偏颇。终点指标是临床试验主要评估指标的最佳选择，主要包括对患者生存或死亡、残障水平或其他一些重要临床事件，如疾病复发等的测量。终点结局指标由于与患者最为相关，因此对临床决策最具参考价值。美国国立卫生研究院替代医学办公室的报告强调：传统/替代疗法的"有效性评价是一个关键和核心的问题"，"其疗效必须用人们认可的终点指标来加以证实"。终点结局指标往往可以用率来表示，例如病死率、治愈率、缓解率、复发率、副反应率、生存率等，通常需要进行长期随访的试验研究来测量这些指标。在终点指标的测量不可行（如需要很长时间）的情况下，就需要采用替代指标来评估干预措施的效果。替代指标一般易于测量，如常用的生物学指标，包括实验室理化检测和体征发现，如血脂、血糖、血压、实体肿瘤体积的缩小等，替代指标不追求新、全，而应是公认的。

证候计分在中医临床研究中也常常应用，能较好地反映中医药的疗效优势，但多为人为制定，主观性强，与疾病的关系有多大尚待明确，西医不理解也不认可，有"自己定规则"之嫌；而且量化的内容多数未经信度、效度等科学性评价，其结果的可信性、客观性仍需进一步研究。如果一种证候的改善没有建立在疾病相关指标及生活质量改善的基础上，那么这种证候改善的临床意义有多大？又如何被国际上认可呢？因此，陈可冀院士认为，证候计分量表的研发应注意与疾病的相关性，并需要经过信度、效度评价，以获得同行的认可；也可以选择能够在一定程度上体现中医优势的国际上公认的量表，如生活质量量表和患者报告的结局指标量表（PRO量表），用"共同的语言"与西医同行交流。

除此之外，病证结合临床研究不应忽视卫生经济学指标和安全性指标。卫生经济学评价主要包括成本 - 效果分析 (cost effectiveness analysis,

第六章

CEA)、成本-效用分析 (cost utility analysis, CUA) 和成本-效益分析 (cost benefit analysis, CBA) 等，可以从另一个角度评价中医药的优势。安全性指标既往在中医药临床试验中未受到应有的重视，这方面有待加强。临床上主要通过观察记录或及时报告不良反应、不良事件（包括严重不良事件）和副作用，对治疗的安全性进行评估。应向受试者告知潜在的风险，提醒受试者报告试验期间发生的所有不良反应，有助于及时地获得有关不良事件的信息。最后，临床研究的实施和报告应参照药物临床试验管理规范 (Good Clinical Practice, GCP) 及 CONSORT (Consolidated Standards of Reporting Trials) 声明 2010 修订版 [2] 及其相关研究报告标准。

参考文献

[1] Li HY, Cui L, Cui M. Hot topics in Chinese herbal drugs research documented in PubMed / MEDLINE by authors inside China and outside of China in the past 10 years：based on co-word cluster analysis. J Altern Complement Med, 2009，15 (7)：779-785.

[2] Schulz KF, Altman DG, Moher D, et al. CONSORT 2010 Statement：updated guidelines for reporting parallel group randomised trials. BMJ, 2010，340：332.

推荐应用全球性心肌梗死新定义 *

陈可冀　蒋跃绒

　　心肌梗死是世界范围内致残和致死的主要疾病之一。传统沿用的心肌梗死定义是 1979 年世界卫生组织 (WHO) 制定的 [1]，主要根据临床症状、心电图改变和以肌酸激酶 (CK) 和肌酸激酶同工酶 (CK-MB) 为主的血清心肌酶学改变进行评定。随着敏感性和特异性更高的心肌坏死生化标志物的推广应用和更加精确的冠状动脉影像显示技术的发展，以及临床实践、医疗保健和临床科研的需求，心肌梗死的定义也逐步修订。2000 年，欧洲心脏病学会 (ESC) 和美国心脏病学会 (ACC) 发布联合共识，对急性心肌梗死进行了再定义 [2]。在此基础上，ESC、ACC、美国心脏协会 (AHA) 和世界心脏联盟 (WHF) 组织由临床、检验、心电图、介入和公共政策等多学科专家组成的心肌梗死再定义工作组，于 2007 年 10 月联合发布了关于"心肌梗死全球统一定义" [3] 的共识，分别发表于《Circulation》、《Joumal of the American College of Candiology》(JACC) 和《European Heart Journal》。我国也有专家应邀参加这一工作。中华医学会心血管病学分会和中华心血管病杂志编辑委员会于 2008 年 10 月发表共识，同意推荐在我国采用心肌梗死全球统一新定义 [4]。

　　新定义的亮点之一是推荐以肌钙蛋白 (cTn) 作为心肌梗死诊断的主要依据，强调心肌坏死的生物标志物首推 cTn（cTnI 或 cTnT），其次是 CK-MB, CK 总值不被推荐。根据该定义 [3]，心肌梗死是指患者具有心肌缺血的临床表现并有心肌坏死的证据，下列任何一项存在诊断即可成立。

　　1．心脏生物标志物（最好是 cTn）升高或升高后降低，至少有一次超过参考值上限 (URL) 99 百分位值，截点变异度 ≤ 10%，再加上至少一项心肌缺血的证据（包括症状、心电图缺血改变、病理性 Q 波或影像学证据），即可诊断。

　　2．突发、未预料到的心脏性死亡，包括心脏停搏，常伴有心肌缺血的症状、推测为新的 ST 段抬高或左束支传导阻滞 (LBBB)、冠状动脉造影或病理有新鲜血栓的证据。死亡发生于可取得血样之前或生物标志物在血中出现之前。

　　3．基线 cTn 正常的经皮冠状动脉介入治疗术 (PCI) 治疗的患者，生物标志物升高超过正常上限的 3 倍定义为与 PCI 相关的心肌梗死。

　　4．基线 cTn 正常的冠状动脉旁路移植术 (CABG) 患者，生物标志物升高超过正常上限的 5 倍加上新的病理性 Q 波或新的 LBBB，或冠状动脉

* 原载于《中国中西医结合杂志》，2009，29 (7)：581-582

造影证实新的移植血管或自身冠状动脉闭塞，或有活力心肌丧失的影像学证据，定义为 CABG 相关的心肌梗死。

5．有急性心肌梗死的病理学发现。

新定义的亮点之二是第一次制定了心肌梗死的亚型，从临床实践出发，将心肌梗死细分为 5 型 6 类。

1 型：自发性心肌梗死，由原发冠状动脉事件如斑块侵蚀和（或）破裂、裂隙或夹层引起。

2 型：继发于缺血的心肌梗死，由于心肌供氧减少或需氧增加引起，如冠状动脉痉挛、冠状动脉栓塞、贫血、心律失常、高血压或低血压。

3 型：突发、未预料到的心脏性死亡，包括心脏停搏，通常有心肌缺血的症状，伴随新的 ST 段抬高或新的 LBBB 或冠状动脉造影和（或）尸检发现冠状动脉有新鲜血栓的证据，但死亡发生于可取得血样之前或血中生物标志物升高之前。

4a 型：伴发于 PCI 的心肌梗死。

4b 型：冠状动脉造影或尸检证实的伴发于支架血栓形成的心肌梗死。

5 型：伴发于 CABG 的心肌梗死。

其中 1 型为经典的心肌梗死；2 型需结合患者具体情况，治疗主要针对原发病，而不是盲目进行介入治疗；3 型危害最大，病死率高，需要加强教育，对高危患者加强预防；4 型和 5 型都与手术操作相关。有时患者可能同时或先后出现 1 种以上类型的心肌梗死。

新定义为心肌梗死流行病学调查、临床研究、临床实践及公共卫生政策制定等提供了一个更为精确且全球统一的标准，具有重要的意义和价值，但也会带来一些问题。首先，以 cTn 测定作为心肌梗死诊断的主要依据，将明显提高心肌梗死诊断的敏感性和特异性。由于 cTn 超过参考值上限 99 百分位再加上 1 项心肌缺血表现即可诊断心肌梗死，许多过去诊断为不稳定型心绞痛的患者，按新定义将诊断为非 ST 段抬高心肌梗死，使更多的人接受冠心病的二级预防，这将对患者的心理状态、医疗保险、就业、驾车驾机执照等产生一定影响，也会影响卫生统计、赔偿率、病离退残疾申请等。而诊断特异性的提高在少数患者可能较特异性较小的 CK-MB 少诊断一些心肌梗死，减少非心肌梗死者住院的人数，减少相关住院费用及二级预防费用。

其次，心肌梗死亚型分类将明显增加诊断的组成，心肌梗死较以往有了更宽的临床谱，如 2 型心肌梗死不会造成预后不良，也可能并不需要正规处方治疗。新的定义应尽快在临床实践中得以应用，并应告知包括医生、临床试验人员、医疗保健机构、人寿保险公司、流行病学家和公共卫生政策制定者等更广泛的人群。

需要指出的是，新定义也并非尽善尽美。很多实验室 cTn 测定的检测精确度达不到新定义中确定的 99% 可信区间变异系数 ≤ 10% 的要求，且不同厂商生产的 cTn 试剂的检测结果可能有较大差异。因此 cTn 测定亟待标准化，临床检验专家们需确保医院实验室能达到要求的诊断精确度。另外，新定义对那些在发病几小时内 cTn 释放之前即致死的病例仍不能覆盖[5]。

为了便于国际交流和与世界接轨，推荐中医界和中西医结合界也应采用心肌梗死的全球统一定义。同时，也应认识到，随着科学的发展，新的诊断方法和技术的出现，心肌梗死的定义将随着变化，该定义在任何时候都不是最终意见。

参考文献

[1] Nomenclature and criteria for diagnosis of ischemic heart disease. Report of the Joint International Society and Federation of Cardiology / World Health Organization task force on standardization of clinical nomenclature. Circulation, 1979, 59 (3)：607-609.

[2] The Joint European Society of Cardiology / American College of Cardiology Committee. Myocardial infarction redefined——a consensus document of the Joint European Society of Cardiology / American College of Cardiology Committee for the redefinition of myocardial infarction. Eur Heart J, 2000, 21 (18)：1502-1513.

[3] Thygesen K, Alpert JS, White HD. On behalf of the Joint ESC / ACCF / AHA / WHF Task Force for the Redefinition of Myocardial Infarction. Universal definition of myocardial infarction. Circulation, 2007, 116 (22)：2634-2653.

[4] 中华医学会心血管病学分会，中华心血管病杂志编辑委员会．推荐在我国采用心肌梗死全球统一定义．中华心血管病杂志，2008，36 (10)：867-869.

[5] 高润霖．心肌梗死全球统一定义的意义及问题．中华心血管病杂志，2008，36 (10)：865-866.

多效药片 (polypill) 的临床应用与中成药的研发 *

陈可冀　蒋跃绒

心血管疾病的预防已由单一危险因素的控制转变为多重危险因素的综合控制。全球迅速增加的心血管病负担要求干预措施对广大人群，尤其是具有主要不良事件高危风险的人有效。已经证明许多药物包括阿司匹林、血管紧张素转换酶抑制剂 (ACEI)、他汀类、β 受体阻滞剂和钙通道阻滞剂等对心血管病的一级或二级预防有效，但这些药物即使在发达国家也没有得到最佳应用，对多种药物治疗的低依从性是常见原因之一。近年来，一些研究者倡导多效药片 (polypill) 的概念，即通过多成分组合药物来降低心血管事件发生率，为现代心血管疾病的防治提供了新的启示和模式 [1]。

1. Polypill 的由来及临床应用

早在 2002 年，Yusuf[2] 在《柳叶刀》的社论中提出可用一种组合药片来预防心血管事件以方便服用的观点。2003 年，Wald 和 Law[3] 两位教授在《英国医学杂志》(BMJ) 上详细阐述了以命名为 "polypill" 的复方药片预防心血管疾病的战略设想。根据国际上发表的随机对照试验和队列研究的 Meta 分析结果，针对高血压、高血低密度脂蛋白胆固醇、高同型半胱氨酸血症和血小板功能亢进 4 种心血管危险因素，设计了由 6 种药物组成的 polypill，包括 1 种他汀（如阿托伐他汀 10mg / d 或辛伐他汀 40mg /d），3 种减半量的降压药（如 1 种噻嗪类利尿降压药，1 种 β 受体阻滞剂，1 种血管紧张素转换酶抑制剂），叶酸 0.8mg / d 和阿司匹林 75mg / d，认为可使心脏事件和卒中发生率降低 80% 以上，且有着良好的安全性。建议已有心血管病的患者及年龄在 55 岁以上的人群使用。该设想的创新之处还在于完全抛弃了高血压和高血脂的概念，对那些血压和血脂在正常水平，但年龄、性别属于心血管病高危人群的个体进行干预。

2009 年 4 月，《柳叶刀》发表了 Yusuf 博士及其同事完成的 TIPS (Indian polycap study) 研究结果 [4]，再次引起了人们对多成分复方药物降低心血管病风险的热烈关注。TIPS 研究是首次针对在中老年健康人群使用 polypill (polycap) 的耐受性以及对心血管危险因素影响的 II 期双盲随机临床试验。该试验由印度 50 家临床中心参与，共纳入 2053 例年龄在 45 ～ 80 岁、具有 1 种心血管病危险因素的健康受试者，随机分为 polycap 组（412 例，polycap 由低剂量双氢氯噻嗪 12.5mg、阿替洛尔 50mg、雷米普利 5mg、辛伐他汀 20mg 和阿司匹林 100mg 组成），及另外 8 个对照组，每组约 200 例，包括单纯阿司匹林组、单纯辛伐他汀组、单纯双氢氯噻嗪组、3 种降压药中任两种降压药组合而成的 3 个治疗组、3 种降压药联合治疗组、或 3 种降压药联合阿司匹林组。观察的主要结局包括低密度脂蛋白水平、血压、心率、尿 11- 脱氢血栓烷 B_2，并以中止治疗的发生率作为安全性指标。采用意向性分析。研究发现，polycap 能降低 62% 的心血管疾病发生风险，48% 的卒中疾病发生风险，其耐受性与其他治疗组相近，且无证据表明随着药片中活性成分的增加不耐受情况增加。认为 polycap 服用方便，能有效降低多种风险因素，降低心血管事件发生率。不过，有关 polycap 所含 5 种药物的组合方案还有待开展更深入的研究，以获得更多的相关数据。另外，该研究仅测试了血压、血脂、血小板等替代指标，而不是主要不良心血管事件。

最近，美国 FDA 刚刚批准了 1 种用于降压的 polypill，名为 Exforge HCT[5]。由 3 种抗高血压药组成，包括钙离子拮抗剂 (CCB) 氨氯地平、血管紧张素受体拮抗剂 (ARB) 缬沙坦和利尿降压剂双氢氯噻嗪，氨氯地平 / 缬沙坦 / 双氢氯噻嗪的剂量从 5mg/160mg/12.5mg 到最大量 10mg/320mg/25mg。不过，与五合一的 polycap 不同的是，FDA 批准 Exforge HCT 仅用于高血压的治疗，而没有被批准用于预防，因为制药公司没有进行预防用药的试验。因此，Exforge HCT 仅适用于已服用这 3 种降压药的患者的替代治疗，或

---

* 原载于《中国中西医结合杂志》，2009，29 (8)：677-679

者服用 3 种中任何 2 种而血压控制不达标的患者。

2. 关于 polypill 的争议

关于能否使用 polypill 来保护和预防心血管疾病的争论由来已久。Polypill 从设想到临床广泛应用，还面临着一系列来自临床医生、患者和药品管理部门等的挑战[6]：(1) 临床医生的认可度：医生们通常喜欢灵活地调整单个药物的剂量，因此，对于固定剂量的组合药片不是很乐于接受。实际上，对于治疗反应不好的患者，医生更倾向于选择其他药物而不是调整剂量。因此，要提高医生对 polypill 的接受度，需对初级保健医生和专科医生进行再教育。(2) 患者的认可度：患者对 polypill 的接受度取决于服用数量、服用时间和间隔，是否易于吞咽，是否可与食物及水同时服用，以及不良反应情况等。非肠溶的阿司匹林与消化不良有关，polypill 中包含阿司匹林可能会导致治疗中断而失去其他药物带来的获益。β 受体阻滞剂在未识别或病史不明的支气管痉挛或哮喘患者可能会引起严重不良反应。因为对糖代谢的不良反应以及与其他新型抗高血压药相比效果较差，老年高血压病患者应用 β 受体阻滞剂也越来越受到质疑。(3) 药品注册机构：如果 polypill 中的组成药物均可买到，关于其安全性和效果的证据大部分可从现有的临床试验和 Meta 分析获得。药品管理机构要求至少有应用替代指标的药效和药代动力学的报告，不要求硬性的终点指标。大规模的发病率和病死率的试验非常昂贵且伦理学上也具有争论。(4) 组方问题：不是所有的药物都适合在 polypill 中使用。候选药物应该是安全的、耐受性良好的、次全量时有效的，且物理和化学性质上与药丸中其他药物是可配伍的。组方时，还要考虑可能会影响生物利用度和（或）功效的药物相互作用。(5) 价格问题：polypill 的最终价格可能会比每种成分相加的价格更贵一些。

支持 polypill 的观点认为，治疗的简化可提高患者的依从性，并改善获益 / 风险比[6,7]。一般认为减少服用药丸的数量可提高服药的依从性。许多老年患者可能混淆、漏服或随意服用他们的药丸或把剂量弄错，1 天 1 片的 polypill 将会一定程度上给这些患者提供帮助。重要的是，polypill 可能因降低健康人群心血管病风险而具有潜在的巨大的公共健康的获益，从而获得更广泛的应用。polypill 可能通过药物之间的相互作用改善 1 种药物的不良反应谱。组合药物与高剂量的单一药物相比同样

有效但安全性更高，或比单一药物更有效，且安全性在可接受的范围内。除减少服用药丸数量外，组合药物可能通过比单一药物治疗更快地达到治疗目标而提高依从性。这一点对那些无症状患者尤为重要，如高血压和血脂异常，他们可能会中断治疗，除非在治疗的最初几个月内取得可测量到的获益。

也有不少学者对 polypill 持反对或怀疑态度[6,8]，比如这样一个药丸是否太大而难以下咽；polypill 中的每个药物可能对一般人群是最好的，但对个体来说不是最佳的。因此，反对不加甄别地使用 polypill。在很多情况下，需要对个别药物的剂量进行调整，这就需要设计不同的 polypill 以覆盖每个组成药物的所有可能剂量。而决定需要多少这样的 polypill 也是一个重要的挑战。另外，应设计不同种类的 polypill 以适应不同的患者谱，如心肌梗死后、高血压、糖尿病、慢性心力衰竭等。关于组方的问题，争论的焦点之一是 polypill 中是否应该包含阿司匹林？因为阿司匹林可能是组分中耐受性最差的，如果由于消化道症状而中止治疗，可能会失去其他耐受性良好的组分的获益，因此，有学者倾向于单独给予阿司匹林。

3. 对中成药研发的借鉴意义

近年来，西方世界正逐渐认识到多成分复方药物治疗的益处。通过使用针对多靶点的多成分组合药物，同时降低多种危险因素而不增加不良反应风险，有助于提高心血管病危险因素的控制，从而减少心血管病的发生。Polypill 的出现，满足了人们希望通过服用一种药物而控制多重危险因素的愿望，为心血管病的预防提供了一种更为方便、安全有效的新选择。

中药复方的临床应用，是中医临床医疗中使用的重要治疗手段之一。由于中药复方大多有效成分不明，作用机制不清，一定程度上限制了其推广应用。尽管中西复方药物大不相同，但也有某些共同的优缺点，从 polypill 引发的各种见解，对于改进和推动复方中成药的完善，不无可借鉴之处[9]：(1) 首先应科学评价复方中成药的临床疗效和安全性。对确有疗效的、常用的复方中成药进行多中心、大样本临床验证，从经验性应用上升到遵循科学证据的应用。重视复方中成药长期用药的安全性评价，尽量避免将明确的毒性较大的药物加入复方中长期使用。(2) 对复方中成药的作用机制按照传统理法方药、君臣佐使的配伍原则给出科学阐

明。中药复方是在辨证审因确定治法后，选择合适的药物酌定用量，按照组成原则妥善配伍而成，其药理作用具有多靶点、多层次的特点。有学者在分子水平阐明中药复方黄黛片治疗急性早幼粒性白血病的多成分、多靶点作用机制，并从生化和分子生物学的角度解释了其君、臣、佐、使的配伍机制，为复方中成药作用机制研究提供了很好的范例[10]。(3) 应对复方中成药有效成分、体内代谢过程及有效成分间相互作用，开展深入研究。复方中成药与polypill 的不同之处，除前者为根据中医学理论辨证组方外，其有效成分的复杂性也远远高于后者，体内代谢过程及相互作用更为复杂。若完全按照西药的标准分析清楚，还有很长的路要走。(4) 在现代药理和药化研究的基础上，优化中成药复方组成，中西医结合，病证结合，开发新复方，明确其有效性和安全性，提高复方中成药临床应用和研究的水平，使复方中成药在心血管疾病等重大疾病的防治中发挥更大作用。

参考文献

[1] Reddy KS. The preventive polypill-much promise, insufficient evidence. N Engl J Med, 2007，356 (3)：212.

[2] Yusuf S. Two decades of progress in preventing vascular disease. Lancet, 2002，360 (9326)：2-3.

[3] Wald NJ, Law MR. A strategy to reduce cardiovascular disease by more than 80%. BMJ, 2003，326 (7404)：1419.

[4] Indian Polycap Study (TIPS), Yusuf S, Pais P, et al. Effects of a polypill (Polycap) on risk factors in middle-aged individuals without cardiovascular disease (TIPS)：a phase Ⅱ, double-blind, randomised trial. Lancet, 2009，373 (9672)：1341-1351.

[5] FDA Approves Triple-Drug Antihypertensive Polypill. [2009-5-15] http：// www. medpagetoday. com /Product Alert / Prescriptions / 14032.

[6] Sleight P, Pouleur H, Zannad F. Benefits, challenges, and registerability of the polypill. Eur Heart J, 2006，27 (14)：1651-1656.

[7] Rastegarpanah M, Malekzadeh F, Thomas GN, et al. A new horizon in prmiary prevention of cardiovascular disease, can we prevent heart attack by "heart polypill"？Arch Iran Med, 2008，11 (3)：306-313.

[8] Stirban AO, Tschoepe D. Should we be more aggressive in the therapy against cardiovascular risk factors? Diabetes Care, 2008，31 (Supp l2)：S226-S228.

[9] 陈可冀. 关于复方中成药的临床应用与研究. 中国中西医结合杂志，2004，24 (4)：293.

[10] Wang L, Zhoug B, Liu P, et al. Dissection of mechanisms of Chinese medicinal formula Realgar-Indigo naturalis as an effective treatment for promyelocytic leukemia . Proc Natl Acad Sci USA, 2008，105 (12)：4826-4831.

心血管病临床治疗中存在的问题探讨 *

赵福海

循证心血管病医学近年来得到国内外迅速的普及和发展，针对心血管疾病防治中的代表性问题，大规模的临床试验结果为指南的更新和临床实践工作提供了支持和挑战。针对常见心血管疾病如冠心病、心房颤动、慢性心力衰竭的新药物、新疗法、新介入方法不断涌现。与此同时，中西医结合学者在该领域也做了相应的探索。但仍有诸多临床医疗问题亟待进一步探索、解决。

1. 冠心病

过去40年来，冠心病病死率下降超过60%，其中50% 以上归功于一级预防和危险因素干预的结果。然而，以心肌损伤标志物为诊断标准的急性心肌梗死 (AMI) 发病率在过去50年中则增高了约2倍，从 1970—1979 年的 38/10 000 人增加到 1990—1999 年的 72/10 000 人[1-4]，当然这与诊断技术的进步和诊断标准的修订有关。但 AMI 并

* 原载于《中国中西医结合杂志》，2010，30 (12)：1320-1324

发心源性休克的发生率却在 1975—1999 年一直稳定在 7.5% 左右，而其住院期间的病死率则高达 65.4% [5]。近年来虽然在冠心病的基础及临床研究方面取得了长足的进步，但仍有诸多问题如急性冠状动脉综合征（ACS）并发微血管栓塞、再灌注损伤、无复流现象、支架内血栓等问题亟待解决。

1.1　冠状动脉微血管栓塞

冠状动脉粥样硬化斑块破裂并不总是导致完全的冠状动脉血流中断及发生心肌梗死。小的粥样硬化斑块破裂在未完全阻断血流的情况下，其碎屑会随血流冲刷到微血管远端而形成栓塞 [6,7]，是急诊经皮冠状动脉介入 (PCI) 术中常见并发症之一。PCI 术中微栓塞的发生率平均为 25% 左右 [8]，这主要与既往的肾功能不全病史、不稳定型心绞痛、病变的复杂程度、支架置入、球囊扩张的次数和持续时间、斑块旋切与旋磨等有关。病理研究发现：从猝死患者冠状动脉微循环常发现动脉粥样硬化斑块成分如胆固醇结晶、透明蛋白和聚集的血小板，这与急诊 PCI 术中远端保护装置中检出成分一致 [9-11]。微栓塞多与易损斑块的侵蚀和破裂有关。但目前尚不清楚为何有的斑块侵蚀/破裂，其碎屑组织冲洗到远端产生微栓塞但仍有血流通过，而有的则会导致冠状动脉血流完全中断？也不清楚是否斑块的生物学特性差异（纤维碎屑混杂胆固醇结晶与新鲜的血栓物质）产生的微栓塞是否会有不同的结局？实验研究表明：冠状动脉微栓塞可造成梗死区心肌收缩功能的进行性丧失，但与心肌梗死面积并无明显关系，2%～5% 的片状微梗死灶即可使心肌收缩功能完全丧失，主要与以白细胞（单核细胞、巨噬细胞）浸润为特征的炎症反应相关 [12,13]。急诊 PCI 术中由于微循环血流受损，0.5%～1% 的患者会发生慢/无复流，临床上常简单地把冠状动脉微栓塞归结为罪魁祸首。但动物实验中常常阻断大的冠状动脉分支，然后恢复其血流，而无复流区仅限于阻塞性毛细血管损害的梗死区域。所以慢/无复流可能是心肌梗死的结局而非原因。慢/无复流和冠状动脉微栓塞可能是两种不同的现象 [14]。他汀类药物具有较强的预防冠状动脉微栓塞作用，机制在于其多效能的抗炎作用而不是稳定斑块的作用。抗血小板药物、抽吸导管应用，以及具有抗血小板作用的活血化瘀方药的应用，是预防和治疗微栓塞和改善微循环的重要手段 [6,15]，但合理掌握抗栓治疗的药物及其剂量选择，或多重抗栓药物应用，监测不良反应，以达到降低各种死亡，仍为最主要目标。

1.2　再灌注损伤 (RI)

对于 ST 段升高的心肌梗死 (STEMI) 患者来说，早期再灌注是治疗的首要目标，否则将导致心肌梗死面积的扩大、室性心律失常、心力衰竭、心源性休克甚至死亡。急诊 PCI 可使 95% 的患者冠状动脉血流恢复到 TIMI 3 级。然而尽管及时开通梗死相关动脉 (IRA)，仍有部分患者不能达到心肌水平再灌注（微循环再灌注）。潜在机制可能是微血管功能失常（如冠状动脉微栓塞、慢/无复流），以及致死性 RI。RI 与微血管栓塞、血小板和粥样斑块、原位血栓、冠状动脉痉挛和（或）炎症反应相关 [7,6]。RI 的病理生理机制可能与再灌注后局部代谢受损、活性氧产生、钙超载、快速纠正体内乳酸堆积以及白细胞介导的炎症反应（细胞黏附分子、活性氧、细胞因子、补体）有关，这些因素导致心肌细胞和内皮细胞坏死，出现致死性 RI。然而针对动物实验模型有效地抗 RI 措施在人类临床实践中并未显示出预期的心脏保护作用。RI 现象在人类真的不存在吗？答案是否定的。因为 STEMI 患者多为高龄动脉粥样硬化患者，缺血周期并不完全相同，往往合并多种疾病，同时应用多种药物，所有这些因素都会干扰或减弱针对 RI 有效的措施。相对于动物实验，临床实践中的许多因素不可控制或无法预测。分析原因，我们认为与一些临床试验药物缺乏严格的临床前期试验，对 STEMI 患者缺血周期入选标准不一（主要是 RI 的相对治疗时间窗较窄），心肌梗死面积的大小，患者是否存在侧支循环，血栓是否自溶有关；此外，RI 往往发生于冠状动脉血流恢复的同时，而心脏保护措施则在 RI 之后，以上诸因素均可影响 RI 的治疗效果。一些基础研究：如再灌注损伤抢救激酶通路 (RISK) 是一种蛋白激酶家族，于再灌注时激活，通过组织心肌细胞钙超载、抑制线粒体膜通透性转变孔 (MPTP) 开放、回复抗凋亡通路发挥心脏保护作用、抑制 MPTP [17]、缺血预适应/缺血后适应等，仍在探索当中。我们的经验是采用益气养阴乃至助阳方药，或应用西洋参总皂苷等防治 AMI，结果表明其可改善 AMI 后心肌缺血、调节糖脂代谢、促进缺血心肌血管新生、抗脂质氧化损伤，似亦可作用于心肌缺血再灌注损伤的多个病理环节 [18]，值得进一步认真探索发展。

1.3　支架内血栓形成

支架内血栓 (ST) 是 PCI 术后少见但致命的不

第六章

良事件，以猝死或 AMI 为主要表现，故应在术前避免血栓风险，并慎重考虑选择支架种类。根据 PCI 时间将 ST 分为急性、亚急性、晚期和极晚期 ST。

1.3.1 急性 ST ACUITY 和 TRITON-TIMI 研究入选中到高危的急性冠脉综合征 (ACS) 患者，急性 ST 的发生率在药物洗脱支架 (DES) 时代高达 1.4%。ISSAR-REACT-3 研究入选低危且稳定的冠心病患者，急性 ST 的发生率在 0.4% 左右。这些结果提示 BMS 与 DES 的急性 ST 发生率相同。其中患者因素（糖尿病史、肾功能不全、左室功能受损）、病变因素（斑块破裂部位血栓负荷过重、微循环障碍致冠状动脉血流受损、斑块坏死核心暴露、斑块脱垂到支架网眼、内皮功能受损、促凝状态、血小板激活抑制不足、多支血管病变、血管直径、支架贴壁不全）以及药物因素（过早停用抗血小板药物）与急性 ST 发生相关[19-21]。

1.3.2 极晚期 ST DES 极晚期 ST 形成可能与血管内皮化延迟或缺乏内皮化；血管壁对聚合物的超敏反应；慢性炎症、血管的正性重构导致支架贴壁不良；动脉瘤形成局部涡流，血流速度减慢，过早停用抗血小板药物或抗血小板药物抵抗相关[22-26]。Stephane Cook 等研究表明：置入 DES 发生极晚期 ST 的患者，73% 的病例显示支架贴壁不良，支架部位血管横截面积 (6.2±2.4) mm²，重构指数 1.6±0.3，提示支架节段血管存在正性重构。组织病理分析显示血栓部位炎性细胞浸润（DES：白细胞 263±149；嗜酸细胞 20±24，雷帕霉素洗脱支架 34±28，紫杉醇洗脱支架 6±6），与自发的 AMI 患者相比，ST 患者支架节段嗜酸性粒细胞计数较高，表明局部存在免疫反应，可能是 Ⅳ 型迟发型高敏反应（雷帕霉素洗脱支架主要是 Ⅳ b 型，以嗜酸性粒细胞增高为主；紫杉醇洗脱支架少见 T 细胞聚集，以非特异性炎症为主）。嗜酸细胞在三层血管壁的分布差异也提示中层和外膜炎症反应较重。嗜酸性粒细胞通过嗜酸颗粒蛋白抑制血栓调节蛋白辅助因子活性，促进局部血栓形成，或者直接通过血小板激活、黏附分子和脂质调节子介导的脱颗粒作用激活凝血瀑布[27-29]。

2. 心房纤颤（Afi）

Afi 是备受关注的健康问题，流行病学资料显示，心房颤动的病死率甚高，在 10 年的随访期间，3085/4618 人死亡。Kaplan-Meier 预计的存活率在 4 个月、1 年、3 年、5 年分别为 83%、

77%、63%、52%[30]，但其确切的发病机制目前尚不清楚。因此心房颤动的治疗目标仍是以减轻症状（转复窦性心律）、预防血栓栓塞卒中、控制心室率（心动过速性心肌病）以及预防心力衰竭为主，降低心房颤动患者的致残率和病死率。目前尚缺乏非常有效的一级预防办法。

2.1 Afi 的机制

电重构：快速心房率时，内向钙离子流显著增加心肌细胞钙负荷，而过高细胞内钙浓度因适应性机制使钙负荷降低，进而钙通道失活和受体下调，最终使内向钙电流减少，动作电位时程缩短，心房不应期缩短，促进 Afi 的功能折返和持续[31]。解剖重构：其特征为心房扩大、间质纤维化。近年来逐渐认识到心房纤维化是致心律失常解剖重构的标志。动物实验表明：心房组织纤维胶原沉积导致组织纤维化，进而使局部传导减慢，传导异质性增加，为 Afi 的发生提供了基质。血管紧张素转换酶和血管紧张素 Ⅱ 作为促纤维化分子的上游调节机制，为临床应用其拮抗剂预防 Afi 提供了理论基础[32]。治疗高血压、睡眠呼吸暂停综合征、肥胖、甲状腺功能亢进症等疾病则是预防心房重构，进而发生 Afi 的关键环节。Afi 一旦发生，及早恢复窦性心律，治疗并存疾病则是阻断心房重构进展的重要步骤。

2.2 节律控制还是心率控制

关于两种治疗策略孰优孰劣还在争论当中，但 Afi 的人群病死率保持不变也是不争的事实。有研究表明，恢复窦性心律可以降低死亡等不良心血管事件的风险[33,34]，由于这些研究要么是回顾性，要么是非随机研究，而且研究周期短，因此不能真正回答其是否能改善长期存活率。但恢复窦性心律确实能减轻症状，改善生活质量。而新发生 Afi 患者由于其全身处于促凝状态，血小板激活，内皮依赖性 NO 合酶表达减少、纤溶酶原激活物抑制剂表达增加，因此近期（4 个月）内死亡风险明显较高。及时转复窦律可以阻止进展为持续性 Afi，减少抗心律失常药物和华法林的应用。对于持续性/永久性 Afi 的患者，合适的心室率控制也是缓解症状的重要措施。有研究[35]表明，无论是严格的静息心率控制 < 80 bpm，还是温和的控制心率在 < 110bpm，随访中死亡、心力衰竭、栓塞、卒中、出血等不良事件两组差异无统计学意义[36]，提示温和的心率控制在带来获益的同时可减少不必要的风险。

2.3　Afi 的导管消融

AFFIRM 研究表明转复窦律带来的获益常被抗心律失常药物的不良反应所抵消。因此导管消融根治心房颤动，恢复窦律成为难治性心房颤动的重要替代手段。虽然导管消融根治心房颤动的临床研究表明[36]：与抗心律失常药物相比，其无心房颤动事件率明显较高，患者生活质量明显改善。但应该明确这些研究所入选人群多为阵发 Afi，年龄较轻，并存疾病较少；而疗效评价，即针对复发的评价多以患者症状为主，缺乏客观可信的评价手段，随访周期短；消融治疗后部分患者表现持续性难治性房性心动过速；而且手术花费较高，复发率各家报道不一，技术复杂，仅能在大的心脏中心进行，在一定程度上限制了此项技术的普及。因此导管消融可做为 Afi 治疗的潜在选择，对阵发性、不能耐受抗心律失常药物不良反应、无器质性心脏病、职业运动员等可考虑导管消融，但对于器质性心脏病合并持续性和（或）永久性 Afi 的患者应审慎选择。

2.4　Afi 的抗凝治疗是目前预防患者发生缺血性脑卒中唯一有效的、不可取代的措施，也是 Afi 治疗的基石

多个对 Afi 患者用华法林抗凝预防缺血性脑卒中的临床试验荟萃分析结果显示，脑卒中发生的危险因素为年龄、高血压、既往短暂性脑缺血发作和脑卒中史以及糖尿病。华法林抗凝治疗使脑卒中的发生率下降 68%、病死率下降 33%、复合终点事件（脑卒中、体循环栓塞和死亡）下降 48%。阿司匹林使 Afi 患者脑卒中的发生率降低 36%。表明华法林抗凝治疗能使非瓣膜性 Afi 患者脑卒中的发生率明显降低。由此确立了华法林抗凝治疗的重要性[37-42]。但出血并发症不容忽视，合适的抗凝强度在预防栓塞事件的同时可有效减少出血事件。正在研究中的直接凝血酶抑制剂达比加群，X 因子抑制剂洛伐沙班、安皮沙班显示了良好的降低卒中风险的效果，对不能耐受华法林不良反应的患者，可考虑应用。由于几乎各类心血管疾病均可引起 Afi，益气活血、化瘀祛浊方药的应用前景都尚待探索，作者过去观察到理气活血方药的应用在一些病例中有一定疗效。

3.　慢性心力衰竭 (CHF)

我国住院病例调查显示，慢性心力衰竭患病率为 1.3% ~ 1.8%，以超声心动图指标统计，则在 3% 左右，慢性心力衰竭住院率占同期心血管病的 20%。有报道 CHF 患病率女性为 1.0%，男性 0.7%[43]。随着年龄增高，患病率明显上升[44]。慢性心力衰竭前 3 位的病因是冠心病 (57.1%)、高血压病 (30.4%)、风湿性心脏病 (29.6%)，在一些地区肺心病也是基层医院慢性心力衰竭的主要病因。

3.1　慢性心力衰竭的治疗原则为纠正血流动力学异常，缓解症状；提高运动耐量、改善生活质量；防止心肌进一步损害，延缓心功能衰竭（简称心衰）发展，提高生存率。治疗上要以抑制左室重构、改善左室功能为主，延缓疾病进展为目标。

3.2　药物治疗当突出"新常规治疗"。β受体阻滞剂适应证最广，长期应用宜从小剂量开始，逐渐加量，但要注意该药的禁忌证。血管紧张素转换酶抑制剂 (ACEI) 是心衰治疗的基石，通过抑制肾素-血管紧张素醛固酮系统 (RAAS) 和缓激肽的降解，提高缓激肽水平而发挥治疗作用。所有慢性心力衰竭患者需长期应用 ACEI，从小剂量开始，逐渐增至靶剂量，其绝对禁忌证是血管神经性水肿、无尿性肾衰竭和妊娠；肾上腺素能受体拮抗剂为 ACEI 不能耐受的替代药；利尿剂是治疗的基础或首选药，目前虽无利尿剂降低死亡率的临床证据，但可减轻液体潴留改善症状，应根据患者体重下降调整剂量，注意电解质失衡；醛固酮拮抗剂适于中重度患者，从小量开始，注意血钾水平；洋地黄制剂用于改善心衰症状，对慢性心力衰竭合并 Afi 的患者适用，非洋地黄类正性肌力药多用于常规治疗无效或终末期慢性心力衰竭，仅限短期使用。

3.3　心脏再同步化治疗是治疗 CHF 的有效方法，需遵循指南，对左室射血分数 (LVEF) ≤ 35%，左室舒张末直径 (LVEDD) ≥ 55 mm，心电图 QRS 宽度 > 120ms，药物治疗无效者可考虑。

3.4　CHF 中医药治疗，注重病证结合，一般概括为"虚"、"瘀"、"水"三个方面。倡导益气温阳利水、活血化瘀，突出活血化瘀治法，认为血不利则为水，慢性心力衰竭患者水液滞留多因血脉不利所致。故欲利其水，应先活其血。血脉调和则水道调畅，小便自利。由于目前临床治疗慢性心力衰竭多用利尿剂，利水过度容易伤阴。适当合用养阴药物，可防止阴伤；同时还要敛心气，避免温阳药耗散心气的作用。中药复方尤其是生脉散制剂及其加减变化制剂研究较多，初步观察表明在改善心功能、利尿、抑制心室重构、调节交感神经等方面

第六章

有一定作用[44-46]，根据辨证，也可选用苓桂术甘汤、真武汤、四逆汤等化裁。

参考文献

[1] Parikh NI, Gona P, Larson MG, et al. Long-term trends in myocardial infarction incidence and case fatality in the national heart, lung, and blood institute's Framingham heart study. Circulation, 2009, 119 (9)：1203-1210.

[2] Guidry UC, Evans JC, Larson MG, et al. Temporal trends in event rates after Q-wave myocardial infarction：the Framingham heart study. Circulation, 1999, 100 (20)：2054-2059.

[3] Rosamond WD, Chambless LE, Folsom AR, et al. Trends in the incidence of myocardial infarction and in mortality due to coronary heart disease, 1987 to 1994. N Engl J Med, 1998, 339 (13)：861-867.

[4] Fox CS, Evans JC, Larson MG, et al. Temporal trends in coronary heart disease mortality and sudden cardiac death from 1950 to 1999：the Framingham heart study. Circulation, 2004, 110 (5)：522-527.

[5] Goldberg RJ, Spencer FA, Gore JM, et al. Thirty-year trends (1975 to 2005) in the magnitude of, management of, and hospital death rates associated with cardiogenic shock in patients with acute myocardial infarction：a population-based perspective. Circulation, 2009, 119 (9)：1211-1219.

[6] Heusch G, Kleinbongard P, Böse D, et al. Coronary microembolization from bedside to bench and back to bedside. Circulation, 2009, 120 (18)：1822-1836.

[7] Prasad A, Stone GW, David R, et al. Reperfusion injury, microvascular dysfunction, and cardioprotection the "dark side" of reperfusion. Circulation, 2009, 120 (21)：2105-2112.

[8] Herrmann J. Peri-procedural myocardial injury：2005 update. Euro Heart J, 2005, 26 (23)：2493-2519.

[9] El-Jack SS, Suwatchai P, Stewart JT, et al. Distal embolization during native vessel and vein graft coronary intervention with a vascular protection device：predictors of high risk lesions. J Interv Cardiol, 2007, 20 (6)：474-480.

[10] Heusch G, Schulz R, Haude M, et al. Coronary microembolization. J Mol Cell Cardiol, 2004, 37 (1)：23-31.

[11] Popma JJ, Cox N, Hauptmann KE, et al. Initial experience with distal protection using the filter-wire in patients undergoing coronary artery and saphenous vein graft percutaneous intervention. Catheter Cardio Interv, 2002, 57 (2)：125-134.

[12] Dorge H, Neumann T, Behends M, et al. Perfusion contraction mismatch with coronary microvascular obstruction：role of inflammatory. Am J Physiol Heart Circ Physiol, 2000, 279 (6)：H2587-H2589.

[13] Dorge H, Schulz R, Belosjorow S, et al. Coronary microembolization：the role of TNF-α in contractile dysfunction. J Mol Cell Cardiol, 2002, 34 (1)：51-62.

[14] Reffelmann T, Kloner RA. The no-flow phenomenon：a basic mechanism of myocardial ischemia and reperfusion. Basic Res Cardiol, 2006, 101 (5)：359-372.

[15] 赵福海，陈可冀 . 关于急性冠脉综合征中无复流现象的防治 . 中国中西医结合杂志，2010，30 (4)：341-342.

[16] Murry CE, Jennings RB, Reimer KA. Preconditioning with ischemia：a delay of lethal cell injury in ischemic myocardium. Circulation, 1986, 74 (5)：1124-1136.

[17] Hausenloy DJ, Yellon DM. The mitochondrial permeability transition pore：its fundamental role in mediating cell death during ischaemia and reperfusion. J Mol Cell Cardiol, 2003, 35 (4)：339-341.

[18] Ma XJ, Zhang XH, Li CM, et al. Effect of postconditioning on coronary blood flow velocity and endothelial function in patients with acute myocardial infarction. Scand Cardiovasc J, 2006, 40 (6)：327-333.

[19] Stone GW, McLaurin BT, Cox DA, et al. The ACUITY Investigators. Bivalirudin for patients with acute coronary syndromes. N Engl J Med, 2006, 355 (21)：2203-2216.

[20] Wiviott SD, Braunwald E, McCabe CH, et al. Intensive oral antiplatelet therapy for reduction of ischaemic events including stent thrombosis in patients with acute coronary syndromes treated with percutaneous coronary intervention and stenting in the TRITON-TIMI 38 trial. Lancet, 2008, 371 (9621)：1353-1363.

[21] Kastrati A, Neumann FJ, Mehilli J, et al. The ISSAR-REACT 3 trial investigators. Bivalirudin versus unfractionated heparin during percutaneous coronary intervention. N Engl J Med, 2008, 359 (7)：688-696.

[22] Joner M, Finn AV, Farb A, et al. Pathology of drug-eluting stents in humans：delayed healing and late thrombotic risk. J Am Coll Cardiol, 2006, 48 (1)：193-202.

[23] Kotani J, Nanto S, Morozumi T, et al. Angioscopic findings of the neo-intimal coverage over the

sirolimus-eluting stent：nine months follow-up study. J Am Coll Cardiol, 2006, 47 (Suppl B)：27B.

[24] Nebeker JR, Virmani R, Bennett CL, et al. Hypersensitivity cases associated with drug-eluting coronary stents：a review of available cases from the research on adverse drug events and reports (RADAR) project. J Am Coll Cardiol, 2006, 47 (1)：175-181.

[25] Virmani R, Guagliumi G, Farb A, et al. Localized hyper sensitivity and late coronary thrombosis secondary to a sirolimus-eluting stent：should we be cautious? Circulation, 2004, 109 (6)：701-705.

[26] Pfisterer M, Brunner-LaRocca HP, Buser PT, et al. For the BASKET-LATE investigators. Late clinical events after clopidogrel discontinuation may limit the benefit of drug-eluting stents. J Am Coll Cardiol, 2006, 48 (1)：2584-2591.

[27] Posadas SJ, Pichler WJ. Delayed drug hypersensitivity reactions. Clin Exp Allergy, 2007, 37 (7)：989-999.

[28] Pichler WJ. Delayed drug hypersensitivity reactions. Ann Intern Med, 2003, 139 (8)：683-693.

[29] Cook S, Ladich E, Nakazawa G, et al. Correlation of intravascular ultrasound findings with histopathological analysis of thrombus aspirates in patients with very late drug-eluting stent thrombosis. Circulation, 2009, 120 (5)：391-399.

[30] Miyasaka Y, Barnes ME, Bailey KR, et al. Mortality trends in patients diagnosed with first atrial fibrillation：a 21-year community-based study. J Am Coll Cardiol, 2007, 49 (9)：986-992.

[31] Gaspo R, Bosch RF, Talajic M, et al. Functional mechanisms underlying tachycardia-induced sustained atrial fibrillation in a chronic dog model. Circulation, 1997, 96 (11)：4027-4035.

[32] Li Y, Li W, Yang B. Effects of cilazapril on atrial electrial, structural and functional remodeling in fibirillation dogs. J Electrocardiol, 2007, 40 (1)：100-106.

[33] Pederson OD, Bagger H, Keller N, et al. Efficacy of dofetilide in the treatment of atrial fibrillation-flutter in patients with reduced left ventricular function：a Danish investigators of arrhythmia and mortality on dofetilide (DIAMOND) substudy. Circulation, 2001, 104 (3)：292-296.

[34] Corley SD, Epstein AE, DiMarco JP, et al. Relationships between sinus rhythm, treatment, and survival in the atrial fibrillation follow-up investigation of rhythm management (AFFIRM) study. Circulation, 2004, 109 (12)：1509-1513.

[35] van Gelder IC, Groenveld HF, Crijns HJ, et al. Lenient versus strict rate control in patients with atrial fibrillation. N Engl J Med, 2010, 362 (15)：1363-1373.

[36] Stabile G, Bertaglia E, Senatore G, et al. Catheter ablation treatment in patients with drug refractory atrial fibrillation：a prospective, multicenter, randomized, controlled study (Catheter ablation for the cure of atrial fibrillation study). Eur Heart J, 2006, 27 (2)：216-221.

[37] Petersen P. Placebo-controlled, randomised trial of warfarin and aspirin for prevention of thromboembolic complications in chronic atrial fibrillation. The Copenhagen AFASAK study. Lancet, 1989, 1 (8631)：175-179.

[38] Stroke prevention in atrial fibrillation investigators：stroke prevention in atrial fibrillation study final results. Circulation, 1991, 84 (2)：527-539.

[39] The Boston Area Anticoagulation Trial for Atrial Fibrillation Investigators. The effect of low-dose warfarin on the risk of stroke in patients with nonrheumatic atrial fibrillation. N Engl J Med, 1990, 323 (22)：1505-1511.

[40] Ezekowitz MD, Bridgers SL, James KE, et al. Wafarin in the prevention of stroke associated with nonrheumatic atrial fibrillation. N Engl J Med, 1992, 327 (20)：1406-1412.

[41] Connolly SJ, Laupacis A, Gent M, et al. Canadian atrial fibrillation anticoagulation (CAFA) study. J AM Coll Cardiol, 1991, 18 (2)：349-55.

[42] 心房颤动抗栓研究协作组. 华法林对非瓣膜病心房颤动抗栓的安全性和有效性研究. 中华内科杂志, 2006, 45 (10)：800-803.

[43] 卫生部心血管病防治中心. 中国心血管病报告 2006. 北京：中国大百科全书出版社, 2008：60-63.

[44] 李立志. 陈可冀治疗充血性心力衰竭经验. 中西医结合心脑血管病杂志, 2006, 4 (2)：136-138.

[45] 赵淳, 叶勇, 吴英, 等. 慢性心力衰竭现代治疗进展及中医诊治思路探讨. 中国中医急症, 2006, 15 (2)：158-159.

[46] 史大卓. 慢性心力衰竭的发病机制及中西医结合治疗. 中国中西医结合杂志, 2008, 28 (11)：1053-1056.

诊治心力衰竭学术思想及临证经验总结 [*]

李立志

1 学术思想

1.1 病名应切中病机且反映临床特点

心力衰竭是所有不同种类心脏病的最终结局及主要并发症。陈可冀老师结合现代医学对该综合征的定义并参照中医历代与其相关的文献描述，认为仍将其按主要症状或体征特点归入中医学的"喘证""肺胀""惊悸""怔忡""水肿""痰饮"及"阴水"等病证中不利于中医药学对心力衰竭的规范化研究。关于心力衰竭的中医病名，虽有"心水""心痹""悸-喘-水肿联证""心衰病"等的探讨，但陈可冀老师认为"心水""心痹"仅突出病机，"悸-喘-水肿联证"只是证候诊断，"心衰病"文字上虽接近心力衰竭，但心力衰竭不是一种独立疾病而是一种临床综合征，所以陈可冀老师认为直接应用"心衰"是较为合理的。"心"反映了中医的主要病位，"衰"概括其主要病机及临床表现，用"心衰"作为中医病名，既不失中医特色，又能在病因病机、病理生理、诊断治疗、病证结合及中西医结合研究等方面与西医找到共同切入点，有助于中医对心力衰竭诊治水平的提高和创新。

1.2 病机研究是全面提高心力衰竭诊疗水平的关键

陈可冀老师认为认识心力衰竭病机，必须紧紧围绕以下两个方面：(1) 以心为中心的内虚观。分析心力衰竭，必须首先抓住其心之阴阳、气血的虚衰这个关键问题。结合中医对气血的来源与功能的认识及气血亏虚的临床表现，陈可冀老师认为心脏是循环系统最重要的器官，本身就是一个耗氧耗能多的器官，而西医所言"心脏不能泵出足够的血液以满足组织代谢需要"及"其特征是左室功能和神经激素调节异常，伴有体力受限、体液潴留和寿命缩短"，恰恰与心之气血阴阳虚衰的表现及实质有异曲同工之妙。陈可冀老师认为诊治心力衰竭，如偏离了以心为中心的内虚观，就可能犯下"虚虚实实"之误，临证不仅会错失最佳治疗时机，还有可能造成严重后果。(2) 气血辨证观。陈可冀老师认为心力衰竭与气血的关系最为密切。心力衰竭的

发病可以突然，也可以隐匿。突出特点是渐进性恶化，直至成为难治性心力衰竭而引起循环衰竭。陈可冀老师认为久病、频发之病当从瘀认识。例如在心肌梗死后或缺血性心肌病引起的心力衰竭中，瘀血已经成为非常突出的病理产物，其在心力衰竭的发生发展中起到了"催化剂"和"接力棒"作用。因此，在气血辨治观基础上，陈可冀老师认为活血化瘀是治疗心力衰竭的重要方法之一。在应用活血化瘀治疗心力衰竭时，强调以气血为纲，从整体上把握心力衰竭的病机特点，方能辨证精当，施治合理，收到佳效。

1.3 病证结合全方位，衷中参西同提高

陈可冀老师认为，虽然中医对心力衰竭的认识和研究有了不断深入和发展，但临床上若能充分利用现代医学的研究成果，在深入了解心力衰竭的病因、病理及其发病机制的基础上，从中西医两方面的理论入手进行分析探讨，寻求互补或结合点，并指导用药，将能取得更好的疗效。同样是心力衰竭，心肌病和冠心病引起者无论是临床表现还是病理生理，都存在着较大区别。即使同是心肌病引起，扩张性心肌病和肥厚性心肌病又有所不同；同样是冠心病，心肌梗死梗后和缺血性心肌病又不能一概而论。在强调"异"的时候，还应注意到各种心力衰竭在病理生理环节上的"同"，如心脏重塑和心肌细胞凋亡等。这种有异有同，为心力衰竭病证结合全方位研究提供了必要性和可能性背景。

陈可冀老师认为，病证结合不可偏废，应兼顾中西医特点。目前的临床研究结果，如温阳逐水活血法、益气利水活血法、益气活血法、益气养阴法等可改善心功能，降低心脏前后负荷，改善冠脉循环及微循环等有一定深度，但总体水平还有待提高。

对心力衰竭的临床研究，注重名医经验、挖掘单方验方固然重要，但从这些研究中真正发现规律性，进而从循证医学水平证实其效果是必走的道路，而且这种效果不能仅仅局限在临床症状的改善，更要追求生活质量的提高及终点事件及长期预

* 原载于《中国中西医结合杂志》，2012，32 (8)：1130-1134

后的改善。在此同时，可在机制研究中下些功夫，如能在关键机制上有所发现，心力衰竭的整体研究突破才可谓实至名归。

2. 临证经验

2.1 参照传统中医思辨特点，执简驭繁，以"虚""瘀""水"统领病机

心力衰竭病程往往较长，早期到终末期，症状、证候演变多，在阴阳、脏腑、气血、津液等多个层次产生很多复杂盛衰虚实变化。但大多数心力衰竭患者的病机演变有较强的规律性，应执简驭繁加以总结。心力衰竭的最根本中医病机为内虚，早期主要为心气心阳亏虚，可兼肺气亏虚，随病情发展及病机变化，心气心阳亏虚致运血无力，瘀血内停；中期脾阳受损，脾虚失运，复加肺气亏虚，水道失其通调，水湿内停；后期肾阳虚衰，膀胱气化不利，水饮泛滥。因此，心衰的病机可用"虚""瘀""水"三者概括。分析中医病证病机时，应遵循简明扼要原则，有益于中医疾病的病机规范化研究。但在理解与运用病机进行分析及遣方用药时，又不能孤立而机械地理解，应运用动态和有机联系的观点去探讨与分析。这样可使治疗前后衔接，总体完整，从而获得最好的疗效。

2.2 病证结合，方中寓法，法中有方，治疗时常中达变

陈可冀老师认为，心力衰竭辨证固然应以中医理论为指导，以望、闻、问、切四诊取得患者的综合信息为基础，但应结合中医证的规范化研究成果及现代医学对心力衰竭病理生理认识进展，即运用病证结合的方法，可使其辨证更趋于合理，体现中西医优势互补。治疗上，施以紧扣中医病机的理法方药，结合现代中药药理学的研究成果，做到病证结合、理效结合、常变有度。

2.2.1 气虚血瘀，加味保元汤

本型主症为：气短心慌，活动时及劳累后突出，可伴胸闷、胸痛、头晕乏力、失眠多梦、两颧暗红、舌质暗或见瘀斑瘀点、苔薄白、脉细涩而数。临证在此主症下据舌脉、心力衰竭原发病、其他伴随症状，可分为心气虚兼血瘀、心阳虚兼血瘀、肺肾气虚兼血瘀、气阴两虚兼血瘀4种亚型。此型患者多见于心力衰竭早期，NYHA心功能分级为Ⅰ级、Ⅱ级，病位主要在心、肺。心力衰竭，从其病理生理来看，未必都存在心排血量的降低。实际上，心室灌注压升高而心排血量尚正常时，心力衰竭诊断便可确定[1]。此

类患者临床症状，除运动能力有所下降外，往往不很明显，结合引起心力衰竭的原发病及运用超声心动图等其他检查，这些心功能处于所谓代偿期的患者应尽早被发现并治疗。另外，其他如慢性肺源性心脏病、缺血性心肌病、扩张性心肌病、风湿性心脏瓣膜病引起的心力衰竭，在血流动力学基本稳定的情况下，以劳力型气促为突出表现者多归属本型。

保元汤出自明代魏桂岩所著的《博爱心鉴》[2]。此方只有人参、黄芪、甘草、肉桂4味，是临床常用补气方剂之一。该方剂主在温阳，温而不燥，补而不滞，但其活血之力稍弱。治疗气虚血瘀型心力衰竭在原方基础上添加丹参、川芎、赤芍，名为加味保元汤，再结合引起心力衰竭之原发病的不同及兼症之区别加减应用。形寒肢冷，并发劳力型心绞痛，尤其是寒冷诱发者，加栝蒌、薤白、干姜，重用肉桂或桂心；肺心病心力衰竭伴轻度肺淤血，肺通气及弥散功能障碍，气短显著者加葶苈子，蛤蚧尾研末冲服；口干渴，盗汗明显者加玉竹、地骨皮，另服生脉饮；高血压性心脏病左室肥厚加红花、地龙，三七粉冲服。

病例1 患者，男，62岁，初诊。主诉劳力性心前区闷痛5年，加重9个月伴气促。在加拿大犹大医院行冠状动脉造影：左前降支在第一对角支发出后完全闭塞，左前降支开口85%狭窄，右冠状动脉中段80%～95%狭窄，建议行经皮冠状动脉介入治疗（PCI）。心脏超声：左心房、左心室扩大，左室前壁、下壁节段性运动异常，左室射血分数（LVEF）51%，左室舒张功能受限；心电图：正常。服用比索洛尔2.5mg，阿司匹林100mg，福新普利10mg，辛伐他汀20mg，单硝酸异山梨酯40mg，每日1次，治疗逾半年，劳力性气促及劳力性心绞痛未改善，怕冷，自汗出。体检：血压90/60mmHg（1mmHg=0.133kPa），心浊音界向左扩大，心尖区Ⅱ-Ⅲ/6级收缩期杂音，心率78次/分，律齐，S₁低钝。舌质淡暗，有瘀斑，舌体胖，边有齿痕，苔薄白，脉细涩。西医诊断：(1) 慢性心力衰竭，心功能Ⅱ级；(2) 恶化劳力型心绞痛，心绞痛分级3级。中医诊断：心力衰竭，气虚血瘀型。治疗：益气活血，加味保元汤主之。红参3g（另煎兑入）、生黄芪40g、桂枝10g、炙甘草10g、防风10g、丹参30g、川芎10g、赤芍10g、益母草20g、栝蒌15g、薤白15g、炒枣仁30g。前14剂为每日1剂，后14剂为隔日1剂。因血压偏低，冠状动脉灌注压不足会损害心

脏收缩及舒张功能，福新普利调整为 5mg，每日 1 次，单硝酸异山梨酯改为硝酸异山梨酯 5mg，每日 3 次。再诊，活动耐量明显增加，自汗减少，舌、脉未见变化。初诊方去防风，加远志 15g，隔日 1 剂，服用 7 个月。三诊，连续上 3 层楼无心绞痛及气促感。上方炼蜜为丸，6g，每日 3 次，长期巩固调理。

按：从患者临床症状及客观检查来看，由于缺血致冬眠心肌所引起的心力衰竭，既有收缩功能障碍，亦有舒张功能不全。以劳力型气促、胸痛为主症，"劳则气耗""不通则痛"，结合舌、脉，气虚血瘀辨证精当。药理学研究证实，保元汤能稳定急性心肌梗死 (AMI) 犬的每搏及每分冠状动脉灌流量，缩小 AMI 家兔心肌梗死范围，改善冠心病患者 ST-T 缺血改变，提高 LVEF 等。陈可冀老师紧密联系病机辨证，构建益气活血治法，处以加味保元汤更加切中病情。除上述几种机制外，还可通过改善心肌供氧及心肌能量代谢，降低心肌氧耗，保护心肌细胞，抑制血小板聚集，清除氧自由基，抑制左室重构及心肌细胞凋亡等多种复合机制，从而延缓或阻止心力衰竭发展，改善血流动力学。目前临床上冠心病心力衰竭患者多依据指南合并应用血管紧张素转换酶抑制剂 (ACEI)、硝酸酯类药物及 β 受体阻滞剂。本例患者应用药物选择及剂量不适，致动脉血压偏低。陈可冀老师予及时调整，改善冠状动脉灌注。治疗前后，如能在严密医疗保护下行运动负荷试验，将有助于心力衰竭疗效进一步的客观判定。

2.2.2 中阳亏虚，水饮内停，苓桂术甘汤加味

本型主症为：心悸气短，形寒肢冷，食欲不振或兼呕恶，小便短少，肝脾肿大，水肿，舌淡、苔白滑，脉沉细。此型多见于心力衰竭发展至中期，或以右心功能不全为主者。NYHA 心功能分级为 Ⅱ - Ⅲ 级，病位主要在心、肺、脾。心力衰竭由左心功能不全之肺淤血（如风湿性心瓣膜病二尖瓣狭窄）进展到右心功能不全致体循环淤血时，引起一系列症状体征时多归为此证。此型心力衰竭由气虚血瘀型心力衰竭进展而来，由较单纯的心气（阳）虚兼血瘀演变为心脾阳虚兼水饮，心功能由 NYHA Ⅰ - Ⅱ 级进展到 Ⅱ - Ⅲ 级。而苓桂术甘汤其组方既无参芪之补气要药，又无麻附等温阳之品，如何能治疗阳虚水停型心力衰竭，陈可冀老师认为，此处切不可以药测证而机械理解。心力衰竭病至此期，心气虚已进展为心阳、脾阳虚，无形或轻

症之瘀已变化为有形之痰饮水气夹瘀，如不阻断则会迅速质变为阳虚水泛甚至阳脱证。故处于此阶段的心力衰竭患者，本虚标实并存。苓桂术甘汤源自《伤寒论》，具温阳健脾利水降逆之功，是脾虚兼水饮的主治方剂。取此方之意，一是突出脾虚湿盛在病机演变中的重要性；二是强调温补而不留邪，化饮活血而不伤正，即张仲景治疗痰饮以"温药和之"的思想。临证当在判断正邪消长的基础上灵活变通。

基本方：茯苓、桂枝、白术、炙甘草、丹参、桃仁。动则气喘或合并心绞痛者加人参、生黄芪；肺淤血显著或伴肺水肿者加葶苈子、苏子；胃肠道淤血心下痞塞，干呕或呕吐明显者加姜半夏、砂仁、陈皮、佩兰；肝脾肿大者加鳖甲、三棱、莪术；水肿明显者加猪苓、泽泻、冬瓜皮。

病例 2 患者，女，41 岁，初诊。主诉胸闷、气短、尿少、水肿反复发作 3 年，加重 9 天伴恶心、呕吐。曾诊断为风湿性心脏瓣膜病，5 年前开始心悸明显，心电图示心房颤动。近 3 年来胸闷、气短、尿少、水肿。检查：血压 100/70 mmHg，慢性消耗性病容，唇发绀，呼吸困难，心尖搏动弥散，可触及猫喘，心浊音界向双侧扩大，心尖区可闻及双期杂音，心率 54 次 / 分，律不齐，双中下肺闻细湿啰音，肝肋下 6cm，质中等度硬，叩击痛 (+)，腹水征 (+)，双下肢凹陷性水肿，双下肢静脉曲张，舌淡黯，苔白滑，脉结代沉细。胸部 X 线摄片：呈肺淤血改变，肺门处增大模糊，心脏扩大呈梨形，主动脉结缩小，肺动脉段及左心耳突出，双侧少量胸腔积液。超声心动图：左心房、右心房、右心室增大，右房上下径及左右径为 68 mm×41 mm，二尖瓣前后叶增厚变形、钙化，交界处黏连，开放受限，瓣口面积 0.8 cm^2，左心房见附壁血栓，双侧少量胸腔积液，少量心包积液；腹部超声提示肝大、腹水；心电图：心房颤动伴频发室性期前收缩，房室传导阻滞；血生化：丙氨酸转氨酶 (ALT) 143.4 U/L，天门冬氨酸转氨酶 (AST) 125.8 U/L，肌酐 164.3μmol/L，B 型尿钠肽 (BNP) 2186 pg/mL，地高辛血药浓度 3.76ng/mL。西医诊断：风湿性心脏瓣膜病，联合瓣膜病变，二尖瓣狭窄并关闭不全，主动脉瓣关闭不全，全心扩大，心律失常 - 心房颤动伴频发室性期前收缩，房室传导阻滞，心功能 Ⅲ 级。中医诊断：心力衰竭，证属心脾阳虚，水饮内停，兼挟瘀血。治宜苓桂术甘汤加味，处方：云茯苓 20g、桂枝 10g、白术 10g、丹参 15g、桃仁 10g、

炙甘草 10g、葶苈子 15g、苏子 10g、姜半夏 10g、砂仁 10g、陈皮 10g、佩兰 15g，7 剂。患者肾功能损害，地高辛清除率下降，长期服用地高辛，临床表现及心电图均支持为蓄积中毒，予停用。过缓性心律失常，停用美托洛尔（倍他乐克）。利尿剂不变。上方服 3 剂后，呕吐已止，恶心亦减，已有食欲，尿量增多，体重下降，气急改善。再服 4 剂，恶心亦除，余症状继续改善，血中地高辛浓度下降至 1.3ng/mL。患者感乏力明显，坐起头晕，首方去葶苈子、半夏、陈皮、佩兰，加党参 15g、黄芪 30g、麦冬 10g、五味子 6g，以增益气养阴之力，再服 10 剂，X 线胸片复查示肺淤血显著改善，心电图示心房颤动，平均心率 74 次 /min，期前收缩及房室传导阻滞消失。BNP 425 pg/mL。腹部超声提示肝明显回缩，腹水仅少量。患者属瓣膜性心脏病，持续心房颤动，左心房见血栓，应抗凝治疗，故三诊时除守二诊方剂继进外，嘱华法林 3.75 mg 口服，每日 1 次，调整剂量，监测凝血国际标准化比值（INR），维持 INR 于 2.0～2.5 水平。另地高辛恢复为 0.125mg，口服，每日 1 次，定期监测血药浓度。

按：本例为典型风湿性心脏瓣膜病（联合瓣膜病变），全心衰伴肝、肾功能损害，地高辛中毒。据症状、体征、舌脉，心脾阳虚与水饮瘀血俱存，属本虚标实。且恶心呕吐、中焦痞满症状尤为突出，故陈可冀老师在苓桂术甘汤的基础上加苏子、半夏、砂仁、陈皮、佩兰化湿止呕降逆，同时固护胃气。呕恶止，胃气实，则中西药物才能吸收奏效。肾功能不全，地高辛清除减少，易引起地高辛中毒，该患者心房颤动伴长 R-R 间期及频发室性期前收缩，血中地高辛浓度显著增高，均支持地高辛中毒。故及时停用地高辛实属重要。地高辛的不足与过量，临床上也有另外一种情况，即体循环胃肠道淤血突出，口服地高辛利用率低下，致血药浓度远达不到理想血药浓度的情况，应注意鉴别。苓桂术甘汤单味药及复方的化学成分分析提示，单味茯苓含有甾体、强心苷等；桂枝含强心苷、挥发油等；甘草含类脂、强心苷。而该复方则具强心、利尿、抗心肌缺血、抑制 ANP 和 ADH 释放，减轻肺水肿、镇静、祛痰、改善消化系统症状的作用。

陈可冀老师运用化浊祛邪之品，中病即止，且适时加入党参、黄芪、麦冬、五味子，取生脉散之意，这也符合"温药和之"原则。BNP 水平被认为与心力衰竭严重程度呈正相关，本例显著升高的 BNP 水平，随病情改善而下降。但 BNP 水平

与中医证型之间有何关系尚不明确。该患者左心房有附壁血栓，陈可冀老师中西合参，予华法林抗凝治疗，体现了严谨、务实的学术风格。

2.2.3 肾阳虚衰，水饮泛滥，真武汤化裁 本型主症为：心悸怔忡，气短喘息，甚至端坐呼吸，或咳粉红色泡沫样痰，形寒肢厥，面色苍白，下肢水肿或重度水肿，尿少或无尿，唇舌紫黯，脉微细欲绝。本型本虚标实皆甚，属危急重症，抢救不力可迅致死亡。心力衰竭进一步发展至重度心力衰竭，NYHA 心功能分级为 Ⅳ 级或终末期心力衰竭多属此证，相当于重度全心力衰竭或心源性休克阶段，病变脏腑波及心、脾、肾、肺，形成数脏同病，气血水交互为患。

真武汤亦出自《伤寒论》，是温阳利水方剂，其心动悸、四肢沉重、身瞤动、小便不利及水肿等症状，与右心衰竭或全心衰竭、NYHA 心功能 Ⅲ - Ⅳ 级者非常吻合。然而，与苓桂术甘汤应用同理，陈可冀老师认为应用真武汤亦必须悉心分析心力衰竭发生发展至此阶段的心脾肾阳虚程度与痰瘀水饮互结之间的消长变化。

此型心力衰竭，陈可冀老师主用基本方为：茯苓、芍药、生姜、白术、附子、丹参、桃仁。少尿或无尿，加猪苓、车前子、冬瓜子、冬瓜皮、泽泻；腹水甚者，并用黑白丑末吞服；肺淤血、肺水肿咯血者，加旋覆花、苏子霜、大小蓟、侧柏叶，并三七粉冲服；胸腔积液或心包积液显著者加己椒苈黄汤；心悸甚合并快速性心律失常如心房颤动、房性心动过速、频发室性期前收缩者，加琥珀末冲服，珍珠母、苦参；过缓性心律失常如病态窦房结综合征时，加用红参另煎兑入；长期大量应用利尿剂引起代谢性碱中毒，出现口烦渴、舌光红无苔、烦躁者加生地、玄参、石斛、芦根；因合并感染长期应用广谱抗生素而引起伪膜性肠炎，患者腹泻频繁难止，是脱证之兆，应并用保元汤加罂粟壳；厥脱既成，心源性休克时静脉应用参附注射液或合用生脉注射液。

病例 3 患者，男，57 岁，初诊。反复咳喘 11 年，近 3 周咳喘气短，尿少水肿不能平卧。既往数次住院诊断为肺源性心脏病心力衰竭。3 周前感冒诱发咳喘，痰多黏稠难咳，咳痰时痰中带血，血色鲜红，尿少，肢肿，心慌心悸，心下痞满，腹胀，不欲饮食。曾在通州接受静脉输液注射头孢哌酮舒巴坦钠及口服呋塞米、氨茶碱等治疗，症状无明显改善。检查：重病容，唇发绀，呼吸急促不能平卧，喉中痰鸣，心界向双侧扩大，心率 120 次 /

min，律不齐，心音强弱不等，两肺闻及广泛湿啰音及哮鸣音，肝右胁下 3 cm，剑突下 6 cm，肝区叩击痛 (+)，轻触痛，腹部膨隆，移动性浊音 (+)，双下肢可凹性水肿，舌体胖大，边有齿痕，苔白腻，根部黄腻，脉结代而数，沉取无力。心电图：心房颤动，肺型 P 波；X 线胸部摄片：右心室段显著延长、膨隆，两肺广泛性索状及斑片状模糊阴影，双侧少量胸腔积液。动脉血气分析：pH 7.31，$PaCO_2$ 71mmHg，PaO_2 51mmHg。西医诊断：(1) 慢性支气管炎合并感染；(2) 阻塞性肺气肿；(3) 慢性肺源性心脏病急性发作，心力衰竭Ⅲ度。中医诊断：心衰，证属脾肾阳虚，水饮泛滥，兼夹瘀血痰热，宜温阳利水，蠲饮活血为治。痰黄难咳，痰中带血，舌根部黄腻，属痰热蕴肺所致，故先佐以清化，以真武汤加味，处方：黑附片 10g、桂枝 6g、茯苓 30g、赤芍 10g、白芍 15g、白术 10g、生石膏 15g、知母 10g、黄芩 10g、鱼腥草 15g、丹参 15g、杏仁 10g、生姜 6g。上方浓煎取汁 150mL，频服。三七粉 1.5g，冲服，每日 3 次。继续应用头孢哌酮舒巴坦钠静脉输注，口服呋塞米 20mg，每日 1 次，氨茶碱片 0.1g，每日 2 次。服药 4 剂，尿量显著增多，每日超过 2000mL，水肿消退明显，咳喘减轻，痰转稀易咳，痰中带血消失，心悸改善。前方去生石膏、知母，加入党参 15g、麦冬 10g、五味子 10g、猪苓 15g、琥珀末 1.5g 冲服，呋塞米改为 20 mg，隔日 1 次，头孢哌酮舒巴坦钠治疗第 8 天停用。再服 7 剂，基本不喘，偶咳白痰，能平卧，水肿消失，食欲改善，腹围减小，体重由 69kg 降至 58kg。动脉血气指标正常，表明心衰临床基本控制。

按：本例为慢性肺源性心脏病急性发作，虽脾肾阳虚，与瘀血水饮并存，然肺之痰热亦盛，故陈可冀老师在真武汤的基础上，重用生石膏、知母、黄芩、鱼腥草清热化痰，痰化热清，肺气宣发肃降有序，通调水道功能复常，水饮才可能有其出路。

真武汤，无论其单味药还是复方研究，均证实其抗心力衰竭作用是多方位的，如强心，利尿，增加心排血量，降低心脏前后负荷，抑制心脏重塑及心肌细胞凋亡，清除氧自由基，提高血浆谷胱肽过氧化物酶 (GSH-Qx) 水平，增强红细胞超氧化物歧化酶 (SOD) 活性，降低血清脂质水平，降低血栓素 A_2 活性等。临床上多用于肺心病引起的右心衰竭或全心衰竭的治疗。但该患者伴发急性肺部感染，已有轻度二氧化碳潴留，如不加强抗感染措施以改善通气，恐会产生肺性脑病致呼吸衰竭。故继续应用抗生素静脉输注，配合解痉药物。心力衰竭重症须中西并用，优势互补，方能体现中西医结合的最大效应。

参考文献

[1] Braunwald E. Heart disease. Philadelphia：W. B. Saunders Company, 1997：445.

[2] 邓中甲 . 方剂学 . 北京：中国中医药出版社，2005：152.

《黄帝内经》体质分型与高血压发病关系初探 *

陈可远　李谡翙　徐超

高血压发病 [1] 与多种危险因素相关，包括遗传因素和家族聚集性、超重、饮酒、高盐等膳食因素及社会经济因素等。同时个体对某种或某些因素的易感素质在高血压发病机制中起到了至关重要的作用。中医体质分型 [2] 的研究，正是以人个体为中心，探讨健康与疾病相互转变的规律。《黄帝内经》（以下简称《内经》）对体质进行了多种不同的分型。各种分型方法自成体系，又相互补充，通过对《内经》体质分型的分析，发现体质类型与高血压发病关系密切。

《灵枢·通天》以人体阴阳的偏颇为依据，并结合个体的行为表现、心理性格及生理功能等将体质分为 5 型，即通常所讲的五态体质分类法：多阴而无阳的太阴之人、多阴少阳的少阴之人、多阳而少阴的太阳之人、多阳而少阴的少阳之人和阴阳和平之人。陈孝银等 [3] 根据此分型法中人格心理

---

* 原载于《中华中医药杂志》，2012，27 (7)：1893-1895

特征部分即 5 种气质类型做进一步分型描述，观察了 252 例肝阳上亢证，进行气质分型，发现其中以太阳型之人最为多见，共 108 例，占 42.9%。说明肝阳上亢证与太阳型人关系密切。郭克锋等[4] 研究发现原发性高血压与个性明显相关，胆汁型气质类型多见，认为中医的太阳之人气质类型与胆汁质气质类型相似，中医辨证分型多为肝火亢盛型、阴虚阳亢型或痰湿壅盛型[1]。可见太阳之人性格精神亢奋，辨证多为肝阳上亢或阴虚阳亢等阳热体质，与高血压发病关系密切。

现代高血压发病观认为心理应激、A 型行为及应对方式是导致高血压发病的重要危险因素。职业紧张是心理应激的典型表现。刘宝英等[5] 在研究中发现，不同个体由于健康状态与遗传特征决定了某器官系统对紧张反应敏感度不同，当个体是职业紧张反应易感者时，在职业紧张作用下，发生高血压、冠心病等心血管疾病的危险性增高。苏丽琼等[6] 研究发现，职业社会心理因素对职业人群健康的影响是通过认知过程、人格特征和对紧张因素评价感知的介导起作用，由于心理特征诸如 A 型行为方式和应对存在很大差异，所以感知紧张的程度则存在差异性。《内经》五态体质分类法认识到人格心理特征与人的形态功能及对外界适应能力、方式等是整体相关的，将人在形态、功能、心理以及对外界适应能力、方式等方面的差异性综合判断，再进行体质分型，既探讨人群中不同个体的体质差异，又重视环境因素对体质的影响，可见《内经》体质分型在研究多因素致高血压发病机制方面占有明显优势。

《灵枢·针经》指出不同体质类型之人对针刺得气反应不同，根据阴阳之气盛衰的差异将体质分为四种类型，即重阳型、重阳有阴型、阴多阳少型和阴阳和调型。章楠《医门棒喝》："故人秉质多有偏胜强弱之殊，或有阳盛阴弱者，或有阴胜于阳者，或有阴阳皆弱者，或有阴阳皆盛者"。阴阳失调，阴虚阳亢，是高血压病中医辨证较多见的。钱岳晟等[7] 将 207 例高血压病患者按中医体质分型为阳亢组 113 例、痰湿组 94 例。宋红普等[8] 对 476 例高血压病患者进行临床调查，结果发现高血压患者近 1/3 具有肾精亏虚的特点。朱克俭等[9] 将高血压病患者病理体质划分为阴虚质、阳虚质、痰湿质、湿热质、气虚质和瘀血质 6 型，发现阴虚质占 49%，认为高血压病患者病理体质主要是阴虚质和痰湿质，可见"多阳而少阴"的体质类型

与高血压发病关系密切。

《灵枢·阴阳二十五人》篇中，主要以五行属性进行体质分类，分为"木、火、土、金、水"5 个主型，每个主型下，又分为 5 个亚型，共 25 种体质类型。特别提出的是《内经》以五行特性分别类比五脏的不同功能，体现了五脏的 5 种体质类型。如《素问·阴阳应象大论》对肾有详尽的论述："北方生寒，寒生水，水生咸，咸生肾……在味为咸……寒伤血，燥胜寒；咸伤血，甘胜咸"。从中可以发现，古人认为饮食五味中的咸味滋养肾脏，咸味伤及血脉。又如《生气通天论》："味过于咸，大骨气劳，短肌，心气抑"。《五脏生成篇》："多食咸，则脉凝泣而变色"。《灵枢·五味》"五味各走其所喜"，"谷味咸，先走肾"，"心病禁咸"。过食咸味，则伤及肾脏，肌肉萎缩，心气抑郁无力，血脉凝涩不畅。从中可以看出，五脏与饮食五味的关系不是简单的一一对应，五脏体质类型可偏盛或偏虚，若肾脏偏弱，则咸味相对"太过"而伤及本脏，若心脏偏弱，则水乘火，咸味伤及心脉。现代医学研究认为，盐与高血压发病关系密切。限盐对高血压患者血压下降有利，但并不是所有高盐摄入人群高血压患病率都增高，在人群中，有一部分人由于遗传因素导致细胞膜离子转运缺陷和肾排钠障碍，对盐的摄入量十分敏感，如果长期进食高盐饮食，就可能引发高血压，这部分人称为盐敏感者。盐敏感者的病理生理特征主要表现为钠的代谢异常、肾潴钠倾向、交感神经系统调节缺陷、胰岛素抗性增加和血管内皮功能失调等一系列引起血压调节的内分泌及生化代谢异常。现代医学正致力于盐敏感者的早期识别，及对盐敏感易感基因及其遗传因素的研究。HC. Deter 等[10] 对正常人群中的盐敏感型与盐抵抗型的两组被试进行了研究，在年龄、身体状况、高血压家族史等方面匹配的条件下，在心理应激情况下，盐敏感组血压、心率、焦虑水平的升高均比盐抵抗组高，而对愤怒的控制力较低，盐敏感组的激惹水平实验前后都相对较高，可见盐敏感人群存在特殊的体质特征。对盐敏感人群与心理应激及与高血压发病关系的认识，《内经》五脏体质类型从五脏与五味、五脏与发病的关系这一宏观角度为我们提供了探求高血压发病机制的方法和思路。

《灵枢·逆顺肥瘦》篇根据形体特征进行体质分类，将体质划分为：肥人、瘦人、常人。《灵枢·卫气失常》篇中，又将肥人划分为：膏、脂、

肉 3 型。肥人多属痰湿体质，《丹溪治法心要》言"肥白人多痰湿"。现代中医学者认为阳亢质和痰湿质均为高血压患者较为常见的体质类型。钱岳晟等[7]研究发现，痰湿质高血压病患者的体重指数 (BMI)、舒张压 (DBP)、空腹血糖 (FBG)、血尿酸 (UA) 明显高于阳亢质高血压患者；带有 α- 内收蛋白 1 (α-ADD1) TT 型基因的痰湿质高血压病患者心脑血管危险因素更多，预后比阳亢质高血压病患者更差，并从分子生物学的角度探讨了体质的差异性。阳亢质、痰湿质两组 122 例原发性高血压病患者血压负荷和血压变异特征比较发现，痰湿质高血压病患者较阳亢质高血压病患者血压昼夜节律减小明显，血压负荷增大，可能容易发生靶器官损害。说明中医体质分型的差异在理化检查中可得到相应的证据。林谦等[11]根据匡调元的中医体质分型理论，将人的病理体质分为晦涩质（瘀滞质）、腻滞质（痰湿质）、燥红质（阴虚质）、迟冷质（阳虚质）、倦晄质（阴阳两虚）。调查发现 371 例原发性高血压患者中各种体质分布差异较大，其中燥红质（阴虚质）和腻滞质（痰湿质）比例最高分别占 35.86% 和 31.27%。燥红质（阴虚质）导致肾素、血管紧张素Ⅱ以及血清过氧化脂质含量明显增高，而血浆一氧化碳和心钠素含量降低；腻滞质（痰湿质）则引起血脂增高，胰岛素的敏感性及 Na^+–K^+–ATP 酶活性降低。上述各种指标的变化均会加重高血压的病情及症状，提示上述两种体质可能对原发性高血压的形成和发展具有某种内在相关性。

从探讨《内经》体质分型与高血压发病关系可以看出，《内经》体质分型以人与自然相统一的整体观为出发点，是对人体的形态结构、生理功能、行为习惯、心理特征、对环境的适应调节能力、对疾病的易患性和倾向性等各方面特征的综合判断，与现代医学探讨高血压发病机制倡导的现代生物、心理、社会、医学模式相吻合，弥补了单一因素致病研究思路的缺陷。《内经》体质分型还具有灵活多变、注重实用的特点，提示我们研究体质分型时应注重与临床结合，以人为主体，以研究

具体疾病为靶点，既需要适合普通人群具有客观性、标准化、规范化的体质分型，同时也需要针对不同疾病或不同年龄等的特定分型方法，从而达到防治疾病的目的。《内经》体质分型涵盖了现代生物、心理、社会、医学模式理念，具有包容性，西医从不断深入的层次探讨每一种致病因素的致病机制的成果，都可以应用于中医体质分型，两者相互补充，相互为用，为体质分型达到防治疾病的目的提供了广阔的发展空间。《内经》中明确提出"治未病"的学术思想，未来的高血压治疗应以预防为主。中医体质分型为全面了解健康状况，获得高血压发病的预测信息提供了理论框架，为调整偏颇体质状态、防治高血压病提供了新的途径和方法。

参考文献

[1] 刘力生 . 高血压 . 北京：人民卫生出版社，2001：20-52，1019-1023.

[2] 王琦 . 中医体质学 . 北京：人民卫生出版社，2005：67-69.

[3] 陈孝银，杨钦河，沈英森，等 . 肝阳上亢证与人体气质关系调查分析 . 陕西中医，2002，23 (2)：124.

[4] 郭克锋，魏建科，关菊香，等 . 原发性高血压患者个性结构与中医辨证分型的关系 . 现代康复，2001，5 (2)：37-38.

[5] 刘宝英，任南，杨华，等 . 职业紧张与多发多种心血管疾病关系的研究 . 卫生研究，2006，35 (4)：489-491.

[6] 苏丽琼，刘宝英，杨华，等 . A 型行为及应对方式与职业紧张的关系 . 海峡预防医学杂志，2007，13 (2)：9-11.

[7] 钱岳晟，张怡，张伟忠，等 . 两种中医体质高血压病患者的表型与 α- 内收蛋白基因多态性分型的关系 . 中国中西医结合杂志，2006，26 (8)：698-701.

[8] 宋红普，何裕民 . 476 例原发性高血压患者体质特点研究 . 上海中医药大学学报，2001，15 (2)：34.

[9] 朱克俭，蔡光先，卢六沙，等 . 高血压病证候及其转化规律研究 . 中国中医药信息杂志，1999，6 (2)：13-14.

[10] Deter HC, Buchhoiz K, Schorr U, et al. Psychophysiologieal reactivity of salt-sensitive normotensive subjects. J. of Hypertension, 1997, 15：839.

[11] 林谦，陈焱，金法，等 . 371 例原发性高血压患者的中医体质辨证研究 . 现代中医药，2004，3 (3)：17-18.

心主血脉与血栓前状态 *

黄　烨　殷惠军　陈可冀

据统计我国每年约有 260 万人死于心脑血管疾病，且呈逐年增长趋势，也就是说平均每 13 秒就有 1 人因此死亡 [1]。血栓形成是心脑血管疾病事件发生发展的关键环节。一旦发病就等于"战争失败了"，所以强调对这类疾病进行一级预防。血栓形成是血管内皮细胞、血小板和凝血 / 纤溶系统等多种因素综合作用的结果，这些因素在血栓形成前已发生了不同程度的变化，呈现出一种易于形成血栓的病理状态，即血栓前状态 (prethrombotic state, PTS)[2]。PTS 是由多种因素引起的机体凝血、抗凝和纤溶系统功能失调并伴有血管内皮功能异常的一种病理过程，常伴有血小板等相关因子的改变以及易导致血栓形成的血液流变学变化 [2]。PTS、血栓形成和血栓栓塞是血栓形成和发展过程中的三个连续病理阶段，而 PTS 是血栓事件发生的前提条件。如何识别这一状态，针对危险因素及时处理，对防止血栓事件无疑具有重要的临床意义。

在规范用药和良好依从性的基础上，仍有患者发生血栓不良事件。多项研究结果显示 [3]，5.5% ~ 61% 人群存在阿司匹林失效，4% ~ 30% 的患者未能从氯吡格雷抗血小板治疗中获益。血栓形成受血管内皮结构和功能、血液成分及血流状态改变、血小板系统及凝血与纤溶系统等多方面的影响，途径复杂，因此防治动脉血栓形成不是抗血小板单一途径能完全奏效的，抗血小板仅仅是防治血栓形成的环节之一。由此可见，寻求多通路抗血小板以及寻求抗血小板以外的多途径抗栓，如抗血管内皮细胞损伤和调节纤溶系统紊乱则是心血管疾病防治的重要研究方向。

PTS 防治与中医"治未病"思想具有高度的一致性。早在《素问·四气调神大论》就有"是故圣人不治已病治未病，不治已乱治未乱，此之谓也"的论断。药理研究证实，中药，尤其是益气、活血中药具有提高心肌收缩力、抑制血小板过度活化、调节凝血 / 纤溶系统功能紊乱、改善血管内皮功能的作用，一定程度上显示了中医"治未病"的特色与优势。中医血瘀证与血栓形成在生理病理认识方面具有很大的相似性，心气充沛、血液充盈和脉道通利是血液正常运行的基本条件，任一环节的异常都会导致血流不畅，乃致血栓形成。作者基于心主血脉理论，对血栓形成的中医认识从理论上进行深入探索，试图为 PTS 的中医药防治提供一定的理论依据。

1. 血栓前状态防治概况

PTS 是一种由复杂因素引起的具有易导致血栓形成的多种血液学变化的病理过程，分为遗传性和获得性两大类。尽管二者的病理改变不尽相同，但都存在着 PTS 发生并发展到血栓形成阶段的关键环节：血管内皮功能失调、血小板过度活化和凝血 / 纤溶系统紊乱 [2]。

PTS 自 20 世纪被认识以来，不少学者致力于寻找有效的检测方法以阻止其向血栓形成阶段发展。在国外，PTS 的全套实验室检测包括全血计数（含血小板形态）、凝血酶原时间及部分凝血活酶时间、结缔组织，活化的蛋白质 C 抵抗性、蛋白质 C 和 S 活性、抗凝血酶Ⅲ抗原及活性狼疮抗凝物、肝素诱导的抗体、同型半胱氨酸水平、亚甲基四氢叶酸还原酶和凝血酶原 G20210A 突变位点 [4]。这些检测指标虽为诊断 PTS 提供参考价值，但因价格昂贵，操作费时，延误治疗，还能给患者带来负面心理影响，而限制了它们在临床中的应用。目前尚没有证据证明，上述检测指标可作为强有效的危险因素用于指导临床治疗 [5]。在我国，目前应用于临床的实验室检查主要是针对血管内皮系统、血小板系统、凝血 / 抗凝系统和纤溶系统 4 个方面，包括血液流变学测定、血小板激活分子标志物测定、血管内皮细胞损伤分子标志物测定以及凝血因子和纤溶系统标志物检测 [6]。这些检测指标虽有可操作性，但缺乏特异性。加之 PTS 形成原因复杂，常涉及多个遗传和环境因素，将上述检测项目作为普通人群筛查 PTS、预测血栓形成的指标既耗时又费力，很有必要寻找廉价、敏感的检测方法 [7]。

* 原载于《中华中医药杂志》，2011，26 (4)：633-636

第六章

防治 PTS 除强调抗血小板、抗凝和抗纤溶治疗外，还包括类固醇激素替代治疗和使用免疫抑制剂等新治疗方法的运用[8]。随着联合用药或药物剂量增加而出现的出血风险，药物治疗窗口期短，治疗剂量的个体差异以及实验室监测以调整药物剂量的繁琐操作等问题局限了抗栓药物的临床应用。尽管现代医学界正在进行包括新型口服凝血酶或 Xa 因子抑制剂的深入研究，但进一步结论尚难预测。

2. 心主血脉的内涵

早在《素问·痿论》就有"心主身之血脉"的论述，这是中医"藏象"学说对心脏生理功能的全面概括，其基本含义是在心的主宰、控制下，以心气为动力，以血脉为基础，血行脉中，濡养五脏六腑、四肢百骸。"脉为心体，血为心用"，心脉、心血互为体用，二者是"心主血脉"功能正常发挥的决定因素。

心在血的生成和运行方面具有重要的地位和作用。《素问·经脉别论篇》云："食气入胃，浊气归心，淫精于脉"，《灵枢·决气》又云："中焦受气取汁，变化而赤，是谓血"，《灵枢·邪客》尚说："营气者，泌其津液，注之于脉，化以为血"。血的化生靠脾运化精微，经心化赤而成，同时亦需肾精化血、肺气调血之清浊等脏腑的协调配合。心在血的化生过程中发挥主导作用，故称"奉心而赤"。源泉不绝之血的正常运行，依赖于脉管的完整和脉气的健旺，其动力主要是宗气。诚如《灵枢·邪客》曰："宗气积于胸中，出于喉咙，以贯心脉，而行呼吸焉"。"宗气贯心脉以行气血"，宗气贯注于心脉之中，助心推动血液循行无端，而心的跳动又鼓动脉道，助血运行于周身脉络，无所不至。《难经·二十二难》有言："血主濡之"。心主血脉功能的正常发挥，使得各脏腑组织器官均得到正常的濡养，才能"肝受血而能视，足受血而能步，掌受血而能握，指受血而能摄"[9]。心与脉在功能上相互依存和协调，约束和推进血液循脉而行，不溢出脉外，使气血周流不息，正常运行。心脏连脉之心系，心是脉之中心总司，脉的功能活动都有赖于心的健全。

现代医学对心血管功能进行的深入研究和重新评价，为"心主血脉"认识提供了理论基础。心脏可根据人体所需调整其他器官血量，松弛血管和影响血压。心脏不仅是动力射血器官和神经-体液作用的效应器官，也是一个内分泌器官；同时血管内皮也不单是一种被动性血管上的覆盖物，也具备内分泌功能，参与体内平衡、炎症免疫反应的调节。心血管系统通过自分泌、旁分泌等方式，能分泌多种生物活性物质和心脏神经递质。它们既有自身调节作用，维持循环系统功能，又参与多种生理病理过程，调节整体的生命活动[10]。

3. 益气活血治则

心、血、脉三者密切关联，构成一个相对独立的系统。该系统的生理功能均由心所主，有赖于心的正常搏动。心脏和脉管作为功能物质场所及载体，在心气的推进和脉道的约束下，血液和生命物质才得以发挥营养和调控的生理效应。气虚、血亏和脉道不利，终将导致血瘀脉中或血溢脉外的血瘀病理状态。早在 1856 年，德国病理学家 Virchow 就提出血栓形成理论，认为血管因素、血液理化性质改变和血流变化与血栓形成有关，许多异常因素最终通过这三环节导致血栓形成[11]。PTS 是多种因素引起的易于形成血栓的病理过程，体现在血管内皮受损、凝血因子活化、纤溶低下及血液流变学改变等方面。

气能行血，血液之所以在脉中运行，环流不息，全赖心气之推动；气能摄血，血液之所以在脉中运行，不溢出脉外，全赖心气之固摄；"气为血帅""血不自行，赖气以动"。益气辅以活血，补气而不壅滞，化瘀配以益气，活血而不耗气，益气活血，相得益彰。清代医家王清任非常重视气血在发病中的重要性，认为"治病之要诀，在明白气血。无论外感内伤，要知初病伤人何物"，"所伤者无非气血"，提出了气虚致瘀理论，倡导"补气活血"，所创制的补气活血名方补阳还五汤，今仍广泛应用于心脑血管疾病的治疗。

现代研究证实益气活血中药具有多种抗血栓药理作用：提高心肌收缩力，保护缺血心肌损伤[12]；抑制血小板活化，调节凝血/纤溶系统功能紊乱从而调整血液循环状态[13]；改善血管内皮细胞功能[14]。这些作用都是对心主血脉中心、血、脉三方面的具体体现。

4. 问题与展望

如何早期识别 PTS，针对危险因素及时处理，对防止血栓事件具有重要的临床意义。目前 PTS 诊断方法特异性差，缺乏预测性。业界尽快达成共识或形成统一的诊断标准，对 PTS 的防治无疑具有重要意义。

无论是以遗传性抗凝缺陷为主的静脉血栓，还是以血管内皮细胞损伤、血小板过度活化及纤溶系统功能紊乱为主的动脉血栓，治疗都应提倡加强修复与重建机体血栓有关系统的平衡状态。基于心主血脉理论，倡导从心、血、脉三方面多途径干预，强调从加强心肌收缩力、改善血液流变异常以及调节血液成分异常、提高血管内皮细胞功能三环节着手，预防血栓形成。

近年来，中药尤其是活血化瘀方药防治血栓形成备受关注，血府逐瘀汤、桃红四物汤、冠心 Ⅱ 号方及川芎、当归、赤芍、丹参、三七等单味中药均已被证实具有一定的抗栓作用，益气和活血中药配伍可通过改善血管内皮细胞损伤、抑制血小板过度活化、调节纤溶系统功能紊乱以及改善血液流变学异常等防治血栓形成，对"心主血脉"理论进行了临床实践的验证，深化了对心主血脉的中医认识。然而，目前尚没有对 PTS 认识的中医系统理论，同时也缺乏符合循证医学的中医药防治 PTS 的临床研究。中医系统理论的形成以及中医药防治 PTS 的循证医学证据，将对中医药防治 PTS 具有重要的里程碑式的意义。

参考文献

[1] 胡大一.转变理念做实我国心血管疾病的预防.中华心血管病杂志，2008，36 (7)：577-580.
[2] Chan MY, Andreotti F, Becker RC. Hypercoagulable states in cardiovascular disease. Circulation, 2008, 118 (22)：2286-2297.
[3] 章靓，陈旺，庞文生，等.血栓形成机制及血小板膜糖蛋白 Ⅱb/ Ⅲa 受体拮抗剂的研究进展.国际药学研究杂志，2009，36 (4)：268-271.
[4] Khor B, Van Cott EM. Laboratory evaluation of hypercoagulability. Clin Lab Med, 2009, 29 (2)：339-366.
[5] Middeldorp S, ban Hylckama Vlieg A. Does thrombophilia testing help in the clinical management of patients? Br J Haematol, 2008, 143 (3)：321-335.
[6] 李士敏.血栓前状态实验室检测.中国医药指南，2008，6 (14)：92-93.
[7] Baglin T. Unraveling the thrombophilia paradox：from hypercoagulability to the prothrombotic state. J Thromb Haemost, 2010, 8 (2)：228-233.
[8] Abramson N, Abramson S. Hypercoagulability：clinical assessment and treatment. South Med J, 2001, 94 (10)：1013-1020.
[9] 颜乾麟，韩鑫冰，韩天雄，等.论气血失衡是心脑血管病的基本病机.中华中医药杂志，2010，7 (25)：1083-1085.
[10] 章薇.心主血脉的内涵考释.中医药学刊，2004，22 (2)：253-254.
[11] Esmon C T. Basic mechanism and pathogenesis of venous thrombosis. Blood Rev, 2009, 23 (5)：225-229.
[12] 张金国，曹勇，董志巨.黄芪在心血管疾病治疗中的应用.医学综述，2009，15 (18)：2838-2840.
[13] 王婕，郭利平，王怡.中药对血小板功能影响的研究进展.北京中医药，2008，27 (11)：893-896.
[14] 宋立群，周延萌，马小茜，等.中药对血管内皮细胞保护作用的研究进展.医药导报，2009，28 (6)：735-736.

Where Are We Going?*

CHEN Ke-ji

The Chinese government has insisted on developing the career of Chinese medicine and pharmacy (CMP) and raised the policy and guidance of realizing the modernization of CMP and promoting the integration of Chinese medicine and Western medicine. Not long ago, the State Council and 16 ministries of China jointly issued CMP Innovation and Developing Project (2006-2020), and further raised the targets of inherition, innovation, modernization, and internationalization. It represents for the willingness of the Chinese nation.

* 原载于 Chinese Journal of Integrative Medicine, 2010, 16 (2)：100-101

1. Absorbing the Essence and Weeding Out the Obsolete and Worthless

CMP, as a magnificent treasure, has made great contributions in guaranteeing the health of the Chinese people, and promoting the reproduction of the Chinese nation.

Now, the existing CMP ancient books have more than 10 thousand kinds and the Chinese materia medica (CMM), medicinal herbs, and available plant drugs amounting to over 10 thousand kinds or so. The invention of artemisinin has been internationally recognized and adopted, and acupuncture has been spreading in various countries all over the world. Integrated Chinese and Western medicine (ICWM) has obtained significant effects on the scientific study of CMP for half a century and has a bright future. The staff engaging in CMP career should have self-esteem, confidence, and self-renewal; they should learn the strategic thoughts outline on the developing and innovation of CMP recently issued by 16 ministries and the State Council, walking an inheritable, innovative, modernized, and internationalized way. There is no need to have any perplexes or doubts. Due to historical reasons, there is certain amount of feudal and superstitious dross in the traditional academics of CMP, or some reasoning gives a strained interpretation. We should confront them, absorb the essence and weed out the obsolete and worthless. We need not ignore it. Neither are we afraid when they are pointed out. We don't need to have any complaints. We insist on the guidance as "making the past serving for the present, making foreign things serving for China, and bringing forth the new from the old".

2. Pure Gold Fears No Fire

The important objective in inheriting and developing CMP is to get rid of pain and diseases for patients using patient-centered CMP technologies and methods and improving the therapeutic efficacy. The safety and effectiveness of relative prophylactic and therapeutic methods should be confirmed. The therapeutic efficacy is a solid foundation for developing medical sciences, and we should have appetite for creation in this aspect.

There are a lot of excellent observatory reports on the clinical efficacy of CMP with good prospective design of clinical trial and rational randomized control, which is able to meet evidence-based medicine and evaluate the therapeutic efficacy and adverse reaction true to the fact. However, there is an essential problem involving the scientific spirits. Now so many clinical articles report only the good news and not the bad. Almost all the recipes and prescriptions show good efficacy after verification. Reports with poor efficacy or negative results are seldom seen. Resorting to deceit cannot report the clinical efficacy true to the fact, even in many doctoral candidates' theses. It is said that the theses cannot pass the examination. Thus, other people cannot obtain the clinical results repeatedly, which greatly affects the opinions on the academics of CMP held by the medical field. So I believe we must advocate seeking the truth from facts as efficacy evaluation, strengthen the scientific and research designs of medical care. Do not resort to deceit. Chinese medicine (CM) and Western medicine (WM) both have their own advantages, but neither is omnipotent; some may be effective in the treatment of some diseases but ineffective in the treatment of some other diseases. It is an inevitable phenomenon and needs our further study. Negative results might be so excellent, which are similarly of essential reference value for disease prevention and treatment.

3. Developing in a Multi-Element Mode

We should treat the CMP academic developing from an international view, advocate tolerance and harmony, open the door wider. We welcome colleagues from different disciplines, and those in modern medical field in particular. Do not hide your face behind the lute in the arms. Do not be ignorantly arrogant. We should advocate learning from each other and improving mutually. As for ICWM, we should advocate team cooperation between CM and WM, exert the superiorities, promote the organic integration, and improve the service quality for patients. "Promoting the organic integration of Chinese medical system and Western medical system" is clearly stipulated in the Regulations of CMP of the P.R. China on April 7, 2003 issued by the State Council. I think, if only it is advantageous to pain and disease relief and beneficial to the inheritance and development of ICMW. The adoptions of traditional inherited mode, modern scientific research mode, ICWM integration mode, and complex scientific systematic and biological research mode should all be welcomed. The present problem is too few innovative new thoughts and new methods. If slightly different from traditional thoughts, they are believed to change a tune, the so-called "westernized", "out of forming", "another kind", so many comments! Comprehensive study on complex prescription, a suite style therapy, study and medical care by a single drug or chemical compositions should be paid enough attention to, only that they have a sparkle of progressive significance in developing CMP. Surgery is the specialty in WM, while perioperative ICWM intervention is the strong point of CMP. The prophylaxis and treatment by CMP sometimes plays a leading role, and sometimes plays a minor role. It is glorious both as a leading role and a minor role.

4. The Three Horse Wagons

Actually, CM and WM exist in China, and this is a condition in China. According to the laws for science developing, the crossing progress and innovation among disciplines is an inevitable developing law. For more than 50 years, the Chinese government has been persisting in advocating the ICWM policy, promoting the unification and cooperation between CM and WM, and taking each other's superiorities for supplement. Great progress has been achieved in scientific connotations of CM and basic studies on the application of recipes and drugs (CM recipes and CMM). The CM, WM, and ICWM exist in China as three medical troops. It is a good thing, better than one central concept. The cooperation of the three troops jointly serves for the medical and health career of China and for the health of the Chinese people as a solid guarantee. This is really marvelous. Someone asks "Will WM substitute for CM?" This is a timid and weak manifestation that is lacking in confidence. The Chinese government is continually strengthening the policy of protecting and developing CMP, as well as the fostering degree. In the WM, it has projects for developing its own medical science, which can be described as "having too full". Where comes the problem of substitution? Premier WEN Jia-bao points out in his inscription that "To carry out the integration of CM and WM, and to develop the traditional CMP". What a feasible proposal!

5. Guiding Rational and Equal Academic Discussions

There were disputes on the existence and abolishment of CMP academics, and they are and will be present. As for these violet disputes, we advocate handling them calmly. It is good to have academic arguments. However, we advocate discussing in an equal way presenting the facts and reasoning things out. We disagree to being frightened by flinging invective and beating sticks. Actually there are a lot of problems worth discussing or arguing in the CMP academics. However, the key point is to have the concept to assist the CMP progressing and the concept to assist the CMP to serve for the people's health better, creating a harmonious environment for arguing. A review recently published in Nature

(July 2007) mentioned "hardness to swallow" CMM decoction. From another aspect, I think whether good medicine tastes bitter. It is advisable to view problems in various aspects.

Therefore, most discussions are beneficial, and I just hope to lessen negative effects. We really need to enhance the study on the convergence of CM and WM.

The Potential Benefit of Complementary/Alternative Medicine in Cardiovascular Diseases[*]

CHEN Ke-ji   HUI Ka Kit   LEE Myeong Soo   XU Hao

Cardiovascular diseases (CVDs) prevalence continues to increase, and it is still the number one killer so far. In 2002, nearly 17 million deaths all over the world were attributable to CVDs, which accounted for almost 30% of the total deaths. Despite treatment with percutaneous coronary inter-vention (PCI) and many other conventional medicines, CVDs patients are still confronted with certain risk of recurrent acute cardiovascular events, readmission to the hospital, and unfavorable quality of life. In recent years, more and more clinicians have successfully applied complementary/alternative medicine (CAM) in CVDs prevention and treatment based on standardized conventional therapy. Nevertheless, the role of CAM in CVDs still needs more clinical evidence and definite mechanism of actions.

In this issue, a collection of several original research articles and reviews are presented that address the clinical application and the mechanism of action of CAM in the treatment of CVDs.These works were submitted by researchers from different parts of the world, including China, Japan, South Korea, Australia, and Sweden. In these studies, the effectiveness of Chinese medicine and some other alternative therapeutic methods in improving symptoms was demonstrated in patients with hypertension, chronic stable coronary artery disease, chronic heart failure, and so forth. Specifically, the use of Chinese herbal medicines was reviewed for the prevention of in-stent coronary restenosis after PCI. The study of Tanshinone II A, a diterpene quinine extracted from the root of salvia miltiorrhiza, a Chinese traditional herb, was presented as a promising cardioprotective agent. The positive effect of Chinese food and herbal medicines in improving certain moderate dyslipidemias was described. The usefulness of Xuezhikang, an extract from Red Yeast Rice, was reviewed in the treatment of coronary heart disease complicated by dyslipidemia. A pharmacological and mechanistic study showed Naoxintong's effect on cytochrome P450 2C19. Further, one study showed the effect of berberine on improving insulin sensitivity by inhibiting fat store and adjusting adipokines profile in human preadipocytes and metabolic syndrome patients.

In the authors' opinion, the clinical research of Chinese medicine and other CAMs for CVDs still faces some major challenges. Issues such as overall quality of medical service and the unmet medical needs in the contemporary society are

* 原载于 Evidence-Based Complementary and Alternative Medicine, 2012, Article ID 125029

common to these medicines. A general guideline is required for practicing Chinese medicine and other CAMs, which should be developed based on solid evidence from well-designed and well- executed clinical studies. Such is the direction that the research of Chinese Medicine and other CAM should follow.

Complementary and Alternative Medicine: Is It Possible to Be Mainstream?*

XU Hao   CHEN Ke-ji

Complementary and alternative medicine (CAM), also known as non-conventional medicine, is used to refer to a broad set of health care practices (such as herbal medicine, acupuncture, Yoga, Taichi, Qigong, meditation, manual therapies, homeopathic medicine, etc.) that are not part of a country's own tradition, or not integrated into its dominant health care system[1]. In fact, CAM is generally used in most developed countries, especially in North America, Europe and Australia, while "traditional medicine (TM)" is more common instead when referring to Africa, Latin America, South-East Asia, and/or the Western Pacific region.

Since the 1990s, the use of CAM has surged in many developed countries. Aging of population, prevalence of chronic diseases and stress-related diseases as well as concern about the adverse reaction of chemical drugs contribute greatly to the worldwide popularity of CAM. According to the 2007 National Health Interview Survey, which gathered information on more than 32,800 Americans, 38.2 percent of adults in the United States aged 18 years and over and nearly 12 percent of children aged 17 years and under used some form of CAM within the previous 12 months[2]. In many parts of the world expenditure on CAM is not only significant, but growing rapidly. In Malaysia, an estimated US $ 500 million is spent annually on this type of health care, compared to about US$ 300 million on allopathic medicine. In the USA, total 1997 out-of-pocket CAM expenditure was estimated at US $ 2.7 billion, while this figure has been up to US $33.9 billion during the 12 months prior to the 2007 National Health Interview Survey[1,2].

Although the use and expenditure of CAM has been increased dramatically, the potential role of CAM in modern clinical practice and health care system seems to be limited, and even be questioned. Many allopathic medicine professionals, even those in countries with a strong history of TM, express strong reservations and disbelief about the claimed benefits of CAM. The efficacy, safety and quality control have been the major concerns in the recognition of CAM and successful integration into the conventional medicine. In most occasions, CAM is just a complement or adjunct to conventional medical care. In this issue, Dr. Abolhassani[3] surveyed the use, capability and satisfaction of CAM in comparison with conventional medicine in Iran. Although the demand for CAM increases, most Iranian patients resort to CAM as a choice at the late stage of the chronic diseases. Therefore, is it possible for CAM to be mainstream rather than only serving as a supporting role in health care system?

Recently, two famous awards honored CAM researchers exemplified the possibility of CAM to be mainstream. In September 2011, the Lasker Clinical Medical Research Award honored Prof.

* 原载于 Chinese Journal of Integrative Medicine, 2012, 18 (6): 403-404

TU You-you who discovered artemisinin and its utility for treating malaria. She and colleagues transformed an ancient Chinese healing method into the most powerful antimalarial medicine currently available that has saved millions of lives across the globe, especially in the developing world. An artemisinin-based drug combination is now the standard regimen for malaria recommended by the World Health Organization (WHO) [4]. On January 24, 2012, Dr. WANG Zhen-yi and Dr. CHEN Zhu have been awarded the 7th Annual Szent-Györgyi Prize for Progress in cancer research for their innovative research that led to the successful development of a new therapeutic approach to acute promyelocytic leukemia (APL). By combining traditional Chinese medicine (arsenic trioxide, As_2O_3) with Western medicine (all-trans retinoic acid, ATRA), Drs. WANG and CHEN have provided dramatic improvement in the 5-year disease-free survival rate of APL patients—from approximately 25 percent to 95 percent—making this therapy a standard of care for APL treatment throughout the world, and turning one of the most fatal diseases into a highly curable one[5].

In this issue, Dr. Park[6] reviewed recent researches into the prevalence, acceptance, accessibility, and recognition of CAM. The results indicated increasing use and acceptance of CAM in the U, S. Practitioners in the U.S. are beginning to be licensed, and insurance companies are beginning to cover some CAM therapies. Many aspects of CAM, especially traditional Chinese medicine and Ayurveda, are becoming mainstream. Acupuncture is a representative CAM therapy which has withstood the test of time and become an accepted treatment for a variety of conditions. At the 1996 WHO conference in Milan, endorsement of acupuncture extended to 64 indications as compared with 43 indications in 1979. In 1997, the U.S. National Institutes of Health (NIH) formally recognized acupuncture as a mainstream medicine healing option with a

statement documenting the procedure's safety and efficacy for treating a range of health conditions. In addition, other CAM Interventions such as hospice care or relaxation and breathing techniques in childbirth that were once considered unconventional are now widely accepted[2].

We have witnessed the development of some CAM therapies and their successful integration into the mainstream medical system. Nevertheless, we still need sufficient scientific evidence from CAM research to clarify their mechanism of action and demonstrate their efficacy and safety. Dr. Micozzi, the founding editor of the Journal of Alternative and Complementary Medicine, has ever said "science should not use the terms 'mainstream' and 'alternative.' Science is science." The benefits of more and more CAM therapies, we believe, will be demonstrated in the future and integrated into the mainstream medicine. This integrative approach will ultimately lead to a safer and more effective patient-centered health care system.

References

[1] World Health Organization. Traditional medicine strategy 2002-2005. 2002. http：//whqlibdoc.who.int/hq/2002/ WHO_EDM_TRM_2002. pdf.

[2] 2007 National health interview survey. http：//nccam.nih.gov/about/plans/2011/introduction.htm.

[3] Abolhassani H, Naseri M, Mahmoudzadeh S. A survey of complementary and alternative medicine in Iran. Chin J Integr Med, 2012, 18：409-416.

[4] Lasker-DeBakey clinical medical research award. http：//www.laskerfoundation.org/awards/2011_c_description.htm

[5] Congratulations to Drs. Zhen-yi wang and Zhu Chen for winning the 7th Annual Szent-Györgyi Prize for progress in cancer research! http：//www.nfcr.org/index.php/asg-prize.

[6] Park JJ, Beckman-Harned S, Cho G, et al. The current acceptance, accessibility and recognition of Chinese and Ayurvedic medicine in the U.S. in the public, governmental, and industrial sectors. Chin J Integr Med, 2012, 18：405-408.

Making Evidence-Based Decisions in the Clinical Practice of Integrative Medicine[*]

XU Hao　CHEN Ke-ji

In 1948，the first clinical paper adopting the protocol of randomized and controlled design was published in British Medical Journal by Bradford Hill, a noted British biostatistician, who introduced rigorous theory of mathematical statistics into clinical design the first time and successfully evaluated the therapeutic effect of streptomycin on tuberculosis[1]. In 1989，clinical trials and systematic review demonstrated that, of 226 maneuvers in obstetrics and childbirth, 20% were beneficial, 30% were harmful or of doubtful value, 50% had no randomized clinical trial evidence available[2]. The result astonished the whole medical community and also brought valuable inspiration for clinical practice. It indicated that experience was unreliable, and all medical interventions should be based on rigorous research evidences. After that, the evidences from a series of systematic researches brought tremendous impacts and challenges to the efficacy, safety and cost-effectiveness of previous accepted strategies of therapeutic, rehabilitative, and preventive regimens. Evidence-based medicine (EBM), a new paradigm for medical practice, emerged[3] and modern medicine has been experiencing a dramatic transition from experience-based medicine to EBM.

There were strong ties between Chinese medicine (CM) and EBM. In the book of "Evidence-based Medicine：How to Practice and Teach EBM", the author Dr. Sackett, one of the pioneers in EBM, said he drew his inspiration for the concept of "Evidence-based medicine" from "textual criticism" in the Qianlong Period of Qing Dynasty, when the texts were used as "evidences" to explain ancient books and records[4]. As a typical traditional medicine, the shortage of objective and quantitative criteria in evaluating therapeutic effect is one of the largest obstacles for CM to move towards the world and received wide recognition. The emergence of EBM provides objective therapeutic evaluation of CM or integrative medicine (IM) with new thinking and method[5-8]. Since both complementary and alternative medicine (CAM) and Western medicine (WM, also known as orthodox medicine in Western countries) have their own superiorities, the integrative medical model of patient-centering care and a combination therapy with both botanical and chemical drugs has been evolving into a new trend of the modern medicine in preventing and treating diseases[9-11]. As the combined applications of CAM and WM are increasing[12-14], more and more concern on their interactions[15] are aroused. As a typical complex intervention[16], whether IM is superior to either CAM or WM, how the combination of CAM and WM play their roles in enhancing efficacy and reducing toxicity from each other, or how to optimize the IM therapeutic regimen, all are not clear. All of these issues warrant further investigation and need more evidences. The introduction of EBM concept brings scientific research and clinical practice of CAM and IM with favorable opportunity and breakthrough point.

EBM is different from prior medical practice, which puts a greater emphasis on the conscientious, explicit, and judicious use

* 原载于 Chinese Journal of Integrative Medicine, 2010，16 (6)：483-485

第六章

of the current best evidence, together with individual clinical expertise, patient values and preferences in making decisions about the care of individual patients[4]. Although the concepts of EBM have been developing since clinical trial publications became available, the formal construction of formulating a clinical question and searching available evidence with a critical eye towards applying it to patient problems have evolved in the recent 20 years. The evidence-based practice (EBP)[4]generally include five steps: converting the need for information into answerable questions; tracking down the best evidence to answer the question (searching related literatures); appraising the evidence for its validity (closeness to the truth), importance (effect size) and applicability (in your own practice); integrating the evidence with your own expertise and the patient's unique biology, values and circumstances; evaluating your effectiveness and efficiency in executing the above steps and seeking ways to improve them. Among these steps, evidence retrieval and use based on PICO (Patients, Intervention, Comparison, Outcome) questions have been given much attention and these are increasingly becoming a basic skill for clinical doctors. With a lot of practicable attempts by many organizations at home and abroad, the EBP methods based on PICO questions have been gradually formulized and popularized internationally, making EBP more and more simplified. However, only in recent years has EBP method based on PICO questions come into domestic people's eyes and has drawn more and more attention. How to conduct an EBP based on PICO questions is still a newborn thing for most doctors, especially for CAM and IM doctors.

Since IM doctors require not only abundant knowledge of CAM but also in-depth understanding and rational application of WM evidence, as well as familiarity with herb-drug interactions between WM and CAM during a combination therapy, it is of vital importance to retrieve relevant evidences. For busy CAM or IM doctors, using PICO question formulation and the corresponding website is a quick way to obtain clinical evidence, which can provide valuable clinical references. In this issue, Dr. Yan, et al introduced an EBP method according to literature retrieval through PICO questions and CAM topics with a practical example of atrial fibrillation[17]. Knowledge of diseases and WM treatment can be acquired by literature retrieval through PICO questions, while searching by CAM topics may provide evidence of CAM. There were a lot of valuable and informative websites or references in this paper, which might be very helpful for CAM and IM doctors. The process from formulation of PICO questions, retrieving website with different characteristics to analyzing, and accepting or rejecting retrieval conclusion, provided CAM or IM clinicians with a very explicit flow path for EBP. The authors held that literature retrieval through both PICO questions and CAM topics was an ideal EBP method for IM.

Nevertheless, the scientificity and reliability of evidences are often relative, which need to be replenished and perfected constantly. Some evidences from authoritative clinical trials were even negated by later studies. Since the standard in CM or CAM evidence hierarchy is still under study, the value of CAM thematic retrieval method remains very limited. During retrieving, conclusions in different evidences may be inconsistent sometimes, just like the evidences for herb-drug interaction between warfarin and Ginkgo in the retrieval conclusion of Dr. Yan, et al[17]. At that time, you have to learn more information in your retrieved evidences about their patient selection criteria, study design and endpoints, and integrate them with patients' specific situation, doctors' clinical experience and pharmacology knowledge of both CAM and WM to analyze and make final choice, so that more objective and accurate evidences can be addressed for a specific clinical decision-making. Although there were few high-ranking evidences on CAM or IM available at present,

第六章

EBP will undoubtedly help us use the best evidence, reduce variation in clinical practice and make us more confident in medical decision-making.

References

[1] Hill AB. B.C.G. in control of tuberculosis. Br Med J, 1948, 1：274.

[2] Chalmers I, Enkin M, Keirse MJ. Effective care in pregnancy and childbirth. Oxford：Oxford University Press, 1989.

[3] Evidence-Based Medicine Working group. Evidence-based medicine. A new approach to teaching the practice of medicine. JAMA, 1992, 268：2420-2425.

[4] Sackett DL, Straus SE, Richardson WS, et al. Evidence based medicine：how to practice and teach EBM. 2nd ed. London：Churchill Livingstone, 2000, 13-27.

[5] Wang JL. A deliberation for evaluating clinical effects in Chinese medicine. Chin J Integr Med, 2010, 16：387-389.

[6] Tang JL. Some reflections on the evaluation of effectiveness of Chinese medicine in China. Chin J Integr Med, 2010, 16：390-391.

[7] Wang JY. Significance of evidence-based medicine in the assessment of Chinese medicine clinical efficacy. Chin J Integr Med, 2010, 16：392-393.

[8] Fang JQ, Liu FB, Hou ZK. Parallel subgroup design of a randomized controlled clinical trial——comparing the approaches of Chinese medicine and Western medicine. Chin J Integr Med, 2010, 16：394-398.

[9] Xu H, Chen KJ. Integrative medicine：the experience from China. J Altern Complem Med, 2008, 14：3-7.

[10] Lu AP, Ding XR, Chen KJ. Current situation and progress in integrative medicine in China. Chin J Integr Med, 2008, 14：234-240.

[11] A Report of the American College of Cardiology Foundation Task Force on Clinical Expert Consensus Documents. Integrating complementary medicine into cardiovascular medicine. J Am Coll Cardiol, 2005, 46：184-221.

[12] Hu XM, Liu F, Zheng CM, et al. Effect and prognostic analysis of treatment for acute myeloid leukemia using Chinese drugs combined with chemotherapy. Chin J Integr Med, 2009, 15：193-197.

[13] Zhang YH, Liu YH. Influence of TCM therapy for supplementing Pi and nourishing Shen on dendritic cell function in patients with chronic hepatitis B treated by lamivudine. Chin J Integr Med, 2009, 15：60-62.

[14] Chen YZ, Li ZD, Gao F, et al. Effects of combined Chinese drugs and chemotherapy in treating advanced non-small cell lung cancer. Chin J Integr Med, 2009, 15：415-419.

[15] Xu H, Chen KJ. Herb-drug interaction：an emerging issue of integrative medicine. Chin J Integr Med, 2010, 16：195-196.

[16] Qiu Y, Xu H, Zhao DY. Therapeutic evaluation on complex interventions of integrative medicine and the potential role of data mining. Chin J Integr Med, 2010, 466-471.

[17] Yan XF, Ni Q, Wei JP, et al. Evidence-based practice of integrative Chinese and Western medicine based on literature retrieval through PICO question and complementary and alternative medicine topics. Chin J Integr Med, 2010, 16：544-550.

Acupuncture：A Paradigm of Worldwide Cross-Cultural Communication[*]

XU Hao　CHEN Ke-ji

On 16 November 2010，an exciting news inspired all traditional Chinese medicine (TCM) practitioners, especially acupuncturists in China. Acupuncture and moxibustion of TCM along with Peking Opera were both inscribed on the Representative List of the Intangible Cultural

* 原载于 Chinese Journal of Integrative Medicine, 2011，17 (3)：163-165

第六章

Heritage of Humanity during the 5th session of the United Nations Educational, Scientific and Cultural Organization (UNESCO) Inter-governmental Committee for the Safeguarding of the Intangible Cultural Heritage Meeting in Nairobi. The Representative List of the Intangible Cultural Heritage of Humanity aims at ensuring better visibility of the intangible cultural heritage and raising awareness of its importance while encouraging dialogue that respects cultural diversity. The Representative List of the Intangible Cultural Heritage of Humanity now comprises 213 elements.

The term "acupuncture" comes from the Latin words "acus" (needle) and "punctura" (to puncture). It refers to the insertion of fine needles into the body at specific points for a therapeutic effect. In a broad sense, "acupuncture" in the literatures may also include moxibustion and other kinds of stimulation to certain points. In its original form, acupuncture was based on the principles of TCM, which defines good health as a balance between two complementary opposites (yin and yang) and free flow of vital force or energy (also spelt "Qi", pronounced "chee") between the organs along channels (meridians), whilst in disease this flow is disrupted causing an imbalance between yin and yang. Needles inserted into specific points along the meridians provide one means of promoting the flow of Qi, redressing imbalances of yin and yang, and hence treat a wide range of ailments.

The practice of acupuncture is rooted in ancient China. It is mentioned in The Yellow Emperor's Classic of Internal Medicine (Huang Di Nei Jing, 黄帝内经), one of the oldest Chinese medical works still in existence and used today as main reference book on acupuncture theory. Acupuncture needles, dating from 4,000 years ago, have been found by archeologists in China. The first needles were made from stone, and gold, silver, bronze and iron needles were used later, until stainless steel needles in modern time. Acupuncture spread into other Asian countries in about A.D. 1000, and was introduced into Europe about A.D. 1700. At the turn of last century, Sir William Osler (1849—1919), a Canadian physician, was using acupuncture to treat low back pain. Although knocked on the door of the world very early, acupuncture's recent popularity in the West dates from the 1970s, as a direct result of James Reston's famous report in the New York Times and President Nixon's visit to China.

James Reston was a reporter for the New York Times. In July 1971, he traveled to Beijing in advance of Dr. Henry Kissinger's famous trip. During his trip, Reston fell ill with appendicitis, and was treated with acupuncture following an emergency operation. Intrigued with the total relief of post-operative pain, Reston wrote of his magical experience following his return to the United States in the New York Times, sparking the mushrooming interest[1]. Reston also told Kissinger about his encounter with acupuncture, and Kissinger passed the story on to President Nixon. The President was so impressed with the story that he even visited a thyroidectomy under the condition of acupuncture anesthesia accompanied by Premier Zhou Enlai during his traveling to Beijing in 1972. He then instituted a program in which traditional Chinese doctors came to the United States to share their medicine, and American doctors were sent to China for the same purpose. In the years following, acupuncture in the United States as well as other Western countries began to take off.

According to the report of World Health Organization (WHO), acupuncture is now used in at least 78 countries and practiced not only by acupuncturists, but also by allopathic practitioners (Figure 1). In Belgium, 74% of acupuncture treatment is administered by allopathic doctors. In Germany, 77% of pain clinics provide acupuncture. In the United Kingdom, 46% of allopathic doctors either recommend patients for acupuncture treatment or treat their patients with acupuncture themselves. Established in

1987, the World Federation of Acupuncture-Moxibustion Societies (WFAS) has nearly 60,000 members from 73 acupuncture organizations from 40 countries in several regions. There are at least 50,000 acupuncturists in Asia. In Europe, there are an estimated 15,000 acupuncturists, including allopathic doctors who also practice as acupuncturists. The USA has 12,000 licensed acupuncturists—the practice of acupuncture is legal in 38 states and six states are developing acupuncture practice policies [2]. Recently, even the New England Journal of Medicine published an article on acupuncture and low back pain [3].

Traditional medicine (TM) /complementary and alternative medicine (CAM) therapies often develop within a very specific cultural environment, and their increasing spreading to other cultural environments is sure to raise safety and efficacy issues. As with all CAM, the absence of a formal system for reporting adverse effects means that acupuncture's safety is difficult to assess. However, it seems to be a relatively safe form of treatment with a low incidence of serious adverse events [2]. In fact, most complications in literatures are preventable not adverse events [4]. To standardize clinical practice of acupuncture, WHO has accordingly worked with experts in acupuncture to propose a standard international nomenclature in 1991 and revised it in 1993. This is now widely accepted. In addition, WHO has also developed guideline on Basic Training and Safety in Acupuncture. These guidelines strongly encourage national health authorities to regulate acupuncture practice.

Acupuncture has been accepted by the general Chinese population as an effective curative method for a wide range of ailments. However, to be acknowledged worldwide, the East have to meet West in term of the methodology of clinical research on acupuncture and provide its efficacy and effectiveness with more evidences. Therefore, WHO developed guidelines for Clinical Research on Acupuncture [5]. In addition, the Standards for Reporting Interventions in Clinical Trials of Acupuncture (STRICTA) reporting guidelines was first published in 2001 [6] and revised in 2010 [7]. These guidelines dramatically improve the design of acupuncture clinical trial and the completeness and transparency of reporting of interventions in controlled trials of acupuncture. At the 1996 WHO conference in Milan, endorsement of acupuncture extended to 64 indications as compared with 43 indications in 1979. In 1997, the U.S. National Institutes of Health (NIH) formally recognized acupuncture as a mainstream medicine healing option with a statement documenting the procedure's safety and efficacy for treating a range of health conditions. Demonstration of other indications under investigation [8-10] will no doubt further extend these lists.

Although a large number of randomized controlled trials have been performed, the acupuncture research has been fraught with problems and challenges all the time [11]. In this issue, Dr. Hopton and MacPherson [12] highlight the importance of assessing blinding in randomized controlled trials to strengthen their internal validities, especially discuss challenges in clinical trials of acupuncture and provide very constructive recommendations. Dr. Witt [13] draws on the experience from large acupuncture trials in recent years to outline the way randomized trials could be used to answer questions on efficacy and effectiveness, and also highlights the controversy over specific and non-specific effects of acupuncture emerging from the results of these trials and puts forward insightful suggestions for future clinical research on acupuncture. Dr. Lin and Chen [14] review the present status of research on mechanism of acupuncture and moxibustion in Taiwan, which is much helpful in understanding the effectiveness of acupuncture and how it works on a scientific basis. Dr. Lee and Ernst [15] summarize Cochrane reviews of acupuncture for a wide range of pain conditions in recent years and provide us with an up-to-date indication list of acupuncture for pain in the principle of evidence-

第六章

based medicine.

Originating in China thousands of years ago, acupuncture is not only an important part of TCM, but also an excellent representative of Chinese national culture. Although there are still many issues existing in respect to standardization of manipulation skill, design of clinical trials, clarification of mechanism and confirmation of safety, acupuncture has withstood the test of time, held up to the scrutiny of scientific method, and become an accepted treatment for a variety of conditions. The development and popularization of acupuncture has no doubt been a paradigm of worldwide cross-cultural communication. During this cultural integration, the East has made tremendous efforts in meeting the West. We thus sincerely call for "the West meets the East" by taking fully the traditional theory of acupuncture and meridians into consideration, and making greater reflection on the TCM pattern differentiation and complex approach. The success of TCM acupuncture in applying for being inscribed on the Representative List of the Intangible Cultural Heritage of Humanity will play an important role in protecting cultural diversity, enhancing inter-cultural dialogue and communication. Acupuncture will also, we believe, make more and more contribution to the healthcare of mankind in the future.

References

[1] Eisenberg D. Reflections on the past and future of integrative medicine from a lifelong student of the integration of Chinese and Western Medicine. Chin J Integr Med, 2011, 17: 3-5.

[2] World Health Organization. Traditional medicine strategy 2002-2005. 2002. http: //whqlibdoc.who.int/hq/2002/ WHO_EDM_TRM_2002.1.pdf.

[3] Berman BM, Langevin HM, Witt CM, et al. Acupuncture for chronic low back pain. New Engl J Med, 2010, 363: 454-461.

[4] Leung PC, Zhang L, Cheng KF. Acupuncture: complications are preventable not adverse events. Chin J Integr Med, 2009, 15: 229-232.

[5] Guidelines for Clinical Research on Acupuncture. Manila, WHO Regional Office for the Western Pacific, 1995 (WHO Regional Publications, Western Pacific Series No. 15).

[6] MacPherson H, White A, Cummings M, et al. Standards for reporting interventions in controlled trials of acupuncture: the STRICTA recommendations. Complement Ther Med, 2001, 9: 246-249.

[7] MacPherson H, Altman DG, Hammerschlag R, et al. Revised Standards for Reporting Interventions in Clinical Trials of Acupuncture (STRICTA): extending the CONSORT statement. PLoS Med, 2010, 7: e1000261.

[8] World Health Organization. 2002. Acupuncture: review and analysis of reports on controlled clinical trials. WHO Geneva.

[9] Zhang CX, Qin YM, Guo BR. Clinical study on the treatment of gastroesophageal reflux by acupuncture. Chin J Integr Med, 2010, 16: 298-303.

[10] Jiang YH, Jiang W, Jiang LM, et al. Clinical efficacy of acupuncture on the morphine-related side effects in patients undergoing spinal-epidural anesthesia and analgesia. Chin J Integr Med, 2010, 16: 71-74.

[11] Kaptchuk TJ, Chen KJ, Song J. Recent clinical trials of acupuncture in the West: responses from the practitioners. Chin J Integr Med, 2010, 16: 197-203.

[12] Hopton AK, MacPherson H. Assessing blinding in randomised controlled trials: challenges and recommendations. Chin J Integr Med, 2011, 17: 173-176.

[13] Witt CM. Clinical Research on Acupuncture-Concepts and guidance on Efficacy and Effectiveness Research. Chin J Integr Med, 2011, 17: 166-172.

[14] Lin JG, Chen YH. The mechanistic studies of the acupuncture and moxibustion in Taiwan. Chin J Integr Med, 2011, 17: 177-186.

[15] Lee MS, Ernst E. Acupuncture for pain: an overview of Cochrane reviews. Chin J Integr Med, 2011, 17: 187-189.

Herb-Drug Interaction: An Emerging Issue of Integrative Medicine[*]

XU Hao   CHEN Ke-ji

With the enhancement of people's awareness of self-care, the voice of human for a return to nature is growing louder and louder. Drugs with natural plants as raw materials are increasingly favored by the people all over the world for their unique advantages in preventing and curing diseases, rehabilitation and health care, especially in Europe, the United States and other Asian countries. According to statistics, in the United States alone, there are more than 15 million people using herbal preparations in varying degrees, including Chinese herbal medicines, as therapy or adjuvant therapy for various diseases at present, with the annual cost of approximately 30 billion U.S. dollars[1].

Because of the integrative medical model of patient-centered healthcare and a combination therapy with both botanical and chemical drugs evolving into a new trend of the modern medicine in preventing and curing diseases, the combined applications of Chinese and Western medicine are also increasing, while their interactions arousing more and more concern. Recently, the *Journal of the American College of Cardiology* published an article saying that patients with cardiovascular diseases consumed a number of botanical products including Chinese herbal medicines while taking the Western medicine, which may increase the risk of cardiac event due to herb-drug interactions[2]. After searching associated literatures of PubMed and Medline databases from 1966 to 2008, it is considered in this article that some botanical products including Chinese herbal medicines such as *Hypericum perforatum Linnaeus, Leohurusu artemisia, Panax ginseng, Ginkgo biloba*, *crataegus pinnatifida, Serenoa serrulata, Salvia mitiorrhiza Bunge, tetrandrine, Bulbus Alli*, and *Aconitum carmichaeli Debx, etc*, may all increase the risk of adverse events in patients with cardiovascular disease through the interactions with other drugs, particularly in those elderly patients taking multiple drugs for comorbid conditions.

However, the results of herb-drug interaction were not consistent. For example, although some studies indicated the interactions between ginkgo biloba and warfarin, a randomized, double-blind, placebo-controlled cross-over trial in 2003 demonstrated that ginkgo biloba did not influence the clinical effect of warfarin[3]. Furthermore, a systematic review of randomised clinical trials in 2005 also did not demonstrate that extract of ginkgo biloba caused significant changes in blood coagulation parameters or had an additive effect to the clinical effects of aspirin or warfarin[4].

In response to this issue, we should take an objective and realistic attitude. According to the clinical experience and research findings of doctors in China, the majority of Chinese herbal medicines is still safe in clinical applications and can have synergistic effects or even reduce the toxic side effects when combined with chemical drugs in most cases, such as the application of many Chinese herbal medicines in relieving clinical symptoms, reducing toxic and side effects of chemotherapy, decreasing drug-resistance of some western medicines as well as assisting

* 原载于 Chinese Journal of Integrative Medicine, 2010, 16 (3): 195-196

第
六
章

the withdrawal of glucocorticoid, which reflect the complementary advantages of integrative medicine[5-8].

Nevertheless, clinicians should pay more attention to consider and distinguish results from evidence-based medicine so as to foster strengths and circumvent weaknesses but not shield the shortcomings of integrative medicine, and give great concern to drug interactions that have already been found in clinical practice to avoid the off-label use, long-term drug overdose and the non-rational combined use of drugs aiming at minimizing the risk of adverse events in patients. For special population such as elderly people taking a variety of chemicals due to comorbidities, children, pregnant women, immunosuppressive patients, perioperative patients as well as those with liver and kidney dysfunction, or taking drugs with narrow therapeutic index such as digoxin or warfarin, we should strengthen monitoring to timely detect adverse effects of potential herb-drug interactions, make detailed, verified records and report to relevant drug administrations for further investigation and analysis, so as to accumulate first-hand knowledge of herb-drug interaction in clinical practice. On this basis, a variety of researches associated with pharmacodynamics, pharmacokinetics, efficacy, toxicity and toxicity-efficacy relevance, as well as the mechanism of herb-drug interaction aiming at drug absorption, distribution, conversion, metabolism and excretion, should be designed scientifically and conducted actively for further promoting the rationally combined use of Chinese and Western medicine. At present, some universities and institutes have established special departments of drug interactions, which is worthy of learning.

In light of the emerging issue in the integrative medicine, *Chinese Journal of Integrative Medicine*, as the first Chinese journal in the field of traditional Chinese medicine and integrative medicine included by Science Citation Index-Expanded (SCI-E) to be the source

magazine, has started a column of "herb-drug interaction" to publish rigorous and well-designed clinical or experimental research articles relating to synergistic effects, reduced toxic or side effects, as well as adverse herb-drug interactions occurring during combined use of Chinese and Western medicine, with a view to provide a more open, timely, and academic exchange platform for researchers of integrative medicine and give more valuable information and objective evidence for herb-drug interactions. This will certainly further standardize the clinical practice in combined use of Chinese and Western medicine, and provide patients with more effective and safe integrative medical services.

Reference

[1] Eisenberg DM, Davis RB, Ettner SL, et al. Trends in alternative medicine use in the United States, 1990-1997: results of a follow-up national survey. JAMA, 1998, 280: 1569-1575.

[2] Tachjian A, Maria V, Jahangir, A. Use of herbal products and potential interactions in patients with cardiovascular diseases. J Am Coll Cardiol, 2010, 55: 515-525.

[3] Engelsen J, Nielsen JD, Hansen KF. Effect of Coenzyme Q10 and ginkgo biloba on warfarin dosage in patients on long-term warfarin treatment. A randomized, double-blind, placebo-controlled cross-over trial. Ugeskr Laeger, 2003, 165 (18): 1868-1871.

[4] Savovic J, Wider B, Ernst E. Effects of ginkgo biloba on blood coagulation parameters: a systematic review of randomised clinical trials. Evidence-Based Integrative Medicine, 2005, 2 (3): 167-176.

[5] Hu XM, Liu F, Zheng CM, et al. Effect and prognostic analysis of treatment for acute myeloid leukemia using Chinese drugs combined with chemotherapy. Chin J Integr Med, 2009, 15 (3): 193-197.

[6] Wug L, Fan YS, Han YM, et al. Effect of Yangyin Jiedu Huoxue Recipe on Hormone Withdrawal and Disease Activity in Patients with Systemic Lupus Erythematosus. Chin J Integr Tradit West Med, 2009, 29 (9): 780-782. Chinese.

[7] Song XR, HOU SX. Research progress in the reversion of traditional Chinese medicine on

第六章

multidrug resistance of tumor. China Journal of Chinese Materia Medica, 2005, 30 (16)：1300-1304. Chinese.

[8] Xu H, Chen KJ. Integrative medicine：the experience from China. J Altern Complem Med, 2008, 14 (1)：3-7.

[9] Sun M, Zhan XP, Jin CY, et al. Clinical observation on treatment of post-craniocerebral traumatic mental disorder by integrative medicine. Chin J Integr Med, 2008, 14 (2)：137-141.

[10] Fu XX, Xiao WJ, Lu J, et al. Retrospective analysis of thrombolysis therapy for 64 cases of acute myocardial infarction with elevated ST segment. Chin J Integr Med, 2009,15 (6)：462-465.

Integrating Traditional Medicine with Biomedicine towards a Patient-Centered Healthcare System[*]

XU Hao　　CHEN Ke-ji

In this new age of scientific developments, biomedicine makes it possible for us to draw precise pictures of the internal workings of the human body, measure tiny metabolic reactions, exchange organs from one person to another, and even grow babies in test tubes. These accomplishments have enabled us to alter successfully and dramatically the natural history of many diseases. Nobody can detract from these achievements, and it is a matter of course for biomedicine to be regarded as conventional medicine or mainstream medicine. However, biomedicine is at its limits nowadays when confronting degenerative diseases, stress-related diseases, and most chronic diseases, which are more related to the way we think and live than to bacteria and viruses. Most notably, biomedicine lacks reference to the self-healing capacity of the human mind and body and focuses on parts rather than the whole, treatment rather than prevention, the suffering disease rather than the diseased person.

Confronted with these problems, more and more far-sighted western scholars began to lay their eyes on traditional medicine (TM).

According to the definition from the World Health Organization (WHO), TM refers to the knowledge, skills, and practices based on the theories, beliefs, and experiences indigenous to different cultures, used in the maintenance of health and in the prevention, diagnosis, improvement, or treatment of physical and mental illnesses. TM therapies include medication therapies—if they involve use of herbal medicines, animal parts, and/or minerals—and nonmedication therapies—if they are carried out primarily without the use of medication as in the case of acupuncture, manual therapies, and spiritual therapies. In countries where the dominant healthcare system is based on biomedicine, or where TM has not been integrated into the national healthcare system, TM is often termed "complementary", "alternative", or "non-conventional" medicine or used interchangeably with TM[1,2].

It is well established that TM plays an important role in healthcare for the majority of the population living in developing countries. In fact, TM was even the only healthcare system available to the prevention and treatment of diseases in different cultures for centuries. For

* 原载于 Chinese Journal of Integrative Medicine, 2011，17 (2)：83-84

example, Chinese medicine (CM) has a history of thousands of years and has made great contributions to the health and well-being of the people and to the maintenance and growth of the population. Currently, more than 90% of the urban and rural Chinese population has sought for CM in their lifetimes[3,4]. In Africa, up to 80% of the population uses TM to help meet their healthcare needs. In Asia and Latin America, populations continue to use TM as a result of historical circumstances and cultural beliefs. Meanwhile, in many developed countries, complementary and alternative medicine (CAM) is becoming more and more popular. The percentage of the population that has used CAM at least once is 48% in Australia, 70% in Canada, 42% in USA, 38% in Belgium, and 75% in France[2]. In addition, information derived from various systems of TM even plays an important role in drug discovery[5], and over 50% of the best-selling pharmaceuticals we are using today are derived from natural products.

TM covers a wide variety of therapies and practices, such as CM, Japan Kampo medicine, Indian Ayurveda medicine, Unani medicine, and various forms of indigenous medicine. In this issue, Dr. Motoo et al.[6] introduce the history and current status of Japan Kampo medicine, from which the experience of integrating Kampo into modern medicine in Japan is quite worthwhile to learn. Dr. Balasubramani et al.[7] review the basics of Rasayana therapy from Ayurveda and the published researches on different Rasayana drugs for specific health conditions, which may provide candidates for the development of antioxidants and immunomodulators. Dr. Yesilada[8] discusses the contribution of Unani medicine or Islamic medicine in the healthcare system of the Middle East. The rich tradition of the Middle East communities in the utilization of herbal remedies as well as diverse spiritual techniques for treating various disorders is very impressive. Dr. Omonzejele et al.[9] show us metaphysical and value underpinnings of TM in

West Africa. His investigation indicated that a large number of Africans consider sicknesses as having both physical and supernatural components. Although the strategies used to checkmate spiritual causes, such as the use of sacrifices and the transference of illnesses to animals and other objects, seem to be a little mysterious and unimaginable, its positive aspects might still be taken as references by modern psychotherapy and mind-body medicine.

It is indisputable that the ultimate goal of any medicine is to improve health of mankind and enhance the therapeutic effect in preventing and treating diseases. In this sense, any medicine should be patient-centered. All kinds of available therapeutic approaches, as long as safe and effective, should be embraced in the same healthcare family. Under this circumstance, the concept and practice of integrative medicine (IM) emerges as the times require[10-12]. TMs are most precious treasures from our ancestors to build a patient-centered healthcare system. WHO has been promoting TM as a source of less expensive, comprehensive medical care, especially in developing countries[2]. However, most TMs have not been successfully integrated into their national healthcare systems. For example, in Africa and Latin America, TMs are completely separated from conventional medicine. There is no communication, no integration.

Worldwide, only China, the Democratic People's Republic of Korea, the Republic of Korea, and Viet Nam can be considered to have attained an integrative system[2]. Especially in China, the integration of CM and western medicine has been explored for more than a century. The experience has exemplified the tolerance, dependence, and assimilation of not only two medicines but also other science disciplines in IM[3], and provided a paradigm for worldwide IM[13,14]. Most importantly, treatment modalities that are not considered part of mainstream medicine equally deserve evaluation and research, and should be considered as opportunities that serve to enrich and perfect conventional medicine rather than be viewed as competitors or disregarded. Some characteristics of CM, such as the concepts of seeing the body as a whole, preventive treatment of disease（Zhi Wei Bing, 治未病）, living in harmony with the environment（Tian Ren Xiang Ying, 天人相应）, treatment based on CM pattern differentiation, and compound prescriptions with synergistic effect, will also provide biomedicine with new perspectives.

Of course, there are still many difficulties in integrating TM into the overall healthcare systems partly due to the insufficient evidence in clinical settings and the problems in safety and quality control. Nevertheless, it is our dream that, in the future, diverse modalities, such as herbal medicine, acupuncture, moxibustion, Tuina bodywork, spiritual therapies, chiropractic, homeopathy, osteopathy, naturopathy, and many other TM therapies, as well as biomedicine can work in conjunction with each other as part of a unified team rather than in competition. This integrative approach will ultimately lead to a safer, more convenient, and effective patient-centered healthcare system.

References

[1] World Health Organization. General guidelines for methodologies on research and evaluation of traditional medicine. 2000. http：//whqlibdoc.who.int/hq/2000/WHO_EDM_TRM_2000.1.pdf.

[2] World Health Organization. Traditional medicine strategy 2002-2005. 2002. http：//whqlibdoc.who.int/hq/2002/WHO_EDM_TRM_2002.1.pdf

[3] Xu H, Chen KJ. Integrative medicine：the experience from China. J Altern Complem Med, 2008，14：3-7.

[4] Lu AP, Ding XR, Chen KJ. Current situation and progress in integrative medicine in China. Chin J Integr Med, 2008, 14：234-240.

[5] Fabricant DS, Farnsworth NR. The value of plants used in traditional medicine for drug discovery. Environ Health Perspect, 2001, 109 (Suppl 1)：69-75.

[6] Motoo Y, Seki T, Tsutani K. Traditional Japanese medicine, Kampo：its history and current status. Chin J Integr Med, 2011, 17：85-87.

[7] Balasubramani SP, Venkatasubramanian P, Kumar SK, et al. Plant based Rasayana drugs from Ayurveda. Chin J Integr Med, 2011, 17：88-94.

[8] Yesilada E. Contribution of traditional medicine in the health care system of the Middle East. Chin J Integr Med, 2011, 17：95-98.

[9] Omonzejele PF, Maduka C. Metaphysical and value underpinnings of traditional medicine in West Africa. Chin J Integr Med, 2011, 17：99-104.

[10] Rees L, Weil A. Integrated medicine. BMJ, 2001, 322：119-120.

[11] Eisenberg D. Reflections on the past and future of integrative medicine from a lifelong student of the integration of Chinese and western medicine. Chin J Integr Med, 2011, 17：3-5.

[12] Weil A. The state of the Integrative Medicine in the U.S. and western World. Chin J Integr Med, 2011, 17：6-10.

[13] Dobos G, Tao I. The model of western integrative medicine：the role of Chinese medicine. Chin J Integr Med, 2011, 17：11-20.

[14] Robinson N. Integrative medicine—traditional Chinese medicine, a model? Chin J Integr Med, 2011, 17：21-25.

第六章

Chinese Medicine Pattern Diagnosis Could Lead to Innovation in Medical Sciences[*]

LU Ai-ping   CHEN Ke-ji

Chinese medicine (CM) is a system with its own rich tradition and over 3000 years of continuous practice and refinement through observation. Pattern diagnosis (Bianzheng or syndrome differentiation) is the hallmark in CM, and CM intervention is based primarily on the pattern classification.

CM pattern is the basic unit in its diagnosis, and it is determined by analysis on all symptoms and signs, including tongue appearances and pulse feelings with CM concepts. Nowadays, CM pattern diagnosis and biomedical diagnosis is integrated, and integrative medicine becomes common model in clinical practice. In the view of integrative medicine CM pattern could be regarded as the summary of the body's condition at a certain stage in a disease process. However, CM pattern is more complicated in defining ill state since CM pattern could change following the CM pattern information (symptoms, signs, tongue appearance, and pulse feelings) and more combined pattern would show up in many cases.

CM pattern classification, as another patient classification approaches, has been incorporated with biomedicine diagnosis in clinical practice in China, and the clinical experience for long time could prove that the integration of biomedicine and CM is better in the treatment of many diseases[1]. Also the research on CM pattern has become a hot topic in CM and integrative field. Since CM pattern diagnosis is completely different from the diagnosis in biomedicine and CM pattern classification has been proven to be an effective way for patient classification, CM pattern diagnosis would lead more scientific new findings for medical sciences. In this paper, how CM pattern diagnosis lead to innovations in medical sciences, including in basic research, clinical research and new drug research and development, is discussed.

1. CM Pattern Diagnosis and Innovation in Basic Research

CM pattern diagnosis, as a classification approach, could be used together with disease diagnosis. At that point, CM pattern diagnosis could lead to some new findings for diagnostics in medical sciences. Some studies of Chinese medicinal herbs used in a specified CM pattern have confirmed a biological basis for CM effect, and the results included the linkage between sex hormones and Kidney deficiency pattern in chronic nephritis[2], linkage between C-reactive protein (CRP) and cold/hot pattern in rheumatoid arthritis (RA)[3], linkage between homeorheology and blood stasis pattern in cardiovascular diseases[4], and linkage between gastric mucosal immune reactions and the CM pattern in chronicgastritis[5]. The correlation analysis between CM pattern information and biomedical parameter is one part of basic research in integrative medicine, which might lead to new findings in medical sciences.

On the other hand, full understanding of the inherent mechanism of the CM pattern in a disease could help further exploration in pathogenesis study for the disease. Yet, it is very difficult to implement the exploration using existing conventional methods[6]. The advances of

* 原载于 Chinese Journal of Integrative Medicine, 2011, 17 (11): 811-817

"Omics" revolution and methodology in modern life science, bioinformatics and systems biology have offered an opportunity to integrate multi-dimensional and various types of data, and capturing these unprecedented opportunities and challenges, bioinformatics and systems biology approaches are expected to open the way to a new convergence of CM pattern information and biomedicine in both concept and methodology. In the exploration on the biological basis of CM patterns, the molecular basis of CM pattern within the context of neuro-endocrine-immune (NEI) system was explored[7]. Our previous studies showed that there were some distinct molecular signatures in discriminating the RA patients with CM cold pattern and heat pattern with related syndrome[8]. Thus more important innovation in basic research might be from the correlation analysis among CM patterns with bioinformatics.

CM pattern diagnosis in a disease also could help find some new ideas for the pathogenesis of the disease. The treatment of RA with CM intervention in the later stage of the disease usually focuses on the blood stasis and deficiency CM pattern[9]. While CM blood stasis pattern shows some linkage with platelet activity[10], the CM deficiency pattern shows some linkage with immune response[11]. Thus it is reasonable to make the hypothesis that there is a positive correlation among IgA (reflecting immune response), platelet and cartilage erosion (severe in late stage) in RA. The changes in peripheral IgA level and platelet number positively correlated with the grade of cartilage damage in active RA patients, thus supporting the hypothesis[12,13]. In the clinical practice, the Chinese herbal medicine with activating blood stasis pattern, and those reinforcing deficiency pattern and containing polysaccharides or animal proteins were used for the treatment [14]. In summary, biomedical sciences not only help identify the scientific basis for CM pattern, but also can improve further clarification of CM pattern.

Another important concept in CM named as "Treating Different Diseases with the Same Therapy" has been applied in CM practice. This means that two patients with different disease diagnoses will receive similar Chinese medical treatments if their Chinese patterns are similar. For instance, some patients with RA and other with coronary heart disease (CHD) can be treated with similar therapies (for example, activation of blood stasis for RA patients with CM pattern of blood stasis). This suggests that there could be something commonly existing between RA and CHD conditions according to CM diagnosis within the context of imbalance in the body functions biological networks or biological basis. Because of the complexity of human being, possible novel and groundbreaking connections between diseases are often missed by researchers even though they can be readily inferred from the existing literatures.[15]

In recent years, data mining methods have been used on large literature databases to extract new and meaningful information, and many researches hare shown that data mining can both model complex biological pathways and serve the purpose of hypothesis generation and biological discovery[16]. Data mining approaches are also used for CM to identify required information more efficiently, discover new relationships which are obscured by merely focusing on biomedicine, and bridge thegaps between biomedicine and CM [17]. In order to substantiate such concepts, there exists a need to search for these interlinking data from reliable databases. Presently in our leading research database the amount of biomedical data is growing rapidly, it is possible toget relevant and meaningful information through the techniques developed in the fields of data mining. Our previous study proposed an hierarchical analysis algorithm called discrete derivatives which is based on the frequencies of co-concurrent "The Medical Subject Headings" (MeSH) terms, we have found some significant results which can support the conce treating different disease with same therapy (TDDST), and also that the biological basis and biological networks commonly existing in RA and CHD. These networks can be affected by the basic Chinese material medica, which are widely used in the CM therapies on both RA and CHD[18]. Also, we retrieved data and calculated the biological networks/basis on biomedicine commonly existed in both RA and ulcerative colitis (UC). RA and UC are both autoimmune disorders. They can be treated with the same CM formula when they are sharing the same CM pattern even though they are different in biomedicine. The results showed that the biological network centered with IgG and CRP is important to both RA and UC[19]. In addition, in a 2010 study, RA, CHD, and diabetes mellitus (DM) were selected to explore the potential biological network shared in these three diseases. By means of association analysis method, four main networks were presented including oxidation reduction, apoptosis, visualization and sex hormone. It suggested that data mining could be the starting for the modern research on pattern in CM[20]. Although the results showed the potential shared network for different diseases and the real study either in animal or hurts are needed for further validation, the sharing same CM pattern in different diseases could lead new findings for those related diseases.

2. CM Pattern Diagnosis and Innovation in Clinical Research

Over the past 50 years, clinical practice in CM hospitals in China has applied both principles of biomedical disease diagnosis and CM pattern classification for intervention/ treatment of patients. A clinical investigation indicated that a more effective treatment rate could be achieved for RA patients when co-diagnosed and treated based on their CM pattern classification[21]. Therefore CM pattern diagnosis could lead to innovation in clinical study, which further helps more specific classification and improvement of efficacy.

Evaluation of CM treatment efficacy should focus on a specific subgroup of patients with a specific disease, or a specific herbal preparation with clinically-proven effectiveness. As CM pattern classification focuses on further classification of the patients into treatment subgroup, the treatment efficacy would be improved if the responsive cases can be clarified from non-responsive cases with their CM patterns. It has been reported that the CM pattern classification can specify the indications for the combination biomedical therapy in the treatment of existing RA patients[22]. The results suggest that it may also be useful in defining specific indications for biomedical therapies used to treat other diseases. Symptoms are diversified, and more attention should be paid to CM symptom study. The extraarticular symptoms are important in CM pattern classification for RA, and the study by Zhang, et al[23] showed that RA patients with "cold intolerance" and "cold joints", which are the extraarticular symptoms that CM practitioners focus on, may show higher American College of Rheumatology (ACR) 20 response. Another important CM sign is tongue appearance. Our previous study explored the associations between the tongue appearances in CM and ACR20 in RA patients treated with CM and biomedical combination therapy. RA patients with white tongue coating showed higher effective rate (ACR20 response) than those patients with yellow tongue coating in the treatment with biomedicine[24].

In addition, CM pattern diagnosis could help find a predictor of the adverse reaction for clinical practice since CM pattern could identify more specific subjects for the intervention. Our previous has explored the risk factors on the gastrointestinal adverse drug reactions (GI ADRs) and hepatic ADRs in the treatment of RA with conventional Western medicine and CM therapy, and the results showed that total ADRs incidence and withdrawal rates were similar in two groups, and in the patients treated with Western medicine, CRP level was negatively related to GI ADRs, dizziness was positively related to GI ADRs, and IgG level and chills were positively related to hepatic ADRs；and in the patients treated with CM, no laboratory measurements were found related with GI ADRs and hepatic ADRs, lassitude and nocturia were risk factors for GI ADRs, cold extremities for hepatic ADRs, respectively[25]. The results suggest that CM related symptoms could be a predictor for ADR events in RA treatment.

CM pattern could help identify the subgroup of patients with a specific disease, and it should be used for identification of subgroup of patients for biomedical therapy. Our previous study explored the role of CM pattern differentiation in defining more specific indications for combination biomedical therapy in the treatment of RA. This study uses data from a multi-center randomized-controlled clinical trial. The total of 194 patients were treated with combination biomedical therapy (diclofenec, methotrexate and sulfasalazine). The results showed that the effective rates in the patients with cold pattern and hot pattern were 51.67% and 29.09%，respectively, after 12-week treatment；88.52% and 55.36%，respectively, after 24 weeks of treatment with the biomedical combination therapy[23]. The results suggest that CM pattern differentiation based on symptoms can help specify the indications for combination biomedical therapy in the treatment of RA. It may also be useful in defining specific indications for biomedical therapies used to treat other diseases.

On the other hand, intervention in different CM patterns might lead to different toxic response, which further leads to better application of the intervention. *Tripferygium Wilfordii Multiglycoside* (GTW), an authorized Chinese patent drug, is used for treatment of RA and other immune disease. We explored whether GTW induced different toxic reactions in adjuvant arthritis rats (AA rats) compared with those in normal rats.

The results showed that the serum aspartate aminotransferase (AST) level was significantly decreased in AA rats under exposure GTW compared with normal rats in the same condition, which indicated that GTW could offer a different liver toxic reaction in normal and AA rats, and the metabolic analysis showed that a clear separation of principal component analysis (PCA) and partial-least-squares discriminate analysis (PLS-DA) score spot in normal rats, but not separation was seen in AA rats perturbed with low dosage GTW, and the biomarker analysis showed that the level of lysophosphatidylcholines (LPC) was down-regulated, but the level of ursodeoxycholic acid (UDCA) and chenodexycholic acid (CDCA) was up-regulated in AA rats compared with normal rats under exposure GTW. We concluded that GTW could induce different toxic reactions between normal and AA rats, and the lipid metabolism might be part of the mechanism for the hepatic lipidosis or the other liver injury[26]. Therefore CM pattern diagnosis could help us apply the intervention correctly.

CM pattern diagnosis also could help design better clinical trial if the trial could be based on the integration of disease diagnosis and CM pattern diagnosis. CM pattern can help choose the most appropriate intervention and could be included in the clinical trial. However, the common randomized controlled trial design has distinct limitations when applied to CM, because CM identifies and treats "CM pattern" rather than only diagnosed diseases. These limitations could be overcome by developing new strategy to evaluate the effect of CM. The idea behind CM pattern-based efficacy evaluation may optimize the clinical trial design by finding out the responsiveness related CM pattern. It can be designed as a two-stage multi-center trial of Chinese herbal medicine for the management of RA[27]. The stage one trial is an open-label trial and aims to explore what groups of CM information (such as symptoms) correlates

第六章

with better efficacy, and the stage two trial is a randomized, controlled, double-blind, double-dummy clinical trial that incorporates the efficacy-related information identified in the stage-one trial into the inclusion criteria. The indication of a Chinese herbal formula is a specific CM pattern and not a single disease and stratifying a disease into several patterns with a group of symptoms is a feasible procedure in clinical trials. Therefore CM pattern diagnosis must help design innovative clinical trial for demonstration of better efficacy of the intervention.

Clinical practice guideline (CPG) is important for clinical practice. and CM pattern diagnosis should be integrated in the process of forming CPG. Take Chinese patent medicine (CPM) for example, there are 1063 kinds of CPMs recorded in the Chinese Pharmacopoeia (2010 edition), and for the treatment of a single disease, there might have more than tens of CPMs marketed in past 30 years. However, there is no higher quality CPG or consensus about CPMs application for the treatment of diseases based on CM pattern diagnosis. In the view of CM, different CPMs must be used for different subsets (CM patterns) of patients. To develop the CPGs for the treatment of disease with CPMs seems to be difficult since lack of high-quality randomized controlled trials recently. On the other hand, in clinical practice, more CPMs are used by biomedical doctors in China, and those doctors did not get well trained in CM, and thus it is difficult to train them in applying CPMs based on CM pattern differentiation theory. Therefore, it is important to form consensus for CPM application in the treatment of disease, and more importantly the guidelines should be illustrated with words both understandable in CM and biomedicine. Fortunately, understandable symptoms are the major evidence for CM pattern classification, and forming an expert consensus is possible if the experts in related fields with rich clinical experience in CPMs application can involve in the consultation. Thus, the expert consensus can be

formed for the treatment of diseases with CPMs, which could help the Western medicine doctors to use CPMs correctly. This is another way to help Western medicine doctors understand CM pattern.

3. CM Pattern Diagnosis and New Drug Discovery

Classical drug discovery is designed to find new chemicals that target a specific disease. It focuses on formulating new drugs. CM considers that all natural products can act as drugs for the treatment of disease when they are found effective in certain patients with specific CM patterns. It focuses on tailoring patients to the drug. It is possible to have a new approach for drug discovery based on such specific criteria for existing drugs. To find "new" drugs by finding the specific indications of existing drugs or natural products can be realized by consecutive clinical trials. More new drugs were denied for marketing since the effectiveness was not higher enough in a classical clinical trial. If we further analyze the clinical data, and find out the differences between the effective cases and non-effective cases based on CM theory by using symptoms and other biomedical markers, the narrowed potential indication for the new drug might be defined. Then we can conduct the next round clinical trial with the new indication. Hopefully the effective rate will be higher enough for marketing.

To find a more specific indication for an existed drug is the first step for making the drug to be a new drug. It would be realized by figuring out what are positively or negatively related to the efficacy. The correlated factors could be obtained by comparing the differences between the effective cases and non-effective cases if there is enough information in the first clinical trial. In a clinical trial, the case report form contains mainly the diagnostic related information; however more information could be obtained from the patients. Many non-diagnostic related symptoms which CM focuses (such as thirst in RA, heavy limbs in diabetes), non-diagnostic related laboratory measurements, and pharmaco-metabolomical, pharmaco-genomicat and pharmaco-proteinomical information aimed to realize the individual therapy should be collected for the comparison between the effective cases and non-effective cases[28]. The next round of randomized clinical trial would have a more specific indication with adding the efficacy-correlated information into the inclusion and exclusion, and the efficacy of the drug in this clinical trial could be higher comparing with the first one since the indication is more specific for the drug. Similarly, more round of clinical trial could be conducted basing on the previous one. The analysis on a clinical trial on an herbal product in RA shows that some non-diagnostic related symptoms correlated with the efficacy of the drug, and the efficacy would be higher if the correlated information were put back to the database[29]. Therefore the way to find a more specific indication for an existed drug might be a new approach for new drug discovery.

Network pharmacology develops rapidly and contribute great progresses in new drug research and development, and it is focusing on disease related drug target based on disease network[30]. We believe that integration of disease network with CM pattern network could lead to further exploration for new drug discovery since CM pattern is another important factor for patient classification. There have enough data for building up a disease network, such as RA network[31], however, we need more data from patients with CM pattern for CM pattern network formation. Our previous study investigated the networks between RA patients with CM cold pattern and hot pattern from a microarray data of CD4 lymphocytes in RA patients with CM cold and hot patterns. Four genes were in higher expression and 21 genes in lower expression were shown in the patients with CM cold pattern comparing with those in the patients with hot

pattern. Four highly-connected regions were obtained from protein-protein interaction network analysis on these differentially expressed genes. The most relevant pathways extracted from these subnetworks for the RA patients with hot pattern were small G protein signaling pathways based on higher expressed TIAM1, fatty acid metabolism based on higher expressed ALOX5, and T cell proliferation increases based on lower expressed EGR1, higher expressed H2AFX and LIG1. We concluded that small G protein signaling pathways, fatty acid metabolism and T cell proliferation might be the key pathogenic factors for RA with CM hot pattern. We believe that screening of herbal products or components in the integration of CM cold or hot pattern network with RA network could help find out more new drug leads for new drug discovery[32].

Another issue in CM pattern based network pharmacology for new drug discovery is that it is hard to build up the network of herbal medicines[33]. In recent years, the available data of CM therapy used to treat some diseases continue to accumulate rapidly, and there are more data mining approaches used for such kind of data analysis. Text mining can retrieve knowledge hidden in text and present the distilled knowledge such as the possible therapeutic network based mechanisms. The therapeutic mechanism of a drug is in fact a biological network comprising hundreds to thousands of gene expressions changed in various affected tissues and effector cells. Systems biology approaches predict biological network, can lead to a deeper understanding of system as a whole. Our previous studies combined text mining with methods of systems biology, to predict functional networks for therapeutic mechanisms of CM. An example is that we combine text mining with methods of systems biology for the first time, to predict functional networks for therapeutic mechanisms of *Salvia miltiorrhiza* in atherosclerosis treatment. The text mining results indicated atherosclerosis highly associated with *Salvia miltiorrhiza*, and six genes associated with both. Protein-protein interaction information for these genes from databases and literature data was searched and visualized using cytoscape. Four highly-connected regions were detected by incremental principal component analysis (IPCA) algorithm to infer significant complexes or pathways in this network. The most relevant functions and pathways extracted from these subnetworks by BINGO tool were related to 1-kappaB kinase/NF-kappaB cascade, regulation of cellular process, regulation of biological process, which were consistent with previously published studies. Interestingly, insulin receptor signaling pathway was also implicated by network-based analysis in our study. The results suggested that therapeutic mechanisms of *Salvia miltiorrhiza* in atherosclerosis should be involved in increasing sensitivity and/or responsiveness to metabolic actions of insulin. Therefore the network based pharmacological exploration would be helpful for clarifying the mechanism of Chinese herbal medicines, and more importantly, herbal medicine network, if integrated with CM pattern network in a disease network, could help find out more new drug leading for new drug discovery.

In conclusion, CM pattern diagnosis is not only a classification approach for patients in CM, but also a resource for innovation in medical sciences, including the innovation in basic research, clinical research and new drug discovery.

References

[1] Lu AP, Chen KJ. Integrative medicine in clinical practice: from pattern differentiation in traditional Chinese medicine to disease treatment. Chin J Integr Med, 2009, 15: 152.

[2] Zhang Q, Wu Z, Fang Y, et al. Levels of sexual hormones in relation with syndrome-differentiation of traditional Chinese medicine in patients of chronic renal failure. J Tradit Chin Med, 1990, 10: 132-135.

[3] Zha QL, He YT, Yu JP. Correlations between diagnostic information and therapeutic efficacy in rheumatoid arthritis analyzed with decision tree model. Chin J Integr Tradit West Med, 2006, 26: 871-876.

[4] Xu H, Chen KJ. Making evidence-based decisions in the clinical practice of integrative medicine. Chin J Integr Med, 2010, 16: 483-485.

[5] Lu AP, Zhang SS, Zha QL, et al. Correlation between CD4, CD8 cell infiltration ingastric mucosa, helicobacterpylori infection and symptoms in patients with chronicgastritis. World J Gastroenterol, 2005, 11: 2486-2490.

[6] Lu AP. Think much of the study on TCM syndrome differentiation of rheumatoid arthritis. Chin J Integr Tradit West Mad, 2007, 27: 587-588.

[7] Li Y, Li S, Lu AP. Comparative analysis via data mining on the clinical features of Western medicine and Chinese medicine in diagnosing rheumatoid arthritis. Chin J Integr Tradit West Med, 2006, 26: 988-991.

[8] Lu C, Zha Q, Chang A, et al. Pattern differentiation in traditional Chinese Medicine can help define specific indications for biomedical therapy in the treatment of rheumatoid arthritis. J Altern Complement Med, 2009, 15: 1021-1025.

[9] Zhou X, Zhou Z, Jin M, et al. Intermediate and late rheumatoid arthritis treated by tonifying the kidney, resolving phlegm and removing blood stasis. J Tradit Chin Med, 2000, 20: 87-92.

[10] Li HX, Han SY, Wang XW, et al. Effect of the carthamins yellow from *Carthamus tinctorius* L. on hemorheological disorders of blood stasis in rats. Food Chem Toxicol, 2009, 47: 1797-1802.

[11] Yuang Q, Jia ZH, Yang HT, et al. Comfortable lifestyle-induced imbalance of neuro-endocrine-immunity network: a possible mechanism of vascular endothelial dysfunction. Chin J Integr Med, 2010, 16: 54-60.

[12] Zha Q, He Y, Lu Y, et al. Relationship between platelet counts and cartilage erosion in 436 cases of rheumatoid arthritis. Clin Chim Acta, 2006, 371: 194-195.

[13] He Y, Zha Q, Liu D, et al. Relations between serum IgA level and cartilage erosion in 436 cases of rheumatoid arthritis. Immunol Invest, 2007, 36: 285-291.

[14] Yang W, Ouyang J, Zhu K, et al. Traditional Chinese medicine treatment for 40 cases of rheumatoid arthritis with channel blockage due to yin deficiency. J Tradit Chin Med, 2003, 23: 172-174.

[15] Swanson DR. Medical literature as a potential source of new knowledge. Bull Med Libr Assoc, 1990, 78：29-37.

[16] Daraselia N, Yuryev A, Egorov S, et al. Extracting human protein interactions from MEDLINE using a full-sentence parser. Bioinformatics, 2004, 20：604-611.

[17] Zhou X, Liu B, Wu Z, F et al. Integrative mining of traditional Chinese medicine literature and MEDLINE for functional gene networks. Artif Intell Med, 2007, 41：87-104.

[18] Zheng G, Jiang M, He X, et al. Discrete derivative：a data slicing algorithm for exploration of sharing biological networks between rheumatoid arthritis and coronary heart disease. BioData Min, 2011, 4：18.

[19] Ding X, Zha Q, Lu A. Seeking potential biological network shared in rheumatoid arthritis and ulcerative colitis through text mining. Bioinformatics and Biomedical Engineering, 2009, ICBBE 2009.

[20] Ding X, Zha Q, Lu A. Getting started in text mining to find the biological network shared with reumatoid arthritis, coronary heart disease and diabetes mellitus. Bioinformatics and Biomedicine Workshops, 2010, BIBMW 2010.

[21] He Y, Lu A, Zha Y, et al. Correlations between symptoms as assessed in traditional Chinese medicine (TCM) and ACR20 efficacy response：a comparison study in 396 patients with rheumatoid arthritis treated with traditional Chinese medicine or Western medicine. J Clin Rheumatol, 2007, 13：317-321.

[22] Van Wietmarschen H, Yuan K, Lu C, et al. Systems biology guided by Chinese medicine reveals new markers for sub-typing rheumatoid arthritis patients. J Clin Rheumatol, 2009, 15：330-337.

[23] Zhang C, Zha QL, He YT, et al. The extraarticular symptoms influence ACR response in the treatment of rheumatoid arthritis with biomedicine：a single-blind, randomized, controlled, multicenter trial in 194 patients. J Tradit Chin Med, 2011, 31：50-55.

[24] Jiang M, Zha Q, Lu C, et al. Association between tongue appearance in traditional Chinese medicine and effective response in treatment of rheumatoid arthritis. Complement Ther Med, 2011, 19：115-121.

[25] Jiang M, Zha Q, He Yi, et al. Risk factors of adverse drug reactions in the treatment of rheumatoid arthritis with biomedical combination and Chinese herbal medicine therapy. J Ethnopharmacol, 2011. In press.

[26] Li J, Lu Y, Xiao C, et al. Comparison of toxic reaction of Tripterygium wilfordii multiglycoside in normal and adjuvant arthritic rats. J Ethnopharmacol, 2011, 135：270-277.

[27] Zhang C, Jiang M, Lu A. A traditional Chinese medicine versus Western combination therapy in the treatment of rheumatoid arthritis：two-stage study protocol for a randomized controlled trial. Trials, 2011, 12：137.

[28] Evans WE, Rolling MV. Moving towards individualized medicine with pharmacogenomics. Nature, 2004, 429：464-468.

[29] He Y, Lu A, Zha Y, et al. Correlations between symptoms and ACR20 efficacy in 396 cases of rheumatoid arthritis. J Ctin Rheumatol, 2007, 13：317-321.

[30] Andrew L Hopkins. Network pharmacology. Nature Biotechnolo, 2007, 25：1110-1111.

[31] Chen G, Liu B, Jiang M, et al. Functional networks for *Salvia mittiorrhiza* and *Panax notoginseng* in combination explored with text mining and bioinformatical approach. JMPR, 2011, 23 [Epub ahead of print].

[32] Lu C, Xiao C, Cheng G, et al. Cold and heat pattern of rheumatoid arthritis in traditional Chinese medicine：distinct molecular signatures indentified by microarray expression profiles in CD4-positive T cell. Rheumatol Int, 2010. （PubMed：20658292] [Epub ahead of print].

[33] Ma XH, Zheng CJ, Han LY, et al. Synergistic therapeutic actions of herbal ingredients and their mechanisms from molecular interaction and network perspectives. Drug Discov Today, 2009, 14：579-588.

第六章

New Findings Validate An Ancient Technique: How Massage Affects the Biochemistry of Inflammation*

Genevieve HSIA   CHEN Ke-ji

Massage is a manual soft tissue manipulation, and includes holding, causing movement, and/or applying pressure to the body defined by American Massage Therapy Association (AMTA). References to massage can be found in many ancient civilizations. The ancient Chinese medical book called *Huangdi's Internal Classic* (Huang Di Nei Jing, 2760 BC) recommended "use massage therapy for treatment of numbness caused by channels blockage".

There is no legal scope of practice for massage professionals in USA. The scope of practice for massage therapy is generally determined by who regulates the profession. In Ontario, the Scope of Practice Statement of Massage Therapists as defined by the Massage Therapy Act, 1991 is: "The practice of massage therapy is the assessment of the soft tissue and joints of the body and the treatment and prevention of physical dysfunction and pain of the soft tissues and joints by manipulation to develop, maintain, rehabilitate or augment physical function, or relieve pain."

Massage is getting popular according to the 2011 AMTA consumer survey, an average of 18 percent of adult Americans received at least one massage between July 2010 and July 2011. Forty-four percent of adult Americans who had a massage between July 2010 and July 2011 received it for medical or health reasons compared to 35 percent the previous year.

Accumulating evidence from clinical and laboratory studies is revealing that massage has measurable, beneficial, biochemical effects. It is not simply an emotional experience or mechanical effect. Implications of these discoveries have immediate relevance.

First, researchers have found that massage promotes mitochondrial biogenesis, specifically- and most interesting-by mitigating the rise in nuclear factor $_\kappa$B (NF-$_\kappa$B) nuclear accumulation and by modulating Peroxisome proliferator-activated receptor gamma coactivator 1 (PGC-1) alpha levels. After exercise-induced muscle damage, Crane, et al[1] found that massage significantly reduced NF-$_\kappa$ B nuclear accumulation. The activation of the NF-$_\kappa$ B pathway has been associated with the pathogenesis of many inflammatory diseases[2]. The key physiological function of NF-$_\kappa$ B appears to be the orchestration of inflammatory responses to both infection and tissue damage[3]. Second, it appears that massage specifically potentiates mitochondrial biogenesis signaling by increasing production of PGC-1alpha[1]. PGC-1alpha is involved in a host of age-related disorders, starting with loss of muscle integrity[4]. Lab testing found PGC-1alpha also promotes recovery after acute kidney injury during systemic inflammation in mice[5], suggesting yet another avenue of research. Multiple sclerosis patients derive benefit from complementary and alternative medicine (CAM) therapies such as acupuncture and massage[6]; if PGC-1alpha is involved in these effects, massage could potentially be used therapeutically for this condition as well. A third, more general lesson to be learned from these specific findings is that massage has complex metabolic effects. With deeper understanding of the underlying

* 原载于 Chinese Journal of Integrative Medicine, 2012, 18 (7): 483-484

biochemical subtleties, treatment of many conditions can be improved. Over centuries, anecdotal evidence supports the use and value of massage. In ancient Chinese texts, massage was mentioned as a treatment modality even before herbs. Recently, massage has been shown effective in: relieving back pain, boosting the immune system, reducing anxiety, lowering blood pressure, treating migraines and tendinopathy, decreasing carpal tunnel symptoms, easing post-operative pain, and alleviating the side effects of cancer. In all of these cases, further study can determine how and to what extent massage can alter the biochemistry to treat-perhaps also to prevent these conditions.

Last but not least, these findings sharply highlight the fact that the commonly held beliefs may not be true. Before these studies, it was widely claimed that massage eased sore muscles by squeezing lactic acid and/or other metabolic waste products out of muscles. There appears to be no scientific evidence for this claim. In what other areas will objective evidence show widely held beliefs to be nothing more than imaginative thinking? Every modality that works, in at least some cases, and especially those that have stood the test of time, need respect and rigorous investigation. CAM therapies such as acupuncture and Chinese herbs have been proven effective in some diseases. The same or similar researches can apply to them to see what the result will be. Those long history treatment experiences may bring surprising discoveries and new applications to get the medical credits with the evidence based researches or clinical trials.

References

[1] Crane JD, Ogborn DI, Cupido C, et al. Massage therapy attenuates inflammatory signaling after exercise-induced muscle damage. Sci Transl Med, 2012, 4 (119): 119ra13.

[2] Mora E, Guglielmotti A, Biondig, Sassone-Corsi P. Bindarit: an anti-inflammatory small molecule that modulates the NF$_K$B pathway. Cell Cycle, 2012, 11: 159-169.

[3] Mohamed RM, McFaddeng. NF$_K$B inhibitors: strategies from poxviruses. Cell Cycle, 2009, 8: 3125-3132

[4] Wenz T, Rossi SG, Rotundo RL, et al. Increased muscle PGC-1alpha expression protects from sarcopenia and metabolic disease during aging. Proc Natl Acad Sci USA, 2009, 106: 20405-20410.

[5] Tran M, Tam D, Bardia A, et al. PGC-1α promotes recovery after acute kidney injury during systemic inflammation in mice. J Clin Invest, 2011, 121: 4003-4014.

[6] Stoll SS, Nieves C, Tabby DS, et al. Use of therapies other than disease-modifying agents, including complementary and alternative medicine, by patients with multiple sclerosis: a survey study. J Am Osteopath Assoc, 2012, 112: 22-28.

Reflections on the Research Status of Kampo Medicine: A Most Rewarding Visit to Japan*

XU Hao　YIN Hui-jun

Traditional medicine in Japan originated from Chinese medicine (CM), on the basis of which the abdominal diagnosis and treatment by differentiation of diseases were developed. It was also called Kampo medicine (KM), natural medicine or oriental medicine. KM had been on

* 原载于 Chinese Journal of Integrative Medicine, 2010, 16 (4): 357-360

the verge of extinction by suffering from serious loss during the Meiji Restoration, and only started to revive in the beginning of the 1950s, and has had considerable progress up to now.

In order to further understand the status of KM in Japan and bring creative thought to the research on CM, on behalf of Academician CHEN Ke-ji (陈可冀)'s research group on the National Major Project for Fundamental Research and Development (973 Project), the authors visited the Institute of Natural Medicine at the University of Toyama and the Oriental Medicine Research Center of the Kitasato Institute in Tokyo consecutively for academic exchanges at the end of 2009. There were some general knowledge and reflections on KM in Japan during the authors' visit to the two famous Japanese KM research institutes, which could be summarized into five aspects as follows.

1. Theoretical Research of Kampo Medicine

Since the Meiji Restoration, traditional medicine in Japan experienced a seriously westernized tendency along with the introduction of Western medicine (WM). For KM, it was basically "wasting medicine and reserving the drug", and the essence of the syndrome differentiated treatment was abandoned, thus there were few studies on theoretical research on KM at that time. However, KM has received much more attention since the end of the 1970s. For example, the Science and Technology Agency formally mapped out a long-term plan for basic and clinical studies on KM, named "Scientific demonstration of syndromes (so-called 'Sho' in Japan) and meridian acupoints, assurance of crude drug resources" within a 5-year period and 1-billion yen funds' investment. Keeping "syndrome" as a key research project and "blood-stasis syndrome" as a principal target, studies on Kampo drugs mainly with the function of activating blood circulation and removing blood-stasis (ABCRBS), the mechanism of action in acupuncture and moxibustion, and assurance of crude drug resources, were conducted at the same time. The diagnostic criteria for the blood-stasis syndrome advanced by Prof. Katsutoshi Terasawa at Toyama Medical and Pharmaceutical University was formulated during this period[1], which not only had great influence on domestic researchers, but also played an active role in promoting the formulation of blood stasis diagnosis criteria in China and international studies on the blood stasis syndrome.

When we visited the Institute of Natural Medicine at the University of Toyama, Prof. Naotoshi Shibahara introduced the relationships between bloodstasis syndrome and bulbar conjunctival microcirculation, blood viscosity, aggregation and deformability of erythrocytes, concentration of fibrinogen as well as the effect of ABCRBS recipes and medicines. Interestingly, they found that *Cortex Cinnamomi* conveys the predominant vasodilation effect in Guizhi Fuling Pills (桂枝茯苓丸)[2,3]. Although the adopted measurements and indices were classical, the studies were very objective.

In addition, Japan has already begun to emphasize the analysis of the pathological changes and characteristics of syndromes by using modern scientific methods such as genetic engineering and immunological techniques, to clarify the syndrome's scientific connotation from its correlation with drug effects. A representative example was the project presided by Prof. Ikuo Saiki of the Pathological Biochemistry Department from the Institute of Natural Medicine at University of Toyama. With the aim of defining the blood stasis syndrome of KM, the method of plasma proteomics, cluster analysis and decision tree were adopted in this project. The results showed that the bloodstasis syndrome of KM had a material basis with regards to protein expression profile, and it could be expected to set up the objective standards of the blood stasis syndrome of KM by combining the methods of proteomics and bioinformatics classification[4].

第六章

2. Clinical Application of Kampo Me-dicine

In the *Medical Practitioners Law* of Japan, there is no setup of KM doctors. There is no formal qualification examination for KM doctors either. The medical practitioners who practice CM are actually WM physicians instead of being independently qualified KM doctors. However, WM physicians can only prescribe KM drugs according to diseases, which departs from the essence of syndrome differentiated treatment in KM. Thus, side effects or unfavorable effects of KM will inevitably occur.

For instance, Japan's Ministry of Health confirmed the effect of Xiaochaihu Decoction (小柴胡汤) on improving liver function and enlisted it in the national pharmacopoeia officially, which led to the spectacular event that tens of thousands of liver disease patients throughout Japan took this decoction concurrently. However, two years later, the side effects of Xiaochaihu Decoction led to interstitial hepatitis in 88 cases of patients with chronic hepatitis, and among them 10 patients died. After that, the sale of Xiaochaihu Decoction decreased by one third and the decoction was even in danger of exclusion from medical insurance. Of course, many patients were also taking WM while receiving KM therapy, so the adverse effects may also be related to the interaction between KM and WM, which had already aroused more and more attention in Japan. As we know, there were special research programs on drug interaction at the Clinical Research Department in the Oriental Medicine Research Center of the Kitasato Institute.

Furthermore, although 70 to 80 percent of physicians in all of Japan have a history of prescribing KM, they only apply KM in the treatment of common diseases and frequently-occurring illnesses, and rarely use it. Only a few hospitals, such as the Kitasato Institute in this visit, have an oriental medicine department. The Oriental Medicine Research Center of the Kitasato Institute consists of a Kampo treatment department and acupuncture treatment department. The Kampo treatment department focuses on the diseases that have poor efficacy by WM, some emotional illness, skin diseases, and gynecological diseases, etc., while the acupuncture treatment department mainly targets patients with a variety of pain or joint diseases. It is a pity that patients in the Oriental Medicine Research Center have to pay their own expenses if they take decoctions, and doctors are also prohibited from prescribing WM there.

3. Basic Research of Kampo Medicine

Compared with theoretical studies on KM, the pharmacy, pharmacokinetics, pharmacodynamics and pharmacology of KM are studied intensively in Japan. For instance, the Institute of Natural Medicine at Toyama University consists of a Department of Medicinal Resources (including a Division of Pharmacognosy, Division of Natural Products Chemistry, and a Division of Metabolic Engineering) and a Department of Bioscience (including a Division of Pharmacology, Division of Pathogenic Biochemistry, and a Division of Gastrointestinal Pathophysiology).

The main research scope of the Division of Pharmacology is field investigation of medicinal plants, developing alternative crude medicines, and promoting the sustainable utility of herbal drug resources. The main research area of the Division of Natural Products Chemistry is the analysis of the components and structure of the world's natural medicines, the influence of KM on drug metabolism enzymes, evaluation methodology for the quality of KM formulas, and studies on the investigation of natural medicines. The Division of Metabolic Engineering mainly conducts studies on the basis of the molecular metabolism that is related to the efficacy of KM. The major focuses of the Division of Pharmacology are the neuropharmacologic studies on the central action of compound drugs and their ingredients, as well as defining the mechanism of action of KM or other drugs. The major purpose at the Division of Pathogenic Biochemistry is to investigate the isolation and identification of effective components from traditional medicines, to examine the regulatory effects of traditional medicines and their components and the molecular mechanisms using biochemical, genetic, and immunological methods, and to elucidate the molecular basis of syndromes in response to traditional medicines by using the advanced technologies of molecular biology and immunology. The Division of Gastrointestinal Pathophysiology mainly targets developing innovative specific treatments including KM for diseases of the digestive tract, especially intestinal autoimmune diseases. It is to be noted here that the areas of advantage of KM have been getting more and more attention. Studies on a variety of intractable diseases (e.g., cancer), senile diseases, and "preventive treatment of disease（治未病）" have all been collaboratively tackling research topics in recent years.

4. Drug Development of Kampo Medicine

Japan's annual drug sales amounts to 6000 billion yen, with 120 billion yen on KM. Along with the aging of the population and the poor efficacy of WM on many chronic and hard-to-treat diseases, KM will be in even greater demand. The management of KM manufacturing authorisation is almost similar to that of WM. However, only 210 prescriptions restricted by the Ministry of Health and Labor are permitted to cover available new drugs, of which 150 are included in medical insurance reimbursement, mainly the prescriptions of *Treatise on Cold Pathogenic and Miscellaneous Diseases*（伤寒杂病论）and representative formulas by well-known physicians of later generations. New drugs should be produced following the compatibility and dose of the original prescriptions, which are mainly granules, tablets and other dosage forms. In Japan, it is almost impossible to

obtain approval for a newly developed Kampo patent medicine. Therefore, there is no Kampo patent medicine in the modern sense in Japan, only the different dosage forms of ancient prescriptions.

It is worth mentioning that the research, development, production and marketing of KM in Japan are very advanced and standardized. For example, at the Pharmacy Department of Kitasato University, the planting of *Radix ginseng* and other precious Chinese herbal medicines has been replaced by production of tissue and cell culture, which can be manufactured in batches with concentrations of active ingredients equal to that of natural or planted ones and achieving considerable benefits.

Moreover, Japan advocates reversion thinking on new drug development, that is, to design target model on which the drug is expected to work according to the results of pathological mechanism research on human diseases at the molecular level, and then to high-throughput screen the chemical structure with computer software. This method makes the research direction and objective of the new drug development more definite, and meanwhile saves a large amount of money and time.

During the visit at the Division of Natural Products Chemistry, the Department of Medicinal Resources at the Natural Medicine Institute of Toyama University, Dr. Suresh Awale introduced a project of this division that screened out 36 species of drugs from the extract of traditional medicines which showed cytotoxic activity against the human pancreatic PANC-1 cancer cell line in a nutrient-deprived condition[5,6], and said that they were the first research group in this field in the world, which was very impressive.

5. Research on Integrative Oriental and Western Medicine

Since the 1980s, a new formulation of "Oriental Medicine and WM Combination" became popular in Japanese medical circles. During a large-scale international academic conference on KM progress held in Tokyo in April 1983，the Japanese scholars openly put forward the viewpoint to establish "the Third Medicine" (also known as the World Medicine) based on the combination of Oriental Medicine and WM. Since 1980，they also put their efforts in this direction in terms of the scientific research plan hosted by the Agency of Science and Technology. Japan has already set it as the ultimate objective to establish a new medical system developing a combination of Oriental Medicine and WM.

In China, as early as 1956，Chairman MAO Ze-dong advocated "to combine the knowledge of CM with WM, so as to create a unified new system of medicine and pharmacy". Developing traditional medicine, laying equal stress on both CM and WM, and integrating CM and WM have always been the important policies and guidelines of China. After development of more than 50 years, the enterprise of integrative CM and WM has changed from small to large, from simple to complex, and has made outstanding achievements. As for integration of the two medical systems, China started earlier than Japan, but should not be self complacent. On the contrary, complex and refractory diseases, the aging society and the concept of "preventive treatment of disease" call for more integration of Oriental Medicine and WM as well as sharing of mutual complementary advantages. We should have a sense of mission and urgency, and go on the path of integrative medicine inflexibly.

In general, KM in Japan still mainly studies KM drug application, while theoretical studies such as zangxiang（藏象），meridians, etiology and pathogenesis, herbal nature and channel tropism, objectification of tongue and pulse diagnosis, are still very insufficient. On the contrary, supported by the National 973 Projects and National Natural Science Foundation, China has invested a large amount of money on studies on CM basic

theories, and won initial success. On the basis of this, we should learn from the successful experiences of Japan in applying modern scientific technology to clarify the basis of syndromes, mechanism of action, and new drug development to work for us. Meanwhile, the lessons of Japan in the clinical application of KM also tell us that we can not walk the road of wasting medicine and reserving the drug. We should uphold the principle of laying equal emphasis on both CM and WM, combining syndrome differentiation and disease differentiation by means of modern science and technology, taking basic theoretical research as a breakthrough, so as to make our contributions towards establishing an innovative medical system and thus benefiting the whole of mankind.

References

[1] Terasawa K, Shinoda H, Imadaya A, et al. The Presentation of Diagnostic Criteria for "Yu-xie" (Stagnated Blood) conformation. Int J Orient Med, 1989, 14：194-213.

[2] Nozaki K, Goto H, Nakagawa T, et al. Effects of keishibukuryogan on vascular function in adjuvant-induced arthritis rats. Biol Pharm Bull, 2007, 30：1042-1047.

[3] Yanaga A, Goto H, Nakagawa T, et al, Cinnamaldehyde induces endothelium-dependent and -independent vasorelaxant action on isolated rat aorta. Biol Pharm Bull, 2006, 29：2415-2415.

[4] Matsumoto C, Kojima T, Ogawa K, et al. A proteomic approach for the diagnosis of "Oketsu" (blood stasis), a pathophysiologic Concept of Japanese Traditional (Kampo) Medicine. Evid Based Complement Alternat Med, 2008, 5：463-474.

[5] Awale S, Li F, Onozuka H, et al. Constituents of Brazilian red propolis and their preferential cytotoxic activity against human pancreatic PANC-1 cancer cell line in nutrient-deprived condition. Bioorg Med Chem, 2008, 16：181-189.

[6] Li F, Awale S, Zhang H, et al. Chemical constituents of propolis from Myanmar and their preferential cytotoxicity against a human pancreatic cancer cell line. J Nat Prod, 2009, 72：1283-1287.

第六章

Profiles of Traditional Chinese Medicine Schools[*]

CHEN Ke-ji   XIE Yuan-hua   LIU Yue

A traditional Chinese medicine (TCM) academic school is a conglomerate of academic ideas revolving around a core of unique medical theory or doctrine, or unique therapeutic methodology and skill. TCM academic schools could be grouped into different types, such as Shicheng Schools (mentor-apprentice system), Geographic Schools and Problem-Oriented Schools, among others. "Academic school" is a classification concept in the academia where different schools compare with each other to demonstrate one's own academic characteristics.

1. The Origin of Traditional Chinese Medicine Academic Schools

Academic schools could be actively formed, or passively classified. At times, the name, extensions and intrinsic characteristics of an academic school only reflect the understanding or perception of the one who classifies the school, which may only represent part rather than whole of the spirit of that academic school. However, conventional wisdom has it that parts make up the whole (school) and once complete, it cannot be partial. Hence it is essential that in the reality of TCM clinical practice, extra attention should always be placed on the complete theoretical viewpoints and treatment based on syndrome differentiations.

A TCM academic school should necessarily have a definitive representative figure and a representative work. Furthermore, this representative figure should be able to demonstrate the academic characteristics which make his school distinctive from others, as well as to demonstrate the origin-inheritance-propagation continuum of the thoughts of the school. It is acknowledged that "academic schools appeared first in Jin and Yuan Dynasties", and before Tang and Song Dynasties, there was no proper classification of the schools as all TCM practitioners simply referred to the classics such as *Plain Questions* (Su Wen) and *Miraculous Pivot* (Ling Shu), and forbearers such as ZHANG Zhong-jing and HUA Tuo as the guiding canons of their practice. For this reason, some scholars have inferred that classics *Huangdi's Internal Classic* (Huang Di Nei Jing), *Treatise on Cold Damage Diseases* (Shang Han Lun), *Synopsis of the golden Chamber* (Jin Gui Yao Lue) and *Shen Nong Herbal Classic* (Shen Nong Ben Cao Jing) should not be consider as academic schools. It was only with the advent of The Four Famous Families in Jin and Yuan Dynasties that TCM academic schools blossomed.

In essence, the multitude of academic schools emerged all descended from the same origin, sharing mainly the fundamental theories and teachings of *Huangdi's Internal Classic*. The branching off from this mainstream teaching leading to emergence of different academic schools was neither forceful nor intentional, but was rather a result of diversity in individual background, geography, and adaptation of therapeutic methodology and formulae.

2. Classification of TCM Academic Schools

In general, TCM academic schools are classified passively, with scholars adopting different classification approaches. If the overall basis of classification of academic schools were

---

* 原载于 Chinese Journal of Integrative Medicine, 2012, 18 (7)：534-538

to be the classic *Huangdi's Internal Classic*, and its representative figures are to be differentiated by their focus of academic pursuit, then for those who focused on fidelity and adherence to classic teachings there are WANG Bing, WU Kun, MA Shi, and ZHANG Zhi-cong, among others; for those who concentrated on classification we have YANG Shang-shan, ZHANG Jing-yue, HUA Shou, LI Zhong-zi and Wang An; and for pursuit of specific topics, the representatives are QIN Yue-ren, ZHANG Zhong-jing, HUA Tuo, HUANG Pu-mi, LIU Wan-su and CHEN Wu-ju. Since there was no clear, or lack of, Shicheng relationship, some scholars didn't even bother to classify them into distinctive academic schools. The situation is the same in the Classic Formula School, as even the concept of formula itself had underwent constant changes throughout history. There were eleven Classic Formula School enumerated in the *Record of Literature and Arts in Hanshu* (Han Shu Yi Wen Zhi). In the period from Six Dynasties to Tang and Song Dynasties, GE Hong's *A Handbook of Prescriptions for Emergency* (Zhou Hou Bei Ji Fang), SUN Si-miao's *Thousandgolden Prescriptions* (Qian Jin Fang), and *Medical Secret of Wai-Tai* (Wai Tai Mi Yao), *Taiping Prescriptions of Supreme Benevolence* (Tai Ping Sheng Hui Fang) and *Taiping Prescriptions of People's Welfare Pharmacies* (Tai Ping Hui Min He Ji Ju Fang) by WANG Tao were regarded as the classics. After Song Dynasty, formulae from *Treatise on Cold Damage Diseases and Synopsis of the Golden Chamber* were recognized as the classics.

The Febrile Disorder School, though lacking a definitive Shicheng relationship, took to ZHANG Zhong-jing and his work *Treatise on Cold Damage Diseases* as the doctrinal canon. However, over the course of history, many TCM practitioners had different perceptions of *Treatise on Cold Damage Diseases*. For instance, the version of *Treatise on Cold Damage Diseases* revised and edited by WANG Shu-he was considered by FANG You-

zhi as to be "disorderly" and have "too many mistakes". Yet the same version was hailed by CHEN Xiu-yuan as a "milestone achievement of TCM" [1]. Various approaches were adopted by different scholars in other attempts to revise *Treatise on Cold Damage Diseases*, where SUN Si-miao advocated "similarity in formulae and syndrome", KE Qin promoted "grouping syndromes according to formulae", YOU Yi "to group syndromes according to treatment methods", SHEN Ji-nao "to group syndromes by symptoms", QING Huang "to group syndromes by pathogenesis" and CHEN Xiu-yuan adopted "grouping of syndromes by Meridians".

Strictly speaking, TCM academic schools that actually met classification requirements only turned up in the period of Jin and Yuan Dynasties (Figure 1). LIU Yuan-su of Jin Dynasty founded the He-Jian School where he condensed the "nineteen articles of pathogenesis" of *Plain Questions* into eleven articles according to the "five evolution phases and six climatic factors" principle and produced the work *Plain Questions on Concept of Original Disease Type* (Su Wen Bing Ji Yuan Bing Shi) where it was put forward that the "six climatic factors could turn into fire". Nine of the "nineteen articles of pathogenesis" were of the fire and heat type, and for such the He-Jian School is also known as the Fire-Heat School. LIU Wan-su expanded on the essential teaching of *Huangdi's Internal Classic* and brought forth new concepts advocating the use

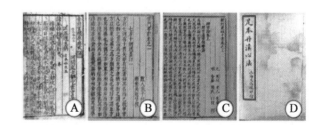

Figure 1　Representative Books of the Famous Four Masters of Jin and Yuan Dynasties

Notes：A：LIU Wan-su's Plain Questions on Concept of Original Disease Type；B：ZHANG Cong-zheng's　Ru Men Shi Qin；C：LI Dong-yuan's　Treatise of Spleen and Stomach；D：ZHU Dan-xi's Dan Xi Xin Fa

of "cool and cold pattern" medications to rectify the inadequacies of "warm and dry" medications of *Taiping Prescriptions of People's Welfare Pharmacies* (Tai Ping Hui Min He Ji Ju Fang) common in use then to treat epidemic diseases of the war-torn periods of the Song and Jin Dynasties.

LIU Wan-su was the mentor of Jing Shan Fu Tu who taught LUO Zhi-di who in turn taught ZHU Dan-xi. ZHU Dan-xi advocated the Xiang Huo theory which focused on yin deficiency and yang excess where the core of his teaching is to "nourish the yin". ZHU Dan-xi likewise had extensive works regarding syndromes of qi, blood, phlegm, gloom and fire and created the famous formula, Yueju Pill (越鞠丸). DAI Si-gong and WANG Lu were disciples, and WANG Ji and WANG Lun followers of ZHU Dan-xi. ZHANG Cong-zheng was a follower of LIU Wan-su and it was recorded in "History of Jin Dynasty" that he "adhered to Liu's teachings and preferred the use of cool and cold medications[2]. To retaliate the blind use of "nourishment" treatment method rampant in Song and Jin Dynasties, Zhang founded the Eliminating Pathogenic Factor School and wrote his signature work "Ru Men Shi Qin". MA Jiu-chou and CHANG De were Zhang's disciples and LI Zi-fan his follower (Figure 2). ZHANG Yuan-su, the founder of Yi-

Shui School, emphasized clinical differentiation using Zang-Fu organs mechanisms and herbs tropism and authored the works *Medical Origins* (Yi Xue Qi Yuan), *Drug Pattern of Zangfu, Biaoben, Hanre and Xushi* (Zang Fu Biao Ben Han Re Xu Shi Yong Yao Shi) and *Pearl Wisdom of Chinese Herbs* (Zhen Zhu Nang). LI Dong-yuan and WANG Hao-gu were ZHANG Yuan-su's disciples. LI Dong-yuan believed that "defective Spleen (Pi) and Stomach (Wei) result in many diseases" and founded the Tonifying Spleen School. Li created numerous therapeutic principles including "replenishing qi and elevating yang", "clearing the heat with sweet-warm medications" and produced the Buzhong Yiqi and Shenyang Yiwei Decoctions and was the author of *Treatise of Spleen and Stomach* (Pi Wei Lun), *Treatise on Identification of Internal Diseases and External Damages* (Nei Wai Shang Bian Huo Lun) and *Lan Cache Room* (Lan Shi Mi Cang). WANG Hao-gu and LUO Tian-yi benefited from Li's teachings and XUE Ji, ZHANG Jing-yue and LI Zhong-zi were Li's followers of latter times.

At the time of late Yuan and early Ming Dynasties when many TCM practitioners followed ZHU Dan-xi blindly and misused the herbs *Cortex Phellodendri Chinensis* and *Anemarrhena asphodeloides*, XUE Ji founded the Warming and Tonifying School where focus was centered on the relationship between Spleen-Stomach and Kidney (Shen, Ming Men, Gate of Life) and warming and tonifying treatment methods were applied to both Spleen and Kidney. ZHAO Xian-ke's theories traced back to XUE Ji and advocated the ultimate importance of kidney-water and life-fire. ZHANG Jing-yue propagated the viewpoint of "concomitant deficiencies of yin and yang" and created the Zuogui Pill (Decoction, 左归丸) and Yougui Pill (Decoction, 右归丸).

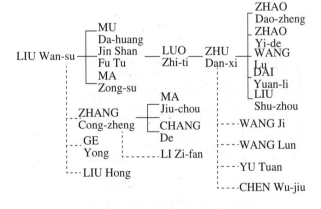

Figure 2 Typical Shicheng Relationship: LIU Wan-su and His Disciples and Followers

Note: ——Disciples (direct student), ······Follower (indirect student)

It is apparent that the rise of each TCM academic schools is closely related to contemporary background. The advent of Warm

第六章

Disease School is a case in point, as it is a product of the calls of the time. At the last years of Ming Dynasty, major epidemic outbreaks erupted in Hubei, Zhejiang and Shandong provinces resulting in countless death. WU You-ke penned the *Treatise on Pestilence* (Wen Yi Lun) promoting the concept that "epidemic pathogens" entering through mouth or nose was the cause of the contagion. It is certainly the precursor of modern epidemiology. YU Shi-yu authored *A View of Epidemic Febrile Diseases* (Yi Zhen Yi De) and created Qingwen Baidu Decoction (清瘟 败毒饮) which contained a large dose of gypsum. YE Tian-shi conceived *Treatise on Epidemic Febrile Diseases* (Wen Re Lun) and initiated TCM differentiation of Wei Qi Ying Xue. XUE Sheng-bai was the author of *Synopsis on Damp-Heat* (Shi Re Bing Pian), while WU Ju-tong wrote Item Differentiation of *Warm Febrile Diseases* (Wen Bing Tiao Bian) illustrating the "differentiation of Triple Energizers" and created Yin Oiao Powder (银翘散) and Sang Ju Decoction (桑菊饮). WANG Meng-ying was the author of *Compendium of Epidemic Febrile Diseases* (Wen Re Jing Wei), a comprehensive work covering various aspects of epidemic febrile disease. It was under this background that Contemporary Formula School made its discrete entrance. It was ZHANG Yuan-su who said that "in unfortunate times of discord, old formulae and new diseases could not co-exist." [2] Up until the time of Qing Dynasty, appropriate and befitting formulae improvised by TCM practitioners to meet the needs in combating diseases were the norm of the time and getting ever popular. Hence the saying by CHEN Xiu-yuan that contemporary formulae began their prevalence after Tang and Song Dynasties[3], as evidenced by the increasing popularity of applying classic, ancient and contemporary formulae as classification criteria since then.

Confluence School is a passive ideological movement resulting from opposition to the shut-in mentality and to the call of wholesale westernization at the time. It advocated that both TCM and Western medicine (WM) had their own merits and advantages, and that one should not be lost at the expense of the other[4]. Early on there were WANG Ang, ZHAO Xue-min, WANG Xue-quan, WANG Oing-ren and CHEN Ding-tai who adopted WM, then WANG Hong-han, ZHU Pei-wen, TANG Zong-hai and ZHANG Xi-chun attempted to merge TCM and WM. Furthermore, there was HUI Tie-qiao who advocated improving TCM and LU Peng-nian's exhortation to make TCM more scientific. Confluence School indeed could be perceived as the precursor of TCM and WM integration.

3. Academic Contention and Development of Academic Schools

With the existence of different academic schools, there bound to have academic contentions. ZHU Dan-xi of Yin Nourishing School stood by the theory that "yang constantly in excess and yin constantly in deficiency", while ZHANG Jing-yue of Warming and Tonifying School insisted on "concomitant Yin and Yang deficiencies". YE Tian-shi elucidated on the patterns and evolution of febrile diseases as well as yin nourishing theories, among others, but failed to gain any recognition from his contemporary Xue Xue, who authored *Medical Records Countering YE Tian-shi* (Sao Ye Shan Zhuang Yi An) to attack and undo Ye's theories. Another famous practitioner, XU Ling-tai, picked through YE Tian-shi's medical records as a guide to Clinical Work (Lin Zheng Zhi Nan Yi An) with more than 260 general and 3,600 specific comments to bluntly point out all its deficiencies and inadequacies. ZHAO Xian-ke authored "Yi Guan" to advocate the "Mingmen Between Kidneys" theory but was negated completely by XU Ling-tai's *Countering Yi Guan* (Yi Guan Bian) which offered opposite views to what Ye proposed. ZHANG Jing-yue in his *New Eight Regimen Formulae* (Xin Fang Ba Zheng) enumerated tonify, harmonize, attack, dissipate, cold, heat, strengthen and yin types of formulae

601

as the eight regimens complete with his collection of 186 original formulae. However, CHEN Xiu-yuan authored *Countering New Eight Regimen Formulae* (Xin Fang Ba Zheng Bian) disputing ZHANG Jing-yue's formulae, calling them vague in concept especially the theories on the nourishing of yin and yang which are inconsistent with the teachings of ZHANG Zhong-jing.

4. Conclusion

In general, the establishment and ensuing proper development of an academic school requires a well-founded hypothesis, logical rationale, free inquiries, and clinical correlation[5]. A viable school should have continuity and consistency and self-initiated pursuit of tradition, fortification and innovation. Furthermore, to be a school entails a multi-system, multi-layer and far-reaching infrastructure, and it should be able to demonstrate clinical efficacy when applied, thus earning the trust and recognition of the community. It should also realized that there are other schools of similar, if not better, merits and it is of advantage to adopt complementary measures in clinical practices. It is also important to avoid blind attachment to other teachings lest foregoing one's own principle and characteristics. In the realm of academic schools, we need to uphold the tradition yet also strive to open up at the same time. In this age of rapid development in life sciences, it is imperative to persist on truth, to think out of one's academic box in order to further sustain, to accommodate and to keep pace with demands of the time. Structures of academic schools likewise need to be constantly enriched to keep up with the time as there is no boundary in progress and innovation. On the face of dissenting views, one needs to keep in mind of the principle of equality and keep the channels of communication open, and stay away from unproductive exchanges. There is no perfect pattern of development; academic schools need to learn to complement each other on their structure as each of these schools has its own merits. To five up to the calls of the time, it is essential to uphold tradition, to stimulate innovation and progress, and to facilitate both localization and globalization of traditional Chinese medicine[6-8]. Hence, equal attention should be paid to Classic TCM Schools, TCM Modernization Schools and Integrative Medicine Schools to achieve development of all.

References

[1] Ren YQ, ed. Doctrines of historical schools. Shanghai: Shanghai Scientific and Technological Educational Publishing House, 1980: 91-118.

[2] Tuo T (Yuan Dynasty). History of Jin Dynasty. Beijing: Zhonghua Book Company, 1975: 2811-2812.

[3] Chen XY (Qing Dynasty). Medicine encyclopedia of Chen Xiuyuan. Beijing: China Press of Traditional Chinese Medicine, 2008: 927.

[4] Qiu PR, Ding GD, eds. Doctrines of historical schools. Beijing: People's Medical Publishing House, 1992: 703.

[5] Gu L. Academic schools and Chinese culture. Soc Sci Chin, 1988, 8 (4): 111-126.

[6] Xu H, Chen KJ. Making evidence-based decisions in the clinical practice of integrative medicine. Chin J Integr Med, 2010, 16: 483-485.

[7] Xu H, Chen KJ. Integrative medicine: the experience from China. J Altern Complem Med, 2008, 14: 3-7.

[8] Liu Y, Chen KJ. Atherosclerosis, vascular aging and therapetic strategies. Chin J Integr Med, 2012, 18: 83-87.

第六章

第七章

综述与系统评价

病证结合的基础研究 *

黄　烨　殷惠军　陈可冀

在不同时代和文化背景下，中医学和西医学分别从不同的角度，采用不同的方式方法研究并探索了人类生命活动的客观规律。其中，中医学着重强调宏观和整体，西医学则注重微观和局部，二者存在着优势互补的可能[1]。尽管先进现代技术已广泛应用，人们对疾病的认识已细化到结构和功能等微观方面，但依然存在冠心病、肿瘤等慢性病的高发生率和高致死率，而使用一些无法定性和量化的中医概念去解释疾病并进行治疗往往能起到一定效果，可见中西医结合是历史的必然和时代的要求[1]。病证结合的临床诊疗和研究模式正是中西医两种医学体系结合的具体体现。

基础研究是在临床取得良好疗效的基础上升华并形成的，同时也将在临床过程中经过反复验证而达到完善，进而指导临床诊疗活动。因此，基础研究在病证结合的研究方面至关重要。

1. 病、证及病证关系

1.1 病

随着中医理论的建立及系统化，病作为一个特定的医学术语才逐渐形成。最早的疾病记录见于殷商时代的甲骨文；随后，在《山海经》中出现了从疾病病理特点和发病情况命名的疾病；至《五十二病方》出现了详细描述的病名和对病用药的方剂。现代中医认为，"病"是以中医学理论为指导，有其自身的特点和理论体系，每一个病都有其各种不同的临床特征，各个不同疾病的发生发展、变化和转归，构成了各个不同疾病的一系列异常变化的全过程，有其病因、病理、病位、辨证分型、治疗方药、预后转归等一整套理论体系。而西医的"病"则建立在西医学理论体系基础上，以研究人体的组织、器官、细胞、分子的结构与功能的病理变化为特点，根据疾病病因及病理的需要，进行相应的药物治疗[2]。就命名而言，中医的"病"往往从整体观出发，或以病因性质命名，如伤风、伤暑之类；或以突出症状命名，如腹泻、眩晕之类；或以病机之所在命

名，如郁证、痰饮之类。而西医多根据物理诊断和实验诊断对疾病进行命名，例如就某种病原体（结核病）、就某种特殊病变的病灶命名（病毒性心肌炎）或就生理上的某种病变命名（糖尿病）。虽然，中西医对病的理解不尽相同，病名不能完全对等，但均反映了疾病发生发展的全过程，体现了以病理学内容为核心的疾病分类体系以及在此基础上的诊断模式。

1.2 证

证是中医学特有的概念，是疾病发生和演变过程中其阶段本质的反映，是疾病某一阶段的病因、病位、病性、病机、病势及邪正虚实等的病理概括。在中医学形成发展早期，并没有"证"的记录，随着中医学理论的形成，"证"才散见于中医学书籍，但该时期的"证"即症状，并无其他特别意义。如《伤寒杂病论》中虽有小柴胡汤证中"但见一证便是"，其"证"也仅仅指症状群（即症状）。新中国成立以后，已故任应秋先生于20世纪50年代提出的"病证结合"才对"证"赋予了另一种含义[3]。现代中医认为，证是指在疾病发展过程中某一阶段的病理概括。其包括病因、病位、病性和邪正关系，反映了疾病发展过程中该阶段病理变化的全面情况[4]。因此，"证"反映疾病过程中某一阶段的病理特征，是以病机为核心的疾病分类体系以及在此基础的诊断模式。

1.3 病、证之间的关系

中医学对疾病的认识和治疗是由"症"到"病"，然后到"证"，多次反复认识、逐渐深化的过程。其中，证是对疾病当前四诊资料的高度概括，反映病的某一特定病理阶段。辨病长于从疾病的全过程、特征上认识疾病的本质，强调始发病因以及病理过程；辨证重在从疾病当前的表现判断病变的位置与性质，强调与疾病有关的各种因素共同作用下的机体整体反应特性。由于病的影响因素复杂多变，在整体上表现的反映特性具有偶发性，同时证又具有动态变化的特征，因此，既不能将证候类型固定，也不存在一种病的固定辨证分型。疾病

* 原载于《中国中西医结合杂志》，2012，32（3）：299-303

与证候虽有其各自侧重，但二者的相互关系可概括为：病的某一病理阶段外在表现为一类证候群；证候是对疾病当前四诊资料的高度概括，故反映的是疾病的某一特定病理阶段。而病证结合就是将疾病概念体系与证候概念体系相结合研究疾病的发生发展规律，指导疾病防治[5]。

2. 病证结合的形式

辨证论治是中医理论体系的特色和中医临床医学的精华，其核心就是病证结合。早在东汉张仲景时期就强调中医辨证论治应"辨证"与"辨病"相结合。经历了漫长的发展历程，辨病辨证结合大体可分为传统病证结合和现代病证结合两类。

2.1　传统病证结合

作为古代医家创建的一种诊疗模式，传统病证结合是指在辨中医之病的基础上，结合辨证施治，以辨病为主题且贯穿在整个诊疗过程中，但又不忽视辨证的重要性。随着不同时期的发展历程，传统病证结合在传承前人的同时又得到了进一步的发展和完善。早在秦汉时期，《黄帝内经》和《五十二病方》就提出多种病名，并针对这些病进行论治，出现了病证结合的雏形。东汉张仲景在《伤寒杂病论》的大多数篇章中以"某某病脉证并治"，且在《金匮要略》中，在诊断上做到脉证合参，既辨病又辨证，如《金匮要略》对百合病的治疗可谓早期辨病论治与辨证论治相结合的典范；同时，在治疗上既有专方，又强调根据具体辨证而选方论药，第一次从真正意义上完善了病证结合治疗理论体系。自晋唐以来，更多医家关注病证结合的重要性，甚至对某些疾病强调了辨病的重要性。岳美中教授认为，"按证候用药是《伤寒》，按病用药是《金匮》"，"余谓中医治病必须辨证论治与专方专药相结合"。上海姜春华教授指出："中医除掉以西医的病为主体外，还要根据中医辨病的原则去辨病，同时也根据中医辨证精神去辨证"[6]。

2.2　现代病证结合

中医的"证"是机体在疾病发展中某一阶段的病理概括，认识疾病过程中的某个横断面；"病"是人体外界致病因素作用下，在体内出现的具有一定发展规律的病理演变全过程，认识整个疾病发生发展。现代病证结合即察西医之病，辨中医之证。首先借助现代科学技术，结合现代医学理论和思维方法对疾病做出明确诊断，弥补中医学在诊断判定和疗效评判标准方面缺乏规范的不足，并在此基础上，运用中医的辨证思维进行分型，确定治则治法、遣方用药，从而达到防治疾病的目的[7]。

3. 病证结合基础研究现状

基于病证结合思路，证候实质的科学内涵得到了深入认识，从而使临床辨证论治更加客观化、更具科学性；通过构建病证结合动物模型，搭建了中医临床研究与基础研究的桥梁，更有效地丰富、拓展了中医基础理论，并对中药有效筛选与机制研究建立了合理的评价体系。

3.1　对证候实质的认识

证候是中医学理论的核心，是对临床现象的概括和总结，也是连接中医基础与临床研究的重要桥梁。"有诸内必形诸外"，证候既然是有规律的病理生理过程，就必然有其规律性的物质基础。证候形之于外的是四诊宏观信息，其内在物质基础是什么尚不清楚[8]。揭示中医证候的实质不仅能使辨证论治更加科学化和客观化，还是实现中医药科学化、现代化的必由之路，而病证结合正是证候实质研究的重要途径之一。

自20世纪80年代以来我国展开了证候的研究工作，近年来随着人类基因图谱的构建，基因组学、蛋白质组学和代谢组学的兴起以及现代磁共振成像、单光子发射体层摄影术技术的广泛应用，拓展了人们认识机体内部结构和功能变化的视野，同时也为证候实质的研究带来了机遇。不少学者基于病证结合的思路和系统生物学基础，分别从生理、生化、组织超微结构以及神经 – 内分泌 – 免疫网络等方面探讨了证候的科学内涵并取得了一定成果。不同证型可能存在不同的基因组学基础和背景，相关基因多态性表达可作为各证型之间不同临床表现的分子遗传学依据[9]。证候与基因表达差异及基因多态性之间存在着密切的内在联系[10]。然而，借助基因组学方法筛选的相关基因仅能反映遗传因素，未能反映环境因素在该证候中的作用。为此，有学者借助蛋白质组学方法寻找差异蛋白质组，发现某些相关基因存在特征的电泳图谱，并发现与该证候相关的某些点，从而较全面地反映遗传和环境因素在该证候中的影响。代谢组学具有整体、动态、综合与分析的特点，能够从代谢网络终端表象的整体角度反映生物体的功能水平，从而更好地与证候实质特征链接，弥补基因组学和蛋白质组学研究的缺陷[11]。

冠心病是由遗传因素和环境因素共同作用的

复杂疾病，其发病率呈逐年增长的趋势，是严重威胁人类健康的常见病和多发病。大量临床和实验研究表明，血瘀证是冠心病最常见的证型之一[12]。大量病证结合研究表明，血瘀证在血液流变学、血小板功能、血管内皮损伤、微循环障碍、炎症反应、免疫调节等方面与疾病的发生发展密切相关[13]。以陈可冀院士为首的课题组分别从基因组学和蛋白组学探讨了冠心病血瘀证的实质并得到了初步认识。一方面，构建了冠心病血瘀证的白细胞差异基因表达谱，从分子水平阐明了冠心病血瘀证与炎症免疫反应的相关性[14]；同时，对筛选出的目标基因白细胞介素 -8（IL-8）和免疫球蛋白 IgG 结晶片段受体ⅢA（FcγRⅢA）分别进行了临床规模验证，并就其参与冠心病血瘀证疾病过程的机制进行了体内外功能分析，发现 IL-8 通过介导血小板活化，FcγRⅢA 通过诱导单核细胞 - 内皮细胞黏附、介导炎症反应影响动脉粥样硬化斑块稳定性进而参与冠心病血瘀证的发生发展过程。另一方面，构建了冠心病血瘀证血小板差异功能蛋白谱，发现部分差异目标分子，初步证实了血小板骨架蛋白在冠心病血瘀证与非血瘀证患者血小板活化进程中发挥了不同作用[15]。基于血瘀证证候实质，为冠心病血瘀证客观化诊断指标群的建立提供了理论依据；同时，以血瘀证目标分子为靶标研究活血化瘀中药的作用机制将为活血化瘀药物防治冠心病的有效筛选和机制研究建立合理的评价体系。

3.2 病证结合动物模型的建立评价与意义

无论是探明中医证候的实质，还是深化对疾病病理机制的研究，动物模型无疑是一个重要的途径与手段，而病证结合动物模型基于探讨疾病病理生理变化与中医证候特征之间的关系，在中医临床与基础之间架起了桥梁，有利于中药的有效筛选、机制研究并满足新药开发的需要，对深层次探讨中西医理论的内在联系具有重要意义[16]。

基于所研究疾病与证候的密切相关性及其发展阶段的同步性，找出二者在临床上的结合点，建立病证结合动物模型。例如发现冠心病与血瘀证在微循环障碍、血流动力学障碍、血液流变学异常以及血管壁损伤等方面密切相关，从而建立微循环障碍模型、血管内凝血模型、动脉粥样硬化模型以及血管管壁结构改变模型等冠心病血瘀证动物模型[17]。目前病证结合模型的造模多采用西医病理造模因素叠加中医证候造模因素的方法。如梁俊清等[18]以 Wistar 大鼠为实验动物，采用高同型半胱

氨酸血症诱发血管内皮功能障碍为基础病理模型，叠加"基础进食和强迫负重游泳"诱发气虚证候，制作络气虚滞型血管内皮功能障碍动物模型。李欣志等[19]采用高脂喂养结合冠状动脉球囊损伤的方法复制出小型猪冠心病痰瘀互结的病证结合模型。采用卵蛋白致敏，结合形寒饮冷与劳倦刺激相结合的方法建立哮喘病寒饮蕴肺证证证结合的大鼠模型[20]。此外，也应用单一物理或化学因素造成病证结合模型的方法。例如，采用 Ameroid 环缩术制备心肌缺血血瘀证小型猪模型[21]、以腹腔注射促红细胞生成素的方法造成继发性红细胞增多症动物模型[22]等都是使用单一造模手段制作病证结合模型的造模方法。这些病证结合动物模型是探究疾病发生机制以及筛选有效治疗中药的关键途径和手段。同时，对病证结合动物模型进行评价以确保模型的可靠性及应用性。评价方法有三：一是通过挖掘动物身上具有诊断意义的信息特征以及能够客观反映证候特征的微观指标，从中医证候角度进行模型评价；二是从病理生化角度对一些脏器组织病变或血液组织液中某些特异性物质的变化对疾病模型进行评价；三是从反映病证关联性的角度出发，侧重寻找相关特定组分的共性加以分析并判断，发现疾病的生物标记物，从而提高诊断的科学化和定量化[23]。

将病证结合动物模型作为中医药研究的对象，既能得到西医对疾病明确的病理组织器官变化和诊断评价的支持，使模型具有良好的可靠性和稳定性，又在模型制备中引入时间观念，动态观察模型动物的宏观表征和微观指标，突出了中医"证"的阶段性和动态性。这更符合临床诊治的实际情况，对探讨疾病病理生理变化与中医证候特征之间的关系有着重要的意义和价值。病证结合动物模型能探讨证候在某一具体疾病上的表现，探讨同病异证机制和同一方药在单纯治病、单纯治证、病证同治中的作用和机制，是中西医结合研究的重要环节[24]。

3.3 基于病证结合，开展中医基础理论研究

辨证论治体现了中医的整体观，重视人体内在抗病能力，强调具体情况具体分析，是阴阳、五行、脏腑、经络、气血、津液等学说在临床上的具体应用。西医以辨病为主，重视局部的器官和功能变化，通过现代科学技术和手段的运用在诊断和治疗方面具有显著优势。因此，把中医的辨证和西医的辨病结合起来，不仅是临床上进行中西医结合的一个重要途径，而且也是中西医基础理论研究的关键方法。

中医学基础理论和西医学基础理论多呈经纬度关系，以西医理论对疾病或各系统器官的认识是"经"，那么中医学理论中的藏象、四诊、八纲、治则、阴阳等都是"纬"，经纬的交叉处可能找到中西医结合点。在不同西医诊断的疾病中，当处于具有中医某个"证"的阶段，采用辨证的治疗而提高疗效。异病既然能同治，必有共同的物质基础。例如作为一种综合性病理状态的血瘀证可见于多种疾病。血瘀证在气虚、气滞、寒凝、血热等多种病因的作用下通过各种复杂机制，最终呈现出多样的临床表现，但却应存在共同的病理特点。近年来，不少学者基于病证结合的思路，结合微循环、血液流变学、凝血和纤溶机制、机体免疫功能、结缔组织代谢等现代病理生理知识，深入探讨了血瘀证的物质基础，利用现代先进技术验证血瘀证中医基础理论的同时深化了血瘀证的科学内涵。这不仅为临床广泛应用活血化瘀治疗原则提供了理论依据，而且拓展了活血化瘀中药在治疗一些难治性病证如系统性红斑狼疮、视网膜中心血管栓塞、急性弥漫性血管内凝血的诊疗思路。

基于病证结合思路，中医基础理论研究在指导思想上继续充分发扬中医的特点与优势，同时在研究手段上大量引进先进的现代医学分子生物学技术，将中医的朴素理论客观化，进一步提出新观点、新思路。这可能是今后中医基础理论现代化发展的趋势。

3.4 基于病证结合，进行中药的有效筛选和作用机制研究

中药（单味、单体、复方）以多靶点、多途径为特点，广泛应用于临床各种疾病的治疗并显示出一定的疗效。然而，普遍存在作用靶点不明、量效关系不清的现象，且中药在临床治疗上过于强调治疗的个体化，从而导致中药对疾病治疗规律难以把握，大大限制了中药的研发和应用。

应用现代科学技术研究方剂药效物质基础，明确药物的作用机制并确定作用靶点，从而有利于中药的临床应用。在以往药效物质基础的研究中形成了对病研究和对证研究两种模式。其中，前者用西医病的诊断标准来评价方剂药效，而后者用中医证的诊断标准来评价方剂药效。然而，这两种模式却存在各自的缺陷：对病研究只注重用西医的病理药理模型，以病的某几个或几组指标来评价方剂的药效，筛选有效成分或部位作为方剂的药效物质基础。这种研究思路忽视了方剂证的本质，结果可能会发现方剂中部分药效（治疗某病）的物质基础，但不能找到整个方剂的药效物质基础。对证研究用单纯证的动物模型来筛选方剂药效物质基础，而没有结合病的因素，导致研究结果只局限于中医药理论内部，不能用来更为广泛指导临床用药，方剂治疗疾病的价值仍难以充分发挥[25]。将对病研究和对证研究相结合，既能突出中医"证"的特色，又能用西医病的标准使中药研究规范化。根据医方中青蒿能截疟的记载进行筛选研究分离出抗疟的有效成分——青蒿素及青蒿琥酯复方治疗耐药恶性疟疾[26]以及中药砒霜（As_2O_3）治疗急性早幼粒细胞性白血病[27]就是基于病证结合思路开发新药以及老药新用的典范。

4. 展望

病证结合研究是在总结中西医结合五十余年来发展的经验与教训基础上，适应医学及科学技术发展趋势而逐渐形成的。尽管这一研究方法在深化中医证候实质的认识，丰富中医基础理论以及推动中药学研究与中药新药创制方面取得了一定的成绩，但仍存在一些问题尚需继续探索与完善。目前已有的"证"的模型是否真正符合中医"证"的本质，尚处于不断探讨和深化的阶段。为了能更准确地反映中医"证"的本质，而考虑到人的整体受到多种影响因素，可根据"证"的临床实验研究得到的某些资料，摸索制备离体器官模型细胞组织模型以及在基础上的分子生物学研究是今后研究的途径和方向之一

参考文献

[1] 陈可冀，宋军. 病证结合的临床研究是中西医结合研究的重要模式. 继续医学教育，2007，1（19）：12-16.

[2] 张方健，陈如泉. 病、证、药结合研究方法是中医药学术发展的重要途径. 中国中医药发展大会，2001：243-245.

[3] 杨勤运，刘春贵. 对症、证、病研究的思考. 亚太传统医药，2007，2：47-49.

[4] 刘保延，王永炎. 证候、证、症的概念及其关系的研究. 中医杂志，2007，48（4）：293-298.

[5] 陈志强. 创新辨证论治 发展现代中医学——对现代中医学辨证论治体系的再思考. 中国中西医结合杂志，2011，1（31）：104-107.

[6] 陈茂盛. 病证结合理论及发展趋势探讨. 中医杂志，2007，10（48）：942-945.

[7] 张笑平. 中西医结合诊治思路与方法. 合肥：安徽科学技术出版社，1995：5.

[8] 崔轶凡，王庆国．病证结合动物模型对中医药研究的意义及建模方法新思路．天津中医药，2009，6：375-379．

[9] 张明，赵英日，李强，等．从基因角度研究中医证候实质的思路．江西中医药，2008，9（39）：68-71．

[10] 薛梅，殷惠军，陈可冀．从基因组学研究证候实质的若干思考．中国中西医结合杂志，2006，1（26）：88-91．

[11] 李运伦．代谢组学是研究证候实质和方剂原理的重要技术平台．山东中医药大学学报，2008，3（32）：187-190．

[12] 张京春，陈可冀．瘀毒病机与动脉粥样硬化易损斑块相关的理论思考．中国中西医结合杂志，2008，28（4）：366-368．

[13] 马晓娟，殷惠军，陈可冀．血瘀证与炎症相关性的研究进展．中国中西医结合杂志，2007，7（27）：669-675．

[14] Ma XJ，Yin HJ，Chen KJ. Differential gene expression profiles in coronary heart disease patients of blood stasis syndrome in traditional Chinese medicine and clinical role of target gene. Chin J Integr Med，2009，15（2）：101-106．

[15] 李雪峰，蒋跃绒，高铸烨，等．冠心病血瘀证血小板差异功能蛋白筛选鉴定及功能分析．中国中西医结合杂志，2010，30（5）：467-473．

[16] 富琦，陈信义．建立病证结合动物模型的新思路．中国中医药信息杂志，2003，10（9）：79-80．

[17] 田金洲，王永炎，徐意，等．血瘀证动物模型的种类评价与研究．北京中医药大学学报，2006，6（29）：396-402．

[18] 梁俊清，孙士然，吴以岭，等．络气虚滞型血管内皮功能障碍病证结合动物模型的建立及通络方药干预研究．山东中医药大学学报，2008，32（1）：52-57．

[19] 李欣志，刘建勋，任建勋，等．痰瘀互结证冠心病小型猪模型的建立．中国中西医结合杂志，2009，3（29）：228-233．

[20] 张艳霞，周红艳，李建生．病证结合模型的研究进展．河南中医学院学报，2008，5（23）：97-100．

[21] 刘蕾，王伟，宋剑南，等．心肌缺血血瘀证小型猪模型差异蛋白质组学研究．中华中医药杂志，2009，24（6）：716-719．

[22] 杨宇飞，马麟麟，许勇刚，等．继发性红细胞增多症血瘀证结合动物模型的建立及清血颗粒的活血化瘀作用．中国中医基础医学杂志，2005，11（6）：446-448．

[23] 纪冬琛，李昌煜．病证结合动物模型的制作评价与展望．浙江中医药大学学报，2010，4（34）：615-620．

[24] 刘蕾，郭淑贞，王伟．中医证候研究的现状及发展趋势．中华中医药杂志，2008，8（23）：661-664．

[25] 刘建勋，任钧国．中药复方作用物质基础研究探讨．中药研究与信息，2004，6（12）：8．

[26] Trampuz A，Jereb M，Muzlovic J，et al. Clinical review：severe malaria．Crit Care，2003，7（4）：315-323．

[27] Soignet SL，Frankel SR，Douer D，et al. United States multicenter study on arsenic trioxide in relapsed acute promyelueytic leukemia．J Clin Oncol，2001，19（18）：3852-3860．

中医和中西医结合临床指南制定的现状与问题 *

陈可冀　蒋跃绒

临床指南是系统发展起来的说明，以帮助在特定临床情况下，对合理的卫生保健做出决策[1]。循证医学的发展给指南的制定带来了根本性的转变，以证据为基础建立的循证指南已在世界迅速兴起。

目前我国已全面启动中医药规范化工作，各类中医或中西医临床指南也在逐渐增多。因此，有必要对我国中医、中西医结合指南制定的现状和问题作一分析。

1. 中医和中西医结合临床指南制定的现状

通过电子检索 2003 年 1 月至 2008 年 9 月发表在中国期刊全文数据库和万方数据库中所有包括共识、建议在内的中医和中西医临床实践指南，并手工收集相关文献作为补充，结果共检索到 11 篇，涉及 7 个指南。其中中医指南 5 个，包括 2003 年《中医杂志》和《中国医药学报》同时发表的传染性非典型肺炎（后称为：严重急性呼

* 原载于《中西医结合学报》，2009，7（4）：301-304

吸综合征，severe acute respiratory syndrome，SARS）中医诊疗指南[2,3]及 2008 年《中医儿科杂志》相继发表的小儿肺炎喘嗽中医诊疗指南[4]、小儿哮喘中医诊疗指南[5]、小儿泄泻中医诊疗指南[6]和流行性腮腺炎中医诊疗指南[7]；中西医结合指南 2 个，包括 2006 年《中西医结合学报》《中国中西医结合杂志》《中西医结合肝病杂志》和《中华肝脏病杂志》同时发表的肝纤维化中西医结合诊疗指南[8-11]及 2007 年《中国中西医结合杂志》发表的慢性前列腺炎中西医结合诊疗指南（试行版）[12]。查阅中华中医药学会、中国中西医结合学会、中华医学会、中国医师协会、国家中医药管理局等相关学会、机构的网站，补充检索到已发布的指南 4 部，包括 2006 年亚健康中医临床指南[13]、2007 年糖尿病中医防治指南[14]、2008 年中医内科常见病诊疗指南[15]和 2008 年血脂康临床应用的中国专家共识[16]。其中前三者均为国家中医药管理局立项，中华中医药学会制定并发布，中国中医药出版社出版发行，后者则为中国医师协会《心血管疾病防治中国专家共识》系列中唯一针对中药临床应用的共识。

目前中华中医药学会正在进行中医肿瘤、中医妇科、中医感染病、中医肛肠科、中医周围血管病、中医皮肤科等各科常见病诊疗指南的编撰工作，部分已完成等待发布。世界卫生组织（WHO）西太区组织编写的传统医学临床实践指南也正在进行，共涉及 27 种疾病，部分疾病已初步完成。

随着对指南质量关注程度的提高，一些指南评价的工具也应运而生。指南研究与评价的评审（Appraisal of Guidelines Research and Evaluation，AGREE）工具和指南标准化会议（Conference on Guideline Standardization，COGS）确定的评价指南的标准就是两个基本得到公认的评价指南方法学质量的工具[17-19]。AGREE 评估系统由来自 13 个国家的研究者共同制定，包括 6 个部分总共 23 个条目：范围和目的、使用事宜、制定的严谨性、清晰性与可读性、应用性、编辑独立。2002 年美国 COGS 会议确定了 18 条评价指南的标准：概述、重点、目标、使用者或背景、目标人群、制定者、资金来源或赞助人、收集证据的方法、建议分级标准、综合证据的方法、发布前评审更新计划、定义、建议、基本原理、潜在利害、患者偏好、运算法则、指南执行中需要考虑的事项。

借鉴上述两大指南质量评估工具初步评价了所收集到的已公开发布的 11 个中医和中西医结合临床指南的质量。结果见表 1。11 篇指南均未描述证据收集的方法，仅有 1 篇粗略描述综合证据的方法，1 篇说明推荐意见的证据质量分级，2 篇描述指南使用的目标人群，4 篇未列详细的参考文献，均未描述指南使用者，未描述卫生经济学情况、患者情况、指南更新、利益冲突、发布前测试等。关于作者情况，均无详细介绍。当然，中医自身特点也应考虑。

2. 中医和中西医结合临床指南制定中存在的问题

2.1 指南编写人员专业背景比较单一

目前的中医或中西医结合指南大多由临床专家根据自身经验和对相关证据的汇总分析后分工编写而成，缺乏多学科专家的参与，尚未充分考虑卫生经济学家、流行病学家、统计学家和患者等的意见，使得制定的指南具有一定的局限性。一些所谓指南实际上是中医或中西医结合有关学科或病种教科书的翻版。

2.2 缺乏高级别的证据，且未根据证据的论证强度注明推荐意见

制订中医、中西医结合临床治疗指南最大的问题是缺乏自己的循证医学研究基础。在许多疾病的治疗上，传统医学目前仍然缺乏高级别的临床证据[20]。中医、中西医结合临床指南引用的证据多以古代文献、专家意见、无对照的病例报告、病例系列、设有对照但管理和控制不好的临床试验和单个小样本随机对照试验等低质量的证据为主，高质量的研究证据如系统评价和多中心、大样本、随机对照试验的文献较少。大多数指南没有说明如何收集证据，证据如何评价，也未根据证据级别注明推荐意见。

另外，还存在指南制作不够规范，循证指南和真正对提高临床疗效具有指导作用的指南较少，以及指南修订不及时等问题。

3. 中医和中西医结合临床指南制定问题的对策

3.1 成立多学科专家组成的指南制定小组

应成立由多学科人员组成的指南制定小组负责指南的制定，下设指南发起小组，挑选和评估证据的研究组和参与形成最终推荐建议的研究组等，

表 1　11 个已公开发布的中医和中西医结合临床指南基本情况

指南名称	制定组织	发表时间	出处	收集证据	综合证据的方法	建议或证据分组标准	使用的目标人群	参考文献
SARS 中医诊疗指南	中华中医药学会	2003 年 10 月	中国医药学报；中医杂志	未描述	粗略描述	未描述	未描述	有
亚健康中医临床指南	中华中医药学会	2006 年 10 月	中国中医药出版社	未描述	未描述	未描述	未描述	有
肝纤维化中西医结合诊疗指南	中国中西医结合学会肝病专业委员会	2006 年 8 月	中西医结合肝病杂志；中国中西医结合杂志；中西医结合学报；中华肝脏病杂志	未描述	未描述	有	有	有
慢性前列腺炎中西医结合诊疗指南（试行版）	中国中西医结合学会男科专业委员会	2007 年 6 月	中国中西医结合杂志	未描述	未描述	未描述	未描述	有
糖尿病中医防治指南	中华中医药学会糖尿病分会	2007 年 7 月	中国中医药出版社	未描述	未描述	未描述	未描述	有
中医内科常见病诊疗指南	中华中医药学会内科分会	2008 年 8 月	中国中医药出版社	未描述	未描述	未描述	未描述	有
血脂康临床应用的中国专家共识	中国医师协会心血管内科医师分会	2008 年 6 月	中国心血管网	未描述	未描述	未描述	有	有
小儿肺炎喘嗽中医诊疗指南	中华中医药学会儿科分会	2008 年 5 月	中医儿科杂志	未描述	未描述	未描述	未描述	未描述
小儿哮喘中医诊疗指南	中华中医药学会儿科分会	2008 年 5 月	中医儿科杂志	未描述	未描述	未描述	未描述	未描述
小儿泄泻中医诊疗指南	中华中医药学会儿科分会	2008 年 7 月	中医儿科杂志	未描述	未描述	未描述	未描述	未描述
流行性腮腺炎中医诊疗指南	中华中医药学会儿科分会	2008 年 9 月	中医儿科杂志	未描述	未描述	未描述	未描述	未描述

由中医或中西医结合临床和基础研究、临床流行病学和循证医学、统计学、卫生经济学、卫生法律和医学决策等多学科专家共同参与，同时纳入管理、撰写、编辑、证据合成、指南制订等方面的人员给予相应的支持和指导，并参考患者代表的意见，以使指南更有实用性。

3.2　结合中医学自身特点，严格遵循循证指南制订的原则和流程

　　循证指南强调在回顾和评价现有临床证据的基础上制定指南，在没有证据的情况下通过严格的讨论共识达成一致性的推荐意见。苏格兰指南制定组织（Scottish Intercollegiate Guideline Network，SIGN）将指南制定过程具体归纳为 9 步[1]：（1）遴选指南题目；（2）陈述临床问题；（3）收集证据；（4）评价证据；（5）将证据整合成指南建议；（6）对指南建议进行分级；（7）考虑患者的意愿；（8）讨论成本效果；（9）更新计划。中医或中西医结合临床指南也应根据自身的特点，规范指南的制定过程和操作程序。

3.3 注重证据的收集、评价、整合、实时更新

从收集证据到将其综合成指南建议是制定指南的核心部分，需要应用系统的方法检索证据，设定合理的入选和排除证据的标准，使用正确的方法对证据的级别进行评分，再根据证据的级别和强度提出推荐意见。当缺乏高质量证据时，由较低质量证据包括专家意见等形成的推荐意见应说明推荐理由，并详细注明证据的等级、专家意见以及形成共识的过程。推荐建议和支持证据之间应当有清楚的联系，提供建议的等级和推荐理由，同时要根据新的证据更新。

例如目前国家批准上市的中成药均有明确的适应证，大多有公开发表的临床研究资料，其证据级别相对较高。临床指南所推荐的中成药也应根据最新的研究数据及时更新，以便临床医生决策时参考。

3.4 建立符合中医文献自身特点的证据评价与证据分级方法

中医学经过数千年的发展，积累了丰富的临床经验，浩如烟海的古籍也记载了大量有效的治法和方药，但这些文献由于缺乏高质量随机对照试验的评价，其证据等级很低，只能列于专家经验。但是，随机对照试验等临床研究方法大都是在以同质性人群为基础的生物医学模式下建立起来的方法，所强调的基线均衡、混杂因素控制等可能正是医生个体化辨证论治的关键。因此，设计实施良好的随机对照试验并不一定能够真实反映中医个体化辨证论治的疗效，大量来自低质量研究证据的经典方药不一定对应较低的推荐强度，需要建立符合中医学自身特点的证据评价与证据分级方法。在借鉴循证医学证据分级体系的基础上，对中医文献中大量的史料记载、名医经验、单方验方等，应根据是否经过临床长期广泛应用（有人建议以使用时间超过30年为准），是否经病例系列研究、病例对照研究、队列研究、非随机对照研究、随机对照研究等不同论证强度的研究的系统验证，划分不同的等级。

3.5 注重中医指南的适用性与指导性，加强对指南质量的评估

疾病千变万化，且中医学治疗疾病强调辨证论治，因人、因地、因时制宜，不同地域在同一疾病的辨证诊断、用药特点和习惯等方面均有所不

同。因此，希望通过一个标准来统一全国是不现实的。在全国各专业委员会组织制定全国指南的基础上，为推广临床指南的应用，各地还可结合当地的经济条件、价值观、医疗资源和医疗水平制定合适的指导意见，方药的选择也要充分考虑地区差异及临床用药习惯，逐步提高中医、中西医结合临床指南的操作性和实用性。同时，还应加强对指南质量的评估。可结合中医或中西医结合临床指南的特点，借鉴目前基本得到公认的评价指南方法学质量的工具 AGREE 和 COGS 等对已制定的中医或中西医结合指南进行评估，对不合要求的指南及时提出改进甚至废止的意见。

参考文献

[1] Scottish Intercollegiate Guidelines Network. SIGN 50：a guideline developer's handbook [2008-11-6]. http：//www. sign.ac.uk/guidelines/fulltext/50/.

[2] 中华中医药学会 . 传染性非典型肺炎（SARS）中医诊疗指南 . 中医杂志，2003，44（11）：865-871.

[3] 中华中医药学会 . 传染性非典型肺炎（SARS）中医诊疗指南 . 中国医药学报，2003，18（10）：579-586.

[4] 汪受传，赵霞，韩新民，等 . 小儿肺炎喘嗽中医诊疗指南 . 中医儿科杂志，2008，4（3）：1-3.

[5] 赵霞，汪受传，韩新民，等 . 小儿哮喘中医诊疗指南 . 中医儿科杂志，2008，4（3）：4-6.

[6] 韩新民，汪受传，虞舜，等 . 小儿泄泻中医诊疗指南 . 中医儿科杂志，2008，4（4）：1-3.

[7] 韩新民，汪受传，虞舜，等 . 流行性腮腺炎中医诊疗指南 . 中医儿科杂志，2008，4（5）：1-3.

[8] 中国中西医结合学会肝病专业委员会 . 肝纤维化中西医结合诊疗指南 . 中西医结合学报，2006，4（6）：551-555.

[9] 中国中西医结合学会肝病专业委员会 . 肝纤维化中西医结合诊疗指南 . 中国中西医结合杂志，2006，26（11）：1052-1056.

[10] 中国中西医结合学会肝病专业委员会 . 肝纤维化中西医结合诊疗指南 . 中西医结合肝病杂志，2006，16（5）：316-320.

[11] 中国中西医结合学会肝病专业委员会 . 肝纤维化中西医结合诊疗指南 . 中华肝脏病杂志，2006，14（11）：866-870.

[12] 中国中西医结合学会男科专业委员会 . 慢性前列腺炎中西医结合诊疗指南（试行版）. 中国中西医结合杂志，2007，27（11）：1052-1056.

[13] 中华中医药学会 . 亚健康中医临床指南 . 北京：中国中医药出版社 . 2006.

[14] 中华中医药学会糖尿病分会 . 糖尿病中医防治指南 . 北

京：中国中医药出版社．2007．

[15] 中华中医药学会内科分会．中医内科常见病诊疗指南．
北京：中国中医药出版社．2008．

[16] 中国医师协会心血管内科医师分会．血脂康临床应用
的中国专家共识 [2008-11-6]. http：//www.365heart.
com/tabloid/2008/05/temp_21227.html.

[17] The AGREE Collaboration. Appraisal of Guidelines
Research and Evaluation（AGREE）instrument
[2008-11-06]. http：//www.agreecollaboration.org.

[18] Shiffman RN, Shekelle P, Overhage JM, 等．
Standardized reporting of clinical practice guidelines：
aproposal from the Conference on Guideline Standardization.
Ann Intern Med, 2003, 139（6）：493-498.

[19] 詹思延．临床指南研究与评价工具简介．中国循证儿科
杂志，2007, 2（5）：375-377.

[20] 宋军，陈可冀．尽早制定传统医学临床治疗指南．中国
中西医结合杂志，2006, 26（7）：581-584.

高血压中西医结合治疗研究的探索 [*]

陈可冀

20 世纪 50 年代后期，我研究了高血压病人弦脉与儿茶酚胺代谢水平关系获进展。我是活血化瘀"冠心 II 号方"复方及芳香温通复方宽胸气雾剂抗心肌缺血及其机制的主要研究者之一，也是益气活血复方治疗心肌梗死的主要设计者之一。我首先应用川芎嗪（四甲基吡嗪）治疗急性缺血性脑血管病并研究其抗血小板机制获显效，现仍在城乡推广应用；我提倡用温通疗法治疗病态窦房结综合征，并是首先应用附子 1 号（去甲乌头碱）治疗该病的主要研究者之一。我研究血府逐瘀汤及芎芍（有效部位）胶囊抗 PTCA 及支架置入术后冠状动脉再狭窄及其对相关基因表达的影响和对内皮素及一氧化氮水平的影响，并取得显著进展。我阐明了血瘀证与血小板超微结构和功能的联系，并在研究复方与证候关系的药物动力学上获得进展。

1. 高血压病人弦脉脉象及其机制的研究

1958—1964 年，中国中医研究院与中国医学科学院阜外心血管病医院（简称阜外医院）协作进行冠心病和高血压病的临床治疗研究。在这一段时间里，我同时对高血压病人常见的弦脉脉象表现和它的有关机制进行探讨。我用中国科学院声学专家马大猷院士帮助设计的酒石酸钾钠压电晶体脉搏描记仪描记高血压病人的所谓"如张弓弦"的弦脉，与心冲击图、心电图及心音图同步描记，将弦脉脉搏波图形分为三级，并与正常脉（平脉）作对照，其程度与血压水平基本相关。在黄宛、张锡钧教授的指导下，对弦脉经治疗后的等级变化与尿内去甲肾上腺素水平（von Euler 荧光法）测定做比较，证明二者确有联系。黄宛教授本来要我和当时在阜外医院工作的吴宁大夫一起总结，但因吴宁大夫临床工作很忙，就经我总结后，再经黄宛教授修改并发表于《中华内科杂志》1962 年第 10 期上。黄宛教授很认真，还专门把我叫他到办公室给予指导，并介绍一本Wiggers CJ 著的 Physiology in Health and Disease给我撰稿时作参考，给我印象深刻。至今我仍对黄宛教授怀有不胜感激之情。

2. 高血压病辨证分型治疗的观察

当年中国中医研究院与阜外医院合作的项目很多。吴英恺、黄国俊教授的食管癌治疗，由名中医蒲辅周和高辉远大夫参与；心血管病由名中医赵锡武、郭士魁参与，我和张家鹏、苗延升、马淑良大夫也参加了这一部分的协作。参加心血管病协作的其他 5 人都已相继故去。1958 年，吴英恺、黄宛、方圻、蔡如升几位阜外医院前辈们都曾到中医研究院开会商讨协作。当年对高血压病治疗盛行用利血平治疗，国产药物则提倡用萝芙木治疗，中医药方面还没有特殊的中成药供临床应用。我记得1981 年随 WHO 组织的访问团访问印度时，印度医学界当时还时常自豪地提到利血平的研发成就。

当年中医辨证论治分型治疗共总结病例 262

---

* 原载于余振球，惠汝太，朱鼎良主编《中国高血压防治历史》，科学出版社，2010，153-164

例，根据老中医的思路和经验，分为8个型，也没有设阳性对照药作比较，是很初步的经验性总结。在阳亢、阴虚阳亢、阴虚、阴阳两虚和阳虚为纲的基础上分为肝热上冲、肝风、怔忡、胸痹、中风等八个证型，分型论治；对症状缓解效果还比较好，但只对轻度高血压病人有效。当时赵锡武老大夫很有想法，他说："把血压计砸了，就没有高血压了！"当然，这是很不切合实际的。这个结果写成论文后，1959年在西安召开的全国心脏血管疾病学术报告会议由我做了大会报告，当时我仅29岁。它激励着我继续努力，探索提高疗效的措施。

3. 血压昼夜变化规律与高血压阴阳辨证联系的探索

我在工作中，注意到了阴阳平衡失调与高血压的关系。进入20世纪80年代，有了动态血压监测仪。我和一个由美来读博士学位的研究生一起对84例高血压病人的24小时昼夜血压变化规律与辨证关系进行了观察。发现偏阳亢型的一般第一高峰出现在辰时，第二高峰出现在酉时，而子时和未时处于低谷。偏阴虚的第一高峰出现在下午，第二高峰出现在上午。

按照传统医学理论，偏阳亢型高血压最高峰值出现在辰时，高于酉时，适逢自然界阳入于阴之后，阳气趋亢，与患者体内阳气相触，因而失去平衡和适应。在动物实验中也注意到，自发性高血压大鼠血压高峰也出现在辰时，很有意思。这一部分工作发表于Chinese Journal of Integrative Medicine 8年第2期（in English）。

4. 北京地区长期素食人群血压水平的观察

1960年前后，我和西苑医院心血管病研究室同事一起对北京地区寺院长期素食的僧尼进行心血管病普查，共96例，平均年龄63.6岁，平均素食34年（女）和44年（男）。结果发现他们的血清总胆固醇水平及肱动脉血压水平与普食人（64例，平均年龄66岁）并无明显差别。考虑长期素食者血脂水平异常及血压的改变与内源性代谢失调及血管本身的老化有关。认为还应该提倡合理的营养和合理防治。这部分工作后来我在1964年在兰州召开的全国第二届心血管病学术会议上作了分组发言。

5. 天麻钩藤饮和清眩调压汤的临床观察

20世纪60年代，中国医学科学院生理学系陈

孟勤教授和药物研究所雷海鹏教授曾经实验研究证实天麻钩藤饮有调节大脑皮质第二信号系统的功用，这与传统医学认为适用于肝风型的高血压病似可相通，对眩晕症状有一定效果。在天麻钩藤饮的基础上，结合我的个人经验，曾制定了一个清眩调压汤（由天麻、钩藤、黄芩、川牛膝、生杜仲、夜交藤、鲜生地、桑叶、菊花、苦丁茶组成），经对轻中度高血压病人做临床观察，证明虽在降压方面较阳性对照药尼群地平明显为弱，但解决相关眩晕等症状却较好，因而宜做进一步探索。

6. 有关中药方剂调节血压的相关机制初探

为了进一步探讨单核苷酸基因多态性与血压幅度及药物疗效的关系，我的课题组对206例汉族高血压病人的血管紧张素Ⅱ的1型受体基因（AT_1R）多态性的关系进行了研究。在高血压病组，AC+CC基因型的频率高于正常血压组，C 66等位基因在高血压组高于对照组，AT_1R在不同证型中未见显著差异；无论是卡托普利，还是清眩调压方，对AA及AC型基因型高血压有类似作用，但与是否携带C1166等位基因则均无关。该论文在《中国中西医结合杂志》2005年第8期发表。

7. 降压中药研究的反省

我国很多学者在寻找降压中药方面做过许多研究，1964年武汉吕富华教授的汉防己甲素（tetrandrine，Tet）的研究应该说是成功的，其口服及血管内应用的药物于20世纪五六十年代曾上市，我曾用过静脉内注射的Tet，60～20mg/次剂量，在多位病例中多次应用，可有效控制高血压危象，可惜长期未能实现人工合成而在市场上消失。不少中草药有效部位或单体，经实验证实有一定降压效应，但多未坚持工作下去，未能过渡到临床应用，包括莲心碱、钩藤碱等。有些成分可能效应不强，但进一步改构，可能尚有研发前景，似乎大家转换医学的观念尚不足吧。现在西药降压药已有长足的进步，大家对中药进行探究的兴趣可能不那么浓了，很是可惜。在中西药合伍的复方方面，20世纪60年代上海的邝安堃教授曾有复方降压片，风行一时。现在市场上还有复方罗布麻片及珍菊降压片，这两种中成药分别在北方及南方流行；近期FDA批准生产的由三种降压药组成的polypill，在综合作用的思路方面似有某些相似。

关于高血压病的中西医结合研究 *

陈可冀

2006 年中国心血管病年度报告指出，我国高血压病的患者数已近 2 亿，是当代我国人口健康和疾病防治中十分严峻的问题和任务；虽然现在人群中高血压病的知晓率和防治率已较往年有明显增加，但控制率仍不甚满意。降压药物的选择虽已有很大的选择余地，包括钙拮抗剂、血管紧张素转化酶抑制剂、血管紧张素受体拮抗剂、利尿剂、β 受体阻滞剂、α 受体阻滞剂、固定复方制剂，以及中成药珍菊降压片、复方罗布麻片等多种中西药物，但由于大多数患者需要终生用药和联合药物治疗，有心、脑、肾并发症以及合并糖尿病等的患者，更需要结合具体病情进行个体化的治疗，其不同程度的不良反应或不合理用药在很多患者身上常有所表现，增加了治疗的难度和不满意度。

单纯中医药治疗对轻度高血压病患者在降低血压方面表现有一定的治疗效果，但对中等度以上的高血压病患者并不满意。不过在调理眩晕、头痛、烦躁、失眠等症状方面，却显示有一定的治疗功效，因而在减轻患者痛苦，减少并发症的发生方面，以及减少西药降压药的用量，减少不良反应方面，中西医结合治疗有一定的优势，应该加强临床及其研究，总结经验和规律，以进一步改善患者的生活质量，延缓或预防其并发症的发生。

本刊本期刊出一组有关高血压病的治疗和研究文章。"痰湿体质高血压病患者脂联素（adiponectin，APN）异常与脂联素基因多态性的相关性研究"一文指出，痰湿体质高血压病患者血清 APN 水平明显低于非痰湿体质患者，而且观察到 APN 基因单核苷酸多态性（SNP）3224 的 T 基因携带者可能是 APN 单核苷酸多态性异常的遗传特征。鉴于 APN 与腹内肥胖、代谢综合征以及心血管功能调节有明显的联系，APN 水平降低更是代谢综合征的一种特征性标志，结合这一认识，提高对高血压病合并有痰湿证型表现患者的病证结合治疗，具有一定的临床指导意义。这也表明，有关祛除痰湿的方药研究和临床应用，在高血压防治中是值得进一步探索、应用和研究的。同时，它也启示我们，其他相关高血压病的中医证型的研究也是值得进一步探索的。本期另一篇有关携带 SLC6A2 基因启动子 3-AG/GG 型可能是高血压病重度血瘀证易患基因，启动子 2-GC/GC、G-C 单倍体可能是血瘀证易患因素之一，相关研究对于本病血瘀证的认识也是一个进步。这些研究对于高血压患者进一步采用"病证结合，方证对应，降压与证候治疗结合，中西医结合防治"看来应是合理的。

在联合药物治疗方面，本期发表的一项临床研究表明，以动脉顺应性及动态血压平滑性为指标，降压协同血脂康胶囊治疗，表明能降低患者动脉血压的脉压（pulse pressure，PP）和脉压指数（pulse pressure index，PPI），并注意到可提高降压药物的血压平滑指数（smooth index，SI）。其治疗后 SI 与 PPI、脉搏波传导速度（pulse wave velocity，PWV）和年龄具有明显的负相关性，这一结果提示必要的联合用药在降压之余，对改善证候或症状会有所帮助。

关于降压中药单味药和复方的研究，自 20 世纪 60 年代开始就有不少学者进行探索，取得了一定进展，其中包括汉防己甲素的口服和血管内应用，以及天麻钩藤饮复方等。我的临床应用也确认汉防己甲素有确切的临床效果，血管内应用对高血压急症有效，起效时间快，该药曾被批准面市，只可惜该药未能实现人工合成，因而限制了其大规模产业化生产而停用。类似药物如莲心碱及钩藤碱等的研究，可惜均未深入下去，多浅尝辄止。希望多学科协作，进一步开展深入的创新性研究，并坚持下去，做出新的业绩，以减少高血压病患者的卒中事件发生率。

* 原载于《中国中西医结合杂志》，2010，30（5）：453

高血压血管内皮机制的中西医研究现状 [*]

陈懿宇 张京春

高血压严重危及人类健康，是引起心脑血管事件的危险因素，开展高血压相关机制的研究从而进行有效的干预意义重大，围绕高血压发生、发展及其预后转归，学术界开展了大量有关内皮功能机制的研究。本文主要分析血管内皮功能障碍和高血压的关系，以及中西医治疗对高血压患者内皮功能的影响。

1. 血管内皮功能障碍和高血压

1.1 血管内皮的生理功能

自 1980 年 Furchgott[1] 发现血管内皮能够释放血管内皮舒张因子（EDRFs）以来，对内皮细胞功能的研究逐渐成为心血管领域研究的热点。血管内皮细胞（vascular endothelial cell，VEC）不仅具有屏障作用，还是体内内分泌器官之一。VEC 可以分泌调节血管张力的相关因子，以及凝血和纤溶系统、炎症反应和血管平滑肌增殖相关因子。其中，EDRFs 有一氧化氮（NO）、前列环素 I_2（PGI_2）、内皮源性超极化因子（EDHF）等，可引起血管舒张[2]；血管收缩因子（EDCF）有内皮素-1（ET-1）、血栓素 A_2（TXA_2）、血管紧张素 Ⅱ（Ang Ⅱ）等，可引起血管收缩；凝血相关因子有血管性假性血友病因子（vW F）、血浆纤溶酶原激活物抑制物-1（PA I-1）、组织因子（TF）等；抗凝相关因子有组织型纤溶酶原激活物（t-PA）、组织因子途径抑制物（TFPI）、抗凝血酶Ⅲ（AT-Ⅲ）；炎症反应相关因子有 C 反应蛋白（CRP）、细胞间黏附分子（ICAM-1）、血管细胞黏附分子-1（VCAM-1）以及白细胞介素 6（IL-6）等[3]，促进血管平滑肌增殖的因子有 ET-1、Ang-Ⅱ、肝细胞生长因子（HGF）等。

1.2 VEC 功能紊乱与高血压

高血压病和 VEC 功能紊乱密不可分，就其病理机制而言，二者可能互为因果[4]，高血压可以引起血管内皮功紊乱，VEC 功能减退促进高血压的发展。

高血压是内皮损伤的始动因素[5]。有研究表明，在未累及靶器官的低、中危组高血压患者 VEC 功能已有轻度受损，在有靶器官损害的极高危患者，VEC 功能损伤更明显[6]。目前普遍认为其机制可能与氧化应激有关[7]。高血压内皮损伤后，自由基产生增多。氧化和抗氧化平稳系统的破坏导致氧化细胞的破坏。超氧化物歧化酶（SOD）是体内合成的氧自由基清除剂之一，能有效地清除超氧阴离子自由基（O_2^-），其活性可反映机体清除自由基的能力。李卫萍[8] 和李小兵等[9] 对高血压患者研究发现，高血压患者 SOD 水平降低。丙二醛（MDA）是生物膜中多价不饱和脂肪酸受自由基作用生成的脂质过氧化代谢产物，可造成生物膜损伤，MDA 含量可以代表自由基的活性。有研究表明 SOD/MDA 值则能更准确地反映机体氧化与抗氧化之间的平衡关系[8,9]。

VEC 功能减退促进高血压的发展。由于内皮功能受损，VEC 因子平衡失调，使得 ET 合成增多，NO 的合成和释放减少，导致血管内皮依赖性舒张功能下降，收缩功能增强，血管壁结构发生变化，血压的升高。有研究表明在血压正常而 VEC 功能受损的人群未来发生高血压的机会与 VEC 功能正常的人群相比明显增加[10]，这提示 VEC 功能不全可能是高血压早期的原发表现。长期血压升高又导致靶器官受损和血管内皮结构改变，发生各种并发症，最终导致这些器官衰竭。

1.3 高血压内皮功能不全的评价方法

目前还没有公认的评价 VEC 功能不全的金标准，常用的方法主要有血管内皮活性相关物质检查、内皮活性相关细胞检查，以及其他方法。

其中实验室检查包括血管活性物质如 NO、ET-1、TXA_2、PGI_2、黏附分子、炎症因子、vWF、PAI-1、AT-Ⅲ、血浆生长素水平（Ghrelin）[11,12]、HGF[13]；内皮相关细胞检查包括循环内皮细

[*] 原载于《中国老年学杂志》，2010，30（20）：3010-3013

胞（CEC）计数及形态检查[14]、内皮细胞微颗粒（endothelialmicroparticles，EMPs）[15]、血管内皮祖细胞（EPCs）[16]等。其他包括目前应用肱动脉超声技术评价前臂血管血流介导的血管舒张（FMD），是临床常用且较为成熟的评价内皮功能的方法[17]；还可以应用心导管方法[18]，但是这一方法具有创伤和一定风险，限制了其临床应用。此外，还有冷加压试验和正电子发射断层显像（PET）技术来评价血管内皮功能[19]。

2. 中西医治疗对高血压患者内皮功能的影响

2.1 西医治疗对高血压患者内皮功能的影响

高血压引起血管内皮功能减退，增加患者心血管事件的发生率。经过对血压的最佳药物治疗后，内皮功能改善者较那些仍异常的患者冠心病事件发生率明显降低[20]。在目前应用的降压药物中，除少数能对内皮起作用的β受体拮抗剂外，一般的β受体拮抗剂无改善血管内皮功能的作用，而钙通道阻滞剂、血管紧张肽转换酶抑制剂（ACEI）、血管紧张素受体拮抗剂（ARB）可改善血管内皮的功能[21]。

2.1.1 肾上腺素β受体（β受体）拮抗剂 一般的β受体拮抗剂无改善血管内皮功能的作用。但是也有研究表明选择性的β_1受体拮抗剂如奈必洛尔（nebivolol）和卡维地洛具有改善血管内皮功能的作用[22]。

2.1.2 钙通道阻滞剂 二氢吡啶类钙通道阻滞剂和非二氢吡啶类钙通道阻滞剂均能改善血管内皮功能。其中二氢吡啶类钙通道阻滞剂的作用更强。钙通道阻滞剂具有一定的抗氧化作用，可使过氧化物浓度降低，使NO破坏减少，同时使血小板释放NO增加。宋月霞等[23]研究非洛地平对原发性高血压患者血管内皮功能的影响，发现治疗后血浆Ghrelin、NO、FMD水平明显升高，ET-1水平降低（$P < 0.01$或$P < 0.05$）。提示非洛地平在降压治疗的同时可提高血浆生长素水平，改善高血压患者的血管内皮功能。另一研究观察到硝苯地平可改善血管内皮功能，而氢氯噻嗪无改善血管内皮功能的作用[24]。

2.1.3 ARB ARB可改善血管内皮功能，使缩血管作用减弱，氧自由基产生减少，NO破坏减少，并促进NO合成。吕纳强等[25]观察AngⅡ受体拮抗剂厄贝沙坦治疗原发性轻中度高血压患者对血浆

ET-1及CECs的影响。结果显示治疗后血压下降的同时，血浆ET-1和CECs显著下降。可见厄贝沙坦在有效降压的同时可改善血管内皮的功能。另有研究发现缬沙坦对内皮功能的改善作用可能优于氨氯地平[26]。还有学者[27]通过测定基线及海捷亚治疗后血清HGF、ET和NO水平，发现高血压患者血清HGF增高，治疗后血清HGF水平下降、血管内皮功能改善。

2.1.4 ACEI Taddei等[22]研究发现，ACEI可以使ATⅡ生成减少，从而减少ATⅡ对NO合成的抑制作用，同时减少氧自由基的产生，减少其对NO破坏。此外，ACEI还可以使缓激肽浓度增加，促进NO的合成[28]。刘妙等[29]研究发现经贝那普利治疗后，原发性高血压患者肱动脉内皮依赖性舒张功能增加，血清NO水平升高，ET、肿瘤坏死因子（TNF）-α、IL-1和IL-6水平降低。同时，苯那普利可有效降低血压，并且不良反应少。但是Sozen等研究发现ACEI和ARB对改善内皮功能有一定作用，但并不持久，3年后内皮功能又回复到治疗前的水平，推测内皮功能损害可能是不可逆的[30]。此外，还有研究发现，钙离子拮抗剂和ACEI类药物合用，可以改善血管内皮功能[31]。

此外，在2006年美国心脏病学会上，Weber教授做了关于口服选择性内皮素A型体拮抗剂辅助治疗顽固性高血压的临床Ⅱ期的报告。该研究收治了115名患者，服用3种足够剂量降压药65例，服用4种降压药50例。降压药包括ACEI、利尿剂、ARB以及其他种类降压药。多中心进行双盲法，采用的内皮素A型受体拮抗剂治疗组与安慰剂组人数比为2：1。治疗组药量从10mg/d开始，逐渐在2周后可增量到50、100、150mg，最后可达到300mg。结果发现治疗组收缩压从治疗第8周后明显降低，并且越严重的顽固性高血压效果越好[32]。

2.2 中医及中西医结合治疗对高血压患者内皮功能的影响

2.2.1 高血压病证候与内皮功能失调 李小兵等[9]通过观察高血压病肝火亢盛、阴阳两虚、阴虚阳亢、痰湿壅盛证患者血中自由基水平及内皮相关舒缩因子，并与正常人对照，探讨了高血压病不同证候与血管自由基损伤的关系及内皮细胞功能失调。结果显示高血压病各证候组的指标与对照组间有显著差异。张臣等[33]探讨了原发性高血压病不同中医证型与血浆ET及血压的关系。通过不同中

医证型各组 ET 浓度变化分析，得出结论为各中医证型组 ET 值及血压较正常对照组明显增高，变化规律为：阴阳两虚型＞肝肾阴虚型＞阴虚阳亢型＞肝阳上亢型＞正常对照组。需要进一步临床研究验证 ET 及血压作为高血压中医辨证分型的客观化指标。

2.2.2　中医治疗对高血压患者内皮功能的影响　目前中医主要通过经方或自拟的降压汤进行相关临床或动物实验研究。谭海彦[34]等用天麻钩藤饮治疗肝阳上亢型高血压患者，对照组服用非洛地平，分别检测两组治疗前后血清谷胱甘肽过氧化物酶（GSH-PX）和过氧化氢酶（CAT）含量。结果显示治疗后，两组 GSH-PX 和 CAT 含量均增加（$P < 0.01$），但治疗组较对照组增加明显（$P < 0.01$）。天麻钩藤饮改善高血压患者内皮功能的机制可能是通过增加 GSH-PX 和 CAT 含量，清除过多的氧自由基，防止血管内皮细胞脂质过氧化，从而改善患者的血管内皮功能。王书梅[35]也选择天麻钩藤饮治疗高血压肝阳上亢型患者，观察对血清 NO、血浆 ET 含量的影响。结果显示天麻钩藤饮组能显著升高血清 NO 水平及降低血浆 ET 水平。

在自拟降压汤的研究方面，主要包括张焱等[36]用化湿利水泄浊合剂治疗后患者的 FMD 明显改善，NO 水平升高（$P < 0.05$），其作用与西拉普利组相似。疗效提示化湿利水泄浊合剂对原发性高血压（EH）患者血管内皮依赖性舒张功能有改善作用。杜立峰等[37]以平肝降压胶囊治疗高血压，结果显示平肝降压胶囊具有明显的降低血压和改善临床症状，可降低血浆 ET、AngⅡ的水平，改善血黏度，从而达到降低血压的作用。陈可冀等[38]曾自拟清眩胶囊治疗阴虚阳亢型轻中度高血压，发现清眩胶囊对治疗轻中度高血压有一定的降压效果，可抑制肾素 - 血管紧张素 - 醛固酮系统（RAAS）活性和下调血管紧张素Ⅱ1型受体（AT1）mRNA 表达和蛋白表达，以及纠正 ET/ 降钙素基因相关肽（CGRP）失衡。

动物实验方面研究也集中在用常用降压方后观察血管相关舒缩因子。刘婷等[39]用桂枝汤观察其对自发性高血压大鼠（SHR）血浆、下丘脑及主动脉中 ET、神经降压素（NT）含量的影响。结果显示桂枝汤可以显著降低 SHR 的 ET 水平，并对抗 NT 的降低，为中药改善内皮功能提供了一定的实验依据。徐树楠等[40]采用 SHR 模型，发现活血降压方能明显降低 SHR 的血压，升高血清中 NO，降低血浆中 ET，还能降低血清胆固醇（CHO）、甘油三酯（TG）和低密度脂蛋白胆固醇（LDL-C），升高高密度脂蛋白胆固醇（HDL-C）。徐树楠[41]等还采用加灌附子汤的方法制备肝阳上亢模型，观察发现潜阳通络方能明显降低肝阳上亢型 SHR 血压，明显降低血浆中 ET 和心钠肽（ANP）的含量，从而改善血管的舒缩功能而达到较好的降压效果。李景新等[42]应用二肾一夹法制备 SHR 模型，结果发现沙苑子总黄酮可使 SHR 血清 ET-1 显著下降，NOS 略有升高。金龙等[43]采用硝基左旋精氨酸（L-NNA）诱导方法造模，显示用络活胶囊可降低 SHR 的血压、改善心率，并可显著降低血浆 ET、AngⅡ水平，升高 NO 含量。陈双厚等[44]对实验肾性高血压大鼠用降压舒心胶囊后，其血清内皮素、血浆血管紧张素Ⅰ和Ⅱ含量的水平均有明显的改善作用。

目前中医治疗对高血压患者内皮功能影响的研究主要以常用的中药降压方治疗后观察常见的血管相关舒缩因子，而对于凝血和纤溶系统、炎症反应以及血管平滑肌增殖相关因子的研究并不多见，同时缺乏大量的可重复研究试验数据，需要日后进一步探索。

2.2.3　中西医结合治疗对高血压患者内皮功能的影响　赵萍等[45]在氨氯地平有效降压的基础上，应用温胆泄浊法，结果发现温胆片组治疗后痰浊积分较安慰剂组有显著性改善、颈动脉内膜中层厚度（IMT）减少、颈动脉斑块积分降低（$P < 0.05$）；颈动脉斑块面积显著性减少（$P < 0.01$），高血压病患者肱动脉内皮依赖性舒张功能与颈动脉 IMT 间呈负相关（$r < -0.596$，$P < 0.05$），治疗后内皮依赖性舒张功能改善；但非内皮依赖性舒张功能两组比较差异无显著性。可见温胆泄浊法对颈动脉斑块和肱动脉内皮依赖性舒张功能异常有较好的改善作用。王晓君等[46]将 60 例 EH 患者随机单盲分为联服川芎素、培哚普利（A）组，单服培哚普利（B）组，结果显示两组治疗 4 周后与治疗前比较，血浆 ET-1、NO 及 BP 均有显著改善（$P < 0.01$ 或 $P < 0.05$），治疗后两组间比较发现各指标 A 组明显优于 B 组。未见有明显药物不良反应。可见联服川芎素、培哚普利在改善血管内皮功能方面具有协同作用。李浩等[47]将 40 只 SHR 随机分为降压胶囊加尼莫地平组、降压胶囊组、尼莫地平组和 SHR 模型组。

连续灌胃给药8周，结果显示与模型组比，降压胶囊联合尼莫地平组有较好的降压效果，且血浆ET、AngⅡ水平显著降低（$P < 0.05$，$P < 0.01$）、血浆降钙素基因相关肽（CGRP）水平显著升高（$P < 0.05$），左室重量及其指数均显著降低（$P < 0.05$）。提示降压胶囊联合尼莫地平能抑制ET、AngⅡ的生物活性，促进CGRP的释放，从而降低血压和减轻左心室肥厚。

VEC作为体内内分泌器官，与高血压关系密切。高血压可以引起血管内皮功能紊乱，血管内皮功能减退促进高血压的发展。内皮源性NO生物利用度降低、血管壁炎性反应增强、促凝物质增多、血小板聚集性增强、管壁增厚和管腔狭窄等，导致重要靶器官如心、脑、肾组织缺血，发生各种并发症，最终导致这些器官衰竭。目前研究的热点主要是高血压内皮损伤的机制，以及相关降压治疗对高血压患者内皮功能的影响，但是以治疗内皮损伤作为主要目的研究目前尚少。西医的降压药物中，钙通道阻滞剂、ACEI、ARB可改善血管内皮功能。中医治疗对高血压患者内皮功能影响的研究主要观察常用的中药降压方治疗后常见的血管相关舒缩因子的改变，而对其他内皮功能相关因子的研究并不多见，同时缺乏大量的可重复研究数据。中医高血压证候与血管内皮细胞功能失调的关系是目前临床研究的一个新领域，但缺乏大规模的临床研究。传统中药制剂与新型西药相结合治疗高血压，研究二者合用对高血压患者内皮功能的影响，是目前较多见的研究方法，但是内皮功能相关指标的选择比较局限。将内皮功能保护机制作为切入点，进一步探讨中西医结合治疗高血压是可行的研究方向。

参考文献

[1] Furchgott RF, Zawadzki JV. The obligatory role of endothelial cells in the relation of arterials mooth muscle by acetylcheoling. Nature, 1980, 288 (5789)：373-376.

[2] Gkaliagkousi E, Douma S, Zamboulis C, et al. Nitric oxide dysfunction in vascular endothelium and platelets：role in essential hypertension. J Hypertens, 2009, 27 (12)：2310-2320.

[3] Androulakis ES, Tousoulis D, Papageorgiou N, et al. Essential hypertension：is there a role for inflammatory mechanisms? Cardiol Rev, 2009, 17 (5)：216-221.

[4] Schiffrin EL. Vascular endothelia in hypertension. Vascu Pharmacol, 2005, 43 (1)：19-29.

[5] Spencer CG, Martin SC, Felmeden DC, et al. Relationship of homocysteine to markers of platelet and endothelial activation in "high risk" hypertensives a substudy of the Anglo-Scandinavian Cardiac Outcomes Trial. Int J Cardiol, 2004, 94 (2-3)：293-300.

[6] 陈明，胡申江，张健，等.不同危险度的高血压病人血管内皮功能.高血压杂志，2006，14（4）：257-260.

[7] de la Sierra A, Larrousse M. Endothelial dysfunction is associated with increased levels of biomarkers in essential hypertension. J Hum Hypertens, 2009, 26.

[8] 李卫萍，孙明，周宏研，等.原发性高血压患者血管内皮功能失调与活性氧的关系及阿托他汀治疗的影响.中国现代医学杂志，2005，15（7）：1096-1103.

[9] 李小兵，冼绍祥，洪永敦.高血压病证候与内皮功能失调及自由基损伤的关系探讨.中国中医基础医学杂志，2005，11（5）：62-64.

[10] Rossi R, Chiurlia E, Nuzzo A, et al. Flow-mediated vasodilation and the risk of developing hypertension in healthy postm enopausal women. J Am Coll Cardio, 2004, 44 (8)：1636-1640.

[11] Shimizu Y, Nagaya N, Teranishi Y, et al.Ghrenlin improves endothelial dysfunction through growth hormone independent mechanisms in rats. Biochem Biophys Res Commun, 2003, 310 (3)：830-835.

[12] Lig Z, Jiang W, Zhao J, et al. Ghrelin blunted vascular calcification *in vivo* and *in vitro* in rats. Regul Pept, 2005, 129 (1-3)：167-176.

[13] Nakamura T, Mizuno S, Matsumoto K, et al. Myocardial protection from ischemia preperfusion injury by endogenous and exogenous HGF. J Clin Invest, 2000, 106 (1 2)：1511-1519.

[14] Makin AJ, Blann AD, Chung NA, et al. Assessment of endothelial damage in atherosclerotic vascular disease by quantification of circulating endothelial cells. Relationship with von Willebr and factor and tissue factor. Eur Heart J, 2004, 25 (5)：371-376.

[15] 王妍，陶军，涂昌，等.高血压患者循环内皮细胞微颗粒水平的变化.中华老年心脑血管病杂志，2006，8（4）：222-224.

[16] de la Pea M, Barcel A, Barbe F, et al. Endothelia function and circulating endothelial progenitor cells in patients with sleep apnea syndrome. Respiration, 2008, 76 (1)：28-32.

[17] 孙妍，王国干，沈磊，等.高血压患者血管内皮功能及颈动脉内-中膜厚度与冠心病事件关系的研究.中国超声医学杂志，2007，23（12）：908-910.

[18] TioRA, Monnink SH, Amorosog, et al. Safety evaluation of routine intracoronary acetylcholine

in fusion in patients undergoing a first diagnostic coronary angiogram. J Investig Med, 2002, 50 (2): 133-139.

[19] Kjaer A, Meyer C, Nielsen FS, et al. Dipyridamole, cold pressor test, and demonstration of endothelial dysfunction: a PET study of myocardial perfusion in diabetes. J Nucl Med, 2003, 44 (1): 19-23.

[20] Modena M, Bonetti L, Coppi F, et al. Prognostic role of reversible endothelial dysfunction in hypertensive postmenopausal women. J Am Coll Cardiol, 2002; 40 (3): 505-510.

[21] 黄震华. 抗高血压药物与血管内皮功能. 中国新药与临床杂志, 2005, 24 (5): 398-401.

[22] Taddei S, Virdis A, Ghiadoni L, et al. Effects of antihypertensive drugs on endothelial dysfunction: clinical implications. Drugs, 2002, 62 (2): 265-284.

[23] 宋月霞, 王希柱, 钟雪莲. 非洛地平对高血压患者血浆生长素水平和血管内皮功能的影响. 中国药房, 2007, 18 (20): 1572-1574.

[24] Muiesan ML, Salvetti M, Monteduro C, et al. Effect of treatment on flow-dependent vasodilation of the brachial artery in essential hypertension. Hypertension, 1999, 33 (1 Pt 2): 575-580.

[25] 吕纳强, 何苒, 宋卫华, 等. 伊贝沙坦对原发性高血压患者血浆内皮素及循环内皮细胞的影响. 中华高血压杂志, 2007, 15 (6): 465-468.

[26] Tzemos N, Lim PO, MacDonald TM. Valsartan improves endothelial dysfunction in hypertension: a randomized, double-blind study. Cardiovasc Ther, 2009, 27 (3): 151-158.

[27] 王邦宁, 胡泽平, 陈大年, 等. 高血压患者血肝细胞生长因子与血管内皮功能的关系及干预研究. 中华高血压杂志, 2007, 15 (3): 219-222.

[28] Galiavich AS, Khamidullina AR, Galiavich RA. Effect of antihypertensive drugs on some humoral parameters of endothelial function. Kardiologiia, 2009, 49 (5): 30-33.

[29] 刘妙, 萧佩玉. 苯那普利对原发性高血压患者内皮功能和血清细胞因子水平的影响. 中山大学学报医学科学版, 2007, 28 (6): 35-37.

[30] Sozen AB, Kayacan MS, Tansel T, et al. Drugs with blocking effects on the renin-angiotensinaldosterone system do not improve endothelial dysfunction long-term in hypertensive patients. J Int Med Res, 2009, 37 (4): 996-1002.

[31] Musikhina NA, Iuferova OV, Gapon LI, et al. Structural-functional properties of the vascular wall in hypertensive patients with coronary heart disease: effects of felodipin and perindopril. Ter Arkh, 2009; 81 (9): 13-16.

[32] 2006 年美国心脏病学会 Weber 教授报告. 顽固性高血压治疗新药 - 内皮素受体拮抗剂. 中华高血压杂志, 2007, 15 (5): 436.

[33] 张臣, 邢之华, 刘卫平, 等. 高血压病中医证型与血浆内皮素及血压的相关性研究. 辽宁中医杂志, 2005, 32 (1): 6-7.

[34] 谭海彦, 朱莉, 邢之华, 等. 天麻钩藤饮改善高血压患者内皮功能的机理研究. 山东医药, 2005, 45 (1): 12-13.

[35] 王书梅, 刘建. 天麻钩藤饮对 66 例高血压患者一氧化氮和内皮素影响的临床研究. 现代预防医学, 2006, 33 (6): 1052-1053.

[36] 张焱, 陈咸川, 何立人, 等. 化湿利水泄浊合剂对高血压病患者血管内皮依赖性舒张功能的影响. 上海中医药杂志, 2005, 39 (6): 14-16.

[37] 杜立峰, 杨杰, 孙师元, 等. 平肝降压胶囊对原发性高血压患者血浆内皮素和血管紧张素 II 的影响. 中国临床康复, 2004, 8 (36): 8250-8251.

[38] 谢元华, 张京春, 蒋跃绒, 等. 陈可冀辨治高血压病医案的数据挖掘分析. 中西医结合心脑血管病杂志, 2008, 6 (2): 135-136.

[39] 刘婷, 张毅, 秦彩玲, 等. 桂枝汤降压作用机制初探——对血浆及组织中 ET、NT 含量的影响. 中国药学杂志, 2005, 40 (6): 421-423.

[40] 徐树楠, 张再康, 冯瑞雪, 等. 活血降压方对自发性高血压大鼠血压及血浆 ET、血清 NO 含量的影响. 中药药理与临床, 2004, 20 (5): 39-40.

[41] 徐树楠, 侯仙明, 王文智, 等. 潜阳通络方对肝阳上亢型高血压病大鼠血压和 ET、ANP 的影响. 中国中医基础医学杂志, 2007, 13 (12): 908-909.

[42] 李景新, 王贞, 王蓉, 等. 沙苑子总黄酮对自发性高血压大鼠血脂及内皮素活性的影响. 中国微循环, 2004, 8 (5): 336-337.

[43] 金龙, 周文泉. 络活胶囊治疗高血压病的实验研究. 中国中西医结合杂志, 2004, 1: 18 -20.

[44] 陈双厚, 刘瑞华, 李世洁. 降压舒心胶囊对实验肾性高血压大鼠血清内皮素、血浆血管紧张素 I、II 含量的影响. 中药药理与临床, 2004, 20 (3): 28-29.

[45] 赵萍, 陈洁, 洪永敦, 等. 温胆泄浊法对痰浊型高血压病患者血管内皮舒张功能与粥样硬化改善作用的超声研究. 中国中西医结合杂志, 2007, 27 (1): 21-24.

[46] 王晓君, 黄文增, 张步延. 联服川芎素、培哚普利与单服培哚普利对高血压患者血管内皮功能和血压的影响. 中华高血压杂志, 2006, 14 (12): 993-996.

[47] 李浩, 郭明冬, 刘剑刚. 降压胶囊联合尼莫地平对自发性高血压大鼠 ET、CGRP 及 Ang II 水平的影响. 中国老年学杂志, 2007, 27 (22): 2178-2180.

西洋参茎叶总皂苷的心血管效应及其机制探讨 *

王　琛　史大卓

1. 历史溯源

西洋参（*Panax quinquefolius* L.）又称花旗参、美国人参，为五加科人参属植物，原产于北美洲加拿大蒙特利尔、魁北克、温哥华山区和美国东部，20世纪70年代在我国吉林、黑龙江和陕西等省引入。西洋参作为传统中药，应用历史悠久，自18世纪在美洲被发现后由法国人传至中国，作为药用，也有300多年的历史。早在清康熙三十三年，当时的医学家汪昂著《补图本草备要》的增补项中首先收载了西洋参，称其"性凉、味苦、甘厚、气薄；补肺降火、生津液、除烦倦，虚而有火者相宜"。

西洋参中的化学成分比较复杂，包括皂苷类、氨基酸类、糖类、挥发油类、无机元素类和脂肪酸类等，其中主要的活性成分为人参皂苷。迄今为止，已从西洋参地下及地上部分分离鉴定出四种类型的皂苷：原人参二醇型、原人参三醇型、齐墩果酸型、奥克梯隆醇型皂苷，其中奥克梯隆醇型皂苷是西洋参中的特有成分，是区别同属植物人参的显著标志。

2. 西洋参的主要活性成分人参皂苷的组成及其生物学活性

徐惠波等[1]对西洋参茎叶总皂苷（*Panax quinquefolius* Saponins，PQS）的静脉注射液及口服制剂的毒理学进行研究。通过对小鼠一次性注射PQS、一天内多次注射PQS及大鼠、犬连续60天口服PQS，结果发现小鼠静脉注射PQS LD_{50}为352.5mg/kg，毒性极低，一天内给药量30g/kg时未见任何毒性反应。以1.5g/kg和0.75g/kg剂量给大鼠60天及2g/kg和1g/kg剂量给犬口服60天后，动物活动正常，状态良好，给药前后心电图、血常规及生化指标无异常改变，脏器指数无明显变化，也无组织病理学改变，以上均说明PQS毒性甚低。

2.1 原人参二醇型皂苷

原人参二醇型皂苷（Protopanaxadiol，PPD），根据C-20的绝对构型不同可分为20（S）和20（R）-原人参二醇型皂苷，如人参皂苷Ra_1、Ra_2、Rb_1、Rb_2、Rc和Rd。现代研究表明，其主要有肝、肾保护作用[2]，抗肿瘤作用[3]，抑制中枢系统，改善小鼠学习记忆能力和脑代谢，减轻脑损伤[4]。并可以改善微循环、抑制血小板聚集[5,6]，减少炎症因子IL-1、IL-6、TNF-α释放以减轻心源性休克、肺水肿等急性心、肺的损伤[7,8]，对缺血再灌注后损伤的心肌及人肾小管细胞具有一定的保护作用[9]。除此以外，人参二醇型皂苷还有降血糖、调节血脂、保护内皮细胞、调节冠状动脉血管张力、增加心肌血流灌注，具有一定的抗动脉粥样硬化作用，并且与化疗药物合用可以增加化疗药物的抗癌效应等[10-12]。

2.2 原人参三醇型皂苷

原人参三醇型皂苷（Protopanaxatriol，PPT）根据C-20位绝对构型不同可分为20（S）和20（R）-原人参三醇型皂苷，如人参皂苷Re、Rg_1、Rf、Rg_2和Rh_1等，其主要作用有改善正常大鼠的学习记忆能力，抗氧化损伤、通过阻滞钙通道从而改善大鼠的心肌收缩功能，增强机体的免疫功能等[13-16]。

2.3 齐墩果酸

目前从人参皂苷仅得到一种齐墩果酸型皂苷，命名为人参皂苷Ro（Ginsenoside Ro）。其主要具有肝、肾保护作用，免疫双调节作用，抑制血小板凝集，以及降血脂、降糖、抗病毒、消炎、抗突变及抗癌等作用[17-19]。

2.4 奥克梯隆醇型皂苷

从人参皂苷中可以得到两种奥克梯隆醇型皂苷：伪人参皂苷F_{11}和RT_5。它主要有促进学习记忆能力，对物理性及化学性损伤造成的急性脑缺氧具有保护作用，对心血管系统既有外周调节又有中枢调节作用，对心肌具有正性肌力作用等[20,21]。

现代药理学研究表明，PQS对机体各个系统

* 原载于《中国中西医结合杂志》，2011，31（6）：825-831

均有广泛的药理学作用，如镇静、抗焦虑、增进学习和记忆能力、抗惊厥、神经保护[22-24]、抗肿瘤[25-28]、降糖、抗肥胖[29-32]，以及增强免疫力、保护肝、增加性功能、抗突变、止吐、抗氧化和抗疲劳等作用[33-39]，以下着重介绍它在心血管系统中的作用及机制。

3. 西洋参茎叶总皂苷的心血管效应及机制研究

西洋参茎叶总皂苷具有抗心肌缺血和保护心肌、抗心律失常、抑制心室重构、抗病毒性心肌炎、降压等作用。

3.1 抗心肌缺血和保护心肌

丁涛等[40]研究显示 PQS 能明显减少冠状动脉结扎犬心肌缺血程度和范围，缩小心肌梗死面积，降低血清中游离脂肪酸（FFA）和丙二醛（MDA）含量，同时还降低急性心肌缺血大鼠血清中乳酸脱氢酶（LDH）、肌酸激酶（CK）、天冬氨酸转氨酶（AST）含量，提高超氧化物歧化酶（SOD）活性，从而起到抗心肌缺血、保护受损心肌作用。研究表明，西洋参叶 20S- 原人参二醇组皂苷（Panax quinquefolium 20S-protopanaxdiol saponins，PQDS）可明显缩小急性心肌梗死（AMI）大鼠的梗死心肌面积，减慢心肌梗死犬心率，降低动脉血压（MAP）、左室内压（LVP）、左室内压变化最大速率（±dp/d$t$max）、左室做功指数（LVMI）、总外周阻力（TPR），降低耗氧量，增加心肌内膜供血，改善缺血区血流供应；降低血清中血管紧张素转化酶（ACE）及血浆肾素（R）的活性；降低血清过氧化脂质（LPO）、去甲肾上腺素（NE）及肾上腺素（E）含量，提高过氧化氢酶（CAT）及谷胱甘肽过氧化酶（GSH-Px）活性；并能使血浆血栓素 A$_2$（TXA$_2$）水平明显下降，前列腺素 I$_2$（PGI$_2$）及 PGI$_2$/TXA$_2$ 比值显著增高；其抗心肌缺血的作用机制是通过增强抗氧化酶活性，减少自由基对心肌的氧化损伤，纠正心肌缺血时 FFA 代谢紊乱和乳酸（LA）堆积及 PGI$_2$/TXA$_2$ 失衡，抑制交感 - 肾上腺髓质过度兴奋，减少儿茶酚胺（CA）大量分泌及其抑制肾素 - 血管紧张素系统（RAS）激活，减少血管紧张素 II（AngII）生成等[41-43]。翟丽杰等[44]研究表明在一定条件下，组织摄取 ^{86}Rb 能力与组织血流量成正比，而 PQDS 可以增加小鼠心肌 ^{86}Rb 摄取率，从而明显增加心肌营养性血流量。卢爱萍等[45]研究显示西

洋参果总皂苷对急性心肌缺血时心电图 ST 段的异常改变有明显改善作用，通过增加冠状动脉血流量，改善心肌供血供氧，缩小急性心梗后梗死心肌面积，从而起到抗心肌缺血、保护受损心肌作用。安钢力等[46]研究显示 PQDS 对皮下注射异丙肾上腺素从而缩短小鼠在长期缺氧状态下的存活时间有明显对抗作用，也可明显减轻静脉注射垂体后叶素诱发的大鼠急性心肌缺血心电图的变化程度。王绚卉等[47]研究显示 PQDS 注射液能明显降低犬 AMI 时结扎前后给药后不同时间各标测点 ST 段升高的总和与结扎前后 ST 段升高 ≥ 2mV 的导联数，缩小梗死面积，对心肌缺血有明显保护作用，并且降低了 AMI 犬全血黏度及血浆黏度。

曹霞等[48]研究显示西洋参茎叶三醇组皂苷（Panax quinquefolium 20S-protopanaxtriol saponins，PQTS）通过抑制心肌收缩力，阻断 Ca^{2+} 通道，维持细胞内 Ca^{2+} 稳态，从而减轻缺血再灌注后由于钙超载对心肌的损伤，提高缺血再灌注损伤心肌氧自由基清除系统 SOD 活性，减少 LPO 含量，从而减轻氧自由基对心肌的损伤。王承龙等[49]研究显示 PQS 可显著升高 AMI 大鼠缺血心肌组织三磷腺苷（ATP）含量及能荷（EC）的储备水平，说明 PQS 具有抑制缺血心肌细胞 ATP 降解或增加 ATP 合成的作用，进而增加心肌细胞的能量储备，对缺血心肌细胞高能磷酸化合物具有明显的保护作用。柳海滨等[50]研究发现 PQDS 作为外源性氧自由基清除剂均能与心肌组织 SOD、GSH-Px 等内源性氧自由基清除剂共同清除心肌缺血再灌注损伤时产生的氧自由基，间接保护内源性 GSH-Px 和 SOD 活性，并减轻脂质过氧化对心肌的损害。殷惠军等[51]研究显示 PQS 能通过增加抗凋亡蛋白 Bcl-2，减少促凋亡蛋白 Fas 的表达，明显抑制缺血心肌细胞的过度凋亡，从而抗心肌缺血损伤。

马琼英等[52]研究显示 PQS 通过抑制中分子物质 MMS III 作用于心肌细胞后导致的心肌细胞内 MDA、总 Ca^{2+} 含量、LDH 漏出率的升高，使线粒体 Ca^{2+} 泵活性降低等生物学活性，从而起到保护心肌的作用。关利新等[53]研究发现 PQS 能明显抑制高钾所致 Ca^{2+} 浓度的增高，从而抑制电压依赖性钙通道（VDC）开放导致的钙内流，最终降低心肌 Ca^{2+} 浓度，起到对心肌的保护作用。

3.2 抗心律失常

PQS 的抗心律失常机制主要与其对钙离子通

道的阻滞作用密切相关的。有研究发现 PQS 可使大鼠心肌细胞动作电位的波幅、波宽、阈点位、最大除极速度减小并能抑制豚鼠心房肌静息电位后增强现象，缩短动作电位时程，延长有效不应期，降低心肌收缩力，其机制与抑制心肌细胞膜 Na^+、Ca^{2+}、K^+ 离子流有关。

3.3 对心室重构的影响

睢大员等[54]研究 PQDS 长期给药能明显升高左心室内压变化最大速率及其校正值，能明显降低左心室舒张末压（LVDEP），可减少重构模型组的左室容积比，显著降低重构心肌 AngⅡ、NE 及 E 含量，一方面通过直接抑制 AngⅡ 进而抑制纤维细胞增殖，减少内皮素生成从而抑制心室重构；另一方面间接抑制心脏交感神经末梢释放儿茶酚胺（CA）从而减少 CA 对 α 受体或 β 受体激活磷酸肌醇代谢系统来抑制心室重构。另外，PQDS 可降低 LPO，增加 SOD、CAT、GSH-Px 的活性从而提高心肌抗氧化能力，改善心室重构。更进一步的研究显示 PQS 可明显降低心室重量、脏器系数及左室舒张末期压力，病理结果显示心肌纤维无明显增粗，排列较整齐，心肌间质内仅见少量结缔组织增生及少量炎性细胞浸润，说明 PQS 可以抑制心室重构的发生与发展，其机制可能与降低心脏负荷，抑制 RAS 激活及内皮素生成，清除体内氧自由基，增加 PGI_2，减少 TXA_2，维持两者的生理平衡，提高体内 NO 含量有关。鞠传静等[55]研究显示 PQDS 可明显升高收缩压、舒张压及平均动脉压，并降低 LVDEP，从而改善心肌梗死后左心收缩和舒张功能以发挥防治心室重构的作用。并在随后的研究中亦证明了 PQDS 通过降低血浆 TXA_2，增加 PGI_2 及 PGI_2/TXA_2 的比值以纠正心室重构时血管内皮细胞的功能失衡，减少 AngⅡ 及内皮素生成，通过以上机制对抗大鼠心室重构。

血管内皮功能恶化导致的血流动力学异常所引起的心脏负荷过大是促发心肌肥厚的主要原因。范宝晶等[56]研究 PQS 对心肌肥厚大鼠血管内皮功能的影响时发现，与心肌肥厚模型组相比，PQS 组 AngⅡ、ET、TXA_2 明显降低，PGI_2 升高，从而改善内皮功能，降低心脏前后负荷，减轻心室壁受到的机械刺激进而抑制心肌肥厚。

3.4 对血管的保护作用

PQS 可对抗由氯化钾、氯化钙和去甲肾上腺素导致的家兔主动脉条血管平滑肌的收缩。其机制与抑制细胞外与细胞内的钙内流的释放有关。

研究表明 PQS 可使缺血心肌血管内皮生长因子（VEGF）、碱性成纤维生长因子（bFGF）表达增强，心肌微血管密度增加，提示 PQS 可以通过促进大鼠 AMI 后缺血心肌内源性 VEGF 和 bFGF 的合成与分泌进而促进心肌血管新生，血管密度增加，改善心肌微循环[57]。血管平滑肌细胞的异常增殖是动脉粥样硬化形成、高血压与血管再狭窄的共同细胞病理基础之一。杜键等[58]研究发现 PQDS 抑制血管平滑肌细胞（VSMC）增殖并诱导其凋亡，其机制为阻滞 Ca^{2+} 内流，减少抗凋亡基因 Bcl-2 及增加促凋亡及基因 bax、fas、p53 的表达。

3.5 抗病毒性心肌炎作用

研究显示西洋参可明显提高病毒性心肌炎小鼠的存活率，使心肌组织病理改变恢复加快，心肌细胞凋亡坏死率减低及外周血 T 细胞亚群比例改善、自身抗体减少，表明其对病毒性心肌炎小鼠有较好的治疗作用[59,60]。在临床应用上用西洋参粉治疗病毒性心肌炎 13 例患者 30 天的临床观察结果证明西洋参粉可逐步改善心功能。

3.6 降压作用

研究表明国产西洋参总黄酮通过对外周阻力血管的扩张，明显降低大鼠的血压和心率[61]。

Stavro PM 等[62]研究显示西洋参有中等强度的降压作用。除此之外，PQS 还有调脂、抗动脉粥样硬化及稳定斑块等作用[31,63]。

4. 西洋参茎叶总皂苷在心血管疾病中的应用前景

由于 PQS 具有多方面的心血管效应，因此它在心血管疾病中的应用也具有多中心、多靶点的特点，现代临床上可以根据其不同的药理作用及机制应用于各种心血管疾病的治疗中，如冠心病、心力衰竭、病毒性心肌炎、高血压及高脂血症等的治疗，有很好的临床应用价值与前景。

5. 问题与展望

近年来，对西洋参皂苷的研究越来越多，并且不断有新的皂苷成分被发现，由于应用部位的不同，其所含的成分及药理作用的侧重亦有所差异。目前对西洋参皂苷的药理学研究也日趋完备，已发现它对神经系统、内分泌系统、血液肿瘤系统等均有一定影响。由于西洋参茎叶皂苷含量明显高于根部，故研究西洋参茎叶总皂苷的药理作用有重要价值，尤其在心血管系统中的作用。研究发现 PQS 具有抗心肌缺血、抗心律失常、保护受损心肌、抗失血性休克及调脂、降压、抗动脉粥样硬化、稳定斑块等作用。近年来越来越多的研究初步证实了 PQS 有改善心室重构、改善心肌缺血再灌注损伤的作用。

虽然目前对于西洋参皂苷的研究愈加深入，但仍存在一些问题有待进一步探索。首先，对于西洋参皂苷的药代学、药效学及毒理学方面的研究较少，有待进一步明确；其次，目前的研究大多着眼于对皂苷成分的研究而对西洋参其他成分如氨基酸类、挥发油类、糖类等的分析较少；最后，在研究 PQS 对改善缺血再灌注心肌损伤方面，我们发现既往研究大多着眼于在体实验，而对细胞层面上的离体实验的机制研究还有待加强。心肌细胞凋亡是缺血再灌注心肌损伤的关键环节，那么除了已知的线粒体凋亡及死亡受体途径外，是否还有其他凋亡相关途径参与了心肌细胞凋亡，比如位于线粒体凋亡及死亡受体途径上游的内质网相关凋亡途径。这些问题将在今后的研究中继续探索。

参考文献

[1] 徐惠波，孙晓波，周继胡，等 . 西洋参茎叶总皂苷毒理学研究 . 中药药理与临床，1999，15（6）：24-26.

[2] 张学武，陈丽艳，崔长旭 . 人参二醇组皂苷对梗阻性黄疸大鼠肝损伤保护作用机理的实验研究 . 时诊国医药，2006，17（5）：771-772.

[3] 张健，张舵舵，张妍，等 . 人参二醇皂苷抑制人乳腺癌细胞增殖的实验研究 . 中国老年学杂志，2008，28（24）：2448-2449.

[4] 孙际童，李洪岩，苏静，等 . 人参二醇组皂苷（PDS）抑制 NOS 和 p38 减轻 LPS 休克脑损伤 . 中国病理生理杂志，2008，24（1）：44-45.

[5] 王秋静，刘芬，刘洁，等 . 人参二醇皂苷对急性血瘀模型大鼠血液流变性及 PGF_{1a}、TXB_2 的影响 . 中国实验方剂学杂志，2009，15（5）：52-54.

[6] 唐笑迪，孙晓霞，王健春 . 人参二醇组皂苷对感染性休克大鼠血液流变性及循环的影响 . 中国老年学杂志，2009，29（23）：3044-3046.

[7] 赵航，陈光，王贵民，等 . 人参二醇皂苷对重症胰腺炎急性肺损伤时水通道蛋白表达的影响 . 中国老年学杂志，2009，29（5）：561-562.

[8] 于振香，刘喜春，赵雪俭 . 人参二醇组皂苷对抗二次打击诱导大鼠急性肺损伤 . 中国病理生理杂志，2008，24（12）：2402-2406.

[9] 古天明，盘强文，冉兵，等 . 人参二醇组皂苷促进缺血

[10] 刘艳波，赵丽娟，郭亚雄，等 . 人参二醇组皂苷增强顺铂对人前列腺癌 DU145 细胞凋亡的效应 . 中国男科学杂志，2009，23（2）：12-16.

[11] 李凤娥，孔繁利，李威 . 人参二醇组皂苷抗动脉粥样硬化作用实验研究 . 北华大学学报（自然科学版），2009，10（6）：498-501.

[12] 刘洁，刘芬，王秋静，等 . 人参二醇组皂苷对心肌梗死犬血清一氧化氮、一氧化氮合酶水平的影响 . 中国实验方剂学杂志，2008，14（4）：46-49.

[13] 刘凯，谢湘林，李晔，等 . 西洋参叶三醇再到对正常大鼠学习记忆的影响 . 中草药，2007，38（11）：1700-1702.

[14] 田志刚，杨贵贞 . 人参三醇皂苷促进人白细胞介素 -1 基因表达 . 中国药理学报，1993，14（2）：159-161.

[15] 江岩，刘伟，王晓明，等 . 人参三醇皂苷对培养心肌细胞的钙通道阻滞作用和抗自由基作用 . 中国药理学报，1996，17（2）：143.

[16] 刘伟宏，龚守良，李新民，等 . 人参三醇组甙对雄性大鼠免疫器官的辐射防护作用 . 白求恩医科大学学报，1994，20（1）：32-34.

[17] 黄敏珊，黄炜，吴其平，等 . 齐墩果酸诱导人乳腺癌细胞凋亡及于细胞内 Ca^{2+} 水平关系的研究 . 中国现代医学杂志，2004，14（16）：58-61.

[18] 刘玉兰，王慧姝 . 齐墩果酸对血小板功能的影响 . 沈阳药学院学报，1993，10（4）：275-278.

[19] 薛芳喜，葛堂栋，王迪迪，等 . 齐墩果酸对 HL60 细胞 bcl-2 和 bax 表达的影响 . 中国老年学杂志，2008，28（5）：437-439.

[20] 李竹，郭月英，吴春福 . 西洋参茎叶皂苷 F_{11} 对学习记忆的影响 . 中药药理与临床，1998，14（2）：12-14.

[21] 张文杰，李红，赵中华，等 . 西洋参皂苷单体 $P-F_{11}$ 对大鼠血流动力学心室肌细胞动作电位的作用 . 人参研究，2002，14（3）：21-23.

[22] Wei XY, Yang JY, Wang JH, et al. Anxiolytic effect of saponins from Panax quinquefolium in mice. J Ethnopharmacol, 2007, 111 (3)：613-618.

[23] Lian XY, Zhang ZZ. Protective effects of ginseng components in a rodent model of neurodegeneration. Ann Neurol, 2005, 57 (5)：642-648.

[24] Lian XY, Zhang ZZ. Anticonvulsant and neuroprotective effects of ginsenosides in rats. Epilepsy Res, 2006, 70 (2)：244-256.

[25] King ML, Murphy LL. Role of cyclin inhibitor protein P21 in the inhibition of HCT116 human colon cancer cell proliferation by American ginseng (*Panax quinquefolius*) and its constituents. Phytomedicine, 2010, 17 (3-4): 261-268.

再灌注性血清致人肾小管细胞损伤后增殖作用研究 . 中药药理与临床，2008，24（4）：28-30.

[26] Peralta EA, Murphy LL, M innis J, et al. American ginseng inhibits induced COX-2 and NF-κB activation in breast cancer cells. J Surg Res, 2009, 157 (2): 261-267.

[27] Miller SC, Delorme D, Shan JJ. CVT-E002 stimulates the immune system and extends the life span of mice bearing a tumor of viralorigin. J Soc Integr Oncol, 2009, 7 (4): 127-136.

[28] Kitts DD, Popovich DG, Hu C. Characterizing the mechanism for ginsenoside-induced cytotoxicity in cultured leukemia (THP-1) cells. Can J Physiol Pharmacol, 2007, 85 (11): 1173-1183.

[29] Xie JT, Wu JA, Mehendale S, et al. Antihyperglycemic effect of the polysaccharides fraction from American ginseng berry extract in ob/ob mice. Phytomedicine, 2004, 11 (2-3) 11: 182-187.

[30] 臧晓峰, 谢湘林, 吴轶川, 等. 西洋参二醇组皂苷对糖尿病肾病大鼠肾脏葡萄糖转运蛋白、尿 β_2- 微球蛋白的影响. 中国病理生理杂志, 2008, 24 (6): 1237-1239.

[31] 殷惠军, 张颖, 蒋跃绒, 等. 西洋参总皂苷对四氧嘧啶高血糖大鼠血脂代谢的影响. 中西医结合心脑血管病杂志, 2004, 2 (11): 647-648.

[32] Liu W, Zheng Y, Han L, et al. Saponins (Ginsenosides) from stems and leaves of *Panax quinquefolium* prevented high-fat diet-induced obesity in mice. Phytomedicine, 2008, 15 (12): 140-145.

[33] 许力军, 段秀梅, 钱东华, 等. 西洋参茎叶皂苷对 CPHD 患者细胞免疫功能的影响. 中国药理学通报, 2004, 20 (8): 901.

[34] 赵玉珍, 刘蕾, 陈立平, 等. 西洋参茎叶皂苷对大鼠实验性肝损伤的影响. 中成药, 2000, 22 (3): 219.

[35] Murphy LL, CadenaRS, ChavezD, et al. Effectof American ginseng (*Panax quinquefolium*) on male copulatory behavior in rat. Physiol Behav, 1998, 64(4): 445-450.

[36] Pawar AA, Tripathi DN, Ramarao P, et al. Protective effects of American ginseng (*Panax quiquefolium*) against mitomycin C induced micronuclei in mice. Phytother Res, 2007, 21 (12): 1221-1227.

[37] Mehendale SR, Aung H. Effects of antioxidant herbs on chemotherapy-induced nausea and vomiting in a rat-picamodel. Am J Chin Med, 2004, 32 (6): 897-905.

[38] Mehendale SR, Wang CZ, Shao ZH, et al. Chronic pre-treatment with American ginseng berry and its polyphenolic constituents attenuate oxidant stress in cardiomyocytes. Eur J Pharmacol, 2006, 553 (1-3): 209-214.

[39] 翟鹏贵, 赵珺彦, 祝铃栋, 等. 西洋参制剂抗疲劳作用的实验研究. 浙江中医药大学学报, 2007, 31 (6): 761-762.

[40] 丁涛, 徐慧波, 孙晓波, 等. 西洋参茎叶总皂苷对心肌缺血的保护作用. 中药药理与临床, 2002, 18 (4): 14-15.

[41] 陆丰, 睢大员, 于晓风, 等. 西洋参叶 20S- 原人参二醇组皂苷对急性心肌梗死大鼠交感神经递质及肾素 - 血管紧张素系统的影响. 中草药, 2001, 32 (7): 619-621.

[42] 刘尚欲, 睢大员, 于晓风, 等. 西洋参叶 20S- 原人参二醇组皂苷对急性心肌梗死犬血流动力学和氧代谢的影响. 中国药学杂志, 2001, 36 (1): 25-29.

[43] 武淑芳, 睢大员, 于晓风, 等. 西洋参叶 20S- 原人参二醇组皂苷抗实验性心肌缺血作用及其机制. 中国药学杂志, 2002, 37 (2): 100-103.

[44] 翟丽洁, 于晓风, 曲绍春, 等. 西洋参叶 20S- 原人参二醇组皂苷对小鼠心肌营养性血流量的影响. 人参研究, 2004, 4 (4): 2-4.

[45] 卢爱萍, 刘金平, 卢丹, 等. 西洋参过总皂苷对冠状动脉结扎犬血流动力学及心肌缺血的影响. 吉林大学学报 (医学版), 2006, 32 (3): 383-386.

[46] 安钢力, 于晓风, 曲绍春, 等. 西洋参叶 20S- 原人参二醇组皂苷对鼠实验性心肌缺血的保护作用. 吉林中医药, 2005, 25 (1): 48-49.

[47] 王绚卉, 徐华丽, 于晓风, 等. 洋参二醇皂苷注射液对犬实验性心肌梗死的保护作用及其机制. 中国药学杂志, 2008, 43 (10): 754-757.

[48] 曹霞, 谷欣权, 陈燕萍, 等. 西洋参茎叶三醇组皂苷对缺血再灌注损伤心肌的保护作用. 中国老年学杂志, 2004, 24 (7): 654-655.

[49] 王承龙, 缪宇, 殷惠军, 等. 西洋参茎叶总皂苷对急性心肌梗死大鼠心肌能量代谢的影响. 中华老年心脑血管病杂志, 2005, 7 (5): 341-343.

[50] 柳海滨, 赵洪序, 张秀和, 等. 西洋参二醇组皂苷对心肌缺血与再灌注损伤保护效果的临床观察. 白求恩医科大学学报, 1999, 25 (1): 47-48.

[51] 殷惠军, 张颖, 蒋跃绒, 等. 西洋参叶总皂苷对急性心肌梗死大鼠心肌细胞凋亡及凋亡相关基因表达的影响. 中国中西医结合杂志, 2005, 25 (3): 232-235.

[52] 马琼英, 周文祥, 高鸣, 等. 西洋参茎叶皂苷对中分子物质损伤心肌的保护作用的实验研究. 中国中西医结合肾病杂志, 2000, 1 (2): 79-81.

[53] 关利新, 衣欣, 杨世杰, 等. 西洋参茎叶皂苷对大鼠心肌细胞 Ca^{2+} 内流的影响. 中国药理与临床, 2004, 20 (6): 8-9.

[54] 睢大员, 于晓风, 曲绍春, 等. 西洋参叶 20S- 原人参二醇组皂苷对大鼠实验性心室重构的影响. 中国药学

杂志，2007，42（2）：108-112.

[55] 鞠传静，张志国，赵学忠，等.西洋参叶二醇组皂苷对大鼠实验性心室重构的保护作用.中国老年学杂志，2007，27（22）：2173-2175.

[56] 范宝晶，裴非，赵学忠.西洋参茎叶总皂苷对心肌肥厚大鼠血管内皮功能的影响.中国老年学杂志，2009，29：811-812.

[57] 王承龙，史大卓，殷惠军，等.西洋参茎叶总皂苷对急性心肌梗死大鼠心肌 VEGF、bFGF 表达及血管新生的影响.中国中西医结合杂志，2007，27（4）：331-334.

[58] 杜键，张治国，李洋，等.西洋参叶二醇组皂苷对血管平滑及细胞增殖及凋亡的影响.中国老年学杂志，2007，27（21）：2085-2088.

[59] 徐海燕，马沛然.西洋参对小鼠病毒性心肌炎的疗效及机制.山东中医药大学学报，2002，26（6）：458.

[60] 林艳，藤清，邢丽君.西洋参粉治疗病毒性心肌炎 13 例.护理研究，2004，18（2）：29613.

[61] 吴捷，于晓江，刘传镐.西洋参茎叶皂苷对离体家兔胸主动脉条的作用.中国药理学与毒理学杂志，1995，9（2）：155-156.

[62] Stavro PM, Woo M. North American ginseng exerts a neutral effect on blood pressure in individuals with hypertension. Hypertension, 2005, 6 (6): 411.

[63] 周明学，徐浩，史大卓，等.西洋参茎叶皂苷对载脂蛋白 E 基因敲除小鼠血脂及脂质代谢相关基因周脂素和 CD36 表达的影响.中国动脉硬化杂志，2007，15（12）：881-884.

病证结合动物模型的研究进展 *

殷惠军　黄　烨

辨证论治的中医特色决定了证候研究的核心地位，证是中医理、法、方、药的关键环节。

中医证候动物模型的建立与研究是连接中医基础和临床的桥梁与纽带，是深化证候物质基础认识的方法，同时也是有效中药的筛选药物作用机制深入研究的手段。证候是对人体疾病变化过程中某一阶段的病理状态的综合描述，换句话说，是疾病一个"横断面"。要想真正把握疾病的全过程必须采用病证结合的模式。近年来有关病证结合动物模型研究取得了一定进展[1]。

1. 中医证候动物模型的研究现状

自 20 世纪 60 年代以来，中医证候模型研究进行了广泛的探索，取得了一定的进展，至今中医动物模型已涉及八纲辨证、脏腑辨证，建立了百余种证的动物模型[2]，形成了 4 种证候动物模型研究思路：病因型模型、症状型模型、病理型模型和病因病理叠加型模型[3]。然而，证候动物模型的不足使得中医证候本质研究进入了瓶颈。由中医病因中非特异性因素较多，致使造模条件不易控制、模型难以评价，加之证候的生物学基础尚未完全揭示、

内在机制尚不清楚，脱离疾病，构建某一证候的动物模型缺乏可行性，进而影响了中医病因模型在证候研究中的应用；通过使用化学或物理刺激方法得到的症状型动物模型往往不是单一证候的体现，难以进行后期研究；西医病理模型缺乏疾病与中医证候的联系，难以体现中医证候的特征；病因病理叠加型模型通常是病因造模与病理造模的简单叠加，但这种 1+1 的模型很难真实反映病证结合的确切含义。基于此，寻找既符合中医学理论、真实反映证候特征，又具有客观性和重现性的动物模型更能反映和满足中医药研究的需要，是中医动物模型研究的必然趋势。构建病证结合动物模型在此基础上应运而生。

2. 病证结合动物模型

2.1　病证结合动物模型的概念

病证结合动物模型是指通过临床调查研究，选择有密切联系的疾病和证候，即寻找两者在临床的结合点，分别或同时复制两者特征用于观察研究的模型动物[4]。

* 原载于《中国中西医结合杂志》，2013，33（1）：8-10

2.2 病证结合动物模型建立的特点

病证结合动物模型是探究疾病发生机制以及筛选有效治疗中药的关键途径和手段，其特点体现在以下方面：（1）以疾病模型为基础模型具有良好的可靠性和稳定性；（2）将时间观念引入模型较好地体现出中医"证"的动态性与阶段性特征，从而体现出中医对疾病发展规律的认识；（3）疾病与证候结合，宏观与微观结合，既能以中医学理论为指导，又能用实验方法加以证实，实用性和操作性较强[5]；（4）病证结合动物模型使很多"证"的不确定因素由于"病"的限制变得更加清晰，更符合临床实际，并更能精确地阐明中医证候的本质[6]。

3. 病证结合动物模型的模式[7]

3.1 多因素复合模型

多因素复合模型是基于中医药理论，结合现代医学理论与实验动物科学知识，分别或同时采用中医学病因复制证候模型和现代医学病因复制疾病动物模型，使模型动物同时表现出疾病和证候的特征[8]。有学者采用高脂饲料喂养后经空腹尾静脉注射链脲佐菌素制备2型糖尿病大鼠模型，同时运用中药四气五味的药性理论，根据辛苦、大苦、大寒、温热药物损伤机体阳气、津液的原理，通过给大鼠灌服不同中药入分别研究阴阳两虚型、阴虚热盛型、气阴两虚型和血瘀气滞型4种临床常见的2型糖尿病动物模型，并通过考察不同行为体征变化和相应客观指标，对模型的合理性进行了药物干预的验证[9]。

3.2 从西医病理判断中医的"证"

单一的病理因素作为病证结合模型疾病与证候共同的造模因素。有学者在采用冠状动脉Ameroid环缩术建立慢性心肌缺血模型基础上通过对四诊信息的采集，在出现宏观体征改变的时间点，从舌质紫暗、心电图提示出现心律失常（脉结代的替代指标）、冠状动脉造影显示冠状动脉狭窄或阻塞、全血黏度增高、心脏彩超观察心尖水平运动消失并伴有室壁膨出，并参照1986年中国中西医结合学会活血化瘀专业委员会制定的血瘀证诊断标准，发现术后4周模型动物即出现血瘀证表现[10]。

3.3 在中医"证"的基础上建立西医的"病"模型

基于传统中医学理论，运用中医特有的六淫、饮食情志和劳倦等为致病因素建立符合中医病因的证候模型，再施以药物或手术等方法建立西医疾病模型。以脾虚胃癌病证结合动物模型为例，有学者根据中医学理论"味过于酸，肝气以津，脾气乃绝"，在过食酸味法建立脾气虚证动物模型基础上，连续灌胃2-乙基亚硝胺120天，通过对动物摄食量、自发活动和体重变化情况以及荷瘤数、荷瘤面积指标验证脾虚胃癌动物模型制备成功[11]。

3.4 基于西医病的模型进行辨证建立模型

在西医疾病模型的基础上，不施加人为干预因素，在疾病模型建立过程中或建成后，观察并检测模型是否具备中医某些"证"的特点。即观察疾病形成过程中"证"的动态演变过程以及疾病模型建成后表现出的中医证型，进而确定某一特定的病证结合模型。

4. 病证结合动物模型的思考

4.1 合理选择造模用动物

病证结合动物模型所用的造模动物既要满足对造模药物敏感、模型特征出现迅速、持续和稳定的要求，又要满足易于造成所要研究的疾病和相应证候特征的要求[12]。不同品系、不同性别的实验动物对造模因素的耐受程度和敏感度不同，进而对同等强度的造模因素作用于不同种系、不同生长阶段的动物上所表现出来的效果也不尽相同。此外，人和实验动物宏观和微观疾病变化规律也不完全一致。例如脾虚证所用动物就有大鼠、小鼠、豚鼠、家兔和驴等，使得造模标准难以统一[13]。因此需要寻找与人体组织器官相似的动物进行模型复制，或者针对某个系统或某个器官相似的动物进行造模。例如实验用小型猪的心脏解剖结构和侧支循环与人类相似，且被毛稀少，皮肤组织结构与人相似，便于观察皮肤变化；可根据中医辨证施治要求进行舌诊观察；体型较大，可反复大量采取血液和其他体液，便于动态观察血液流变学及其他生化指标[14]。

4.2 优化病证结合动物模型造模因素，鼓励双因素或多因素造模

目前病证结合动物模型造模的因素很多，存在同一证候多种造模方法的问题。以脾虚证模型为例，不少学者根据中医传统病因思路，形成了苦寒泻下、限制营养、饮食失节、耗气破气等单因素或复合因素建造的脾虚模型，再加上用现代医学方法建立的模型，使脾虚证造模方法多达24种[15]，何种造模因素更能符合临床实际，造出较为典型的中

医证型，目前尚未建立统一的造模方法评价体系。因此，建立中医证候动物模型时，首先必须分清临床上导致证候出现的主次原因，根据中医发病规律优化造模因素，尽可能采用复合因素造模，使动物模型既符合中医的致病因素，又符合临床自然发病的实际过程。同时，对同一证多种造模方法应进行比较鉴别研究，从中筛选出一个能反映证候特征的最佳造模因素和模型构建方法[16]。

4.3 建立符合中医学理论和临床实际的病证结合动物模型

证候的存在，必然有其赖以确立的关键物质基础。病证结合动物模型必然要基于疾病和证候的规范化诊断标准，才能体现中医特色并符合临床实际。然而目前，绝大多数模型是在西医疾病模型基础上利用人为干预手段采用化学药物或物理、化学和机械性刺激方法使动物的生活环境、条件改变（进食量改变、温度改变、活动改变等），造成同时兼有证的模型。这种动物模型中证候的表现多是化学药物干预后的毒性反应或机械损伤，出现的病理状态和中医的某个证候生拉硬套，难以等同于人体的某一证候；同时这种模型虽然客观指标符合相应疾病和证候的外在表现，但动物体内的功能状态和病理生理可能已经发生较大变化，难以采用客观手段检测[17]。因此，应在中医基础理论指导下，从病因、病机入手，根据动物自身的特性及相关疾病选择最适的动物复制中医证候动物模型。例如慢性疲劳复制虚证动物模型；苦寒泻下复制脾虚证动物模型；助阳伤阴复制阴虚证动物模型以及膏粱厚味伤脾加大肠埃希菌感染复制的温病湿热证动物模型等基本都是能够真正揭示中医证候实质的中医证候动物模型[18]。

4.4 规范病证结合动物模型的评价体系

病证结合动物模型建立成功与否，其评判标准如何，是一个极具价值的关键问题。目前，证候动物模型缺乏合理的评价标准和评价方式。大部分中医证候动物模型主要是通过病理改变、解剖形态学指标来衡量，这本身就与中医"证"的实质存在明显的差异。针对这种现状，建立病证结合模型评价体系应着眼于以下关键环节[19]：（1）基于中医学理论指导。在中医病因、病机藏象理论指导下，在中医人体证候规范化基础上，在动物身上复制出符合人体证候的动物模型，从而较好地反映中医病因病机理论特点；（2）着重症状和体征。将临床证候诊断标准中的部分内容赋予具有同等生物学意

义的动物，注重挖掘动物身上具有诊断意义的信息特征，对模型进行恰当的辨证诊断，确定专门评判动物证候的标准，为建立证候模型评价指标体系群提供基础；（3）结合实验室指标。基因芯片技术目前在中医药研究中得到广泛应用。当使用证的动物模型，或在疾病模型基础上通过辨证区分出不同的证，可利用基因芯片技术观察有关病变组织基因的变异，从而了解证与证以及证与病之间的差异[20]。使用科学准确、微观量化的现代分子生物学客观指标来标示证候，为证候模型评价的客观化提供支持；（4）重视药物反证。根据"有是证用是方"的治疗思路，基于方证相应理论，采用药物的反证治疗能加强病证结合模型建立的合理性和科学性。

5. 展望

自20世纪60年代邝氏成功地塑造了首例中医阳虚动物模型至今，不少学者通过深入探索，采用190余种方法，建立了40多类中医证候的动物模型，为揭示中医"证"的物质基础进而提高临床诊疗水平起到了至关重要的作用。然而病证结合动物模型在中医证候研究中仍存在不少不足或者可探索之处。基于中医学理论，坚持中医特色，领悟中医本质，同时又掌握先进科学技术并灵活运用于科研工作，不断完善病证结合动物模型评价体系，建立既符合中医学理论和临床实际，又能充分体现证候实质的动物模型将是中西医学者探求和努力的方向，可以说是任重而道远。

参考文献

[1] 黄烨，殷惠军，陈可冀．病证结合的基础研究．中国中西医结合杂志，2012，32（3）：299-303．

[2] 刘丽梅，王瑞海，陈琳等．病证结合方证相应在证候动物模型研究中的应用．中国中医基础医学杂志，2010，16（1）：88-90．

[3] 赵慧辉，王伟．病证结合证候模型研究基本思路．中华中医药杂志，2006，21（12）：762-766．

[4] 黄碧燕．关于病证结合动物模型研究现状的思考．中国中医药信息杂志，2010，17（1）：4-8．

[5] 赵辉，王健．试论多因素复合制作病证结合动物模型思路．安徽中医学院学报，2001，20（5）：57-59．

[6] 白云静，申洪波，孟庆刚等．基于复杂性科学的中医学发展取向与方略．中国中医药信息杂志，2005，12（1）：2-5．

[7] 吴同玉，高碧珍，林山等．病证结合动物模型的模式探讨．中国中医药信息杂志，2009，16（12）：6-8．

[8] 康洁, 高碧珍. 病证结合动物模型研究概况. 中华中医药学刊, 2009, 27 (11): 2357-2359.

[9] 李敬林, 王太一, 王禄增等. 2型糖尿病证结合动物模型的研究. 中国比较医学杂志, 2007, 17 (8): 473-475.

[10] 郭淑贞, 王伟, 刘涛等. 小型猪冠心病心肌缺血血瘀证模型血液流变学及超生评价. 中华中医药学刊, 2007, 25 (4): 702-705.

[11] 张宏, 林代华, 余成浩, 等. 脾虚胃癌病证结合动物模型的建立. 四川动物, 2007, 26 (3): 699-701.

[12] 陈奇. 中药药理研究方法学. 北京人民卫生出版社, 2006: 176-178.

[13] 易杰, 李德新. 脾虚证动物模型研究思路和方法探析. 上海中医药杂志, 2001, 5 (3): 40-42.

[14] 许文玉, 王伟, 郭淑贞等. 小型猪心肌缺血血瘀证动物模型的复制方法. 中西医结合学报, 2008, 6 (4): 409-413.

[15] 郭书文, 孟庆刚, 王硕仁. 中医动物模型研究存在的问题. 中国中医基础医学杂志, 2001, 7 (2): 63-65.

[16] 郭书文, 孟庆刚, 王硕仁. 病证结合模型的研究思路. 中医药学报, 2001, 29 (1): 2-6.

[17] 富琦, 陈信义. 建立病证结合动物模型的新思路. 中国中医药信息杂志, 2003, 10 (9): 79-81.

[18] 赵宗江, 张新雪, 牛建昭. 中医证候动物模型存在的问题与对策. 中国中医药信息杂志, 2002, 9 (6): 5-6.

[19] 张艳霞, 周红艳, 李建生. 病证结合模型的研究进展. 河南中医学院学报, 2008, 23 (5): 97-99.

[20] 肖芸, 方肇勤. 中医证候动物模型的研究进展. 内蒙古中医药, 2008, 5 (3): 64-66.

动脉粥样硬化及其中西医结合防治新策略 *

汪 杰 刘 玥 蒋跃绒

近年来随着我国经济发展步伐的加快、人民生活方式的改变, 冠心病、缺血性卒中、外周血管病等心脑血管疾病的发病率与病死率急剧上升, 已成为危害人类健康的重大杀手。因此, 控制心血管疾病的大面积蔓延成为提高人类健康水平、延长寿命的重中之重。

动脉粥样硬化 (atherosclerosis, AS) 是多种心脑血管疾病的病理生理基础, 以动脉内膜下脂质沉积, 并伴有平滑肌细胞和纤维基质成分的增殖, 逐步发展形成动脉粥样硬化斑块为主要病变特征的一种疾病。动脉粥样硬化斑块的突然破裂可导致血小板的激活和血栓形成, 继而引起动脉局部闭塞或远端栓塞, 其病变广泛, 主要可累及冠状动脉、脑动脉、下肢动脉、颈动脉等, 严重危害着人类健康。因此, 如何防治AS成为全球医学界的研究焦点之一。20世纪90年代以来, 随着对AS危险因素的深入了解和积极控制, 冠心病的一级预防取得了令人鼓舞的成果, 积极控制危险因素成为近半个世纪以来心血管病防治的重心。芬兰、美国等国家近年来心血管病死率大幅下降、人均寿命延长均与控制危险因素密切相关[1]。但近年来的研究表明, 即使积极干预心血管危险因素, 仍有60%以上的患者AS斑块在进展, 这迫使我们在现有认识的基础上, 对动脉粥样硬化的病因病机及其中西医结合防治策略进行更为深入的分析和思考[2]。

1. 从重视"阳微阴弦"到"血瘀致变"再到"瘀毒从化"的转变

中医学历代文献虽未出现"动脉粥样硬化"的病名, 从临床表现方面可将其归属于中医的"胸痹心痛"范畴。《金匮要略·胸痹心痛短气病》指出胸痹心痛的病因病机为"阳微阴弦。即胸痹而痛, 所以然者, 责其极虚也。今阳虚知在上焦, 所以胸痹心痛者, 以其阴弦故也"。认为本病是胸阳极虚, 阴寒痹阻产生的正虚邪实证。20世纪60年代以前, 中医药临床治疗冠心病最常用的治法即是宣痹通阳法或芳香温通法, 但从临床疗效来看并不十分理想, 因此近20年来有学者从其他方面探寻其发病的可能机制, 如有从血瘀论者、湿热论者, 有从痰浊论者, 有从络风内动论者等[3～6]。随着研究的逐渐深入, 目前对冠心病病因病机的认识逐渐趋于统一, 认为本病属于本虚标实之证, 本虚为气、血、阴、阳亏虚, 标实为气滞、血瘀、痰浊、寒凝, 而尤以血瘀被公认为最重要的病因病机之

* 原载于《医学研究杂志》, 2012, 41 (5): 9-11

第七章

一，贯穿于冠心病发生发展的全过程，临床上以活血化瘀法为主治疗冠心病，创制了一系列活血化瘀方药，使临床疗效进一步得到提高[3]。

病机的发现和创新是永无止境的，临床急性心血管事件的高发生率和严重危害性促使我们继续对其中西医结合病机的研究与时俱进。AS 的西医发病机制过去主要为脂质浸润学说、血栓形成学说和损伤反应学说。近年来研究发现，AS 具有慢性炎症病理的基本表现形式（变性、渗出和增生），随着炎症细胞和炎症介质的不断被检出，AS 通常已不再被认为是单纯的动脉壁脂质堆积的疾病，而是进展性炎症反应。国外学者 Ross[7] 明确提出 AS 是一种炎症性疾病，这已是大多数专家的共识。从 AS 的病生理特点并结合其炎症反应的新认识，虽然血瘀及活血化瘀机制涉及了血小板聚集、活化、凝血活性、血栓形成等诸多方面，但却不能很好地解释冠心病 AS 病理过程中的炎症介质、内皮损伤、氧化应激、组织坏死等现象。因此有学者在"血瘀"的基础上进一步提出了"瘀毒致变""瘀毒从化"的新的冠心病 AS 发病学说，认为血瘀是贯穿于冠心病发展过程的中心环节，也是稳定期患者的基础病理状态[8,9]。若瘀久化热、酿生毒邪，或从化为毒，可致瘀毒内蕴。如迁延日久、失治误治，则正消邪长，一旦外因引动、蕴毒骤发，则蚀肌伤肉，进而毒瘀搏结、痹阻心脉，导致病情突变，出现不稳定型心绞痛、急性心肌梗死、心源性猝死等急危重症，这是稳定期冠心病发生急性心血管事件的主要病因和关键病理机转。并且认为"活血解毒法"为冠心病稳定期瘀毒内蕴高危患者的治疗大法，这也正是中医"未病先防、既病防变"的优势所在。

2. 从重视"易损斑块"到重视"易损患者"的转变

动脉粥样硬化斑块破损导致的血栓形成是急性心血管事件发生的共同病理过程，而斑块的不稳定性或易损性被视为导致本病的主要因素。"易损斑块"是指所有易于发生血栓，以及可能快速进展从而成为罪恶斑块的粥样病变，其形态学特征具有大量炎症细胞浸润、纤维帽较薄、脂质核心较大、内皮功能不良和凝血机制增强等特点。

易损斑块可能导致临床事件，然而导致临床事件的发生除斑块以外还有其他因素，例如易形成血栓的血液（易损血液），易于发生威胁生命的

心律失常的心肌（易损心肌），因此有学者提出了"易损患者"的概念，指以斑块、血液或心肌易损性为基础，易发生急性冠状动脉综合征或心源性猝死的患者[10,11]。临床上及早对"易损患者"进行识别、干预无疑对降低急性心血管疾病的发生率具有重大意义。这种认识上的转变暗含中医"防重于治"的理念。研究表明血管老化通常出现在动脉粥样硬化血管性疾病发生之前，提示血管老化可能是致动脉粥样硬化形成的始动环节。血管老化不仅容易进展为动脉粥样硬化，而且易诱发多种心脑血管疾病，尽早对血管老化进行预防干预能够延缓 AS 的发病及进展，降低"易损患者"的形成率[12]。这种认识上的改变反映在临床治疗上就是从"规范化治疗"到"个体化治疗"的转变。众所周知，现代医学规范化诊疗方案的制定都是基于"病"的特点通过大样本临床流行学的客观资料而获得的，并没有考虑人的差异性。药物治疗也只关注于"靶向治疗"而不关注整体、个性化治疗。用药标准也只是能使"一般人"在"通常情况下"减轻痛苦的平均剂量，但"一般人"与"通常情况"很难界定，规范化治疗方案的临床疗效差异性非常大。传统的危险评估策略可预示大宗人口的长期结果，然而缺乏预示个体将来发生事件的可能性。这种把斑块、心肌、血液三者的易损性联系起来，综合评价患者心血管事件发生"易损性"的策略，不但符合中医的"整体观念"和"防重于治"的理念，而且这种由局部到整体、由微观到宏观的转变也是现代医学在治疗理念及方法学上向传统中医学回归的一个缩影，亦是心血管疾病临床预防策略的进一步完善[13]。

3. 从单纯关注"危险因素"到综合干预血管的转变

自从 1961 年美国 Framingham 研究提出"危险因素"的概念以来，其在 AS 及心血管疾病的预防中具有举足轻重的作用。危险因素又分为不可改变的（如年龄、性别、种族等）和可改变的（如吸烟、肥胖、高血压、血脂异常等）两大类。对 AS 危险因素的积极控制成为近半个世纪以来心血管病防治的重心。近 30 年来美国心脑血管疾病发病率大幅度下降，得益于完成了"三大任务"，即成功的戒烟、高血压监测评估干预计划的实施（JNC1 ~ JNC7）、推行美国成人胆固醇教育计划（ATP Ⅰ ~ ATP Ⅲ）。

那么是否单纯控制危险因素就能完全阻断 AS 的进展，避免心血管疾病的发生呢？答案是否定的。最新研究表明，即使积极控制危险因素，仍有 60% 的患者 AS 斑块在进展，斑块进展患者发生心血管事件的风险是斑块未进展患者的 2.1 倍[2]。单纯关注危险因素的局限性越来越受到重视，许多冠状动脉事件在没有任何预警的情况下发生，Framingham 危险评分虽然依据危险因素，但多种影响动脉粥样进展的因素并未包含在内，也未被干预，如炎症标志物的升高、ECG 阳性改变、精神压力以及血管造影发现等，并且其危险评分个体针对性不强，尤其对女性及年轻人[14]。因此 2010 年美国中风学会杂志《Stroke》载文提出"全面干预血管比只关注危险因素更重要"的 AS 临床防控新策略[2]。新策略主要着眼于对血管的全面干预，不局限于仅对 AS 危险因素的防控，即对于 AS 人群重在综合指标的评价，无论胆固醇、血压血糖水平是否在正常范围之类，只要还存在诸如颈动脉中内膜厚度（cMIT）、炎症标志物或 ECG 的阳性变化等存在异常，就需要对血管进行强化干预，阻止斑块的进一步进展，继而降低心血管事件的发生率。

他汀类药物的出现是 AS 防治史上的里程碑，其对 LDL-C 的降低、稳定 AS 斑块方面具有显著效果，其结合抗血小板等药物构成了 AS 治疗的一道坚强防线。但随着以上几类药物的大量使用，临床上亦出现了诸如肝酶异常、肌溶解以及出血、抗血小板药物抵抗等不良事件。中医药具有全面调节机体功能和多途径、多靶点干预的优势，且不良反应小，在防治 AS 方面应当大有可为。许多中药对脂质代谢有良好的调节作用，祛除痰湿、调理肝脾肾、活血化瘀法为中医治疗血脂异常的主要原则。血脂康、活血调脂颗粒、红花黄色素注射液、丹参注射液、脉络宁注射液等一大批中药在调节 AS 脂质代谢方面发挥重要的作用[15]。近年来，一些具有抗血小板作用同时不良反应较小的中药提取物或复方引起了人们的重视，如白藜芦醇、银杏叶提取物、丹酚酸 A、复方丹参滴丸、芎芍胶囊等具有降低血小板黏附性、抑制血小板聚集、降低血小板释放反应等作用而发挥抗血小板效果[16~20]。

4. 从基于经验到基于证据再到以患者为中心的中西医结合临床诊疗模式的转变

基于个人临床经验的诊疗模式一直是中医临床的主流方式。但在过去的 30 年间，这种模式的局限性逐渐显现，传统中医药存在临床主观意识强、疗效难以客观评价的缺陷，这也成为中医药走向世界的一个很大阻碍。循证医学（EBM）目前已经成为全世界范围内评价一种药物或治疗手段有效性的一个金标准，在中国许多从事中西医结合医学的学者们已经逐渐意识到 EBM 的重要性，也尝试将 EBM 的理念和研究方法用于中西医结合防治 AS 的临床研究当中，取得了一定的进展。冠心病二级预防（CCSPS）研究就以中药血脂康为研究药物的一个纳入中国 65 家医院、4870 名冠心病患者的随机、双盲、安慰剂对照的循证医学研究，研究结果显示，与安慰剂相比，血脂康能显著降低冠心病患者非致命性心肌梗死和心源性死亡等心血管事件的发生率。XS0601 是一种由川芎和赤芍有效组分配伍的中药制剂，为评价其在冠心病介入术后再狭窄防治方面的安全性和有效性，学者们设计了一个纳入 355 名冠心病患者的随机、双盲、安慰剂对照的临床试验。初级临床终点为经冠状动脉造影证实的介入术后再狭窄。研究结果表明，服用 XS0601 超过 6 个月可以显著降低冠心病患者冠状动脉介入术后再狭窄的发生率。同样，学者们为评价长期（超过 6 个月）口服麝香保心丸对冠心病稳定型心绞痛的治疗有效性和安全性，设计了纳入 200 名冠心病患者的临床随机对照试验。研究结果亦证实了长期服用麝香保心丸对于冠心病稳定型心绞痛患者具有明显的疗效和较好的安全性。为了评价通心络胶囊对冠心病患者治疗的有效性和安全性，学者们通过医学数据库搜集了所有已经发表的涉及通心络胶囊治疗冠心病的临床随机对照试验（RCTs），一共有 13 项研究，共涉及冠心病患者 1496 例。Meta 分析结果表明，与异山梨酯（消心痛）或单硝酸异山梨酯相比，在对冠心病患者心电图指标的改善方面，通心络胶囊并不显示出优势，但通心络胶囊的不良反应发生率很低，还需要设计时间更长的随访研究来评估其远期疗效和安全性。

近年来，随着个体化诊疗模式理念的逐渐回归，医学家们慢慢认识到以患者为中心的中西医结合临床诊疗模式的优势和重要性所在。我们相信随着研究的深入和研究结果的不断积累，必将在全世界范围内形成一个更加安全、更加有效的基于患者个体化的结合医学健康诊疗模式。

5. 结语

基于患者的结合医学诊疗模式以及植物药和化学药联合使用的不断出现必将发展成为防治疾病的一个新的医学趋势。中医中药配合西药对于 AS 的防治起了重大作用，尽管目前已经涌现出许多中药制剂防治 AS 的临床循证研究以及相关的系统评价，但仍然存在缺乏大样本、前瞻性、规范化的研究，缺乏明确的循证医学证据。未来我们应该将理论研究、实验研究、临床研究三驾马车齐头并进，加快实验研究成果向临床实际应用的转化，为中西医结合防治 AS 做出更大贡献。相信未来随着越来越多的临床以及实验研究证据的不断积累，将进一步验证中西医结合医学的优势及智慧所在。

参考文献

[1] Laatikainen T, Critchley J, Vartiainen E, et al. Explaining the decline in coronary heart disease mortality in Finland between 1982 and 1997. Am J Epidemiol, 2005, 162 (8): 764-773。

[2] David S, Daniel G, Hackam. Treating arteries instead of risk factors: a paradigm change in management of atherosclerosis. Stroke, 2010, 41 (6): 1193-1199.

[3] 林培政，杨开清. 动脉粥样硬化中医湿热病机再认识. 新中医，2006，38（3）：5-6.

[4] 贾连群，杨关林. 动脉粥样硬化中医痰浊血瘀证候的现代生物学基础研究. 中西医结合心脑血管病杂志，2010，8（1）：95-96.

[5] 王显. 有关冠心病诊疗及研究的思考———动脉粥样硬化"络风内动"假说与实践. 中国中西医结合杂志，2011，31（3）：310-312.

[6] 陈可冀，李连达，翁维良. 血瘀证与活血化瘀研究. 中西医结合心脑血管病杂志，2005，3（1）：1-2.

[7] Ross R. Atherosclerosis: an inflammatory disease. N Engl J Med, 1999, 340 (2): 115-126.

[8] 徐浩，史大卓，殷惠军，等."瘀毒致变"与急性心血管事件：假说的提出与临床意义. 中国中西医结合杂志，2008，28（10）：934-938.

[9] 史大卓，徐浩，殷惠军，等."瘀毒从化"心脑血管血栓性疾病病因病机. 中西医结合学报，2008，6（11）：1105-1108.

[10] Naghavi M, Libby P, Falk E, et al. From vulnerable plaque to vulnerable patient: a call for new definitions and risk assessment strategies: Part Ⅰ. Circulation, 2003, 108 (14): 1664-1672.

[11] Naghavi M, Libby P, Falk E, et al. From vulnerable plaque to vulnerable patient: a call for new definitions and risk assessment strategies: Part Ⅱ. Circulation, 2003, 108 (14): 1772-1778.

[12] Clarkson TB. Nonhuman primate models of atherosclerosis. Lab Animal Sci, 1998, 48 (6): 569.

[13] 周明学，徐浩. 浅谈从"人易患的病"到"易患病的人"治疗思路的演变. 中医药学刊，2006，24（12）：2213-2215.

[14] Johnson KM, Dowe DA. The detection of any coronary calcium outperforms Framingham risk score as a first stepinscreening for coronary atherosclerosis. American Journal of Roentgenology, 2010, 194 (5): 1235-1243.

[15] 任勇才. 中药制剂治疗血脂异常概况. 广西中医学院学报，2004，7（4）：64-66.

[16] 杨雨民，王兴祥，王世君，等. 白藜芦醇在体外对 ADP 诱导人血小板聚集的抑制作用及其机制. 药学学报，2008，43（4）：356-360.

[17] 衡亮，宦梦蕾. 银杏叶提取物抗实验性血栓模型大鼠的作用及机制. 现代生物医学进展，2009，9（10）：1835-1837

[18] Fan HY, Fu FH, Yang MY, et al. Antiplatelet and antithrombotic activities of salvianolic acid A. Thrombosis Research, 2010, 126 (1): e17-e22.

[19] 刘培良，沈菀真，靖涛，等. 复方丹参滴丸及阿司匹林对老年 ACS 患者血小板聚集功能及 PKB 活性变化的影响. 中国新药杂志，2009，18（10）：900-902

[20] 李立志，刘剑刚，马鲁波，等. 芎芍胶囊对兔动脉粥样硬化模型脂质代谢及血小板聚集的影响. 中国中西医结合杂志，2008，28（12）：1100-1103.

患者报告结局在中医药防治心血管系统疾病疗效评价中的应用与思考 *

董国菊　李立志

患者报告结局（patient-reported outcome，PRO）是直接来源于患者个人的感受，体现患者最关心的症状和问题，是临床结局评价的重要手段，在现代医学中得到越来越多的重视和应用，尤其在心血管疾病领域，近年来有很大的发展。现将 PRO 在国内外心血管领域的发展做一概括，并对 PRO 在中医药防治心血管疾病领域中的应用与发展提出几点粗浅的想法，供大家借鉴。

1. PRO 的含义

PRO 是一种直接来源于患者，没有医生或其他任何人对于患者反应的解释，对患者健康状况的各个方面进行评定的量表[1]，它可以体现患者最关心的症状和问题，可以捕捉最细微、最微妙的心理变化和功能改变，作为临床疗效的补充。

2. PRO 作为临床结局评价的重要手段之一与中医药临床疗效评价体系具有强关联性

PRO 的应运而生是生物医学模式发展的必然，以前在相当长的时间里，西医学对疾病的疗效标准着重于评价病因、病理、生化等指标的改变。但临床常会遇到患者"病"的指标恢复正常，而主观不适症状仍然存在的现象，因此对于疾病的疗效评价，只重视疾病的生物学指标是不够的，还应该重视患者"人"的一面。PRO 应该作为临床疗效评价的终点指标之一，是临床结局评价的重要手段[2]。PRO 这种"以人为本"的理念与中医学不谋而合。几千年来，中医学在维护人类健康、防治疾病中"效"不可没，但西方医学不认同我们的"效"，因为我们的疗效主要是基于患者的自我感受，而不是客观的生化指标，缺乏"量化"和"客观化"的东西，这也是困扰中医药走向世界的关键瓶颈。PRO 的提出，不仅将患者的主观感受引进了临床疗效评价，以确定治疗的好处是否多于伤害，而且将其量化，让患者"说话"，将患者的主

观感受客观化，更好地服务于患者，服务于临床，尤其适合中医药临床疗效评价模式。

3. PRO 在心血管疾病疗效评价中的发展和应用现状

3.1 国际上 PRO 在心血管疾病疗效评价中的发展与应用现状

心血管系统疾病患者，尤其是慢性病程的患者，往往在客观指标有了改善以后，自我症状缓解不明显，自我感觉比较差，因此心血管疾病系统一直是 PRO 应用活跃而广泛的领域。如评价心力衰竭的明尼苏达心衰量表（Minnesota living with heart failure questionnaire，MLHFQ）[3]、堪萨斯城心肌病量表（Kansas City cardiomyopathy questionnaires，KCCQ）[4]、具体活动量表[5]、左心功能不全量表（left ventricular dysfunction 36，LVD 36）[6] 等都是从不同侧重点对患者的症状报告、衣食住行等功能状态、运动耐量、社交、心理等多个方面进行评价，根据患者的自我反应评估患者的生活质量，评价临床治疗效果，预测患者的预后，是经济有效的临床疗效评价工具。评价冠心病的西雅图心绞痛量表（Seattle angina questionnaire，SAQ）[3]、心绞痛生命质量量表（angina pectoris quality of life，APQOL）[7] 等都具有良好的临床反应性，在多个国家广泛应用于疗效评价。Szende A 等[8] 对 1995 年至 2003 年欧洲药监局批准的新药的疗效评价进行了回顾性分析。结果发现，在疗效评价中引进健康相关量表（health-related quality of life，HRQL）和 PRO 的研究逐渐增多，尤其在肿瘤、心力衰竭等慢性病中，超过一半研究引用了 HRQL 或 PRO。

3.2 国内 PRO 在心血管疾病疗效评价中的发展与应用现状

国内的 PRO 在心血管领域尚处于初步阶段，临床疗效测评多是应用国外量表的中文版，如

* 原载于《中国中西医结合杂志》，2011，31（2）：260-263

SAQ、MLHFQ。由于国情、语言、表达、理解等多种因素干扰，国外量表在翻译过程中难免会失真，所以临床应用或多或少存在不足。针对此种情况，国内也开始研制基于中国国情和中国心血管疾病患者群的量表。如杨瑞雪等[9]采用程序化决策方式，结合我国语言和文化背景进行慢性病患者生活质量测定量表体系中的高血压量表（quality of life instruments for chronic disease-hypertention，QLICD-HY）开发和研制，可以作为我国高血压患者生活质量的测评工具。徐伟等[10]采用形成条目库并进行条目分析和因子分析以选取合适条目构成多维度量表的方法，编制和检验适合国情、符合老年原发性高血压特点的生活质量评定工具，可作为老年原发性高血压患者生活质量评定工具。刘江生等[11]对中国20个城市28所医院进行了"中国心血管患者生活质量评定问卷"的测定，得出了适合中国国情，同时涵盖了冠心病、高血压和心力衰竭三种常见心血管疾病的评定问卷。

4. PRO在中医药防治心血管疾病疗效评价中的发展和应用现状

中医药是调节式的治疗，而西医是对抗式的治疗，所以中医药的优势是能有效改善患者的主观症状，而西医则能有效改善客观指标。因此，患者症状群的改善是中医药疗效评价不可缺少的内容。PRO正是将患者自我感受进行量化的测评工具，所以近年来，很多知名的量表如MLHFQ、SAQ等广泛被引入中医药防治心血管系统疾病的疗效评价中。如苏慧敏[12]利用MLHFQ评价芪苈强心胶囊治疗慢性充血性心力衰竭的疗效，结果表明，中药组患者MLHFQ积分和功能等各项指标均明显优于对照组。再如荆鲁等[13]利用SAQ评价血府逐瘀汤及其拆方治疗稳定型心绞痛的临床疗效，结果表明，中药各组SAQ评分均优于对照组。

目前，具有中医特色的PRO研制尚处于探索阶段。由刘保延[14]进行的8类（后扩至10类）系统疾病患者自我感受的量表已经初步结题，其中笔者作为子课题组进行了基于心血管系统（冠心病、高血压和慢性心力衰竭）患者的自我感受测量，形成了初步量表，有较好的信度和效度[15]，进一步的临床应用正在进行，有望对量表进一步完善，并对于其适应人群、前后测评时间、前后测评分值的评价提供依据。林谦等[16]按照国际通用原则和程序，拟制定符合我国国情，并能反映中医特色的心力衰竭生活质量量表，最终共筛选出6个领域共36个合格条目，构成正式量表，并经过统计分析表明有良好的信度和效度。

5. PRO在中医药防治心血管疾病疗效评价中应用的几点建议

5.1 编制符合国情PRO量表

中国仍属于不发达国家，受教育程度相对较低，医疗保险不健全，各地区经济条件不一致，这些均影响了中国心血管患者的生活质量[11]。我们在量表的研制过程中也发现，医疗保险的有无直接影响了患者对治疗的依从性，影响了疗效，影响了患者的生活质量。受教育程度的高低直接影响患者对疾病本身的认知、对治疗的理解，同样影响治疗效果。因此，国内PRO量表要能代表和涵盖东南西北中各个区域、各级医院患者共同关注的健康以及与健康相关的问题。

5.2 编制符合中医药临床疗效评价特点的PRO量表

理论上讲，患者是不分"中医"和"西医"的，所以来自患者的报告如何体现中医特色是目前争论的焦点。陈薇等[17]提出建立中医特色的量表评价体系，使中医药疗效评价达到客观化和定量化，促进中医药事业的发展，这固然是好，可是如何体现？中医问诊虽然有"十问歌"，但那是医生问，而非患者报告，不能将两者混淆。因此，笔者认为，不在于研制能体现中医特色的PRO量表，因为中医证的变化、舌苔脉象不是患者能够表述清楚的，而且治疗前如果评分提示是气虚证，治疗后评分提示为阴虚证，又如何评价治疗效果？所以关键在于编制符合中医药临床疗效评价特点的PRO量表，比如可以将患者关注的症状、体征赋值加大，对于社会心理等因素赋值可相对小，充分体现中医药的疗效。

5.3 选择适宜病种作为切入点，严格遵循PRO研制国际标准与技术

量表研制的成功与否很大程度上取决于是否选择了一个合适的患者群，换言之，是否选择了具有某些共同特征的一种疾病或一类疾病。如慢性颈肩腰腿痛、慢性盆腔痛、慢性心力衰竭等。而且PRO量表的研制过程需要临床医生、量表专家、统计人员等多方参与，不仅要遵循PRO国际标准进行，而且要通过信度、效度、区分度、临床反应度等测量。因此，构建一个优秀的PRO量表并推

广应用，需要有合适的切入点，并严格按 PRO 标准化方法进行。

5.4 研制 PRO 过程中的几点体会

在国家科技部基金资助项目支撑下，本课题组进行了基于心血管系统疾病患者自我感受的测量，有如下几点体会：（1）无论选择哪一种或一类疾病，此种或此类疾病应该具有共同的困扰患者的症状群。如果不具备这一条，研制的量表可能固然普适性强，但临床对单病种的区分度不强，对临床治疗反应性不高；（2）患者自我感受的测量，要尽可能除去医生和家属给患者带来的干扰，给患者一个安静舒适的环境，无论是面对面访谈还是问卷调查，都给患者最大的作答空间。比如，生病/住院以来，你最关注什么？这样可以得到尽可能多的信息；（3）反复修改，完善量表。没有最好，只有更好，用在 PRO 的研制上非常合适，每一个条目都需要反复修改、增删：这一条是不是患者很关心的？能否反应患者的自我感受？语言表述是否通俗易懂？答案采取几分法作答更合适？（4）专家共识：PRO 虽然反应的是患者的自我感受，最终还是医生将其总结、归纳，因此面对患者众多的感受，如何提炼、凝练，需要专家的参与指导，充分讨论，达成共识。

6. 合理使用 PRO 进行中医药临床疗效评价

随着医学模式和疾病谱的改变，现代医学逐渐认识到患者自身感受在临床疗效中的意义，在完善现代临床评价体系的过程中，如果应用合适的量表，建立基于患者报告的结局评价指标量化测量体系来评价临床疗效，将会解决临床疗效评价中的模糊性和不确定性问题。PRO 的引入，可以丰富和完善中医药临床疗效评价体系，更好地服务于中医药事业。

参考文献

[1] U. S. Department of Health and Human Services FDA Center for Drug Evaluation and Research；U. S. Department of Health and Human Services FDA Center for Biologics Evaluation and Research；U. S. Department of Health and Human Services FDA Center for Devices and Radiological Health. Guidance for industry patient-reported outcome measures：use on medical product development to support labeling claims, draft guidance. Health Qual Life Outcomes,

2006, 11 (4)：79.

[2] Willke RJ, BurkeLB, Erickson P. Measuring treatment impact: a review of patient-reported outcomes and other efficacy end points in approved product labels. Control Clin Trials, 2004, 25 (6): 535-552.

[3] Guyattg H. Measurement of health-related quality of life in heart failure. J Am Coll Cardiol, 1993, 22 (4Suppl A)：185A-191A.

[4] Faller H, Steinbuchel T, Stork S, et al. Impact of depression on quality of life assessment in heart failure. Int J Cardiol, 2010, 142 (2): 133-137.

[5] Rankin SL, Briffa TG, Morton AR, et al. A specific activity questionnaire to measure the functional capacity of cardiac patients. Am J Cardiol, 1996, 77 (14): 1220-1223.

[6] C JOcLeary, PW Jones. The left ventricular dysfunction questionnaire (LVD-36): reliability, validity and responsiveness. Heart, 2000, 83 (6): 634-640.

[7] Mauquis P, Fayol C, Joire JE，et al. Psychometric properties of a specific quality of life questionnaire in angina pectoris patients. Qual Life Res, 1995, 4 (6): 540-546.

[8] Szende A, Leidy NK, Revicki D. Health-related quality of life and other patient-reported outcomes in the European centralized drug regulatory process：a review of guidance documents and performed authorizations of medicinal products 1995 to 2003. Value Health, 2005, 8 (5): 534-548.

[9] 杨瑞雪，潘家华，万崇华，等. 高血压患者生命质量量表研制及评价. 中国公共卫生，2008，24（3）：266-269.

[10] 徐伟，王吉耀，Phillips M，等. 老年原发性高血压患者生活质量量表编制的商榷. 实用老年医学，2000，14（5）：242-245.

[11] 刘江生，马琛明，涂良珍，等. "中国心血管患者生活质量评定问卷"常模的测定. 心血管康复医学杂志，2009，18（4）：305-309.

[12] 苏慧敏. 芪苈强心胶囊对慢性充血性心力衰竭患者生活质量的影响. 中国中西医结合心脑血管病杂志，2007，5（10）：917-918.

[13] 荆鲁，王阶，王停. 西雅图量表评价血府逐瘀汤及其拆方治疗冠心病稳定型心绞痛的疗效观察. 中国中西医结合杂志，2007，27（1）：18-20.

[14] 刘保延. 有关辨证论治临床评价若干问题的思考. 中医杂志，2007，48（1）：680-682.

[15] 李立志，董国菊，王承龙，等. "基于心血管疾病患者报告的临床疗效评价量表"的研制及统计学分析. 中西医结合心脑血管病杂志，2008，6（7）：757-759.

[16] 林谦，农一兵，万洁，等．慢性心力衰竭中西医结合生存质量量表的临床研究．中国中西医结合急救杂志，2008，15（3）：131-134.

[17] 陈薇，刘建平．临床疗效研究中的患者报告结局．中国中西医结合杂志，2009，29（8）：746-749.

抗血小板药物抵抗 *

吴彩凤　殷惠军　王景尚

动脉粥样硬化斑块破裂处过多血小板黏附、聚集和释放，启动血栓形成，导致冠状动脉高度狭窄或者完全闭塞，伴或不伴有远端微循环栓塞，从而发生急性冠状动脉综合征（acute coronary syndrome，ACS），是造成心血管疾病患者死亡的重要原因之一[1]。无论是作为冠状动脉内斑块破裂及局部炎症反应加重的继发现象，还是作为原发现象，血小板活化、黏附、聚集以及血小板因子的释放都是触发 ACS 的核心环节。随着人们对血小板在动脉血栓形成以及心血管疾病发展进程中的关键作用和地位认识的不断深入，抗血小板药物治疗已经成为 ACS 和冠状动脉介入术（PCI）患者预防和治疗的基石[2]。此类药物不断涌现并在临床广泛应用，包括阿司匹林、噻氯吡啶类和血小板糖蛋白（GPⅡb/Ⅲa）受体拮抗剂均为抗栓防栓治疗的基础用药。但在规范用药和良好依从性的基础上，仍有患者发生血栓不良事件，这就是备受人们关注的抗血小板药物抵抗现象。

1. 抗血小板药物抵抗的定义与检测

抗血小板药物抵抗，目前尚没有明确的概念，主要倾向于从反映血小板功能的多种实验室指标检测和临床再发血栓事件情况两个方面来定义抗血小板药物抵抗：（1）抗血小板药物作为心脑血管病的二级预防，未能减少栓塞及其他缺血事件的发生；（2）服用抗血小板药物者体外试验中血小板聚集功能未受抑制[3]。从抵抗发生机制的角度，国内外学者根据各自临床或实验室研究方法的不同分别给出了不同的定义，但大多数学者倾向于是一种药物低反应，并非真正抵抗或完全无反应，而是一种药物反应的差异性。所谓药物低反应是指药物在某些因素作用下，未能到达药物作用靶点或虽到达但未能与药物作用靶点充分有效地结合，且能被实验室检测出[4]。这种抗血小板药物抵抗现象与血小板多通路活化所造成的某一种抗血小板药物的治疗失败略有区别。

随着抗血小板药物抵抗现象研究的不断深入，抗血小板药物抵抗的检测方法也在不断地完善。光学检测法测定血小板聚集率的方法应用比较广泛，且与临床结果相关性较良好，曾一度被认为是血小板功能检测的金标准，但是存在重复性和特异性较差、样本需求量大且操作要求也很高的缺陷[5]。血小板功能分析仪（PFA-100）检测法操作简单、便捷、样本量小，但同样存在特异性差的问题[6]。Verify now 快速血小板功能检测法（The Ultegra Rapid Platelet Function Assay，RPFA-Verify-Now）可以通过 RPFA-Verify-Now ASA 和 RPFA-Verify-Now P2Y12 特异性地进行花生四烯酸（arachidonic acid，AA）通路和 P2Y12 通路的检测[7]，分别应用于阿司匹林抵抗和氯吡格雷抵抗的研究，虽然具有简便、快速、半自动化和特异性的特点，但是其检测费用较高，且仅具有一定的敏感性和特异性[8]。流式细胞术的检测方法的出现也使得血小板功能检测具有样本需求量小、重复性和特异性较好（如对氯吡格雷抵抗的特异性较高的检测——VASP 的检测[9]），但这些费用较高，临床上尚未得到广泛应用。这些检测方法的不断改进为进一步的研究提供了更可靠的证据。

2. 抗血小板药物抵抗的机制

抗血小板药物抵抗的发生是多因素的，主要包括药物的生物学特性、多通路的血小板活化、受

* 原载于《中国中西医结合杂志》，2010，30（2）：221-224

体的基因多态性以及药物之间的相互作用。

2.1 阿司匹林抵抗的机制

2.1.1 环氧化酶 -1（COX-1）生物特性的因素

环氧化酶（COX）是阿司匹林抗血小板作用的靶点，有两种亚型 COX-1 和 COX-2。阿司匹林为非选择性的 COX 抑制剂，对二者均有不可逆的抑制作用，但阿司匹林对 COX-1 的抑制作用是 COX-2 的 170 倍。血小板是无核细胞，除自身的 COX-1 外，没有再生 COX-1 的能力，所以阿司匹林不可逆地抑制了 COX-1 的活性，从而抑制了血栓素 A_2（TXA_2）的生成，但血小板在血液中是持续生成的，且有核细胞具有再生 COX-1 的能力，后者能生成前列腺素类物质，导致 24h 内血小板活化功能的恢复，而且有核细胞生成的 COX-1 对阿司匹林的敏感性低于血小板源性的 COX-1，这可能是阿司匹林抵抗的一个原因[10]。有学者[11]认为，有核细胞如单核细胞、血管内皮细胞能够直接向血小板提供前列腺素 H_2（PGH_2），而不需要血小板 COX-1 的催化作用，经血小板血栓素合成酶作用生成 TXA_2；有核细胞本身也富含大量的血栓素合成酶，能够利用 PGH_2 合成其自身的 TXA_2，这两种来源的 TXA_2 均可诱导血小板聚集。

2.1.2 COX-1 的基因多态性

目前，研究发现 COX-1 基因存在 20 多个变异体，大多数变异体并不常见，且几乎都是同义的，也就是说 COX-1 可能是高度保守的蛋白。关于 COX-1 与阿司匹林对血小板反应性的影响的关系，学者们做了大量的实验研究。Feher G 等[12]对 101 例行冠状动脉介入术患者每天服用阿司匹林（100mg）2 周以上的心血管病患者进行 COX-1 基因序列检测，发现发生突变最常见的基因，分别为 A842G、C22T、G128A、C644A 和 C714A，且证实 A842G 与另一变异体 C50T 是完全不对等的。在 AA 诱导血小板聚集增多和血浆 TXB2 升高的患者，COX-1 的单倍体更多的是包含 -842G 等位基因的突变而不是 A842- 等位基因的突变。这些研究结果显示 -842G 等位基因突变的患者对阿司匹林抵抗的敏感性差。

2.1.3 可能与环氧化酶 -2（COX-2） 有关

COX-2 在炎症和细胞生长过程中有着重要的作用，其结构与 COX-1 相似。COX-2 为诱导型酶，大多数细胞不表达这种酶，仅主要存在于单核细胞、巨噬细胞和血管内皮细胞，在血小板膜上仅有不同的数量的表达。在动脉粥样硬化的慢性炎症过程中，炎症刺激因子如趋化因子、内毒素和生长因子可诱导并调节血液循环中的单核细胞和巨噬细胞的 COX-2 表达[13]。Cambria-Kiely JA 等[14]对人血管内皮细胞 COX-1 和 COX-2 源性的前列腺素进行检测，发现白介素 -1β 诱导 COX-2 表达上调，使得 TXA_2 生成量增加 2 倍。COX-2 的上调和过量表达增强其催化 AA 生成 PGH_2 以及 TXA_2 的作用。同时，单核细胞和巨噬细胞内含有大量的血栓素合成酶，促进 TXA_2 的合成，且单核细胞、巨噬细胞以及内皮细胞均能合成 PGH_2，从而转化为血小板强激动剂 TXA_2，诱导血小板聚集，而阿司匹林对 COX-2 的抑制作用很弱，仅为对 COX-1 抑制的抑制作用 1/170[15]。

2.1.4 药物之间的相互作用

AA 以磷脂的形式存在于细胞膜中，多种刺激因素可激活磷脂酶 A，使 AA 从膜磷脂中释放出来。游离的 AA 在 COX 作用下转变成前列腺素 G_2（PGG_2）和前列腺素 H_2（PGH_2）。后者在前列腺素合成酶的作用下，转化生成血 TXA_2。TXA_2 是血小板强聚集剂，活化血小板，使其释放和聚集。而阿司匹林可使 COX 丝氨酸位点乙酰化，从而阻断 COX 催化位点与底物的结合，导致 COX 永久地不可逆地失活。而非甾体类抗炎药如布洛芬，也能抑制 COX 的活性，但其对 COX 的作用是可逆的。所以同时服用阿司匹林和布洛芬时，布洛芬与阿司匹林可竞争性地抑制 COX 活性，从而大大影响阿司匹林的抗血小板作用。

2.2 氯吡格雷抵抗的发生机制

2.2.1 药物之间的相互作用

氯吡格雷作为一种噻氯吡啶类前体药，只有经过肝 P450 酶系（CYP3A4、CYP3A5 和 CYP2C19）代谢后才能转化为活性物质，后者通过不可逆地选择性地抑制 ADP 与其血小板膜受体 P1Y12 结合，从而阻断下游的信号传导，发挥其抗血小板聚集作用[15]。由于 P450 酶系的代谢活性存在差异，造成氯吡格雷的作用存在异质性。Hulot JS 等[16]研究发现，服用氯吡格雷的患者中 CYP3A5 表达者对氯吡格雷的反应性要高于 CYP3A5 表达缺失者，且行冠状动脉介入患者中 CYP3A5 表达者的心血管不良事件的发生率也高于 CYP3A5 表达缺失者。而 CYP2C19 等位基因表达缺失者对氯吡格雷的反应性比此等位基因正常表达者要低，致使患者对氯吡格雷的反应存在差异[17]。Kim KA 等[18]对 CYP2C19 在氯吡格雷的药代动力学中的作用进行

第七章

研究并评价了其基因多态性造成的氯吡格雷反应的差异性，结果显示 CYP2C19 等位基因的缺失及其基因多态性，使得酶活性异常，是造成氯吡格雷反应个体差异的一个重要因素。

同样经过 P450 酶系 CYP3A 代谢的药物如脂溶性他汀类药物，可能通过竞争性地抑制了氯吡格雷的活性，从而影响氯吡格雷的药效。Lau WC 等[19]研究证实急性心肌梗死患者服用氯吡格雷后血小板功能的抑制存在差异性，同时发现氯吡格雷治疗的差异性与其 CYP3A 代谢活性的差异相关。而大环内酯类药物如红霉素作为 CYP3A 抑制药，影响了 CYP3A 的活性，从而削弱氯吡格雷的抗血小板聚集作用。

2.2.2　P1Y12 基因多态性　血小板膜上的 ADP 受体 -P1Y12 为氯吡格雷作用主要靶点，其主要有两种亚型——H1 和 H2。H2 与健康者 ADP 诱导的血小板聚集具有相关性[20]。Fontana P 等[21]研究发现 P1Y12 的 H2 基因型虽然只占少数（14%），却具有很强血小板聚集作用，而氯吡格雷对其反应却比较差，这大大削弱了氯吡格雷的抗血小板作用。凝血酶、TXA_2 和胶原诱导受体 P1Y12 的激活，也可能是抵抗的一个因素[22]。这些研究结果显示了氯吡格雷抵抗与 P1Y12H2 相关的可能性。但是一些研究者对此研究却得出一些相反的结论。Cuisset T 等[23]研究发现从 ADP 诱导的血小板聚集率、VASP 磷酸化和 P- 选择素的表达水平并未发现 P1Y12 的 T744C 基因多态性与氯吡格雷反应性具有明显相关性。这还有待于进行进一步研究。

3. 抗血小板药物抵抗的治疗措施及存在问题

抗血小板药物抵抗和实验室检查方法还有待于进一步完善和确立，其临床治疗也尚没有确切有效的治疗方案，主要通过加大阿司匹林或氯吡格雷使用剂量和联合用药来改善抗血小板药物抵抗，或寻求更有效的抗血小板药物，降低急性心血管事件发生率。

发生 AR 的患者可通过阿司匹林与其他类抗血小板药物联合服用来改善和克服 AR，这种联合应用的方法要优于直接取代阿司匹林。发生 AR 患者其血小板对 ADP 的敏感性以及 ADP 水平是显著增高的，还有这些患者呈现对 ADP 受体 P1Y12 拮抗剂 - 氯吡格雷较好的敏感性[24,25]。Yusuf S[26]

对 16562 例非 ST 抬高的急性冠状动脉综合征的患者进行研究，治疗组采用氯吡格雷 300mg 和阿司匹林 75 ~ 325mg 联合应用，对照组采用安慰剂和阿司匹林，结果显示联合治疗组使心血管疾病的病死率降低 20%。

最近研究显示，600mg 负荷量氯吡格雷对血小板抑制的强度和速度都有所提升，持续服用 600mg 负荷量氯吡格雷对血小板的抑制作用要强于初用 600mg 负荷量，继而每天 75mg 维持量的患者，氯吡格雷抵抗的发生率也会降低[27,28]。但行 PCI 的患者术前服用 600mg 氯吡格雷仍有 5% ~ 11% 发生氯吡格雷抵抗，且继续增大剂量也不能改善氯吡格雷抵抗的发生[29]。尽管双重抗血小板药物联合应用似乎是 AR 最有效的治疗方案，但是 CR 的迅速出现甚至阿司匹林 - 氯吡格雷抵抗的出现，使得人们不得不寻求更有效的抗血小板药物治疗，新的 ADP 受体拮抗剂如普拉格雷就应运而生，呈现更快速、有力和持久的血小板抑制作用，且能改善氯吡格雷反应的差异性[30]。

目前采用联合用药或加大药物使用剂量和寻求新的抗血小板药物来解决抗血小板药物抵抗的问题，但前者虽在一定程度上能改善了 AR 或 CR，但存在一定的安全性问题。加大药物剂量或联合用药会增加出血的危险，且对于用于一级预防的患者，阿司匹林的疗效取决于血栓危险和出血危险二者之间的评估，对于血管事件低危的患者（≤ 1%），收益与出血并发症相抵消；在心血管或脑血管合并症高危的患者（3%/ 年），收益明显大于风险[31]。有研究[32]显示药物加大到一定剂量，药物抵抗得不到继续改善，最终并未降低血管不良事件的发生率。

4. 中医药的研究现状

鉴于抗血小板药物抵抗现象的出现以及目前解决策略的所存在的局限性，中医中药在此方面也展开了有益的探索。刘新灿等[33]研究发现通心络胶囊联合阿司匹林有一定改善 AR 的作用；张妍等[34]应用脑心通胶囊联用阿司匹林同样发现具有改善一定改善 AR 的疗效。也有中药单体对 AR 的有效性报道，李彬等[35]采用三七总苷联合阿司匹林治疗 AR 1 个月后，血小板聚集率联合治疗组较单用阿司匹林治疗组数值上有所降低，但两组比较无统计学意义（$P > 0.05$）。这些研究虽初步证实中药复方或中药单体对 AR 的有效性，但是其具体作用环节、靶点和发挥作用的机制还有待学者们进一步研究。

5. 展望

随着血小板活化机制的研究的不断深入，了解到血管内皮损伤引起的血小板活化、血栓形成是多方面、多途径的，主要包括血小板黏附、聚集和释放。参与黏附的主要黏附蛋白和受体有：纤维蛋白原、玻连蛋白、血管性血友病因子（von Willebrand factor，vWf）、纤维连接蛋白、GPⅠb、GPVI、GPⅠa-Ⅱa和GPⅡb-Ⅲa。血小板聚集激动剂如凝血酶、TXA_2、AA、ADP、胶原、肾上腺素等都是活化血小板的诱导剂，这些通路最终都作用于它们的共同通路GPⅡb/Ⅲa，从而活化血小板。这些主要的血小板激动剂和黏附受体在血小板活化、黏附、聚集和血栓形成过程中起到重要作用[1]。正是随着对血小板活化和血栓形成的分子机制的深入研究，使得这些激动剂和活化受体成为探索更有效的抗血小板药物的靶点和突破点，也为未来抗血小板药物治疗从单靶点到多靶点，从某一种药物独立治疗到两种或多种药物联合治疗提供了可能性[36]。

中药具有多环节发挥作用的特点，国内相关的研究初步显示了中药在抗血小板方面的良好前景。那么在规范使用抗血小板药物基础上联合应用中药是否可以减少或减轻AR或CR，甚至可以减少抗血小板基础用药量，并最终减少事件发生率，乃是中医药研究领域努力的方向。但目前，存在作用靶点不清晰、作用机制不明了、量效关系不明确的问题。那么如何建立中药抗血小板功效的合理评价体系就是摆在我们面前亟待解决的问题。"方（药）证对应"是中医药功效研究的核心问题，以"证"作为切入点，结合代谢组学、基因组学和蛋白组学等现代生物学方法寻找病证状态下血小板功能特异性的标志分子群，从而建立不同中药抗血小板的指标体系。目前，抗血小板中药多集中在活血化瘀中药或复方，因此有关冠心病血瘀证的实质研究有望为活血化瘀中药抗血小板的深入研究提供了可能。

参考文献

[1] Jackson SP, Schoenwaelder SM. Antiplatelet therapy：in search of the "magic bullet". Nat Rev Drug Discov, 2003, 2 (10): 775-789.

[2] Angiolillo DJ, Suryadevara S, Capranzano P, et al. Prasugre L：a novel platelet ADP P2Y12 receptor antagonist. A review on its mechanism of action and clinical development. Expert Opin Pharmacother, 2008, 9 (16): 2893-2900.

[3] Patrono C, Coller B, Dalen JE, et al. Platelet active drugs: the relationships among dose, effectiveness, and side effects. Chest, 2001, 119 (1): 39S-63S.

[4] Cattaneo M. Laboratory detection of "aspirin resistance"：what test should we use (if any). Eur Heart J, 2007, 28 (14): 1673-1675.

[5] Eikelboom JW, Hirsh J, Weitz JI, et al. Aspirin-resistanct thromboxane biosynthesis and the risk of myocardial in farction, stroke, or cardiovascular death in patients at high risk for cardiovascular events. Circulation, 2002, 105 (14): 1650-1655.

[6] Hankey GJ, Emery J, Baglin T, et al. Narrative review：a spirin resistance and its clinical implications. Ann Intern Med, 2005, 142 (5): 370-380.

[7] Von Beckerath N, Pogatsa-Murrayg, Wieczorek A, et al. Correlation of a new point-of-care test with conventional optical aggregometry or the assessment of clopidogrel responsiveness. Thromb Haemos, 2006, 95 (5): 910-911.

[8] Zimmermann N, Hohlfeld T. Clinical implication of aspirin resistance. Thromb Hemost, 2008, 100 (3): 379-390.

[9] Cattaneo M. Resistance to antiplatelet drugs：molecular mechanisms and laboratory detection. J Thromb Haemost, 2007, 5 (1): 230-237.

[10] Gladding P, Webster M, Ormiston J, et al. Antiplatelet drug nonresponseness. Am Heart J, 2008, 155 (4): 591-599.

[11] Tran HA, Anand SS, HankeygJ, et al. Aspirin resistance. Thromb Res, 2007, 120 (3): 337-346.

[12] Feher G, Feher A, Puschg, et al. The genetics of antiplatelet drug resistance. Clin Genet, 2009, 75 (1): 1-18.

[13] Lau WC, Gurbel PA. Antiplatelet drug resistance and drug-drug interactions：role of cytochrome P450 3A4. Pharm Res, 2006, 23 (12): 2691-2708.

[14] Cambria-Kiely JA, Gandhi PJ. Aspirin resistance and genetic polymorphisms. J Thromb Thrombolysis, 2002, 14 (1): 51-58.

[15] Fitzgerald DJ, Maree A. Aspirin and clopidogrel resistance. Hematology (Am Soc Hematol Educ Program), 2007: 114-120.

[16] Hulot JS, Bura A, Villard E, et al. Cytochrome P450

2C19 loss-of-function polymorphism is a major determ inant of clopidogrel responsiveness in healthy subjects. Blood, 2006, 108 (7): 2244-2247.

[17] Brandt JT, Close SL, Iturria SJ, et al. Common polymorphisms of CYP2C19 and CYP2C9 affect the pharmacokinetic and pharmacodynamics response to clopidogrel but not prasugrel. J Thromb Haemost, 2007, 5 (12): 2429-2436.

[18] Kim KA, Park PW, Hong SJ, et al. The effect of CYP2C19 polymorphism on the pharmacokinetics and pharmacodynamics of clopidogrel：a possible mechanism for clopidogrel resistance. Clin Pharmacol Ther, 2008, 84 (2): 236-242.

[19] Lau WC, Gurbel PA, Watkins PB, et al. Contribution of hepatic cytochrome P450 3A4 metabolic activity to the phenomenon of clopidogrel resistance. Circulation, 2004, 109 (2): 166-171.

[20] Gachet C. Regulation of platelet functions by P2 receptors. Annu Rev Pharmacol Toxicol, 2006, 46: 277-300.

[21] Fontana P, Reny JL. Frequently asked questions on clopidogrel treatment：indications, resistance, and biological evaluation in vascular patients. Rev Med Suisse Romande, 2008, 4 (143): 360-363.

[22] Wiviott SD, Antman EM. Clopidogrel resistance: a new chapter in a fast-moving story. Circulation, 2004，109 (25): 3064-3067.

[23] Cuisset T, Frere C, Quilici J, et al. Role of the T744C polymorphism of the P2Y12 gene on platelet response to a 600mg loading dose of clopidogrel in 597 patients with non-ST-segment elevation acute coronary syndrome. Thromb Res, 2007, 120 (6): 893-899.

[24] Borna C, Lazarowski E, van Heusden C, et al. Resistance to aspirin is increased by ST-elevation myocardial in farction and correlates with adenosine diphosphate levels. Thromb J, 2005, 26 (3): 10.

[25] Eikelboom JW, Hankeyg J, Thom J, et al. Enhanced antiplatelet effect of clopidogrel in patients whose platelets are least inhibited by aspirin: a randomized crossover trial. J Thromb Haemost, 2005, 3 (12):

2649-2655.

[26] Yusuf S, Zhao F, Mehta SR, et al. Effects of clopidogrel in addition to aspirin in patients with acute coronary syndromes without ST-segment elevation. N Engl J Med, 2001, 345 (7): 494-502.

[27] Gurbel PA, Bliden KP, Zaman KA, et al. Clopidogrel loading with eptifibatide to arrest the reactivity of platelets study. Circulation, 2005, 111 (9): 1153-1159.

[28] Kastrati A, von Beckerath N, Joost A, et al. Loading with 600mg clopidogrel in patients with coronary artery disease with and without chronic clopidogrel therapy. Circulation, 2004, 110 (14): 1916-1919.

[29] Gurbel PA, Bliden KP, Hayes KM, et al. The relation of dosing to clopidogrel responsiveness and the incidence of high post-treatment platelet aggregation in patients undergoing coronary stenting. J Am Coll Cardi, 2005, 45 (9): 1392-1396.

[30] Gasparyan AY, Watson T, LipgY. The role of aspirin in cardiovascular prevention：implications of aspirin resistance. J Am Coll Cardiol, 2008, 51 (19): 1829-1843.

[31] 李小鹰. 阿司匹林在动脉硬化性心血管疾病中的临床应用：中国专家共识（2005）. 中华心血管病杂志，2006，34（3）：281-284.

[32] Chew DP, Bhatt DL, Sapp S, et al. Increased mortality with all platelet glycoprotein Ⅱb/Ⅲa antagonists：a meta-analysis of phase Ⅲ multicenter randomized trials. Circulation, 2001, 103 (2): 201-206.

[33] 刘新灿，胡宇才，朱明军. 通心络胶囊对冠心病病人阿司匹林抵抗的影响. 中西医结合心脑血管病杂志，2006，4（6）：545.

[34] 张妍，梁静，周玉杰，等. 脑心通胶囊对阿司匹林抵抗的影响. 山东中医杂志，2008，27（1）：13-15.

[35] 李彬，毛静远，王强，等. 三七总苷对阿司匹林抵抗影响的临床观察. 中西医结合心脑血管病杂志，2007，5（7）：579-581.

[36] Xiang YZ, Xia Y, Gao XM, et al. Platelet activation, and antiplatelet targets and agents：current and novel strategies. Drugs, 2008, 68 (12): 1647-1664.

第
七
章

关于急性冠状动脉综合征中无复流现象的防治 *

赵福海　陈可冀

冠状动脉介入术（percutaneous coronary intervention, PCI）作为急性冠状动脉综合征（acute coronary syndrome, ACS）重要而有效的治疗策略，挽救了大量垂危患者的生命。但令人遗憾的是，急诊 PCI 术中有高达 12% ～ 30% 的无复流（no-reflow）现象[1]，使心肌组织有效灌注严重受损，导致心功能恶化及远期效果不良等心血管事件增加，因而正确认识无复流的发生机制并建立有效的防治策略，至关重要。

无复流是指冠状动脉闭塞再通后，在无明显残余狭窄、夹层、痉挛或血栓形成等造成冠状动脉前向血流减少的情况下，却无心肌组织有效灌注的现象。心肌梗死溶栓试验（thrombolysis in myocardial infarction, TIMI）血流分级 ≤ Ⅰ 级者为无复流，TIMI 血流分级 2 级者为慢血流。Eeckhout E 等[2]根据发生情况不同将无复流现象分为 3 类：（1）实验性无复流（experimental no-reflow）：指实验条件下诱发的无复流；（2）心肌梗死再灌注无复流（myocardial infarction repefusion no-reflow）：指急性心肌梗死（AMI）时经药物和（或）机械性血管再通时产生的无复流；（3）血管造影无复流（angiographic no-reflow）：指 PCI 期间血管造影显示的无复流。Galiuto L[3]根据形态学和功能学研究将无复流分为两类：（1）解剖型：指微血管解剖结构受到破坏，导致不可逆心肌细胞损坏，对药物治疗无反应；（2）功能型：指开放的、解剖结构完整的微血管由于痉挛和（或）微栓塞而受损，具有动态时相性和可逆性，经处理可改善。

无复流的发生机制复杂，目前尚不十分明确，共同的病理生理基础是微血管水平血流受阻和微循环功能障碍。其中微栓子栓塞主要在急性冠状动脉综合征的无复流发生中起作用，微栓子主要来源于冠状动脉不稳定病变中的富含坏死脂质核心的斑块。急诊 PCI 过程中粥样斑块机械性破裂，产生碎片栓塞冠状动脉远端，导致无复流发生。最近研究发现除微血栓外，罪犯血管中斑块成分如脱落坏死核心碎屑、富含脂质的巨噬细胞、纤维蛋白与无复流现象发生明显相关[4]。血管内超声（intra vascular ultra sound, IVUS）研究提示血栓形成、血管壁正性重构、斑块负荷过重、PCI 术后减少的斑块容积是 ACS 发生无复流的独立预测因素。此外，微血管痉挛，缺血再灌注后细胞黏附和炎症因子水平变化，内皮的缺血损伤和心肌细胞水肿，微血管损伤，血小板激活并聚集，氧自由基释放，无复流区大量白细胞聚集也参与了无复流的发病过程。

冠状动脉无复流可产生严重心肌缺血，危及患者的生命，甚至发生心血管而导致崩溃而导致立即死亡。因此及早识别、迅速作出诊断十分关键。患者此时往往突发急剧胸痛，随后发生血流动力学紊乱。严重者即刻出现低血压、心源性休克、心力衰竭甚至死亡。冠状动脉造影见对比剂滞留在冠状动脉内。心肌标志物：再灌注后心肌组织灌注情况也可以部分通过心肌标志物（如肌球蛋白、肌钙蛋白、肌酸磷酸激酶同功酶）的变化进行评价。再灌注后 60min 与基线值的比值以及随后上升的斜率反映心外膜冠状动脉再通情况的同时，也反映了微循环及组织灌注的情况。心电图显示：AMI 患者再灌注治疗后，抬高的 ST 段是否完全回落至等电位线可作为心肌灌注或无复流的替代指标。如 PCI 后 1h 抬高 ST 段无回落，对判断微血管灌注或无复流准确性较高。冠状动脉造影：冠状动脉无夹层、痉挛或阻塞情况下，TIMI 血流分级 < 2 级，校正 TIMI 血流帧数（CTFC）> 40；心肌灌注血流分级（TMPG）< 2 级；心肌呈色分级（MBG）< 2 级[5]；心肌声学造影（MCE）相应供血区未见微气泡流入或心肌内微气泡反常持续存在，以上征象均提示无复流发生。IVUS 及其虚拟组织学显像显示：罪犯斑块中超声衰减、大的坏死核心、大的斑块负荷、薄壁纤维帽的易损斑块（thin fibrous cap atheroma, TFCA）、重构指数升高常预示无复流的发生[4]。

临床上预防无复流发生是关键问题，应力图减少心肌缺血时间，现代医学一般在介入术前负荷

* 原载于《中国中西医结合杂志》，2010，30（4）：341-342

剂量抗血小板药物应用及强化他汀类药物治疗，及时识别高危ACS人群，选择性替罗非班/阿昔单抗预处理等，可有效降低无复流发生率，而改善心肌水平的微循环灌注则是治疗无复流现象的根本策略，中医药疗法的合理结合使用是值得研发的领域。针对ACS中微血栓形成的关键环节，抑制血小板激活、聚集，减少血管活性物质和趋化因子释放，降低血小板微血栓形成。血小板膜糖蛋白GPⅡb/Ⅲa受体抑制剂如替罗非班/阿昔单抗冠状动脉内注射，在无复流治疗中已取得较肯定的循证医学证据，但仍有部分患者无法从其治疗中获益。本期刊载的"冠状动脉内注射血塞通对ST段抬高型急性心肌梗死介入术中缓再流现象的影响"，对替罗非班伍用三七总皂苷的临床应用价值，在中西医结合治疗无复流方面作出了有益的探索和尝试[6]；鉴于三七总皂苷系在血管内应用，建议在进一步完善有关这类中药注射剂药物代谢和药物动力学及免疫毒理学的基础上，讲求药品质量控制要求，科学合理应用，以达到真正活血通瘀的效果，更好地做到安全和有效。三七总皂苷的生产企业不下十余家，进一步选择应用时，应严格要求。针对微栓子栓塞环节应用远端保护装置和血栓抽吸导管[7,8]，多个临床试验验证其应用价值；此外，血管扩张剂如硝普钠、硝酸甘油、腺苷、尼卡地尔、合心爽以及他汀类药物在无复流的治疗和预防中也显示了一定效果。有研究证实主动脉内气囊泵（intraaortic balloon pump，IABP）应用可纠正合并血流动力学障碍的梗死相关动脉的无复流；无复流的发病机制复杂，多因素参与其发病过程，目前尚未完全阐明。有学者提出临床应作出有针对性的个体化治疗策略[9]。应该清楚地认识到冠状动脉血运重建并不等同于心肌水平的再灌注。无复流现象重在预防，进一步研究其病理生理机制，并探索中西医结合治疗方法的可操作性，相信会使相当一部分患者从中获益。

参考文献

[1] Piana RN, Paikg Y, Moscucci M, et al. Incidence and treatment of no-reflow after percutaneous coronary intervention. Circulation, 1994, 89 (6): 2514-2518.

[2] Eeckhout E, Kern MJ. The coronary no-reflow phenomenon：a review of mechanisms and therapies. Eur Heart, 2001, 22 (9): 729-739.

[3] Galiuto L. Optimal therapeutic strategies in the setting of post-infarct no reflow：the need for a pathogenetic classification. Heart, 2004, 90 (2): 123-125.

[4] Higashikuni Y, Tanabe K, Tanimoto S, et a1. Impact of culprit plaque composition on the no-reflow phenomenon in patients with acute coronary syndrome——an intravascular ultrasound radio frequency analysis. Circ J, 2008, 72 (8): 1235-1241.

[5] Keuy RV, Cohen MG, Runge MS, et al. The no-reflow phenomenon in coronary arteries. J Thromb Haemest, 2004, 2 (11): 1903-1907.

[6] 甘立军，张春卉，张猛，等．冠状动脉内注射血塞通对ST段抬高型急性心肌梗死介入术中缓再流现象的影响．中国中西医结合杂志，2010，30（4）：348-351.

[7] Yan HB, Wang J, Li N, et al. Diver CE versus guardwire plus for thrombectomy in patients with inferior myocardial infarction：a trial of aspiration of thrombus during primary angioplasty for inferior myocardial infarction. Chin Med J, 2007, 120 (7): 557-561.

[8] Ikari Y, Sakurada M, Kozuma K, et al. VAMPIRE investigators. Upfront thrombus aspiration in primary coronary intervention for patients with ST-segment elevation acute myocardial infarction：report of the VAMPIRE（Vacuum as piration thrombus removal）trial. JACC Cardiovasc Interv, 2008, 1 (4): 424-431.

[9] Niccolig, Burzotta F, Galiuto L, et al. Myocardial no-reflow in humans. J Am Coll Cardiol, 2009, 54 (4): 281-292.

莪术及其提取物的心血管药理研究进展 *

钱 伟 赵福海 史大卓

莪术为姜科植物蓬莪术或温郁金的干燥根茎，主要成分为挥发油和姜黄素类。研究发现莪术及其提取物具有抗癌、抗早孕、抗癫痫和保肝等作用，此外，还具有抗凝、抗血小板、抗氧化、调脂等广

* 原载于《中国中西医结合杂志》，2012，32（4）：575-576

泛的心血管药理作用[1-3]。本文就莪术及其提取物的心血管相关药理研究进展综述如下。

1. 抗血小板聚集作用

夏泉等[4]在研究莪术二酮抑制血小板聚集作用的实验中，对 ADP 诱导的兔血小板聚集模型进行体外对比实验，发现当莪术二酮的血浆浓度从 0 增加到 1.634 mmol/L 时，其 5min 内血小板聚集抑制率逐渐升高，并于 1.634 mmol/L 时达到最大聚集抑制率（38.49%），此后随着血浆浓度的增加，5min 内聚集抑制率无明显增加，仅在一定范围内波动（30%～40%），表明莪术二酮对 ADP 诱导的兔血小板聚集具有抑制作用。

2. 抗血管内皮细胞增生作用

叶兰等[5]观察莪术对人工皮下移植海绵内新生肉芽组织生长及其新生血管的影响，通过免疫组化法进行内皮细胞特异性Ⅷ因子、血管内皮细胞生长因子（vascular endothelial growth factor, VEGF）染色，RT-PCR 检测 VEGF mRNA 表达。证实莪术可抑制海绵内新生肉芽组织的血管新生，其机制可能与抑制新生血管表达 VEGF 有关。Chen W 等[6]在活体及体外实验中研究莪术油抗血管再生作用，发现 20 及 40μg/mL 莪术油在鸡胚胎膜形成血管的离体实验中表现出显著的抑制血管增生作用；且不同浓度莪术油在灌胃黑色素瘤模型小鼠 34 天后，小鼠瘤体内的血管生成显著减少，黑色素瘤的肺转移也相应减少，提示黑色素瘤生长受到抑制，可能与巨噬细胞分泌基质金属蛋白酶（metalloproteinases, MMPs）的表达下调有关。高承贤等[7]在姜黄素对牛血清促进的牛内皮细胞及人肝癌细胞 SGC-7901 增殖的影响研究中证实：姜黄素具有抗血管生成作用，潜在机制可能是抑制内皮细胞增殖和迁移，表明姜黄素是一种特异性血管生成抑制剂。

3. 调整血脂作用

Kim M[8]对高脂肪喂养的雄性大鼠进行实验研究，通过测定胆固醇 7α- 羟化酶（一种胆汁酸合成限速酶），从 mRNA 水平研究姜黄素对心血管疾病的预防和保护作用。表明姜黄素通过上调 CYP7A1 基因水平，从而达到降脂效果。谢海波等[9]在探讨活血、破血中药对动脉粥样硬化大鼠血脂、血液流变学影响的实验中发现：莪术能降低

大鼠血清 TC、TG 水平及全血黏度（低切、中切、高切）和血浆黏度。王舒然等[10,11]对高脂血症模型大鼠的实验研究表明姜黄素通过降低 apoB 水平，进而抑制 LDL-C 代谢，可能是姜黄素降血脂的机制之一。孙玉凤等[12]对高脂血症模型大鼠进行实验，证实姜黄素可增加前列环素含量，减少缩血管物质 TXA$_2$ 的分泌，防止血栓形成，延缓动脉粥样硬化的形成。董月等[13,14]也通过实验证实了姜黄素固体分散体对高脂血症模型大鼠具有调节血脂作用。另有实验表明姜黄素可以延缓或减轻高脂血症对组织造成的损伤[15]。

4. 对血液流变学的影响

和岚等[16]在观察莪术对血液流变影响的研究中，将莪术组 SD 大鼠与空白对照组、模型组、三棱组进行对比，结果发现：莪术组在不同切变率下全血黏度 η_{a5}、η_{a30}、η_{a200} 降低，红细胞变形指数明显提高，平均血小板容积（mean platelet volume, MPV）明显降低，表明莪术可对不同血液流变学指标产生影响。苗明三等[17]通过探讨姜黄素对血瘀性脑缺血大鼠模型的作用特点，在实验中发现与模型组比较姜黄素可显著降低全血高、低切黏度、红细胞聚集指数以及全血高、低切还原黏度及红细胞刚性，可显著降低脑匀浆乳酸含量，可显著提高脑匀浆乳酸脱氢酶水平及胆碱酯酶水平，表明姜黄素可显著改善大鼠血瘀性脑缺血模型血液流变学及脑匀浆生化指标。

5. 抗氧化作用

孙非等[18]研究莪术油对小鼠血液超氧化物歧化酶（superoxide dismutase, SOD）、谷胱甘肽过氧化物酶（glutathione peroxidase, GSH-Px）和丙二醛（malondialdehyde, MDA）含量的影响，与对照组比较，发现莪术油可明显提高小鼠血液 SOD、GSH-Px 活性，同时降低 MDA 含量。欧阳英英等[19]研究血红素氧化酶-1（heme oxygenase-1，HO-1）在姜黄素拮抗乙醇所致大鼠肝细胞氧化损伤过程中所起的作用，发现姜黄素能够诱导 HO-1 的活性，且 HO-1 的活性和表达与肝细胞的抗氧化水平明显相关。其他实验也表明姜黄素固体分散体对高脂血症模型大鼠具有抗组织氧化的作用[13,14]。王关林等[20]通过对健康雏鸡的实验，将莪术多糖组与正常对照组、环磷酰胺组、环磷酰胺加莪术多糖组进行对比，证实莪术多糖

对 -OH 和 O_2^- 有明显的清除作用，表明莪术多糖具有一定的抗氧化能力，能够提高机体免疫力，修复组织损伤。

6. 其他相关研究

一个利用犬冠状动脉模型验证莪术油洗脱支架抑制再狭窄的动物实验表明：与裸支架和涂层支架比较，莪术油洗脱支架减少了新生内膜厚度、新生内膜面积、管腔面积狭窄率（$P < 0.01$），增加了管腔面积（$P < 0.01$），说明莪术油洗脱支架具有抑制再狭窄作用[21]。唐家驹等[22]以可降解高分子材料聚乳酸 - 乙醇酸共聚物（PLGA）为载体分别制备了三种浓度（3wt%、5wt%、8wt%）的姜黄素复合薄膜，采用傅立叶变换红外光谱研究了复合薄膜的组成成分，结果表明姜黄素 /PLGA 复合薄膜的抗凝血性在实验药物浓度范围内，随着药物含量的增加逐步提高。

Kim TH 等[23]使用白蛋白捆绑技术，静脉注射人血清白蛋白装载的姜黄素纳米颗粒（curcumin-human serum alnumin-particles, CCM-HSA-NPs），观察到 CCM-HSA-NPs 的水溶解度及在血管中的积累量是 CCM 的 300 倍，生物活性作用只有很少损失。CCM-HSA-NPs 在注射 1h 后作用于肿瘤细胞局部，姜黄素含量约为直接注射姜黄素的 14 倍，与血管内皮细胞的结合增加了 5.5 倍，通过单层血管细胞的运输能力增高了 7.7 倍。在体内抗肿瘤实验中 CCM-HSA-NPs 显示出了较好的治疗效果，50% ～ 60% 的肿瘤细胞生长受到了抑制。CCM-HSA-NPs 强大的抗肿瘤作用源于其在血管内皮细胞内的高水溶性和积累能力。

莪术及其提取物的多效能药理作用被越来越多的研究所证实，但研究多集中在对莪术油、姜黄素等粗组分的水平。未来研究应集中对莪术进行分离、纯化、鉴定，在细胞、分子、基因水平研究莪术单体的药理作用，对阐明其多效能药理作用机制会大有帮助。

参考文献

[1] 钟锋，顾健，张亮亮，等 . 莪术药理作用的现代研究进展 . 中国民族民间医药，2010，19（13）：67-68.

[2] 曹利娟，刘华钢，刘丽敏，等 . 莪术油近五年的研究进展 . 医学综述，2010，16（3）：447-450.

[3] 龙明智，陈磊磊 . 姜黄素的药理作用 . 国外医学 . 中医中药分册，2003，25（5）：270-287.

[4] 夏泉，董婷霞，詹华强，等 . 莪术二酮对 ADP 诱导的兔血小板聚集的抑制作用 . 中国药理学通报，2006，22（9）：1151-1152.

[5] 叶兰，徐晓玉，李荣亨，等 . 三棱莪术对大鼠皮下移植人工海绵新生血管的影响研究 . 中国药房，2008，19（21）：1610-1612.

[6] Chen W, Lu Y, Gao M, et al. Anti-angiogenesis effect of essential oil from *Curcuma zedoaria in vitro* and *in vivo*. J Ethnopharmacol, 2010, 133 (1): 220-226.

[7] 高承贤，丁志山，梁冰冰，等 . 姜黄素对血管生成影响的实验研究 . 中药材，2003，26（7）：499-502.

[8] Kim M, Kim Y. Hypocholesterolemic effects of curcumin via up-regulation of cholesterol 7a-hydroxylase in rats fed a high fat diet. Nutr Res Pract, 2010, 4 (3): 191-195.

[9] 谢海波，莫新民，罗尧岳 . 活血药、破血药对动脉粥样硬化大鼠血脂、血液流变学的影响 . 湖南中医药大学学报，2010，30（3）：20-22.

[10] 王舒然，陈炳卿，王朝旭，等 . 姜黄素降血脂及抗氧化作用的研究 . 中国公共卫生学报，1999，18（5）：263-265.

[11] 王舒然，陈炳卿，孙长颢 . 姜黄素对大鼠调节血脂及抗氧化作用的研究 . 卫生研究，2000，29（4）：240-242.

[12] 孙玉凤，陈志强，丁奇峰，等 . 姜黄素对高脂血症大鼠 TXB_2、6-Keto-PG$_{F1\alpha}$ 的影响 . 河北中医，2008，30（5）：533-535.

[13] 董月，韩刚，原海忠，等 . 姜黄素固体分散体对高脂血症大鼠血脂代谢的影响 . 中药材，2009，32（6）：951-953.

[14] 姚国贤，傅静波，韩刚 . 姜黄素与辛伐他汀降血脂及抗氧化作用比较 . 中国医院药学杂志，2010，30（3）：204-206.

[15] 李慧，王永钧，柴可夫，等 . 姜黄素防治大鼠高脂血症致肾脏损害的实验研究 . 中华中医药学刊，2007，25（9）：1878-1881.

[16] 和岚，毛腾敏 . 三棱莪术对血瘀证模型大鼠血液流变性影响的比较研究 . 安徽中医学院学报，2005，24（6）：35-37.

[17] 苗明三，陈元朋，吴巍 . 姜黄素对大鼠血瘀性脑缺血模型血液流变学及脑匀浆 LD、LDH 和 TchE 水平的影响 . 中药药理与临床，2010，26（1）：29-31.

[18] 孙非，刘建伟，刘志屹，等 . 莪术油对小鼠血液 SOD、GSH-Px 和 MDA 的影响 . 中国老年学杂志，2005，25（4）：445-446.

[19] 欧阳英英，李珂，荣爽，等 . HO-1 在姜黄素拮抗乙醇所致肝细胞氧化损伤过程中的作用 . 华中科技大学学报（医学版），2010，39（1）：82-86.

[20] 王关林，宋扬，罗红梅．莪术多糖对雏鸡抗氧化能力和免疫功能的影响．畜兽医学报，2006，37（11）：1184-1188.

[21] 赵军礼，孙宝贵，温沁竹，等．莪术油洗脱支架防治犬冠状动脉支架术后再狭窄的实验研究．中国中西医结合杂志，2008，28（4）：326-329.

[22] 唐家驹，王进，潘长江，等．姜黄素聚乳酸 - 乙醇酸共聚物复合薄膜的制备及抗凝血研究．生物医学工程学杂志，2008，25（1）：113-116.

[23] Kim TH, Jiang HH, Youn YS, et al. Preparation and characterization of water-soluble albumin-bound curcumin nanoparticles with improved antitumor activity. Int J Pharm, 2010, 403 (2011): 285-291.

延胡索碱治疗快速性心律失常的研究进展 *

张　萍　徐凤芹　马晓昌　陈可冀

快速性心律失常是临床常见病、多发病，见于各种心血管疾病，可影响血流动力学，诱发或加重心功能不全，甚至死亡。其临床常见症状有心慌心悸、心跳剧烈，伴胸闷气短、乏力、汗出、烦躁、头晕等，舌质淡或暗红，有瘀斑、瘀点，苔薄白或少苔，脉象多见促、结、代、数、涩等。属于中医"心悸""怔忡"等范畴。中医学对"心悸""怔忡"等病因病机的认识与治疗有着丰富的经验。目前多数医家经临床研究认为其病因为外邪侵袭、情志失调、饮食劳倦及先天禀赋不足、大病久病失养等，导致机体出现虚实两大证候。实证多为气滞血瘀、痰湿阻滞、肝经郁火等；虚证多为气阴两虚、阳气虚衰、阴血不足等。实证心神扰乱而动，虚证心失所养而悸是本病的病机关键。治疗上，虚证主要有养血、补气、滋阴、温阳基础上加养心安神；实证主要有祛痰、化饮、清火、行瘀基础上加重镇安神。如安神定志丹、天王补心丹、朱砂安神丸、炙甘草汤、黄连阿胶汤、血府逐瘀汤等治疗各种证候心悸的代表方。近些年来，随着新的研究技术方法的出现和中医理论体系的完善，中医药治疗快速性心律失常有了长足的发展，不仅仅涌现出许多疗效确切的中成药，如稳心颗粒、参松养心胶囊等，同时，单味中药提取有效成分治疗心律失常的研究也备受关注。

延胡索又名元胡、玄胡索等，为罂粟科紫堇属植物延胡索（*Corydalis yanhusuo* W.T.Wang）的干燥块茎，是著名的"浙八味"之一，主产于浙江省东阳、磐安一带，河北、山东等地亦有栽培。延胡索味辛、苦，性温，归心、肝、脾经。具有活血、行气、镇痛等功用，用于胸胁疼痛、脘腹疼痛、经闭痛经、产后瘀阻等。现在临床主要集中用于心律失常、心绞痛、气滞血瘀诸痛。其主要成分是延胡索碱。研究发现的延胡索碱有 20 余种，主要分为叔胺碱和季胺碱。其中叔胺碱类主要包括原小檗碱型的紫堇碱（即延胡索甲素）、dl- 四氢巴马汀（即延胡索乙素）、l- 四氢黄连碱（延胡索丁素）、dl- 四氢黄连碱（延胡索戊素）、l- 四氢非洲防己胺（延胡索己素、子素和丑素）；阿朴菲型的 d- 南天竹啡碱、d- 去甲海罂粟碱等；原托品碱型的原阿片碱（即延胡索丙素）、别隐品碱（延胡索寅素）等。季胺碱类主要包括小檗碱型的黄连碱、小檗碱、脱氢紫堇碱（又名去氢紫堇碱、脱氢延胡索碱、脱氢延胡索甲素）、非洲防己胺（又名非洲防己碱）和巴马汀；阿朴菲型的 pontevedrine 等。研究发现它们具有镇痛、镇静、抗心肌缺血、抗心律失常等作用。现主要就其抗心律失常的研究进展综述如下。

1. 临床研究

1983 年马胜兴、陈可冀等[1] 最先开始研究延胡索抗心律失常的作用。在延胡索碱治疗期前收缩的临床研究中发现，延胡索碱Ⅰ（延胡索总碱中水溶性部分）对室性期前收缩，延胡索碱Ⅱ（延胡索总碱中水不溶部分）对房性期前收缩、交界性期前收缩的疗效在不同剂量组均明显优于安慰剂，且随着剂量增加，有效例数增多。延胡索碱Ⅱ能够引起心电图 P、QRS 波增宽和 P-R、Q-T 间期延长，与奎尼丁对心电图的影响颇为相似；而延胡索碱 I 则具有与胺碘酮相似的延长 Q-T 间期、使 T 波变形、心率减慢和扩张血管及降低血压等作用[1]。根据季胺碱比较易溶于水，而叔胺碱几乎不溶或者难溶于水的特点，推测碱 I 可能属于季铵碱部分，碱 II 可能属于叔胺碱部分[2]。而此研究成果激起了对延胡索碱抗心律失常作用机制的研究热潮，且随着膜片钳等技术的出现，不少研究开始从离子通道和分子水平来阐述延胡索碱的抗心律失常机制。

汪大金等[3]研究表明，静脉注射罗痛定（左旋延胡索乙素）对快速型室上性心律失常有明显的转复和减慢心率作用，特别是快速心房颤动的转复成功率较高，用药后心率减慢，与用药前比较差异有统计学意义（$P < 0.01$），且无严重副反应。同时研究还显示罗痛定明显延长房室传导系统有效不应期（AVCERP）、心房有效不应期（AERP），减慢房室传导，有防止程序电刺激诱发阵发性室上性心动过速（PSVT）的作用。同时抑制折返环路正向和（或）逆向传导，取消或缩短折返带，对折返性室上性心动过速有效。另有研究发现[4]该药明显延长预激综合征伴快速室上性心律失常患者 A-H 间期、房室结有效不应期和房室结文氏周长，对窦房结无明显影响，延长旁路前传时间及旁路前传有效不应期，明显延长心房有效不应期，防治程序电刺激诱发室上性心动过速（SVT）有效率达 77.8%。

唐召力[5]研究发现左旋四氢巴马汀治疗预激综合征合并的快速室上性心律失常有效；韩凤波[6]通过研究同样证实左旋四氢巴马汀可以有效治疗预激综合征并发室上性心动过速。且发现该药静脉注射后 0～5 min 抗心律失常作用最好，5～10 min 仍有较好的疗效，此后作用逐渐减弱，40～60 min 基本恢复到用药前水平。

2. 基础电生理研究

2.1 延胡索碱可延长有效不应期和动作电位时程（APD），降低自律性

姚伟星等[7]研究发现四氢巴马汀（THP）的衍生物 7-氯苄基四氢巴马汀可以使 2 种标本动作电位的振幅及 V_{max} 下降，使跨膜动作电位的有效不应期及 APD 延长。从实验模型及电生理特性角度分析改构物，发现其作用性质相似于 I a 类药奎尼丁，即对 Na^+ 通道有阻滞作用，并能延迟复极，

但似乎优于奎尼丁。且 7-氯苄基四氢巴马汀能明显消退左甲状腺素引起大鼠心肌肥厚及左心室质膜 Na^+-K^+-ATPase 酶活力的增高[8]。7-氯苄基四氢巴马汀的抗心律失常作用可能与其延长功能性不应期、降低自律性和减慢心率有关[9]。

张桂清等[10]利用单相动作电位技术，观察 THP 对氯化铯诱发家兔在体心脏早期后除极（EAD）和触发性室性心律失常的影响，观察到氯化铯明显延长动作电位时限，加用 THP 后这一延长作用更为明显，单向动作电位复极 50%（$MAPD_{50}$）由（130 ± 21）ms 延长到（154 ± 13）ms，单向动作电位复极 90%（$MAPD_{90}$）由（172 ± 28）ms 延长到（226 ± 25）ms，说明 THP 有平行延长 $MAPD_{50}$ 和 $MAPD_{90}$ 的作用，而 $MAPD_{50}$ 相当于动作电位 2 相平台期，此期又称复极前期。复极前期处于有效不应期中，其延长有抗心律失常的作用。同时，THP 对 I_{Ca-L} 呈剂量依赖性的抑制作用，对延迟整流钾电流（I_K）有显著抑制作用，而对内向整流钾电流（I_{K1}）无影响，大剂量时对 I_{Na} 亦有抑制作用。THP 能明显降低早期后除极振幅和由 EAD 所引起的触发性室性心律失常的发生率，推测其作用机制可能是通过 THP 对 I_{Ca-L} 和 I_K 的抑制作用，导致内向电流减少所致。同时曾秋棠等[11]也观察到 THP 可以降低哇巴因诱发家兔在体心脏延迟后除极振幅，从而减少由延迟后除极所引起的触发性室性心律失常的发生。

杨宝峰等[12]发现 THP 的衍生物 7-溴化乙氧苯四氢巴马汀（EBP）能降低离体豚鼠乳头状肌 APD_{20} 与 APD_{90} 及右房自律性，延长不应期，对小鼠乌头碱、豚鼠哇巴因、兔肾上腺素诱发的心律失常均有明显对抗作用，对大鼠冠状动脉结扎和再灌注引起的心律失常有保护作用。

2.2 延胡索碱可以作用钾离子通道，抑制 I_K、I_{K1} 及尾电流

杨宝峰等[13]首次用膜片钳技术研究了 EBP 对豚鼠左房单细胞膜电流的影响，发现 EBP 具有频率和浓度依赖性抑制尾电流和 I_k，对慢钙和保持电流无明显作用，能明显延长 APD_{90}，认为主要出于其电压依赖性抑制外向尾电流和 I_k，并通过电压钳技术证实 EBP 有明显的剂量依赖性的延长豚鼠乳头状肌 APD 的作用，并能明显抑制 K^+ 的外向电流，从而降低自律性，减少异位节律活动，这是 EBP 抗心律失常作用的重要机制[14]。

曾维忠等[15]应用细胞内标准微电极方法及

双微电极电压钳技术研究发现苄基四氢帕马汀（BTHP）能阻滞羊浦氏纤维延迟整流电流，大剂量 BTHP 可抑制豚鼠心肌收缩力，阻滞犬浦氏纤维慢内向电流，依赖浓度地延长豚鼠心肌细胞 APD，提示 BTHP 阻滞钾通道是其抗心律失常的重要机制。

刘玉梅等[16]通过酶解法分离豚鼠单个心室肌细胞，应用全细胞膜片钳技术，研究显示延四氢帕马汀可明显抑制 I_K 和 I_{K1}，并呈剂量依赖性，使 APD 和有效不应期延长从而发挥其抗心律失常作用。亦有研究显示 I_{K1} 还参与 3 期复极过程，THP 抑制 I_{K1} 可以使 3 相末期复极化速率减慢[17]，使 APD 延长发挥其抗心律失常作用。

2.3 延胡索碱可以作用钙离子通道，抑制钙电流，降低钙超载

程龙献等[18]采用全细胞膜片钳技术研究罗痛定对酶解分离的豚鼠心室肌细胞膜钙通道电流（$I_{Ca^{2+}}$）的影响，结果显示罗痛定 $1 \sim 100\ \mu mol/L$ 可浓度依赖性抑制 $I_{Ca^{2+}}$，10、30 $\mu mol/L$ 分别使 I_{Ca} 峰值从 $-(1135\pm224)$ Pa 降至 $-(832\pm216)$ Pa（$P < 0.01$），从 $-(1174\pm216)$ 降至 $-(452\pm71)$ Pa（$P < 0.01$），抑制百分率分别为 27%、61%，冲洗后可部分恢复，提示罗痛定对 $I_{Ca^{2+}}$ 的抑制为其主要的抗心律失常作用机制之一。

赵昕等[19]采用离体豚鼠心脏 Langendorff 法灌注，用荧光指示剂方法（Fure-2/AM）标记心肌（$[Ca^{2+}]_i$）变化，并观察低氧后在营养液、脱氢紫堇碱（dehydeocorydaline, DHC）液及维拉帕米液中心肌 $[Ca^{2+}]_i$ 的变化。结果显示，DHC 100 $\mu mol/L$ 可显著减少正常氧和缺氧后心肌 $[Ca^{2+}]_i$，说明 DHC 通过降低钙超载，从而对心肌缺血有保护作用。本研究还证实了其作用与经典的钙通道阻断剂维拉帕米作用相似。

2.4 延胡索碱可降低血浆内皮素 -1（ET-1）及去甲肾上腺素（NE），阻止氧自由基的损害作用及迟后除极，减少再灌注心律失常的发生

许多研究发现，心肌缺血及再灌注时血浆 ET-1、NE 水平明显升高。血浆 ET-1 浓度升高，可与心肌细胞上内皮素 A（ETA）受体结合，通过激活磷脂酶 C，使磷脂酰胺醇 4,5 二磷酸水解，生成三磷酸肌醇和二酰基甘油，促进细胞内储存钙释放。ET-1 还可通过其受体直接打开电压依赖性钙通道，促进细胞外 Ca^{2+} 内流，提高胞浆 Ca^{2+} 浓度，促进缺血及再灌注时心肌细胞钙超载。ET-1

引起的室性心律失常不仅与其收缩冠状动脉，减少灌注血流有关，而且与其能通过二氢吡啶敏感性钙通道促发的早期后除极的形成有关[20]。血浆 NE 浓度升高引起缺血再灌注 VA 的机制可能与其刺激心肌缺血再灌注时增多的 α_1 肾上腺素能受体数目，从而激活慢钙通道和通过第二信使环磷酸腺苷（cAMP）促进 Ca^{2+} 依赖的迟后除极有关。马建群等[21,22]利用硫喷妥钠静脉麻醉开胸犬结扎左前降支冠状动脉 40 min，继以再灌注 40 min 模型，研究表明颅痛定能显著降低缺血再灌注性室性心律失常的发生率和血浆 ET-1 及 NE 浓度。

汪永孝等[23]研究发现 THP 5 ~ 15 mg/kg 静脉滴注明显降低大鼠心肌缺血再灌注心律失常的发生率和心肌脂质过氧化物的含量。THP 10 $\mu mo/L$ 能显著抑制缺氧再给氧所致豚鼠离体心室肌的迟后除极和触发活动，表明 THP 有良好的抗缺血再灌注心律失常的作用，其机制是阻止氧自由基的损害作用和迟后除极的产生。

2.5 延胡索碱可以抗心肌缺血，保护心功能

闵清等[24]研究发现 1-THP 可明显改善垂体后叶素所致心肌缺血。在异丙肾上腺素所致心肌缺血大鼠，1-THP 10 mg/kg 可显著抑制心肌肌酸激酶（CK）和乳酸脱氢酶（LDH）的释放和血清 CK 和 LDH 的升高。同时还发现 1-THP 治疗组丙二醛（MDA）的含量较缺血再灌组明显降低，超氧化物歧化酶（SOD）的含量较缺血再灌组明显增高，提示外源性 1-THP 可进入细胞内，减少氧自由基的生成，加快氧自由基的清除，保护缺血后再灌注心肌，促进心功能的恢复[25]。因此，抑制自由基生成或清除氧自由基作用可能是 1-THP 参与大鼠心肌缺血再灌注损伤心功能保护作用的机制之一。

综上所述，延胡索碱抗心律失常作用主要是通过作用钾离子通道，抑制 I_K、I_{K1} 及尾电流，延长 APD 和有效不应期，降低自律性；作用钙离子通道，抑制钙电流，降低钙超载等。同时其改善心肌缺血、保护心功能、阻止氧自由基损害及迟后除极，也是其抗心律失常的作用机制。在临床研究方面，不少研究已经表明延胡索碱对房性期前收缩、室性期前收缩、心房颤动和预激综合征有一定作用。尽管目前对延胡索碱的实验及临床研究报道较多，但大多数实验研究多是通过测定各个离子通道的电流改变来推测其抗心律失常作用机制，而对其离子通道蛋白及调控蛋白的酶学如 Na^+-K^+-ATP 酶、Ca^{2+}-Mg^{2+}-ATP 酶等方面的研究相对较少，还

需要多方面综合对其作用机制进行更深入广泛的研究，为研制和开发抗心律失常中药有效成分奠定基础。临床方面，目前对延胡索碱制剂的研究存在样本量小，观察疗效指标不统计，研究设计不严谨，研究心律失常类型杂而多，研究目的缺乏针对性等问题，希望有大样本、多中心、随机双盲对照研究来增加其疗效力度及强度。

参考文献

[1] 马胜兴，陈可冀，王荣金.延胡索碱治疗过早搏动的临床研究.中华心血管病杂志，1983，11（1）：6-9.

[2] 马胜兴，陈可冀，马玉玲，等.延胡索抗心律失常作用的初步实验.中药通报，1985，10（11）：41-42.

[3] 汪大金，毛焕元，黄从新.植物性钙拮抗剂颅痛定的抗心律失常临床疗效及其电生理作用.同济医科大学学报，1993，22（5）：322-324.

[4] 汪大金，毛焕元，黄从新，等.罗通定在预激综合征病人中的临床电生理作用.中华心血管病杂志，1993，21（5）：286.

[5] 唐召力.颅痛定治疗预激综合征所合并的快速室上性心律失常.急诊医学，1999，8（6）：399-400.

[6] 韩凤波.硫酸罗通定注射液治疗快速室上性心律失常.天津药学，2002，14（1）：44-45.

[7] 姚伟星，夏国瑾，曾维忠，等.7-氯苄基四氢巴马汀的抗心律失常作用.中国药理学与毒理学杂志，1995，9（3）：220-223.

[8] 闵清，吴基良，罗德生，等.7-氯苄基四氢巴马汀对L2甲状腺素诱发大鼠心肌肥厚及左心室肌原纤维 Na$^+$-K$^+$-ATPase 活力的影响.咸宁学院学报（医学版），2004，18（6）：385-387.

[9] 闵清，白育庭，吴基良，等.7-氯苄基四氢巴马汀对豚鼠离体心房的作用.咸宁学院学报，2000，14（2）：97-99.

[10] 张桂清，曾秋棠，曹林生，等.四氢巴马汀对氯化铯诱发家兔在体心脏早后除极和触发性室性心律失常作用的研究.中华心律失常学杂志，2000，4（3）：208.

[11] 曾秋棠，张桂清，曹林生，等.四氢帕马汀抗触发性室性心律失常作用机制的研究.中华内科杂志，2000，39（10）：667-669.

[12] 杨宝峰，姚伟星，夏国瑾，等.7-溴化乙氧苯四氢巴马汀的抗心律失常作用.中国药理学与毒理学杂志，1990，4（2）：95-98.

[13] 杨宝峰，陈庆文，张永春，等.7-溴化乙氧苯四氢巴马汀抑制外向钾电流和尾电流.中国药理学通报，1994，10（5）：352-354.

[14] 杨宝峰，宗贤刚，王刚，等.7-溴化乙氧苯四氢巴马汀抗心律失常作用的机理.药学学报，1990，25（7）：481-484.

[15] 曾维忠，夏国瑾，姚伟星，等.苄基四氢巴马汀对心肌动作电位及浦氏纤维跨膜钾、钙离子流的影响.中国药理学报，1990，11（4）：314-317.

[16] 刘玉梅，周宇宏，单宏丽，等.延胡索乙素对豚鼠单个心室肌细胞钾离子通道的影响.中国药理学通报，2005，21（5）：599-601.

[17] Miake J, Marban E, Nuss HB. Functional role of inward rectifier current in heart probed by Kir2-1 overexpression and dominant-negative suppression. J Clin Invest, 2003, 111 (10): 1529-1536.

[18] 程龙献，毛焕元，戴水平，等.颅痛定对单个豚鼠心室肌细胞膜钙通道电流的影响.临床心血管病杂志，1995，11（3）：170-172.

[19] 赵昕，汤浩，王亚杰，等.脱氢紫堇碱对正常和低氧豚鼠心肌细胞内钙的影响.中国应用生理学杂志，2003，19（3）：222-225.

[20] 黄亚莉，陆彤，蒋文平.内皮素对豚鼠心室肌细胞触发电活动的影响.中华心血管病杂志，1995：23（5）：381-383.

[21] 马建群，毛焕元，曹林生，等.颅痛定对心肌缺血-再灌注性室性心律失常及血浆内皮素-1浓度的影响.中国危重病急救医学，1993，10（1）：7-9.

[22] 马建群，毛焕元，曹林生，等.颅痛定对心肌缺血再灌注性室性心律失常及血浆去甲肾上腺素浓度的影响.中国实用内科杂志，2002，22（8）：485-486.

[23] 汪永孝，郑云敏，谭月华.四氢巴马汀抗缺血再灌注心律失常的作用及其机理.中国药理学通报，1993，9（5）：358-361.

[24] 闵清，白育庭，吴基良，等.罗通定对大鼠心肌缺血的保护作用.医药导报，2001，20（9）：554-555.

[25] 闵清，白育庭，舒思洁.四氢巴马汀对大鼠心肌缺血再灌注损伤的保护作用.中国误诊学杂志，2007，7（23）：5462-5464.

川芎嗪的心脑血管系统药理作用及临床应用研究进展 *

蒋跃绒　陈可冀

川芎嗪（Ligustrazine）是从伞形科藁本属植物川芎（*Ligusticum chuanxiong* Hort）中提取的生物碱，即四甲基吡嗪（tetramethylpyrazine, TMP），是川芎的有效成分之一。自20世纪70年代陈可冀首先将其应用于缺血性卒中至今[1]，已有近40年的历史。川芎嗪有保护血管内皮、抗血小板、抗缺血再灌注损伤、抗氧化应激等多种心脑血管药理作用，除传统广泛用于冠心病、脑血栓、脉管炎等闭塞性心脑血管疾病外，近年来还被报道应用于肺心病、心力衰竭、冠心病、肾病、门脉高压及冠心病支架术后再狭窄等多种疾病的治疗[2-9]。目前临床常用的有磷酸川芎嗪片、注射用磷酸川芎嗪、盐酸川芎嗪注射液等。

1. 心脑血管药理作用

1.1 保护血管内皮、抗动脉粥样硬化

川芎嗪可减少动脉粥样硬化大鼠循环内皮细胞数，提高总抗氧化能力和超氧化物歧化酶活性，减少MDA生成，减轻血管内皮损伤，通过减轻氧化应激和改善血脂异常而抑制大鼠动脉粥样硬化的发生和肝脂肪积聚[10]。

血管内皮细胞（VECs）的功能状态与血栓栓塞性疾病的发生发展及其预后密切相关。凝血酶具有多种生物学作用，除参与凝血反应外，还参与炎症反应，加重VECs损伤[11]。研究发现，在给予凝血酶之前30min用TMP预处理ECV304细胞，TMP可呈剂量依赖式地抑制凝血酶诱导ECV304细胞促凝血活性（PCA）和组织因子（TF）mRNA增加，减轻内皮细胞的损伤[12]。

多项研究认为川芎嗪的保护血管内皮作用机制与丝裂原活化的蛋白激酶（MAPK）通路有关。Li XY[13]等研究认为，川芎嗪可抑制脂多糖（LPS）诱导的人脐静脉内皮细胞（HUVEC）IL-8mRNA和蛋白水平升高，减少LPS诱导的U937单核细胞和HUVEC黏附，抑制ERK1/2和p38的磷酸化水平以及核因子（NF）-κB（p65）活性，提示TMP通过NF-kappaB介导的通路以及ERK和p38 MAPK通路对内皮细胞发挥抗炎作用。Zhai L[14]等研究也发现，川芎嗪通过MAPK和Caspase-3途径发挥抗氧化和抗凋亡的作用，从而预防H_2O_2诱导的HUVEC损伤。

1.2 抗心肌缺血再灌注损伤、抗心肌肥厚和心肌纤维化

研究认为，川芎嗪通过磷脂酰肌醇3-激酶/蛋白激酶B（PI3K/Akt）途径发挥抗心肌缺血再灌注损伤和抗凋亡作用[15]。内皮型一氧化氮合酶（eNOS）的磷酸化及一氧化氮（NO）生成是重要的下游效应子，明显增强TMP的心肌保护作用。

川芎嗪还可抑制肥大心肌细胞Jak激酶/信号转导转录活化因子（JAK-STAT）信号通路，减少心肌细胞（ANP）mRNA表达，降低pJAK2、pJAK1、pSTAT3蛋白水平，提示其可临床应用于心肌肥厚的治疗[16]。扩张型心肌病（DCM）是心力衰竭最常见的原因之一。川芎嗪可通过降低心肌肥厚的标志物BNP和ACTA1的蛋白表达水平，减少间质胶原沉积和心肌纤维化标志物Col1a1和Col3a1的蛋白表达，减轻cTnT（R141W）表达引起的心肌超微结果破坏，减少结构性蛋白如肌收缩蛋白和钙粘蛋白的表达等，显著抑制cTnT（R141W）转基因小鼠DCM模型的心脏扩大和心功能不全的发展，降低病死率54%[17]。而人参皂苷Rb1和TMP在减轻cTnT（R141W）转基因扩张型心肌病小鼠心室扩张、收缩功能障碍、间质纤维化和超微结构变性等方面有协同作用[18]。

此外，有报道川芎嗪对柯萨奇病毒3（CVB3）感染的大鼠心肌细胞有保护作用，机制可能与其减少乳酸脱氢酶（LDH）活性和NF-κB表达有关[19]。川芎嗪可抑制血管紧张素Ⅱ诱导的大鼠心肌成纤维细胞的增殖，减少Ⅰ型胶原的分泌与合成[20]，是其抗心肌纤维化的作用机制之一。

1.3 抗炎、抗氧化应激

川芎嗪是活性氧（ROS）的拮抗剂。体内和

* 原载于《中国中西医结合杂志》，2013，33（5）：707-711

体外实验均表明，TMP 可保持线粒体结构和功能的完整性，维持线粒体膜电位，该作用与其作为还原剂或抗氧化剂减少 ROS 生成、抑制脂质过氧化、保护谷胱甘肽过氧化物酶和谷胱甘肽还原酶等有关，从而对氧化损伤发挥保护作用[21]。川芎嗪可减轻缺氧诱导的肺血管通透性增加，其机制与清除细胞内 ROS 和抑制缺氧诱导的因子 1（HIF-1）和 VEGF 蛋白水平增加有关[22]。川芎嗪对 H_2O_2 诱导的 HUVEC 氧化损伤具有保护作用，川芎嗪预先孵育 24 小时，可降低丙二醛水平、细胞内 NO 和 NOS 水平，并减少 HUVEC 细胞凋亡[23]。

川芎嗪二苯甲基哌嗪（TMPDP），由川芎嗪分子结构杂交和生物电子等排取代而成。TMPDP 可明显增强 H_2O_2 诱导的 HUVEC 活性，减少细胞 LDH 释放，减少脂质过氧化，增强内源性抗氧化酶超氧化物歧化酶（SOS）和谷胱甘肽过氧化物酶（GSH）活性，减少 ROS 生成，减少细胞内 Ca^{2+} 浓度。提示 TMPDP 可通过清除 ROS，调节细胞内钙离子浓度而保护 HUVEC 免受氧化损伤[24]。

1.4 钙拮抗作用

万海同[25]等研究了川芎嗪对体外培养海马神经元糖氧剥夺损伤模型细胞内钙离子的影响，结果表明，川芎嗪具有钙拮抗作用，提示川芎嗪对脑组织具有保护作用，为川芎嗪作为新型钙通道阻滞剂提供了体外实验依据。川芎嗪可抑制抑制钙/钙调蛋白/钙调蛋白依赖的蛋白激酶（Ca/CaM/CaMKII）通路[18]。张晓丹[26]等采用腹主动脉缩窄法建立舒张型心力衰竭（DHF）大鼠模型，结果发现川芎嗪给药 4 周显著降低左心室舒张末期内压（LVEDP），显著升高左室内压最大下降速率（-dp/dtmax），显著缩短左室松弛时间常数（T）；明显减轻心肌超微结构的损害；显著降低心肌细胞内荧光值；心肌细胞线粒体中 Ca^{2+}-ATPase 活力明显增加。认为中、低剂量的 TMP 可明显减轻 DHF 所致的心肌损伤，改善 DHF 大鼠心功能及心肌细胞内 $[Ca^{2+}]_i$，提高心肌线粒体 ATP 酶活性，拮抗钙超载。

1.5 抗脑缺血再灌注损伤，发挥神经保护作用

川芎嗪被认为是治疗神经细胞缺血-再灌注损伤的有效药物。大鼠脑缺血再灌注 4 小时内应用川芎嗪治疗，可减轻大鼠脑缺血再灌注损伤，其神经保护机制部分与其上调硫氧还蛋白（thioredoxin）有关[27]。Xiao X[28]等采用大脑中动脉闭塞造成局灶性脑缺血大鼠模型，研究认为川芎嗪可明显缩小梗死面积，促进缺血诱发的细胞增生和分化，其机制可能与减少神经元型一氧化氮合酶（nNOS）表达有关。川芎嗪可促进缺氧状态下大鼠脑神经干细胞增殖和分化为神经元，增强 ERK1/2 的磷酸化，降低 p38 的磷酸化，ERK 抑制剂可部分抑制这一效应，说明 MAPK 通路参与了这一作用机制[29]。川芎嗪还可抑制脂多糖诱导的 N9 小胶质细胞 NO 和 iNOS 的过度生成，其机制与抑制 NF-κB 从胞浆转位至细胞核，阻止 p38 MAPK、ERK1/2、c-Jun 氨基末端激酶（JNK）和 Akt 的磷酸化，抑制细胞内 ROS 生成有关[30]。

川芎嗪由于在周围环境中性质稳定，可通过血脑或血眼屏障，且给药方便，在中枢神经系统和周围神经网络均发挥神经保护作用，从而成为一种非常有前景的神经保护药物。动物实验显示皮下注射川芎嗪可阻止海马神经元变性，对阿茨海默病或其他脑损伤均有较强的神经保护作用。虽然其神经保护的分子机制尚不十分清楚，现有证据表明其与抗氧化应激、拮抗钙超载、抑制促炎因子等有关[31]。

川芎嗪有血管舒张作用，有报道川芎嗪可增加家兔脑血管痉挛模型基底动脉 eNOS 和 NO 表达，减少磷酸二酯酶（PDE-V）表达，引起剂量依赖性内皮细胞内 Ca^{2+} 增加，其血管舒张效应至少部分是通过调节一氧化氮/环鸟苷酸（NO/cGMP）信号通路发挥作用的[32]。

1.6 抗血小板作用

20 世纪 70 年代，西苑医院用电镜观察到川芎嗪有降低血小板表面活性和聚集性的作用。对 20 例冠心病患者用川芎嗪治疗后，扩大聚集型血小板数由（40.40±11.52）%，降为（30.40±12.54）%（$P < 0.05$）；血小板聚集数由（149.20±72.56）个，降为（84±39.65）个（$P < 0.01$）。川芎嗪对 ADP、胶原、凝血酶诱导的血小板聚集均有明显的抑制作用，并对已聚集的血小板有解聚作用；能对抗凝血酶诱导的单核细胞与血小板之间的聚集，其作用机制包括调节 TXA_2-PGI_2 系统、抑制 cAMP 磷酸酯酶活性、降低血小板内的 Ca^{2+} 浓度、影响磷脂酰肌醇代谢[33]。近年来，国内有学者以川芎嗪和阿魏酸为先导物，按生物电子等排原理和药物拼合原理，用川芎嗪基替代咪唑基，将川芎嗪与阿魏酸通过醚键进行拼合而合成的化合物（E）-3-{ 4-[（3,5,6- 三甲基吡嗪 -2- 基）甲氧基]-3- 甲氧基苯基 } 丙烯酸；Ⅰ 的体外抗血小板聚集实验

结果显示，对 ADP 诱导的血小板聚集具有较好的抑制活性，是奥扎格雷的 5.7 倍，是川芎嗪阿魏酸盐的 192 倍。并以阿魏酸及其类似物为原料，设计并合成了 6 个新型的川芎嗪阿魏酸衍生物，初步药理活性测试结果显示，部分化合物的血小板抑制率较高 [34,35]。

2 临床应用

2.1 预防冠心病支架术后再狭窄、治疗急性冠状动脉综合征

陈丽娟 [36] 等研究发现川芎嗪药物洗脱支架可抑制猪冠状动脉新生内膜形成，通过减少血管平滑肌增殖和促进血管平滑肌凋亡而减少支架内再狭窄，为川芎嗪洗脱支架的临床应用提供了实验依据和良好的前景。

刘丽梅 [37] 回顾性分析了 92 例采用川芎嗪口服预防冠心病支架术后再狭窄的患者，并与同期 92 例采用复方丹参滴丸的患者进行对照，结果两组观察期间不良事件发生率组间比较无显著差异，两组均未发生明显不良反应，认为川芎嗪用于预防冠心病支架术后再狭窄值得临床推广。郭景源 [38] 将 120 例不稳定型心绞痛患者随机分为常规对照组和常规治疗加川芎嗪治疗组，结果表明川芎嗪治疗组疗效优于常规对照组。

2.2 缺血性脑卒中

陈可冀等最早于 1974 年 12 月至 1975 年 9 月对 28 例急性闭塞性脑血管病应用由北京制药工业研究所制备的川芎一号碱（川芎嗪）为主进行治疗，结果发现以川芎嗪治疗急性闭塞性脑血管病有一定效果，且所有有效的病例一般发生效果都较快，也无明显的毒、副作用，是一个值得进一步研究推广应用的疗法 [39]。后经北京、天津等地近 20 个医院治疗 545 例急性闭塞性脑血管患者，有效率达 80% 以上 [40]。近 40 年来，川芎嗪被城乡广泛应用于缺血性脑卒中和眩晕的治疗。陈瑶 [41] 等收集了 2003 年 1 月以前有关川芎嗪治疗脑梗死的文献 441 篇，经筛选符合纳入标准的试验 7 个，4 例报道了不良反应，没有关于川芎嗪治疗脑梗死远期疗效的研究，Meta 分析认为川芎嗪可能降低治疗期末的神经功能缺损评分（RR 为 0.34，95%CI 0.25-0.48），但由于文献质量较低，尚不能推荐临床常规使用川芎嗪治疗脑梗死，应开展设计严格的随机双盲安慰剂对照试验。李可建共查及 2005 年以前关于川芎嗪治疗缺血性脑卒中急性期的文献

122 篇，共 4 项符合纳入标准，系统评价结果显示川芎嗪注射液治疗缺血性脑卒中急性期有效，由于纳入研究质量较低，降低了系统评价的可靠性 [42]，建议开展大样本、多中心、随机双盲安慰剂对照试验，为川芎嗪治疗缺血性脑卒中的进一步临床推广应用提供高级别的证据。

2.3 肺心病、肺动脉高压

川芎嗪有助于肺心病患者肺动脉高压的缓解，其机制可能与保护肺血管内皮细胞、重建血管活性因子平衡有关 [37]。程少冰 [2] 等将 100 例慢性肺心病急性发作患者随机分为川芎嗪加常规治疗组和单纯常规治疗组，两组治疗后右室射血前期时间与肺动脉血流加速时间（RVPEP/AT）比值、血浆血管性血友病因子（vWF）和内皮素 -1（ET-1）含量均低于治疗前，而血浆 NO 高于治疗前（$P < 0.01$），所有这些变化均以川芎嗪组的变化程度更明显（$P < 0.01$）。慢性肺源性心脏病（CPHD）患者血清趋化因子（fractalkine，FKN）和肿瘤坏死因子 α（TNF-α）水平升高，在西医常规治疗的基础上加用川芎嗪可明显降低血清 FKN 和 TNF-α 水平，降低平均肺动脉压（mPAP）[43]。川芎嗪用于治疗多种血管疾病，如缺血性脑卒中和继发于慢性阻塞性肺病的肺动脉高压。

2.4 慢性心力衰竭

方诚 [3] 等认为川芎嗪对风湿性心脏病慢性心力衰竭致重度瘀血性肝硬化的近期治疗作用效果显著，在肝下界上移、肝功能改善、黄疸消退、肝区痛缓解的时间、住院时间短于对照组，差异有显著性意义。游红利 [44] 将 128 例慢性充血性心力衰竭患者随机分为常规对照组和卡托普利与川芎嗪注射液联合治疗组，结果表明卡托普利与川芎嗪注射液联合治疗组疗效优于常规治疗组。陈阵 [5] 等认为黄芪与川芎嗪注射液联合治疗对慢性充血性心力衰竭患者，可增加心力衰竭患者心脏的心肌收缩力和心排血量，明显改善心力衰竭症状。认为川芎嗪是一种新型的钙离子拮抗剂，可抑制内皮素及去甲肾上腺素的释放，对抗血管紧张素 II 和血管加压素等神经体液因子的缩血管效应，以阻断心力衰竭的发病环节，达到强心作用；同时，具有抗自由基和抑制血小板聚集、扩张冠状动脉，改善心肌缺血等作用。

2.5 其他

此外，川芎嗪还广泛用于治疗眩晕综合征、椎基底动脉供血不足、紧张型头痛等方面，具有很好的对症处理疗效，能迅速缓解症状并且疗效平稳

持久，具有临床推广的价值[45-47]。此外，还有报道将川芎嗪用于小儿病毒性心肌炎、慢性肾衰竭、肝纤维化、门脉高压、肿瘤、糖尿病肾病等的治疗[8,48-50]。

川芎嗪是活血理气中药川芎的一种生物碱，近40年来，经我国城乡临床广泛应用于治疗缺血性心脑血管疾病等多系统疾病，取得了良好的效果，积累了相当丰富的实践经验，具有广阔的应用前景。但相关临床报道以小样本临床观察为主，缺乏高级别的循证医学证据支持，一定程度上阻碍了其进一步推广应用。应选择疗效较好的病种，开展大样本、多中心、随机双盲安慰剂对照试验，为川芎嗪的临床应用提供依据。另外，因川芎嗪有代谢快、半衰期短、生物利用度低等缺点，国内外学者也致力于以川芎嗪为先导药物，通过对其母核或侧链的结构改造和修饰，开发出一系列的川芎嗪衍生物[9]，以期从中得到更加高效低毒的药物。深入开展川芎嗪及其衍生物药理作用及临床应用研究具有重要的理论和实际意义。

参考文献

[1] 陈可冀，钱振淮，张问渠，等. 川芎Ⅰ号碱（川芎嗪）治疗急性闭塞性脑血管病疗效观察. 北京地区川芎嗪协作会议报告，1975.

[2] 程少冰，卢康荣，王达安. 川芎嗪对肺心病患者肺动脉压及血管内皮细胞功能的影响. 中药材，2011，31（1）：161-163

[3] 方诚. 川芎嗪对风湿性心脏病慢性心力衰竭致重度瘀血性肝硬化的影响. 江西中医药，2010，41（325）：30-31.

[4] Huang YT, Chang FC, Chen KJ, et al. Acute hemodynamic effects of tetramethylpyrazine and tetrandrine on cirrhotic rats. Planta Med, 1999,65(2)：130-134.

[5] 陈阵，周发祥. 黄芪与川芎嗪注射液治疗慢性充血性心力衰竭疗效观察. 医药论坛杂志，2011，32（6）：149-150.

[6] 徐红. 川芎嗪在治疗慢性肾功能衰竭中的作用. 中医杂志，2010，51（suppl）：165-166.

[7] 薛现中. 大剂量川芎嗪对2型糖尿病PAI-1活性水平影响的研究. 第二军医大学学报，2003，24（8）：568.

[8] 田春娟，程春瑞，熊奕，等. 川芎嗪治疗糖尿病肾病的系统评价. 中国药房，2012，23（19）：1794-1799.

[9] 董雪娇，姜伊鸣，于暕辰，等. 川芎嗪衍生物及其药理活性研究进展. 中南药学，2012，10（4）：294-299.

[10] Jiang F, Qian J, Chen S, et al. Ligustrazine improves atherosclerosis in rat via attenuation of oxidative stress. Pharm Biol, 2011, 49 (8): 856-863.

[11] Strukova S. Coagulation-dependent inflammation and inflammation-dependent thrombosis. Front Biosci, 2006, 11: 59-80.

[12] 成春英，孙勇，文志斌，等. 川芎嗪对凝血酶诱导血管内皮细胞组织因子表达的影响. 南方医科大学学报，2009，29（8）：1743-1747.

[13] Li XY, He JL, Liu HT, et al. Tetramethylpyrazine suppresses interleukin-8 expression in LPS-stimulated human umbilical vein endothelial cell by blocking ERK, p38 and nulear factor-kappa B signaling pathways. J Ethnopharmacol, 2009, 125 (1): 83-89.

[14] Zhai L, Zhang P, Sun RY, et al. Cytoprotective effects of CSTMP, a novel stilbene derivative, against H_2O_2-induced oxidative stress in human endothelial cells. Pharmacol Rep, 2011, 63 (6): 1469-1480.

[15] Lu L, Jiang SS, Xu J, et al. Protective effect of ligustrazine against myocardial ischaemia reperfusion in rats：the role of endothelial nitric oxide synthase. Clin Exp Pharmacol Physiol，2012，39 (1): 20-27.

[16] 高美华，张丽，李冰，等. 川穹嗪对AngⅡ诱导的大鼠心肌肥大细胞JAK-STAT通路作用. 细胞与分子免疫学杂志，2011，27（5）：519-521，524.

[17] Zhao HP, Lu D, Zhang W, et al. Protective action of tetramethylpyrazine phosphate against dilated cardiomyopathy in cTnT (R141W) transgenic mice. Acta Pharmacol Sin, 2010, 31 (3): 281-288.

[18] Lu D, Shao HT, Ge WP, et al. Ginsenoside-Rb1 and tetramethylpyrazine phosphate act synergistically to prevent dilated cardiomyopathy in cTnTR141W transgenic mice. J Cardiovasc Pharmacol, 2012，59 (5): 426-433.

[19] 钱招昕，黄寒，林晓娟. 川芎嗪对柯萨奇B3病毒感染乳鼠心肌细胞的保护作用及信号转导机制研究. 中国当代儿科杂志，2009，11（8）：687-690.

[20] 张冬梅，秦英，吕浠滢，等. 川芎嗪对血管紧张素Ⅱ诱导的大鼠心肌成纤维细胞增殖及Ⅰ型胶原合成的影响. 中西医结合学报，2009，7（3）：232-236.

[21] Li SY, Jia YH, Sun WG, et al. Stabilization of mitochondrial function by tetramethylpyrazine protects against kainate-induced oxidative lesions in the rat hippocampus. Free Radic Biol Med, 2010, 48 (4): 597-608.

[22] Zhang L, Deng M, Zhou S. Tetramethylpyrazine inhibits hypoxia-induced pulmonary vascular

leakage in rats via the ROS-HIF-VEGF pathway. Pharmacology, 2011, 87 (5-6): 265-273.

[23] Li WM, Liu HT, Li XY, et al. The effect of tetramethylpyrazine on hydrogen peroxide-induced oxidative damage in human umbilical vein endothelial cells. Basic Clin Pharmacol Toxicol, 2010, 106 (1): 45-52.

[24] Ou Y, Guo XL, Zhai L, et al. TMPDP, a tetramethylpyrazine derivative, protects vascular endothelial cells from oxidation damage by hydrogen peroxide. Pharmazie, 2010, 65 (10): 755-759.

[25] 万海同, 王玉, 杨洁红, 等. 体外培养海马神经元糖氧剥夺损伤模型的建立及川芎嗪对其胞内钙离子的影响. 中国中西医结合杂志, 2007, 27 (3): 234-236

[26] 张晓丹, 刘旺, 周嘉辉, 等. 川芎嗪对 DHF 大鼠心肌损伤的保护作用及其机制研究. 中国中药杂志, 2009, 34 (21): 2808-2812.

[27] Jia J, Zhang X, Hu YS, et al. Protective effect of tetraethyl pyrazine against focal cerebral ischemia/reperfusion injury in rats: therapeutic time window and its mechanism. Thromb Res, 2009, 23 (5): 727-730.

[28] Xiao X, Liu Y, Qi C, et al. Neuroprotection and enhanced neurogenesis by tetramethylpyrazine in adult rat brain after focal ischemia. Neurol Res, 2010, 32 (5): 547-555.

[29] Tian Y, Liu Y, Chen X, et al. Tetramethylpyrazine promotes proliferation and differentiation of neural stem cells from rat brain in hypoxic condition via mitogen-activated protein kinases pathway in vitro. Neurosci Lett, 2010, 474 (1): 26-31.

[30] Liu HT, Du YG, He JL, et al. Tetramethylpyrazine inhibits production of nitric oxide and inducible nitric oxide synthase in lipopolysaccharide-induced N9 microglial cells through blockade of MAPK and PI3K/Akt signaling pathways, and suppression of intracellular reactive oxygen species. J Ethnopharmacol, 2010, 129 (3): 335-343.

[31] Tan Z. Erratum: neural protection by naturopathic compounds——an example of tetramethylpyrazine from retina to brain. J Ocul Biol Dis Infor, 2009, 2 (3): 137-144.

[32] Shao Z, Li J, Zhao Z, et al. Effects of tetramethylpyrazine on nitric oxide/cGMP signaling after cerebral vasospasm in rabbits. Brain Res, 2010, 1361: 67-75.

[33] 陈可冀主编. 川芎嗪的化学、药理与临床应用. 北京: 人民卫生出版社, 1999: 56-58.

[34] 盛日正, 李家明, 张飞龙, 等. 新型川芎嗪阿魏酸衍

生物的合成及其抗血小板聚集活性. 合成化学, 2011, 19 (2): 157-161.

[35] 李家明, 赵永海, 马逢时, 等. 川芎嗪芳酸醚类衍生物的合成及抗血小板聚集活性. 有机化学, 2008, 28 (9): 1578 -1583.

[36] 陈立娟, 冯毅, 丁澍, 等. 川芎嗪药物涂层支架预防猪冠状动脉再狭窄的实验研究. 中华心血管病杂志, 2008, 6 (9): 843-846.

[37] 刘丽梅. 川芎嗪预防冠心病患者支架术后再狭窄的临床研究. 中国现代药物应用, 2011, 5 (1): 111-112.

[38] 郭景源. 川芎嗪治疗不稳定型心绞痛的临床观察. 中外医学研究, 2011, 9 (10): 1532-1534.

[39] 陈可冀, 钱穆英, 管汀鹭. 川芎一号碱对冠心病患者血小板影响的电子显微镜观察. 中华内科杂志, 1976, 新1 (2): 89-91.

[40] 林求诚. 中西医结合诊疗手册. 福州: 福建科学技术出版社, 1989: 349.

[41] 陈瑶, 刘鸣. 川芎嗪治疗脑梗死: 疗效及安全性的系统评价. 2004, 8 (7): 1299-1301.

[42] 李可建. 川芎嗪注射液治疗缺血性中风急性期随机对照试验的系统评价. 时珍国医国药, 2006, 17 (10): 1874-1876.

[43] 李略, 王良兴, 董央庆, 等. 川芎嗪对慢性肺源性心脏病患者趋化因子 Fractalkine 及肿瘤坏死因子 -α 表达的影响. 中国中西医结合杂志, 2010, 30 (4): 373-375.

[44] 游红利. 卡托普利与川芎嗪联用治疗慢性充血性心力衰竭的疗效观察. 亚太传统医药, 2010, 6 (6): 75-76.

[45] 吴伟文. 川芎嗪、胞磷胆碱钠联合盐酸苯海拉明治疗眩晕综合征的临床疗效. 药物与临床, 2011, 18 (4): 51, 55.

[46] 李新生, 陈永生. 川芎嗪治疗紧张型头痛的疗效观察. 中国实用神经疾病杂志, 2010, 13 (18): 64-65.

[47] 董明霞, 李颖, 葛楠, 等. 清眩汤联合川芎嗪注射液治疗椎基底动脉供血不足的疗效观察. 北京中医药, 2011, 30 (1): 8-10.

[48] 彭湘兰. 川芎嗪注射液治疗小儿病毒性心肌炎的效果观察. 右江民族医学院学报, 2010, 3: 376-377.

[49] Chang FC, Chen KJ, Lin JG, et al. Effects of tetramethylpyrazine on portal hypertensive rats. J Pharmacy Pharmacol, 1998, 50 (8): 881-884.

[50] 李柳宁, 徐凯, 刘宇龙, 等. CT 引导经皮穿刺放射性粒子植入配合川芎嗪治疗晚期恶性肿瘤 20 例. 陕西中医, 2008, 29 (5): 542-544.

转化医学与中西医结合的研究和发展 *

蒋跃绒 陈可冀

转化医学（translational medicine），或称为转化研究（translational research），是近年来国际医学科学领域出现的新概念，通常是指打破基础医学与药物研发、临床医学之间的屏障，把基础医学研究成果快速有效地转化为疾病预防、诊断治疗及预后评估的技术、方法和药物，即"从实验台到病床，再从病床到实验台"（bench to bedside and bedside to bench，简称 B2B）的一种连续过程[1]，这一过程的实现是双向的。很多人用"连接缺口"（bridging the gap）来形容转化医学。

1. 转化医学的概念与背景

1992 年，美国《Science》杂志首次提出"Bench to Bedside"（B-to-B）的概念[2]。"转化研究"这一术语 1993 年首次出现在 PubMed，当时人们建议将实验室发现的乳腺癌易感基因（BRCA1）和其他癌基因用于癌症早期检测和治疗[3]。于是，将实验室获得的研究成果作为临床治疗参考和手段的"转化研究"应运而生。1996 年，英国《Lancet》杂志正式提出"转化医学"这一名词[4]，文章指出，可将分子生物学发现的与特定肿瘤相关的基因突变应用于临床，使患者受益。2000 年美国国家科学院医学研究院（The US Institute of Medicine）召开临床研究圆桌会议，将转化研究提上日程，之后相关论文迅速增多。2003 年 10 月，美国国立卫生研究院（NIH）主任 Elias Zerhouni 在《Science》上发表 NIH 路线图计划（The NIH Roadmap）[5]，率先提出要整合各种资源建立区域性的转化研究中心，并设立国家基金。之后，转化医学日益受到医学界的广泛关注。

当前，医学科学进入一个医疗保健费用迅速上升，人类基因组序列产生大量生物学数据，先进的高通量技术研究健康和疾病的分子网络逐步深入的革命性时期。这一独特时期为基于精确的分子知识鉴别个体疾病风险和进行干预提供了前所未有的机会[6]。一方面基础医学与临床医学、药物研发相

对自成体系，都在各自快速地扩展，相互之间缺乏足够的转化整合；另一方面随着人类基因组计划的长足进步和后基因组时代的路线图计划及其向临床医学的广泛渗透，基础研究获得的知识、成果完全有可能快速转化为临床诊断和治疗的新方法、新手段。NIH 路线图为实现这一变化提供了重要的媒介——该计划的一个重要部分是重建国家临床研究事业，这要求转化临床科学（translational clinical science）的转变和新的整合方法。转化医学可看做是后基因组时代基因组学和生物信息学革命的结果，是分子医学与宏观临床医学相结合的产物。

将研究成果转化为临床实践的过程需要克服两个障碍，第一个障碍（T1）是实验室获得的疾病机制的新理解转化为诊断、治疗和预防的新方法以及在人体的初步测试，第二个障碍（T2）是临床研究结果转化到日常临床实践和卫生决策的制定[7]。

转化医学还包含医学科学研究理念的转变。进入新世纪后，医学进入一个崭新的"3P"时代，即预测性（predictive）、预防性（preventive）和个体化（personalized）[8]，代表了医学发展的终极目标和最高阶段。新近提出的"6P"医学还包括了 Promotive、Protective、Prewarning 等健康促进和健康保护的重要内容。转化医学通过利用各种组学方法以及分子生物学数据库，筛选各种生物标志物，用于疾病危险评估、诊断与分型，进行基于分子分型的个体化治疗，治疗反应和预后评估，以及治疗方法和新药物的开发等，从而有利于推动 3P 医学的进步。

2. 转化医学的发展现状

美国 NIH 于 2006 年实施了临床和转化科学奖励计划（clinical and translational science awards，CTSA）资助转化研究，目的是整合不同学科的队伍，鼓励新的方法和信息工具，培训新的研究者。预计 2012 年将建立 60 个临床和转化科学

* 原载于《中国中西医结合杂志》，2010，30（10）：1017-1020

中心（clinical and translational science centers, CTSCs），每年资助研究经费约5亿美元[9]。现在，美国已经在38所大学（包括哈佛大学、耶鲁大学、斯坦福大学等世界名校）建立了转化医学研究中心。CTSC-s将取代临床研究中心（general clinical research centres, GCRCs），以包括基础科学家、临床医生、生物信息学家、工程师和工业专家等在内的大型多学科团体的形式，重塑基础科学和临床之间的密切联系。美国国家心肺和血液研究所（National Heart, Lung, and Blood Institute, NHLBI）在2007年完成了一项未来5～10年的科学工作战略计划，整个计划特别强调了转化研究——包括从实验室到床旁及从床旁到社区[7]。

转化研究在英国也得到了政府的大力推动[9]。2008年4月英国国家健康研究院（National Institute for Health Research, NIHR）在国家医疗服务系统和大学里建立了12个生物医学研究中心（Biomedical Research Centres, BRCs），每年资助经费达100万英镑，以促进生物医学创新发现向临床实践的转化。英国卫生部近来颁布了一项称为"最好的健康，最好的研究"的战略计划[10]，陈述了转化研究的定义，以达到病患照顾的真正改善。转化研究也可从分享患者数据库中获益。例如，在英国，NIHR提出了一项电子健康议程，为电子病历提供研究界面，使得它们能够用于临床试验、前瞻性研究和跟踪不良事件。

在亚洲，2008年新加坡国立大学依托其附属医院，也开始建立他们的第一个转化医学中心。国际出版界也先后创办了Journal of Translational Medicine、American Journal of Translational Research、Science Translational Medicine等转化医学的专业期刊。Pubmed中发表的有关转化医学的论文已达68 000余篇。转化医学越来越受到世界的关注，已经成为世界医学研究的一个新的着力点。

尽管转化医学在发达国家已初具规模，但在我国尚处于起步阶段，中国转化医学的发展仍面临体制、思路等方面的制约。目前我国在创建研究型医院、开展转化医学学术研讨和转化医学研究、成立转化医学中心等方面已进行了一些初步工作，如湘雅医院成立了中南大学转化医学研究中心，"健康中国2020"科技支撑也提出动态性、系统性转化整合战略，将建立基础、临床、预防、药物一体化的国家转化整合中心纳入新的科技支撑体系框架。但真正意义上的大型转化医学中心还属空白，需要相应的资金、人才和相关体制政策的配合。

3. 转化医学与中西医结合研发

长期以来，中医和中西医结合研究存在着先"床旁"后"实验台"、基础研究与临床应用相对脱节的状况。转化医学的兴起为中医学的发展提供了新的时代契机，将有利于中医理论的传播和新的诊疗技术的推广应用。转化医学在中西医结合研发中的应用，大致有两种模式可供借鉴：一种是从临床经验到基础研究再到临床及社区应用；另一种是从古典文献到基础研究再到临床及社区应用。

中国学者从中医治疟草药黄花蒿中分离出来的抗疟新药青蒿素，可看做是从"古典文献到基础研究再到临床应用"的转化研究范例。青蒿素的研究始于20世纪60年代中期，针对当时疟疾防治的需求，在"523"紧急军工项目系统工程的安排之下，由全国多部门、多学科、军民研究单位尽心协作、相互配合，取得了重大成果。从20世纪80年代中期起，国内又开始研制青蒿素衍生物及复方，其中蒿甲醚、青蒿琥酯和蒿甲醚-本芴醇复方得到了世界医疗卫生组织的公认，分别在1997年、2002年和2003年由世界卫生组织（WHO）先后列入了第9、11和12版基本药物目录（Essential Medicine List）[11]，是对人类的重大贡献。而上海血液学研究所关于"三氧化二砷通过直接结合PML控制癌蛋白PML-RARα的命运"[12]的研究，经历了"从临床到基础再到临床"的过程，为砷剂治疗急性早幼粒细胞性白血病提供了有力证据，也成为我国中西医结合肿瘤治疗领域转化性医学研究的典范。

目前，我国的疾病谱已从急性病转向以慢性病为主，慢性病的防治已成为重要的课题。以高血压为例，其带来的高心血管疾病风险，已成为主要的全球性健康问题。一项在中国≥40岁的169 871例具有代表性的样本中进行的前瞻性队列研究显示[13]，高血压及高血压前期与全因死亡和心血管性死亡的增加显著相关。2005年，中国233万例心血管性死亡可归因于血压升高，127万过早死亡（男性在72岁以前、女性在75岁以前死亡）可归因于血压升高。一项最新心脏性猝死流行病学调查结果显示[14]：我国心脏性猝死（SCD）发生率为41.84例/10万人。若以13亿人口推算，我国SCD总人数高达54.4万例/年，位居全球各国之首。中国SCD防治工作任务艰巨。

为了提高血压控制率，中国高血压联盟联合中国医师协会心血管内科医师分会，共同发起"中国高血压控制现状调查"（China STATUS），被认为是进行了转化医学的第一步，即了解现状，同时通过教育将指南转化为社区医生可执行的措施，将有效的疾病防治措施切实地应用于临床实践。2010年、2011年中医药行业科研专项慢性病项目建议框架也指出，对我国人民群众健康水平危害较大的慢性病，在集成既往研究成果的基础上开展技术方法、方案及制剂等的系统研究，并促进转化应用。

借鉴以往青蒿素研究从实验室走向临床应用的成功案例，参考发达国家转化医学研究的先进经验和国内慢性病转化医学研究的初步探索，中医药和中西医结合研究应以临床问题和社会需求为导向，临床疗效为重点，加强基础与临床研究的沟通与合作，实现基础研究成果到临床应用再到社区的转化。为了探索中医学和中西医结合转化研究的模式，提出下列几点建议以供讨论。

3.1 建设中医药与中西医结合转化医学研究机构

有条件的大学、研究型医院或国家中医临床研究基地应把握先机，采用加盟或联合方式进行资源整合，建立以基础、临床和药物研发为主体，结合中医古籍传承研究的跨学科中西医结合转化研究中心，吸引企业共同参与，以平台管理方式进行统一部署和联合攻关，加强团队建设，构建转化链，建立临床-基础-产业-人才一体化模式和运行机制，大力开展转化性研究模式探索，促进中医药与中西医结合转化医学研究。

3.2 加强转化医学教育和转化型人才培养

转化医学注重研究成果的临床可行性，倡导以患者为中心，从临床中发现和提出问题。长久以来，基础医学研究已逐步形成了自身规律，晋升和奖励主要基于研究者发表在顶级杂志上的论文，而不是在多大程度上促进了医学，临床医生则缺乏时间和动力去阅读复杂的基础文献，这极大地限制了知识和假说在床旁和实验室之间的转化。要改变现状，就应该加强转化医学教育，倡导临床医生同基础医学研究人员合作进行深入研究，促进科研成果快速转化到临床应用。一方面对转化医学有兴趣的临床医生积极参与基础科学研究；另一方面，涉及转化医学的基础研究人员要掌握基本的临床知识，多学科组成课题攻关小组，发挥各自优势。同时，要特别注重中医临床思维和经验的深化。

3.3 加强基础研究的科学性

实验室研究结果的真实性、可靠性及可重复性是基础研究成果进入转化的绝对前提。事实上，国内外许多已发表的基础研究类论文，被重复检查和验证的只是少数。应在加强基础研究与临床应用相互沟通、合作的基础上，继续加强基础研究，提高自主创新能力，为实现中医药和中西医结合基础研究的创新成果成功应用于临床，奠定坚实的基础。

3.4 加大资金支持和政策引导

应以足够的资金资助中医药和中西医结合转化医学研究和奖励研究成果，以增强基础研究和临床医学的沟通。政策上应重点支持有一定基础的、临床确有疗效的多学科交叉的转化性研究项目，培育新的增长点。科研成果从实验室向临床的转化过程需要很高的转化成本，且回报周期长。另外，缺乏政策支持和积极主动的参与、实验室建设与医疗单位经济效益之间存在的冲突等也是经常遇到的问题。

我国传统医学有着数千年的临床经验积累和浩瀚的医籍记载，这些宝贵的经验如通过循证医学证实临床疗效，再转入基础研究，而后再从基础到临床应用，就会获益更大。总之，中医和中西医结合转化研究的关键是从临床实际需求出发，构建基础与临床相结合的"转化平台"，从体制、资金、人才及政策导向进行整合和试点。其核心是"转化"，重点是"效率"，关键是"行动"。

参考文献

[1] Marincola FM. Translational medicine: a two-way road. J Transl Med, 2003, 1 (1): 1.

[2] Choi DW. Bench to bedside：the glutamate connection. Science, 1992, 258 (5080): 241-243.

[3] Butler D. Translational research：crossing the valley of death. Nature, 2008, 453 (7197): 840-842.

[4] geraghty J. Adenomatous polyposis coli and translational medicine. Lancet, 1996, 348 (9025): 422.

[5] Zerhouni E. Medicine. The NIH Roadmap. Science, 2003, 302 (5642): 63-72.

[6] Zerhouni EA. US biomedical research：basic, translational and clinical sciences. JAMA, 2005, 294 (11): 1352-1358.

[7] Lauer MS, Skarlatos S. Translational research for cardiovascular diseases at the National Heart, Lung,

and Blood Institute moving from bench to bedside and from bedside to community. Circulation, 2010, 121 (7): 929-933.

[8] Hudson TJ. Personalized medicine：a transformative approach is needed. Can Med Assoc J, 2009, 180 (9): 911-913.

[9] Adams JU. Building the bridge from bench to bedside. Nat Rev Drug Discov, 2008, 7 (6): 463-464.

[10] Snape K, Trembath RC, Lord GM. Translational medicine and the NIHR biomedical research centre concept. QJM, 2008, 101 (11): 901-906.

[11] 吴毓林. 青蒿素——历史和现实的启示. 化学进展,

2009，21（11）：2365-2371.

[12] Zhang XW, Yan XJ, Zhou ZR, et al. Arsenic trioxide controls the fate of the PML-RAR alpha oncoprotein by directly binding PML. Science, 2010, 328 (5975): 240-243.

[13] He J, Gu D, Chen J, et al. Premature deaths attributable to blood pressure in China：a prospective cohort study. Lancet, 2009, 374 (9703): 1765-1772.

[14] Hua W, Zhang LF, Wu YF, et al. Incidence of sudden cardiac death in China：analysis of 4 regional populations. J Am Coll Cardiol, 2009, 54 (12): 1110-1118.

波动性高血糖与心血管并发症的关系 [*]

夏城东　殷惠军　陈可冀

1. 糖尿病与心血管疾病

心血管疾病（cardiovascular disease, CVD）的发生（尤其是加速发展的动脉粥样硬化）是糖尿病患者高致残率和死亡率的主要原因。与无糖尿病的人群相比，男性糖尿病患者的 CVD 危险升高 2～3 倍，女性糖尿病患者升高 3～5 倍，高血糖与 CVD 密切相关。糖化血红蛋白（HbA_{1c}）每升高 1%，1 型和 2 型糖尿病（DM）患者的 CVD 相对危险性分别增加 15% 和 18%[1,2]。糖尿病控制和并发症试验（The Diabetes Complications and Control Trial, CCT）确立了 HbA_{1c} 作为糖尿病血糖控制的金标准。$HbA_{1c} \leq 7\%$ 被认为是减少血管并发症的合适水平，然而在强化治疗组和常规治疗组 HbA_{1c} 没有明显差别，可是随着时间的进展后者的视网膜病变进展却更加明显，说明可能除了 HbA_{1c} 外，血糖的变异性对糖尿病长期并发症的发展也至关重要[3]。糖尿病慢性并发症的发生、发展不仅与血糖整体水平升高有关，而且与血糖的波动性也有密切关系，血糖稳态受损（impaired glucose homeostasis）可能是发生 CVD 的主要危险因素之一。DECODE 研究（Diabetes Epidemiology：Collaborative Analysis Of Diagnostic Criteria in Europe） 和心脏健康 Framingham 后续研究（Cardiovascular Health Study and the Framingham Offspring Study）均表明餐后高血糖是糖尿病患者心血管事件发生与死亡的独立预测因素[4]。餐后 2h 血糖增高的非糖尿病人群的 CVD 死亡率是血糖正常人群的 2 倍，无论是否确诊糖尿病，餐后高血糖都是危险因素[5]。血糖的控制指标不仅应包含 HbA_{1c}、空腹血糖、餐后 2h 血糖，还应包含血糖的波动幅度[6]。

2. 糖尿病与内皮功能异常

血管内皮功能异常是动脉粥样硬化的始动环节，也是糖尿病血管病变的病理生理基础。大量的体内外研究证实，高血糖能损伤多种血管功能，培养的内皮细胞暴露于高浓度葡萄糖介质，与正常葡萄糖介质相比，单核细胞结合增多，内皮素-1 产生增加，细胞间通透性增高，内皮型一氧化氮合成酶表达减少。在高糖状态下，一些内皮细胞的主要功能，如血管舒缩功能、凝血和纤溶功能、血管通透性、血管形成等可能都会发生改变[7]。高血糖可致多元醇通路激活，竞争性消耗 NADPH，细胞内氧化还原状态改变；通过糖酵解增加葡萄糖代谢，引起二酰甘油从头合成增加，增加蛋白激酶 C

* 原载于《心血管病学进展》，2009，30（1）：99-101

（protein kinase C，PKC）亚型在细胞膜上的易位和活化，增加由 NADPH 氧化酶介导的氧自由基生成，增多的氧化产物通过影响氧化还原反应敏感的信号途径和降低一氧化氮生物利用度来影响内皮功能，通过磷酸化细胞靶点调节细胞生长、迁移、收缩、基因表达和代谢；高血糖还能在蛋白质与脂质的伯铵与葡萄糖之间形成希夫碱而增加非酶糖基化，通过糖基化终末产物（AGE）及其内皮特殊受体（RAGE）的相互作用，介导氧自由基生成增加，激活多种细胞因子如核因子 κB 等，引起血管功能异常；高血糖通过线粒体电子传递链介导的超氧化物增多，活性氧产生增加，致使脂质、蛋白质、氨基酸及 DNA 发生氧化性损伤，参与多种途径激活导致内皮损伤[8]。

3. 波动性高血糖与内皮功能异常

波动性高血糖损伤血管内皮细胞的机制至今尚未阐明。目前认为，血糖波动通过不同代谢途径产生的活性氧（reactive oxygen species，ROS），可诱导细胞内氧化应激反应，使对氧化应激敏感的核因子 κB 等多种细胞因子激活，通过启动和调节一些炎性因子如化学趋化因子、金属蛋白酶、黏附分子等的基因转录，介导血管内皮的损伤，导致血管收缩、白细胞黏附、血小板激活，发生有丝分裂、血栓形成、血管炎症，最终加速动脉粥样硬化的发展。Monnier 等[9]发现，平均 24h 尿游离 8-异前列腺素 F2α（8-iso prostaglandin F2α，8-iso PGF2α）排泄率在糖尿病患者中显著增加，平均血糖波动幅度（mean amplitude of glycemic excursions，MAGE）、餐后血糖波动（应用餐后与餐前血糖增量曲线下面积描述）[mean postprandial in cremental area under the curve（AUCpp）]与尿 8-iso PGF2α 有显著关系，说明餐后期间或者更广泛的血糖波动比慢性持续高血糖更能加强氧化应激。对 SD 大鼠注射葡萄糖 30min 后血糖升高，单核细胞对胸主动脉内皮细胞的黏附数增加，120min 后才恢复正常，同时血糖也回至正常，注射奥曲肽抑制内源性胰岛素分泌并不能阻止这种效应，说明暂时性血糖升高能够导致单核细胞对胸主动脉内皮细胞的黏附数增加[10]。Watada[11]应用链脲菌素（streptozotocin，STZ）诱导糖尿病模型大鼠每日两次喂食造成餐后高血糖，与随意喂食的模型大鼠比较，虽然前者有较低的 HbA$_{1c}$，却有更加显著的单核细胞对胸主动脉的

黏附数目。活体实验说明餐后高血糖促进单核细胞对内皮细胞的黏附比稳定性高血糖严重。Mita 等[12]应用每日两次喂食 apo-E 基因缺陷大鼠麦芽糖诱导餐后高血糖，喂食 1 周后巨噬细胞对胸主动脉内皮细胞的黏附数目增加，5 周后动脉硬化损伤面积增加，同时应用米格列醇可以阻止这种变化。显示血糖的波动性可以加速动脉硬化，并不依赖于血浆胆固醇水平的变化。Quagliaro 等[13]在培养人脐静脉内皮细胞（human umbilical vein endothelial cells，HUVEC）时，分别给予正常葡萄糖浓度（5mmol/L）、稳定高糖浓度（20mmol/L）和波动性糖浓度（5mmol/L 和 20mmol/L 每 24h 交替）的培养环境，2 周后发现在稳定性高血糖，细胞间黏附分子 -1（intercellular adhesionmolecule-1，ICAM-1）、血管细胞黏附分子 -1（vascular cell adhesion molecule-1，VCAM-1）和 E- 选择素含量和 mRNA 表达增加，在间断性高血糖这种效应更加明显，相比稳定性高血糖，波动性高血糖 PKC 活性增加，PKCβ Ⅰ、β Ⅱ、δ 亚型高表达，应用 PKC 抑制剂 BIM Ⅰ -I（bisindolyl maleimide- Ⅰ）和特异性 PKCβ 抑制剂 LY379196 可以减少 ICAM-1、VCAM-1 和 E- 选择素的表达，8-OH dG（8-Hydroxydeoxyguanosine）（一种对 DNA 氧化损伤的指示剂）也同样被观察到类似现象，加入线粒体复合物 Ⅱ 抑制剂噻吩甲酰三氟丙酮（thenoyltrifluoroacetone，TTFA）和超氧化物歧化酶（SOD）类似物 MnTBAP[Mn（Ⅲ）tetrakis（4-benzoic acid）porphyrin chloride]，所有的黏附分子、PKC 亚型表达和 8-OH dG 都正常化。说明间断性高血糖比稳定性高血糖有更强的黏附分子表达，与 PKCβ 激活有关，但这种效应完全依赖于线粒体自由基的过表达。采用类似的实验设计，还发现间断性高血糖激活多聚 ADP 核糖聚合酶（poly ADP ribose polymerase，PARP），加速黏附分子表达和炎症反应，促进硝基酪氨酸合成，诱导细胞间黏附分子和白介素 -6 表达[14]。Piconi 等[15]通过观察细胞内硝基酪氨酸和 8-OH dG 的变化，检测 Bcl-2 和细胞凋亡蛋白酶 3（caspase-3）表达和活性发现，持续性和间断性高血糖通过线粒体转运链 ROS 的大量合成，增强氧化应激，诱导内皮细胞凋亡。

4. 波动性高血糖的临床评价与治疗

过去血糖控制的评价以 HbA$_{1c}$ 为唯一金标准，

随着对血糖波动性的逐渐认识，近年来不断完善的动态血糖检测技术也为精确评估血糖稳定性提供了条件。该技术评估日内和日间血糖的波动程度，同时还包括针对餐后血糖反应进行评估。主要评估参数有：血糖水平的标准差、最大血糖波动幅度、平均血糖波动幅度、M 值、低血糖指数、空腹血糖变异系数、日间血糖平均绝对差、餐后血糖峰值与达峰时间，及餐后血糖波动的幅度、时间与曲线下面积增值等[16,17]。

糖尿病患者血糖波动过大的主要原因与未经合理控制的餐后高血糖和治疗不当导致的低血糖有密切关系，减少血糖波动的主要策略有两种：其一，调节葡萄糖从肠道吸收和进入血液循环的速度，通过改变饮食结构，兼顾总热量控制与葡萄糖指数的合理性，或者应用 α- 糖苷酶抑制剂通过竞争性抑制小肠上皮细胞表面的 α- 糖苷酶活性，延缓葡萄糖的消化吸收，降低餐后血糖，减少血糖波动；其二，调节恢复胰岛素的合理利用与分泌，应用人胰岛素类似物甘精胰岛素与速效胰岛素（赖脯胰岛素、天门冬氨酸胰岛素）提供缓慢持续释放的基础量和进餐时的快速利用胰岛素，平稳控制血糖；或者应用格列奈类胰岛素促泌剂通过快速阻断 ATP 敏感的钾通道，增加胰岛内源性 β 细胞分泌胰岛素，吸收迅速，起效快，持续时间短，与促胰岛素分泌的受体快速结合与解离，更快刺激胰岛素第一时相分泌胰岛素，降低餐后血糖[18,19]。

5. 结 语

虽然英国前瞻性糖尿病研究（United Kingdom prospective diabetes study, UKPDS）和 DCCT 回答了控制血糖的疑问，但正如对高血压动态血压监测的认识深入一样，对糖尿病血糖波动性的认识也必将随着动态血糖检测技术的发展而进一步深入，如何开展血糖波动性的评价及其对糖尿病本身和并发症的影响研究，如何从流行病学、治疗学和基础研究等方面进行深入的研究可能是未来方向之一，对血糖波动的正确认识、评价和治疗可能对糖尿病合并心血管并发症的研究具有重要意义。

参考文献

[1] Rydn L, Standl E, Bartnik M, et al. Guidelines on diabetes, pre-diabetes, and cardiovascular diseases：executive summary. The Task Force on Diabetes and Cardiovascular Diseases of the European Society of Cardiology (ESC) and of the European Association for the Study of Diabetes (EASD) . Eur Heart J, 2007, 28 (1): 88-136.

[2] Buse JB, Ginsberg HN, BakrisgL, et al. Primary prevention of cardiovascular diseases in people with diabete smellitus：a scientific statement from the American Heart Association and the American Diabetes Association. Circulation, 2007, 115 (1): 114-126.

[3] Hirsch IB, Brownlee M. Should minimal blood glucose variability become the gold standard of glycemic control? J Diabetes Complications, 2005, 19 (3): 178-181.

[4] Gao W, Qiao Q, Tuomilehto J. Post-challenge hyperglycaemia rather than fasting hyperglycaemia is an independent risk factor of cardiovascular disease events. Clin Lab, 2004, 50 (9-10): 609-615.

[5] Ceriello A, Davidson J, Hanefeld M, et al. Postprandial hyperglycaemia and cardiovascular complications of diabetes：an update. Nutr Metab Cardiovasc Dis, 2006, 16 (7): 453-456.

[6] Monnier L, Colette C, Boegner C, et al. Continuous glucose monitoring in patients with type 2 diabetes：Why? When? Whom? Diabetes Metab, 2007, 33 (4): 247-452.

[7] Cersosimo E, DeFronzo RA. Insulin resistance and endothelial dysfunction：the road map to cardiovascular diseases. Diabetes Metab Res Rev, 2006, 22 (6): 423-436.

[8] Kim JA, Montagnani M, Koh KK, et al. Reciprocal relationships between insulin resistance and endothelial dysfunction: molecular and pathophysiological mechanisms. Circulation, 2006, 113 (15): 1888-1904.

[9] Monnier L, Mas E, Ginet C, et al. Activation of oxidative stress by acute glucose fluctuations compared with sustained chronic hyperglycemia in patients with type 2 diabetes. JAMA, 2006, 295 (14): 1681-1687.

[10] Otsuka A, Azuma K, Lesaki T, et al. Temporary hyperglycaemia provokes monocyte adhesion to endothelial cells in rat thoracic aorta. Diabetologia, 2005, 48 (12): 2667-2674.

[11] Watada H, Azuma K, Kawamori R. Glucose fluctuateon on the progression of diabetic macroangiopathy——new findings from monocyte adhesion to endothelial cells. Diabetes Res Clin Pract, 2007, 77 (suppl1): S58-61.

[12] Mita T, Otsuka A, Azuma K, et al. Swings in blood glucose levels accelerate atherogenesis in

第七章

apolipoprote in E-deficient mice. Biochem Biophys Res Commun, 2007, 358 (3): 679-685.

[13] Quagliaro L, Piconi L, Assaloni R, et al. Intermittent high glucose enhances ICAM-1, VCAM-1 and E-selectin expression in human umbilical vein endothelial cells in culture: the distinct role of prote in kinase C and mitochondrial superoxide production. Atherosclerosis, 2005, 183 (2): 259-267.

[14] Piconi L, Quagliaro L, Da Ros R, et al. Intermittent high glucose enhances ICAM-1, VCAM-1, E-selectin and interleuk in-6 expression in human umbilical endothelial cells in culture: the role of poly (ADP-ribose) polymerase. J Thromb Haemost, 2004, 2 (8): 1453-1459.

[15] Piconi L, Quagliaro L, Assaloni R, et al. Constant and intermittent high glucose enhances endothelial cell apoptosis through mitochondrial superoxide overproduction. Diabetes Metab Res Rev, 2006, 22 (3): 198-203.

[16] Kovatchev BP, Clarke WL, Breton M, et al. Quantifying temporal glucose variability in diabetes via continuous glucose monitoring: mathematical methods and clinical application. Diabetes Technol Ther, 2005, 7 (6): 849-862.

[17] Mc Donnell CM, Donath SM, Vidmar SI, et al. A novel approach to continuous glucose analysis utilizing glycemic variation. Diabetes Technol Ther, 2005, 7 (2): 253-263.

[18] Gerich JE, Odawara M, Terauchi Y. The rationale for paired pre- and postprandial self-monitoring of blood glucose: the role of glycemic variability in micro and macro vascular risk. Curr Med Res Opin, 2007, 23 (8): 1791-1798.

[19] Carroll MF, Izard A, Riboni K, et al. Control of postprandial hypergly cemia: optimal use of short-acting insulin secretagogues. Diabetes Care, 2002, 25 (12): 2147-2152.

Atherosclerosis: An Integrative East-West Medicine Perspective[*]

XU Hao   SHI Da-zhuo   CHEN Ke-ji

1. Introduction

Atherosclerosis (AS) is the most common type of arteriosclerosis. It mainly involves the large and middle muscular arteries, especially aorta, coronary and cerebral arteries, which often leads to serious outcomes such as sudden cardiac death, unstable angina pectoris, acute myocardial infarction, stroke, and intermittent claudication due to vessel obliteration or plaque rupture and subsequent thrombosis. In the beginning of the 21st century, we are facing serious challenges of cardiovascular disease (CVD). Although it is becoming less lethal, CVD prevalence is incessantly increasing, and it is still the most common cause of death. How to prevent AS and reduce the incidence and mortality of CVD have been one of the most important health-related issues all the time.

However, biomedicine is at its limits nowadays when confronting degenerative diseases, stress-related diseases, and most chronic diseases. It lacks reference to the self-healing capacity of the human mind and body and focuses on parts rather than the whole, treatment rather than prevention, the suffering disease rather than the diseased person. Confronted with these problems, more and more farsighted Western scholars began to lay their eyes on

* 原载于 Evidence-Based Complementary and Alternative Medicine, 2012, Article ID 148413

traditional Chinese medicine (TCM) [1-3]. Drugs with Chinese herbal medicines as raw materials are increasingly favored by people all over the world for their unique advantages in preventing and curing diseases, rehabilitation, and health care. The benefit of TCM in CVD was also demonstrated in several multicenter clinical trials in recent years [4-7]. More importantly, the unique theory of TCM might also have some implications for the renewal of thinking in fighting against CVD [8]. Therefore, we reviewed traditional understanding and shifted concepts on AS pathophysiology along the track of previous studies and read these transitions taking full advantage of TCM theory together with our experimental and clinical studies in recent years, so as to provide an integrative East-West medicine perspective for future AS prevention and treatment.

2. Updated Concept of Atherosclerosis

2.1 From Emphasizing "Luminal Stenosis" to Highlighting "Vulnerable Plaques"

With the deep understanding and active control of AS risk factors, dramatic advances have been made in primary prevention of chronic cardiovascular diseases since 1990s. However, there is still lack of effective measure to prevent acute cardiovascular events (ACEs), which cause 20 million deaths worldwide per year. Most of the victims die suddenly without any prior symptoms.

The previous studies focused on the severity of coronary stenosis, taking coronary heart disease (CHD) as an example of AS, and highlighted detection of severe luminal stenosis and subsequent treatment of percutaneous coronary intervention (PCI). The development or improvement of coronary stenosis is also regarded as an important indicator to evaluate the state of illness or therapeutic effect. However, angiographic studies on patients before myocardial infarction showed that the majority of subsequent events involved sites with less than 70% obstruction. It indicated that the severity of

stenosis was not the main cause of ACEs [9].

In 1989, Muller and his colleagues used the word "vulnerable" to describe rupture-prone plaques, with characteristics of a large lipid pool, a thin cap, and macrophage-dense inflammation on or beneath its surface [10], as the underlying cause of most clinical coronary events. More and more studies suggested that ACEs were triggered by thrombosis associated with rupture of vulnerable atherosclerotic plaques [11]. The change of plaque from its stable state to an unstable one was not related to the plaque size, quantity, or position or the severity of stenosis. Although PCI improves significant stenosis, it cannot influence the biological course of vulnerable plaque, thus the problem of "unstable" plaque is still unresolved.

In recent years, many clinical trials showed that statins could reduce ACEs significantly yet only improve the luminal size slightly [12]. Experimental researches have proved that statins have potential effects on stability of AS plaques [13]. Stenting (including drug-eluting stents) reduces restenosis and repeated intervention, but does not reduce mortality or myocardial infarction [14]. Therefore, it is necessary for us to reevaluate the benefits of active medicinal treatment and invasive PCI treatment in chronic myocardial ischemia. Based on in-depth understanding of AS pathogenesis, the vascular pathophysiological research has turned to new direction of stabilizing vulnerable plaque and inhibiting thrombosis after plaques rupture. The secondary prevention of CHD also focused on intervention of vulnerable plaque instead of treating luminal stenosis of coronary artery [15,16].

2.2 From Predominant Theory of "Lipid Deposit" to General Acknowledgment of "Inflammatory Reaction" Theory

"Lipids deposit" theory of AS has been put forward for over 100 years based on the causal relation between hyperlipidemia and AS [17]. This theory holds that lipids deposition on the artery wall leads to the AS plaques and has played a very important role in AS pathogenesis for a long period.

In recent years, some researches indicated that AS had the basic manifestation of inflammation: degeneration, exudation, and proliferation. The cell-cell interaction is similar to other chronic inflammation diseases such as rheumatoid arthritis, chronic pancreatitis, and hepatic cirrhosis. With continuous detection of inflammatory cells and mediators, AS was no longer regarded as a simple disease of lipid deposition on vessel wall but also an advancing inflammatory reaction. Recent advances in basic science have established a fundamental role for inflammation in mediating all stages of this diseases from initiation through progression and, ultimately, the thrombotic complications of AS.

In 1999, based on his famous "injury reaction" theory, Ross declared that AS is one of the inflammatory disease [18]. AS is a process of active inflammatory reaction inside the vessel wall rather than a process of passive lipid deposit onto the vessel wall. This theory initiates a new epoch of AS treatment and it leads to deep understanding of cardiovascular diseases: inflammation fuels the development and progression of atherosclerosis as well as causes certain plaques to rupture and subsequent thrombosis, leading to such atherosclerotic complications as heart attack and stroke. High-sensitivity C-reactive protein (hs-CRP) and other blood inflammatory markers may be useful in the estimation of prognosis, risk level in AS patients, and even be a potential target of AS treatment and prevention [19]. Despite regulating blood lipids metabolism, statins should be recommended for their anti-inflammation and other protective effects on cardiovascular diseases. Aspirin can not only inhibit platelet aggregation but also prevent the malfunction of endothelial cells through its anti-inflammation effects [16]. Anti-inflammation has been one of the most important issues of AS research and several strategies that intervene

with inflammation reaction are under study.

2.3 New Concept from "Vulnerable Plaque" to "Vulnerable Patient"

Plaque rupture is the most common type of plaque complication, accounting for nearly 70% of fatal acute myocardial infarctions and/or sudden coronary deaths. Vulnerable plaque is the main, but not the unique, cause for ACEs. The position of plaque rupture, the size and amount of plaques, coronary spasm, hypercoagulable state, collateral circulation, and the degree of myocardial damage should also be considered. In 2003, an article named "From vulnerable plaque to vulnerable patient: a call for new definitions and risk assessment strategies" was published on Circulation written by over fifty of the most famous cardiovascular experts of the world [20,21]. The new concept of "vulnerable plaque" to "vulnerable patients" has led in a new direction to the prevention of ACEs.

The term "vulnerable patient" is proposed to define subjects susceptible to an acute coronary syndrome or sudden cardiac death based on plaque, blood, or myocardial vulnerability (1-year risk ≥ 5%). Extensive efforts are needed to quantify an individual's risk of an event according to each component of vulnerability (plaque, blood, and myocardium). Such a comprehensive risk-stratification tool capable of predicting acute coronary syndromes as well as sudden cardiac death would be very useful for preventive cardiology. The new concept of "vulnerable plaque" to "vulnerable patients" stresses evaluating patients as a whole and thus further optimizes overall assessment of cardiovascular risks, and prevents ACEs by early intervention of vulnerable patients.

3. An Integrative East-West Medicine Perspective for Future AS Management

The transitions in understanding AS, from local plaques to entire coronary tree and patient as a whole, from passive lipid deposit process to an active inflammatory reaction and cell interaction process, innovate strategies of prevention and treatment for AS and CHD from coronary stenosis-targeted invasive PCI treatment to vulnerable patient-targeted comprehensive assessment, early-detection and preventive medication strategies, happen to mirror "holism concept" "living in harmony with the environment" "preventive treatment of disease" and "treatment based on syndrome differentiation or pattern diagnosis" advocated by TCM. They can also help us fully understand the two different medical systems, Western medicine (WM) and TCM, as well as make the best of the advantages of both of them.

The previous researches have shown that Chinese medicines of activating blood circulation (ABC) could treat AS by multiple ways such as lowering blood lipid, inhibiting platelet adhesion and aggregation, and improving blood viscosity and inhibiting SMC proliferation. In 2003, based on AS models of ApoE-deficient mice, we studied the effects of six ABC herbs (Radix Salviae Miltiorrhizae, Radix Paeoniae Rubra, Rhizoma Chuanxiong, Radix Notoginseng, Semen Persicae, Wine steamed Radix, and Rhizoma Rhei) and a compound preparation (consisting of Chuanxingol and Paeoniflorin) on stabilizing AS plaque and their potential mechanisms. The results indicated that most ABC herbs showed multiple effects on different links of AS, such as regulating blood lipids, influencing collagen metabolism, and anti-inflammatory reaction, thus had potential effect on stabilizing AS plaque [22,23]. Although the final effect of ABC herbs on stabilizing plaque was slightly less than that of simvastatin, they showed better effects on certain links such as increasing high-density lipoprotein cholesterol (HDL-C), which exhibited the superiorities of Chinese medicine in overall regulation by influencing multiple targets [8]. The superior effect of the compound preparation to either herbal extractive component [24] indicated the synergetic effect based on TCM compatibility theory. Therefore, Chinese herbal medicines, especially compound prescriptions, warrant further investigation and might be an complementary or alternative therapy to statins in stabilizing vulnerable plaque through a synergistic and multitargeted effect.

The new concept of "vulnerable patient" also provides TCM with new opportunity in detecting high-risk CHD patients and further reducing ACEs by early intervention. Under the guidance of TCM holism concept and thought of treatment based on syndrome differentiation, we conducted a multicenter cohort study, enrolling stable CHD patients and documenting one-year follow-up cardiovascular endpoint events. Prognosis-related factors, including past medical history, symptoms, body signs, biochemical indicators, and tongue manifestations, were identified to establish an integrative risk-assessment system for detecting high-risk CHD patients [25-27]. A large-scale randomized controlled trial aiming at early intervening high-risk CHD patients based on this integrative risk assessment system is about to start soon. Given the convergence of both the East and the West conceptualization of AS, it is hopeful that this integrative East-West strategy will facilitate early detection and more effective treatment for the vulnerable patients with CHD and other AS-related diseases.

References

[1] Dobos G, Tao I. The model of Western integrative medicine: the role of Chinese medicine. Chinese Journal of Integrative Medicine, 2011, 17 (1): 11-20.

[2] Robinson N. Integrative medicine-traditional Chinese medicine, a model. Chinese Journal of Integrative Medicine, 2011, 17 (1): 21-25.

[3] Xu H, Chen KJ. Integrating traditional medicine with biomedicine towards a patient-centered healthcare system. Chinese Journal of Integrative Medicine, 2011, 17 (2): 83-84.

[4] Chen KJ, Shi DZ, Xu H,et al. XS0601 reduces the incidence of restenosis: a prospective study of 335 patients undergoing percutaneous coronary intervention in China. Chinese Medical Journal, 2006, 119 (1): 6-13.

[5] Shang QH, Xu H, Lu XH, et al. A multi-center randomized double-blind placebo controlled trial of Xiongshao Capsule in preventing restenosis after percutaneous coronary intervention: a subgroup analysis of senile patients. Chinese journal of integrative medicine, 2011, 17 (9): 669-674.

[6] Gao ZY, Xu H, Shi DZ, et al. Analysis on outcome of 5284 patients with coronary artery disease: the role of integrative medicine. Journal of Ethnopharmacology. In press.

[7] Lu Z, Kou W, Du B,et al. Effect of Xuezhikang, an extract from red yeast Chinese rice, on coronary events in a Chinese population with previous myocardial infarction. American Journal of Cardiology, 2008, 101 (12): 1689-1693.

[8] Wen C, Xu H, The new strategy for modulating dyslipidemia:consideration from updated understanding on highdensity lipoprotein. Chinese Journal of Integrative Medicine, 2011,17 (6) 467-470.

[9] Smith SC. Risk-reduction therapy: the challenge to change. Circulation, 1996, 93 (12): 2205-2211.

[10]Muller JE, Tofler GH, Stone PH. Circadian variation and triggers of onset of acute cardiovascular disease. Circulation, 1989, 79 (4): 733-743.

[11] Conti CR. Updated pathophysiologic concepts in unstable coronary artery disease. American Heart Journal, 2001, 141 (2): S12-S14.

[12] Dupuis J. Mechanisms of acute coronary syndromes and the potential role of statins. Atherosclerosis Supplements, 2001, 2 (1): 9-14.

[13] Koh KK. Effects of statins on vascular wall: vasomotor function, inflammation, and plaque stability. Cardiovascular Research, 2000, 47 (4): 648-657.

[14] Serruys PW, Kutryk MJB, Ong ATL. Coronary artery stents. New England Journal of Medicine, 2006, 354 (5): 483-495.

[15] Kullo IK, Edwards WD, Schwartz RS. Vulnerable plaque: pathobiology and clinical implications. Annals of Internal Medicine, 1998, 129 (12): 1050-1060.

[16]Ozer K, Cilingiroglu M. Vulnerable plaque: definition,detection, treatment, and future implications. Current Atherosclerosis Reports, 2005, 7 (2): 121-126.

[17] Steinberg D, Joseph L, Witztum JL. Lipoproteins and atherogenesis. Current concepts. Journal of the American Medical Association, 1990, 264 (23): 3047-3052.

[18] Ross R. Atherosclerosis—an inflammatory disease. New England Journal ofMedicine, 1999, 340 (2) 115-126.

[19] Wilson AM, Ryan MC, Boyle AJ. The novel role of C-reactive protein in cardiovascular disease: risk marker or pathogen. International Journal of Cardiology, 2006, 106 (3): 291-297.

[20]Naghavi M, Libby P, Falk E ,et al. From vulnerable plaque to vulnerable patient: a call for new definitions and risk assessment strategies: Part Ⅰ. Circulation, 2003, 108, (14): 1664-1672.

[21]Naghavi M, Libby P, Falk E,et al. From vulnerable plaque to vulnerable patient: a call for new definitions and risk assessment strategies: part Ⅱ. Circulation,2003, 108 (15), 1772-1778.

[22] Wen C, Xu H, Huang QF. Effect of drugs for promoting blood circulation on blood lipids and inflammatory reaction of atherosclerotic plaques in ApoE gene deficiency mice. Chinese Journal of Integrated Traditional and Western Medicine, 2005, 25 (4): 345-349, 2005.

[23] Wen C, Xu H, Huang QF. Effects of herbs for promoting blood circulation and Xiongshao Capsule on collagen deposition and metabolism of atherosclerotic plaques in ApoE gene deficient mice. Chinese Journal of Pathophysiology, 2005, 21 (8): 1640.

[24] Xu H, Wen C, Chen KJ. Study on the effect of rhizoma Chuanxiong, radix paeoniae rubra and the compound of their active ingredients, Xiongshao Capsule,on stability of atherosclerotic plaque in ApoE (-/-) mice. Chinese Journal of Integrated Traditional and Western Medicine, 2007, 27 (6): 513-518.

[25]Xu H, Qu D, Zheng F,et al. Clinical manifestations of "blood-stasis and toxin" in patients with stable coronary heart disease. Chinese Journal of Integrated Traditional and Western Medicine, 2010, 30 (2): 125-129.

[26] Feng Y, Xu H, Qu D, et al. Study on the tongue manifestations for the blood-stasis and toxin syndrome in the stable patients of coronary heart disease. Chinese Journal of Integrative Medicine, 2011, 17 (5): 333-338.

[27] Chen KJ, Shi DZ, Xu H, et al. The criterion of syndrome differentiation and quantification for stable coronary heart disease caused by etiological toxin of Chinese medicine. Chinese Journal of Integrated Traditional and Western Medicine, 2011, 31 (3): 313-314.

第七章

Atherosclerosis, Vascular Aging and Therapeutic Strategies*

LIU Yue   CHEN Ke-ji

Lifespan is the maximum amount of time an organism has been observed to survive from birth to death. It is typically measured by age. The maximum lifespan in humans is believed to be between 100 to 120 years. Of the recognized factors that affect health and lifespan, personal health and heredity only account for 15% of lifespan, while factors such as social economic environment, life style, mental state and access to medical care account for 60%. Unlike premature aging and lifespan shortening caused by genetic diseases such as Werner syndrome and Hutchinson-Gilford progeria syndrome, where no treatment is currently available, diseases that are significantly influenced by lifestyle, such as coronary artery disease and type II diabetes mellitus, have a much brighter outlook in terms of disease prevention and disease control.

1. Cardiovascular Diseases and Atherosclerosis

Cardiovaslular diseases (CVD) is the number one killer in China with annual deaths of more than 3,000,000 from 1990 to 2010[1]. China also has a high incidence of sudden cardiac death (SCD). A survey across four major regions in China（Beijing, Guangzhou, Kelamayi, and Yuxian）showed a SCD incidence of 41.8 per 100,000 per year[2]. This would translate to an estimated annual incidence of 500,000 SCD in China based on a population of 1.33 billion. China is also one of the countries with more prevalent ischemic stroke with an incidence well above that of the developed countries. At the same time, the age-adjusted prevalence of total diabetes and pre-diabetes are 9.7% and 15.5%，respectively, accounting for 92.4 million adult Chinese with diabetes and 148.2 million with pre-diabetes[3]. Diabetes is recognized as a major risk factor for CVD and those diagnosed with diabetes or pre-diabetes will contributed to the prevalence of CVD in the next 10-20 years.

Atherosclerosis is the common pathological mechanism of coronary artery diseases, stroke, and peripheral vascular disease, and it mostly affects the medium and large arteries. The elasticity and flexibility of healthy arteries are fundamental to the delivery of oxygen and nutrients to the body. Over time, however, the thickening of arterial walls and stiffness of arteries may occur and may sometimes restrict blood supply to organs and tissues. This process is called arteriosclerosis, or hardening of the arteries. Atherosclerosis occurs when fat, cholesterol and other substances build up inside the arteries and leads to the formation of plaques, narrowing of the lumen, hardening of the arterial walls and ultimately blockade of the blood flow. Clinically, occlusion of the coronary arteries due to atherosclerosis manifests as chest pain, shortness of breath, and other serious symptoms indicating the acute onset of cardiovascular events[4]. Atherosclerotic plaques are classified into stable and unstable (also called vulnerable) plaques. Stable atherosclerotic plaques, which tend to be asymptomatic, are rich in extracellular matrix and smooth muscle cells. Unstable or vulnerable plaques are rich in macrophages and foam cells and the fibrous cap separated from the

---

* 原载于 Chinese Journal of Integrative Medicine, 2012，18（2）：83-87

wall by a large lipid pool is particularly unstable and prone to rupture. Ruptured plaques induce thrombus formation and thromboembolism, both lead to cardiocelebrovascular events.

2. From Treating Risk Factors to Treating Arteries

CVD is typically preventable and controllable. The Framingham Heart Study was the first prospective study with the objective of identifying the common risk factors or characteristics that contribute to CVD by following its development over a long period of time in a large group of participants who had not yet developed overt symptoms of CVD or suffered from a heart attack or stroke[5]. A risk factor is defined as a measurable characteristic that is causally associated with increased disease frequency and is a significant independent predictor of an increased risk presenting with the disease[6]. Risk factors are either modifiable (e.g., obesity, hypertension, dyslipidemia and smoking) or unmodifiable (e.g., age, gender, race and family history). In the past 50 years, active control of the risk factors has been the focus of CVD prevention and treatment. Both Finland and USA that were once high CVD risk countries have demonstrated a sharp decrease in CVD incidence in recent years, indicating the essential role of primary CVD prevention[7,8]. Experiences from other countries have also consistently confirmed that the risk factor control could dramatically cut down the mortality of coronary disease[8].

Although reduction in CVD incidence was demonstrated, the effectiveness of risk factor control has been limited. Virtually all positive randomized trials of cardiovascular prevention in high-risk patients showed relative risk reductions in the range of 9% to 30%, which means that 70% to 80% of events are not prevented by guideline-advocated therapies[9]. In a long-term, intensive, multi-factorial intervention study in diabetic subjects, only 50% of cardiovascular events were prevented during a follow-up of

14 years[10]. Efforts have been made to identify other parameters that can better predict and treat CVD. For instance, the area of carotid plaque was used in identifying and managing the high-risk vascular patients[11]. While cardiovascular events were reported in 30% of subjects with a high Framingham risk score, 70% of those with the events were in the top quartile of total plaque area (TPA)[11]. TPA strongly predicted cardiovascular risk, and that plaque progression despite treatment according to guidelines further predicted cardiovascular risk[12]. The recognition that treatment according to consensus guidelines was failing half of the patients necessitates a shift in the strategy for patient management from treating risk factors to treating arteries[9,13].

3. Atherosclerosis and Vascular Aging

Vascular aging is different from atherosclerosis. As Sir William Osler (1849-1919), a legendary physician and one of the founders of Johns Hopkins University, stated in his textbook, "A man is as old as his arteries". Vascular aging has become a focus for prevention and treatment of CVD in recent years. Vascular aging and atherosclerosis are distinct pathological processes, but are often mistakenly used interchangeably. The large- and medium-sized arteries in elderly people show varying degrees of intimal and medial changes, which are known as vascular aging or age-related intimamedial degeneration and sclerosis[14]. Clinically, the assessments of vascular aging include carotid intima-media thickness (cIMT), pulse wave velocity (PWV) and ankle-brachial index (ABI). The detrimental effect of aging on the vascular system is considered in terms of potential mechanisms involved in endothelial dysfunction and age-related atherosclerosis[15]. The cellular and molecular basis of vascular aging is unclear, but is shown to be related with oxidative stress and endothelial dysfunction[15,16], vascular inflammation[17,18], increased arterial stiffness[19], impaired angiogenesis[20], defective vascular repair[21], endothelial replicative senescence[22]and impaired endothelial progenitor cell recruitment[23]. Understanding the mechanisms underlying the age-induced vascular pathophysiological alterations[24]may shed light on therapeutic strategies for reducing cardiovascular mortality in an aging population.

4. Therapeutic Strategies to Treat Athero-sclerosis and Delay Vascular Aging

Therapeutic strategies to treat athero-sclerosis and delay vascular aging include regular exercise[25,26], caloric restriction[27], lowering cholesterol[28], anti-inflammation[29,30]and growth hormone (GH) /insulinlike growth factor-1 (IGF-1) supplementation[31].

Progress has been made in research and development of Chinese medicine (CM) for the treatment of atherosclerosis and delaying vascular aging. According to the Chinese medicine theory, qi deficiency and blood stasis are the basic characteristics in the pathogenesis of CVD. Tonifying deficiency and removing stasis are the fundamental treatment principle for selection of herbal medications. Ginseng, Notoginseng and *Ligusticum Rhizoma* are the main Chinese medicines used for anti-aging treatment and have been shown to delay vascular aging in experimental studies[32,33]. Xiongshao Capsule (芎芍胶囊, XSC) is developed from Xue Fu Zhu Yu Decoction (血府逐瘀汤), which is the classic formula used for promoting blood circulation and removing blood stasis. Clinical studies showed that XSC can effectively prevent restenosis after percutaneous coronary intervention (PCI)[34,35]. XSC was shown to enhance the protective effect of ischemic post-conditioning on rat with myocardial ischemic reperfusion injury, and this action may be related to its inhibition of MCP-1 and TNF-α expression as well as inflammatory cell infiltration[36]. XSC was also shown to stabilize atherosclerotic plaque by suppressing inflammation and the expression of FcγR Ⅲ A[37]. These findings indicate that XSC

may affect multiple molecular targets and possibly multiple signaling cascades. It is likely that these effects act together to exert clinical benefit of anti-restenosis. The study of XSC exemplifies the multi-component, multi-pathway and multiple-target characteristics of Chinese herbal medicine, and such treatment strategy may have great advantage over conventional single-target approach in treating the complex processes of atherosclerosis and vascular aging.

5. Conclusion

According to the lasted report[38], the global population is expected to hit 7 billion later in 2011. People over the age of 60 accounts for a big proportion of the toal population and the aged population is growing. Population aging is taking place globally and further acceleration of the process is anticipated for this century. Increase in longevity and decline in fertility are the two main demographic effects that result in population aging. An increase in longevity raises the average age of the population by increasing the number of surviving older people. With the extended lifespan, it is important to ensure that the growing older population living the extra years of life in a good health among other social and economic issues. Atherosclerosis and vascular aging are the key influencing factor of lifespan. Vascular aging, which proceeds atherosclerosis, marks the first sign of cardiovascular system degeneration[39]. Despite some progress in preventing atherosclerosis and vascular aging, the mechanism of pathogenesis requires further investigation and effective therapeutic interventions await to be developed. Therapeutic strategies focus on comprehensive, multi-target interventions rather than the single target therapy may hold great potential. The holistic approach and long history of human use make Chinese herbs and formulae the ideal candidates for the development of therapeutic interventions for this purpose.

References

[1] National Center for Cardiovascular Diseases of China. Report on cardiovascular diseases in China (2010). Beijing: Encyclopedia of China Publishing House, 2011: 1.

[2] Hua W, Zhang LF, Wu YF, et al. Incidence of sudden cardiac death in China: analysis of 4 regional populations. J Am Coll Cardiol, 2009, 54: 1110-1118.

[3] Yang WY, Lu JM, Weng JP, et al. Prevalence of diabetes among men and women in China. N Engl J Med, 2010, 362: 1090-1101.

[4] Fuster V. Atherosclerosis, thrombosis, and vascular biology. // Goldman L, Ausiello D, eds. Cecil Medicine. 23rd ed. Philadelphia, Pa: Saunders Elsevier, 2007, chap 69.

[5] Kannel WB, Dawber TR, Kagana, et al. Factors of risk in the development of coronary heart disease-six year follow-up experience. The Framingham Study. Ann Intern Med 1961, 55: 33-50.

[6] O' Donnell CJ, Elosuak. Cardiovascular risk factors. Insights from framingham heart study. Rev Esp Cardiol, 2008, 61: 299-310.

[7] Laatikainen T, Critchley J, Vartiainen E, et al. Explaining the decline in coronary heart disease mortality in Finland between 1982 and 1997. Am J Epidemiol, 2005, 162: 764-773.

[8] Ford ES, Ajani UA, Croft JB, et al. Explaining the decrease in U.S. deaths from coronary disease, 1980-2000. N Engl J Med, 2007, 356: 2388-2398.

[9] Spence JD, Hackam DG. Treating arteries instead of risk factors: a paradigm change in management of atherosclerosis. Stroke, 2010, 41: 1193-1199.

[10] Gaede P, Lund-Andersen H, Parving HH, et al. Effect of a multifactorial intervention on mortality in type 2 diabetes. N Engl J Med, 2008, 358: 580-591.

[11] Spence JD. Point: uses of carotid plaque measurement as a predictor of cardiovascular events. Prev Cardiol, 2005, 8: 118-121.

[12] Spence JD, Eliasziw M, DiCicco M, et al. Carotid plaque area: a tool for targeting and evaluating vascular preventive therapy. Stroke, 2002, 33: 2916-2922.

[13] Spence JD. Technology insight: ultrasound measurement of carotid plaque-patient management, genetic research, and therapy evaluation. Nat Clin Pract Neurol, 2006, 2: 611-619.

[14] Sawabe M. Vascular aging: from molecular mechanism to clinical significance. Geriatr Gerontol Int, 2010, 10 (Suppl): S213-S220.

[15] Donato AJ, Eskurza I, Silver AE, et al. Direct evidence of endothelial oxidative stress with aging in humans: relation to impaired endothelium dependent dilation and upregulation of nuclear factor-kappaB. Circ Res, 2007, 100: 1659-1666.

[16] Csiszar A, Wang M, Lakatta EG, et al. Inflammation and endothelial dysfunction during aging: role of NF-{kappa} B. J Appl Physiol, 2008, 105: 1333-1341.

[17] Franceschi C, Bonafè M, Valensin S, et al. Inflamm-aging. An evolutionary perspective on immunosenescence. Ann N Y Acad Sci, 2000, 908: 244-254.

[18] Wang M, Zhang J, Jiang LQ, et al. Proinflammatory profile within the grossly normal aged human aortic wall. Hypertension, 2007, 50: 219-227.

[19] Jiang L, Wang M, Zhang J, et al. Increased aortic calpain-1 activity mediates age-associated angiotensin II signaling of vascular smooth muscle cells. PLoS One, 2008, 3: e2231.

[20] Rivard A, Fabre JE, Silver M, et al. Age-dependent impairment of angiogenesis. Circulation, 1999, 99 (1): 111-120.

[21] Weinsaft JW, Edelberg JM. Aging-associated changes in vascular activity: a potential link togeriatric cardiovascular disease. Am Jgeriatr Cardiol, 2001, 10 (6): 348-354.

[22] Erusalimsky JD. Vascular endothelial senescence: from mechanisms to pathophysiology. J Appl Physiol, 2009, 106: 326-332.

[23] Chang EI, Loh SA, Ceradini DJ, et al. Age decreases endothelial progenitor cell recruitment through decreases in hypoxia-inducible factor 1 alpha stabilization during ischemia. Circulation, 2007, 116: 2818-2829.

[24] Ungvari Z, Kaleyg, de Cabo R, et al. Mechanisms of vascular aging: new perspectives. J Gerontol A Biol Sci Med Sci, 2010, 65: 1028-1041.

[25] Sindler AL, Delp MD, Reyes R, et al. Effects of aging and exercise training on eNOS uncoupling in skeletal muscle resistance arterioles. J Physiol, 2009, 587: 3885-3897.

[26] Taddei S, Galetta F, Virdis A, et al. Physical activity prevents age related impairment in nitric oxide availability in elderly athletes. Circulation, 2000, 101: 2896-2901.

[27] Ungvari Z, Parrado-Fernandez C, Csiszar A.

Mechanisms underlying caloric restriction and lifespan regulation: implications for vascular aging. Circ Res, 2008, 102: 519-528.

[28] Okazaki S, Yokoyama T, Miyauchi K, et al. Early statin treatment in patients with acute coronary syndrome: demonstration of the beneficial effect on atherosclerotic lesions by serial volumetric intravascular ultrasound analysis during half a year after coronary event: the ESTABLISH Study. Circulation, 2004, 110 (9): 1061-1068.

[29] Csiszar A, Ungvari Z, Edwards JG, et al. Aging-induced phenotypic changes and oxidative stress impair coronary arteriolar function. Circ Res, 2002, 90: 1159-1166.

[30] Bruunsgaard H, Skinhoj P, Pedersen AN, et al. Ageing, tumour necrosis factor-alpha (TNF-alpha) and atherosclerosis. Clin Exp Immunol, 2000, 121: 255-260.

[31] Sonntag WE, Ramsey M, Carter CS. Growth hormone and insulinlike growth factor-1 (IGF-1) and their influence on cognitive aging. Ageing Res Rev, 2005, 4: 195-212.

[32] Lei Y, Yang J, Zhao H, et al. Experimental study on extracts from Ginseng, Notoginseng and Chuanxiong for delaying vascular aging in senescent Mice. Chin J of Integr Tradit West Med, 2010, 30: 946-951.

[33] Yang J, Lei Y, Fang SP, et al. Study on acting mechanism of extracts from Ginseng, Notoginseng and Chuanxiong for delaying the aging of

endothelial cells induced by angiotensin II. Chin J of Integr Tradit West Med, 2009, 29: 524-528.

[34] Lu XY, Shi DZ, Xu H, et al. Clinical study on effect of Xiongshao Capsule on restenosis after percutaneous coronary intervention. Chin J of Integr Tradit West Med, 2006, 26: 13-17.

[35] Chen KJ, Shi DZ, Xu H, et al. XS0601 reduces the incidence of restenosis: a prospective study of 335 patients undergoing percutaneous coronary intervention in China. Chin Med J, 2006, 119: 6-13.

[36] Zhang DW, Zhang L, Liu JG, et al. Effects of Xiongshao Capsule combined with ischemic postconditioning on monocyte chemoattractant protein-1 and tumor necrosis factor-α in rat myocardium with ischemic reperfusion injury. Chin J of Integr Traditi West Med, 2010, 30: 1279-1283.

[37] Huang Y, Yin HJ, Ma XJ, et al. Correlation between FcγR III A and aortic atherosclerotic plaque destabilization in apoE knockout mice and intervention effects of effective components of Chuanxiong rhizome and red peony root. Chin J Integr Med, 2011, 17: 355-360.

[38] David E. Bloom. 7 billion and counting. Science, 2011, 333: 562-569.

[39] Boos CJ, Goon PK, Lipgy. Endothelial progenitor cells in the vascular pathophysiology of hypertension: arterial stiffness, ageing and more. J Hum Hypertens, 2006, 20: 475-477.

Systematic Review of Compound Danshen Dropping Pill: A Chinese Patent Medicine for Acute Myocardial Infarction [*]

LUO Jing   XU Hao   CHEN Ke-ji

1. Introduction

Acute myocardial infarction (AMI) is a serious type of coronary heart disease (CHD) and a major cause of death worldwide with an estimated annual incidence rate of seven million people [1]. As a result of coronary artery

* 原载于 Evidence-Based Complementary and Alternative Medicine, 2013, Article ID 808076

thrombotic occlusion from plaques rupture or erosion, AMI usually leads to death if complicated by severe heart failure, malignant ventricular arrhythmia, or cardiac rupture [1,2]. Despite the application of percutaneous coronary intervention (PCI) and conventional western medicine, AMI patients remain at certain risk of in-hospital death and complications as well as recurrent acute cardiovascular events [2-4]. With more and more clinicians successfully applied traditional Chinese medicine (TCM) in CHD prevention and treatment based on conventional therapy, the effects of TCM for CHD have drawn more and more attention [5-8].

Compound Danshen dropping pill (CDDP, also known as the "Dantonic Pill"), a Chinese oral patent medicine, has been widely used for cardiovascular diseases, including AMI, in China and some Asia countries. The phase II clinical trial of CDDP to treat chronic stable angina

(http：//clinicaltrials.gov/，NCT00797953) had been completed in the United States in 2010. Moreover, this drug has been approved by the Australian Therapeutic Goods Administration for use and is widely available in Australia [9]. CDDP consists of three compositions, namely, *Radix Salviae Miltiorrhizae*, *Radix Notoginseng*, and *Borneolum Syntheticum*. These compositions and their pharmacological actions [10-15] are listed in Table 1 with common, pinyin, and Latin names. Previous pharmacologic studies and randomized clinical trials have indicated the potential benefit of CDDP for patients with AMI [16-21]. Recent systematic reviews [22-24] also revealed potential benefits of CDDP for angina pectoris. The efficacy and safety of CDDP for AMI, however, have not been systematically evaluated. The aim of this study was to assess the efficacy and safety of CDDP on the treatment of AMI patients.

Table 1　Compositions of Compound Danshen Dropping Pill

Common name	Pinyin name	Latin name	Pharma. actions
Danshen root	Danshen	*Radix Salviae Miltiorrhizae*	Dilates coronary vessels and antimyocardial ischemia inhibit platelet aggregation and thrombosis, decrease cholesterol and endothelial damage, scavenge free radicals, antilipid peroxidative, and antiatherosclerosis, and reduce myocardial ischemia-reperfusion injury, anti-inflammatory [10,11].
Sanchi root	Sanqi	*Radix Notoginseng*	Dilates blood vessel increases blood platelet number to promote hemostasis, inhibits platelet aggregation and thrombosis, and reduces viscosity of whole blood, decreases the heart rate and myocardial ischemia-reperfusion injury, inhibits proliferation of vascular smooth muscle cell, decreases cholesterol and antiatherosclerosis, antioxidation [12,13].
Borneol	Bingpian	*Borneolum Syntheticum*	Analgesia and sedation boost other drugs' bioavailability, anti-inflammatory, and decreases the heart rate and myocardial oxygen consumption [14,15].

2. Methods

2.1 Inclusion and Exclusion Criteria

Randomized controlled trials (RCTs) comparing CDDP with no intervention, placebo, or conventional western medicine were sought regardless of their publication status. Participants of any gender, age, or ethnic origin with AMI meeting with one of the past or current definitions of AMI [25-29] were included. Those without description of diagnostic criteria but stated patients with definite AMI were also considered. Quasirandomized trials and animal experiments were excluded. Trials with CDDP as adjunctive therapy or with duration less than four weeks were also excluded.

Primary outcomes consisted of all-cause mortality, cardiac mortality, recurrent myocardial infarction (RMI), and revascularization, including PCI and coronary artery bypass graft (CABG). Secondary outcomes included heart failure, readmission, left ventricular ejection fraction (LVEF), recurrent angina, adverse events and health-related quality of life measured by a validated tool.

2.2 Source of Literature and Search Strategy

2.2.1 Electronic Searches. We searched the following databases up to October 2012 for the identification of RCTs both published and unpublished：Pubmed, The Cochrane Library, Chinese Biomedical Database (CBM), Chinese VIP Information (VIP), China National Knowledge Infrastructure (CNKI), Wanfang Databases, China Proceedings of Conference Full-text Database (CPCD), Chinese Doctoral Dissertations Full-text Database (CDFD), and Chinese Master's Theses Full-text Database (CMFD). Search strategy in Table 2 was used in the Cochrane Library and adapted appropriately for other databases.

In addition, we searched databases of ongoing trials：ClinicalTrials.gov (http：// clinicaltrials.gov/) and Current Controlled Trials (http：//www.controlled-trials.com/).

2.2.2 Additional Searches. We also searched the reference lists of studies included in this systematic review and of other relevant reviews to identify missing relevant articles.

Table 2　Search Strategy for the Cochrane Library

Strategy
No. 1 Danshen pill
No. 2 salvia pill
No. 3 compound Danshen
No. 4 compound salvia
No. 5 composite Danshen
No. 6 composite salvia
No. 7 Dantonic pill
No. 8 CDDP
No. 9 CSDP
No. 10 FFDS
No. 11 myocardial infarction [MeSH]
No. 12 coronary disease [MeSH]
No. 13 coronary artery disease [MeSH]
No.14 acute coronary syndrome[MeSH]
No. 15 myocardial infarct
No.16 AMI
No. 17 MI
No. 18 acute coronary syndrome
No. 19 （1，2，3，4，5，6，7，8，9，or 10）
No. 20 （11，12，13，14，15，16，17，or 18）
No. 21 （19 and 20）

2.3　Study Identification and Data Extraction

Two authors (Jing Luo, Hao Xu) independently screened the titles and abstracts of references for potentially relevant RCTs. Full texts of potentially eligible articles were retrieved for further identification according to the inclusion and exclusion criteria. Any disagreement was resolved by consensus.

Two authors (Jing Luo, Hao Xu) independently extracted data using a preset data extraction form. Characteristics of RCTs including methods, participants, interventions, comparisons, and outcomes were extracted. We obtained missing information from the original authors whenever possible and resolved any disagreement through discussion or consulting the third author (Keji Chen).

2.4　Assessment of Risk of Bias and Quality of Evidence

Two authors (Jing Luo, Hao Xu) independently assessed the methodological quality of each of the included studies using the Cochrane "risk of bias" criteria [30], which covers the following items：random sequence generation,

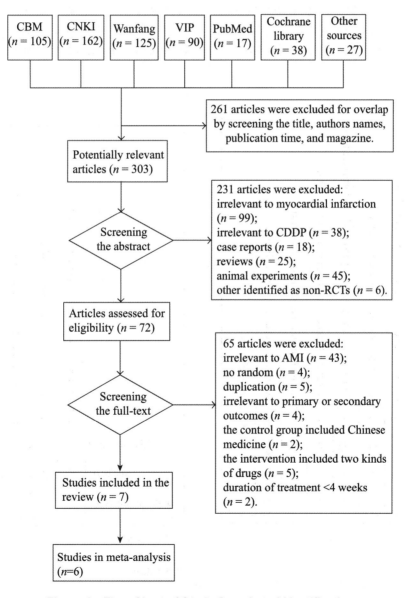

Figure 1　Flow Chart of Study Search and Identification

allocation concealment, blinding of participants and personnel, blinding of outcome assessment, incomplete outcome data, selective reporting, and other bias. Disagreements were resolved by consensus. For each item, a low risk was considered when we judged a "Yes, " conversely, a "No" for a high risk, and otherwise for an unclear risk.

We also evaluated the quality of evidence of each outcome using the Grading of Recommendations Assessment, Development and Evaluation (GRADE) approach [31], as recommended by the Cochrane Collaboration. Patient important outcomes in the main comparison were judged across five factors: limitations in study design and execution, inconsistency of results, indirectness of evidence,

imprecision, and publication bias. Accordingly, we graded the quality of evidence in this review as very low, low, moderate, or high.

2.5　Data Analysis

We used RevMan 5.1 software for data analyses.

Studies were stratified by the different types of comparisons. We performed intention-to-treat analysis (ITT) for dichotomous data and presented outcome data as risk ratio (RR) with corresponding 95% confidence interval (CI). We calculated mean difference (MD) with its 95% CI for continuous outcomes. Fixed effect model was used to analyze data with low heterogeneity ($I^2 \leqslant 50\%$); random effects model was applied if heterogeneity is significant ($50\% < I^2 < 75\%$).

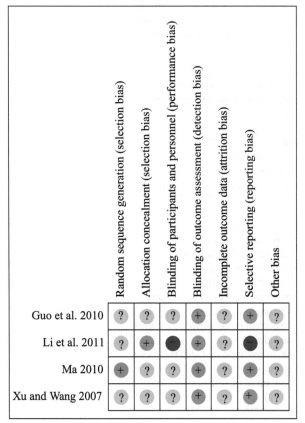

+　Low risk
−　High risk
?　Unclear

Figure 2　Risk of Bias Summary—All-cause Mortality

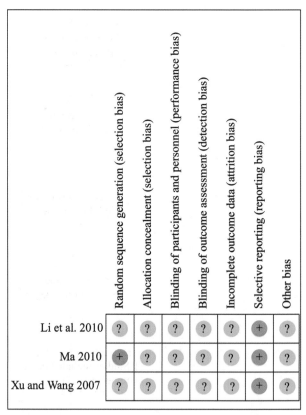

+　Low risk
−　High risk
?　Unclear

Figure 3　Risk of Bias Summary—Cardiac Mortality

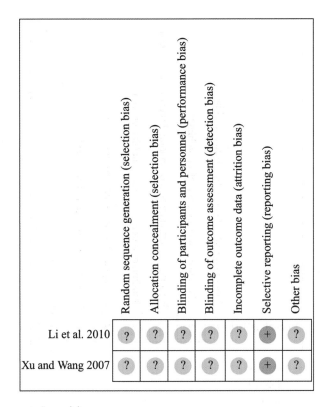

+ Low risk
− High risk
? Unclear

Figure 4　Risk of Bias Summary—Recurrent Myocardial Infarction

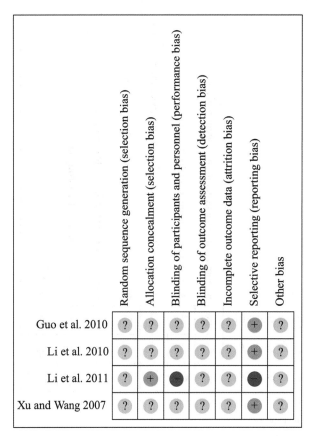

+ Low risk
− High risk
? Unclear

Figure 5　Risk of Bias Summary—Heart Failure

Results were not pooled for data with high heterogeneity ($I^2 \geqslant 75\%$)[32], in which case we explored potential causes of heterogeneity by conducting subgroup analyses based on the characteristics of intervention (dosage, duration) and the types of conventional therapy (PCI versus thrombolysis). We also performed sensitivity analyses on studies with lower methodological quality, in order to investigate whether the inclusion of such studies altered the conclusion of the meta-analysis. Possible publication bias was checked using funnel plots when the number of included studies of any particular outcome is greater than eight.

3. Results

3.1　Study Identification

A total of 564 references were found according to search strategy, of which 261 were excluded for duplicates among databases. After screening the abstract, we excluded 231 articles. 72 potentially eligible studies were retrieved for further identification, of which 65 were excluded because they did not meet the prespecified inclusion criteria described in the methods. At last, seven eligible RCTs [19-21,33-36] were included. No ongoing trial was found. Please refer to Figure 1 for a more detailed illustration of the data screening process.

3.2　Description of Included Studies

The characteristics of the included seven studies [19-21,33-36] are summarized in Table 3. Each of the studies was conducted in China. One postgraduate dissertation [35] was unpublished in 2010，and the others were published from 2006 to 2011. One study[19] was of multicenter design,

第七章

673

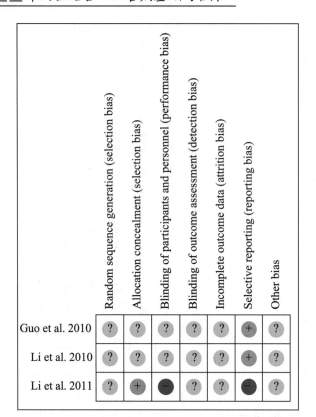

+ Low risk
− High risk
? Unclear

Figure 6   Risk of Bias Summary—Recurrent Angina

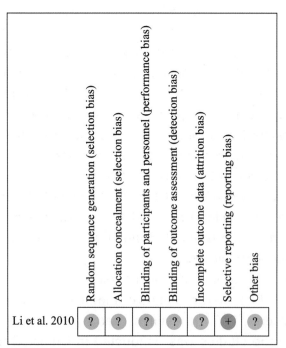

+ Low risk
− High risk
? Unclear

Figure 7   Risk of Bias Summary—Readmission

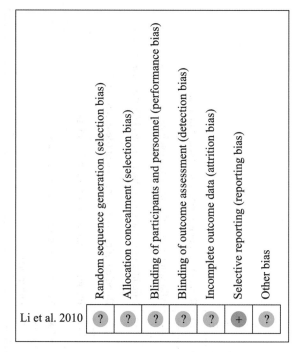

+ Low risk
− High risk
? Unclear

Figure 8   Risk of Bias Summary—QOL

but the others were of single centre trials.

The number of participants in the individual study ranged from 45 to 500，with a total of 1215 in this review (583 in intervention groups and 632 in control groups). There were 863 males and 352 females included in the review, with mean age, where given [19,20,34-36]，ranging from 52 to 66 years. All of the participants were diagnosed with AMI by different diagnostic criteria：two studies [20,21] used the WHO diagnostic criteria；one study [33] used ACC/AHA diagnostic criteria；four studies [19,34-36] without specified diagnostic criteria but mentioned "patients with AMI were eligible to include". Two studies [19,35] only included patients with ST-elevation myocardial infarction (STEMI), one study excluded AMI without Q wave [21]，and the others did not introduce the types of AMI (four studies) [20,33,34,36].

All participants in the intervention groups were treated with CDDP, 10 pills three times a day (tid) orally based on conventional therapy

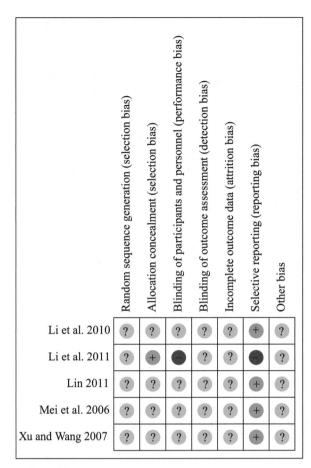

+ Low risk
− High risk
? Unclear

Figure 9　Risk of Bias Summary—LVEF

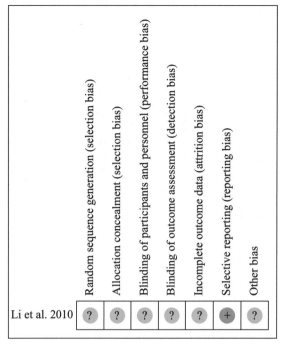

+ Low risk
− High risk
? Unclear

Figure 10　Risk of Bias Summary—Adverse Events

since the day of diagnosis [19,20,33-36]. Only one study [21] began the CDDP treatment four to five weeks later after diagnosis and changed the dosage from 10 pills tid to five pills tid after 60 days of treatment.

The duration of treatment was mainly as same as the length of follow up, ranging from four weeks to 12 months. One study [21] was designed as three groups with two comparisons including CDDP versus no intervention and CDDP versus propranolol. Six studies consisted of two groups (one study [36] compared CDDP with placebo and the others [19,20,33-35] focused on CDDP compared with no intervention). In total, there were three comparisons in the review：（1）CDDP plus conventional therapy versus conventional therapy (six studies)[19-21,33-35]；（2）CDDP plus conventional

therapy versus placebo plus conventional therapy (one study)[36]；（3）CDDP plus conventional therapy versus propranolol plus conventional therapy (one study)[21].

Five studies [19-21,35,36] reported mortality including all-cause mortality (four studies) [19-21,35] and cardiac mortality (three studies) [21,35,36]. Two studies provided numerical information on RMI [21,36], but the data could not be pooled for the different comparisons. Four studies [19-21,36] reported heart failure. Three studies [19,20,36] provided the number of patients having recurrent angina. Besides the incidence of readmission and adverse events (narrative introduction), one study[36] also assessed the QOL by questionnaire score, and the questionnaire was designed referring to Treatment of Mild Hypertension Study (TOMHS) and Medical Outcomes Study 36-Item Short-Form Health Survey (SF-36). Five studies [19,21,33,34,36] assessed the LVEF with the aim of evaluating the heart function. None of the included studies mentioned revascularization.

第七章

第七章

Table 3　Characteristics of Included Studies

ID	Sample size (I/C)	Age (y, I/C)	Diagnostic criteria of AMI	Type of AMI	Intervention	Control	Duration of treatment	Follow up	Outcomes	Baseline report
Li et al. 2011[19]	500 (252/248)	60.10±9.60/ 56.70±7.80	Not specified	STEMI	CDDP 10 pills tid + CT (the same as control)	CT (western medicines +PCI)	30 days	30 days	All-cause mortality, shock, arrhythmia, LVEF%, HF, angina, myocardial enzyme.	Yes
Lin 2011[33]	90 (46/44)	43-75/36-72	ACC/AHA 2004	Unclear	CDDP 10 pills tid + CT (the same as control)	CT (western medicines)	6 weeks	6 weeks	LVEF%, WBC, CRP, Chinese symptoms.	Yes (narrative only)
Ma 2010[35]	163 (78/85)	62.55±11.95/ 66.02±11.40	Not specified	STEMI	CDDP 10 pills tid + CT (the same as control)	CT (western medicines or plus PCI/thrombolysis)	1 month	3 months	All-cause mortality, IL-6, cardiac mortality, hs-CRP, MACEs, MMP-9, TNF-α.	Yes
Li et al. 2010[36]	63 (42/21)	58.40±11.60	Not specified	Unclear	CDDP 10 pills tid + CT (the same as control)	Placebo + CT (western Medicines + thrombolysis).	4 months	4 months	Cardiac mortality, LVEF%, readmission, QOL, RMI, HF, angina, adverse events.	Yes (narrative only)
Guo et al. 2010[20]	136 (76/60)	55.60±12.5/ 51.80±13.60	WHO	Unclear	CDDP 10 pills tid + CT (the same as control)	CT (western medicines + thrombolysis)	4 weeks	4 weeks	All-cause mortality, shock, HF, recanalization, angina, myocardial enzyme.	Yes
Xu and Wang 2007[21]	218 (66/72/80)	36-75/37-78 /32-79	WHO	With Q-wave	CDDP 10 pills d1-60, then 5 pills tid + CT (the same as control)	Propranolol 10～15 mg tid + CT (no detail); CT (no detail)	12 months	12 months	All-cause mortality, RMI, cardiac mortality, HF, arrhythmia, LVEF%.	Yes (narrative only)
Mei et al. 2006[34]	45 (23/22)	56.11±11.13	Not specified	Unclear	CDDP 10 pills tid + CT (the same as control)	CT (western medicines)	6 months	6 months	LVEF%, SV, CO	Unclear

Notes: CT: conventional therapy; HF: heart failure; AHA: American heart Association; ACC: American College of Cardiology; CRP: C-reactive protein; hs-CRP: high sensitive C-reactive protein; WBC: white blood cell; MACEs: major adverse cardiac events; WHO: World Health Organization; TNF-α: tumor necrosis factor-alpha; MMP-9: matrix metalloproteinase-9; IL-6: interleukin-6; SV: stroke volume; CO: cardiac output; tid: three times a day.

3.3 Quality of Included Studies

3.3.1. Risk of Bias in Included Studies. Risk of bias summaries for each outcome in the included RCTs at the study level are presented in Figures 2-10. No study was felt to have a low risk of bias. Of the seven studies, one [35] introduced the random sequence being generated from a random number table, and the others just mentioned "patients were randomly allocated" without the method of randomization. Only one study [19] reported allocation concealment. None of the studies described blinding of participants and personnel although one study [36] used placebo. All of the studies did not report blinding of outcome assessment. Neither withdrawals nor losses to follow up were reported in the studies. One study [19] had incomplete outcome data. Five studies [20,21,33,35,36] reported the comparability of the baseline among groups, but four of them did not provide baseline data [20,21,33,36]. The multicenter study[19], with other similar baselines, reported that the rate of diabetes patients in the intervention group was higher than the control group. In addition, no study mentioned prior sample size estimation or ITT analysis for any outcome.

After we contacted with the original authors by telephone and email, only one author [19] told us that there was no blinding of participants or personnel in their study, and the randomization was designed by public health statistics teaching and research section of Tianjin Medical University; he did not know any other details. In fact, due to a number of unsuccessful contacts and some unclear or unavailable replies, most of our questions were not resolved.

3.3.2 Quality of Evidence in Included Studies. The quality of evidence for each outcome in the main comparison (CDDP versus no intervention) was ranged from "low" to "moderate" (Table 4). Quality assessment of the evidence in accordance with the GRADE approach showed some limitations of the study design and execution, inconsistency, indirectness, and imprecision. Due to the low number of included studies for each outcome, we could not create funnel plots to detect publication bias. For each outcome, there were one or two serious limitations among the five factors. For example, because of the serious risk of bias and imprecision for all-cause mortality in the main comparison, we downgraded the quality rating by two levels, thus the quality of evidence for this outcome was low. The quality of evidence was moderate for cardiac mortality and heart failure, low for all-cause mortality, RMI, recurrent angina, and LVEF.

3.4 Effect of Interventions (Table 5 to Table 7)

3.4.1 All-Cause Mortality (Table 5). Four studies [19-21,35] reported all-cause mortality in two different comparisons. Meta-analysis of the four studies showed no statistically significant difference in the risk of all-cause death between CDDP and no intervention (RR 0.65；95%CI 0.37 to 1.14；n=945). Sensitive analysis, excluding the lower quality study [19], found that CDDP was associated with a statistically significant reduction in the risk of all-cause death compared with no intervention without heterogeneity (RR 0.51；95%CI 0.27 to 0.98；three studies, n= 445；I^2=0%) [20,21,35]. A single study reported that there was no statistical difference in reducing all-cause mortality between CDDP and propranolol on the basis of conventional therapy (RR 0.65；95%CI 0.16 to 2.63；n=138) [21]. The associated risk of bias is presented in Figure 2. The quality of evidence in the main comparison (CDDP versus no intervention) was low (Table 4) .

3.4.2 Cardiac Mortality (Table 5). Three studies [21,35,36] assessed cardiac mortality in three different comparisons. Meta-analysis of two studies [21,35] showed that CDDP was associated with a statistically significant reduction in the risk of cardiac death compared with no intervention without heterogeneity (RR 0.43；95%CI 0.20 to 0.95；n=309；I^2=0%). Compared with placebo on the basis of conventional therapy, CDDP had no statistically significant advantage in reducing cardiac mortality (RR 0.50；95%CI 0.03 to 7.60；

Table 4 GRADE Analysis: Summary of Findings for the Main Comparison

Compound Danshen dropping pill versus no intervention for acute myocardial infarction

Patient or population: patients with acute myocardial infarction
Settings: inpatients and outpatients
Intervention: compound Danshen dropping pill (CDDP)

Outcomes	Illustrative comparative risks* (95% CI)		Relative effect (95% CI)	None of participants (studies)	Quality of the vidence (GRADE)	Comments
	Assumed risk Control	Corresponding risk CDDP				
All-cause mortality Follow-up: 4 weeks–12 months	*Study population*		RR 0.65 (0.37-1.14)	945 (4 studies)	⊕⊕⊖⊖ low[1,2]	
	63 per 1000	41 per 1000 (23-72)				
	Moderate					
	104 per 1000	68 per 1000 (38-119)				
Cardiac mortality Follow-up: 3-12 months Moderate	*Study population*		RR 0.43 (0.2-0.95)	309 (2 studies)	⊕⊕⊕⊖ moderate[3,4]	
	127 per 1000	55 per 1000 (25-121)				
	Moderate					
	127 per 1000	55 per 1000 (25-121)				
Recurrent myocardial infarction Follow-up: mean 12 months	*Study population*		RR 0.30 (0.07-1.38)	146 (1 study)	⊕⊕⊖⊖ low[5]	
	100 per 1000	30 per 1000 (7-138)				
	Moderate					
	100 per 1000	30 per 1000 (7-138)				
Heart failure Follow-up: 4 weeks-12 months	*Study population*		RR 0.41 (0.22-0.75)	782 (3 studies)	⊕⊕⊕⊖ moderate[1]	
	85 per 1000	35 per 1000 (19-64)				
	Moderate					
	150 per 1000	62 per 1000 (33-112)				

第七章

Compound Danshen dropping pill versus no intervention for acute myocardial infarction

Outcomes	Illustrative comparative risks (95%CI)		Relative effect (95%CI)	No of Participants (studies)	Quality of the evidence (GRADE)	Comments
	Assumed risk	Corresponding risk				
	Study population					
Recurrent angina Clinical diagnosis based on patients complaint Follow-up: 4weeks-30days	211 per 1000	70 per 1000 (21-217)	RR 0.33 (0.1-1.03)	636 (2 studies)	⊕⊕⊝⊝ low[1,6,7]	
	Moderate:					
	201 per 1000	66 per 1000 (20-207)				
Left ventricular ejection fraction Measured with echocardiogram. Scale from 30% to 75%. Duration of treatment: 4-6 week	The mean left ventricular ejection fraction in the control groups was 50.48%[9]	The mean left ventricular ejection fraction in the intervention groups was 5.71% higher (4.38%-7.04% higher)		590 (2 studies)	⊕⊕⊝⊝ low[1,8]	Higher score indicates improvement
Left ventricular ejection fraction Measured with echocardiogram. Scale from: 30% - 75%. Duration of treatment: 6-12 months	The mean left ventricular ejection fraction in the control groups was 49.71%[9]	The mean left ventricular ejection fraction in the intervention groups was 3.82% higher (2.46%-5.19% higher)		191 (2 studies)	⊕⊕⊝⊝ low[3,8]	Higher score indicates improvement

*The basis for the assumed risk (e.g., the median control group risk acrossstudies) is provided in footnotes. The corresponding risk (and its 95%confidence interval) is based on the assumed risk in the comparison group and the relative effect of the intervention (and its 95%CI).

CI: confidence interval; RR: risk ratio; GRADE Working group grades of evidence:

High quality: further research is very unlikely-change our confidence in the estimate of effect.

Moderate quality: further research is likely-have an important impact on our confidence in the estimate of effect and may change the estimate.

Low quality: further research is very likely-have an important impact on our confidence in the estimate of effect and is likely-change the estimate.

Very low quality: we are very uncertain about the estimate.

[1] One study had selective reporting. For the other studies, the overall risk of bias was felt-be unclear.

[2] 95%CI includes possibility of both benefits and harms, and the sample size was not the optimal information size. After sensitive analysis excluding the lower quality study, the result suggested benefit, but the sample size was still small.

[3] The overall risk of bias of the studies was unclear. The sample size was not the optimal information size.

[4] 95% CI included only benefit, so we were cautious about downgrading the imprecision although the sample size was less than the optimal information size.

[5] Unclear risk of bias and only 146 patients enrolled. 95%CI included possibility of both benefits and harms.

[6] The heterogeneity (I²=61%) can be explained by the major differences of conventional therapy and sample size between the two studies, and this outcome is not so important affect the decision-making; therefore, we did not downgrade for this factor.

[7] 95% CI suggested benefit as well as no benefit.

[8] This is an indirect outcome for AMI patients.

[9] Final measurements at the end of the study.

one study, n=63)[36]. A single study reported a similar result between CDDP and propranolol (RR 0.81；95%CI 0.17 to 3.76；n=138)[21]. Figure 3 presents the associated risk of bias. The quality of evidence in the main comparison (CDDP versus no intervention) was moderate (Table 4).

3.4.3 Recurrent Myocardial Infarction (Table 5). Two studies [21,36] reported RMI in three different comparisons. None of the comparisons, however, presented a statistically significant difference in the risk of RMI：CDDP versus no intervention (RR 0.30；95% CI 0.07 to 1.38；one study, n=146)[21]；CDDP versus placebo (RR 0.50；95% CI 0.11 to 2.27；one study, n=63)[36]；CDDP versus propranolol (RR 0.73；95%CI 0.13 to 4.22；one study, n=138)[21]. The associated risk of bias is presented in Figure 4. The quality of evidence in the main comparison (CDDP versus no intervention) was low (Table 4).

3.4.4. Heart Failure (Table 6). Four studies [19-21,36] reported heart failure in three different comparisons. Meta-analysis of three studies [19-21] found that CDDP was associated with a statistically significant reduction in the risk of heart failure compared with no intervention with no heterogeneity (RR 0.41；95%CI 0.22 to 0.75；n=782；I^2=0%). Sensitive analysis, excluding the lower quality study [19], got a similar conclusion (RR 0.30；95%CI 0.14 to 0.65；two studies, n=282；I^2=0%) [20,21]. Compared with propranolol on the basis of conventional therapy, CDDP still presented a statistical difference in reducing heart failure (RR 0.26；95% CI 0.07 to 0.99；one study, n=138)[21]. Nevertheless, compared with placebo on the basis of conventional therapy, CDDP showed no effect in the reduction of heart failure (RR 0.63；95% CI 0.19 to 2.09；one study, n=63) [36]. The associated risk of bias is presented in Figure 5. And the quality of evidence in the main comparison (CDDP versus no intervention) was moderate (Table 4).

3.4.5 Recurrent Angina (Table 6). Three studies [19,20,36] assessed the number of patients

Table 5 Analyses of Primary Outcomes

Outcomes （comparisons）	Treatment （n/N）	Control （n/N）	Weight （%）	RR	95% CI
（1）*All-cause mortality*					
（1.1）CDDP + conventional therapy versus conventional therapy					
Guo et al. 2010 [20]	5/76	5/60	19.10	0.79	[0.24，2.60]
Li et al. 2011 [19]	6/252	4/248	13.80	1.48	[0.42，5.17]
Ma 2010 [35]	5/78	11/85	36.10	0.50	[0.18，1.36]
Xu and Wang 2007 [21]	3/66	10/80	31.00	0.36	[0.10，1.27]
Total（FEM，I^2= 0%）			**100.00**	**0.65**	**[0.37，1.14]**
Sensitive analysis					
Guo et al. 2010 [20]	5/76	5/60	22.20	0.79	[0.24，2.60]
Ma 2010 [35]	5/78	11/85	41.80	0.50	[0.18，1.36]
Xu and Wang 2007 [21]	3/66	10/80	35.90	0.36	[0.10，1.27]
Total（FEM，I^2=0%）			**100.00**	**0.51**	**[0.27，0.98]**
（1.2）CDDP + conventional therapy versus propranolol + conventional therapy					
Xu and Wang 2007 [21]	3/66	5/72	100.00	0.65	[0.16，2.63]
（2）*Cardiac mortality*					
（2.1）CDDP + conventional therapy versus conventional therapy					

Outcomes（comparisons）	Treatment（n/N）	Control（n/N）	Weight（%）	RR	95% CI
Ma 2010 [35]	5/78	11/85	53.80	0.50	[0.18，1.36]
Xu and Wang 2007 [21]	3/66	10/80	46.20	0.36	[0.10，1.27]
Total（FEM，I²=0%）			**100.00**	**0.43**	**[0.20，0.95]**
(2.2) CDDP + conventional therapy versus placebo + conventional therapy					
Li et al. 2010 [36]]	1/42	1/21	100.00	0.50	[0.03，7.60]
(2.3) CDDP + conventional therapy versus propranolol + conventional therapy					
Xu and Wang 2007 [21]	3/66	4/72	100.00	0.81	[0.17，3.76]
(3) *Recurrent myocardial infarction*					
(3.1) CDDP + conventional therapy versus conventional therapy					
Xu and Wang 2007 [21]	2/66	8/80	100.00	0.30	[0.07，1.38]
(3.2) CDDP + conventional therapy versus placebo + conventional therapy					
Li et al. 2010 [36]	3/42	3/21	100.00	0.50	[0.11，2.27]
(3.3) CDDP + conventional therapy versus propranolol + conventional therapy					
Xu and Wang 2007 [21]	2/66	3/72	100.00	0.73	[0.13，4.22]

Table 6 Analyses of Secondary Outcomes

Outcomes（comparisons）	Treatment（n/N）	Control（n/N）	Weight（%）	RR	95% CI
(1) *Heart failure*					
(1.1) CDDP + conventional therapy versus conventional therapy					
Xu and Wang 2007 [21]	3/66	12/80	32.40	0.30	[0.09，1.03]
Guo et al. 2010 [20]	5/76	13/60	43.40	0.30	[0.11，0.80]
Li et al. 2011 [19]	6/252	8/248	24.10	0.74	[0.26，2.10]
Total（FEM，I²=0%）			**100.00**	**0.41**	**[0.22，0.75]**
Sensitive analysis					
Xu and Wang 2007 [21]	3/66	12/80	57.30	0.30	[0.09，1.03]
Guo et al. 2010 [20]	5/76	13/60	42.70	0.30	[0.11，0.80]
Total（FEM，I²=0%）			**100.00**	**0.30**	**[0.14，0.65]**
(1.2) CDDP + conventional therapy versus placebo + conventional therapy					
Li et al. 2010 [36]	5/42	4/21	100.00	0.63	[0.19，2.09]
(1.3) CDDP + conventional therapy versus propranolol + conventional therapy					
Xu and Wang 2007 [21]	**3/66**	**11/72**	**100.00**	**0.26**	**[0.07，0.99]**
(2) *Recurrent angina*					
(2.1) CDDP + conventional therapy versus conventional therapy					
Guo 2010 [20]	2/76	11/60	33.40	0.14	[0.03，0.62]
Li et al. 2011 [19]	27/252	54/248	66.60	0.49	[0.32，0.75]
Total（REM，I²= 61%）			100.00	0.33	[0.10，1.03]
(2.2) CDDP + conventional therapy versus placebo + conventional therapy					
Li et al. 2010 [36]	12/42	11/21	100.00	0.55	[0.29，1.02]
(3) *Readmission*					
CDDP + conventional therapy versus placebo + conventional therapy					
Li et al. 2010 [36]	3/42	4/21	100.00	0.38	[0.09，1.52]

having recurrent angina in two different comparisons. While meta-analysis of two studies showed that CDDP was associated with a statistically significant reduction in the risk of recurrent angina compared with no intervention; the heterogeneity was significant (RR 0.43; 95%CI 0.29 to 0.64; n=636; I^2=61%) [19,20]. We, hence, examined the data and looked over the papers carefully. We found that besides the types of conventional therapy, the sample sizes between the two studies were also of big differences. Furthermore, one study was high risk of bias [19]. Random effects model, therefore, was used and got a different result without statistical difference (RR 0.33; 95%CI 0.10 to 1.03; n=636). Compared with placebo on the basis of conventional therapy, CDDP still showed no effect in the reduction of recurrent angina (RR 0.55; 95% CI 0.29 to 1.02; one study, n=63)[36]. Figure 6 presents the associated risk of bias. The quality of evidence in the main comparison (CDDP versus no intervention) was low (Table 4).

3.4.6　Readmission (Table 6). Only one study reported readmission in the comparison of CDDP plus conventional therapy versus placebo plus conventional therapy (RR 0.38; 95%CI 0.09 to 1.52; n=63)[36]. The associated risk of bias is presented in Figure 7.

3.4.7　Quality of Life (Table 7). One study assessed QOL by questionnaire score. The questionnaire

Table 7　Analyses of Secondary Outcomes

Outcomes (comparisons)	Treatment			Control			Weight (%)	MD	95% CI
	Mean	SD	N	Mean	SD	N			
(4) LVEF%									
(4.1) CDDP + conventional therapy versus conventional therapy									
Mei et al. 2006 [34]	60.80	7.20	23	59.20	6.80	22	10.50	1.60	[-2.49, 5.69]
Xu and Wang 2007 [21]	51.20	4.30	66	47.10	4.60	80	34.60	4.10	[2.65, 5.55]
Li et al. 2011 [19]	57.10	8.70	252	51.90	9.90	248	31.70	5.20	[3.57, 6.83]
Lin 2011 [33]	54.50	6.80	46	47.80	3.90	44	23.30	6.70	[4.42, 8.98]
Total (REM, I^2=51%)							100.00	4.79	[3.31, 6.28]
Subgroup analysis (according to duration of treatment)									
(4.1.1) 30 days-6 weeks									
Li et al. 2011 [19]	57.10	8.70	252	51.90	9.90	248	33.90	5.20	[3.57, 6.83]
Lin 2011 [33]	54.50	6.80	46	47.80	3.90	44	17.40	6.70	[4.42, 8.98]
Subtotal (FEM, I^2=9%)							51.30	5.71	[4.38, 7.04]
(4.1.2) 6 months-12 months									
Mei et al. 2006 [34]	60.80	7.20	23	59.20	6.80	22	5.40	1.60	[-2.49, 5.69]
Xu and Wang 2007 [21]	51.20	4.30	66	47.10	4.60	80	43.30	4.10	[2.65, 5.55]
Subtotal (FEM, I^2=22%)							48.70	3.82	[2.46, 5.19]
(4.2) CDDP + conventional therapy versus placebo + conventional therapy									
Li et al. 2010 [36]	55.69	9.34	42	50.21	7.83	21	100.00	5.48	[1.10, 9.86]
(4.3) CDDP + conventional therapy versus propranolol + conventional therapy									
Xu and Wang 2007 [21]	51.20	4.30	66	49.60	5.00	72	100.00	1.60	[0.05, 3.15]
(5) *Quality of life (score)*									
CDDP + conventional therapy versus placebo + conventional therapy									
Li et al. 2010 [36]	110.28	19.33	42	97.68	17.13	21	100.00	12.60	[3.23, 21.97]

was designed referring to TOMHS and SF-36. Compared with placebo group on the basis of conventional therapy, patients in the group treated with CDDP had higher scores (MD 12.60；95%CI 3.23 to 21.97; n=63)[36]. The associated risk of bias is presented in Figure 8.

3.4.8 Left Ventricular Ejection Fraction (Table 7).

Five studies [19,21,33,34,36] assessed LVEF in three different comparisons. Meta-analysis (random effects model) of four studies [19,21,33,34] found that CDDP was associated with a statistically significant increase in LVEF compared with no intervention (MD 4.79%；95%CI 3.31 to 6.28；n=781). For the significant heterogeneity (I^2=51%) among the studies, we examined the data and looked over the papers carefully. We found that there was a significant difference in the duration of treatment among the studies. Therefore, we conducted a subgroup analysis according to the duration of treatment. In the subgroup analysis of patients with 30 days to six weeks treatment [19,33] versus six months to 12 months treatment [21,34], the test effect still had statistical significant but without significant heterogeneity：MD 5.71% (95% CI 4.38 to 7.04；two studies, n=590；I^2=9%) for 30 days to six weeks treatment versus MD 3.82% (95%CI 2.46 to 5.19；two studies, n=191；I^2=22%) for six months to 12 months treatment. Compared with placebo on the basis of conventional therapy, CDDP also presented a statistical difference in the increase of LVEF (MD 5.48%；95%CI 1.10 to 9.86；one study, n=63) [36]. In addition, a single study reported a similar result between CDDP and propranolol (MD 1.60%；95%CI 0.05 to 3.15；n=138) [21]. Figure 9 presents the associated risk of bias. The quality of evidence in the main comparison (CDDP versus no intervention) was low (Table 4).

3.4.9 Adverse Events.

One of the seven studies reported adverse events [36]. The authors described that there were mild adverse events in the CDDP group such as blushing (1/63 patient), abdominal distention (2/63 patients)，dizziness, and distention of head (2/63 patients). However, all of the adverse events remitted spontaneously. There were no significant differences between the two groups in blood glucose, hepatic function, and renal function after treatment. The associated risk of bias is presented in Figure 10.

4. Discussion

Seven RCTs including 1215 participants were included in this review. CDDP presented statistically significant benefit on the incidence of cardiac death and heart failure as compared with no intervention based on conventional therapy for AMI. Compared with propranolol, CDDP showed the similar effect on heart failure. In addition, the benefit of CDDP on LVEF was statistically significant both in short-term (30 days to six weeks) and long-term (six months to 12 months) treatment compared with no intervention, placebo, or propranolol. CDDP was also associated with a statistically significant improvement in QOL compared with placebo on the basis of conventional therapy. However, it was not associated with a statistically significant effect on RMI, readmission, or recurrent angina. Unfortunately, no data was available to assess the effect of CDDP on revascularization.

The discrepancy between the effect on all-cause mortality before and after sensitive analysis might be related to the lower quality study [19]. Although CDDP was found to be beneficial for the reduction of all-cause mortality after sensitive analysis, the effect still need to be demonstrated due to the low quality of the evidence.

When we mention TCM, often natural products with fewer side effects come to mind. In fact, systematic reviews [22-24] do indicate fewer mild side effects of CDDP for angina pectoris. A latest parallel double blind randomized placebo-controlled trial also showed no significant adverse effects of CDDP for hypercholesterolemia patients [9]. However, in this review, only one study with small simple size described mild adverse events of CDDP with spontaneous remission. Due to the insufficient data, it is too early to evaluate the safety of CDDP for AMI patients at present. We, therefore, suggest detailed description of adverse events in the future studies of CDDP.

We have to consider a number of limitations in this review before recommending the conclusion to clinical practitioners. (1) We might miss some unpublished relevant studies since we only searched unpublished studies from CPCD, CDFD, and CMFD. What is more, we could not create a funnel plot to check for possible publication bias for each outcome due to the low number of included studies. Publication bias might exist in our results. (2) None of the included studies was assessed to be at low risk of bias. The main reasons are as follows: firstly, the method of random sequence generation was unclear in most of the studies, and only one study reported allocation concealment; most of the studies might have selection bias; secondly, no study described double blind method as well as the blinding of outcome assessment; both selection bias and detection bias might exist in the conclusion; thirdly, neither withdrawals nor losses to follow up was reported in each study; this could lead to a high risk of attrition bias; fourthly, one study [19] had selective reporting on cardiac mortality and RMI which should be reported in accordance with its study plan, this could induce reporting bias. In addition, all of the included studies did not mention ITT analysis, which might lead to some other bias. (3) Most of the durations of follow up were short; the reliability and validity of some outcomes such as mortality could be influenced. (4) The small number of included studies and the different comparisons among the studies precluded us from conducting subgroup analyses to explore effect modifiers such as duration of intervention and type of conventional therapy. (5) For some

outcomes, only single study provided data and most of the studies did not meet the calculated optimal information size. This might influence the precision of results, which could downgrade the quality of evidence. (6) We assessed the quality of evidence for each outcome according to the GRADE approach with caution. However, the overall quality of evidence in the main comparison was poor, which can weaken the strength of recommendation.

Although this systematic review suggests some benefits of CDDP for AMI patients, the recommendation of findings was limited due to the poor quality studies. Therefore, rigorously designed clinical trials are warranted to further demonstrate the effectiveness and safety of CDDP for AMI. Moreover, we suggest that researchers of RCTs provide complete, clear, and transparent information on their methodologies and findings in the future. This is important for readers or reviewers to assess and use RCTs accurately. Thus, we expect that more RCTs of TCM will be appropriately designed, conducted, and reported according to the CONSORT statement [37] or the CONSORT statement for herbal interventions [38].

5. Conclusion

This systematic review found the following potential benefits from CDDP added to conversional therapy in AMI patients: reduction of cardiac death and heart failure, improvement of QOL and LVEF. However, the benefits should be considered due to the poor quality of evidence. In addition, the safety of CDDP has not been confirmed for the deficiency of available studies. More high quality evidence from high quality RCTs is needed to support the clinical use of CDDP for AMI patients.

References

[1] White HD, Chew DP. Acute myocardial infarction. The

Lancet, 2008,372(9638):570-584.

[2] Libby P. Current concepts of the pathogenesis of the acute coronary syndromes. Circulation, 2001,104(3):365-372.

[3] Ma XJ, Yin HJ, Chen KJ. Appraisal of the prognosis in patients with acute myocardial infarction treated with primary percutaneous coronary intervention. Chinese Journal of Integrative Medicine, 2009,15(3): 236-240.

[4] Chen KJ, Hui KK, Lee MS. The potential benefit of complementary/alternative medicine in cardiovascular diseases. Evidence-Based Complementary and Alternative Medicine, 2012, 2012, Article ID 125029,1 page.

[5] Dobos G, Tao I. The model of Western integrative medicine: the role of Chinese medicine. Chinese Journal of Integrative Medicine, 2011,17(1):11-20.

[6] Ferreira AS, Lopes AJ. Chinese medicine pattern differentiation and its implications for clinical practice. Chinese Journal of Integrative Medicine, 2011,17(11):818-823.

[7] Xu H, Chen KJ. Integrating traditional medicine with biomedicine towards a patient-centered healthcare system. Chinese Journal of Integrative Medicine, 2011,17 (2) :83-84.

[8] Chen KJ, Lu AP. Situation of integrative medicine in China: results from a National Survey in 2004. Chinese Journal of Integrative Medicine, 2006, 12 (3): 161-165.

[9] O' Brien KA, Ling SH, Abbas E et al. A Chinese herbal preparation containing radix salviae miltiorrhizae, radix notoginseng and borneolum syntheticum reduces circulating adhesion molecules. Evidence-based Complementary and Alternative Medicine, 2011,Article ID 790784.

[10] Ji XY, Tan BKX, Zhu ZY. Salvia miltiorrhiza and ischemic diseases. Acta Pharmacologica Sinica, 2000, 21 (12): 1089-1094.

[11] Wing-Shing CD, Koon CM, Ng CF,et al. The roots of Salvia miltiorrhiza (Danshen) and Pueraria lobata (Gegen) inhibit atherogenic events: a study of the combination effects of the 2-herb formula. Journal of Ethnopharmacology, 2012, 143 (3): 859-866.

[12] Leng J, Fu CM, Wan F. Research progress on chemical compositions and pharmacological effects of panaxatriol saponins. West China Journal of Harmaceutical Sciences, 2011, 26 (1): 83-86.

[13] Yang ZG, Chen AQ, Yu SD. Research progress of pharmacological actions of Panax notoginseng. Shanghai Journal of Traditional Chinese Medicine, 2005, 39(4): 59-62.

[14] Wu SR, Cheng G, Feng Y. Progress in studies on pharmacology of borneol. Chinese Traditional and Herbal Drugs, 2001, 32 (12): 90-92.

[15] Liu Y, Zhang BL, Hu LM. General view on pharmacological research of borneol. Tianjin Journal of Traditional Chinese Medicine, 2003, 20 (4): 85-87.

[16] Lu Y, Jia MJ. Pharmacological and clinical research of Compound Danshen Dropping Pill in coronary heart disease. Chinese Heart Journal,2000, 12 (5): 418-419.

[17] Sun J, Huang SH, Tan BKH,et al. Effects of purified herbal extract of Salvia miltiorrhiza on ischemic rat myocardium after acute myocardial infarction. Life Sciences, 2005. 76 (24): 2849-2860.

[18] Ji X, Tan BKH, Zhu YC, et al. Comparison of cardioprotective effects using ramipril and DanShen for the treatment of acute myocardial infarction in Rats. Life Sciences,2003, 73 (11): 1413-1426.

[19] Li GP, Zheng XT, Wang HZ,et al. Multicenter investigation of Compound Danshen Dripping Pills on short-term clinical events in patient with ST elevation myocardial infarction undergoing primary PCI, (MICD-STEMIPCI). Chinese Journal of Interventional Cardiology, 2011, 19 (1): 24-28.

[20] Guo HY, Lin SF, Kang XZ. Effects of Compound Danshen Dripping Pills on reperfusion injury after intravenous thrombolytic therapy in acutemyocardial infarction. Journal of Chinese Physician, 2010, 38 (7): 49-50.

[21] Xu H, Wang J. Effects of Compound Danshen Dripping Pill on survival rate of patients with acute myocardial infarction. Proceeding of Clinical Medicine, 2007, 6 (6): 429-430.

[22] Guo YM, Zhang C, Cha QL, e t al. Compound Salvia Droplet Pill for treatment of coronary heart disease: a systematic review. Journal of Shanghai University of Traditional Chinese Medicine, 2012, 26 (3): 24-31.

[23] Zhang J, Zhang MZ, Wang L. The systematic review of compoud Danshen dripping pills in treatment of coronary heart disease. Chinese Journal of New Drugs, 2009, 18 (6): 465-468.

[24] Chen W, Qin LM, Liu ZH, et al. The systematic review of Compound Danshen Dropping Pills in treatment

of stable angina pectoris. Journal of Shandong University of Traditional Chinese Medicine, 2012, 36 (4): 287-291.

[25] Chinese Society of Cardiology of Chinese Medical Association and Editorial Board of Chinese Journal of Cardiology. Guideline for the diagnosis and treatment of patients with acute myocardial infarction. Chinese Journal of Cardiology, 2001, 29 (12): 9-24.

[26] Braunwald E, Antman EM, Beasley JW, et al. ACC/AHA guidelines for the management of patients with unstable angina and non-ST-segment levationmyocardial infarction: executive summary and recommendations: a report of the American College of Cardiology/American Heart Association task force on practice guidelines (committee on the management of patients with unstable angina). Circulation, 2000,102 (10): 1193-1209.

[27] Chinese Society of Cardiology of Chinese Medical Association and Editorial Board of Chinese Journal of Cardiology. Guideline for diagnosis and treatment of patientswith unstable angina and non-ST-segment elevation myocardial infarction. Chinese Journal of Cardiology, 2007,3 5 (4): 295-304.

[28] Chinese Society of Cardiology of Chinese Medical Association and Editorial Board of Chinese Journal of Cardiology. Recommendation of the application of universal definition of myocardial infarction in China. Chinese Journal of Cardiology, 2008, 36 (10): 867-869.

[29] Chinese Society of Cardiology of Chinese Medical Association and Editorial Board of Chinese Journal of Cardiology. Guideline for diagnosis and treatment of patients with ST-elevation myocardial infarction. Chinese Journal of Cardiology, 2010, 38 (8): 675-687.

[30] Higgins JPT, Green S. Cochrane Handbook for Systematic Reviews of Interventions, Version 5.1.0, The Cochrane Collaboration, 2011, http://handbook. cochrane.org/.

[31] Brozek J, Oxman A, H. Schünemann. GRADEpro. [Computer program]. Version 3.2 for Windows." 2008,http://ims.cochrane. org/revman/other-resources/gradepro.

[32] Higgins JPT, Thompson SG, Deeks JJ. Measuring inconsistency in meta-analyses. British Medical Journal, 2003, 327 (7414): 557-560.

[33] Lin XD. Clinical trial of Compound Danshen Dripping Pill on ventricular remodeling after acute myocardial infarction.World Chinese Medicine, 2011, 6 (2): 111-112.

[34] Mei FG, Zhang YQ, Wang ZL, et al. Effects of Compound Danshen Dripping Pill on BNP and left ventricular function in patients with acute myocardial infarction. Heilongjiang Journal of Traditional Chinese Medicine, 2006, 6:4-6.

[35] Ma YM.Relationship between serum level of tumor necrosis factor-alpha, matrix metalloproteinase-9 and interleukin-6 and clinical prognosis and the effects of Compound Danshen Dripping Pill on STEMI. Tianjin Medical University, Tianjin, China, 2010.

[36] Li XF, Liu F, Jiang TL, et al. Efficacy of compound Danshen Drop Pill 42 patients with early acute myocardial infarction. Chinese Journal of New Drugs, 2010, 19 (18): 1699-1702.

[37] Schulz KF, Altman DG, Moher D. CONSORT 2010 statement: updated guidelines for reporting parallel group randomized trials. Annals of Internal Medicine, 2010, 152 (11): 726-732.

[38] Gagnier JJ, Boon H, Rochon P, et al. Reporting randomized, controlled trials of herbal interventions: an elaborated CONSORT statement. Annals of Internal Medicine, 2006, 144 (5): 364-367.

第七章

Chronic Intermittent Hypoxia and Hypertension: A Review of Systemic Inflammation and Chinese Medicine[*]

WU Chun-xiao LIU Yue ZHANG Jing-chun

Obstructive sleep apnea syndrome (OSAS) is a common disease, affecting about 2%-4% of the general population and characterized by repetitive upper airway collapse, frequent arousals and sleep disruption[1]. Data convincingly show a high correlation between OSAS and cardiovascular disorders such as hypertension, coronary artery disease, arrhythmia and stroke [2]. Great strides have been made in establishing OSAS as an independent risk factor for hypertension[3]. The high correlation between OSAS and hypertension was first discovered in the 1970s; scholars reported an improvement in blood pressure (BP) after surgical intervention for a variety of sleep disorder-related breathing problems[4-6]. In the past several decades, a number of studies have found a relationship between OSAS and hypertension. Additionally, hypertension has been observed in 40% of OSAS patients. Meanwhile, OSAS is found in 30%-40% of patients with hypertension. These results indicate that OSAS and hypertension are intimately related [7]. However, the mechanism of OSAS-related hypertension remains unclear. Because of upper airway obstruction, disordered breathing events lead to the intermittent occurrence of hypoxia throughout the sleep period. This phenomenon is called chronic intermittent hypoxia (CIH) [8]. CIH is different from continuous hypoxia. The former is distinguished by periods of low oxygen between periods of normal oxygen. However, both of them independently lead to inflammation. While the underlying mechanisms of OSAS-related hypertension are poorly understood, systemic inflammation may play a key role in the process.

Indeed, the circulating levels of C-reactive protein (CRP), tumor necrosis factor-α (TNF-α), interleukin (IL) -6 and IL-8 are elevated in patients with OSAS[9-12], suggesting that CIH may be pivotal in systemic inflammation. Inflammation has been receiving a fair amount of attention as the etiology for the initiation and progression of hypertension. In brief, endothelial dysfunction develops at an early stage in response to the afore-mentioned inflammatory cytokines. This process leads to the up-regulation of intercellular adhesion molecules, which promote leukocyte adherence to and extravasation into the endothelium [13]. This is a potential mechanism leading to hypertension.

Few studies have evaluated the potential interactions among OSAS, hypertension and systemic inflammation in the development of these disorders. The objectives of this paper are, first, to review the correlation between systemic inflammation caused by CIH and the pathogenesis of hypertension, including biochemical/molecular mechanisms; and second, to review the progress of interventions with Chinese medicine in treating OSAS-hypertension. CM interventions could provide a useful alternative treatment to prevent cardiovascular complications after hypertension.

* 原载于 Chinese Journal of Integrative Medicine, 2013, 19 (5): 394-400

1. CIH and Inflammatory Activation Pathways

1.1 CIH and Nuclear Factor-Kappa B

Recent studies exploring the relationship between hypertension and OSAS have focused on the role of the transcription factor nuclear factor-kappa B (NF-κB). Many studies have revealed the complex regulation by NF-κB of genes involved in cell growth, survival, and division, as well as in apoptosis, stress, hypoxia, and the immune system [14-16]. CIH increases the expression of NF-κB, which then up-regulates the expression of inflammatory factors, including chemokines, adhesion molecules, cytokines, nitric oxide synthase, tissue factor and blood coagulation factor Ⅷ [17]. Ryan, et al[18] found higher NF-κB expression in intermittent hypoxia (IH) mice, in accordance with recent studies showing NF-κB activation in cardiovascular tissue from hypoxic mice[17] and in cells cultured under IH [19]. IH-induced NF-kB activation could underlie the inflammatory alterations in OSAS patients.

IH-induced activation of NF-κB could also improve the survival rate of polymorphonuclear neutrophils (PMNs) [20]. The long-term presence of a growing number of PMNs may lead to hypertension by causing endothelial dysfunction. After apoptosis, PMNs are unresponsive to inflammatory stimuli. Simultaneously, apoptosis improves the clearance of PMNs from the blood [21,22]. Apoptosis is thus considered a fundamental mechanism for halting inflammation.

NF-κB can provide a strong anti-apoptotic signal in PMNs [23]. The up-regulation of NF-κB under CIH, which suppresses PMN apoptosis, was confirmed by using the NF-κB inhibitors-gliotoxin[24] and parthenolid [25,26]. Interestingly, parthenolid has been shown to increase apoptosis only in PMNs exposed to CIH and it did not affect the apoptosis of PMNs under normoxia [27]. NF-κB is clearly implicated in the survival of PMNs under CIH conditions.

Expression of the downstream survival gene IL-8, induced by NF-κB, may activate the inflammatory pathways [20]. CIH induces the activation of NF-κB p65, after which levels of Bcl-2 and IL-8 are elevated, and PMN apoptosis is suppressed. IL-8, one of the most important survival cytokines [28,29], has been shown to increase PMN survival [30,31]. IL-8 transduces its signals through interactions with chemokine receptors (CXCR) 1 and 2 [32]. The expression of CXCR2 is down-regulated during PMN apoptosis, and up-regulation of CXCR2 during activation protects PMNs from apoptosis [30,33]. CIH-induced expression of IL-8 thus parallels the up-regulation of CXCR2 expression and increased PMN survival.

1.2 CIH and p38 Mitogen-activated Protein Kinase

P38 mitogen-activated protein kinase (MAPK) belongs to a serine/threonine kinase family that is involved in a variety of cellular stress responses[34]. P38 MAPK was reported to increase the number of PMNs[35] and to improve PMN survival under continuous hypoxi [36]. Furthermore, a study by Dyugovskaya[37] found that the anti-PMN-apoptosis role of p38 MAPK signaling pathways is more significant under IH than under normoxia. The question arises whether p38 MAPK and NF-κB result in the same ongoing inflammatory response. Therefore, the possibility of p38 MAPK elevating the number of PMNs through interactions with NF-κB and TNF-α is discussed follow.

Further connecting p38 MAPK and NF-κB, p38 MAPK plays an important role in the IH-induced activation of NF-κB. The p38 MAPK inhibitor SB203580 increased apoptosis and decreased NF-κB expression, and using siRNA to degrade p38 MAPK can significantly attenuate the IH-induced activation of NF-κB [38].

Furthermore, important interactions occur between p38 MAPK and TNF-α in the development of inflammation. TNF-α-stimulated PMN survival is entirely IL-8-dependent [29], but the expression of IL-8 requires p38 MAPK [21].

Exposure of PMNs to TNF-α results in phosphorylation of IκBα, which leads to the activation of NF-κB. It is widely accepted that two main TNF-α receptors are involved in PMN apoptosis: TNF receptor 1 (TNFR1) and TNFR2. Both independently mediate the activation of NF-κB, thereby promoting PMN survival [39,40]. Together, these results suggest that CIH, and therefore TNF-α, suppress PMN apoptosis [41].

2. CIH and Oxidative Stress

Oxidative stress and inflammation have a close relationship: each appears capable of triggering the other. Under normal conditions, oxidizing agents and endogenous anti-oxidants maintain a balanced state. Once this homeostasis is disrupted, cell damage and inflammatory responses follow because of an increasingly oxidative environment [42,43].

Is there an increased incidence of oxidative stress in CIH? Though scholars have demonstrated that inflammation can be activated by oxidative stress, the molecular events upstream of the oxidative stress biomarkers remain unknown. The only mechanism discovered so far is that reactive oxygen species (ROS) are produced by a protein enzyme called xanthine oxidase [44]. Studies have shown that CIH contributes to an increase in oxidative stress markers, providing strong reasons to explore the activation of oxidative stress combined with CIH in the pathophysiology of OSAS. Discussions of clinical trials, animal experiments and treatments affecting oxidative stress follow.

Currently, small-scale clinical studies have proved that systemic oxidative stress is enhanced in OSAS patients [45-47]. Oxidative stress biomarkers, such as advanced oxidation protein products, ferric reducing antioxidant power, superoxide radicals, serum nitrate and nitrite levels, are significantly different between OSAS patients and matched controls [48]. Serious OSAS patients even appear to have decreased resistance to oxidation [46].

Sleep-disordered breathing is related to many other factors, such as obesity, awakening stimuli and sympathetic nervous system problems, all of which promote oxidative stress [49]. If CIH really plays a key role in the oxidative stress response, increases in oxidative stress markers would also be expected among animal models of hypoxia. Xu, et al [50]. found increased levels of protein oxidation, lipid peroxidation and nucleic acid oxidation in hypoxic mouse brain cortex. Liu, et al. and Nair, et al. exposed mice to an IH environment, and observed a significant elevation in superoxide dehydrogenase activity and nicotinamide adenine dinucleotide phosphate oxidase [51,52].

Many studies have shown that continuous positive airway pressure (CPAP) treatment, for either a long or a short time, can relieve oxidative stress [53-55]; the production of oxidative stress markers, including asymmetrical dimethylarginine, lipid peroxide, superoxide dismutase and thiobarbituric acid reactive substances [56], is inhibited by this OSAS treatment. Del, et al [57]. observed 138 OSAS patients and found that oxidative stress markers were reversed after CPAP treatment for 6 months. Together, these findings suggest an important inhibitory role of CPAP in oxidative stress caused by CIH.

3. Chinese Medicine Interventions: Clinical and Experimental Evidence

The Chinese medicines (CM) ligustrazine, rauwolfia and kudzu vine have been shown to reverse hypertension and improve related symptoms [58]. There is evidence of CM reversing endothelial injury. Repairing endothelial damage also has antihypertensive effects [59]. This has led to investigations designed to clarify whether CM interventions can protect endothelial function and reduce BP by blocking the activation of proinflammatory pathways. Is it possible for CM to make an impact on inflammatory processes? Could this propensity of inflammatory mediators to induce endothelial injury and hypertension be decreased by CM treatment? Some clinical trials found that the production and migration of inflammatory mediators, including NF-κB, TNF-α, high-sensitive (hs) -CRP and IL-6，are favorably modified by treatment with herbal preparations[60,61].

NF-κB is a central activating factor of the inflammatory cascade. Thus, research has been undertaken to investigate whether CM antihypertensive agents reduce NF-κB levels. Zhang, et al[62] used different concentrations of astragalus polysaccharide (APS) to affect the lipopolysaccharide (LPS) -induced activation of NF-κB in human umbilical venous endothelial cells. LPS-induced I-κBa mRNA degradation was significantly inhibited by APS, leading to inhibition of NF-κB in a dose-dependent manner. Sun, et al[60]. explored the effects of puerarin on NF-κB expression in kidneys of spontaneously hypertensive rats (SHR) by dividing 24 SHR into three groups：control group, puerarin group and benazepril group. Results showed that NF-κB was expressed by SHR, and NF-κB expression decreased remarkably in the benazepril group and puerarin group compared with the control group. Puerarin significantly inhibited NF-κB.

A common inflammatory marker, high-sensitivity hs-CRP, has been considered one of the risk factors for cardiovascular disease in recent years by the European hypertension guidelines[63]. A variety of CM preparations can reduce hs-CRP, including Xuezhikang Capsule[61], Qingxuan Tiaoya Recipe (清眩调压方) [64], and calming Liver and restraining Yang formula[65]. These treatments showed favorable effects in depressing blood pressure and decreasing the hs-CRP levels in patients.

The level of hs-CRP has been reported to be increased significantly in cases of excess syndrome combined with deficiency syndrome compared with cases of deficiency syndrome[66]. The hs-CRP level was statistically higher in yin deficiency and overwhelming yang patients than in yin and yang deficiency or overwhelming

liver fire patients[67,68]. Furthermore, a small-scale randomized clinical trial showed that Jiangya Capsule (降压胶囊), a CM preparations having the efficacy of calming Liver yang) could improve the blood pressure and control the increase in serum hs-CRP in hypertensive patients[69].

As noted above, CM interventions reversed hypertension and inflammation, but the mechanism by which they act is unclear. However, an excess accumulation of blood stasis or a hyperactivity of yang and phlegm may indicate a higher risk of hypertension and other cardiovascular events[70]. Phlegm and stasis was positively correlated with IL-6 and hs-CRP levels[71]. These findings imply that CM solved the pathological factors and the corresponding inflammatory factors were also suppressed. Wang, et al[72]. divided 60 hypertension patients into excessive accumulation of phlegm dampness type cases and non-excessive accumulation of phlegm dampness type cases. The former patients received Tanreqing Injection (痰热清注射液) plus telmisartan and the latter cases received telmisartan only. Six weeks later, compared with control patients, the levels of hs-CRP, TNF-α and IL-6 were significantly increased in hypertensive patients. After treatment, levels of the three inflammatory factors aforementioned were significantly reduced in the excessive accumulation of phlegm dampness group.

Overall, the data indicate that CM reduced BP and inhibited NF-κB, TNF-α and IL-6. These findings imply that CM interventions are more effective than Western medicine in improving the inflammatory response in patients with hypertension. CM treatment against hypertension was also shown to improve the apnea hypopnea index (AHI) of OSAS patients[73]. Together, these results strengthen the need for early CM intervention in apneic individuals at risk for hypertension, and suggest new therapeutic options for these patients.

4. Conclusions and Perspectives

Despite the high correlation between OSAS and hypertension, little evidence is available regarding their pathophysiological and clinical outcomes. Most information involves cross-sectional analyses of selected clinical cohorts and there are no long-term follow-up studies. Future research into the relationship between CIH and hypertension needs to include matched control subjects, more consistent definitions and stricter criteria for outcomes. The finding that CIH-induced hypertension mainly involves systemic inflammation needs to be confirmed.

Although there is evidence in CIH and hypertension of overlapping mechanisms involving inflammation, oxidative stress and leukocyte dysfunction, there may be differences in the magnitude and consequences of these responses. Furthermore, the role of inflammatory markers in predicting hypertension in OSAS is unclear and lacks longterm prospective studies. If systemic inflammation is important in CIH and hypertension, studies in overlapping patients should provide insights regarding the nature and significance of these responses. These findings are clinically relevant because systemic inflammation may contribute to the pathogenesis of hypertension, and the molecular pathways involved are similar in OSAS. Studies of patients with OSAS and hypertension should provide insights into the mechanisms of systemic inflammation and help to develop new therapies. Great strides have been made in establishing obstructive sleep apnea as a target for therapy in hypertensive patients. Additionally, CM interventions have shown some advantages in controlling OSAS-related hypertension. In the future, based on the relationship between CIH, inflammation and hypertension, further clinical and animal experimental studies of integrative medicine will be needed to offer high quality evidence for the prevention and control of OSAS-related hypertension.

References

[1] Young T, Palta M, Dempsey J, et al. The occurrence of sleep-disordered breathing among middle-aged adults. N Engl J Med, 1993, 328: 1230-1235.

[2] Parish JM, Somers VK. Obstructive sleep apnea and cardiovascular disease. Mayo Clin Proc, 2004, 79: 1036-1046.

[3] Manciag, De Backerg, Dominiczak A, et al. 2007 Guidelines for the management of arterial hypertension: the Task Force for the Management of Arterial Hypertension of the European Society of Hypertension (ESH) and of the European Society of Cardiology (ESC). Eur Heart J, 2007, 28: 1462-1536.

[4] Lugaresi E, Coccagna, G, Mantovani M, et al. Effects of tracheostomy in two cases of hypersomnia with periodic breathing. J Neurol Neurosurg Psychiatry, 1973, 36: 15-26.

[5] Coccagna G, Mantovani M, Brignani F, et al. Tracheostomy in hypersomnia with periodic breathing. Bull Physiopathol Respir (Nancy), 1972, 8: 1217-1227.

[6] Motta J, Guilleminault C, Schroeder JS, et al. Tracheostomy and hemodynamic changes in sleep-inducing apnea. Ann Intern Med, 1978, 89: 454-458.

[7] Das AM, Khayat R. Hypertension in obstructive sleep apnea: risk and therapy. Expert Rev Cardiovasc Ther, 2009, 7: 619-626.

[8] Adedayo AM, Olafiranye O, Smith D, et al. Obstructive sleep apnea and dyslipidemia: evidence and underlying mechanism. Sleep Breath, 2012, Aug 18. [Epub ahead of print]

[9] Karamanli H, Ozol D, Ugur KS, et al. Influence of CPAP treatment on airway and systemic inflammation in OSAS patients. Sleep Breath 2012, Sep 4. [Epub ahead of print]

[10] Svensson M, Venge P, Janson C, et al. Relationship between sleep-disordered breathing and markers of systemic inflammation in women from the general population. J Sleep Res, 2012, 21: 147-154.

[11] Kaviraj B, Bai SC, Su L, et al. Effect of obstructive sleep apnea syndrome on serum C-reactive protein level, left atrial size and premature atrial contraction. J Southern Med Univ, 2011, 31: 197-200.

[12] Chen J, Zhang JC, Chen YY. Relationship between hs-CRP and obstructive sleep apnea in hypertension patients. Chin J Integr Med Cardio-/Cerebrovascular Dis, 2012, 3: 280-282.

[13] McNicholas WT. Chronic obstructive pulmonary

disease and obstructive sleep apnea: overlaps in pathophysiology, systemic inflammation, and cardiovascular disease. Am J Respir Crit Care Med, 2009, 180: 692-700.

[14] Rauch DA, L Ratner. Targeting HTLV-1 activation of NF-kappa B in mouse models and ATLL patients. Viruses, 2011, 3: 886-900.

[15] Barnes PJ. Pathophysiology of allergic inflammation. Immunol Rev, 2011, 242: 31-50.

[16] Dejean E, Foisseau M, Lagarrigue F, et al. ALK+ALCLs induce cutaneous, HMGB-1-dependent IL-8/CXCL8 production by keratinocytes through NF-kappa B activation. Blood, 2012, 119: 4698-4707.

[17] Greenberg H, Ye X, Wilson D, et al. Chronic intermittent hypoxia activates nuclear factor-kappa B in cardiovascular tissues in vivo. Biochem Biophys Res Commun, 2006, 343, 591-596.

[18] Ryan S, Taylor CT, McNicholas WT. Selective activation of inflammatory pathways by intermittent hypoxia in obstructive sleep apnea syndrome. Circulation, 2005, 112: 2660-2667.

[19] Li S, Qian XH, Zhou W, et al. Time-dependent inflammatory factor production and NF-kappa B activation in a rodent model of intermittent hypoxia. Swiss Med Wkly, 2011, 14: w13309.

[20] Walmsley SR, Print C, Farahi N, et al. Hypoxia-induced neutrophil survival is mediated by HIF-1 alpha-dependent NF-kappaB activity. J Exp Med, 2005, 201: 105-115.

[21] Dunican AL, Leuenroth SJ, Grutkoski P, et al. TNF alpha-induced suppression of PMN apoptosis is mediated through interleukin-8 production. Shock, 2000, 14: 284-289.

[22] Maianski AN, Kuijpers TW, Roos D. Apoptosis of neutrophils. Acta Haematol, 2004, 111: 56-66.

[23] Ward C, Walker A, Dransfield I. Regulation of granulocyte apoptosis by NF-kappa B. Biochem Soc Trans, 2004, 32: 465-467.

[24] Pahl HL, Krauss B, Schulze-Osthoff K. The immunosuppressive fungal metabolite gliotoxin specifically inhibits transcription factor NF-kappa B. J Exp Med, 1996, 183: 1829-1840.

[25] Magni P, Ruscica M, Dozio E, et al. Parthenolide inhibits the LPS-induced secretion of IL-6 and TNF-alpha and NF-kappa B nuclear translocation in BV-2 microglia. Phytother Res, 2012, 1405-1409.

[26] Dyugovskaya L, Polyakov A, Ginsberg D, et al. Molecular pathways of spontaneous and TNF (alpha)-mediated neutrophil apoptosis under intermittent hypoxia. Am J Respir Cell Mol Biol, 2011, 45: 154-162.

[27] Hehner SP, Hofmann TG, Droge W. The antiinflammatory sesquiterpene lactone parthenolide inhibits NF-kappa B by targeting the I kappa B kinase complex. J Immunol, 1999, 163: 5617-5623.

[28] Luo HR, Loison F. Constitutive neutrophil apoptosis: mechanisms and regulation. Am J Hematol, 2008, 83: 288-295.

[29] Cowburn AS, Deighton J, Walmsley SR, et al. The survival effect of TNF-alpha in human neutrophils is mediated via NF-kappa B-dependent IL-8 release. Eur J Immunol, 2004, 34: 1733-1743.

[30] Glynn PC, Henney E, Hall IP. The selective CXCR2 antagonist SB272844 blocks interleukin-8 and growth-related oncogene-alpha-mediated inhibition of spontaneous neutrophil apoptosis. Pulm Pharmacol Ther, 2002, 15: 103-110.

[31] Acorci MJ, Dias-Melicio LA, Golim MA. Inhibition of human neutrophil apoptosis by Paracoccidioides brasiliensis: role of interleukin-8. Scand J Immunol, 2009, 69: 73-79.

[32] Javor J, Bucova M, Cervenova O, et al. Genetic variations of interleukin-8, CXCR1 and CXCR2 genes and risk of acute pyelonephritis in children. Int J Immunogenet, 2012, 39: 338-345.

[33] Allegretti M, Bertini R, Cesta MC, et al. V2-Arylpropionic CXC chemokine receptor 1 (CXCR1) ligands as novel noncompetitive CXCL8 inhibitors. J Med Chem, 2005, 48: 4312-4331.

[34] Alvarado-Kristensson M, Melander F, Leandersson K, et al. p38-MAPK signals survival by phosphorylation of caspase-8 and caspase-3 in human neutrophils. J Exp Med, 2004, 199: 449-458.

[35] Villunger A, O'Reilly LA, Holler N, et al. Fas ligand, Bcl-2, granulocyte colony-stimulating factor, and p38 mitogen-activated protein kinase: regulators of distinct cell death and survival pathways ingranulocytes. J Exp Med, 2000, 192: 647-658.

[36] Leuenroth SJ, Grutkoski PS, Ayala A, et al. Suppression of PMN apoptosis by hypoxia is dependent on Mcl-1 and MAPK activity. Surgery, 2000, 128: 171-177.

[37] Dyugovskaya L, Polyakov A, Lavie P, et al. Delayed neutrophil apoptosis in patients with sleep apnea. Am J Respir Crit Care Med, 2008, 177: 544-554.

[38] Ryan S, McNicholas WT, Taylor CT. A critical role

for p38 map kinase in NF-kappa B signaling during intermittent hypoxia/reoxygenation. Biochem Biophys Res Commun, 2007, 355: 728-733.

[39] Murray J, Barbara JA, Dunkley SA, et al. Regulation of neutrophil apoptosis by tumor necrosis factor-alpha: requirement for TNFR55 and TNFR75 for induction of apoptosis in vitro. Blood, 1997, 90: 2772-2783.

[40] Cabrini M, K Nahmod, Jgeffner. New insights into the mechanisms controlling neutrophil survival. Curr Opin Hematol, 2010, 17: 31-35.

[41] Kilpatrick LE, Sun S, Mackie D, et al. Regulation of TNF mediated antiapoptotic signaling in human neutrophils: role of delta-PKC and ERK1/2. J Leukoc Biol, 2006, 80: 1512-21.

[42] Chen SJ, Yen CH, Huang YC, et al. Relationships between inflammation, adiponectin, and oxidative stress in metabolic syndrome. PLoS One, 2012, 7: e45693.

[43] Sesti F, Tsitsilonis OE, Kotsinas A, et al. Oxidative stress-mediated biomolecular damage and inflammation in tumorigenesis. In Vivo, 2012, 26: 395-402.

[44] Murata M, Fukushima K, Takao T, et al. Oxidative stress produced by xanthine oxidase induces apoptosis in human extravillous trophoblast cells. J Reprod Dev, 2012, Sep 14. [Epub ahead of print].

[45] Baysal E, Taysi S, Aksoy N, et al. Serum paraoxonase, arylesterase activity and oxidative status in patients with obstructive sleep apnea syndrome (OSAS). Eur Rev Med Pharmacol Sci, 2012, 16: 770-774.

[46] Simiakakis M, Kapsimalis F, Chaligiannis E, et al. Lack of effect of sleep apnea on oxidative stress in obstructive sleep apnea syndrome (OSAS) patients. PLoS One, 2012, 7: e39172.

[47] Ntalapascha M, Makris D, Kyparos A, et al. Oxidative stress in patients with obstructive sleep apnea syndrome. Sleep Breath, 2012, May 18. [Epub ahead of print].

[48] Mancuso M, Bonanni E, LoGerfo A, et al. Oxidative stress biomarkers in patients with untreated obstructive sleep apnea syndrome. Sleep Med, 2012, 13: 632-636.

[49] Williams A, Scharf SM. Obstructive sleep apnea, cardiovascular disease, and inflammation—is NF-kappa B the key? Sleep Breath, 2007, 11: 69-76.

[50] Xu W, Chi L, Row BW, et al. Increased oxidative stress is associated with chronic intermittent hypoxia-mediated brain cortical neuronal cell apoptosis in a mouse model of sleep apnea. Neuroscience, 2004, 126: 313-323.

[51] Liu JN, Zhang JX, Lu G, et al. The effect of oxidative stress in myocardial cell injury in mice exposed to chronic intermittent hypoxia. Chin Med J, 2010, 123: 74-78.

[52] Nair D, Dayyat EA, Zhang SX, et al. Intermittent hypoxia-induced cognitive deficits are mediated by NADPH oxidase activity in a murine model of sleep apnea. PLoS One, 2011, 6: e19847.

[53] Barcelo A, Miralles C, Barbe F, et al. Antioxidant status in patients with sleep apnoea and impact of continuous positive airway pressure treatment. Eur Respir J, 2006, 27: 756-760.

[54] Minoguchi K, Yokoe T, Tanaka A, et al. Association between lipid peroxidation and inflammation in obstructive sleep apnoea. Eur Respir J, 2006, 28: 378-385.

[55] Alzoghaibi MA, Bahammam AS. The effect of one night of continuous positive airway pressure therapy on oxidative stress and antioxidant defense in hypertensive patients with severe obstructive sleep apnea. Sleep Breath, 2012, 16: 499-504.

[56] Oyama J, Yamamoto H, Maeda T, et al. Continuous positive airway pressure therapy improves vascular dysfunction and decreases oxidative stress in patients with the metabolic syndrome and obstructive sleep apnea syndrome. Clin Cardiol, 2012, 35: 231-236.

[57] Del Ben M, Fabiani M, Loffredo L, et al. Oxidative stress mediated arterial dysfunction in patients with obstructive sleep apnoea and the effect of continuous positive airway pressure treatment. BMC Pulm Med, 2012, 12: 36.

[58] Liu LS, Chen MQ, Zeng GY, et al. A forty-year study on hypertension. Acta Acad Med Sini, 2002, 24: 401-408.

[59] Chen YY, Zhang JC. Research status of endothelial mechanism in high blood pressure of traditional Chinese and Western medicine. Chin Jgerontol, 2010, 30: 3010-3013.

[60] Sun WC, Zhou HP. The effects of puerarin on renal arterial NF-κB expression in spontaneous hypertensive rats. J Emerg Tradit Chin Med, 2008; 17: 965-966.

[61] Xiong IH, Wang M, Zhang RL, et al. Observation on the intervention efficacy of Xuezhikang Capsule on

levels of CRP and IL-6 in hypertension patients with different complications. Liaoning J of Tradit Chin Med, 2012, 39: 1337-1340.

[62] Zhang JZ, Chen LG, Hu XQ, et al. Influence of astragalus polysaccharide on the expression of Toll-like receptor 4 and nuclear transcription factor-κB in essential hypertension patients with blood stasis syndrome. J Traditi Chin Med, 2011, 52: 1286-1304.

[63] Whitworth JA. 2003 World Health Organization (WHO) / International Society of Hypertension (ISH) statement on management of hypertension. J Hypertens, 2003, 21: 1983-1992.

[64] Tao LL, Ma XC, Chen KJ. Clinical study on effect of Qingxuan Tiaoya Recipe in treating menopausal women with hypertension. Chin J Integr Tradit West Med, 2009, 8: 680-684.

[65] Zhong GW, Luo YH, Xiang LL, et al. Clinical efficacy study on calming Liver and restraining Yang formula in treating patients with mild or moderate degree of essential hypertension. Chin J Chin Mate Med, 2010, 35: 776-781.

[66] Suo HL, Wang SR, Wu AM, et al. Risk stratification of EH and correlation between TCM syndromes of EH and high-sensitivity C-reactive protein in clinic. J Beijing Univ Tradit Chin Med, 2009, 32: 265-269.

[67] Qing Y, Zhang ZZ, Yang LY. Connection between pattern of traditional Chinese medicine syndrome in primary hypertension and C-reactive protein. Jguangxi Tradit Chin Med Univ, 2008, 11: 18-19.

[68] Zhang ZB, Zhou CG, Lu S. Distribution of TCM syndrome types of essential hypertension and their relationship to biochemical indicators. Liaoning J Tradit Chin Med, 2010, 37: 969-971.

[69] Li H, Zhao WM, Han YX. Effect of a integrative medical regimen on levels of vascular endothelial function and hypersensitive C-reactive protein in elderly patients with isolated systolic hypertension. Chin J Integr Tradit West Med, 2009, 29: 115-119.

[70] Fu DY, Zu LH, Xin XY, et al. Analysis of cardiovascular vulnerable factors among 409 cases of EH patients with different pattrens of TCM. Univ Tradit Med Sin Pharmacol Shanghai, 2009；23: 15-18.

[71] Liu LL, Guo RJ, Zhang YL. Relationship between syndrome factor of hypertension and interleukin-6, highly sensitive C-reactive protein and matrix metalloproteinase-9. Chin J Tradit Chin Med Pharm, 2011, 26: 1583-1586.

[72] Wang X, Li WQ. The expression and the intervention of Tanreqing Injection of the pulse pressure and the levels of serum inflammatory factors in hypertensive patients of excessive accumulation of phlegm dampness type. J Emerg Tradit Chin Med, 2009, 18: 1389-1414.

[73] Zhang JC, Chen YY, Chen J, et al. The impact of Qingxuan Granule on endothelial function in hypertensive patients with and without obstructive sleep apnea. Chin J Gerontol, 2012, 23: 672-675.

Chinese Herb and Formulas for Promoting Blood Circulation and Removing Blood Stasis and Antiplatelet Therapies[*]

LIU Yue   YIN Hui-Jun   SHI Da-zhuo   CHEN Ke-ji

1. Introduction

Cardiovascular and cerebrovascular events have become the major killer of people's health and life all over the world. Rupture of atherosclerotic plaque in an artery wall and the

* 原载于 Evidence-Based Complementary and Alternative Medicine，2012，Article ID 184503

ensuing thrombotic events are the triggers for acute ischemic injury. Activated platelets play a pivotal role in the formation of pathogenic thrombi underlying acute clinical manifestations of vascular atherothrombotic disease. Oral antiplatelet drugs are a milestone in the therapy of cardiovascular atherothrombotic diseases and provide the primary and secondary prevention strategy to combat these diseases. Efficient antiplatelet therapy can make the death rates of heart disease and stroke decline by about 25% [1,2]. Commonly used oral antiplatelet drugs include cyclooxygenase inhibitor aspirin, the glycoprotein IIb/IIIa inhibitor ReoPro, and the P2Y12 inhibitor clopidogrel, et al. Many clinical studies show that dual antiplatelet therapy with aspirin and clopidogrel is currently the standard of drugs for prevention of adverse cardiovascular events in most patients at high risk owing to acute coronary syndromes or recent placement of a stent.

But along with prolonging of treatment by dual or triple antiplatelet drugs, the effectiveness and security have garnered particular attention in clinic. Despite their proven benefit, recurrent cardiovascular events still occur in those taking antiplatelet drugs. This has led to the concept of antiplatelet resistance [3], most commonly aspirin resistance as this drug is the cornerstone of most regimens. Although there are some debates on definition and mechanism of antiplatelet resistance [4,5], it cannot be denied that it has important clinical significance. At the same time, numerous adverse reactions including serious bleeding risk (digestive and nervous systems) and combination with PPIs and statin [6,7], which limit the clinical practice of antiplatelet drugs. So developed novel classes of antiplatelet agents possess high efficiency, and fewer adverse effects have been always the research focus for prevention of cardiovascular disease. Modern medicine and pharmacology has done a lot of valuable exploration, newer agents are in development recent years that include prasugrel, cangrelor, ticagrelor, and vorapaxar, et al[8].

Study on the blood stasis syndrome (BSS) and promoting blood circulation and removing blood stasis (PBCRBS) is the most active field of research of integration of traditional and western medicine in China. During the past 50 years, much significant progress has been made from theory, experiments to clinic fields based on the inherit, and innovation of thoughts in traditional Chinese medicine [9], to clarify the treatment regulations and principles of PBCRBS, which has already got consensus in medical community in China. A lot of formulas for PBCRBS (see Table 1) have showed great antiplatelet effect in clinic, and most of them are the Chinese patent drugs. On the prevention of atherosclerosis or vulnerable plaque, Chinese and Western medicine have the consensus that stabling plaque and promoting blood circulation. Based on the agreed thoughts of the Eastern and Western worlds, the application of Chinese herb and formulas for PBCRBS has valuable significance in the exploration of reducing the risk of cardiovascular event [10].

Blood-stasis syndrome has the status of platelet activation, and it has high correlation [11,12]. As early as the last century of 1970s, there were scholars who had made pilot study to observe the mechanism of Chinese herb and formulas for PBCRBS on platelet function [13]. BSS has the definite diagnostic criteria [14] from 1991 in China, and during the past 5 years, diagnosis criteria have improved by scholars [15] and keep pace with the development of TCM. There is a special focus on natural compounds present in dietary and medicinal plants exhibiting antiplatelet/ thrombotic properties. Now we know that platelet mainly was regulated by three kinds of substance, one kind is generated out of platelet such as catecholamine, collagen, thrombin, and prostacyclin; the second kind is generated from platelet and acts on the platelet membrane glycoproteins such as ADP, PGD2, PGE2, and 5-HT; the last kind is generated from platelet and acts on the platelet such as TXA2, cAMP, cGMP, and Ca^{2+}, et al. Some of these substances have

Table 1　The Ingredient of Frequently Used Formulas for Promoting Blood Circulation and Removing Blood Stasis

Names of formulas	Ingredients of formulas	Label
Xiongshao capsule	*Szechuan Lovage Rhizome*，*Red Paeony Root*	Chinese patent drug
Compound danshen dripping pills	*The root of red-rooted salvia*，*Panax Notoginseng*，*Borneol*	Chinese patent drug
Buyanghuanwu decoction	*Radix Astragali Bunge*，*Peach Seed*，*Safflower*，*Szechuan Lovage Rhizome*，*Angelica sinensis*，*Red Paeony Root*，*earthworm*	
Xuesaitong capsule	*Panax Notoginsenosides*	Chinese patent drug
Tongxinluo capsule	*Sanguisuge*，*Scorpio*，*centipede*，*ground beeltle*，*cicada slough*，*et al.*	Chinese patent drug
Danhong injection	*The root of red-rooted salvia*，*safflower*	Chinese patent drug
Taohongsiwu decoction	*Peach Seed*，*Safflower*，*Szechuan Lovage Rhizome*，*Angelica Sinensis*，*White Paeony Root*，*Radix Rehmanniae Praeparata*	
Xue Fu Zhu Yu decoction	*Hovenia dulcis*，*Radix Achyranthis Bidentatae*，*Peach Seed*，*Safflower*，*Szechuan Lovage Rhizome*，*Angelica sinensis*，*White Paeony Root*，*Radix Rehmanniae Praeparata*，*Radix Bupleuri*，*Platycodon Grandiflorum*，*et al.*	

been identified as effective target of antiplatelet. Owing to the many problems of effectiveness and security of current antiplatelet drugs, a great need now arises to develop both efficacious and pharmaceutical medicines to combat these diseases. Screening the highly efficiency and fewer adverse effects of antiplatelet drugs from Chinese herb and formulas for PBCRBS attracts great attention of researchers, and the study of target or mechanism of Chinese herb and formulas for PBCRBS to be the hot topic of research and development of antiplatelet drugs. It had been approved that antiplatelet mechanism of Chinese herb and formulas for PBCRBS involves the following aspects.

2. Antiplatelet Mechanism of Chinese Herb and Formulas of Promoting Blood Circulation and Removing Blood Stasis

2.1　Inhibition of Platelet Aggregation

Platelet aggregation means the clumping together of platelets in the blood, which is the main function of platelet and has key role in the physiological hemostasia and pathogenesis of atherothrombosis. Platelet activates when it adheres to breakage of vessel or has been induced by activator. Activated platelet membrane glycoprotein (GP) IIb/ IIIa exposes its fibrinogen receptor with the participation of Ca^{2+}, one fibrinogen can bind to at least two GP IIb/ IIIa at the same time, and platelet clump together with fibrinogen by GP IIb/ IIIa. The typical aggregation is induced by different activators, which included the following two aspects, one is chemical agents such as ADP, collagen, thrombin, AA, and PAF, et al.；the other is shear stress. It is now taken that platelet aggregation rate (PAR) is the evaluation criterion of the intensity. Born [16] designed the platelet aggregation analyzer in 1962 by the turbidimetry principle which to accelerate the understanding of platelet aggregation. Now PAR was considered as the marker of antiplatelet efficacy evaluation and was used intensively in medical research of platelet. Studies show that the vast majority of Chinese herb and formulas for PBCRBS such as *Xiongshao Capsule*[17], *Compound Danshen dripping pills*[18], *Buyanghuanwu Decoction*[19], *Xuesaitong Capsule* [20], *DaHuang Zhe Chong pill* [21], *and Tongxingluo Capsule* [22], et al. can reduce the PAR of patients or animal model of thromboembolic diseases significantly. Active principles such as ferulic acid[23], ligustrazine[24], propylgallate[25], resveratrol[26], curdione[27], Total flavone in Sanguis Draconis[28], Salvianolic acid B[29], Hirulog[30], and Safflower flavin[31] et al. can inhibit the platelet aggregation induced by AA, ADP, PAF, collagen, and thrombin to some extent, bringing out the superior antiplatelet effect.

2.2　Inhibition of Platelet Release Reaction

Platelet release reaction means that many substances stored in α-granules, densegranule, and lysosome in platelet are released out of platelet upon different activator. These substances including CD62p (P-selection), GP IIb/ IIIa compound, PKC, β-TG, PF-4, and Ca^{2+}, which has been considered as the usual evaluation indicator of screening the effective antiplatelet drug from Chinese herb and formulas for PBCRBS.

2.2.1　CD62P. CD62p (P-selection) is a 140 kD glycoprotein which is present in the granules of platelets and translocates rapidly to the cell surface after platelet activation and is generally considered to be the gold marker of platelet activation [32,33]. Clinical research indicates that the expression of CD62p increases markedly in the different types of cardiovascular patients (including patients with stable angina and ACS) [34-36] and has found high positive correlation between CD62p level and blood stasis syndrome (BSS) [37]. So making the increased expression of CD62p after platelet activation dropped is taken for the one of the antiplatelet mechanisms and scientific measurements of Chinese herb and formulas for PBCRBS. According to the current studies, *Danhong injection*[38], *Ligustrazine injection* [39], *Compound Danshen dripping pills*[40], *Taohongsiwu Decoction*[41], and *Tongxinluo capsule*[42] can reduce the CD62p expression after platelet activation significantly and inhibit platelet activation *in vivo,* to show satisfactory effect of antiplatelet.

2.2.2　GPII b/ IIIa Compound　The detection of PAC-1 is considered as the sensitive and important marker of platelet activation [43], PAC-1 is the specific monoclonal IgMK, which only

binds to activating platelet GPIIb/IIIa compound, while it has no recognition capability for resting one. The activation of GPIIb/IIIa depends on the platelet activation which makes the former change its configuration to have strong affinity with receptors. Using the flow cytometry to detect PAC-1 which has the characteristic of specific fast sensitive, and has splendid future in the study on screening antiplatelet drugs from Chinese herb and formulas for PBCRBS.

Da Huang Zhe Chong pill is the earliest formula of PBCRBS and is widely used for atherothrombotic disease treatment. Research shows that it has better antiplatelet aggregation ability than aspirin [44], the further study indicates that it can reduce the level of PAC-1 after ADP induced platelet activation and of patients with coronary heart disease and cerebral infarction in clinic, which also has superior antiplatelet activation than aspirin [21] and is an ideal antithrombotic drug. Other study [45] found that *Xue Fu Zhu Yu decoction* can inhibit the ADP-induced expression of GPIIb/IIIa compound significantly and restrain the ADP induced platelet activation, which provides experimental evidence to long-term treatment of coronary heart disease, and no symptoms of myocardial ischemia, et al.

2.2.3　PKC　Protein kinase C (PKC), a ubiquitous protein kinase found in a variety of animal tissues, has been implicated in the regulation of many cellular processes and plays a central role in signal transduction. In platelets, the PKC is an important signaling mediator required for activation, secretion of granule contents, and aggregation [46]. During the process of platelet activation, close relationship between translocation of PKC in platelet and platelet function has been found. PKC has both cytosolic and plasma membrane-bound forms, and the former is the most abundant under resting conditions. The cytosolic form can translocate to the plasma membrane upon cell stimulation and elevation of cellular Ca^{2+}, one particular and important aspect of PKC activation is the intracellular redistribution of the enzyme from the cytosol to the cell membrane [44]. Now translocation or redistribution of PKC from the cytosolic form to the plasma membrane can be taken for an indicator of PKC activation [47].

Resveratrol (*RESV*), a well-known polyphenolic compound of, was extracted from *Polygonum Cuspidatum*, which was a Chinese herb for PBCRBS and has been efficaciously used in traditional Chinese medicine to treat several diseases, including thromboembolic diseases for over hundreds of years. In recent years, pharmacological studies have found that RESV possesses multifaceted cardiovascular benefits, but the mechanism is not clear. Recent research[48] shows that PKC distributed mostly across the cytosol of platelets in resting platelets and redistributed to the membrane later to be activated by ADP. If pretreated by *RESV*, PKC translocation to the membrane was partially inhibited in the platelets activated by ADP. These results suggested that *RESV* inhibited the PKC-mediated signal transduction pathway in platelets, and it might act as an inhibitor on PKC activity in platelets and serve as a novel antithrombotic agent.

2.2.4 PF-4 and β-TG It is thought that PF-4 and β-TG are the specific indicators of platelet release reaction [49]. Both increases of PF-4 and β-TG indicate the height of platelet release reaction, which is common in thromboembolic disease and prethrombotic state. On the contrary, both decreases of PF-4 and β-TG indicate the suppression of platelet release reaction. β-TG can make the PGI_2 concentration and adenylate cyclase activity reduction, and then make cAMP decrease which bring about weak inhibition and enhance the aggregation of platelet [50,51]. PF-4 can reduce the anticoagulation of heparan sulphate in endothelial cell and enhance the metabolism of membrane phospholipid and AA, to produce TXA_2, also PF-4 can promote precipitation and polymerization of fibrin

monomer and accelerate platelet aggregation [52]. Research has found that *Salvia miltiorrhiza Bunge* injection [53] can reduce the PF-4 and β-TG concentration markedly to inhibit platelet aggregation.

2.2.5 Ca^{2+} Calcium ion plays a vital role in the development of platelet activation. The transformation, aggregation, and release reaction of platelet are triggered by the increase of free calcium ion concentration of platelet ($[Ca^{2+}]_i$), which is the essential mechanism of thrombosis [54]. Studies have found that the increase of $[Ca^{2+}]_i$ in patient with CHD, meanwhile calcium antagonist can reduce $[Ca^{2+}]_i$ of platelet accompanied by inhibiting platelet aggregation [55].

Studies [56] have indicated that some Chinese herbs, such as *Salvia Miltiorrhiza*, *Ligusticum wallichii Franch*, *Carthamus tinctorius*, *Radix Paeoniae Rubra*, and some active constituents as Ligustrazine (see Figure 1), Tanshinone ⅡA (see Figure 2), et al. have the certain effect of calcium channel antagonists and have good results of inhibit platelet aggregation and activation. Another research [57] shows that Safflor yellow

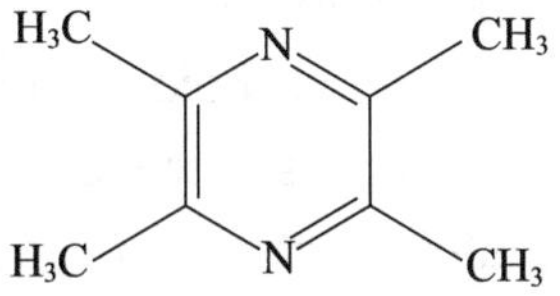

Figure 1   Chemical Structures of Ligustrazine

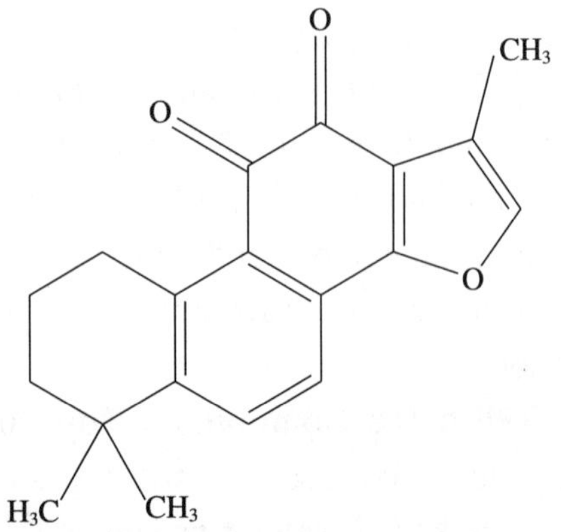

Figure 2   Chemical Structures of Tanshinone ⅡA

(a kind of soluble natural pigment of *Carthamus tinctorius*) can inhibit platelet release of 5-HT and Ca^{2+}, which has similar effect to Ginkgolides (admitted PAF receptor antagonist), which means that Safflor yellow might suppress the platelet activation via inhibition of PAF and calcium influx.

2.3　Influence of the Process of Platelet Metabolism

2.3.1　Influence of the Metabolic System of Arachidonic Acid (AA)　TXA_2 and PGI_2 are the metabolites of AA, which have the strong bioactivity of PG, and have a short halflife, quickly degrade to the TXB_2 and 6-keto-PGF1α, the latter make further metabolizes to the 6-keto-PGE.

It is now thought that many cardiovascular diseases such as atherosclerosis, thrombosis, coronary spasm, acute myocardial infarction, and hypertension have close relationship with the disequilibrium of TXA_2/PGI_2[58]. TXA_2, which is synthesized and released by platelet microsome and has the function of promoting platelet aggregation and thrombosis, is one of the strong inducers of platelet aggregation and vasoconstrictor. TXA_2 promotes the Ca^{2+} of density tube system free to make dense bodies contracting and releasing ADP and 5-HT, which result in platelet aggregation. PGI_2 is the main metabolite of AA and is the strong endogenous inhibitor of platelet aggregation；it has the function of antiplatelet aggregation and vasorelaxant and is considered as the vascular protection factor. Under normal physiological state, TXA_2 and PGI_2 have the balance condition and keep the platelet internal environment stable. Out of balance of TXA_2 and PGI_2 in plasma or tissue is one of the reasons of platelet aggregation, vasospasm, and thrombosis. Studies show that influence of TXA_2/PGI_2 has been closely related to antiplatelet mechanism of Chinese herb and formulas for PBCRBS, such as *Total saponins of paeonia*[59] can reduce the ADP-induced platelet maximum aggregation rate and plasma TXB_2 concentration, meanwhile, increase the plasma

6-keto-PGF1α concentration, which means it can promote the release of PGI_2, inhibit the produce of TXA_2, improve the balance of $TXA2/PGI_2$, and reach the aim of antithrombotic therapy. The same results have been found in the following drugs: *Guanxin* II[60], *Taohongsiwu Decoction*[61], *Notoginsenoside*[62], *salvianolic acid A*[63], *Honghua injection*[64], et al.

2.3.2　Influence of the Metabolic System of cAMP and cGMP　cAMP and cGMP in platelet are the second messengers of signal transmission, which make the different platelet activators acting on the specific receptor, then resulting in platelet aggregation and activation. Studies[65,66] show that drugs which make the level of cAMP and cGMP increase can inhibit platelet aggregation owing to promoting the intake of calcium ions, lowering the level of Ca^{2+}, and having close relation with the phosphorylation of myglobulin. So whether can affect the metabolic system of cAMP and cGMP has been taken as the main point of antiplatelet mechanism of Chinese herb and formulas for PBCRBS. Research[19] shows that *BuYang HuanWu decoctioncan* inhibit the ADP induced platelet aggregation and the decrease of cAMP and cGMP after the platelet aggregation, which suggested that its antiplatelet aggregation may be related to inhibiting the decrease of cyclic nucleotide in platelets after the aggregation. *Compound Danshen dripping pills*[67] and *pseudoginseng*[68] have the same mechanism of antiplatelet.

2.4　Influence of the Signal Transduction in Platelet

There is a series of signal transductions in platelet, which has close relationship with platelet activation. Upon agonist stimulation, specific receptor of membrane binds to the ligand to make the conformational changes and to activate the key enzymes action, which produces or releases the signal molecules and led to adhesion, aggregation, and reaction release to form thrombus at last. The mechanism of transmembrane signal transduction in platelet is unclear owing to more than one receptor bound by platelet agonist and the activated platelet release α-granules as secondary agonist to bring about amplification effect [69]. Platelet signal transduction pathway usually includes several aspects [70]: PI3-K pathway, PLC-β pathway, PTK pathway, MARK pathway, cAMP-PKA pathway, and PLA$_2$ pathway. At present, most researches are about Phosphoinositide 3-kinase (PI3K). PI3K is a critical transmitter of intracellular signaling during platelet activation. The PI3K family is divided into three classes (I , II , and III). Depending on differences in the heterodimerization of catalytic subunits and regulatory subunits, class I is further divided into I A (PI3Kα, PI3Kβ, and PI3Kγ) and I B (PI3Kδ), PI3Kβ and PI3Kγ are crucial in platelet signaling[71]. Akt phosphorylation can be used as an indicator of PI3K pathway activation [72,73].

In recent years, with the further study of antiplatelet mechanism of Chinese herb and formulas for PBCRBS, there are studies involving signal transduction in platelet to investigate the mechanism. Salvianolic acid A (SAA, Figure 3) is a water-soluble component from the root of *Salvia miltiorrhiza Bunge*, a herb that is widely used for

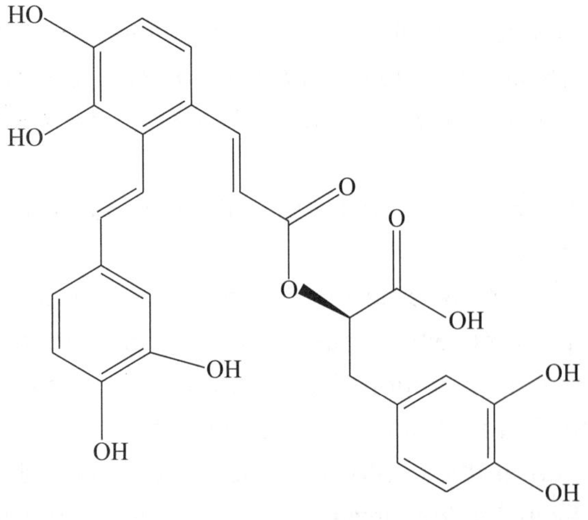

Figure 3   Chemical Structures of Salvianolic Acid A

atherothrombotic disease treatment in China. New study [74] shows that SAA could inhibit platelet spreading on fibrinogen, a process mediated by outside-in signaling. Western blot analysis showed that SAA, like the PI3K inhibitors LY294002 and TGX-221, potently inhibited PI3K, as shown by reduced akt phosphorylation, which indicates that the target spot may be the PI3Kβ. The *in vitro* findings were further evaluated in the mouse model of arterial thrombosis, in which SAA prolonged the mesenteric arterial occlusion time in wild-type mice. Interestingly, SAA could even counteract the shortened arterial occlusion time in Ldlr [tmlHer] mutant mice. And for the first defined the fact [74] that SAA inhibits platelet activation via the inhibition of PI3K and attenuates arterial thrombus formation *in vivo*. The results suggest that SAA may be developed as a novel therapeutic agent for the prevention of thrombotic disorders.

3. Discussion and Perspective

From above mentioned, during the past 30 years, research of antiplatelet and antithrombotic therapy of Chinese herb and formulas for PBCRBS has made rapid progress, but there are still some problems existing. In the clinical research, at present many studies limited to small sample of curative effects, lack of multicenter, prospective, large sample, and control study which made the clinical practice of Chinese herb and formulas for PBCRBS be short of definite clinical evidence. And Chinese scholars has begun to attempt to study like above and got to some good results [75]. But those which deserve attention are, in the practical use of clinical medicine, we should comply with the principle of differentiation of symptoms and signs, minimize the potential abuse, and improve on the clinical practical effects. In the experimental research, many studies mainly focused on the mechanism on one aspect of a certain Chinese herb and formulas for PBCRBS, the experimental design owes rigor, and only a few studies were equipped with *in vitro* and *in vivo* at the same design. It is generally known that platelet activation is a complex, multifactor process, which involves adhesion, aggregation, and reaction release. For example, there are different platelet activation stimulators, which have the different mechanism of platelet aggregation and signal transduction. It is necessary to take a systematic study on the mechanism of Chinese herb and formulas for PBCRBS inhibiting platelet aggregation by different stimulators in the future and making further study on the signal transduction in platelet. Now Chinese scholars[74] have made good study and publish the paper on the well-famous journal.

Proteomics technology has been successfully applied to platelet research, contributing to the emerging field of platelet proteomics which led to the identification of a considerable amount of novel platelet proteins, many of which have been further studied at functional level [76]. During the last 3 years, a rapid development of two-dimensional gel electrophoresis and mass spectrometry-based proteomic approaches has been used to profile alterations in platelet pro-teins [77-79]. Using differential proteomics of platelet, our previous studies found many different platelet proteins [37,80] between CHD patients of blood stasis syndrome (BSS) and non-BSS patients, and healthy controls, which indicate that the platelet cytoskeleton may play an important role in the development in BSS of CHD. Based on the Chinese medicine principle of "prescription and syndrome are corresponding", these platelet differential proteins may be the new target spots or target group. Getting intensive study on it, we believe that we can develop many new antiplatelet and antithrombolytic drugs possess definite curative effect and target, clear mechanism.

References

[1] Antiplatelet Trialists' Collaboration. Collaborative overview of randomised trials of antiplatelet therapy— Ⅰ: prevention of death, myocardial infarction, and stroke by prolonged antiplatelet therapy in various categories of patients. British Medical Journal, 1994, 308 (6921): 81-106.

[2] Antithrombotic Trialists' Collaboration. Collaborate meta analysis of randomized trials of antiplatelet therapy for prevention of death,myocardial infarction, and stroke in high risk patients. British Medical Journal, 2002,324 (7329): 71-86.

[3] Rafferty M, Walters MR, Dawson J. Anti-platelet therapy and aspirin resistance—Clinically and chemically relevant? Current Medicinal Chemistry, 2010, 7(36): 4578-4586.

[4] Pena A, Collet JP, Hulot JS,et al. Can we override clopidogrel resistance? Circulation, 2009,119 (21): 2854-2857.

[5]Gorog DA, Sweeny JM, Fuster V. Antiplatelet drug "resistance". Part 2: laboratory resistance to antiplatelet drugs fact or artifact? Nature Reviews. Cardiology, 2009, 6 (5): 365-373.

[6] Juurlink DN, Gomes T, Ko DK, et al. A population-based study of the drug interaction between proton pump inhibitors and clopidogrel. Canadian Medical Association Journal, 2009, 180, (7): 713-718.

[7] Mega JL, Close SL, Wiviott SD, et al. Cytochrome P-450 polymorphisms and response to clopidogrel. New England Journal of Medicine, 2009, 360 (4): 354-362.

[8]Choi J, Kermode JC. New therapeutic approaches to combat arterial thrombosis: better drugs for old targets, novel targets, and future prospects. Molecular Interventions, 2011, 11 (27): 111-123.

[9] Chen KJ, Li LD, Weng WL, et al. Blood stasis and research of activating blood circulation and eliminating stasis. Zhong Xi Yi Jie He Xin Nao Xue Guan Bing Za Zhi, 2005, 1: 1-2.

[10] Chen KJ. Exploration on the possibility of reducing cardiovascular risk by treatment with Chinese medicine recipes for promoting blood-circulation and relieving blood-stasis. Zhong Xi Yi Jie He Xin Nao Xue Guan Bing Za Zhi, 2008, 28 (5): 389.

[11] Chen KJ, Xue M, Yin HJ. The relationship between platelet activation related factors and polymorphism of related genes in patients with coronary heart disease of blood-stasis syndrome. Shoudu Yi Ke Da Xue Xue Bao, 2008, 29 (3): 266-269.

[12] Xue M, Chen KJ, and Yin HJ. Relationship between platelet activation related factors and polymorphism of related genes in patients with coronary heart

disease of blood-stasis syndrome. Chinese Journal of Integrative Medicine, 2008, 14 (4): 267-273.

[13] Wang Z. Mechanism on modulating platelet function of activating blood circulation and removing stasis herbs. Zhong Xi Yi Jie He Xin Nao Xue Guan Bing Za Zhi, 1992, 12 (9): 567-570.

[14] Society of Cardiology and Chinese Association of the Integration of Traditional and Western Medicine. The diagnostic criteria of TCM in coronary heart disease. Chinese Journal of Integrated Traditional and Western Medicine, 1991, 11 (5): 257.

[15] Fu CG. The study of diagnostic criterion on blood stasis for patients with coronary heart disease. Doctor Dissertation, Beijing:Beijing University of Chinese Medicine, 2011.

[16] Li JZ, He SL, Wang HL. Thrombosis Epidemiology. Beijing: Science Press, 1998.

[17] Xu FQ, Chen KY, Ma XC, et al. Clinical observation on effect of xiongshao capsule on coronary heart disease with angina pectoris. Zhongguo Zhong Xi Yi Jie He Za Zhi, 2003,23 (1): 16-18.

[18] Feng J，Wang SL. Effect of Fufang Danshen Diwan to Platelet Aggregation Function. Chinese Journal of Misdiagnostics, 2006,6 (12): 2261-2263.

[19] Jiang JB, Yang J, Deng CQ. Effect of Buyang huanwu decoction and its active fraction alkaloid and glycoside on platelet aggregation and cyclic nucleotide in rats. Zhong Nan Yao Xue,2008,6 (4): 388-391.

[20] Wang J, Xu J, Zhong JB. Effect of Radix notoginseng saponins on platelet activating molecule expression and aggregation in patients with blood hyper viscosity syndrome. Zhong Xi Yi Jie He Xin Nao Xue Guan Bing Za Zhi, 2004, 24 (4): 312-316.

[21] Wang DS, Chen FP, He SL,et al. Mechanism study on Dahuangzhechong pill anti-platelet activation. Zhonghua Zhong Yi Yao Za Zhi, 2008,23 (9): 818-821.

[22] Liu F, Li J, Wang XD. Effect of tongxinluo capsule on platelet aggregation in patients with cerebral infarction. Zhongguo Zhong Xi Yi Jie He Za Zhi, 2008, 28 (4): 304-306, 2008.

[23] Li JM, Zhao JY, Zhong GC,et al. Synthesis of ferulic acid derivatives and their inhibitory effect on platelet aggregation. Yao Xue Xue Bao, 2011, 46 (3): 305-310.

[24] Shu B, Zhou CJ, Ma YH, et al. Research progress on pharmacological activities of the available compositions in Chinese medicinal herb Ligusticum chuanxiong. Chinese Pharmacological Bulletin, 2006,22 (9): 1043-1047.

[25] Jiang YR, Yin HJ, Li LZ. Treatment of non-ST-elevation acute coronary syndrome with propyl gallate. Zhongguo Zhong Xi Yi Jie He Za Zhi, 2008,28(9):839-842.

[26] Chen P, Yang LC, Lei W, et al. Effects of polydatin on platelet aggregation and platelet cytosolic calcium. Tianran Chan Wu Yan Jiu Yu Kai Fa, 2005, 17 (1) 21-25.

[27] Xia Q, Dong TX, Zhan HQ,et al. Inhibition effect of curdione on platelet aggregation induced by ADP in rabbits. Chinese Pharmacological Bulletin, 2006, 22 (9): 1151-1152, 2006.

[28] Ma JJ, Song Y, Jia M, et al. Effect of total flavone in sanguis draconis on platelet aggregation, thrombus formation Evidence-Based Complementary and Alternative Medicine 7 and myocardial ischemia. Zhong Cao Yao, 2002, 33 (11): 1008-1010.

[29] Yao Y, Wu WY, Liu AH,et al. Interaction of salvianolic acids and notoginsengnosides in inhibition of ADP-induced platelet aggregation. American Journal of Chinese Medicine, 2008, 36 (2): 313-328.

[30] Jiang ZW, Zhao LJ, Zhang H, et al. Effect of hirudin injecton on antithrombosis in rats. Ji Lin Da Xue Xue Bao (Yi Xue Ban), 2003, 29 (4): 417-418.

[31] Guo ZQ, Chen Z, Li L, et al. Effect of administration of Safflower yellow injection on the platelet aggregate rate and transforming growth factor-β1 in patients without ST elevation acute myocardial infarction. Journal of Clinical Cardiology, 2010, 26 (8): 591-593.

[32] Hsu-Lin SC, Berman CL, Furie BC. A platelet membrane protein expressed during platelet activation and secretion. Studies using a monoclonal antibody specific for thrombin-activated platelets. Journal of Biological Chemistry, 1984, 259 (14): 9121-9126.

[33] Michelson AD，Furman MI. Laboratory markers of platelet activation and their clinical significance. Current Opinion in Hematology, 1999, 6 (5): 342-348.

[34] Ikeda H, Takajo Y, Ichiki K,et al. Increased soluble form of P-selectin in patients with unstable angina. Circulation,1995,92 (7): 1693-1696.

[35] Shimomura H, Ogawa H, Arai H, et al. Serial changes in plasma levels of soluble P-selectin in patients with acute myocardial infarction. American Journal of Cardiology, 1998,81 (4): 397-400.

[36] Furman MI, Benoit SE, Barnard MR,et al. Increased

platelet reactivity and circulating monocyte-platelet aggregates in patients with stable coronary artery disease. Journal of the American College of Cardiology, 1998, 31 (2): 352-358.

[37] Liu Y, Yin HJ, Jiang YR,et al. Research on the correlation between platelet gelsolin and blood-stasis syndrome of coronary heart disease. Chinese Journal of Integrative Medicine, 2011,17 (8): 587-592.

[38] Chen ZQ, Hong L, Wang H. Effect of danhong injection on platelet activation and inflammatory factors in patients of acute coronary syndrome after intervention therapy. Zhongguo Zhong Xi Yi Jie He Za Zhi, 2009, 29 (8): 692-694.

[39] Chen ZQ, Hong L, Wang H. Effect of tetramethylpyrazine on platelet activation and vascular endothelial function in patients with acute coronary syndrome undergoing percutaneous coronary intervention. Zhongguo Zhong Xi Yi Jie He Za Zhi, 2007, 27 (12): 1078-1081.

[40] Xiong P，Zhou L. Effect of compound danshen droplet pill on plasma endothelin and platelet α-granule membrane protein-140 in patients with unstable angina pectoris. Zhong Xi Yi Jie He Xin Nao Xue Guan Bing Za Zhi, 2009, 7 (5); 5100-511.

[41] Han L, Peng D Y, Xu F,et al. Studies on anti-platelet activation effect and partial mechanisms of Taohong Siwu decoction. Zhongguo Zhong Yao Za Zhi, 2010, 35 (19): 2609-2612.

[42] Luo HM, Fu DY, Ren M.Z, et al. Clinical study on tongxinluo capsule affecting activity of platelet's GP IIb/ IIIa receptor in patients with coronary heart disease. Zhong Cheng Yao, 2007, 27 (2): 181-183 .

[43] Kasirer-Friede A, Cozzi MR, Mazzucato M, et al. Signaling through GP Ib-IX-V activates αIIbβ3 independently of other receptors. Blood, 2004, 103 (9): 3403-3411.

[44] Wang DS, Chen FP, He SL et al. Comparative research between plasma pharmacology and serum pharmacology of dahuang zhe chong pill. Xue Shuan Yu Zhi Xue Xue, 2005, 11 (1): 5-8.

[45] Li YL. Research progress in the treatment of cardiovascular diseases by Xue Fu Zhu Yu Tang. Beijing Zhong Yi Yao, 2008, 27 (3): 228-230.

[46] Yacoub D, Théorêt JF, Villeneuve L,et al. Essential role of protein kinase C δ in platelet signaling, αIIb β3 activation, and thromboxane A$_2$ release. Journal of Biological Chemistry, 2006, 281 (40): 30024-30035.

[47] Nishizuka Y. Intracellular signaling by hydrolysis of phospholipids and activation of protein kinase C. Science, 1992, 258 (5082): 607-614.

[48] Yang YM, Wang XX, Chen JZ, et al. Resveratrol attenuates adenosine diphosphateinduced platelet activation by reducing protein kinase C activity. American Journal of Chinese Medicine, 2008, 36 (3): 603-613.

[49] Kaplan KL, Owen J. Plasma levels of β-thromboglobulin and platelet factor 4 as indices of platelet activation in vivo. Blood, 1981, 57 (2): 199-202.

[50] Pumphrey CW Dawes J. Plasma beta-thromboglobulin as a measure of platelet activity. Effect of risk factors and findings in ischemic heart disease and after acute myocardial infarction. American Journal of Cardiology, 1982, 50 (6): 1258-1261.

[51] Slungaard A. Platelet factor 4: a chemokine enigma. International Journal of Biochemistry and Cell Biology, 2005, 37 (6): 1162-1167.

[52] Hope W, Martin TJ, Chesterman CN, et al. Human β-thromboglobulin inhibits PGI$_2$ production and binds to a specific site in bovine aortic endothelial cells. Nature, 1979, 282 (5735): 210-212.

[53] Kong YQ, Yao Z, Yun ML, et al. Effect of danshen on angina pectoris and platlet function. Gao Xue Ya Za Zhi, 2002, 10 (5): 451-453.

[54] Yoshimura M, Oshima T, Hiraga H,et al. Increased cytosolic free Mg^{2+} and Ca^{2+} in platelets of patients with vasospastic angina. American Journal of Physiology, 1998, 274 (2): R548-R554.

[55] Fujinishi A, Takahara K, Ohba C, et al. Effects of nisoldipine on cytosolic calcium, platelet aggregation, and coagulation/fibrinolysis in patients with coronary artery disease. Angiology, 1997, 48 (6): 515-521.

[56] Zhang RX, Lian XF, Lian N. Study progress of calcium antagonist of Chinese medicine on cardiovascular diseases. Shanxi Zhong Yi Xue Yuan Xue Bao, 1999, 22 (4): 52-54.

[57] Chen WM, Jin M, Wu W, Study of Safflor yellow inhibit the PAF-induced platelet activation, Zhongguo Yao Xue Za Zhi, 2000, 35 (11): 741.

[58] Chen C, Yang TL. TXA^2/PGI^2 and cardiovascular diseases. Xian Dai Sheng Wu Yi Xue Jin Zhan, 2008, 8 (11): 2166-2172.

[59] Xu HM, Liu QY, Dai M, et al. Effect of total glucosides of radix paeoniae rubra on platelet function of rats. Hefei Gong Ye Da Xue Xue Bao (Zi Ran Ke Xue

Ban), 2003, 26 (1): 141-144.

[60] Gao HL, Li YK, Tong Y, Li LD. Comparative study on the protective effects of different Guanxin Ⅱ formula on 8 Evidence-Based Complementary and Alternative Medicine acute myocardial ischemia in dogs. Zhong Yao Yao Li Yu Lin Chuang, 2007, 23 (5): 1-4.

[61] Lan ZX, Wang WZ, Ma YN, et al. Experimental research on the influence of Taohong Siwu decoction on the TXB_2,6-keto-PGF1α in the blood stasis syndrom of rats. Hua Xi Yao Xue Za Zhi, 2008, 23 (6): 687-688.

[62] Wu Y, Guo HB, Wang TJ, et al. Comparative study on effects of active ingredients of several traditional Chinese medicines on rabbit platelet aggregation in vitro. Zhong Yao Lin Chuang Yao Li Xue Yu Zhi Liao Xue, 2007, 12 (9): 1047-1051.

[63] Yu WG, Xu LN. Effects of acetylsalvianolic acid A on arachidonic acid metabolism in platelets". Yao Xue Xue Bao, 1998, 33 (1): 62-63.

[64] Yuan SJ, Zhang ZW, Gao TH, et al. Mechanism research of Honghua injection antithrombotic function. Zhongguo Zhong Yao Za Zhi, 2011, 36 (11): 1528-1529.

[65] Wang ZY, Li JZ, Ruan CG. Basic theory and clinical of thrombosis and hemostasis. Shanghai Scientific and Technical Publishers, Shanghai, China, 2004.

[66] Xu SH, Cyclic nucleotides and blood platelet function. Sheng li Ke Xue Jin Zhan, 1992, 23 (4): 318-322.

[67] Zhu GG, Luo RZ, Guo ZX, Advance of cardiotonic pill on inhibiting platelet activation and aggregation. Zhongguo Xin Xue Guan Za Zhi, 2007, 12 (2): 149-151.

[68] Yan J, Qin CL. Brief review on effects of Fufangdanshen prescription, Dan-shen and San-qi on the platelet functions. Zhongguo Shi Yan Fangji Xue Za Zhi, 2003, 9 (2): 59-62.

[69] Pei HY, Han Y, Platelet activation through signal transduction-review. Zhongguo Shi Yan Xue Ye Xue Za Zhi, 2004, 12 (5): 704-707.

[70] Lu J, Yu YN, Xu RB. Receptor Signaling System and Diseases. Shandong Science and Technology Press, Shandong, China, 1999.

[71] Cosemans JMEM, Munnix ICA, Wetzker R, et al. Continuous signaling via PI3K isoforms β and γ is required for platelet ADP receptor function in dynamic thrombus stabilization. Blood, 2006, 108 (9): 3045-3052.

[72] Li Z, zhang G, Le Breton GC, et al. Two waves of platelet secretion induced by thromboxane A_2 receptor and a critical role for phosphoinositide 3-kinases. Journal of Biological Chemistry, 2003, 278 (33): 30725-30731.

[73] Kroner C, Eybrechts K, and Akkerman JWN. Dual regulation of platelet protein kinase B. Journal of Biological Chemistry, 2000, 275 (36): 27790-27798.

[74] Huang ZS, Zeng CL, Zhu LJ, et al. Salvianolic acid A inhibits platelet activation and arterial thrombosis via inhibition of phosphoinositide 3-kinase. Journal of Thrombosis and Haemostasis, 2010, 8 (6): 1383-1393.

[75] Chen KJ, Shi DZ, Xu H, et al. XS0601 reduces the incidence of restenosis: a prospective study of 335 patients undergoing percutaneous coronary intervention in China. Chinese Medical Journal, 2006, 119 (1): 6-13.

[76] García A. Clinical proteomics in platelet research: challenges ahead. Journal of Thrombosis and Haemostasis, 2010, 8 (8): 1784-1785.

[77] Thiele T, Steil L, Gebhard S, et al. Profiling of alterations in platelet proteins during storage of platelet concentrates: Transfusion, 2007, 47 (7): 1221-1233.

[78] Banfi C, Brioschi M, Marenzi G, et al. Proteome of platelets in patients with coronary artery disease. Experimental Hematology, 2010, 38 (5): 341-350.

[79] Senzel L, Gnatenko DV, Bahou WF. The platelet proteome. Current Opinion in Hematology, 2009, 16 (5): 329-333.

[80] Li XF, Jiang YR, Wu CF, et al. Study on the correlation between platelet function proteins and symptom complex in coronary heart disease. Zhongguo Fen Zi Xin Zang Bing Xue Za Zhi, 2009, 9(6): 326.

Outcome Measures of Chinese Herbal Medicine for Coronary Heart Disease: An Overview of Systematic Reviews[*]

Jing Luo　Hao Xu

1. Introduction

Coronary heart disease (CHD) is the most common cause of death in western countries. With the infectious diseases controlled and improvement of people's living, the morbidity of CHD increases year by year in many developing countries. Acute myocardial infarction (AMI) and angina pectoris are the most important two types of CHD. Chinese herbal medicine (CHM) has a 3000-year-old history with unique theories for concepts of etiology and systems of diagnosis and treatment [1]. The interest in CHM is growing rapidly beyond China [2-5]. In recent years, some researchers have reported the effect of CHM on clinical symptoms, biomarkers and mortality in CHD patients. However, the evidence of CHM needs to be reviewed systematically and appraised critically.

High-quality systematic reviews (SRs) of randomized controlled trials (RCTs) are the sources of the best evidence [6]. Currently, there is an increasing number of SRs on studies of CHM, but few of them concluded that CHM was definitely effective for CHD due to the weak evidence. In addition to rigorous clinical design and standard reporting, the selection of outcome measures also plays an important role in drawing a more persuasive conclusion. The aim of this overview was to summarize the outcome measures of CHM as the treatment of CHD based on available SRs, so as to display the current situation and evaluate the potential benefits and advantages of CHM on CHD.

2. Methods

Electronic literature searches were performed to identify the maximum possible number of systematic reviews/meta—analyses of CHM for CHD. The following electronic databases were searched: (1) The Cochrane Database of Systematic Reviews (Issue 10 of 12, Oct 2011); (2) MEDLINE (2001 to 2011); (3) Chinese Biomedical Database (CBM, 2001 to 2011); (4) China National Knowledge Infrastructure (CNKI, 2001 to 2011); (5) Wanfang Databases (2001 to 2011); (6) Chinese VIP Information (VIP, 2001 to 2011). CBM, CNKI, Wanfang, and VIP were databases in Chinese. We searched databases in Chinese because CHMs were researched in china mostly. And we searched papers from 2001 to 2011 for high-quality RCTs and SRs mainly focusing in recent ten years.

The strategy below was used to search The Cochrane Library and adapted appropriately for use in different electronic bibliographic databases: #1 herb*；#2 medic*；#3 (#1 and #2); #4 Chinese；#5 (#3 or #4); #6 cardiac；#7 heart；#8 circulation；#9 (#6 or #7 or #8); #10 (#5 and #9). To determine which article was we want, we scanned the title and abstract of each record independently by two reviewers (J. Luo and H. Xu). If the information included a systematic

---

* 原载于 Evidence-Based Complementary and Alternative Medicine，2012，Article ID 927392

review or a meta-analysis of CHM for CHD, the full paper was obtained for further assessment. Papers were excluded when problems occurred with: repeat publication; methodological studies; quality assessment report; the interventions in the control groups were other Chinese herbs; research on acupuncture, qigong, massage, or other treatments (Figure 1).

We divided the outcome measures into primary endpoints and secondary endpoints [50,51]. Primary endpoints include the mortality, AMI, restenosis after percutaneous coronary intervention (PCI), and recanalization. Secondary endpoints mainly indicate surrogate endpoints and laboratory measures, which include angina pectoris, arrhythmia, heart failure, consumption of nitroglycerine, electrocardiogram (ECG), ultrasonic cardiogram (UCG), level of blood lipids, plasma endothelin, nitric oxide, myocardial enzyme, hemorheology, heart rate variability, and traditional Chinese medicine (TCM) syndrome.

In addition, we used PRISMA (preferred reporting items for systematic reviews and meta-analyses) as assessment tool to estimate the quality of the included reviews. This checklist includes 27 items of 7 key areas. And it describes the preferred way to present the abstract, introduction, methods, results, and discussion sections of a systematic review and a meta-analysis paper. It requires authors of each review to include a flow diagram that provides information about the number of studies identified, included, and excluded and the reasons for excluding them [52]. Information on each of the included reviews was imported into PRISMA statement for analysis. All data were extracted independently by two authors using predefined criteria. Disagreements were resolved by discussion between the authors. All inconsistencies were revised after a consensus was reached.

3. Results

46 articles were included (7 in English and 39 in Chinese). 39 SRs from the Chinese databases were published between 2004 and 2011. Since 2007, the number of SR increased markedly. 5 SRs from the Cochrane Database were published between 2006 to 2011 [8,13,26,36,44]. 2 SRs from MEDLINE were published between 2006 to 2011 [14,45].

7 SRs were concerned with myocardial infarction (MI), 38 SRs were related to angina pectoris, and one SR was concerned with preventing and treating restenosis after PCI. The trials in SRs were mainly originated from china. The original trials included were called "RCTs" or "quasi-RCTs", but only a few of them were

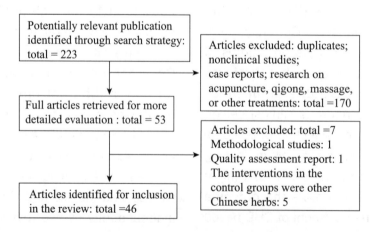

Figure 1   Flow-Chart of SRs Selection

Table 1　Outcome Measures of CHM for CHD in Systematic Reviews

Outcome measures (number of SR)	Condition (number of SR)	CHM	First author	Number of RCTs/total	Conclusion	Risk of publication bias
Primary Endpoints						
Mortality (7)	MI (6)	Shenmai injection	Zeng (2010) [7]	13/13	A	H
		Danshen preparations	Wu (2008) [8]	6/6	B	NA
		Shengmai injection	Gao (2008) [9]	4/4	A	NA
		Yiqi huoxue patent medicine	Zhang (2008) [10]	9/28	B	NA
		Herbal injection products	Zhen (2007) [11]	5/15	A	H
		Herbal products	Lin (2006) [12]	4/8	B	L
	Angina pectoris (1)	Tongxinluo capsule	Wu (2006) [13]	1/18	B	H
AMI (6)	MI (2)	Yiqi huoxue patent medicine	Zhang (2008) [10]	1/28	B	NA
		Herbal products	Lin (2006) [12]	2/8	A	L
		Compound salvia pellet	Zhang (2008) [14]	1/17	B	H
	Angina pectoris (4)	Puerarin	Wang (2008) [15]	1/11	B	H
		Tongxinluo capsule	Wu (2006) [13]	3/18	B	NA
		Dengzhanhua injection	Cao (2005) [16]	1/8	A	NA
Restenosis after PCI (1)	CHD (1)	Herbal products	Ren (2008) [17]	17/17	A	H
Recanalization (2)	MI (2)	Yiqi huoxue patent medicine	Zhang (2008) [10]	7/28	B	NA
		Herbal injection products	Zhen (2007) [11]	15/15	A	NA
Secondary Endpoints (ECG)						
ECG (34)	CHD (4)	Shuyu zaogan tablets	Zhang (2011) [18]	29/32	A	L
		Kudiezi injection	Zuo (2011) [19]	15/16	A	H
		Sodium tanshinone ⅡA Sulfonate	Wang (2011) [20]	17/29	A	H
	Angina pectoris (30)	Danhong injection	Xu (2011) [21]	19/19	A	H
		Tongxinluo capsule and compound salvia pellet	Jia (2011) [22]	65/58	A	L
		Xuefuzhuyu Decoction	Cui (2011) [23]	8/10	A	H

Continued

Outcome measures (number of SR)	Condition (number of SR)	CHM	First author	Number of RCTs/total	Conclusion	Risk of publication bias
		Shengmai injection	Zhang (2010)[24]	8/13	A	H
		Safflower Injection	Wu (2010)[25]	2/6	B	NA
		Herbal products	Zhuo (2010)[26]	3/3	A	NA
		Tongxinluo capsule	Hao (2010)[27]	18/20	A	L
		Gingko	Zha (2010)[28]	36/50	A	L
		Gingko	Zhao (2010)[29]	9/23	A	L
		Xuefuzhuyu decoction	Song (2010)[30]	3/3	A	H
		Xinkeshu	Chen (2010)[31]	12/18	A	H
		Yiqihuoxue	Long (2009)[32]	25/30	A	H
		Compound salvia pellet	Zhang (2009)[33]	5/8	A	L
		Compound salvia pellet	Zhang (2008)[14]	10/17	A	H
		Shexiang baoxin wan	Lin (2008)[34]	20/22	A	L
		Puerarin	Wang (2008)[15]	6/11	A	H
ECG (34)	Angina pectoris (30)	Suxiao jiuxin wan	Wang (2008)[35]	14/14	A	L
		Suxiao jiuxin wan	Duan (2008)[36]	3/15	A	H
		Tong xin luo Capsule	He (2007)[37]	12/17	A	H
		Compound salvia pellet	Jiang (2007)[38]	26/34	A	H
		Danshen preparations	Li (2007)[39]	7/13	A	L
		Compound preparation of salvia miltiorrhiza	Zhang (2007)[40]	30/33	A	H
		Danshen preparations	Li (2007)[41]	20/21	A	H
		Rhodiola L.	Wang (2006)[42]	7/8	A	L
		Tetramethylpyrazine	Zhang (2006)[43]	10/10	A	L
		Tongxinluo capsule	Wu (2006)[13]	10/18	A	NA
		Puerarin injection	Wang (2006)[44]	17/20	A	H
		Compound salvia pellet	Wang (2006)[45]	27/27	A	L
		Dengzhanhua injection	Cao (2005)[16]	8/8	A	NA

Continued

Outcome measures (number of SR)	Condition (number of SR)	CHM	First author	Number of RCTs/total	Conclusion	Risk of publication bias
		Compound salvia pellet	Wang (2004)[46]	17/17	A	L
		Compound salvia pellet	Zhang (2004)[47]	19/22	A	L
Secondry Endpoints (Angina Pectoris)						
Angina pectoris (30)	CHD (3)	Shuyu zaogan tablets	Zhang (2011)[18]	21/22	A	L
		Shengmai injection	Zhang (2010)[24]	10/13	A	H
		Compound salvia pellet	Zhang (2009)[33]	8/8	A	L
		Sodium tanshinone IIA Sulfonate	Wang (2011)[20]	29/29	A	H
		Danhong injection	Xu (2011)[21]	19/19	A	H
		Tongxinluo capsule and compound salvia pellet	Jia (2011)[22]	65/65	A	L
		Kudiezi injection	Zuo (2011)[19]	16/16	A	H
		Shuxuetong	Li (2010)[48]	11/13	A	L
		Herbal products	Zhuo (2010)[26]	3/3	B	NA
		Tongxinluo capsule	Hao (2010)[27]	20/20	A	L
		Xinkeshu	Chen (2010)[31]	16/18	A	H
Angina pectoris (30)	Angina pectoris (26)	Xuefuzhuyu decoction	Song (2010)[30]	3/3	A	H
		Gingko damo injection	Zha (2010)[28]	46/50	A	L
		Ginkgo extract	Zhao (2010)[29]	22/23	A	L
		Suxiao jiuxin wan	Duan (2008)[36]	1/15	A	H
		Puerarin	Wang (2008)[15]	10/11	A	H
		Suxiao jiuxin wan	Wang (2008)[35]	14/14	A	L
		Compound salvia pellet	Zhang (2008)[14]	11/17	A	H
		Compound salvia pellet	Jiang (2007)[38]	34/34	A	H
		Compound preparation of salvia miltiorrhiza	Zhang (2007)[40]	32/33	A	H
		Danshen preparations	Li (2007)[41]	21/21	B	H

Outcome measures (number of SR)	Condition (number of SR)	CHM	First author	Number of RCTs/total	Conclusion	Risk of publication bias	Continued
		Tetramethylpyrazine	Zhang (2006)[43]	8/10	A	L	
		Rhodiola L.	Wang (2006)[42]	5/8	A	L	
		Tongxinluo capsule	Wu (2006)[13]	5/18	A	NA	
		Compound salvia pellet	Wang (2006)[45]	27/27	A	L	
		Puerarin injection	Wang (2006)[44]	18/20	A	H	
		Dengzhanhua injection	Cao (2005)[16]	8/8	A	NA	
		Compound salvia pellet	Wang (2004)[46]	17/17	A	L	
		Compound salvia pellet	Zhang (2004)[47]	20/22	A	L	
	CHD after PCI (1)	Herbal products	Ren (2008)[17]	15/17	A	H	

Secondry End points (Others)

Outcome measures (number of SR)	Condition (number of SR)	CHM	First author	Number of RCTs/total	Conclusion	Risk of publication bias	Continued
Consumption of nitroglycerine (5)	Angina pectoris (5)	Herbal products	Zhuo (2010)[26]	2/3	A	NA	
		Suxiao jiuxin wan	Duan (2008)[36]	1/15	A	H	
		Rhodiola L.	Wang (2006)[42]	1/8	A	L	
		Puerarin injection	Wang (2006)[44]	6/20	A	H	
		Tongxinluo capsule	Wu (2006)[13]	1/18	A	NA	
Level of blood lipids (4)	Angina pectoris (3)	Shuxuetong	Li (2010)[48]	4/13	A	H	
		Compound salvia pellet	Zhang (2008)[14]	8/22	B	L	
		Compound salvia pellet	Zhang (2004)[47]	4/8	A	L	
	CHD (1)	Compound salvia pellet	Zhang (2009)[33]	4/17	A	L	
Hemorheology (2)	Angina pectoris (1)	Safflower Injection	Wu (2010)[25]	2/6	A	NA	
	CHD (1)	Shengmai injection	Zhang (2010)[24]	5/13	A	H	

第七章

Continued

Outcome measures (number of SR)	Condition (number of SR)	CHM	First author	Number of RCTs/total	Conclusion	Risk of publication bias
Heart failure (3)	MI (3)	Yiqi huoxue patent medicine	Zhang (2008) [10]	7/28	B	NA
		Danshen preparations	Wu (2008) [8]	1/6	B	NA
		Herbal products	Lin (2006) [12]	3/8	A	L
Arrhythmia (2)	MI (2)	Yiqi huoxue patent medicine	Zhang (2008) [10]	2/28	B	NA
		Herbal products	Lin (2006) [12]	2/8	B	L
UCG (2)	MI (2)	Yiqi huoxue herbal products	Song (2008) [49]	3/3	A	NA
		Herbal products	Lin (2006) [12]	4/8	A	L
Myocardial enzyme (1)	Angina pectoris (1)	Tongxinluo capsule	Wu (2006) [13]	1/18	B	NA
Level of plasma endothelin (2)	Angina pectoris (2)	Puerarin injection	Wang (2006) [44]	2/20	A	H
		Tongxinluo capsule	Wu (2006) [13]	4/18	A	NA
Level of nitric oxide (1)	Angina pectoris (1)	Tongxinluo capsule	Wu (2006) [13]	2/18	A	NA
Heart rate variability (1)	CHD (1)	Compound salvia pellet	Zhang (2009) [33]	3/8	A	L
TCM syndrome (1)	Angina pectoris (1)	Safflower Injection	Wang (2006) [25]	3/8	A	L

Notes: Yiqi huoxue: supplementing qi and activating blood circulation to patients with qi-deficiency and blood-stasis syndrome;
A: CHM may be or appears to be effective; B: The evidence is insufficient, inconclusive;
H: high; L: low; NA: not mentioned.

第七章

711

typical RCTs. Most of the trials in the SRs were of low quality, only 14 RCTs were high quality: one was concerned with MI, 12 were related to angina pectoris, and one was about preventing and treating restenosis.

20 kinds of CHM were reviewed, including injections, capsules, tablets, pellets, and herbal decoction as follows: Danshen preparations (n= 13) [8,14,20-22,33,38-41,45-47], 7 of them were compound salvia pellet [14,22,33,38,45-47]; Tongxinluo Capsule (n=4) [13,22,27,37]; Yiqi huoxue (supplementing qi and activating blood circulation) products (n= 3) [10,32,49]; Xuefu zhuyu decoction (n = 2) [23,30]; herbal products (n = 4) [11,12,17,26]; Shengmai injection (n =2) [9,24]; Suxiao jiuxin wan (n = 2) [35,36]; Gingko(n= 2) [28,29]; Acanthopanax(n = 2) [53,54]; Puerarin (n =2) [15,44]; Shexiang baoxin wan (n = 2) [34,55]; Shenmai injection (n = 1) [7]; Tetramethylpyrazine (n = 1) [43]; Shuxuetong (n = 1) [48]; Xinkeshu (n = 1) [31]; Safflower injection (n = 1) [25]; Rhodiola (n = 1) [42]; Kudiezi injection (n=1) [19]; Shuyu zaogan tablets (n= 1) [18]; Dengzhanhua injection (n = 1) [16].

11 SRs analyzed primary endpoints and the others all focused on secondary endpoints to evaluate CHM for CHD (Table 1). This was mainly based on whether there were available data in the original trials or not. Four primary endpoints were analyzed in the SRs including mortality, nonfatal myocardial infarction, restenosis after PCI, and recanalization. None of these SRs analyzed the quality of life. Angina pectoris was the most common secondary endpoint in the SRs. There was one SR without clear outcome measures [53], and 2 SRs only used "marked effective", "effective", "ineffective" as comprehensive outcome measures involving symptoms improvement and ECG changes [19,54]. Many CHMs appear to have significant effect on improving symptoms, ECG, and level of blood lipids and reducing the consumption of nitroglycerine, and so forth. Some SRs also reflected that CHM may be effective to reduce the risk of subsequent MI, heart failure,

and arrhythmia. However, most SRs failed to draw a definite conclusion of the effectiveness of CHM for CHD due specifically to the poor evidence.

Adverse effects, which are important when evaluate a medicine, should be regarded as an essential outcome measure in clinical trials. However, only a few of the trials in the SRs had long-term data on adverse effects. Most of adverse effects of CHM were mentioned as "low adverse effect" or "none obvious". The adverse events reported majorly were abdominal complaints, nausea, and dyspepsia. One review reported more adverse reactions in treatment groups than in control groups [44]. Recently, several reviews have highlighted adverse reactions of CHM [56,57].

Compared the usage of outcome measures between Cochrane and non-Cochrane reviews, we found that outcome measures of the included papers in Cochrane are more comprehensive. Every Cochrane review took primary endpoints, secondary endpoints, and safety as outcome measures. However, primary endpoints and safety are seldom taken as outcome measures in most of the non-Cochrane reviews. None of reviews analyzed quality of life or pay attention to medical economics.

According to PRISMA statement, we found that most of the included reviews are of low quality. The deficiencies are as follows: review methods in the abstracts and rationales for review were not well reported; only about half of the SRs reported the characteristics of included trials; just 5 SRs provided flow chart in the article, 2 in Chinese [22,29], and 3 in English [8,14,26]; potential biases were not described well in the reports; most SRs lack in persuasive outcome measures.

4. Discussion

Our overview shows that primary endpoints and secondary endpoints are all used to evaluate the effect of CHM for CHD. Secondary endpoints are most commonly adopted in clinical trials due to their feasibility in small sample size and short-term clinical trials. They may signify future cardiovascular event to some extent and are sure to be valuable as surrogate endpoints. But it is clearly that primary endpoints are more persuasive in RCT of cardiovascular diseases. However, most of the outcome measures in the included SRs are angina pectoris and ECG. Primary endpoints such as mortality and major cardiovascular events are not used widely. Adverse effects, quality of life, and medical economics, which are also important when evaluate a medicine, should be taken as outcome measures too. All of these are the reasons why neither the trials nor the SRs of CHM for CHD could meet a sufficiently high standard to be broadly accepted by the Western medical community.

SRs of CHM with poor methodology and reporting quality have been reported [58]. According to PRISMA statement, we found that most of the included reviews have poor quality. Reviewers were not good at reporting how they avoided bias in selecting primary studies, how they extracted data, and how they evaluated the validity of the primary studies. Also, most of the reviewers chose less persuasive outcome measures, which reduced the persuasion of the interventions. So if reviewers did not master the method of performing SR, they could produce inaccurate or misleading conclusions for current clinical practice and even the future research. Although it appeared that CHM was effective for CHD in clinical use, such as compound salvia pellet, shengmai injection, suxiao jiuxin wan, and gingko, puerarin, most SRs were inconclusive that CHM had a definite effect for CHD owing to the poor evidence.

Before recommending the conclusion, we have to consider the following weaknesses in this overview. Firstly, data were abstracted from SRs instead of the original trials, and most of the included SRs have poor quality. Secondly, most

of the RCTs in the SRs included are also of low quality due mainly to unclear randomization and blinding method, incomplete outcome reporting, publication bias, and so forth. Thirdly, we only selected SRs published in Chinese and English. SRs of CHM for CHD published in other language or originated from other countries might be omitted. Fourthly, we did not identify unpublished studies, thus negative trial might not be reported and could induce publication bias.

In conclusion, primary and secondary endpoints were all used to evaluate the effectiveness of CHM for CHD, but primary endpoints were not used widely. Although it appeared that CHM was effective for CHD in terms of some outcome measures, most SRs failed to draw a definite conclusion for the effectiveness of CHM in CHD patients due to the poor evidence. The benefits of CHM for CHD still need to be confirmed in the future with RCTs of more persuasive primary endpoints and high-quality SRs.

References

[1] Chen KJ, Xu H. The integration of traditional Chinese medicine and Western medicine. European Review, 2003, 11(2): 225-235.

[2] Robinson N. Integrative medicine—traditional Chinese medicine, a model? Chinese Journal of Integrative Medicine, 2011, 17(1): 21-25.

[3] Dobos G, Tao I. The model of western Integrative medicine: the role of Chinese medicine. Chinese Journal of Integrative Medicine, 2011, 17(1): 11-20.

[4] Tindle HA, Davis RB, Phillips RS et al. Trends in use of complementary and alternative medicine by US adults: 1997-2002. Alternative Therapies, Health and Medicine, 2005, 11(1): 42-49.

[5] Eisenberg D. Reflections on the past and future of integrative medicine from a lifelong student of the integration of Chinese and western medicine. Chinese Journal of Integrative Medicine, 2011, 17(1): 3-5.

[6] Medical Research Library of Brooklyn, The Evidence Pyramid, http://library.downstate.edu/EBM2/2100.htm.

[7] Zeng YJ, Wang J, Zhou YC et al, Effect of shenmai injection on mortality rate of patients with acute myocardial infartion: a systematic review. Modern

Journal of Integrated Traditional Chinese and Western Medicine, 2010, 19 (28): 3555-3558.

[8] Wu T, Ni J, Wu J. Danshen (Chinese medicinal herb) preparations for acute myocardial infarction. Cochrane Database of Systematic Reviews, 2008, (2): CD004465.

[9] Gao ZY, Guo CY, Shi DZ, et al. Effect of Shengmai injection on the fatality rate of patients with acutemyocardial infarction: a systematic review. Chinese Journal of Integrated Traditional and Western Medicine, 2008, 28 (12): 1069-1073.

[10] Zhang JH, Shang HC, Zhang BL, et al. Systematic review of randomized controlled trials on treatment of myocardial infarction with Yiqi Huoxue Chinese Patent medicine. China Journal of Traditional Chinese Medicine and Pharmacy, 2008, 23 (4): 300-306.

[11] Zhen L, Liu HX, Shang JJ. Effect of herbal injection products as adjutant treatment on mortality rate and recanalization rate of patients with acute myocardial infartion: a meta analysis. Journal of Emergency in Traditional Chinese Medicine, 2007, 16(7): 859-862.

[12] Lin Q, Nong YB, Duan WH. Meta analysis of clinical research literature on Chinese materia medica for acute myocardial infarction. China Journal of Traditional Chinese Medicine and Pharmacy, 2006, 21 (9): 529-556.

[13] Wu T, Harrison RA, Chen X, et al. Tongxinluo (Tong xin luo or Tong-xin-luo) capsule for unstable angina pectoris. Cochrane database of systematic reviews (Online), 2006, (4): CD004474.

[14] Zhang JH, Shang HC, Gao XM, et al. Compound salvia droplet pill, a traditional Chinese medicine, for the treatment of unstable angina pectoris: a systematic review. Medical Science Monitor, 2008, 14 (1): RA1-RA7.

[15] Wang J, Tian Y, Feng C, et al. Effect of Puerarin injection for unstable angina pectoris: a systematic review. Guangming Journal of Chinese Medicine, 2008, 23 (4): 399-403.

[16] Cao W, Lan D, Zhang T, Tang C, et al. Effect of Dengzhanhua Injection for angina pectoris: a systematic review. Chinese Journal of Evidence-Based Medicine, 2005, 5 (4): 317-322.

[17] Ren Y, Chen KJ, Ruan XM. Systematic review of randomized controlled trials on preventing and treating restenosis after percutaneous coronary intervention with Chinese medicine. Chinese Journal of Integrated Traditional and Western Medicine, 2008, 28 (7): 597-601.

[18] Zhang ZH, Chen ZJ, Sheng YC, et al. Systematic evaluation of Shuyu Zaogan tablets for coronary heart disease. World Clinical Drugs, 2011, 32 (3): 159-164.

[19] Zuo ZJ, Huang QM. A systematic review of Kudiezi injection in the treatment of angina pectoris. China Medical Herald, 2011, 8 (4): 32-35.

[20] Wang CI, Gu F, Wang SL. Meta-analysis on randomized controlled trials for treatment of angina pectoris by sodium tanshinone IIA sulfonate. Chinese Journal of Integrative Medicine on Cardio/Cerebrovascular Disease, 2011, 9 (6): 644-647.

[21] Xu GL, Lin SM, Xu H, et al. Meta-analysis of Danhong injection for unstable angina pectoris. Li Shizhen Medicine and MateriaMedica Research, 2011, 22 (3): 765-767.

[22] Jia YL, Zhang SK, Bao FF, et al. Indirect Comparison of Tongxinluo capsule and Danshen dripping pill for angina pectoris: a systematic review. Chinese Journal of Evidence-Based Medicine, 2011, 11 (8): 919-931.

[23] Cui HJ, He HY, Xing ZH. System evaluation and meta analysis of Xuefuzhuyu Decoction on unstable angina pectoris. Journal of Emergency in Traditional Chinese Medicine, 2011, 20 (7): 1071-1074.

[24] Zhang Q, Jin RM. Meta-analysis of Shengmai injection and conventional therapy for coronary heart disease. Chinese Journal of New Drugs and Clinical Remedies, 2010, 29(4): 310-314.

[25] Wu FB, Xu T, Li J, et al. Meta Analysis on Efficacy and Safety of Safflower Injection in Treating unstable angina pectoris. China Pharmaceuticals, 2010, 19 (17): 4-5.

[26] Zhuo Q, Yuan Z, Chen H, et al. Traditional Chinese herbal products for stable angina. Cochrane database of systematic reviews (Online), 2010, (5): CD004468.

[27] Hao CH, Zhang JY. Meta-analysis of Tongxinluo Capsule for coronary heart disease angina. China Modern Docter, 2010, 48 (14): 6-9.

[28] Zha Y, Li L. Systematic Evaluation of Yinxing Damo injection in the treatment of angina pectoris. China Pharmacy, 2010, 21(44): 4143-4147.

[29] Zhao W, Xiang JS, Ye K. Systematic Review on Randomized Controlled Trials for treatment of UAP by Ginkgo extract. Journal of Liaoning University of Traditional Chinese Medicine, 2010, 12(11): 216-220.

[30] Song XM. Effect of Xuefuzhuyu decoction as adjutant

treatment to isosorbide dinitrate and aspirin for coronary angina pectoris: a meta-analysis. The Journal of Practical Medicine, 2010, 26 (14): 2633-2635.

[31] Chen XT, Guo SE, Guo Y. Effect of Xinkeshu for coronary angina pectoris: a meta-analysis. Journal of Changchun University of Traditional Chinese Medicine, 2010, 26 (3): 357-359.

[32] Long Y, Jin X, Shao ZJ et al. Systematic review on randomized controlled trials for qisupplementing and blood-quickening treatment of angina pectoris due to qi-deficiency and blood stasis. China Heart Journal, 2009, 21 (1): 54-59.

[33] Zhang MZ, Zhang J. Meta-analysis of Compound salvia pellet for coronary heart disease. Li Shizhen Medicine and Materia Medica Research, 2009, 20(4): 1007-1008.

[34] Lin H, Tang WP. Systematic review of randomized controlled trials on treating CHD with Shexiang baoxin wan, First National Middle-Aged MD Forum Proceedings of Integrative Medicine on Cardiovascular Disease, 2008, 147-152.

[35] Wang XJ, Xu BN, Meta analysis on treating angina pectoris with Suxiao jiuxin pill. Shaanxi Journal of Traditional Chinese Medicine, 2008, 29 (9): 1249-1251.

[36] Duan X, Zhou L, Wu T, et al. Chinese herbal medicine suxiao jiuxin wan for angina pectoris. Cochrane Database of Systematic Reviews, 2008, (1): CD004473.

[37] He SZ, Wu WK, Deng ZS, et al. Systematic Review on Randomized Controlled Trials for treatment of coronary heart disease by Tong xin luo Capsul. Journal of Sun Yat-Sen University, 2007, 28(5): 573-577.

[38] Jiang SY, Tong JC, Shun RY, et al. Meta-analysis of compound salvia pellet for coronary angina pectoris. Practical Pharmacy and Clinical Remedies, 2007, 10 (6): 334-337.

[39] Li KJ. A systematic review on Randomized Controlled Trials for treatment of unstable angina pectoris with Danshen preparations. Guangming Journal of ChineseMedicine, 2008, 22 (2): 37-40.

[40] Zhang JH, Shang HC, Gao XM et al. Systematic evaluation of compound preparation of salvia miltiorrhiza in treating stable angina in a randomized controlled trial. Tianjin Journal of Traditional Chinese Medicine , 2007, 24(3): 195-200.

[41] Li KJ. A systematic review on randomized controlled trials for treatment of stable angina pectoris with Danshen preparations. Herald of Medicine, 2007, 26(4): 383-386.

[42] Wang X, Zhu YY, Hu LS. A systematic review of Rhodiola L. for treating angina. Progress in Modern Biomedicine, 2006, 6 (2): 42-45.

[43] Zhang YC, Zhi FC, Tan QX, et al. Treating unstable angina with tetramethylpyrazine: a systematic review. Chinese Journal of Clinical Rehabilitation, 2006, 10 (27): 102-104.

[44] Wang Q, Wu T, Chen X, et al. Puerarin injection for unstable angina pectoris. Cochrane Database of Systematic Reviews, 2006, (3): CD004296.

[45] Wang G, Wang L, Xiong ZY, et al. Compound salvia pellet, a traditional Chinese medicine, for the treatment of chronic stable angina pectoris compared with nitrates: a meta-analysis. Medical Science Monitor, 2006, 12 (1): SR1-SR7.

[46] Wang L, Xiong ZY, Wang G. Systematic assessment on randomized controlled trials for treatment of stable angina pectoris by compound salvia pellet. Chinese Journal of Integrated Traditional and Western Medicine, 2004, 24 (6): 500-504.

[47] Zhang MZ, Wang L, Chen BJ, et al. Meta analysis of document on compound danshen dropping pills (DSP) in treatment of patients with stable angina. Chinese Journal of Integrative Medicine Cardio/ Cerebrovascular Disease, 2004, 2(6): 311-314.

[48] Li XY, Du F, Cheng WL, et al. Systematic review on randomized controlled trials for treatment of unstable angina pectoris by Shuxuetong. Modern Journal of Integrated Traditional Chinese and Western Medicine, 2010, 19 (18): 2231-2233.

[49] Song QG, Du WX, Liu M, et al. Effect of Yiqi Huoxue herbal products for ventricular remodeling after acute myocardial infarction: a meta-analysis. Liaoning Journal of Traditional ChineseMedicine, 2008, 35 (3): 323-325.

[50] European Medicines Agency (EMA). Committee for medicinal products for human use, guideline on the evaluation of medicinal products for cardiovascular disease prevention London, 2008, http://www.ema.europa.eu/ema/index/.

[51] Yusuf S, Mehta S, Anand S, et al. The Clopidogrel in unstable angina to prevent recurrent events (CURE) trial programme: rationale, design and baseline characteristics including a meta-analysis of the effects

第七章

of thienopyridines in vascular disease. European Heart Journal, 2000, 21 (24): 2033-2041.

[52] Moher D, Liberati A, Tetzlaff J, et al. The PRISMA Group I. Preferred reporting items for systematic reviews and meta-analyses: the PRISMA statement. PLOS Med, 2009, 6 (7): e1000097.

[53] Wang P, Xu YG, and Gao ZY. Effect of Acanthopanax Senticosus injection for coronary angina pectoris: a meta-analysis, Lishizhen Medicine and Materia Medica Research, 2007, 18 (9): 2243-2244.

[54] Zhong ZH, Li WH. A meta analysis on randomized controlled trials for treatment of coronary angina pectoris with Acanthopanax Senticosus injection. China Pharmaceuticals, 2007, 16 (15): 5-6.

[55] Zhou XG, Wang HW, Yu GB. Meta analysis on

treating unstable angina pectoris with Shexiang baoxin wan. Chinese Traditional Patent Medicine, 2004, 26(supplement): 1-6.

[56] Guo LM, Feng YG. Adverse reaction of puerarin injection. Chinese Magazine of Clinical Medicinal Professional Research, 2003, 69: 11495-11497.

[57] Zhi LM, Zhang ZQ. Review on the adverse reactions of puerarin injection. Hebei Traditional Chinese Medicine, 2002, 24 (7): 555-556.

[58] Zhang JH, Shang HC, Gao XM. et al. Methodology and reporting quality of systematic review/meta-analysis of traditional Chinese medicine. Journal of Alternative and Complementary Medicine, 2007, 13 (8): 797-805.

Astragalus Injection for Hypertensive Renal Damage: A Systematic Review[*]

Sun Tian   Xu Hao   Xu Feng-qin

1. Introduction

Hypertensive renal damage has been defined as being characterized by the changes in renal structure and function which was caused by hypertension. Renal damage is one of three hypertensive complications. Hypertension could cause renal damage in early stage, and the renal damage often happens insidiously and persists many years without any typical clinical symptoms. In the past ten years, the incidence of end-stage renal disease (ESRD) was rising at an annual rate of 9% and 28% was caused by hypertension [1]. In recent years, the incidence of ESRD caused by hypertension was also increased in China [2].

At present, antihypertensive drugs have been shown to be effective in lowering blood pressure and thus reducing morbidity and mortality of cardiovascular diseases. Angiotensin-converting enzyme inhibitors (ACEI) or angiotensin II receptor blocker (ARB) could also exert kidney protective effect by dilating efferent arterioles more than afferent arteriole, decreasing urinary albumin, and inhibiting the glomerulosclerosis. However, the treatment of hypertensive renal damage still needs to be further improved even on the basis of ACEI or ARB. Astragalus injection is a preparation of an extract of Radix Astragali. The major components are astragalosides [3], and the other pharmacological ingredients include polysaccharides, flavones, and amino acids. Modern pharmacological research has indicated that astragalus injection could enhance myocardial contractility, improve circulation, protect myocardial cells and regulate immune function [4,5]. Recent reviews [6-8] further indicated the potential benefit of astragalus injection in the treatment of

---

* 原载于 Evidence-Based Complementary and Alternative Medicine，2012，Article ID 929025

hypertensive renal damage. The following systematic review aims to test whether astragalus injection is effective and safe in treating hypertensive renal damage.

2. Methods

2.1 Database and Search Strategies

We searched MEDLINE, China National Knowledge Infrastructure (CNKI), Chinese VIP Information, China Biology Medicine (CBM), and Chinese Medical Citation Index (CMCI). The date of search was from the first of database start to August 2011. No language restrictions were applied. We used the terms "hypertensive renal damage", "hypertensive renal injury", "astragalus injection", and "Huangqi injection". Various combinations of the terms were used, depending on the database searched.

2.2 Inclusion Criteria

(1) Randomized controlled trials (RCT); (2) male or female patients, of any age or ethnic origin, who had hypertensive renal damage. Hypertensive renal damage was diagnosed on the basis of: (i) a history of essential hypertension, (ii) persistent proteinuria, (iii) hypertensive retinopathy, (iv) primary renal diseases or other secondary renal disease was excluded；(3) the intervention measure was astragalus injection, astragalus injection plus placebo, or astragalus injection plus antihypertensive drugs；(4) all trials had to report clinically relevant outcome measures of hypertensive renal damage；(5) the treatment should be at least two weeks. Outcome measures include results of blood pressure, renal function, clinical comprehensive effect, and Traditional Chinese medicine (TCM) syndrome differentiation. Duplicated publications reporting the same groups of participants were excluded.

2.3 Data Extraction and Quality Assessment

Two reviewers (T. Sun, H. Xu) extracted data independently. We assessed the methodological quality of all included trials by using the table

of risk of bias provided by RevMan 5.1.0. The scale consists of seven items pertaining to description of random sequence generation, allocation concealment, blinding of participants and personnel, blinding of outcome assessment, incomplete outcome data, selective reporting, and other bias.

2.4 Data Synthesis

We used RevMan 5.1.0 provided by Cochrane Collaboration to analyse the data. Dichotomous data were expressed as relative risk (RR) and continuous outcomes as weighted mean difference (WMD), both with 95% confidence intervals (CI). Heterogeneity was assessed using the I^2 test with the significance level set at I^2 over 50% or $P < 0.1$. In the absence of significant heterogeneity, we pooled data using a fixed-effect model ($I^2 < 50\%$), otherwise we using random effects model ($I^2 > 50\%$) [9].

3. Results

3.1 Description of Included Trials

Our search identified 32 references. We excluded 27 of these articles. Flow diagram of the article selection for this study is shown in Figure 1.

The search yielded 5 eligible trials, which were all conducted and published in China. A total of 429 participants with renal damage induced by hypertension were included in the 5 trials. The proportion of male participants was 66.8%. All the trials included inpatients, and the average size of the trials was 86 patients (ranging from 48 to 127 participants). Five trials enrolled patients with renal damage induced with hypertension. The diagnostic criteria of trials were based on the guidelines for prevention and treatment of hypertension in China [4,5], clinical manifestations, and laboratory tests[3,6,7]. Three trials were astragalus injection combined with antihypertensive drugs against antihypertensive drugs, one trial was astragalus injection against placebo, and one trial was astragalus injection against prostaglandin.

第七章

Table 1　Characteristics of Included Studies

Study ID	Gender male/female	Base-line information	Average age (years)	Interventions	Control	Duration of treatment (days)	Outcome measures
Ji and Yin 2006 [10]	59/35	Age, sex, condition	45.2	Astragalus injection (250 mL i.d, qd)	5% glucose injection	30	β_2-MG, mAlb
Hua et al. 2009 [17]	84/43	Age, sex, blood pressure, duration	44.3	Astragalus injection (250 mL i.d, qd) calcium channel blockers (CCB), ACEI/ARB, thiazine diuretics	CCB, ACEI/ARB, thiazine diuretics	20	Twenty-four hours urinary protein content, blood pressure, urinalysis, renal function
Xu et al. 2008 [11]	28/20	Age, sex, blood pressure	63.6±14.2	Astragalus injection (250 mL i.d, qd) Telmisartan, Plendil	Telmisartan, Plendil	21	Twenty-four hours urinary protein content, blood pressure, mAlb, serum potassium, pulse pressure, estimated glomerular filtration rate (eGFR)
He 2004 [12]	78/18	Age, sex	74.2	Astragalus injection (500 mL i.d, qd)	Prostaglandin (PGE1)	15	BUN, Scr, Ccr
Yao et al. 2002 [13]	38/26	Age, sex, blood pressure	64.7±13.7	Astragalus injection (250 mL i.d, qd) Lotensin, Plendil	Lotensin, Plendil	21	Twenty-four hours urinary protein content

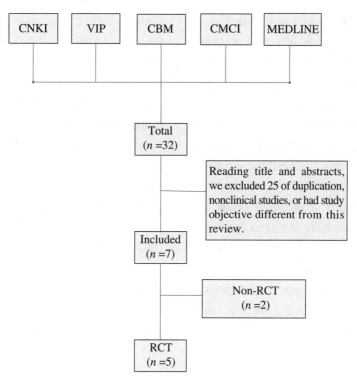

Figure 1　Flow Diagram of the Article Selection for This Study

Table 2　The Analysis of Improvement of Renal Damage Indices

Renal damage indices and comparison between the groups	No. of studies	WMD [95% CI]	P value
β_2-MG			
Astragalus versus glucose injection [10]	1	−15.14 [−21.61, −8.67]	$P < 0.00001$
mAlb			
Astragalus versus glucose injection [10]	1	−28.4 [−47.67, −9.15]	$P = 0.004$
Astragalus plus Telmisartan, Plendil versus Telmisartan, and Plendil [11]	1	−4.20 [−7.47, −0.93]	$P = 0.01$
eGFR			
Astragalus plus Telmisartan, Plendil versus Telmisartan, and Plendil [11]	1	4.10 [−2.38, 10.58]	$P = 0.21$
pulse pressure			
Astragalus plus Telmisartan, Plendil versus Telmisartan, and Plendil [11]	1	−7.00 [−11.56, −2.44]	$P = 0.003$
SBP			
Astragalus plus Telmisartan, Plendil versus Telmisartan, and Plendil [11]	1	−21.70 [−31.24, −12.16]	$P < 0.00001$
DBP			
Astragalus plus Telmisartan, Plendil versus Telmisartan, and Plendil [11]	1	−4.20 [−11.02, 2.62]	$P = 0.23$
serum potassium			
Astragalus plus Telmisartan, Plendil versus Telmisartan, and Plendil [11]	1	−0.08[−0.28, 0.12]	P=0.44
twenty-four hours urinary protein content			
Astragalus plus Telmisartan, Plendil versus Telmisartan, and Plendil [11]	1	−0.05 [−0.07, −0.04]	$P < 0.00001$
Astragalus plus Lotensin, Plendil versus Lotensin, and Plendil [13]	1	−0.21 [−0.50, 0.08]	P =0.15
BUN			
Astragalus versus prostaglandin [12]	1	−7.39 [−9.83, −4.95]	$P < 0.00001$
Scr			
Astragalus versus prostaglandin [12]	1	−3.37 [46.05, 39.31]	$P = 0.88$
Ccr			
Astragalus versus prostaglandin [12]	1	6.84 [4.57, 9.11]	$P < 0.00001$

No trial reported outcomes of the incidence of complications, health economic costs, quality of life, or adverse effects. The outcomes that were reported included twenty-four hours urinary protein content, microalbuminuria (mAlb), β_2-microglobulin (β_2-MG), blood urea nitrogen (BUN), serum creatinine (Scr), and creatinine clearance rate (Ccr). Characteristics of included studies were shown in Table 1.

3.2 Methodological Quality of Included Trials

The methodological quality of all the five trials was very low (Figure 2): none of trials reported sample calculation, the sample size of trials was small. These trials provided limited information on allocation concealment and blinding, and they were all lack of description of the allocation sequence generation. All the trials did not mention followup. We contacted the author for further information but regrettably no information has been provided to date.

3.3 Effect of Interventions

Three trials [3,5,7] gave biochemical indices to analyse the effective of astragalus injection. One trial [4] only gave the number of patients who had symptomatic improvement, and one trial [6] gave both biochemical indices and the number of patients who had symptomatic improvement. All were showed in Tables 2 and 3.

3.3.1 The Analysis of Improvement of Renal Damage Indices   It was not possible to pool the data on renal damage indicators, since the results describing varied indicators to prove the curative effect of astragalus injection.

In the Ji trial [10], the experimental group used astragalus injection (n=54), while glucose injection was administered in the control group. Astragalus injection showed significant effect on indicators of β_2-MG (MD –15.14, 95%CI –21.61 to –8.67) and mAlb (MD –28.41, 95%CI 47.67 to –9.15).

Xu trial [11] used astragalus injection combined with Telmisartan and Plendil in the experimental group (n=26), while Telmisartan and Plendil were administered in the control group.

Only indicators of pulse pressure (MD –7.00, 95%CI –11.56 to –2.44), systolic blood pressure (SBP) (MD –21.70, 95%CI –31.24, –12.16), and twenty-four hours urinary protein content (MD –0.05, 95%CI –0.07, –0.04) showed significant differences.

In He trial [12], the experimental group used astragalus injection (n = 50), and prostaglandin was used in the control group. Astragalus injection showed significant effect on indicator of BUN (MD –7.39, 95%CI –9.83, –4.95) and Ccr (MD 6.84, 95%CI 4.57, 9.11)

In Yao trial [13], there was no significant difference between astragalus injection plus Lotensin and Plendil group and Lotensin and Plendil group, according to indicator of twenty-four hours urinary protein content.

3.3.2. Symptoms and Signs   There were only two trials who reported the improvement on symptoms and signs (Table 3). However, they were all for comprehensive therapeutic effect. We cannot obtain the number of patients with individual symptoms and the data of individual symptoms improvement after treatment. So we cannot get the analysis of comparison between groups.

3.4 Final Indicator at Endpoint

None of the trial reported the mortality rate or the incidence of complication.

3.5 Sensitivity Analysis, Subgroup Analysis, and Publication Bias

The number of trials was too small to conduct any sufficient additional analysis of sensitivity, subgroup, and publication bias.

3.6 Adverse Reaction

None of the trial reported the observation of side effects.

4. Discussion

Our systematic review suggested that astragalus injection may be effective on laboratory indices of renal damage (β_2-MG, mAlb, pulse pressure, SBP, BUN, Ccr) or improvement of symptoms and signs. However, according

Table 3 The Analysis of Comprehensive Therapeutic Effect.

Symptom and sign	No. of studies	Intervention (*n/N*)	Control (*n/N*)	RR [95%CI]	*P* value
Astragalus plus thiazine diuretics versus thiazine diuretics	1	10/64	32/64	0.18 [0.08，0.41]	*P* < 0.00001
Astragalus versus prostaglandin	1	2/50	13/46	0.11 [0.02，0.50]	*P* = 0.005

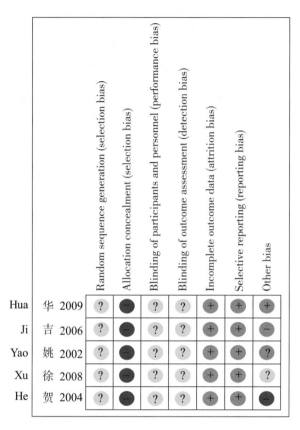

Figure 2 Risk of Bias Summary

to potential publication bias and low-quality trials, available data are not adequate to draw a definite conclusion of astragalus injection in treating renal damage induced by hypertension. More specifically, the positive findings should be interpreted conservatively due to the following facts.

The five trials included in this paper had risk of bias in terms of design, reporting, and methodology. They provided only limited descriptions of study design, allocation concealment, and baseline data. All the five RCTs prohibited us from performing meaningful sensitivity analysis. The included trials were heterogeneous in the populations (adults, elderly people) and the reported outcomes. All the

included trials were not multicenter, large scale RCTs.

The primary goal of treatment for renal damage induced by hypertension is to prevent death or progression to complications. The outcomes from all the included trials are mainly laboratory indices and symptom improvement. There is a lack of data from all the trials on clinically relevant outcomes such as the mortality, incidence of complications, and quality of life.

Nevertheless, astragalus injection is administered for treating renal damage induced by hypertension in China. We have identified more than 30 randomized trials on this topic until now. However, most of them are not eligible for the review due to inadequate design, conducting, and reporting of the trials. Chinese researchers must be aware of the need to design and use appropriate statistical methods in future RCTs of astragalus injection and to measure clinical outcomes rather than physiological (surrogate) outcomes.

All the five trials did not report that adverse events. A conclusion about the safety of astragalus injection cannot be made. In China, it is widely believed that it is safe to use herbal medicines for various conditions. All the trials did not report that adverse events may reflect current situation. However, the safety of herbal medicines needs to be monitored carefully and reported appropriately in the future clinical trials. In fact, we found that some reports [14-16] indicated that astragalus injection had adverse outcomes.

Although we conducted comprehensive searches, we only identified and included trials published in Chinese. Most of the trials are small sample with positive findings. We tried to avoid language bias and location bias, but we cannot exclude potential publication bias. We have conducted extensive searches for unpublished material, but at the same time we cannot neglect the fact that trials with negative findings remain unpublished.

Based on this systematic review, the effectiveness and safety of astragalus injection in patients with hypertensive renal damage is uncertain. The evidence is inconclusive due to poorly designed and low-quality trials. There is a need for additional RCTs that emphasize not only good clinical design but also more elaborated description of the intervention and clinically relevant outcomes including the mortality, incidence of complications, and quality of life.

References

[1] Ruilope LM. The kidney as a sensor of cardiovascular risk in essential hypertension. Journal of the American Society of Nephrology, 2002, 13 (3): S165-S168.

[2] Liu LS. Hypertension. People's Medical Publishing House Press, 2001.

[3] Zhang Y, Zhang Q, Wang HX. Research development of TCM for treating renal damage induced by hypertension. Journal of Integrated Traditional and Western Medicine, 2010, 5 (6): 549-551.

[4] Jiang KL，Dai XH. Research development of TCM for treating renal damage induced by hypertension. Clinical Journal of Traditional ChineseMedicine, 2011, 23 (6): 554-555.

[5] Bao Zhang Island Pharmaceutical Co, Huangqi Injection, Chinese science and technology achievements database, 2007.

[6] Fu T, Ji Y, He M. Industrialized research and development of Huangqi Injection. Chinese science and technology achievements database, 2006.

[7] Jining Medical College Hospital. The clinical research on the effects of Huangqi Injection for blood plasma apoptosis correlation factor of chronic heart failure patients. Chinese science and technology achievements database, 2007.

[8] Bi ZJ. Astragalus injection in lowering urine protein of eldly patients with hypertensive renal damage, Chinese Journal of Integrative Medicine on Cardio-/ Cerebrovascular Disease, 2007, 5 (12): 1235.

[9] Higgins JPT，Green S. Corchrane Reviewers' Handbook 5.1.0 [updated March 2011]. Review Manager (RevMan) [Computer program]. Version 5.1.0.

[10] Ji Y, Yin WH. Influence of Astragalus Injection in treating with renal damage induced by hypertension. Journal of Emergency in Traditional Chinese Medicine, 2006, 15 (11): 1237-1238.

[11] Xu GH, Yuan L, Li Y, et al. Clinical observation of Astragalus Injection in treatment of renal injury in patients with primary hypertension. Journal of Chinese Integrative Medicine, 2008, 6 (5): 530-532.

[12] He XG. Astragalus injection in the treatment of senile renal damage induced by hypertension, Practical Journal of Medicine & Pharmacy, 2004, 21 (8): 712-713.

[13] Yao GL, Gui BS, MLQ. et al. Astragalus Injection in the reduction of protein content of patients with renal damage induced by hypertension. Journal of Herald of Medicine, 2010, 3 (5): 12-14.

[14] Lai Y, Wang P. Analysis of adverse outcomes of Astragalus Injection in 71 cases of patients with renal damage induced by hypertension. Journal of Herald of Medicine, 2006, 25 (2): 23-25.

[15] Zhao H, Li JC. Adverse outcomes of Astragalus Injection. Journal of Chinese Misdiagnostics, 2005, 5 (7): 14-16.

[16] Yang LZ. Adverse outcomes of Astragalus Injection in 1 cases of patients with renal damage induced by hypertension. Journal of Herald of Medicine, 2007, 8(5): 27-29.

[17] Hua J, Zhang AL, Chen GX. Clinical observation on Astragalus Injection in the treatment of 64 cases of renal damage induced by hypertension、Journal of Traditional Chinese Medicine, 2010, 32(1): 45-46.

A Systematic Review of Xuezhikang, An Extract from Red Yeast Rice, for Coronary Heart Disease Complicated by Dyslipidemia[*]

SHANG Qing-hua   LIU Zhao-lan   CHEN Ke-ji   XU Hao   LIU Jian-ping

1. Introduction

Coronary heart disease (CHD) is one of the most serious diseases with high incidence and mortality. Dyslipidemia contributes greatly to the formation and progression of atherosclerosis (AS), which plays a dominant role in leading to CHD. Patients with CHD are also commonly complicated with dyslipidemia. Modulating dyslipidemia actively, especially lowering low-density lipoprotein-cholesterol (LDL-C) by statins, has been demonstrated to be very crucial to prevent AS and reduce the morbidity and mortality of CHD. Most recently, the updated ESC/EAS guidelines for management of dyslipidemia [1] further highlighted the aggressive lipid-lowering strategy in subjects with documented coronary vascular disease (CVD) or previous myocardial infarction (MI). However, the application of statins might be restricted by the adverse effect on the liver function and creatine kinase, especially in patients with old age, multiple comorbid diseases, high-dose statins, or a combination lipid-lowering therapy. Thus it is of great clinical significance to find an effective but safer alternative therapy in CHD patients complicated by dyslipidemia.

Xuezhikang is a partially purified extract of fermented red yeast rice (Monascus purpureus). It is composed of 13 kinds of natural statins,

unsaturated fatty acids, ergosterol, amino acids, flavonoids, alkaloid, trace element, and so forth. The health enhancing qualities of this yeast have been introduced and used in China for over two thousand years. At latest systematic review indicated the beneficial effects of Xuezhikang in the treatment of hyperlipidemia [2]. Therefore, Xuezhikang has been recommended in a guideline for China adult dyslipidemia prevention [3]. Recently, clinical benefits of Xuezhikang were also found in CHD patients combined with dyslipidemia in some randomized controlled trials [4-6]. This systematic review aims to evaluate the benefit and side effect of Xuezhikang, a potential alternative drug of statins, for CHD patients complicated by dyslipidemia, and thus provide further evidence for clinical application.

2. Methods

2.1 Inclusion Criteria

Randomized controlled trials (RCTs) comparing Xuezhikang with placebo, no intervention, or established lipid-lowing agents in English or Chinese were considered. Quasirandomized trials were excluded, and the duration of the intervention was no less than four weeks. Participants of all age with CHD complicated by dyslipidemia meeting. with at least

* 原载于 Evidence-Based Complementary and Alternative Medicine，2012，Article ID 636547

one of the current or past definitions or guidelines of CHD [including acute coronary syndrome (ACS)] [7-13] and dyslipidemia (treatment goal as the lower limit, see Table 1) [14-20] were considered. Those who did not introduce diagnostic criteria in the text but stated patients with definite CHD or dyslipidemia were also included. Secondary dyslipidemia, high serum lipid level after meal, serious heart failure, and serious hepatic or renal failure were excluded.

Outcome measures include primary outcomes (including all-cause mortality, CHD mortality, incidence of MI, revascularization, and rehospitalization for unstable angina) and secondary outcomes [including serum total cholesterol (TC), triglyceride (TG), LDL-C, and-high density lipoprotein cholesterol (HDL-C)].

2.2 Search Strategy

Two reviewers searched the following databases up to September 2011 independently for the identifications of trials (publication or nonpublication): The Cochrane Library, Pubmed, Chinese Biomedical Database (CBM), China National Knowledge Infrastructure (CNKI), Chinese VIP Information (VIP), and Wanfang Databases. We used the terms as follows: coronary heart disease, CHD, coronary artery disease, angina pectoris, myocardial infarction, acute coronary syndrome, cardi*, and Xuezhikang, red yeast rice, monascus. Because of different characteristics of various databases,

Table1　Definition of Dyslipidemia or Treatmentgoal of Patients with CHD or Equivalents on Serum Lipid Level

Orgination	Definition of dyslipidemia or treatmentgoal of Patients with CHD or equivalents on serum lipid level
ATP Ⅰ 1988 [14]	Ideal lipid level：TC < 5.17 mmol/L (200 mg/dL)；LDL-C < 3.36 mmol/L (130 mg/dL) . Patients with HDL-C < 0.9 mmol/L (35 mg/dL) were defined unmoral. The definition of dyslipidemia was according to the level of LDL-C
ATP Ⅱ 1993 [15]	Treatment goal：LDL-C ≤ 2.6 mmol/L (100 mg/dL)
Ministry of Health of the People's Republic of China 1993 [8]	The treatment goal was not introduced
CADPS 1997 [16]	Treatmentgoal：TC < 4.68 mmol/L (180 mg/dL)；TG < 1.7 mmol/L (150 mg/dL)；LDL-C < 2.6 mmol/L (100 mmol /L)
ATP Ⅲ 2001 [17]	Treatmentgoal：LDL-C < 2.6 mmol/L (100 mg/dL)
Implication of ATP Ⅲ 2004 [18]	Treatmentgoal：LDL-C < 2.6 mmol/L (100 mg/dL)；the optionalgoal：LDL-C < 1.8 mmol/L (70 mg/dL)
AHA/ACCguideline 2006 [19]	Treatmentgoal：LDL-C < 2.6 mmol/L (100 mmol/L)，and it is seasonal for lower than 1.8 mmol/L (70 mg/dL)
CADPG 2007 [3]	Treatmentgoal：TC < 4.14 mmol/L (160 mg/dL) and LDL-C < 2.59 mmol/L (100 mg/dL) for CHD or equivalents Treatmentgoal：TC < 3.11 mmol/L (120 mg/dL)；LDL-C < 2.07 mmol/L (80 mg/dL) for ACS or ischemic cardiovascular disease complicated with diabetes mellitus Suitable scope of HDL-C：≥ 1.04 mmol/L (40 mg/dL)；suitable scope of TG：< 1.7 mmol/L (150 mg/dL)
ESC/EAS 2011 [1]	In patients at very high CV risk (established CVD，type 2 diabetes，type I diabetes with target organ damage，moderate to severe CKD or a score level ≥ 10%)，the LDL-C goal is < 1.8 mmol/L (70 mg/dL) and/or ≥ 50% LDL-C reduction when target level cannot be reached (Ⅰ A recommendation)

MeSH terms and free text terms were used regardless of the report types in full text, title, keyword, subject terms, or abstract.

2.3 Data Extraction and Quality Assessment

Two reviewers (Shang QH, Liu ZL) independently extracted data according to a data extraction form made by the authors. Disagreements were resolved by consensus or consultation from a third reviewer (Liu JP). The methodological quality of trials was assessed independently using criteria from the Cochrane Handbook for Systematic Review of Interventions, Version 5.0.1 (Shang QH, Liu ZL) [20]. We contacted with the authors if there was any doubt in randomization and blinding method. The items included random sequence generation (selection bias), allocation concealment (selection bias), blinding of participants and personnel (performance bias), blinding of outcome assessment (detection bias), incomplete outcome data (attrition bias), selective reporting (reporting bias), and other bias. We judged each item from three levels ("Yes" for a low of bias, "No" for a high risk of bias, "Unclear" otherwise), and then we assessed the trials and categorized them into three levels: low risk of bias (all the items were in low risk of bias), high risk of bias (at least one item was in high risk of bias), unclear risk of bias (at least one item was in unclear).

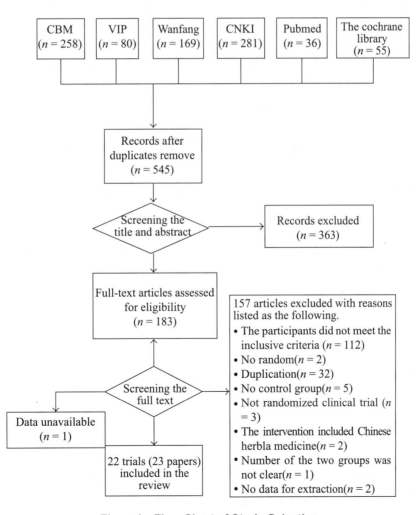

Figure1 Flow Chart of Study Selection

2.4 Data Synthesis.

We used Revman 5.1 software provided by the Cochrane Collaboration for data analyses. Studies were stratified by the types of comparisons. We will express dichotomous data as risk ratio (RR) and its 95% confidence intervals (CI). Continuous outcome will be presented as mean difference (MD) and its 95% CI. Heterogeneity was recognized significant when $I^2 \geqslant 50\%$. Fixed effects model was used if there is no significant heterogeneity of the data; random effects model was used if significant heterogeneity existed ($50\% < I^2 < 85\%$). Publication bias was explored using a funnel plot.

3. Results

3.1 Description of Included Trials

22 RCTs (23 papers) [4-6,21-39] were included, 21 papers were published in Chinese, one paper published in English, and one was unpublished as a postgraduate dissertation. The whole process of trials selection was demonstrated in Figure 1. The characteristics of included trials were listed in Table 2.

6520 Participants were included (3264 in intervention group and 3256 in control group). Two of the trials did not report the gender, and 4905 male and 1538 female were included in the other 20 trials. A total of 7 criteria of CHD (including ACS) were selected, but 6 trials did not introduce criteria of CHD but mentioned "patients with CHD were eligible to include". 3 criteria of dyslipidemia were used for 11 trials, and the other 11 trials only reported the serum lipid levels, which were categorized to dyslipidemia according to the previous and current definitions and guidelines Table 1. One trial [4] included patients with MI; five of the trials [5,27,28,34,39] included patients with unstable angina; two of the trials [6,38] included patients with ACS; three of the trials [21,22,31] included patients with stable angina. The other 11 trials [23-26,29,30,32,33,35-37] did not introduce the types of CHD or all types were included.

Patients in 19 trials prescribed Xuezhikang 600 mg QD (regulation was conducted for adverse events), one trial used Xuezhikang 600 mg TID if the serum TC or TG still higher after having been prescribed for 6 weeks (600 mg BID in previous 6 weeks) [30], one trial [37] prescribed Xuezhikang 300 mg TID, and one trial [31] prescribed Xuezhikang 1200 mg QN. The duration of treatment ranged from 4 weeks to 7 years.

There were five comparisons in the review according to various control groups. (1) Xuezhikang and conventional therapy versus conventional therapy (8 trials) [5,6,24,29,33,34,38,39]; (2) Xuezhikang and conventional therapy versus placebo and conventional therapy (2 trials) [4,35]; (3) Xuezhikang and conventional therapy versus statin and conventional therapy (9 trials) [21-23,25,26,28,31,37,39]; (4) Xuezhikang and statin and conventional therapy versus statin and conventional therapy (2 trials) [27,36]; (5) Xuezhikang and aspirin versus inositol nicotinate and aspirin (1 trials) [32]. One trial [39] was designed as three groups with two comparisons and Xuezhikang and conventional therapy versus conventional therapy; Xuezhikang and conventional therapy versus atorvastatin and conventional therapy.

3.2 Methodological Quality of Included Trials

According to the criteria introduced above, no trial was evaluated as having a low risk of bias. Only one trial of the 22 trials reported the method to generate the allocation sequence (random number table) in the paper [6]. After we contacted with the authors, six trials announced a correct method for allocation sequence [4-6,31,33,35]. One trial was assessed as having adequate concealment [35]. Two trials applied double-blinding [4,35], and two trials used single-blinding but did give us objective to be blinded [25,37]. One trial blinded the outcome assessors [4]. One trial reported prior sample size estimation and mentioned intention-to-treat analysis [4]. Five trials reported information on withdrawal/dropout [4,6,22,29,32]. 18 trials [4-6,22-27,29,31-33,35-39] provided baseline data for the comparability among groups. The results of the assessment of risk of bias are presented in a "risk of bias summary" figure produced by Revman 5.1 automatically Figure 2.

3.3 Effect Estimates of Outcomes (Tables 3 and 4)

3.3.1 All-Cause Mortality There was only 1 trial [4] reported the all-cause mortality in the comparisons of Xuezhikang and conventional therapy versus placebo and conventional therapy [RR 0.67；95% CI 0.54 to 0.83；1 trial, n=4870].

3.3.2 Mortality of CHD. There were 5 studies [4,22,27,28,32] that presented the effect of Xuezhikang in reducing the mortality of CHD. Compared to placebo on the basis of conventional therapy, Xuezhikang showed a reduction of mortality of CHD (RR 0.69；95% CI 0.54 to 0.89；1 trial, n =4870) [4]. Compared to simvastatin on the basis of conventional therapy, Xuezhikang showed no significant difference in mortality of CHD (RR 0.26；95% CI 0.06 to 1.21；2 trial, n =220) [22,28]. Compared to no treatment on the basis of simvastatin and conventional therapy, Xuezhikang showed no effect in reducing mortality of CHD (RR 0.33；95% CI 0.01 to 7.80；1 trial, n = 48) [27]. Compared with inositol nicotinate on the basis of aspirin, Xuezhikang showed no significant difference in mortality of CHD (RR 0.15；95% CI 0.02 to 1.18；1 trial, n=122) [32].

3.3.3 Incidence of MI There were 3 studies reporting CHD events in 3 different comparisons. Compared with placebo on the basis of conventional therapy, Xuezhikang showed a reduction of morbidity of MI (RR 0.39；95% CI 0.28 to 0.55；1 trial, n=4870) [4]. Compared with simvastatin on the basis of conventional therapy, Xuezhikang showed no significant difference (RR 0.95；95% CI 0.30 to 3.05；1 trial, n=84) [28]. In comparisons of Xuezhikang and simvastatin and conventional therapy versus simvastatin and conventional therapy, Xuezhikang showed no effect in reducing incidence of MI (RR 0.20；95% CI 0.01 to 3.96；1 trial, n=48) [27].

	Random sequence generation (selection bias)	Allocation concealment (selection bias)	Blinding of participants and personnel (performance bias)	Blinding of outcome assessment (detection bias)	Incomplete outcome data (attrition bias)	Selective reporting (reporting bias)	Other bias
CCSPS 2005	+	?	+	+	+	+	?
Dai 1999	+	?	−	?	+	+	?
Gao 2003	?	?	?	?	?	?	?
Guan 2010	?	?	?	?	+	+	?
Huang 2005	?	?	?	?	?	?	?
Huang 2009	?	?	?	?	?	+	?
Jiang 2001	?	?	?	?	+	+	?
Li 2011	?	?	?	?	+	+	?
Lin 2009	?	?	?	?	+	?	?
Lou 2008	?	?	?	?	+	+	?
Ma 2005	?	?	?	?	?	?	?
Qi 2001	?	?	?	?	?	?	?
Shang 2007	+	?	?	?	+	+	?
Wang 2000	?	?	?	?	+	?	?
Wang 2004	+	?	?	?	+	+	+
Xu 2005	?	?	?	?	+	+	?
Yan 2006	?	?	?	?	?	?	?
Yan 2007	+	?	?	?	?	?	?
Yu 2002	+	+	+	?	?	+	?
Zhang 2010	?	?	?	?	?	−	?
Zhang 2011	?	?	?	?	?	?	?
Zhou 2003	?	?	?	?	?	+	?

Note
+ Low risk
− High risk
? Unclear

Figure 2 Risk of Bias Summary.

3.3.4 Revascularization Revascu larization included percutaneous coronary intervention (PCI) and coronary artery bypass graft (CABG). There were 2 studies [4,28] reporting revascularization in 2 different comparisons. Compared with placebo on the basis of conventional therapy, Xuezhikang showed a significant reduction of revascularization (RR 0.67; 95% CI 0.50 to 0.89; 1 trial, n=4870) [4]. Compared with simvastatin on the basis of conventional therapy, Xuezhikang showed no significant difference (RR 1.14; 95% CI 0.38 to 3.46; 1 trial, n=84) [28].

3.3.5 Rehospitalization for Unstable Angina There were 2 trials [27,28] reporting rehospitalization in 2 different comparisons. Compared with simvastatin on the basis of conventional therapy, Xuezhikang showed no significant difference in the number of rehospitalization (RR 1.02; 95% CI 0.57 to 1.84; 1 trial, n=84) [28]. Compared with no treatment on the basis of simvastatin and conventional therapy, Xuezhikang showed no effect in reducing rehospitalization (RR 0.20; 95% CI 0.03 to 1.59; 1 trial, n=48) [27].

3.3.6 Serum TC Level There were 21 studies that reported the level of total cholesterol Table 4, but one trial only reported the serum lipid level of the treatment group [30]. (1) Compared to no treatment with cointervention of conventional therapy, Xuezhikang showed a reduction of TC level (MD−0.97 mmol/L; 95% CI −1.24 to −0.71; 8 trials, n=500) [5,6,24,29,33,34,38,39]. (2) There were two trials that reported Xuezhikang versus placebo on the basis of conventional therapy, meta-analysis was not used for significant difference, and, in this comparison, Xuezhikang showed a reduction of TC level (MD −0.57 mmol/L; 95% CI −0.61 to −0.53; 1 trial, n=4870) [4] and (MD −2.62 mmol/L; 95% CI −2.98 to −2.26; 1 trial, n = 62) [35]. (3) There was no significant difference on serum TC level of Xuezhikang comparing to statins on the basis of conventional therapy (MD 0.19 mmol/L; 95% CI −0.22 to 0.59; 8 trial, n=633) [21,23-25,28,31,37,39]. Since there was significant heterogeneity in the

comparison, we examined the data carefully and found that data of two trials deviated from the others. After looking over the papers, one of the two trial [26] with an unclear conventional therapy and the other used Xuezhikang 300 mg tid in the whole trial [37]. Sensitive analysis was used and got a similar conclusion (MD 0.02 mmol/L; 95% CI −0.03 to 0.06; 6 trial, n=489) after excluded the two trials [26,37]. (4) Compared with no treatment on the basis of statins and conventional therapy, Xuezhikang showed a reduction of TC level (MD−0.96 mmol/L; 95% CI−1.33 to −0.58; 2 trial, n=108) [27,36]. (5) Compared to inositol nicotinate on the basis of aspirin, Xuezhikang showed a significant difference in the reduction of TC level (MD −1.05 mmol/L; 95% CI −1.46 to −0.64; 1 trial, n=105) [32].

3.3.7 Serum TG Level There were 20 studies that reported the level of TG (seeTable 4), but one trial only reported the serum lipid level of the treatment group [30]. (1) Compared to no treatment with cointervention of conventional therapy, Xuezhikang showed a reduction of TG level (MD −0.49 mmol/L; 95% CI −0.58 to −0.39; 7 trial, n=412) [5,6,24,29,33,38,39]. (2) There were two trials that reported Xuezhikang versus placebo on the basis of conventional therapy, meta-analysis was not used for significant difference, and, in this comparison, Xuezhikang showed a reduction of TG level (MD−0.17 mmol/L; 95% CI−0.22 to−0.12; 1 trial, n=4870) [4] and (MD−1.29 mmol/L; 95% CI−1.57 to−1.01; 1 trial, n=62) [35]. (3) There was no significant difference on serum TG level of Xuezhikang comparing to statins on the basis of conventional therapy (MD −0.05 mmol/L; 95% CI −0.12 to 0.02; 8 trial, n=633) [21,23-25,28,31,37,39]. (4) Compared with no treatment on the basis of fluvastatin and conventional therapy, Xuezhikang showed a reduction of TG level (MD −0.27 mmol/L; 95% CI−0.35 to−0.19; 1 trial, n=60) [36]. (5) Compared to inositol nicotinate on the basis of aspirin, Xuezhikang showed a significant difference in the reduction of TG level (MD −0.60 mmol/L; 95% CI −0.95 to −0.25; 1 trial, n =

Table 2　Characteristics of Included Trials

ID	Diagnostic criteria of CHD (ACS)	Diagnostic criteria of dyslipidemia	Types of CHD	Sample size (I/C)	Age (y, I/C)	Interventions group	Control group	Duration of treatment	Outcomes evaluation	Balance report of baseline
CCSPS 2005[4]	Not specified	TC: 4.40-6.47	MI	2441/2429	(Male: 58.1±9.9; female: 62.9±6.7)/(male: 58.0±9.7; female: 62.6±7.4)	Xuezhikang 600 mg BID + conventional therapy (no detail)	Placebo + conventional therapy (no detail)	4 year in average	Serum lipid level (TC, TG, LDL-C, HDL-C), all-cause mortality, cardiovascular events, serum lipid level (TC, TG, HDL-C, LDL-C), ADs	Yes
Dai et al. 1999[5]	WHO 1979 and Gao 1994	Ministry of Health of the People's Republic of China 1993	Unstable angina	33/25	(57±9)/(56±8)	Xuezhikang 600 mg, BID + control	Nitrate esters 10 mg BID + nifedipine GIFTS 30 mg QD/diltiazem 30 mg TID +metoprolol 12.5 mg BID + aspirin 50 mg QD	8 weeks	erum lipid level (TC, TG, HDL-C, LDL-C), ADs	Yes
Gao and Liao 2003[21]	Not specified	TC ≥ 5.2 mmol/L, LDL-C ≥ 3.12 mmol/L, TG ≥ 1.7 mmol/L	Stable Angina	30/30	53-85, 67.5 in average	Xuezhikang 600 mg BID + conventional therapy (no detail)	Fluvastatin (Lescol see fluvastatin) 20 mg QD + conventional therapy (no detail)	4 weeks	Serum lipid level (TC, TG, LDL-C, HDL-C)	Unclear
Guan 2010[22]	Not specified	TC > 7.08 mmol/L; TG > 3.34; LDL-C > 4.2; HDL < 0.93. Two items of the above were included	Stable Angina	72/64	49-76, 62 in average	Xuezhikang 600 mg BID	Simvastatin 10 mg QN	1 year	CHD mortality, ADs	Yes
Huang et al. 2005[23]	WHO 1979	CADPS 1997	OMI and UA	45/63	44-72	Xuezhikang 600 mg BID	Simvastatin 20 mg QN	6 weeks	Serum lipid level (TC, TG, LDL-C, HDL-C)	Yes
Huang et al. 2009[24]	WHO 1979	CADPS 1997	Unclear	43/42	65.78±4.62	Xuezhikang 600 mg, BID + control	Nitroglycerine 20 mg BIDIV + 10% KCL + insulinIV QD	12 weeks	Serum lipid level (TC, TG, HDL-C, LDL-C)	Yes

Continued

ID	Diagnostic criteria of CHD (ACS)	Diagnostic criteria of dyslipidemia	Types of CHD	Sample size (I/C)	Age (y, I/C)	Interventions group	Control group	Duration of treatment	Outcomes evaluation	Balance report of baseline
Jiang and Cai 2001[25]	Not specified	CADPS 1997	Unclear	30/45	51±8	Xuezhikang 600 mg BID + conventional therapy (as same as B)	Simvastatin 10 mg QN + conventional therapy (nitrate esters 10 mg TID, aspirin 100 mg QD or anticoagulation drugs or thrombolytic drug or hypoglycemic)	8 weeks	Serum lipid level (TC, TG, LDL-C, HDL-C), ADs	Yes
Li et al. 2011[26]	References [12, 13]	As same as Guan 2010	Unclear	32/32	(46.9±14.5) / (50.7±15.1)	Xuezhikang 600 mg BID	Lovastatin 40 mg QD (20 mg QD if the ALT or AST was 3 times higher than the normal)	8 weeks	Serum lipid level (TC, TG, LDL-C, HDL-C), ADs	Yes
Lin et al. 2009[27]	Chinese Society of cardiology 2000	TC ≥ 4.68 mmol/L or LDL-C ≥ 2.6 mmol/L	Unstable angina	24/24	35-71, 55.4 in Average	Xuezhikang 600 mg, BID + control	Simvastatin 60 mg QN + conventional therapy (nitrate esters, β adrenergic blocking agent, CCB, aspirin, low molecular heparin and et al.)	6 months	Serum lipid level (TC, LDL-C), CHD events	Yes
Lou et al. 2008[28]	Chinese society of cardiology 2000	TC > 3.64 mmol/L and TG > 3.9 mmol/L and LDL-C > 2.6	Unstable angina	43/41	65±10	Xuezhikang 600 mg BID + conventional therapy (as same as B)	Simvastatin 20 mg QD + conventional therapy (anticoagulation drugs, nitrate esters, β adrenergic blocking agent, ACEI, CCB and et al.)	6 months	Serum lipid level (TC, TG, LDL-C, HDL-C), Cardiovascular events, ADs	Unclear
Ma and Teng 2005[29]	WHO 1979	CADPS 1997	Unclear	29/28	(62.7±6.5) / (61.2±7.1)	Xuezhikang 600 mg BID + control	Conventional therapy (nitrate esters, β adrenergic blocking agent, ACEI, CCB and et al.)	8 weeks	Serum lipid level (TC, TG)	Yes
Qi et al. 2001[30]	WHO 1979	TC > 6.0 mmol/L	Unclear	60/60	60.6±12.3	Xuezhikang 600 mg, BID (600 mg TID if the lipid level was still higher than the treatment goal) + control	Conventional therapy (nitrate esters, β adrenergic blocking agent, ACEI, CCB, and et al.)	12 weeks	Serum lipid level (TC, TG), ADs	Unclear

Continued

ID	Diagnostic criteria of CHD (ACS)	Diagnostic criteria of dyslipidemia	Types of CHD	Sample size (I/C)	Age (y, I/C)	Interventions group	Control group	Duration of treatment	Outcomes evaluation	Balance report of baseline
Shang 2007[31]	WHO 1979	CADPS 1997	Stable Angina	65/65	(51±10)/(55±10)	Xuezhikang 1200 mg QN +conventional therapy (as same as control group)	Atorvastatin 10 mg QN + conventional therapy (aspirin, nitrate esters, β adrenergic blocking agent, ACEI, and et al.)	2 months	Serum lipid level (TC, TG, LDL-C, HDL-C)	Yes
Wang and Xiao 2000[32]	WHO 1979	CADPS 1997	MI, UA, CHD with no symptoms	65/57	49-76, 62 in average	Xuezhikang 600 mg BID + aspirin 50 mg QD	Inositol niacinate 400 mg TID + aspirin 50 mg QD	1 year	Serum lipid level (TC, TG, LDL-C, HDL-C), cardiovascular evnets, ADs	Yes
Wang et al. 2004[6]	ACC/AHH 2000	CADPS 1997	ACS	26/26	(60.1±8.9)/(59.7±8.6)	Xuezhikang 600 mg BID + control	Conventional therapy (aspirin, nitrate esters, β adrenergic blocking agent, ACEI, and et al.)	12 weeks	Serum lipid level (TC, TG, LDL-C, HDL-C), ADs	Yes
Xu 2005[39]	Chinese Society of cardiology 2000	Not specified	UA	12/13/10	Unclear	Xuezhikang 600 mg BID + control group (1)	(1) Conventional therapy (isosorbide dinitrate 10 mg tid, betaloc 25-50 mg BID/TID, aspirin 50-150 mg QD, low molecular heparin 0.4-0.6 mL Q12H or diltiazem 30 mg TID/QID, or plendil 5 mg QD/BID or captopril 12.5-25 mg TID or nitroglycerine) (2) Conventional therapy (as same as (1)) and atorvastatin 20 mg QN	1month	Serum lipid level (TC, TG, LDL-C, HDL-C)	Yes

Continued

ID	Diagnostic criteria of CHD (ACS)	Diagnostic criteria of dyslipidemia	Types of CHD	Sample size (I/C)	Age (y, I/C)	Interventions group	Control group	Duration of treatment	Outcomes evaluation	Balance report of baseline
Yan 2006[34]	Chinese Society of cardiology 2000	LDL-C: 1.84-4.12 mmol/L	UA	44/44	56.8±8.6	Xuezhikang 600 mg BID + control	magnesium polarizing liquor IV + heparin IH + Aspirin, Nitrate esters, β adrenergic blocking agent, CCB and et al.	8 weeks	Serum lipid level (TC, TG, LDL-C, HDL-C), ADs	Unclear
Yan and Li 2007[33]	WHO 1979	CADPS 1997	Unclear	28/28	(66.68±4.23) / (66.79±4.48)	Xuezhikang 600 mg, BID + control	Nitroglycerine 20 mg BID.iv + 10% KCL + insulin IV QD	8 weeks	Serum lipid level (TC, TG, LDL-C, HDL-C)	Yes
Yu et al. 2002[35]	WHO 1979	CADPS 1997	Unclear	32/30	(53.5±10.8) / (50.6±6.7)	Xuezhikang 600 mg, BID + conventional therapy (as same as control)	Placebo + conventional therapy (aspirin, nitrate esters, CCB and et al.)	8 weeks	Serum lipid level (TC, TG, LDL-C, HDL-C)	Yes
Zhang 2010[36]	Reference[8]	CADPS 1997	Unclear	30/30	(58-80, 72.3 in average) / (59-82, 73.1 in average)	Xuezhikang 600 mg, BID + control	Fluvastatin 40 mg QD	4 weeks	Serum lipid level (TC, TG, LDL-C, HDL-C)	Yes
Zhang 2011[37]	Unclear	CHOL > 5.72 mmol/L or LDL-C > 3.64 mmol/L complicated with high TG level	Unclear	40/40	(50±13) / (45±15)	Xuezhikang 300 mg TID	Atorvastatin 20 mg/d QD	8 weeks	Serum lipid level (TC, TG, LDL-C), ADs	Yes
Zhou et al. 2003[38]	Unclear	TC > 6.0 mmol/L and (or) LDL-C > 4.2 mmol/L complicate with > 1.92 mmol/L	ACS		60.8±10.6	Xuezhikang 600 mg BID + control	Conventional therapy (nitrate esters, β adrenergic blocking agent, CCB, anticoagulation drugs, thrombolytic drug, PTCA and et al.)	8 weeks	Serum lipid level (TC, TG, LDL-C)	Yes

第七章

105)[32].

3.3.8　Serum LDL-C Level　There were 21 studies that reported the level of LDL-C (see Table 4), but one trial only reported the serum lipid level of the treatment group [30]. (1) Compared to no treatment with cointervention of conventional therapy, Xuezhikang showed a reduction of LDL-C level (MD −0.78 mmol/L；95% CI −1.19 to −0.38；7 trial, n=444) [5,6,24,33,34,38,39]. (2) There were two trials that reported Xuezhikang versus placebo on the basis of conventional therapy, meta-analysis was not used for significant difference, and, in this comparison, Xuezhikang showed a reduction of LDL-C level (MD −0.57 mmol/L；95% CI −0.62 to −0.52；1 trial, n=4870) [4] and (MD −1.82 mmol/L；95% CI −2.01 to −1.63；1 trial, n=62) [35]. (3) There was no significant difference on serum LDL-C level of Xuezhikang comparing to statins on the basis of conventional therapy (MD 0.03 mmol/L；95% CI −0.10 to 0.25；8 trial, n=633) [21,23-25,28,31,37,39]. Because there was significant heterogeneity in the comparison, we examined the data carefully and found that data of two trials deviated from the others. After looking over the papers, one of the two trials [26] with an unclear conventional therapy and the other used Xuezhikang 300 mg tid in the whole trial [37]. Sensitive analysis was used and got a similar conclusion (MD 0.05 mmol/L；95% CI −0.09 to 0.19；6 trial, n=489) after excluded the two trials [26,37]. (4) Compared with no treatment on the basis of statins and conventional therapy, Xuezhikang showed a reduction of LDL-C level (MD −0.44 mmol/L；95% CI −0.57 to −0.31；2 trial, n=108) [27,36]. (5) Compared to inositol nicotinate on the basis of aspirin, Xuezhikang showed a significant difference in the reduction of LDL-C level (MD −0.88 mmol/L；95% CI −1.27 to −0.48；1 trial, n=105) [32].

3.3.9　Serum HDL-C Level　There were 19 studies that reported the level of HDL-C (see Table 4), but one trial only reported the serum lipid level of the treatment group [30]. (1) Compared to no treatment with cointervention

Table 3　Analysis of Clinical Events

Outcomes（comparisons）	Treatment group（n/N）	Control group（n/N）	RR	95% CI
（1）*All-cause mortality*				
Xuezhikang capsule and conventional therapy versus placebo and conventional therapy				
CCSPS 2005[4]	126/2429	189/2441	0.67	[0.54，0.83]
（2）*Mortality of CHD*				
（2.1）Xuezhikang capsule and conventional therapy versus placebo and conventional therapy				
CCSPS 2005[4]	92/2429	134/2441	0.69	[0.54，0.89]
（2.2）Xuezhikang and conventional therapy versus simvastatin and conventional therapy				
Guan 2010[22]	1/72	6/64	0.15	[0.02，1.20]
Lou et al. 2008[28]	1/43	1/41	0.95	[0.06，14.75]
	Overall（FEM, I^2=13%）		0.26	[0.06，1.21]
（2.3）Xuezhikang and simvastatin and conventional therapy versus simvastatin and conventional therapy				
Lin et al. 2009[27]	0/24	1/24	0.33	[0.01，7.8]
（2.4）Xuezhikang and aspirin versus inositol nicotinate and aspirin				
Wang and Xiao 2000[32]	1/65	6/57	0.15	[0.02，1.18]
（3）*Myocardial infarction*				

第七章

Continued

Outcomes（comparisons）	Treatment group（n/N）	Control group（n/N）	RR	95% CI
（3.1）Xuezhikang and conventional therapy versus placebo and conventional therapy				
CCSPS 2005 [4]	47/2429	120/2441	0.39	[0.28，0.55]
（3.2）Xuezhikang and conventional therapy versus simvastatin and conventional therapy				
Lou et al. 2008 [28]	5/43	5/41	0.95	[0.30，3.05]
（3.3）Xuezhikang and simvastatin and conventional therapy versus simvastatin and conventional therapy				
Lin et al. 2009 [27]	0/24	2/24	0.2	[0.01，3.96]
（4）Revascularization				
（4.1）Xuezhikang capsule and conventional therapy versus placebo and conventional therapy				
CCSPS 2005 [4]	73/2429	110/2441	0.67	[0.50，0.895]
（4.2）Xuezhikang and conventional therapy versus simvastatin and conventional therapy				
Lou et al. 2008 [28]	6/43	5/41	1.14	[0.38，3.46]
（5）Rehospitalization				
（5.1）Xuezhikang and conventional therapy versus simvastatin and conventional therapy				
Lou et al. 2008 [28]	15/43	14/41	1.02	[0.57，1.84]
（5.2）Xuezhikang and simvastatin and conventional therapy versus simvastatin and conventional therapy				
Lin et al. 2009 [27]	1/24	5/24	0.2	[0.03，1.59]

of conventional therapy, Xuezhikang showed a beneficial effect of HDL-C level (MD 0.24 mmol/L；95% CI 0.08 to 0.40；6 trial, n=364) [5,6,24,33,34,39]. (2) There were two trials that reported Xuezhikang versus placebo on the basis of conventional therapy, meta-analysis was not used for significant difference, and, in this comparison, Xuezhikang showed a beneficial effect of HDL-C level (MD 0.05 mmol/L；95% CI 0.03 to 0.07；1 trial, n =4870) [4] and (MD 0.48 mmol/L；95% CI 0.37 to 0.59；1 trial, n =62) [35]. (3) There was a lower effect on serum HDL-C level of Xuezhikang comparing to statins on the basis of conventional therapy (MD-0.10 mmol/L；95% CI -0.19 to -0.01；8 trial, n =633) [21,23-25,28,31,37,39]. Because there was significant heterogeneity in the comparison, we examined the data carefully and found that data of one trials deviated from the others. After looking over the papers, we found that the trial used Xuezhikang 300 mg tid [37]. Sensitive analysis was used and got a similar conclusion (MD –0.10 mmol/L；95% CI –0.11 to –0.08；7 trial,

n=553) after excluded the trial [37]. (4) Compared with no treatment on the basis of fluvastatin and conventional therapy, Xuezhikang showed a beneficial of HDL-C level (MD 0.15 mmol/L；95% CI 0.05 to 0.25；1 trial, n=60) [36]. (5) Compared with inositol nicotinate on the basis of aspirin, Xuezhikang showed no significant difference on HDL-C level (MD 0.17 mmol/L；95% CI –0.21 to 0.55；1 trial, n=105) [32].

3.4　Publication Bias

A funnel plot analysis of the 8 trials in comparison of Xuezhikang and conventional therapy versus conventional therapy on serum TC level was conducted and shown in Figure 3.

3.5　Adverse Events

There were 17 trials that reported adverse events (Ads); see Table 5.4 of the 17 trials [5,24,33,37] indicated no Ads in the duration of treatment, and 2 trials[23,34] only introduced that there was no difference of the two groups. The most commonly reported Ads in the 10 trials were intestinal disturbance (abdominal distension,

Table 4 Analysis of Serum Lipid Level

Serum lipid level (comparison)	Intervention group		Control group		Weight (%)	MD	95% CI
	Mean	SD	Mean	SD			
(1) *TC* (*mmol/L*)							
(1.1) Xuezhikang and conventional therapy versus conventional therapy							
Dai et al. 1999 [5]	5.41	0.87	6.54	0.89	11.40	−1.13	[−1.59, −0.67]
Huang et al. 2009 [24]	4.98	0.79	5.99	0.87	13.30	−1.01	[−1.36, −0.66]
Ma and Teng 2005 [29]	5.30	1.30	6.30	1.00	9.00	−1.00	[−1.61, −0.39]
Wang et al. 2004 [6]	4.33	0.96	6.30	0.79	11.10	−1.97	[−2.45, −1.49]
Xu 2005 [39]	5.49	1.12	6.20	0.93	6.60	−0.71	[−1.52, 0.10]
Yan 2006 [34]	4.90	0.10	5.50	0.20	17.30	−0.60	[−0.67, −0.53]
Yan and Li 2007 [33]	4.90	0.13	5.93	0.23	17.00	−1.03	[−1.13, −0.93]
Zhou et al. 2003 [38]	4.30	0.54	4.84	0.78	14.30	−0.54	[−0.83, −0.25]
Overall (REM, I^2=92%)					100	−0.97	[−1.24, −0.71]
(1.2) Xuezhikang and conventional therapy versus placebo and conventional therapy							
CCSPS 2005 [4]	4.65	0.67	5.22	0.88	—	−0.57	[−0.61, −0.53]
Yu et al. 2002 [35]	4.10	0.58	6.72	0.85	—	−2.62	[−2.98, −2.26]
(1.3) Xuezhikang and conventional therapy versus statin and conventional therapy							
(1.3.1) Xuezhikang and conventional therapy versus lovastatin and conventional therapy							
Li et al. 2011 [26]	4.57	1.42	5.32	1.72	9.5	−0.75	[−1.52, 0.02]
(1.3.2) Xuezhikang and conventional therapy versus simvastatin and conventional therapy							
Huang et al. 2005 [23]	4.62	0.63	4.36	0.60	13.8	0.26	[0.02, 0.50]
Jiang and Cai 2001 [25]	5.19	0.90	4.91	0.66	12.8	0.28	[−0.10, 0.66]
Lou et al. 2008 [28]	5.4	0.12	5.40	0.11	14.4	0.00	[−0.05, 0.05]
Subgroup Overall (REM, I^2=69%)						0.14	[−0.08, 0.35]
(1.3.3) Xuezhikang and conventional therapy versus fluvastatin and conventional therapy							
Gao and Liao 2003 [21]	4.05	0.74	3.63	0.59	13.1	0.42	[0.08, 0.76]
(1.3.4) Xuezhikang and conventional therapy versus atorvastatin and conventional therapy							
Shang 2007 [31]	4.65	0.79	4.88	0.85	13.5	−0.23	[−0.51, 0.05]
Xu 2005 [39]	5.49	1.12	5.50	0.92	8.8	−0.01	[−0.86, 0.84]
Zhang 2011 [37]	4.51	0.38	4.00	3.35	14.1	1.16	[0.99, 1.33]
Subgroup Overall (REM, I^2=97%)						0.33	[−0.77, 1.43]
After sensitive analysis Subgroup Overall (FEM, I^2=0%)						−0.21	[−0.48, 0.06]
Total Overall (REM, I^2=96%)						0.19	[−0.22, 0.59]
After sensitive analysis Total Overall (REM, I^2=66%)						0.02	[−0.032, 0.06]
(1.4) Xuezhikang and statin and conventional therapy versus statin and conventional therapy							
(1.4.1) Xuezhikang and simvastatin and conventional therapy versus simvastatin and conventional therapy							
Lin et al. 2009 [27]	4.30	0.71	5.00	0.81	35.6	−0.70	[−1.13, −0.27]
(1.4.2) Xuezhikang and fluvastatin and conventional therapy versus fluvastatin and conventional therapy							

Continued

Serum lipid level (comparison)	Intervention group		Control group		Weight (%)	MD	95% CI
	Mean	SD	Mean	SD			
Zhang 2010[36]	4.60	0.10	5.70	0.24	64.4	−1.10	[−1.19, −1.01]
	Total	Overall (REM, I^2=68%)				−0.96	[−1.33, −0.58]

(1.5) Xuezhikang and aspirin versus inositol nicotinate and aspirin

Wang and Xiao 2000[32]	5.20	0.80	6.00	0.70	—	−1.05	[−1.46, −0.64]

2. *TG（mmol/L）*

(2.1) Xuezhikang and conventional therapy versus conventional therapy

Dai et al. 1999[5]	1.84	0.68	2.30	0.87	5.50	−0.48	[−0.87, −0.05]
Huang et al. 2009[24]	1.49	0.31	1.97	0.37	44.40	−0.48	[−0.63, −0.33]
Ma and Teng 2005[29]	1.70	0.40	2.30	0.70	10.50	−0.60	[−0.90, −0.30]
Wang et al. 2004[6]	1.88	0.5	2.2	0.76	7.70	−0.32	[−0.67, 0.03]
Xu 2005[39]	2.70	0.92	2.52	1.67	0.90	0.18	[−0.87, 1.23]
Yan and Li 2007[33]	1.54	0.10	2.02	0.59	19.10	−0.48	[−0.70, −0.26]
Zhou et al. 2003[38]	1.20	0.66	1.80	0.61	12.10	−0.60	[−0.88, −0.32]
		Overall (FEM, I^2=0%)			100%	−0.49	[−0.58, −0.39]

(2.2) Xuezhikang and conventional therapy versus placebo and conventional therapy

CCSPS 2005[4]	1.58	0.78	1.75	0.88	50.80	−0.17	[−0.22, −0.12]
Yu et al. 2002[35]	2.22	0.71	3.51	0.36	49.20	−1.29	[−1.57, −1.01]

(2.3) Xuezhikang and conventional therapy versus statin and conventional therapy

(2.3.1) Xuezhikang and conventional therapy versus lovastatin and conventional therapy

Li et al. 2011[26]	3.75	1.17	3.82	1.29	1.3	−0.07	[−0.67, 0.53]

(2.3.2) Xuezhikang and conventional therapy versus simvastatin and conventional therapy

Huang et al. 2005[23]	1.85	0.81	1.92	0.72	5.5	−0.07	[−0.37, 0.23]
Jiang and Cai 2001[25]	1.9	0.72	2.11	0.91	3.5	−0.21	[−0.58, 0.16]
Lou et al. 2008[28]	3.1	0.2	3.2	0.33	35.2	−0.11	[−0.21, 0.00]
	Subgroup	Overall (FEM, I^2=0%)			44.3	0.11	[−0.21, −0.00]

(2.3.3) Xuezhikang and conventional therapy versus fluvastatin and conventional therapy

Gao and Liao 2003[21]	1.01	0.63	1.42	0.46	6.2	−0.41	[−0.69, −0.13]

(2.3.4) Xuezhikang and conventional therapy versus atorvastatin and conventional therapy

Shang 2007[31]	1.61	0.53	1.57	0.55	14.1	0.04	[−0.15, 0.23]
Xu 2005[39]	2.7	0.92	2.22	0.73	1.0	0.48	[−0.21, 1.17]
Zhang 2011[37]	1.64	0.33	1.61	0.21	33.0	0.03	[−0.09, 0.15]
	Subgroup	Overall (FEM, I^2=0%)			48.1	0.04	[−0.06, 0.14]
	Total	Overall (FEM, I^2=45%)			100	−0.05	[−0.12, 0.02]

(2.4) Xuezhikang and statin and conventional therapy versus statin and conventional therapy

Zhang 2010[36]	1.58	0.20	1.85	0.10	—	−0.27	[−0.35, −0.19]

Serum lipid level (comparison)	Intervention group		Control group		Weight（%）	MD	95% CI
	Mean	SD	Mean	SD			
（2.5）Xuezhikang and aspirin versus inositol nicotinate and aspirin							
Wang and Xiao 2000 [32]	1.70	0.90	2.30	0.90	—	−0.60	[−0.95, −0.25]
（3）LDL-C（mmol/L）							
（3.1）Xuezhikang and conventional therapy versus conventional therapy							
Dai et al. 1999 [5]	3.42	0.96	3.93	0.81	13.50	−0.51	[−0.97, −0.05]
Huang et al. 2009 [24]	2.88	0.91	3.96	0.96	14.10	−1.08	[−1.48, −0.68]
Wang et al. 2004 [6]	2.21	0.4	3.87	0.56	15.20	−1.66	[−1.92, −1.40]
Xu 2005 [39]	2.82	0.95	3.7	0.95	10.50	−0.88	[−1.63, −0.13]
Yan 2006 [34]	2.89	0.44	2.9	0.6	15.50	−0.01	[−0.23, 0.21]
Yan and Li 2007 [33]	2.97	0.10	3.88	0.20	16.20	−0.91	[−0.99, −0.83]
Zhou et al. 2003 [38]	3.22	0.6	3.68	0.71	15.00	−0.46	[−0.75, −0.17]
	Overall（REM，I^2=94%）				100	−0.78	[−1.19, −0.38]
（3.2）Xuezhikang and conventional therapy versus placebo and conventional therapy							
CCSPS 2005 [4]	2.66	0.85	3.23	0.85	50.30	−0.57	[−0.62, −0.52]
Yu et al. 2002 [35]	2.48	0.39	4.30	0.39	49.70	−1.82	[−2.01, −1.63]
（3.3）Xuezhikang and conventional therapy versus statin and conventional therapy							
（3.3.1）Xuezhikang and conventional therapy versus lovastatin and conventional therapy							
Li et al. 2011 [26]	2.45	0.72	3.25	0.84	10.6	−0.80	[−1.18, 0.42]
（3.3.2）Xuezhikang and conventional therapy versus simvastatin and conventional therapy							
Huang et al. 2005 [23]	2.68	0.55	2.52	0.49	13.9	0.16	[−0.04, 0.36]
Jiang and Cai 2001 [25]	3.1	0.41	2.90	0.90	12.2	0.20	[−0.10, 0.50]
Lou et al. 2008 [28]	2.8	0.09	2.9	0.1	15.7	−0.10	[−0.14, −0.06]
Subtotal	Overall（REM，I^2=79%）				41.8	0.06	[−0.17, 0.28]
（3.3.3）Xuezhikang and conventional therapy versus fluvastatin and conventional therapy							
Gao and Liao 2003 [21]	2.13	0.58	2.08	0.61	12.2	0.05	[−0.25, 0.35]
（3.3.4）Xuezhikang and conventional therapy versus atorvastatin and conventional therapy							
Shang 2007 [31]	2.54	0.56	2.44	0.52	14.2	0.10	[−0.09, 0.29]
Xu 2005 [39]	2.82	0.95	2.93	0.52	6.9	−0.11	[−0.74, 0.52]
Zhang 2011 [37]	3.04	0.48	2.51	0.32	14.3	0.53	[0.35, 0.71]
	Subtotal	Overall（REM，I^2=84%）			35.4	0.23	[−0.14, 0.60]
After sensitive analysis	Subtotal	Overall（FEM，I^2=0%）				0.08	[−0.10, 0.26]
	Total	Overall（REM，I^2=90%）				0.03	[−0.10, 0.25]
After sensitive analysis	Total	Overall（REM，I^2=64%）				0.05	[−0.09, 0.19]
（3.4）Xuezhikang and statin and conventional therapy versus statin and conventional therapy							
（3.4.1）Xuezhikang and simvastatin and conventional therapy versus simvastatin and conventional therapy							
Lin et al. 2009 [27]	2.10	0.78	2.60	0.80	8.4	−0.50	[−0.95, −0.05]

Continued

Serum lipid level (comparison)	Intervention group		Control group		Weight (%)	MD	95% CI
	Mean	SD	Mean	SD			
(3.4.2) Xuezhikang and fluvastatin and conventional therapy versus fluvastatin and conventional therapy							
Zhang 2010 [36]	2.87	0.32	3.30	0.20	91.6	−0.43	[−0.57, −0.29]
Total	Overall (FEM, I^2=0%)					−0.44	[−0.57, −0.31]
(3.5) Xuezhikang and aspirin versus inositol nicotinate and aspirin							
Wang and Xiao 2000 [32]	2.70	0.70	3.40	0.90	100	−0.88	[−1.27, −0.48]
(4) HDL-C (mmol/L)							
(4.1) Xuezhikang and conventional therapy versus conventional therapy							
Dai et al. 1999 [5]	1.71	0.42	1.04	0.49	14.60	0.67	[−0.43, 0.91]
Huang et al. 2009 [24]	1.12	0.3	0.82	0.2	19.50	0.3	[0.19, 0.41]
Wang et al. 2004 [6]	1.44	0.38	1.31	0.27	17.00	0.13	[−0.05, 0.31]
Xu 2005 [39]	1.67	0.51	1.68	0.75	7.10	−0.01	[−0.51, 0.49]
Yan 2006 [34]	1.04	0.10	1.04	0.20	20.60	0.00	[−0.07, 0.07]
Yan and Li 2007 [33]	1.09	0.09	0.80	0.07	21.10	0.29	[0.25, 0.33]
	Overall (REM, I^2=93%)				100	0.24	[0.08, 0.40]
(4.2) Xuezhikang and conventional therapy versus placebo and conventional therapy							
CCSPS 2005 [4]	1.24	0.31	1.19	0.31	50.80	0.05	[0.03, 0.07]
Yu et al. 2002 [35]	1.45	0.25	0.97	0.19	49.20	0.48	[0.37, 0.59]
(4.3) Xuezhikang and conventional therapy versus statin and conventional therapy							
(4.3.1) Xuezhikang and conventional therapy versus lovastatin and conventional therapy							
Li et al. 2011 [26]	1.12	0.38	1.06	0.36	11.4	0.16	[−0.33, 0.65]
(4.3.2) Xuezhikang and conventional therapy versus simvastatin and conventional therapy							
Huang et al. 2005 [23]	1.85	0.81	1.92	0.72	6.4	−0.09	[−0.47, 0.29]
Jiang and Cai 2001 [25]	1.16	0.17	1.21	0.12	19.0	−0.05	[−0.12, 0.02]
Lou et al. 2008 [28]	0.8	0.03	0.9	0.03	21.4	−0.10	[−0.11, −0.09]
	Overall (FEM, I^2=0%)					−0.10	[−0.11, −0.09]
(4.3.3) Xuezhikang and conventional therapy versus fluvastatin and conventional therapy							
Gao and Liao 2003 [21]	1.14	0.27	1.30	0.45	11	−0.16	[−0.35, 0.03]
(4.3.4) Xuezhikang and conventional therapy versus atorvastatin and conventional therapy							
Shang 2007 [31]	1.45	0.41	1.44	0.33	14.9	0.01	[−0.12, 0.14]
Xu 2005 [39]	1.67	0.51	1.53	0.48	3.8	0.14	[−0.27, 0.55]
Zhang 2011 [37]	1.09	0.48	1.62	0.27	12.1	−0.53	[−0.70, −0.36]
	Subtotal	Overall (REM, I^2=93%)			30.9	−0.15	[−0.57, 0.28]
After sensitive analysis	Subtotal	Overall (FEM, I^2=0%)				0.01	[−0.10, 0.14]
	Total	Overall (REM, I^2=79%)				−0.10	[−0.19, −0.01]
After sensitive analysis	Total	Overall (FEM, I^2=35%)				−0.10	[−0.11, −0.08]

Continued

Serum lipid level (comparison)	Intervention group		Control group		Weight（%）	MD	95% CI
	Mean	SD	Mean	SD			
（4.4）Xuezhikang and fluvastatin and conventional therapy versus fluvastatin and conventional therapy							
Zhang 2010 [36]	0.97	0.28	0.82	0.06	100	0.15	[0.05，0.25]
（4.5）Xuezhikang and aspirin versus inositol nicotinate and aspirin							
Wang and Xiao 2000 [32]	0.95	0.22	0.91	0.25	100	0.17	[-0.21，0.55]

Note：FEM：fixed effects model；REM：random effects model.

constipation, and diarrhea), dizziness, high serum alanine aminotransferase (ALT), high serum creatine kinase (CK), high serum creatinine, high blood urea nitrogen (BUN), and skin itch. All of Ads were not significantly different between the Xuezhikang group and control group. One trial [4] reported that there was significant difference between the two groups on sexual dysfunction (P =0.0253) in the paper, but after we import the data into Revman 5.1, there was no difference (RR 0.09, 95% CI [0.01, 1.64]) between the two groups. CCSPS [4] reported the clinical total Ads number (intestinal disturbance, allergy and et al.) in each group (treatment group 43；control group 39), and there was no significant difference between the two groups, this trial also reported death in other reason, which was introduced in all cause mortality, and the difference between the two groups was not significant.

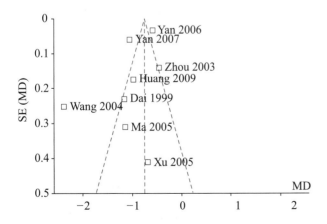

Figure 3 The Funnel Plot for Assessing Reporting Bias
Note：The funnel plot presented 8 trials in the comparison of Xuezhikang and conventional therapy versus conventional therapy on the effect of TC

4. Discussion

This systematic review included 22 randomized trials and a total of 6520 participants. Xuezhikang showed significant benefit on the incidence of all-cause deaths, CHD deaths, myocardial infarction, and revascularization as compared with placebo or no intervention based on conventional treatment for CHD. It remarkably lowered TC, TG, and LDL-C as compared with the placebo or inositol nicotinate group, which was similar to statins group. Xuezhikang also significantly raised HDL-C compared to placebo or no intervention, which was similar to inositol nicotinate and slightly inferior to statins. The incidence of adverse events did not differ between the Xuezhikang and control group. The results showed the comprehensive lipid-regulating effect of Xuezhikang and indicated that it was safe and effective in reducing cardiovascular events in CHD patients complicated by dyslipidemia.

Due to the potential side effects of statins, natural products have raised more and more attention worldwide. The health-enhancing qualities of red yeast rice have been introduced and used in China for over two thousand years. A meta-analysis of randomized controlled trials on Chinese red yeast rice for primary hyperlipidemia showed a significant reduction in serum levels of TC, TG, LDL-C, and an increase

Table 5　Adverse Events

Ads/ID	Comparison	Treatment group (n/N)	Control group (n/N)	RR	95% CI
Loss of followup					
Guan 2010 [22]	Xuezhikang versus simvastatin	16 (72)	15 (64)	0.95	[0.51, 1.76]
CCSPS 2005 [4]	Xuezhikang and conventional therapy versus placebo and conventional therapy	37 (2441)	28 (2429)	1.31	[0.81, 2.14]
Ma and Teng 2005 [29]	Xuezhikang and conventional therapy versus conventional therapy	1 (29)	No report		
Intestinal disturbance					
Guan 2010 [22]	Xuezhikang versus simvastatin	5 (72)	2 (64)	2.22	[0.45, 11.06]
Ma and Teng 2005 [29]	Xuezhikang and conventional therapy versus conventional therapy	2 (29)	No report		
Wang et al. 2004 [6]	Xuezhikang and conventional therapy versus conventional therapy	2 (26)	No report		
Jiang and Cai 2001 [25]	Xuezhikang and conventional therapy versus simvastatin and conventional therapy	0 (30)	1 (45)	0.49	[0.02, 11.75]
Shang 2007 [31]	Xuezhikang and conventional therapy versus atorvastatin and conventional therapy	No report	1 (65)		
Wang and Xiao 2000 [32]	Xuezhikang and aspirin versus inositol nicotinate and aspirin	5 (65)	2 (57)	2.19	[0.44, 10.87]
Headache					
Jiang and Cai 2001 [25]	Xuezhikang and conventional therapy versus simvastatin and conventional therapy	1 (30)	0 (45)	4.45	[0.19, 105.77]
Dizziness					
Guan 2010 [22]	Xuezhikang and conventional therapy versus simvastatin and conventional therapy	0 (72)	10 (64)	0.04	[0.00, 0.71]
Jiang and Cai 2001 [25]	Xuezhikang and conventional therapy versus simvastatin and conventional therapy	1 (30)	1 (45)	1.5	[0.10, 23.07]
		Overall (REM, I^2=72%)		0.26	[0.01, 10.49]
Skin itech					
Guan 2010 [22]	Xuezhikang versus simvastatin	0 (72)	3 (64)	0.13	[0.01, 2.42]
Wang and Xiao 2000 [32]	Xuezhikang and aspirin versus inositol nicotinate and aspirin	0 (65)	3 (57)	0.13	[0.01, 2.38]
Sexual dysfunction					
CCSPS 2005 [4]	Xuezhikang and conventional therapy versus placebo and conventional therapy	0 (1996)	5 (1990)	0.09	[0.01, 1.64]
High serum ALT					
CCSPS 2005 [4]	Xuezhikang and conventional therapy versus placebo and conventional therapy	15 (2441)	22 (2429)	0.68	[0.35, 1.30]
Lou et al. 2008 [28]	Xuezhikang and conventional therapy versus simvastatin and conventional therapy	No report	1 (41)		
High serum CK					
CCSPS 2005 [4]	Xuezhikang and conventional therapy versus placebo and conventional therapy	0 (2441)	3 (2429)	0.14	[0.01, 2.75]
High serum CR					
CCSPS 2005 [4]	Xuezhikang and conventional therapy versus placebo and conventional therapy	104 (2441)	89 (2429)	1.16	[0.88, 1.53]
High BUN					
CCSPS 2005 [4]	Xuezhikang and conventional therapy versus placebo and conventional therapy	124 (2441)	131 (2429)	0.94	[0.74, 1.20]

in HDL-C levels compared with placebo. The lipid modification effects appeared to be similar to pravastatin, simvastatin, atorvastatin, lovastatin, or fluvastatin[40]. A latest systematic review also indicated the beneficial effects of Xuezhikang in the treatment of hyperlipidemia [2]. The lipid-regulating effects of Xuezhikang in these reviews were similar to our findings. In addition, some cardioprotective effects of Xuezhikang have been investigated in recent years [41-43]. We further demonstrated the benefit of Xuezhikang in reducing cardiovascular events in CHD patients complicated by dyslipidemia, or even CHD with normal blood lipid level but failed to reach the lipid-lowering goal. However, current evidence comparing the effectiveness and Ads between Xuezhikang and statins in CHD patients was not enough to draw the conclusion.

It is worth mentioning China Coronary Secondary Prevention Study (CCSPS) [4], which was the largest RCT included in this review. This multicenter, randomized, and placebo-controlled study aimed to demonstrate the longterm therapeutic effect and safety of Xuezhikang in the second prevention of CHD. 4870 cases in 66 medical centers were enrolled and followed up for an average of 4.5 years. The results showed that Xuezhikang significantly decreased the recurrence of coronary events and the occurrence of new cardiovascular events and deaths, improved lipoprotein regulation, and was safe and well tolerated [4]. The study was the first large-scale clinical trial in eastern population who suffered from mild or moderate degree of hyperlipidemia and previous MI. The CCSPS study is quite comparable with (Cholesterol and Recurrent Events) CAREs study [44] in terms of the target population, sample size, baseline lipid and follow-up time. However, Xuezhikang in CCSPS lowered less lipid level as compared with pravastatin in CARE but seemed to gain more benefit in reducing the cardiovascular events. Since the effect of Xuezhikang is partially attributed to the presence of statins, it has been

hypothesized that relatively high concentrations of unsaturated fatty acids and other natural compounds found in Xuezhikang may work in concert with the statins to provide additional health benefits [45]. Therefore, a large-scale RCT comparing directly the effectiveness and safety of long-term use of Xuezhikang and statins is warranted.

Before recommending the conclusion of this review to clinical practicers, we have to consider the following weaknesses in this review. (1) Firstly, the "randomization" was not clear in most of the trials for insufficient reporting of generation methods of the allocation sequence and allocation concealment. Most trials stated only that patients were randomly assigned. (2) Secondly, most of trials did not introduce double blind in this review, and only one trial introduced blinding of outcome assessment, therefore, in non-placebo-controlled and non-double-blind trials, placebo effects may add to the complexity of interpreting the conclusion. (3) Most of the trials did not introduce the study plan, attrition bias and selective reporting bias might exist in this conclusion. (4) Thirdly, funnel plot indicated that publication bias would exist in this review. The reasons are as follows. We only selected trials published in Chinese and English, and trials published in other language or originated from other countries might be omitted; we only identified unpublished studies from conference paper or academic thesis, and negative trials might not be reported and induced publication bias.

Therefore, further rigorously designed trials are still needed before Xuezhikang could be recommended to patients with CHD complicated by dyslipidemia, especially as an alternative to statins. Whether or not long-term medication of Xuezhikang could provide similar benefit to statins for CHD secondary prevention with less adverse events? Is it related to the target lipid value? All of these need to be answered in the future investigation.

5. Conclusion

Xuezhikang showed a comprehensive lipid-regulating effect and was safe and effective in reducing CHD mortality, the incidence of myocardial infarction and revascularization in CHD patients complicated by dyslipidemia. However, the small sample size and potential bias of most trials influence the convincingness of this conclusion. Before recommending Xuezhikang as an alternative to statins in CHD patients, more rigorous trials with high quality are needed to give high level of evidence, especially for comparing the effectiveness and safety between Xuezhikang and statins.

References

[1] The Task Force for the Management of Dyslipidemias of the European Society of Cardiology (ESC) and the European Atherosclerosis Society (EAS). ESC/EAS guidelines for the management of dyslipidemias. European Heart Journal, 2011, 32: 1769-1818.

[2] Liu ZL, Liu JP, Zhang AL et al. Chinese herbal medicines for hypercholesterolemia. Cochrane Database of Systematic Reviews, 2011, (7): CD008305.

[3] Joint Commission on China Adult Dyslipidemia Prevention Guildeline. China adult dyslipidemia prevention guildeline. Chinese Journal of Cardiology, 2007, 35 (5): 390-419.

[4] Lu Z, Kou W, Du B et al. Effect of Xuezhikang, an extract from red yeast Chinese rice, on coronary events in a Chinese population with previous myocardial infarction. The Evidence-Based Complementary and Alternative Medicine 17 American Journal of Cardiology, 2008, 101 (12): 1689-1693.

[5] Dai XH, Zhuo XZ, Xue XY, et al. Xuezhikang capsule for unstable angina pectoris. Traditional Chinese Drug Research & Clinical Pharmacology, 1999, 10 (4): 202-204.

[6] Wang WH, Zhang H, Yu YL, et al. Effect of Xuezhikang for patients with acute coronary syndrom complicated with different serum lipid levels. Chinese Journal of Integrative Medicine, 2004, 24 (12): 1073-1076.

[7] Ye RG and Lu ZY. Internal Medicine. Beijing: People's Medical Publishing House, 6th edition, 2005.

[8] Bureau of Drug Administration of People's Republic of China. Cardiovascular medicine clinical research guilding principles, 1993.

[9] Gao RS, Chen ZJ. Further improving the understanding of unstable angina pectoris. Chinese Journal of Cardiology, 1994, 22 (4): 243.

[10] Chinese Society of Cardiology. Diagnosis and treatment recommendation for unstable angina pectoris. Chinese Journal of Cardiology, 2000, 28(6): 409-412.

[11] Braunwald E, Antman EM, Beasley JW et al. ACC/AHA guidelines for the management of patients with unstable angina and non-ST-segment elevation myocardial infarction: executive summary and recommendations: a report of the American College of Cardiology/American Heart Association task force on practice guidelines (committee on the management of patients with unstable angina). Circulation, 2000, 102(10): 1193-1209.

[12] Zheng YY. Chinese Herbal Medicine Clinical Research Guilding Principles (for trial implementation). Beijing: Chinese Medicine and Technology Publishing House, 2002.

[13] Chen HZ. Practice Internal Medicine. 10th edition. Beijing: The People's Medical Publishing House, 2005.

[14] Goodman DS, Hulley SB, Clark LT et al. Report of the national cholesterol education program expert panel on detection, evaluation, and treatment of high blood cholesterol in adults. Archives of Internal Medicine, 1988, 148 (1): 36-69.

[15] Grundy SM, Bilheimer D, Chait A et al. Summary of the second report of the National Cholesterol Education Program (NCEP) Expert Panel on Detection, Evaluation, and Treatment of High Blood Cholesterol in Adults (Adult Treatment Panel II). JAMA, 1993, 269 (23): 3015-3023.

[16] Fang X, Wang ZL, Ning TH et al. Prevent and treatment recommendation for dyslipidemia. Chinese Journal of Cardiology, 1997, 25 (3): 169-175.

[17] Cleeman JI. Executive summary of the third report of the National Cholesterol Education Program (NCEP) expert panel on detection, evaluation, and treatment of high blood cholesterol in adults (adult treatment panel III). JAMA, 2001, 285 (19): 2486-2497.

[18] Grundy SM, Cleeman JI, Bairey Merz CN et al. Implications of recent clinical trials for the national cholesterol education program adult treatment panel

Ⅲ guidelines. Circulation, 2004, 110 (2): 227-239.

[19] Smith SC, Allen J, Blair SN et al. AHA/ACC guidelines for secondary prevention for patients with coronary and other atherosclerotic vascular disease: 2006 Update. Circulation, 2006, 113 (19): 2363-2372.

[20] Higgins JPT, Green S. Cochrane handbook for systematic reviews of interventions, version 5.0.2 [updated September 2009]. The Cochrane Collaboration, 2009, http://www.cochrane-handbook.org/.

[21] Gao LS, Liao Y. Clinical observation of Xuezhikang and fluvastatin sodium capsules on serum lipid. Modern Journal of Integrated Traditional Chinese and Western Medicine, 2003, 12 (23): 2528.

[22] Guan SQ. Long-term effect of Xuezhikang for patients with coronary heart diseae complicated with hyperlipidemia. Guide of China Medicine, 2010, (1): 62-63.

[23] Huang ST, Chen XL, Zhang J. Clinical observation of Xuezhikang for patients with coronary heart disease complicated with hyperlipidemia. Proceeding of Clinical Medicine, 2005, (3): 193-195.

[24] Huang SX, Yin JZ, Pan M, et al. Effect of Xuezhikang for aged patients with angina pectoris complicated with dyslipidemia. Contempoary Medicine, 2009, 13: 128-129.

[25] Jiang WH, Cai ZD. Clinical observation of simvastatin for 45 patients with hyperlipidemia. Medical Information, 2001, (10): 699-700.

[26] Li B, Hu SY, Wu X, et al. Effect of Xuezhikang for patients with coronary heart disease on anti-oxidation and anti-imflammation. Progress in Modern Biomedicine, 2011, (12): 2289-2291.

[27] Lin H, Yang L S, Zheng D R. Effect of simvastatin and Xuezhikang for patients with unstable angina pectoris. China Medical Herald, 2009, 6 (23): 58-59.

[28] Lou DQ, Liu B, Yan WG, et al. Effect of Xuezhikang for patients with unstable angina pectoris. Clinical Medicine, 2008, 28 (3): 23-24.

[29] Ma W, Teng YX. Effect of Xuezhikang for patients with coronary heart disease complicated with hyperlipidemia on endothelial function and C response protein. Liaoning Yi Yao, 2005, 20 (2): 22-24.

[30] Qi BL, Zhang GJ, Suo XX. Efficiency rate of Xuezhikang for angina pectoris. Chinese Journal of Primary Medicine and Pharmacy, 2001, 8 (6): 547.

[31] Shang XB. Clinical observation of Xuezhikang and atorvastatin for patients with coronary heart disease complicated with dyslipidemia on serum lipid and hemorheology. Guangxi Medical Journal, 2007, 29 (8): 1158-1159.

[32] Wang J, Xiao MY. Long term effect of Xuezhikang and aspirine for 65 patients with coronary heart disease complicated with hyperlipidemia. New Medicine, 2000, 31 (10): 596-597.

[33] Yan L, Li XM. Effect of Xuezhikang for aged patients with coronary heart disease complicated with dyslipidemia on serun lipid modification, Sichuan Medical Journal. 2007, 28 (11): 1232-1233.

[34] Yan XD. Clinical observation of Xuezhikang for 88 patients with unstable angina pectoris. Chinese Community Doctors. Comprehensive Edition, 2006, 8 (15): 37.

[35] Yu H, Cui YL, Wang SY, Han B. Effect of Xuezhikang for patients with coronary heart diseae complicated with hyperlipidemia on fibrinolytic function. Chinese Journal of Coal Industry Medicine, 2002, 5 (1): 61-62.

[36] Zhang HY. Efficiency of fluvastatin and Xuezhikang for coronary heart disease. China Practical Medicine, 2010, (22): 115-116.

[37] Zhang X. Clinical effect of atorvastatin calcium tablets for coronary heart disease complicated with hyperlipidemia. Hebei Medical Journal, 2011, 33 (6): 882-883.

[38] Zhou CS, He WZ, Liu R, et al. Effect of Xuezhikang for patients with acute coronary syndrome on vascular endothelial function. Chinese Magazine of Clinical Medicinal Professional Research, 2003, (71): 44.

[39] Xu M. Clinical comparative study on treatment of unstable angina pectoris disease with lipid-reducing hongqu Xuezhikang and atorvastatin. Shandong University of Traditional Chinese Medicine, 2005.

[40] Liu J, Zhang J, Shi Y, et al. Chinese red yeast rice (Monascus purpureus) for primary hyperlipidemia: a meta-analysis of randomized controlled trials. Chinese Medicine, 2006, 1: 4.

[41] Gong C, Huang SL, Huang JF et al. Effects of combined therapy of Xuezhikang Capsule and Valsartan on hypertensive left ventricular hypertrophy and heart rate turbulence. Chinese Journal of Integrative Medicine, 2010, 16 (2): 114-118.

[42] Lu L, Zhou JZ, Wang L, et al. Effects of Xuezhikang and Pravastatin on circulating endothelial progenitor cells in patients with essential hypertension. Chinese Journal of Integrative Medicine, 2009, 15 (4): 266-

271.

[43] Fan XF, Deng YQ, Ye L et al. Effect of Xuezhikang Capsule on serum tumor necrosis factor-α and interleukin-6 in patients with nonalcoholic fatty liver disease and hyperlipidemia. Chinese Journal of Integrative Medicine, 2010, 16 (2): 119-123.

[44] Pfeffer MA, Sacks FM, Moyé LA et al. Cholesterol and recurrent events: a secondary prevention trial for normolipidemic patients. The American Journal of Cardiology, 1995, 76 (9): 98C-106C.

[45] Lu ZL. Advance in basic and clinical research of Xuezhikang Capsule: a commentary on the Chinese coronary secondary prevention study. Chinese Journal of Integrative Medicine, 2006, 12 (2): 85-87.

Natural Polypill Xuezhikang: Its Clinical Benefit and Potential Multicomponent Synergistic Mechanisms of Action in Cardiovascular Disease and Other Chronic Conditions[*]

FENG Yan   XU Hao   CHEN Ke-ji

1. Introduction

In the beginning of the 21st century, the population is facing the serious challenge of cardiovascular diseases (CVD). Although it is becoming less lethal, the prevalence of CVD continues to increase and it is still the number one killer [1]. In fact, ground may be being lost on the advancements in developed countries because of increasing risk factors in the population. The major risk factors such as blood pressure, cholesterol, blood glucose, body-mass index, smoking, and others are significantly correlated with the morbidity of CVD. Multiple interventions resulted in dramatic reductions in CVD, which was more effective than interventions targeting a single risk factor [2]. Furthermore, the combination of several drugs in low dose could not only improve efficacy and reduce adverse reactions of drugs, but also increase the compliance of patients and reduce the cost of treatment [3]. Then, is it a possible treatment regimen to put multiple drugs into one pill? Furthermore, is it a feasible way in real-world clinical practice?

2. The Conception of Polypill

In 2003, Wald and Law quantified the efficacy and adverse effects of the proposed formulation: one statin drug (atorvastatin 10mg/d or simvastatin 40mg/d); three antihypertensive drugs (thiazide, β-blocker, angiotensin-converting enzyme inhibitor, each at half standard dose); folic acid (0.8mg/d); aspirin (75mg/d) from published meta-analysis and cohort studies (including over 750 trials with 400,000 participants), and first introduced a polypill concept in the *British Medical Journal*. If taken by people above age 55 years, this polypill regimen could

* 原载于 The Journal of Alternative and Complementary Medicine, 2012，18（4）：318-328

第七章

reduce CVD by 80% with acceptable safety [4]. The accompanying editorial called it "one of the boldest claims for a new intervention." [5] This new concept immediately stirred up a worldwide discussion and raised a variety of debates and concerns [6,7]. Although the composition and reasonableness of this polypill and its clinical benefits still need further verification, the focus on intervention of multiple risk factors in modern medicine has no doubt been the trend of combination therapies for complicated diseases. Recent trials supported the recommendation that such multidrug regimens would be quite cost-effective in reducing the burden of CVD [8,9].

3. *Xuezhikang*, a Natural Polypill with Multicomponents

Xuezhikang is a partially purified extract of fermented red yeast rice (*Monascus purpureus*). The health-enhancing qualities of this yeast have been known and used in China for over 2000 years. *Xuezhikang* is composed of 13 kinds of natural statins, unsaturated fatty acids, ergosterol, amino acids, flavonoids, alkaloid, trace element, and others [10] (Figure 1), and thus could be regarded as a natural polypill. Evidence showed that fermented red yeast rice lowered cholesterol levels moderately compared to other statin drugs, but with the added advantage of causing fewer adverse effects [11,12]. To demonstrate the long-term therapeutic effect and safety of *Xuezhikang* in prevention of a second coronary heart disease (CHD) event, a multicenter, randomized, placebo-controlled study (CCSPS, China Coronary Secondary Prevention Study) was conducted in China. The results showed that *Xuezhikang* significantly decreased the recurrence of coronary events and the occurrence of new cardiovascular events and deaths, improved lipoprotein regulation, and was safe and well tolerated [13]. The study was the first large-scale clinical trial in an Eastern population who suffered from a mild or moderate degree of hyperlipidemia and

previous myocardial infarction. CCSPS was thus included in the Chinese Guidelines on Prevention and Treatment of Dyslipidemia in Adults [14]. The CCSPS study is quite comparable with CARE (the Cholesterol and Recurrent Events) study[15] in terms of the target population, sample size, baseline lipid level, and follow-up time. However, *Xuezhikang* in CCSPS lowered lipid levels less as compared with provastatin in CARE, but seemed to gain more benefit in reducing the cardiovascular events. Since the effect of *Xuezhikang* is partially attributed to the presence of statins, it has been hypothesized that relatively high concentrations of unsaturated fatty acids and other natural compounds found in *Xuezhikang* may work in concert with the statins to provide additional health benefits [16].

Xuezhikang is composed of 13 kinds of natural statins, unsaturated fatty acids, ergosterol, amino acids, flavonoids, alkaloid, trace elements, and so on.

4. Clinical Benefits of *Xuezhikang* and Its Potential Synergetic Mechanism Modulation of Overall Lipid Profiles

A meta-analysis of randomized controlled trials on Chinese red yeast rice for primary

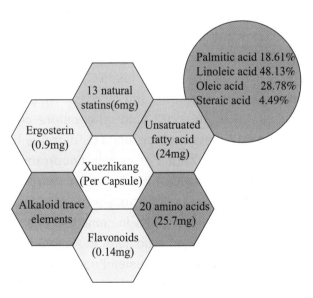

Figure 1　Active Ingredients in *Xuezhikang*

hyperlipidemia showed a significant reduction in serum levels of total cholesterol (TC), triglycerides (TG), low-density lipoprotein-cholesterol (LDL-C), and an increase in high-density lipoprotein-cholesterol (HDL-C) levels compared with placebo. The lipid modification effects appeared to be similar to those of pravastatin, simvastatin, atorvastatin, lovastatin, or fluvastatin [12].

Incontrovertibly, the main lipid-lowering mechanism of *Xuezhikang* is the component of statins, especially lovastatin as a 3-hydroxy-3-methylglutaryl-coenzyme A (HMG-CoA) reductase inhibitor, which can reduce endogenous cholesterol synthesis, and increase the activity of LDL receptor on the surface of liver cells to promote the clearance of LDL through feedback mechanisms.

As another major component in *Xuezhikang*, polyunsaturated fatty acids (PUFAs) can decrease TG [17], reduce the rate of lipid shuttle driven by cholesteryl ester transfer protein, increase HDL, reduce small LDL production, and get the cholesterol out of the vessel wall. As for α-linolenic acid and γ-linolenic acid, their effects on serum levels of TC, TG, and HDL-C were significant [18]. The OPTILIP study found that an increased intake of n-3 long-chain PUFAs caused a reduction in plasma triacylglycerol and favorable changes in LDL size [19]. Furthermore, a diet enriched in eicosapentaenoic acid (EPA) and docosahexaenoic acid (DHA) can reduce blood levels of neutral lipids, TC, LDL, very-low-density lipoprotein, and increase HDL [18]. The intake of omega-3-acid ethyl esters can significantly decrease serum TG, along with plasma concentrations of certain lipoproteins up to 45% [20]. The COMBOS study confirmed significant improvements across a range of lipid indicators by taking PUFAs in combination with statins [21]. In addition, ergosterol in *Xuezhikang* can compete with the cholesterol absorption site to interfere with the absorption of cholesterol, reducing exogenous cholesterol. Moreover, most flavonoids can reduce levels of TG, TC, and LDL [22].

All of the abovementioned components might be involved in the mechanism of *Xuezhikang* to modulate overall lipid profiles.

5. Antiatherosclerosis Effects

Xuezhikang can not only reduce the proportion of atherosclerotic substance in the plaque, but also effectively improve endothelial function through its potent anti-inflammatory and lipid-lowering effects [23,24] to set more mature collagen and more stable fibrous cap. Anti-inflammatory action of *Xuezhikang* plays an important role in early-stage treatment of atherosclerosis. *Xuezhikang* can inhibit the serum levels of inflammatory factors such as tumor necrosis factor-α (TNF-α) and interleukin-6 (IL-6) [25], serum oxidized LDL, C-reactive protein (CRP) [26] and fibrinogen [27], high-sensitivity C-reactive protein (Hs-CRP), matrix metalloproteinase-9 (MMP-9) [28], and regulate the balance between thromboxane and prostacyclin [29] in patients.

Lovastatin in *Xuezhikang* is an inhibitor of endothelial HMG-CoA reductase. It was reported that it could upregulate endothelial constitutive nitric oxide synthase (ecNOS) expression predominantly by post-transcriptional mechanisms, suggesting that the HMG-CoA reductase inhibitor may have beneficial effects in atherosclerosis beyond that attributed to the lowering of serum cholesterol by increasing ecNOS activity [30]. Furthermore, upregulation and activation of ecNOS in endothelial cells will increase the secretion of plasma NO, which may play an important role in vasodilation, antivascular smooth-muscle cell proliferation, and inhibition of platelet aggregation.

The metabolites of N-3 PUFA, another main component of *Xuezhikang*, can directly or indirectly play a role in the immune system, and contribute to slowing the progression [31] of atherosclerosis by modulating inflammation, platelet activation, endothelial functions, and so on [32]. The dietary intake of long-chain n-3 PUFAs

Table1　Clinical Benefits of Xuezhikang in Cardiovascular Disease and Other Chronic Conditions

No.	Clinical benefits	Study	Design	Sample	Control	Duration	Effect of Xuezhikang
1	Lipid profiles modulation	Liu J 2006[12]	Meta-analysis	99 Randomized trials	—	—	The lipid modification effects appeared to be similar to pravastatin, simvastatin, lovastatin, atorvastatin, or fluvastatin
2	Anti-atherosclerosis	Zhao SP 2004[23]	Randomized control trial (RCT)	50 Coronary heart disease patients	placebo	6 weeks	Reducing proportion of atherosclerotic substance in the plaque
		Lu L 2009[24]	RCT	88 Essential hypertensive (EH) patients	Antihypertensive drug and pravastatin	8 weeks	Improving endothelial function through its potent anti-inflammatory and lipid-lowering effects to set more mature collagen and more stable fibrous cap
		Fan XF 2010[25]	RCT	84 Patients with nonalcoholic fatty liver disease and hyperlipidemia	Polyene-phosphatidylcholine capsule	24 weeks	Lowering the serum levels of inflammatory factors such as tumor necrosis factor-alpha and interleukin-6 (IL-6)
		Liu JD 2006[26]	RCT	90 patients with unstable angina (UA)	Blank	3 days	Reducing the serum levels of serum oxidized low-density lipoprotein-cholesterol (ox-LDL), and C-reactive protein (CRP)
		Yao QH 2003[27]	RCT	103 patients with UA (69 male) 69 patients with	Vitamin E	4 months	Lowering the serum levels of fibrinogen
		Huang J 2006[28]	Case-control trial	acute coronary syndrome and 30 healthy people	Blank	2 weeks	Reducing the serum levels of high-sensitivity CRP, matrix metalloproteinase-9
		Jian J 1999[29]	RCT	91 patients with hyperlipidemia	Gemfibrozil	8 weeks	Regulating the balance between thromboxane and prostacyclin
3	Liver protection	Yao ZL 2006[47]	RCT	62 patients with fatty liver	Blank	14 months	Relieving clinical syndromes and improving liver function
4	Anti-cancer	CCSPS[13]	RCT	4870 patients	Placebo	4.5 years	Reducing the risk of death for cancer
5	Improving insulin resistance	Dai XH 2000[62]	RCT	64 patients with hypertension and dyslipidemia	Efamol	2 months	Lowering levels of fasting serum insulin and C peptide, raising

第七章

Continued

No.	Clinical benefits	Study	Design	Sample	Control	Duration	Effect of Xuezhikang
6	Inhibiting ventricular remodeling	Wang JM 2000[69]	RCT	42 patients with hypertention and left ventricular hypertrophy (LVH)	Enalapril	8 weeks	Reversing hypertensive LVH and improving heart function in patients with hypertension
		Gong C 2010[70]	RCT	90 patients with hypertention and LVH	Valsartan	2 years	Improve LVH and heart rate turbulence parameters, and lessening the damage on the autonomous nervous system
		Ye P 2009[71]	RCT	55 hypertensive patients with normal blood LDL-C level	Placebo and blank	72 weeks	Improving left ventricular diastolic function, probably mediated through antifibrotic and anti-inflammatory effects
7	Kidney protection	Cao ZX 2007[78]	RCT	58 patients with nephritic syndrome and hyperlipidemia	Blank	8 weeks	Regulating the levels of lipid and had potential effects of kidney protection
		Liu ZX 2007[79]	RCT	94 patients with youth obesity	Blank	8 weeks	Strengthening the efficacy and controlling the progression of proteinuria and glomerular lesion effectively
8	Others	Lu L 2009[83]	RCT	88 EH patients	Antihypertensive drug and pravastatin	8 weeks	Combined use of Xuezhikang with the antihypertensive therapy could lead to benefits independent of pressure-lowering effects

第七章

748

Table 2　Potential Synergetic Mechanism by Pharmacological Effects of Different Components in *Xuezhikang*

No.	Effective components	Clinical benefits	Study	Study type	Results
1	Natural statins	Overall lipid profiles modulation	Huang Z 2010[a]	Review	Statins, especially lovastatin, can reduce endogenous cholesterol synthesis, and increase the activity of low-density lipoprotein (LDL) receptor on the surface of liver cells to promote the clearance of LDL through feedback mechanisms
		Anti-atherosclerosis	Laufs U 1998[30]	*In vitro*	Lovastatin could upregulate endothelial constitutive nitric oxide synthase (ecNOS) expression predominantly by post-transcriptional mechanisms
		Anticancer	Hong MY 2008[53]	*In vivo*	Not only *Xuezhikang* and lovastatin had inhibitory effects on tumor cells, but also product after removal of lovastatin (PG) had, which demonstrated that the antitumor effect in *Xuezhikang* is a synergetic result of lovastatin and other useful elements
		Inhibiting ventricular remodeling	Ye P 2009[71]	*In vivo*	The mechanism of the protective effect on ventricular remodeling might be mainly from natural lovastatin in *Xuezhikang*
		Kidney protection	Patel S 2006[80]	*In vitro*	Lovastatin was demonstrated to have the effects of renal fibrosis prevention through the activation of ρGTPases
		Bone formation	Marini H 2008[85]	*In vivo*	Statins have been shown to promote bone formation, thus it may be possible to influence peak bone and to decrease the risk of osteoporosis in later life
2	Unsaturated fatty acids	Overall lipid profiles modulation	Phillipson BE 1985[17]	*In vivo*	Polyunsaturated fatty acids (PUFAs) can decrease triglycerides (TG), reduce the rate of lipid shuttle driven by cholesteryl ester transfer protein, increase high-density lipoprotein (HDL), reduce small LDL production, and get the cholesterol out of the vessel wall
			Dai Y 2009[18]	*In vivo*	α-Linolenic acid and γ-linolenic acid, their effects on serum levels of total cholesterol (TC), TG, and high-density lipoprotein-cholesterol (HDL-C) were significant
			OPTILIP[19]	*In vivo*	An increased intake of n-3 long-chain PUFAs caused the reduction in plasma triacylglycerol and favorable changes in LDL size
			Dai Y 2009[18]	*In vivo*	Diet enriched in eicosapentaenoic acid (EPA) and docosahexaenoic acid (DHA) can reduce blood levels of neutral lipids, TC, LDL, very low-density lipoprotein, and increase HDL
			Sadovsky R 2009[20]	*In vivo*	Intake of omega-3-acid ethyl esters can significantly decrease serum TG, along with plasma concentrations of certain lipoproteins up to 45%

Continued

No.	Effective components	Clinical benefits	Study	Study type	Results
			COMBOS 2008[21]	In vivo	Significant improvements were confirmed across a range of lipid indicators by taking PUFAs in combination with statin
	Unsaturated fatty acids	Anti-atherosclerosis	Arntzenius AC 1985[31]	In vivo	N-3 PUFAs, another main component of *Xuezhikang*, can directly or indirectly play a role in the immune system, and contribute to slowing the progression of atherosclerosis
			Carpentier YA 2006[32]	In vivo	N-3 PUFAs modulate inflammation, platelet activation, endothelial functions, and so on
			He K 2009[33]	In vivo	The dietary intake of long-chain n-3 PUFAs was inversely associated with concentrations of interleukin-6 (IL-6), matrix metalloproteinase-3
			Vedin I 2008[34]	In vivo	Reduced the release of interleukin-1β (IL-1β), granulocyte colony-stimulating factor
			He K 2008[35]	In vivo	Reflecting lower levels of inflammation and endothelial activation for a lower prevalence of subclinical atherosclerosis
			Hilpert KF 2007[36]	In vitro	Unsaturated fatty acids differentially affected concentrations of apoB-containing lipoprotein subclasses to attenuate the impairment of endothelial function
			Zhao G 2007[37]	In vivo	Increased intakes of α-linolenic acid exerted anti-inflammatory effects by inhibiting IL-6, IL-1β, and TNF-α production in cultured peripheral blood mononuclear cells
			Djoussé L 2003[38]	In vivo	Higher consumption of total linolenic acid was associated with the lower prevalence odds of carotid plaques and with lesser thickness of segment-specific carotid intimamedia thickness
			Bouwens M 2009[39]	In vivo	The intake of EPA and DHA for 26 weeks could alter the gene expression profiles of peripheral blood mononuclear cells (PBMCs) to a more anti-inflammatory and anti-atherogenic status
2	Unsaturated fatty acids	Anticancer	Hardman WE 2004[54]	In vitro	The efficacy of cancer chemotherapy drugs such as doxorubicin, epirubicin, irinotecan (CPT-11), 5-fluorouracil, and tamoxifen, and of radiation therapy has been improved when the diet included n-3 fatty acids
			Jiang WG 1998[55]	In vivo	PUFAs could also promote the absorption and storage of anticancer drugs, and enhance anticancer drug concentration in tumor cells to increase their efficacy
			Mehta SP 2008[56]	In vivo	Supplementation with EPA significantly reduced cyclooxygenase 2 concentrations, which also had beneficial effects for cancer prevention

Continued

No.	Effective components	Clinical benefits	Study	Study type	Results
2	Unsaturated fatty acids	Improving insulin resistance	Carpentier YA 2006[63]	In vivo	N-3 PUFAs can regulate the activity of key transcription factors to regulate gene expression in lipid metabolism and improve insulin sensitivity of type 2 diabetes mellitus to prevent diabetic complications
			Stirban A 2010[64]	In vivo	Six weeks of supplementation with n-3 PUFAs reduced the postprandial decrease in macrovascular function and meanwhile improved postprandial microvascular function
		Neural regulation	Tian F 2009[74]	In vitro	Enhancing protein synthesis in hippocampal neurons and increasing cell differentiation, α-linolenic acid-enriched diet has certain effects on nutrition and health care for brain
			Féart C 2008[75]	In vivo	Higher plasma EPA was associated with a lower severity of depressive symptomatology in elderly subjects, especially those taking antidepressants
			Pan YH 2001[76]	In vivo	γ-Aminobutyric can reduce damage of brain neurons caused by massive release of glutamate
		Kidney protection	Qian JL 2009[81]	In vivo	n-3 PUFAs can slow down the progression of kidney diseases by lipid-lowering, anti-inflammation, inhibition of oxidative stress, improving hemodynamics, intervention of cell proliferation, and signal transduction
			Wang J 2004[82]	In vitro	α-Linolenic acid can improve kidney function, reduce urinary calcium excretion, inhibit calcium oxalate crystal formation in kidney
		Anti-atrial fibrillation	Virtanen JK 2009[88]	In vivo	An increased concentration of long-chain n-3 PUFAs in serum, especially DHA, may protect against atrial fibrillation
3	Flavonoids	Overall lipid profiles modulation	Jahromi MAF 1993[22]	In vitro	Most flavonoids can reduce levels of TG, TC, and LDL
		Anti-atherosclerosis	Xiao LZ 2004[40]	In vitro	Protecting blood vessels though inhibiting platelet aggregation, anti-inflammatory, and antioxidant effects
			Loke WM 2008[41]	In vivo	Dietary flavonoids, such as quercetin and epicatechin, can augment nitric oxide status and reduce endothelin-1 concentrations and may thereby improve endothelial function
		Anti-atherosclerosis	Fuchs D 2007[42]	In vivo	Flavonoids-enriched diet could reduce the levels of soluble vascular cell adhesion molecule-1 and increase the anti-inflammatory response in blood mononuclear cells
			Nasca MM 2008[43]	In vivo	Flavonoids caused an improvement in endothelial function that may reflect an overall improvement in the underlying inflammatory process underlying atherosclerosis

第七章

Continued

No.	Effective components	Clinical benefits	Study	Study type	Results
3	Flavonoids	Liver protection	Tipoe GL 2010[50]	In vitro	Flavonoids have different levels of protection effects on liver damage caused by a variety of reasons, and the protective mechanism was related to antioxidant function of enzyme
			Kim MH 2010[51]	In vitro	It inhibited the release of TNF-α, and the role of cell apoptosis
		Anticancer	Zhu RX 2010[57]	Review	Some natural flavonoids and chalcone derivates can reverse the multidrug resistance of tumor cells
			Zeng S 2009[58]	Review	Activating and up-regulating caspase-3, modulating Bax/Bcl-2 expression level and intracellular Ca^{2+} level, decreasing the mitochondrial transmembrane potential and promoting the release of cytochrome C are involved in the induction of apoptosis in cancer cells by the compounds, which is associated with the regulatory factors, such as p53, eukaryotic protein kinases (EPK), nuclear factor kappa-B (NF-κB), and so on
		Improving insulin resistance	Liu ZM 2010[65]	In vivo	Flavonoids also have a significant effect in the improvement of insulin resistance, and many associated drugs have already been put into clinical practice
		Bone formation	Marini H 2008[85]	In vivo	Flavonoids have been shown to promote bone formation, and decrease the risk of osteoporosis in later life
4	Trace element: magnesium	Anti-atherosclerosis	Li JJ 2003[44]	Review	Many animal experiments show that magnesium has an anti-atherosclerosis effect, the mechanisms of which may be reducing lipemia, protecting blood vessels, decreasing free radical and lipid peroxide, and affecting the level of hormone
		Improving insulin resistance	Barbagallo M 2007[66]	Review	Magnesium deficiency can lead to reduction of insulin sensitivity affecting the stability of glucose metabolism
			Kim DJ 2010[67]	Review	Increasing the intake of magnesium plays an important role in prevention of non-insulin-dependent diabetes mellitus and its complications
		Neural regulation	Tymianski M 1996[77]	In vitro	Magnesium can significantly reduce the mortality in patients with injury of ischemic brain, and promote the recovery of neurological function. In acute state of cerebral infarction, magnesium is a neural-protective agent of high clinical value
5	Trace element: selenium	Anti-atherosclerosis	Yun BS 2002[46]	In vivo	Selenium supplementation increases the activity of anti-oxidative glutathione peroxidase 1 in endothelial cells of patients, which may also protect against the progress of arteriosclerosis
		Liver protection	Aaseth J 1980[52]	Review	Selenium may have some preventive effects in alcoholic cirrhosis

第七章

Continued

No.	Effective components	Clinical benefits	Study	Study type	Results
5	Trace element: selenium	Anticancer	Shen DL 2008[59]	Review	Selenium's anti-cancer mechanisms are multifaceted, including anti-oxidative damage, regulation of gene expression and cell cycle to promote apoptosis of cancer cells, stabilizing the structure of DNA and enhancing immune function against cancer as well as intermediary in the metabolism of certain chemical carcinogens
		Improving insulin resistance	Zhang M 2009[68]	In vitro	Selenium also has inhibitory effects on complications of diabetes such as osteoporosis and retinopathy
		Bone formation	InCHIANTI study[87]	In vivo	Low plasma selenium is independently associated with poor skeletal muscle strength in community-dwelling older adults
6	Ergosterol	Overall lipid profiles modulation	Subbiah MT 1973[60]	Review	Ergosterol can compete with the cholesterol absorption site to interfere with the absorption of cholesterol, reducing exogenous cholesterol
		Anticancer	Kahols K 1989[61]	In vitro	Ergosterol proved to be active against Walker 256 carcinosarcoma and MCF-7 breast cancer cell lines
7	Sterins	Anti-atherosclerosis	Yun BS 2002[46]	In vitro	Anti-oxidative effects of sterins may also have some value in atherosclerosis prevention

aHuang Z, Li DD. Recent advances in the studies of lovastatin. Chin J Biochem Pharmaceutics, 2010, 31: 144.

第七章

was inversely associated with concentrations of IL-6, matrix metalloproteinase-3 (MMP-3)[33], and reduced the release of interleukin-1β (IL-1β), granulocyte colony-stimulating factor[34], reflecting lower levels of inflammation and endothelial activation for a lower prevalence of subclinical atherosclerosis [35]. The study by Hilpert et al. suggested that unsaturated fatty acids differentially affected concentrations of apolipoprotein B-containing lipoprotein subclasses to attenuate the impairment of endothelial function [36], whereas increased intakes of α-linolenic acid exerted anti-inflammatory effects by inhibiting IL-6, IL-1β, and TNF-α production in cultured peripheral blood mononuclear cells [37]. Higher consumption of total linolenic acid was associated with lower prevalence odds of carotid plaques and with lesser thickness of segment-specific carotid intima-media thickness [38], and the intake of EPA and DHA for 26 weeks could alter the gene expression profiles of peripheral blood mononuclear cells to a more anti-inflammatory and anti-atherogenic status [39].

As for flavonoids, they protect blood vessels through inhibiting platelet aggregation, and by anti-inflammatory and antioxidant effects [40]. Some scholars found that dietary flavonoids, such as quercetin and (−)-epicatechin, can augment nitric oxide status and reduce endothelin-1 concentrations and may thereby improve endothelial function [41]. Many other studies showed that a flavonoids-enriched diet could reduce the levels of soluble vascular cell adhesion molecule-1 and increase the anti-inflammatory response in blood mononuclear cells [42], which suggested an improvement in endothelial function that may reflect an overall improvement in the inflammatory process underlying atherosclerosis [43].

Furthermore, many animal experiments show that magnesium has an anti-atherosclerosis effect, the mechanisms of which may be reducing lipemia, protecting blood vessels, decreasing

free radicals and lipid-peroxide, and affecting the level of hormone [44]. Selenium supplementation increases the activity of antioxidative glutathione peroxidase 1 in endothelial cells of patients[45], which may also prevent the progress of arteriosclerosis. In addition, antioxidative effects of sterins in *Xuezhikang* may also have some value in atherosclerosis prevention [46].

6. Liver Protection Effects

It was reported that combining other therapies with *Xuezhikang* in the treatment of fatty liver could have the effects of relieving clinical syndromes and improving liver function[47]. Another study also showed that *Xuezhikang* may have potential clinical application in the treatment of nonalcoholic fatty liver disease for its function of reversing aminotransferase abnormalities, and the common therapeutic mechanism of *Xuezhikang* is likely to be involved in the inhibition of hepatic expression of TNF-α [48]. Thus, *Xuezhikang* has been recommended in attempting to treat those patients with hyperlipidemia intolerant to other statins or with elevated liver/muscle enzymes induced by other statins [49].

In the *Xuezhikang*, flavonoids have different levels of protection effects on liver damage caused by a variety of reasons, and the protective mechanisms were related to enzyme antioxidant function[50], inhibiting the release of TNF-α [51], and the role of cell apoptosis. Furthermore, selenium may have some preventive effects in alcoholic cirrhosis [52]. A large number of research reports in China and abroad indicate that selenium is closely related to the emergence, development, and prognosis of liver disease.

7. Anticancer Effects

The CCSPS study found that *Xuezhikang* could reduce the risk of death from cancer [13]. After observing the effects of *Xuezhikang*, the product after removal of lovastatin (PG [product after]), and lovastatin on the inhibition of colon carcinoma *in situ* and metastatic tumor cells, researchers in David Geffen School of Medicine Center for Human Nutrition from the University of California found that not only *Xuezhikang* and lovastatin had inhibitory effects on tumor cells, but also PG had these effects, which demonstrated that the antitumor effect in *Xuezhikang* is a synergetic result of lovastatin and other useful elements [53].

Supplementing the diet of tumor-bearing mice or rats with oils containing n-3 fatty acids can slow the growth of various types of cancers, including lung, colon, mammary, and prostate. The efficacy of cancer chemotherapy drugs such as doxorubicin, epirubicin, irinotecan (CPT-11), 5-fluorouracil, and tamoxifen, and of radiation therapy has been improved when the diet included n-3 fatty acids. Some potential mechanisms for the activity of n-3 fatty acids against cancer include modulation of eicosanoid production and inflammation, angiogenesis, proliferation, susceptibility to apoptosis, and estrogen signaling. In humans, n-3 fatty acids have also been used to suppress cancer-associated cachexia and to improve the quality of life [54]. PUFAs could also promote the absorption and storage of anticancer drugs, and enhance anticancer drug concentration in tumor cells to increase their efficacy [55]. Supplementation with EPA significantly reduced cyclooxygenase 2 concentrations [56], which also had beneficial effects for cancer prevention.

Moreover, recent studies showed that flavonoids can exhibit significant antitumor activities, and the combination treatment with some active flavones can change the antitumor effects. Some natural flavonoids and chalcone derivates can reverse the multidrug resistance of tumor cells [57]. Activating and upregulating caspase-3, modulating Bax/Bcl-2 expression level and intracellular Ca^{2+} level, decreasing the mitochondrial transmembrane potential, and promoting the release of cytochrome C are involved in the induction of apoptosis in cancer cells by the compounds, which is associated with

the regulatory factors, such as p53, eukaryotic protein kinases (EPK), nuclear factor κ-β, and so on [58]. In addition, some flavonoids-enriched diets can modulate immune function and appear to be protective against DNA damage.

Furthermore, another component of *Xuezhikang*, selenium, is one of the trace elements with the effects of anticancer and preventing cancer. Its mechanisms are multifaceted, including antioxidative damage, regulation of gene expression and cell cycle to promote apoptosis of cancer cells, stabilizing the structure of DNA, and enhancing immune function against cancer as well as being intermediary in the metabolism of certain chemical carcinogens [59]. In addition, ergosterin has already been known to have antitumor effects [60,61].

8. Improving Insulin Resistance

Xuezhikang can significantly lower levels of fasting serum insulin and C peptide, and raise insulin sensitivity index in patients with hypertension complicated with dyslipidemia, suggesting it can improve insulin sensitivity for patients with hypertension during lipid-lowering therapy [62].

As main components in *Xuezhikang*, n-3 PUFAs can regulate the activity of key transcription factors to regulate gene expression in lipid metabolism and improve insulin sensitivity of type 2 diabetes mellitus to prevent diabetic complications [63]. Six weeks of supplementation with n-3 PUFAs reduced the postprandial decrease in macrovascular function and meanwhile improved postprandial microvascular function [64]. Furthermore, flavonoids also have a significant effect in the improvement of insulin resistance [65], and many associated drugs have already been put into clinical practice. Also, it was reported that magnesium deficiency can lead to reduction of insulin sensitivity [66] and affect the stability of glucose metabolism. Thus, increasing the intake of magnesium plays an important role in prevention of non-insulin-dependent diabetes mellitus and its complications [67]. Moreover, selenium reduces the production of oxygen free radicals in the body by glutathione peroxidase to prevent further oxidative damage in the body and the insulin A, B between the two peptide chains for ensuring the complete molecule structure and function of insulin to play a role in lowering blood glucose. In addition, selenium also has inhibitory effects on complications of diabetes such as osteoporosis and retinopathy [68].

9. Inhibiting Ventricular Remodeling

Xuezhikang has shown beneficial effects on reversing hypertensive left ventricular hypertrophy (LVH) and improving heart function in patients with hypertension [69]. Combined therapy with *Xuezhikang* and valsartan can improve LVH and heart rate turbulence parameters, and lessen the damage on the autonomous nervous system [70]. Long-term therapy with *Xuezhikang* remarkably improved left ventricular diastolic function, probably mediated through antifibrotic and anti-inflammatory effects [71]. The mechanism of the protective effect on ventricular remodeling might be mainly from natural lovastatin [72] in *Xuezhikang*.

10. Neural Regulation and Protection Effects

Xuezhikang significantly reduced the infarct volume and improved the functional recovery compared to vehicle, and significantly decreased the malondialdehyde (MDA) accumulation after reperfusion. NG-nitro-L-arginine methyl ester partially inhibited the protective effect of *Xuezhikang* but nearly completely abolished the protective effect of simvastatin. The beneficial effects are partly due to the statins and other components in *Xuezhikang* [73].

Since it enhances protein synthesis in hippocampal neurons and increasing cell differentiation, an α-linolenic acid-enriched diet has certain effects on nutrition and health care

for the brain [74]. Furthermore, higher plasma EPA was associated with a lower severity of depressive symptomatology in elderly subjects, especially those taking antidepressants [75]. For other components, γ-aminobutyric acid can reduce damage of brain neurons caused by massive release of glutamate [76]. Magnesium can significantly reduce mortality in patients with ischemic brain injury, and promote the recovery of neurological function. In an acute state of cerebral infarction, magnesium is a neural-protective agent of high clinical value [77].

11. Kidney Protection Effects

The efficacy of *Xuezhikang* has been investigated in patients with nephritic syndrome and hyperlipidemia, and the results found that *Xuezhikang* could regulate the levels of lipid and had potential effects of kidney protection [78]. Adding *Xuezhikang* in routine therapy could strengthen the efficacy and control the progression of proteinuria and glomerular lesion effectively [79].

Lovastatin, the main component of *Xuezhikang*, was demonstrated to have the effect of renal fibrosis prevention through the activation of Rho GTPases [80]. It has been also reported that n-3 PUFAs can slow down the progression of kidney diseases by lipid-lowering, anti-inflammation, inhibition of oxidative stress, improving hemodynamics, intervention of cell proliferation, and signal transduction [81]. α-Linolenic acid can improve kidney function, reduce urinary calcium excretion, and inhibit calcium oxalate crystal formation in kidney, which may have some value in the prevention and treatment of urolithiasis [82].

12. Others

Combined use of *Xuezhikang* with antihypertensive therapy could increase the circulating endothelial progenitor cells and improve their function in essential hypertensive patients with blood pressure controlled by antihypertensive drugs, leading to benefits independent of pressure-lowering effects [83]. *Xuezhikang* stimulated new bone formation in bone defects *in vivo* and increased bone cell formation *in vitro* [84]. Flavonoids and statins have been shown to promote bone formation, and thus may influence peak bone and decrease the risk of osteoporosis in later life [85,86]. In addition, the In-CHIANTI study [87] showed that low plasma selenium is independently associated with poor skeletal muscle strength in community-dwelling older adults. Another study demonstrated that an increased concentration of long-chain n-3 PUFAs in serum, especially docosahexaenoic acid, may protect against atrial fibrillation [88].

The clinical benefits of *Xuezhikang* in cardiovascular disease and other chronic conditions as well as potential synergetic mechanism by pharmacological effects of different components in *Xuezhikang* are summarized in Tables 1 and 2.

The controversy on polypill has never stopped since the first conception in 2003 [89]. As a natural compound medicine, the remarkable clinical benefits and multicomponents synergetic mechanism of *Xuezhikang* make it a successful paradigm of polypill. Although lovastatin is the main component in lowering blood lipid, other ingredients in *Xuezhikang* also work together to reach the goal of overall lipid regulation and additional clinical benefits. In fact, the concept of polypill happens to coincide with the theory of compound prescription in Traditional Chinese Medicine (TCM), which originated in China more than 2000 years ago. It is one of the representative characteristics and strengths of TCM to treat patients by compound prescription through the "monarch, minister, assistant, and guide" compatibility of various herbal medicines to achieve multitarget intervention with efficacy-enhancing and toxicity-reducing effects. The compound prescription based on TCM pattern diagnosis contains a wealth of ideas about "individualized medicine", which might have valuable implications for future development of an individualized polypill.

There might be some limitations in this review. Since most studies reported positive results here, the publication bias could not be excluded. However, this article focused on the synergistic mechanisms of different components in *Xuezhikang* to contribute multiple clinical benefits as a natural polypill, rather than a systematic review on the available clinical evidences of *Xuezhikang*. With the progress of indepth research, it is believed, there will be more clinical benefits of *Xuezhikang* to be discovered, and polypill is anticipated to be a more effective and feasible way for treating complicated diseases.

References

[1] World Health Organization. The World Health Report 2003—Shaping the Future. Online document at: www.who.int/whr/2003/en/ Accessed April 2, 2012.

[2] Emberson J, Whincup P, Morris R, et al. Eur Heart J, 2004, 25: 484-491.

[3] Dezii CM. A retrospective study of persistence with single-pill combination therapy *vs.* concurrent two-pill therapy in patients with hypertension. Manag Care 2000, 9 (suppl): S2-S6.

[4] Wald NJ, Law MR. A strategy to reduce cardiovascular disease by more than 80%. BMJ, 2003, 326: 1419.

[5] Rodgers A. A cure for cardiovascular disease? BMJ, 2003, 326: 1407-1408.

[6] Willis J. Polypill debate continues: concept is a fascinating thought experiment. BMJ, 2004, 328: 289.

[7] Reddy KS. The preventive polypill: much promise, insufficient evidence. NEJM, 2007, 356: 212.

[8] Gaziano TA, Opie LH, Weinstein MC. Cardiovascular disease prevention with a multidrug regimen in the developing world: a cost-effectiveness analysis. Lancet, 2006, 368: 679-686.

[9] Soliman EZ, Mendis S, Dissanayake WP, et al. A Polypill for primary prevention of cardiovascular disease: a feasibility study of the World Health

Organization. Trials, 2011, 12: 3.

[10] Zhang ML, Duan ZW, Xie SM. Study on the active ingredient of Xuezhikang. Chin J New Drugs, 1998, 7: 213-214.

[11] Journoud M, Jones PJ. Red yeast rice: a new hypolipidemic drug. Life Sci, 2004, 74: 2675.

[12] Liu J, Zhang J, Shi Y, et al. Chinese red yeast rice (Monascus purpureus) for primary hyperlipidemia: a meta-analysis of randomized controlled trials. Chin Med, 2006, 1: 4.

[13] Lu Z, Kou W, Du B, et al. Effect of Xuezhikang, an extract from red yeast Chinese rice, on coronary events in a Chinese population with previous myocardial infarction. Am J Cardiol, 2008, 101: 1689-1693.

[14] Joint Committee for Developing Chinese Guidelines on Prevention and Treatment of Dyslipidemia in Adults. Chinese Guidelines on Prevention and Treatment of Dyslipidemia in Adults. Chin J Cardiol, 2007, 35: 390-419.

[15] Pfeffer MA, Sacks FM, Moyé LA, et al. Cholesterol and recurrent events: a secondary prevention trial for normolipidemic patients. CARE Investigators, Am J Cardiol, 1995, 76: 98C-106C.

[16] Lu ZL, Xu ZM, Kou WR, et al. Advance in basic and clinical research of Xuezhikang Capsule. Chin J Integr Med, 2006, 12: 85-93.

[17] Phillipson BE, Rothrock DW, Connor WE, et al. Reduction of plasma lipids, lipoproteins, and apoproteins by dietary fish oils in patients with hypertriglyceridemia. NEJM, 1985, 312: 1210-1216.

[18] Dai Y, Yan HH, Wang F. Effects of α-linolenic acid and γ-linolenic acid on the blood-lipid levels in hyperlipidemia people. Prog Mod Biomed, 2009, 9: 4492-4495.

[19] Griffin MD, Sanders TA, Davies IG, et al. Effects of altering the ratio of dietary n-6 to n-3 fatty acids on insulin sensitivity, lipoprotein size, and postprandial lipemia in men and postmenopausal women aged 45-70 y: The OPTILIP Study. Am J Clin Nutr, 2006, 84: 1290-1298.

[20] Sadovsky R, Kris-Etherton P. Prescription omega-3-acid ethyl esters for the treatment of very high triglycerides. Postgrad Med, 2009, 121: 145-153.

[21] Barter P, Ginsberg HN. Effectiveness of combined statin plus omega-3 fatty acid therapy for mixed dyslipidemia. Am J Cardiol, 2008, 102: 1040-1045.

[22] Jahromi MAF, Ray AB. Antihyperlipidemic effect of flavonoids from Pterocarpus marsupium. J Nat Prod, 1993, 56: 989-999.

[23] Zhao SP, Liu L, Cheng YC, et al. Xuezhikang, an extract of cholestin, protects endothelial function through antiinflammatory and lipid-lowering mechanisms in patients with coronary heart disease. Circulation, 2004, 110: 915-920.

[24] Lu L, Zhou JZ, Wang L, et al. Effects of Xuezhikang and pravastatin on circulating endothelial progenitor cells in patients with essential hypertension. Chin J Integr Med, 2009, 15: 266-271.

[25] Fan XF, Deng YQ, Ye L, et al. Effect of Xuezhikang capsule on serum tumor necrosis factor-alpha and interleukin-6 in patients with nonalcoholic fatty liver disease and hyperlipidemia. Chin J Integr Med, 2010, 16: 119-123.

[26] Liu JD, Liu ZQ, Cui LQ, et al. Short-term application of Xuezhikang on plasma levels of C-reactive protein in perioperative percutaneous coronary intervention. Chin J Cardiol, 2006, 34: 406.

[27] Yao QH, Cui CC, Wang JK. Effect of xuezhikang on blood lipids, serum oxidized low density lipoprotein, C-reactive protein and fibrinogen in patients with unstable angina pectoris. Chin J Integr Tradit West Med, 2003, 23: 750-752.

[28] Huang J, Wang MH, Peng XP, et al. Effects of Xuezhikang on serum levels of high sensitive-C reactive protein, matrix metalloproteinase-9 and lipoprotein in patients with acute coronary syndrome. Chin J Integr Tradit West Med, 2006, 26: 221-223.

[29] Jian J, Hao X, Deng C, et al. The effects of Xuezhikang on serum lipid profile, thromboxane A_2 and prostacyclin in patients with hyperlipidemia. Chin J Intern Med, 1999, 38: 517-519.

[30] Laufs U, La Fata V, Plutzky J, et al. Upregulation of endothelial nitric oxide synthase by HMG CoA reductase inhibitors. Circulation, 1998, 97, 1129-1135.

[31] Arntzenius AC, Kromhout D, Barth JD, et al. Diet, lipoproteins, and the progression of coronary atherosclerosis: The Leiden Intervention Trial. NEJM, 1985, 312: 805-811.

[32] Carpentier YA, Portois L, Malaisse WJ. n-3 fatty acids and the metabolic syndrome. Am J Clin Nutr, 2006, 83 (6 suppl): 1499S-1504S.

[33] He K, Liu K, Daviglus ML, et al. Associations of

第七章

dietary long-chain n-3 polyunsaturated fatty acids and fish with biomarkers of inflammation and endothelial activation (from the Multi-Ethnic Study of Atherosclerosis [MESA]). Am J Cardiol, 2009, 103: 1238-1243.

[34] Vedin I, Cederholm T, Freund Levi Y, et al. Effects of docosahexaenoic acid-rich n-3 fatty acid supplementation on cytokine release from blood mononuclear leukocytes: the OmegAD study. Am J Clin Nutr, 2008, 87: 1616-1622.

[35] He K, Liu K, Daviglus ML, et al. Intakes of long-chain n-3 polyunsaturated fatty acids and fish in relation to measurements of subclinical atherosclerosis. Am J Clin Nutr, 2008, 88: 1111-1118.

[36] Hilpert KF, West SG, Kris-Etherton PM, et al. Postprandial effect of n-3 polyunsaturated fatty acids on apolipoprotein B-containing lipoproteins and vascular reactivity in type 2 diabetes. Am J Clin Nutr, 2007, 85: 369-376.

[37] Zhao G, Etherton TD, Martin KR, et al. Dietary alphalinolenic acid inhibits proinflammatory cytokine production by peripheral blood mononuclear cells in hypercholesterolemic subjects. Am J Clin Nutr, 2007, 85: 385-391.

[38] Djoussé L, Folsom AR, Province MA, et al. Dietary linolenic acid and carotid atherosclerosis: The National Heart, Lung, and Blood Institute Family Heart Study. Am J Clin Nutr, 2003, 77: 819-825.

[39] Bouwens M, van de Rest O, Dellschaft N, et al. Fish-oil supplementation induces anti-inflammatory gene expression profiles in human blood mononuclear cells. Am J Clin Nutr, 2009, 90: 415-424.

[40] Xiao LZ, Xu X, Lai SY, et al. Protective effects of soy isoflavones on atherosclerosis in ovariectomized rabbits and possibly involved mechanism. South China J Cardiovasc Dis, 2004, 10: 144-145.

[41] Loke WM, Hodgson JM, Proudfoot JM, et al. Pure dietary flavonoids quercetin and (-)-epicatechin augment nitric oxide products and reduce endothelin-1 acutely in healthy men. Am J Clin Nutr, 2008, 88: 1018-1025.

[42] Fuchs D, Vafeiadou K, Hall WL, et al. Proteomic biomarkers of peripheral blood mononuclear cells obtained from postmenopausal women undergoing an intervention with soy isoflavones. Am J Clin Nutr, 2007, 86: 1369-1375.

[43] Nasca MM, Zhou JR, Welty FK. Effect of soy nuts on adhesion molecules and markers of inflammation in hypertensive and normotensive postmenopausal women. Am J Cardiol, 2008, 102: 84-86.

[44] Li JJ, Zhang ZY. The progress of anti-atherosclerosis of magnesium. Stud Trace Elem Health, 2003, 20: 49-51.

[45] Schnabel R, Lubos E, Messow CM, et al. Selenium supplementation improves antioxidant capacity in vitro and in vivo in patients with coronary artery disease: The Selenium Therapy in Coronary Artery disease Patients (SETCAP) Study. Am Heart J, 2008, 156: 1201.e1-11.

[46] Yun BS, Cho Y, Lee IK, et al. Sterins A and B, new antioxidative compounds from Stereum hirsutum. J Antibiot, 2002, 55: 208-210.

[47] Yao ZL, Zhu CC, Wan XQ. Clinical research of Xuezhikang joint sport in treatment of steatohepatitis who had symptoms. Chin J Modern Med, 2006, 16: 253-256.

[48] Hong XZ, Li LD, Wu LM. Effects of fenofibrate and xuezhikang on high-fat diet-induced non-alcoholic fatty liver disease. Clin Exp Pharmacol Physiol, 2007, 34: 27-35.

[49] China Consensus Group on the Clinical Application of Xuezhikang Capsule. China consensus on the clinical application of Xuezhikang capsule. Chin J Intern Med, 2009, 48: 171-174.

[50] Tipoe GL, Leung TM, Liong EC, et al. Epigallocatechin-3-gallate (EGCG) reduces liver inflammation, oxidative stress and fibrosis in carbon tetrachloride (CCl4) -induced liver injury in mice. Toxicology, 2010, 273: 45-52.

[51] Kim MH, Kang KS, Lee YS. The inhibitory effect of genistein on hepatic steatosis is linked to visceral adipocyte metabolism in mice with diet-induced non-alcoholic fatty liver disease. Br J Nutr, 2010, 104: 1333-1342.

[52] Aaseth J, Thomassen Y, Alexander J, et al. Decreased serum selenium in alcoholic cirrhosis. NEJM, 1980, 303: 944-945.

[53] Hong MY, Seeram NP, Zhang Y, et al. Anticancer effects of Chinese red yeast rice versus monacolin K alone on colon cancer cells. J Nutr Biochem, 2008, 19: 448-458.

[54] Hardman WE. (N-3) fatty acids and cancer therapy. J Nutr, 2004, 134: 3427S.

[55] Jiang WG, Bryce RP, Horrobin DF, et al. Regulation of tight junction permeability and occludin expression by polyunsaturated fatty acids. Biochem Biophys Res

第
七
章

Commun, 1998, 244: 414-420.

[56] Mehta SP, Boddy AP, Cook J, et al. Effect of n-3 polyunsaturated fatty acids on Barrett's epithelium in the human lower esophagus. Am J Clin Nutr, 2008, 87: 949-956.

[57] Zhu RX, Zhang SL, Jin YS. Recent advances in the study on antitumor effects of flavonoids. Drugs Clinic, 2010, 25: 5-10.

[58] Zeng S, Yang Y, Guo QL. Mechanism of flavonoids-induced apoptosis in cancer cells and related experimental researches: a review. Prog Pharm Sci, 2009, 33: 402-407.

[59] Shen DL, Li B, Li JG, et al. Anticancer mechanism of selenium: recent progress. Chin J Cancer Biother, 2008, 15: 598-600.

[60] Subbiah MT. Dietary plant sterols: current status in human and animal sterol metabolism. Am J Clin Nutr, 1973, 26: 219-225.

[61] Kahols K, Kangas L, Hiltunen R. Ergosterol peroxide, an active compound from Inonutus radiatus. Planta Med, 1989, 55: 389-390.

[62] Dai XH, Xue XY, Wang L, et al. The effects of Xuezhikang on insulin sensitivity for patients with hypertension complicated with dyslipidemia. Chin J Cardiol, 2000, 20: 692-693.

[63] Carpentier YA, Portois L, Malaisse WJ. N-3 fatty acids and the metabolic syndrome. Am J Clin Nutr, 2006, 83 (6 suppl): 1499S-1504S.

[64] Stirban A, Nandrean S, Götting C, et al. Effects of n-3 fatty acids on macro- and microvascular function in subjects with type 2 diabetes mellitus. Am J Clin Nutr, 2010, 91: 808-813.

[65] Liu ZM, Chen YM, Ho SC, et al. Effects of soy protein and isoflavones on glycemic control and insulin sensitivity: a 6-mo double-blind, randomized, placebo-controlled trial in postmenopausal Chinese women with prediabetes or untreated early diabetes. Am J Clin Nutr, 2010, 91: 1394-401.

[66] Barbagallo M, Dominguez LJ, Resnick LM. Magnesium metabolism in hypertension and type 2 diabetes mellitus. Am J Ther, 2007, 14: 375-385.

[67] Kim DJ, Xun P, Liu K, et al. Magnesium intake in relation to systemic inflammation, insulin resistance, and the incidence of diabetes. Diabetes Care, 2010, 33: 2604-2610.

[68] Zhang M. Hypoglycemic effect of selenium-enriched compound SOD green tea in diabetic rats. Parenter Enteral Nutr, 2009, 16: 109.

[69] Wang JM, Lv XY. Effects of Xuezhikang on left ventricular and remodeling for patients with hypertension. Clin Focus, 2000, 15: 645-646.

[70] Gong C, Huang SL, Huang JF, et al. Effects of combined therapy of Xuezhikang Capsule and Valsartan on hypertensive left ventricular hypertrophy and heart rate turbulence. Chin J Integr Med, 2010, 16: 114-118.

[71] Ye P, Wu CE, Sheng L, et al. Potential protective effect of long-term therapy with Xuezhikang on left ventricular diastolic function in patients with essential hypertension. J Altern Complement Med, 2009, 15: 719-725.

[72] Ramasubbu K, Mann DL. The emerging role of statins in the treatment of heart failure. J Am Coll Cardiol, 2006, 47: 342-344.

[73] Zhou FY, Zhang J, Song T, et al. Effects of xuezhikang and simvastatin on cerebral ischemia-reperfusion injury in rat. China J Chin Mater Med, 2006, 31: 1447-1450.

[74] Tian F, Qi XX, Zheng ZH. α-linolenic acid on learning and memory function and hippocampal neurons of rats. Chin J Geriatrics, 2009, 29: 664-666.

[75] Féart C, Peuchant E, Letenneur L, et al. Plasma eicosapentaenoic acid is inversely associated with severity of depressive symptomatology in the elderly: Data from the Bordeaux sample of the Three-City Study. Am J Clin Nutr, 2008, 87: 1156-1162.

[76] Pan YH, Zhao QJ, Feng HL, et al. γ-Hydroxybutyric acid on focal cerebral ischemia-reperfusion injury. Chin J Neurol, 2001, 34: 319.

[77] Tymianski M, Tator CH. Normal and abnormal calcium homeostasis in neuron: A basis for the pathophysiology of traumatic and ischemic CNS injury. Neurosurgery, 1996, 38: 1176-1195.

[78] Cao ZX, Liao PY. Treatment of Xuezhikang on nephotic syndrome for children in hyperlipidemia with 30 cases. Chin J Cardiol, 2007, 27: 855-856.

[79] Liu ZX, Lin Z, Wu YX, et al. Effects of Xuezhikang on microalbuminuria in patients with youth obesity. World J Integr Tradit West Med, 2007, 12: 719-721.

[80] Patel S, Mason RM, Suzuki J, et al. Inhibitory effect of statins on renal epithelial-to-mesenchymal transition. Am J Nephrol, 2006, 26: 381-387.

[81] Qian JL, Zhang MF. Progress of n-3 polyunsaturated fatty acids on chronic kidney disease. Chin J Integr

Tradit West Nephrol, 2009, 1095-1097.

[82] Wang J, Liang Y, Zhang YC, et al. Experimental study of α –linolenic acid inhibitory effect on calcium oxalate crystalization in rats. Chin J Urol, 2004, 25: 163-165.

[83] Lu L, Zhou JZ, Wang L, et al. Effects of Xuezhikang and pravastatin on circulating endothelial progenitor cells in patients with essential hypertension. Chin J Integr Med, 2009, 15: 266-271.

[84] Wong RW, Rabie B. Chinese red yeast rice (Monascus purpureus-fermented rice) promotes bone formation. Chin Med, 2008, 3: 4.

[85] Marini H, Bitto A, Altavilla D, et al. Breast safety and efficacy of genistein aglycone for postmenopausal bone loss: A follow-up study. J Clin Endocrinol Metab, 2008, 93: 4787-4796.

[86] Mundy GR. Nutritional modulators of bone remodeling during aging. Am J Clin Nutr, 2006, 83: 427S-430S.

[87] Lauretani F, Semba RD, Bandinelli S, et al. Association of low plasma selenium concentrations with poor muscle strength in older community-dwelling adults: The In-CHIANTI Study. Am J Clin Nutr, 2007, 86: 347-352.

[88] Virtanen JK, Mursu J, Voutilainen S, et al. Serum long-chain n-3 polyunsaturated fatty acids and risk of hospital diagnosis of atrial fibrillation in men. Circulation, 2009, 120: 2315-2321.

[89] Wald NJ, Wald DS. The polypill concept. Heart, 2010, 96: 1-4.

Traditional Chinese Herbal Products for Coronary Heart Disease: An Overview of Cochrane Reviews*

QIU Yu   XU Hao SHI   Da-zhuo   SHI Da-zhuo

1. Introduction

Coronary heart disease (CHD) is one of the most dangerous threats to human health, manifested by different clinical types such as angina pectoris, myocardial infarction, heart failure, cardiac arrhythmia, and so forth. Although treated with intensive medication or revascularization therapy, uncontrolled angina and recurrent acute cardiovascular events are still the major problems confronting modern medicine. Traditional Chinese medicine (TCM) has a history of thousands of years and has made great contributions to the health and well-being of the people and to the maintenance and growth of the population [1]. Currently, more than 90% of the urban and rural Chinese population has sought for TCM in their lifetimes [2]. TCM has been studied extensively and seems to be safe and effective in treating CHD [3,4]. Recently, the potential benefit of integrative Western and Chinese medicine regimen has also been indicated in a large-scale registry study in China [5]. Cochrane reviews are regarded as the highest standard of evidence [6]. They adopt transparent and comprehensive methods of finding all of the relevant evidence. Their quality and reliability are generally higher than any other systematic review because they employ a predefined, rigorous, and explicit methodology. Cochrane reviews are also reviewed and published in advance. Therefore, conclusion made from the overview of Cochrane reviews is more credible. Some Cochrane systematic reviews of traditional Chinese herbal products (TCHPs) for CHD have been conducted in recent years. These reviews provide preliminary evidence of TCHPs benefits

---

* 原载于 Evidence-Based Complementary and Alternative Medicine，2012，Article ID 417387

第七章

to certain CHD patient populations, which call for a comprehensive evaluation on the effectiveness of TCHPs in CHD patients. This overview aims to evaluate and summarize all Cochrane reviews of TCHP as a treatment of CHD critically.

2. Methods

We searched the titles and abstracts of all reviews in September 2011 of the Cochrane Database of Systematic Review. The search terms were "Herb* and medic* and heart" and "Herb* and medic* and cardiac" and "Herb* and medic* and circulation" and "Chinese and heart" and "Chinese and cardiac" and "Chinese and circulation". We read the title and abstract of each retrieved review in order to confirm that the review was relevant. Articles were included if they related to any type of TCHP as a treatment of CHD. Data were extracted according to predefined inclusion criteria by two independent reviewers (Qiu Y. and Xu H.). Disagreements were resolved by discussion between the authors.

We also searched the Cochrane Central Register of Controlled Trials (CENTRAL) in The Cochrane Library Issue 4 of 4, Oct 2011. Studies of TCHP as the treatment of any type of CHD were included. Studies without results were excluded. The methodological quality was assessed using the Cochrane Collaboration risk of bias criteria with 6 domains [7]: (1) random, (2) blinding of participants, doctor, and outcome assessors, (3) allocation concealment, (4) incomplete outcome data, (5) free of the suggestion of selective outcome reporting, and (6) informed consents. Discrepancies were resolved by consensus through discussion between the two reviewers.

3. Results

Six articles met our inclusion criteria (Table 1) [8-13]. The Cochrane reviews included were published between 2006 and 2011. The studies in these reviews mainly originated from China. They included between 3 and 18 primary studies. Four

reviews were concerned with angina pectoris (unstable or stable) [9,11-13], one review was concerned with heart failure [10] (heart failure was primary caused by CHD), and one review was concerned with acute myocardial infarction[8].

Four Cochrane reviews concluded positively that TCHP may be or appears to be effective. Two reviews showed that the evidence is too weak to make conclusion. No reviews made definite conclusion. All reviews indicated that high-quality trials are required to assess the efficacy and safety of TCHP for CHD and the finding should be interpreted with care because of the very low methodological quality of studies and potential publication bias.

There are 69 studies in the six reviews. Two studies were reported from 1981 to 1985; one study was reported from 1986 to 1990; three studies were reported from 1991 to 1995; twenty-six studies were reported from 1996 to 2000; thirty-five studies were reported from 2001 to 2005; only two studies were reported from 2006 to 2011. Therefore, the most likely reason for the weak evidence of TCHP for CHD is the previous poor methodology.

The randomized clinical trials (RCTs) contained in four Cochrane reviews [8-10,12] were mainly on the basis of conventional western medicine. But the basic treatment is not unchangeable. The RCTs listed in two Cochrane reviews [11,13] directly contrasted one TCHP with western medicine or other TCHP. Two Cochrane reviews [8,13] summarized different TCHP for CHD. The TCHP mentioned in these RCTs were injection (e.g., Shengmai Injection, Puerarin), oral Chinese patent medicine (e.g., Yi Xin Mai, Bao Xin Bao, Li Nao Xin, Shengmai Oral Liquid, Suxiao Jiuxin Wan, Tong Xin Luo), or Chinese herbal decoction. Four Cochrane reviews [9-12] summarized single TCHP for CHD.

In order to assess the status of the quality of the studies of TCHP, we also searched the CENTRAL in The Cochrane Library Issue 4 of 4 Oct 2011. Eight studies were included (Table

第七章

Table1 Cochrane Reviews of TCHP for CHD

First author	TCHP	Control group	Condition	Number of RCTs	Participants	Conclusion
Wu et al. [8]	Danshen as part of decoction	Different basic treatment	Acute myocardial infarction	6	2368	B
Wang et al. [9]	Puerarin	Different basic treatment	Unstable angina pectoris	20	1240	A
Zheng et al. [10]	Different forms of Shengmai	Different basic treatment	Heart failure	6	440	A
Duan et al. [11]	Suxiao jiuxin wan	Isosorbide dinitrate or nitroglycerin or other TCHP	Angina pectoris	15	1776	A
Wu et al. [12]	Tongxinluo	Different basic treatment	Unstable angina pectoris	18	1413	A
Zhuo et al. [13]	Different herbal products	Isosorbide dinitrate or other TCHP	Stable angina	3	216	B

Notes：RCT：randomized clinical trial.

A：TCHP may be or appears to be effective.

B：The evidence is insufficient，reliable conclusions could not be drawn.

2) [14-21]. These studies primary originated from China. These studies were all making an explicit statement that the participants were randomly assigned to different groups, but two were not describing the details. Only four RCTs adopted the application of blinding: one did not report details [18] and three reported that the participants and doctors were blind [14,19,21]. One of the trials adopted allocation concealment [14]. Trials with inadequate blinding and inadequate allocation concealment may result in limited evidence. Six trials did well in the incomplete outcome data adequately addressed [14-16,18,19,21]. Only one trial did well in the free of the suggestion of selective outcome reporting [18]. Not every trial made explicit statement that the participants signed the informed consents [16,17,19]. These RCTs had more participants than usual RCTs. They usually have 60 to 100 participants [15-18,20,21]; only 1 RCT has 35 participants [19] and 1 RCT has 859 participants [14]. These shortcomings highlight the importance of following CONSORT procedures in the future studies [22]. Anyway, the quality of primary studies was better than before, and we still need further progress.

4. Discussion

The current Cochrane reviews indicated the potential benefit of TCHP in treating CHD, but none of them drew a definite conclusion because of the poor quality of primary studies. Although Cochrane reviews have the reputation for being more transparent and rigorous than other systematic reviews, the conclusion needs further discussion. The RCTs listed in two reviews [8,13] were not the same TCHP. The treatments in the control groups, and the durations of the RCTs were also varied. In addition, different TCHP applys to different syndrome according to TCM theory. All of these reviews did not involve this question.

Therefore, four reviews [9-12] about single TCHP are more persuasive. They all made the conclusion of "A", indicating the TCHP may be or appears to be effective. The other two reviews made the conclusion of "B". One review about "Danshen for acute myocardial infarction" concerned with the herb Danshen, but Danshen was not the only part of the treatment. Thus the heterogeneity of included RCTs cannot be

Table2　Registered Studies of TCHP for CHD in the Cochrane Central Register of Controlled Trials

First author	TCHP	Condition	Participants	Random	Blinding of participants, personnel, or outcome assessors	Allocation concealment	Incomplete outcome data adequately addressed	Free of the suggestion of selective outcome reporting	Informed consents	Conclusion
Chu et al. [14]	Xuefu Zhuyu capsule	Unstable anginal patients after percutaneous coronary intervention	90	Yes but no details	Participants and doctor	Yes	Yes	Unclear	Yes	A+
Li et al. [15]	Specific TCHP	Myocardial perfusion in AMI patients after revascularization	80	Yes	Not mentioned	Not mentioned	Yes	Unclear	Yes	A+
Li et al. [16]	Specific TCHP	Ventricular wall motion in AMI patients after revascularization	80	Yes	Not mentioned	Not mentioned	Yes	Unclear	Unclear	A
Hu et al. [17]	Shenfu injection	Heart function in patients with chronic heart failure	63	Yes but no details	Not mentioned	Not mentioned	Unclear	Unclear	No	A+
Tam et al. [18]	Salvia miltiorrhiza and Pueraria lobata	Vascular function and structure in coronary patients	100	Yes	Double-blind but no details	Not mentioned	Yes	Yes	Yes	A+
Qiu et al. [19]	Specific TCHP	The clinical symptoms and quality of life of the AMI patients undergoing PCI	35	Yes	Participants and doctor	Not mentioned	Yes	No	Unclear	A+
Fan et al. [20]	Qihong decoction	Rehabilitation of patients after coronary artery bypass	72	Yes	Not mentioned	Not mentioned	No	No	No	A+
Wang et al. [21]	Shenshao tablet	The quality of life for CHD patients with UA	66	Yes	Participants and doctor	Not mentioned	Yes	Unclear	No	A+

Notes: A+: TCHP has definitely effect.

A: TCHP may be or appears to be effective.

第七章

ignored. The other review of "herbal products for stable angina" is concerned with three different TCHPs comparing with isosorbide dinitrate [13]. It also made the conclusion of "B", indicating the evidence is insufficient and reliable conclusions could not be drawn.

In conclusion, although some Cochrane reviews have shown the potential benefit of TCHP in treating CHD, more evidence from high-quality trials is needed to support the clinical use of TCHP. However, well-designed randomized clinical trials of TCHP with rigorous methodology are in progress or have been completed at several institutions around the world [6]. We hope that the effectiveness and safety of TCHP can be confirmed in the near future.

References

[1] Xu H, Chen KJ. Integrating traditional medicine with biomedicine towards a patient-centered healthcare system. Chinese Journal of Integrative Medicine, 2011, 17 (2): 83-84.

[2] Lu AP, Ding XR, Chen KJ. Current situation and progress in integrative medicine in China. Chinese Journal of Integrative Medicine, 2008, 14 (3): 234-240.

[3] Chen KJ, Shi DZ, Xu H et al. XS0601 reduces the incidence of restenosis: a prospective study of 335 patients undergoing percutaneous coronary intervention in China. Chinese Medical Journal, 2006, 119 (1): 6-13.

[4] Shang QH, Xu H, Lu XY, et al. A multi-center randomized double-blind placebo controlled trial of Xiongshao Capsule in preventing restenosis after percutaneous coronary intervention: a subgroup analysis of senile patients, Chinese Journal of Integrative Medicine, 2011, 17 (9): 669-674.

[5] Gao ZY, Xu H, Shi DZ, et al. Analysis on outcomeof 5284 patients with coronary artery disease: the role of integrative medicine. Journal of Ethnopharmacology. In press.

[6] The Cochrane Collaboration. Cochrane reviews, 2011, http://www.cochrane.org/ cochrane-reviews/.

[7] Higgins JPT, Green S. Cochrane handbook for systematic reviews of interventions, version 5.0.2 [updated September 2009], The Cochrane Collaboration, 2009, http://www.cochranehandbook.

org/.

[8] Wu T, Ni J, Wu J. Danshen (Chinese medicinal herb) preparations for acute myocardial infarction. Cochrane Database of Systematic Reviews, 2008, (2): 004465.

[9] Wang Q, Wu T, Chen X et al. Puerarin injection for unstable angina pectoris. Cochrane Database of Systematic Reviews, 2006, (3): 004196.

[10] Zheng H, Chen Y, Chen J, et al. Shengmai (a traditional Chinese herbal medicine) for heart failure. Cochrane Database of Systematic Reviews, 2011, (2): 005052.

[11] Duan X, Zhou L, Wu T et al. Chinese herbal medicine suxiao jiuxin wan for angina pectoris. Cochrane Database of Systematic Reviews, 2008, (1): 004473.

[12] Wu T, Harrison RA, Chen X et al. Tongxinluo (Tong xin luo or Tong-xin-luo) capsule for unstable angina pectoris. Cochrane Database of Systematic Reviews, 2006, (4): 004474.

[13] Zhuo Q, Yuan Z, Chen H, et al. Traditional Chinese herbal products for stable angina. Cochrane Database of Systematic Reviews, 2010, (5): 004468.

[14] Chu FY, Wang J, Sun XW et al. A randomized double blinded controlled trial of Xuefu Zhuyu Capsule on short term quality of life in unstable anginal patients with bloodstasis syndrome after percutaneous coronary intervention. Journal of Chinese Integrative Medicine, 2009, 7 (8): 729-735.

[15] Li YQ, Jin M, Qiu SL et al. Effect of Chinese drugs for supplementing qi, nourishing yin and activating blood circulation on myocardial perfusion in patients with acute myocardial infarction after revascularization. Chinese Journal of Integrative Medicine, 2009, 15 (1): 19-25.

[16] Li YQ, Jin M, Qiu SL. Effect of Chinese herbal medicine for benefiting qi and nourishing yin to promote blood circulation on ventricular wall motion of AMI patients after revascularization. Chinese Journal of Integrated Traditional and Western Medicine, 2009, 29 (4): 300-304.

[17] Hu YH, Wu HQ, Qi X. Influence of shenfu injection on heart function and bone marrow stem cell mobilization in patients with chronic heart failure of coronary heart disease. Chinese Journal of Integrated Traditional and WesternMedicine, 2009, 29 (4): 309-312.

[18] Tam WY, Chook P, Qiao M et al. The efficacy and tolerability of adjunctive alternative herbal medicine (Salvia miltiorrhiza and Pueraria lobata) on vascular function and structure in coronary patients. Journal of

Alternative and Complementary Medicine, 2009, 15 (4): 415-421.

[19] Qiu SL, Jin M, Yi JH, et al. Therapy for replenishing qi, nourishing yin and promoting blood circulation in patients with acute myocardial infarction undergoing percutaneous coronary intervention: a randomized controlled trial. Journal of Chinese Integrative Medicine, 2009, 7 (7): 616-621.

[20] Fan H, Wang XF, Gao W, Effect of Qihong decoction on rehabilitation of patients after coronary artery bypass. Chinese Journal of Integrated Traditional and Western Medicine, 2009, 29 (3): 215-218.

[21] Wang J, He QY, Zhang YL. Effect of Shenshao tablet on the quality of life for coronary heart disease patients with stable angina pectoris. Chinese Journal of Integrative Medicine, 2009, 15 (5): 328-332.

[22] Begg C, Cho M, Eastwood S et al. Improving the quality of reporting of randomized controlled trials: the CONSORT statement. Journal of the American Medical Association, 1996, 276 (8): 637-639.

Tanshinone ⅡA: A Promising Natural Cardioprotective Agent[*]

SHANG Qing-hua　　XU Hao　　HUANG Li

1. Introduction

Salvia miltiorrhiza Bunge (Danshen) belongs to the Labiatae family of the plant kingdom. It is considered to have the function of activating blood circulation and removing blood stasis, entering the "heart", "pericardium", and "liver" channels according to the theory of traditional Chinese medicine (TCM). Danshen has been widely used in oriental countries, especially China, to treat various circulatory disturbancerelated diseases for its special pharmacological actions, including vasodilatation, anticoagulation, anti-inflammation, and free radical scavenging. In recent years, traditional medicines have been playing more and more important roles in the maintenance of health, the prevention and treatment of diseases, as well as plant-based drug discovery [1,2]. Although many practitioners are used to prescribing nature products, more and more doctors and researchers are fascinated in chemical compounds of Salvia miltiorrhiza Bunge.

There are two main active compounds: the lipophilic (Tanshinone Ⅰ, ⅡA, ⅡB; crypto Tanshinone; other related compounds) and the hydrophilic (polyphenolic acids, danshensu, protocatechuic aldehyde, and protocatechuic acid). Tanshinone ⅡA (Tan ⅡA), which is a member of the major lipophilic components extracted from Salvia miltiorrhiza Bunge, has indicated significant therapeutic effects on various diseases *in vivo* and *in vitro*. Since Tan ⅡA is not easy to be absorbed through intestinal pathway, sodium tanshinone ⅡA sulfonate (STS) was developed to raise the bioavailability. The chemical structure of STS is shown in Figure 1. In this paper, the pharmacology of Tan ⅡA and STS in the treatment for cardiovascular diseases was reviewed.

2. Cardiovascular Pharmacology

2.1 Vasodilative Effect

Cheng et al. [3] demonstrated that Tan ⅡA produced a concentration-dependent relaxation

* 原载于 Evidence-Based Complementary and Alternative Medicine，2012，Article ID 716459

in isolated spontaneously hypertensive rat (SHR) aortic rings precontracted with phenylephrine or potassium chloride (KCl) through ATP-sensitive K (+) channel to lower [Ca (2+)]$_i$. Wu et al. [4] investigated the effects of Tan IIA on isolated rat coronary arteriole and the underlying mechanisms. The results showed that endothelium denudation, inhibition of nitric oxide synthase (NOS), inhibition of the cytochrome P450 epoxygenase, and blockade of the large conductance Ca (2+) -activated potassium channels (BKca) significantly decreased the vasodilation elicited by Tan IIA, which indicated that Tan IIA induces an endothelium-dependent vasodilation in coronary arterioles; nitric oxide (NO) and cytochrome P450 metabolites contribute to the vasodilation; activation of BKca channels plays an important role in the vasodilation. Kim et al. [5] concluded that topical Tan IIA increased both normalized arteriolar diameter and periarteriolar NO concentration in the two-kidney, one-clip renovascular hypertension model. N (G) -monomethyl-L-arginine inhibited Tan IIA-induced vasodilation. Tan IIA prevented the hypertension-induced reduction of endothelial NOS (eNOS) and increased eNOS expression to levels higher than sham-operated control. Topical Tan IIA increased normalized arteriolar diameter more in the cremaster muscle of control mice than that in cremasters of eNOS knockout mice. In ECV-304 cells transfected with eNOS-green fluorescent protein, Tan IIA significantly increased eNOS protein expression and eNOS phosphorylation. The results also indicated that eNOS stimulation was one mechanism by which Tan IIA induced vasodilation and reduces blood pressure.

2.2 Inhibition of Left Ventricular Hypertrophy

Accumulative studies had demonstrated that Tan IIA could inhibit left ventricular hypertrophy (LVH) with different mechanisms. Overwhelming postloading is a main factor promoting LVH, therefore controlling hypertension is very important in LVH inhibition. Tan IIA has

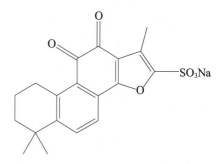

Figure 1　The Chemical Structure of STS

shown vasodilatation effect through adenosine triphosphate (ATP) -sensitive K (+) channel to lower the concentration of Ca^{2+} in myocytes, regulate the condition of hypertension, and inhibit the formation of hypertrophy [3]. Tan IIA could also prevent LVH through inhibiting angiotensin receptor (ATR) expression or blocking free Ca^{2+} influx in rats with hypertrophic myocardium caused by abdominal aorta constriction, and its effect on lowering hypertension had no significant difference compared with Valsartan [6,7]. Additionally, Tan IIA has been reported to block the transforming growth factor (TGF) beta1/Smads signal pathway and inhibit the formation of myocardial hypertrophy [7], attenuate enhanced collagen type I expression and collagen synthesis as well as depressed matrix metalloproteinase-1 (MMP-1) expression and activity by angiotensin II (Ang II) [8]. Furthermore, Tan IIA depressed the intracellular generation of reactive oxygen species (ROS), nicotinamide adenine dinucleotide phosphate (NADPH) oxidase activity, and subunit p47 (phox) expression, which are the factors inducing LVH. Fang et al. [9] concluded that Tan IIA conferred its beneficial effects on the collagen metabolism probably through its regulation of transcript levels of the MMPs/tissue inhibitor of metalloproteinases (TIMPs) balance. Although the balance regulation had no difference as compared with Valsartan, Tan IIA showed slight improvement in attenuating cardiac dysfunction. At least three studies assessed proto-oncogene c-fos mRNA expression of cardiocytes when investigated the mechanism of Tan ⅡA, indicating that Tan ⅡA could prevent LVH induced by Ang Ⅱ, which might be related to its inhibition of proto-oncogene expression [10-12]. Similar conclusion was drawn by Tu et al. [13] that Tan ⅡA had the definite function in preventing LVH by its action on the protein kinase B (PKB/Akt) signaling pathway, which could regulate the expression of proto-oncogene c-fos. Two *in vitro* studies [14,15] had demonstrated that Tan ⅡA dose-dependently inhibited the increment of the total protein level induced by Ang Ⅱ and the p-extracellular signal regulatory kinase (ERK) 1/2 expression stimulated by Ang Ⅱ, which indicated the mechanism that Tan ⅡA inhibited the myocardial cell hypertrophy induced by Ang Ⅱ may be associated with the inhibition of p-ERK1/2.

2.3 Restraining Smooth Muscle Cell Proliferation and Intimal Hyperplasia.

Tan ⅡA could significantly decrease intimal thickening, suppress cell proliferation and migration, inhibit the expression of various growth factors, induce the differentiation, maturity, and apoptosis of the vascular smooth muscle cell (VSMC), and ameliorate the function and condition of vascular smooth muscle [16]. Since there are so many beneficial effects on VSMC, Tan Ⅱ is playing an important role in the treatment of arteriosclerosis, restenosis after angioplasty or stenting, brain arteriovenous malformations, and pulmonary hypertension. However, the mechanism of Tan Ⅱ has not been very clear. Various studies [17-21] had found that Tan ⅡA could suppress cell proliferation and BrdU incorporation into DNA, block cell cycle in G0/G1 phase, and inhibit ERK1/2 phosphorylation and c-fos expression. Initial proliferation might be inhibited by blocking mitogen-activated protein kinase (MAPK) signaling pathway and downregulating c-fos expression. Pan et al.[22] demonstrated that Tan ⅡA could significantly inhibit the proliferation of VSMCs in a dose-dependent manner, and the mechanism might be related to the downregulation of calponin (CaN)

activities and the inhibition on calcineurin mRNA and proliferating cell nuclear antigen (PCNA) expressions. Jin et al. [23] illuminated that Tan ⅡA exhibited multiple effects on inhibiting human aortic SMCs migration, the mechanisms of which might inhibit Ikappa B alpha phosphorylation and p65 nuclear translocation through inhibition of Akt phosphorylation, suppress tumor necrosis factor-alpha (TNF-α) -induced ERK and c-jun phosphorylation, and block nuclear factor-kappa B (NF-κB) and activator protein-1 (AP-1) DNA-binding; all these factors played important roles in human aortic SMCs migration.

2.4 Attenuation of Atherosclerosis

In addition to VSMC proliferation and intimal hyperplasia, injury of vascular endothelium, lipid deposition, oxidative stress, and inflammatory reaction also play important roles in the formation and progression of atherosclerosis. Endothelial cells can secrete two kinds of substances with opposite functions, one can induce VSMC apoptosis (such as NO), and the other can inhibit VSMC apoptosis (such as endothelin-1 (ET-1), Ang Ⅱ, and growth factors). Unbalance between them decides whether endothelium is injured. NO is the key factor in signal transduction, it can relax blood vessels and activate genes relative to VSMC apoptosis. Li et al. [24] and Huang et al. [25] concluded that Tan ⅡA could inhibit the negative effect of Ang Ⅱ on NO production and eNOS expression in porcine aortic endothelial cells. Another *in vitro* study showed that Tan Ⅱ might inhibit ET-1 production and cell apoptosis, inducing protective effect on vessel endothelium [26]. Tan ⅡA could also reduce plaque area in endothelium, decrease lipid deposition, and significantly inhibit the formation of atherosclerosis, although the level of total cholesterol (TC), triglyceride (TG), low-density lipoprotein cholesterol (LDL-C), and high-density lipoprotein cholesterol (HDL-C) in serum had not been changed by Tan ⅡA [27].

To verify the antioxidant effect on atherosclerosis formation, at least five experiments [28-32] had been established. Tang et al. [28] demonstrated that Tan ⅡA could attenuate atherosclerotic lesion in apolipoprotein E (apoE) (-/-) mice, which might be attributed to its properties of both antioxidation and downregulation of scavenger receptors. Furthermore, antagonism of peroxisome proliferators-activated receptor gamma (PPARγ) might be involved in the downregulation of CD36 by Tan ⅡA. Fang et al. [29] found that the superoxide dismutase (SOD) activity was significantly increased while the level of malondialdehyde (MDA) was decreased in Tan ⅡA group, which showed that antioxidant effect of Tan ⅡA might be a potential mechanism involved in antiatherosclerosis. Tang et al. [30] suggested that Tan ⅡA significantly attenuated the atherosclerosis in rat model, which might be attributed to its inhibition of oxidized low density lipoprotein (oxLDL) production, independent of the serum levels of lipids, calcium, and 25-OH Vitamin D. Increasing of Cu/Zn SOD activity as well as mRNA and protein expression by Tan ⅡA might protect LDL against oxidation induced by superoxide anion in vessel. Active oxygen free radical is a major factor inducing endothelial injury; hydrogen peroxide can promote the formation of free radicals, which can penetrate cell membrane, combine with Fe^{2+} or Cu^{2+}, induce lipid peroxidation, and lead to endothelium injury and formation of atherosclerosis finally. Lin et al. [31,32] indicated that Tan ⅡA could protect ECV-304 cell damage induced by hydrogen peroxide through its anti-oxidant effect and CD40 anti-inflammatory approach.

Inflammatory effect can induce endothelium injury, foam-cell appearance, and leukocytes adhesion, all of which play important roles in the formation of atherosclerosis. At least two studies [29,33] had verified that Tan ⅡA could decrease inflammatory effect and attenuate atherosclerosis of vessels. Fang et al. [29] indicated that expression reduction of CD40 and MMP-2 activity might be the potential mechanisms of antiatherosclerosis effect of Tan ⅡA. Fang et al. [33] demonstrated

that Tan ⅡA could dose-dependently inhibit atherosclerotic lesion through downregulation of protein expression and activities of MMP-2 and MMP-9 as well as serum VCAM-1 and interleukin (IL) -1β in rabbits fed highfat diet.

Platelet activation and aggregation can accelerate the formation of atherosclerosis. Jiang et al. [34] indicated that Tan ⅡA could inhibit the increasing P-selectin expression of thrombin-activated platelets in a concentration-dependent manner, which may also be a mechanism of Tan ⅡA to inhibit atherosclerosis.

2.5　Lipid-Lowering Effect

Kang et al. [35] demonstrated that human HepG2 cells treated with Tan ⅡA for 24 h exerted a dose-dependent inhibitory effect on apolipoprotein B (apoB) secretion together with TG. However, another secretory protein, albumin, was unaffected by Tan-ⅡA treatment, indicating that the effect of Tan ⅡA is specific for apoB secretion. Tan ⅡA decreased the transcription level of microsomal TG transfer proteingene, suggesting that lipoprotein assembly is likely to be involved in the inhibited ApoB secretion. Gong et al. [36] reported that Tan ⅡA inhibited 3T3-L1 preadipocyte differentiation and transcriptional activities of full-length PPARγ and PPARγ ligand-binding domains. The effects of Tan ⅡA are mediated through its property as a natural antagonist of PPARγ. Tan ⅡA treatment reduced adipose mass and body weight, improved glucose tolerance, and lowered the LDL/HDL ratio without changing the food intake in a high-fat-diet-induced obese animal model.

2.6　Inhibitory Effect on the Inflammatory Responses

Various studies demonstrated that inflammatory response was involved in the process of myocardial infarction (MI), endothelium injury, atherosclerosis, and cardiovascular hypertrophy [23,29,33,37,38], which have been mostly introduced in the former paragraphs. However, mechanisms underlying this effect have not been fully understood. NF-κB activation by NF-κB-inducing kinase (NIK) -IkappaB alpha kinase (IKK) pathway and MAPKs pathway is known to be involved in the inflammatory response. Jang et al. [39] determined the inhibitory effect of Tan ⅡA on the activation of NF-κB and IkappaB alpha phosphorylation and also examined phosphorylation of NIK and IKK as well as the activation of MAPKs such as p38 MAPK (p38), ERK1/2, and c-Jun Nterminal kinase (JNK) in RAW 264.7 cells stimulated with Lipopolysaccharides (LPS). The result suggested that Tan ⅡA might inhibit LPS-induced Ikappa B alpha degradation and NF-κB activation via suppression of the NIK-IKK pathway as well as the MAPKs (p38, ERK1/2 and JNK) pathway in RAW264.7 cells, and these properties might provide a potential mechanism which could explain the anti-inflammatory activity of Tan ⅡA. Another *in vitro* study [40] suggested that Tan ⅡA had a similar structure with 17 beta estradiol (E₂) and the result indicated Tan ⅡA exerted anti-inflammatory effects by inhibition of inducible NOS (iNOS) gene expression and NO production, as well as inhibition of inflammatory cytokine (IL-1β, IL-6, and TNF-α) expression via estrogen receptor-dependent pathway. Therefore, it could serve as a potential selective estrogen receptor modulator (SERM) to treat inflammation-associated neurodegenerative and cardiovascular diseases without increasing the risk of breast cancer. Similar results were demonstrated by other studies [41,42].

2.7 Antioxidant Effect

Oxidation reaction was involved in various pathological mechanisms, inducing different diseases including MI, angina pectoris, and restenosis after PCI, LVH, and so on. Tan ⅡA can inhibit these reactions, which have been mentioned in the above experiments [8,28-32]. To test the hypothesis that Tan ⅡA can alter the expression and/or activity of specific antioxidant enzymes to prevent cells from oxidant damage, at least three experiments [38,43,44] were conducted

and demonstrated that the cell protective effect of Tan ⅡA was mediated primarily by induction of glutathione peroxidase (GPx) gene expression and activity, as well as other antioxidant enzyme activities in the heart. At least four experiments [44-47] indicated that Tan ⅡA could scavenge the free radicals produced in the superoxide approach, which might be one of the important mechanisms in myocardiocyte damage. Other studies [30,48] suggested that Tan ⅡA significantly attenuates myocardiocyte or vasculocyte damage, which might be attributed to its inhibition of oxLDL production.

2.8 Antiplatelet, Anticoagulant, and Antithrombotic Effect

Tan ⅡA can decrease the blood viscosity obviously, inhibit the activation of thrombin, and promote fibrin degradation; it can inhibit the function of platelets and the formation of thrombus. Li et al. [49] showed that Tan ⅡA could significantly decrease the platelet number, with efficacy similar to aspirin. Jiang et al. [34] also found that Tan ⅡA could reduce the number of blood platelets by inhibiting P-selectin expression in a concentration-dependent manner. Li et al. [50] demonstrated that Tan ⅡA could inhibit the thrombus formation and platelet aggression in *in vivo* study, and it exerted more significant effect on antiplatelet than anticoagulation.

To investigate the effects of Tan ⅡA on procoagulant activity (PCA) of human ECV304 cells induced by acute promyelocytic leukemia cell line NB4 cells, Zhang et al. [51] showed that the conditional media of NB4 cells treated with Tan ⅡA (Tan ⅡA-NB4-CM) can increase the levels of PCA and tissue factor (TF) activity of ECV304 cells through some unidentified factor; however, Tan ⅡA can obviously decrease the PCA and TF activity of ECV304 cells induced by Tan ⅡANB4-CM.

CD41 and CD62p are two of the most important inflammatory factors, which can induce platelets aggregation and promote blood

第七章

coagulation. Jia et al. [52] found that Tan IIA could decrease the expression of CD41 and CD62p, which might inhibit platelet aggregation and blood coagulation.

2.9 Antiarrhythmia Effect

Jia et al. [52] indicated that Tan IIA could decrease the expression of adhesion molecule in blood platelet to prevent arrhythmia. In addition, high-conductance Ca^{2+}-activated K^+ channels (BK_{Ca}) in vascular smooth muscle also play important roles in controlling the vascular tone by determining the level of membrane potential and Ca^{2+} influx through voltage-gated Ca^{2+} channels. Agents that can alter the activity of Ca^{2+} channels or BK_{Ca} thus affect the vascular tone in both physiological and pathological conditions. Experiments [53,54] showed that Tan IIA could block L-type Ca^{2+} channel, decrease concentration of intracellular Ca^{2+}, ameliorate calcium overload in myocardiocytes, and prevent or even treat arrhythmia finally. Except for Ca^{2+} and K^+, microRNA-1 (miR-1) level is also one of the important factors in ischemic arrhythmia. Shan et al. [55] indicated downregulation of miR-1 and consequent recovery of Kir2.1 might account partially for the efficacy of Tan IIA in suppressing ischemic arrhythmia and cardiac mortality. These findings support the proposal that miR-1 could be a potential therapeutic target for the prevention of ischemic arrhythmias. On gene level, Sun et al. [56] indicated that Tan IIA could activate human cardiac KCNQ1/KCNE1 potassium channels (I_{Ks}) in HEK 293 cell directly and specifically through affecting the channels' kinetics, which would be a promising therapeutic medicine in arrhythmia.

2.10 Antimyocardial Hypoxia

Reducing oxygen consumption and increasing the tolerance in hypoxygen of myocardiocytes are beneficial to coronary heart disease. Huang et al. [57] detected the left ventricle end diastole pressure (LVEDP) after ligating coronary artery of dogs, the result indicated Tan IIA could decrease LVEDP and heart volume and reduce myocardial oxygen consumption.

Shao et al. [58] demonstrated that the activation of ATP enzyme in myocardium was decreased in patient with hyperthyroidism; however, Tan IIA could protect it and increase the tolerance in hypoxygen of the myocardiocytes. Various studies [4,59,60] have suggested that Tan IIA might dilate coronary artery, inhibit vascular contraction, increase coronary blood flow and reduce oxygen consumption of myocardiocytes with different mechanisms. Sun et al. [61] suggested that Tan IIA could decrease intracellular calcium overload and K^+ outflow, inhibit Na^+ inflow, keep the balance of membrane potential, and therefore protect myocardiocyte in hypoxia.

2.11 Reduction of Myocardial Infarct Size

Tan IIA can dilate coronary artery and increase coronary blood flow, which is beneficial for reducing MI size. Various experiments [62-65] have demonstrated that Tan IIA might recover cardiac function and reduce MI size significantly with different mechanisms. Zhang et al. [62] indicated that the possible mechanism responsible for the effect of Tan IIA was associated with the phosphatidylinositol 3-kinase (PI3K/Akt) -dependent pathway, which was accompanied with decreased cardiac apoptosis and inflammation. In addition, Tan IIA was found to reduce MI size by $53.14 \pm 22.79\%$ as compared to that in the saline control, simultaneously, and significantly prolonged the survival of cultured human saphenous vein endothelial cells rather than human ventricular myocytes *in vitro* (these cells were separately exposed to xanthine oxidase (XO) -generated oxyradicals), which may suggest that Tan IIA could reduce MI size through prolonging survival of endothelial cells [63]. Xu et al. [64] have assessed the effect of Tan IIA on endothelial cells of MI in rats, and they suggested that Tan IIA could reduce MI size and myocardial ischemia injury through promoting angiogenesis and upregulating vascular endothelial growth factor (VEGF) expression. Jiang et al. [65] found that Tan IIA might establish extensive collateral circulation and increase blood flow in ischemic area.

2.12　Inhibiting Ischemia Reperfusion Injury

Ischemia reperfusion (IR) exerts disturbance of microcirculation and leads to many diseases, including myocardial stunning and reperfusion arrhythmia. Production of oxygen free radicals, calcium overload in myocytes, endothelial cell injury, adhesion of leukocyte, energy supply reduction, mitochondrial damage, and myocardiocytes apoptosis are considered to be involved in this process. Tan ⅡA can inhibit the activation of proteases and ameliorate calcium overload in myocytes, which have been introduced in the previous paragraph [53,54,61]. In addition, Tan ⅡA can increase the SOD content in the injured myocytes, decrease the MDA concentration, and influence electron transfer reaction in mitochondria, thus scavenge the free acids, reduce the lipid peroxidation, and protect myocytes and vascular endothelial cells in the IR process [45-47]. ET, which can induce constriction of the vessel, increases significantly in IR, and Tan ⅡA can inhibit the production and release of ET, promote secretion of NO, and decrease IR injury of the heart [24-26]. Jiang et al. [34] indicated that Tan A could inhibit HL-60 cell adhesion to human umbilical vein endothelial cells through concentration dependently inhibiting TNF-alpha and ameliorate microcirculation disturbance. Fu et al. [46] suggested that Tan ⅡA might markedly inhibit H_2O_2-induced oxidation *in vitro*, significantly inhibit IR-induced cardiomyocyte apoptosis by attenuating morphological changes and reducing the percentage of terminal transferase dUTP nick end-labeling (TUNEL) -positive myocytes and caspase-3 cleavage, as well as ameliorate IR injury by upregulating Bcl-2/Bax ratio.

3.　Final Comments

In the beginning of 21st century, we are facing serious challenges of cardiovascular diseases (CVDs). Although it is becoming less lethal, CVD prevalence is incessantly increasing and it is still the most common cause of death. As a representative of complementary and alternative medicines, TCM has a history of thousands of years and has made great contributions to the health and wellbeing of the people and to the maintenance and growth of the population. It provides us with great treasure of herbal medicines or natural products, which can be served as lead compound or new drug candidates in the battle against CVDs.

Herbal medicines with the function of activating blood circulation (ABC) have been investigated extensively and made remarkable achievements in recent years [66,67]. Salvia miltiorrhiza Bunge is the most common used ABC herb in China for treating CVDs and other circulatory disturbance-related diseases. Tan ⅡA, which is a member of the major lipophilic components extracted from Salvia miltiorrhiza Bunge, has indicated significant therapeutic effects and multiple pharmacological actions including vasodilative, antithrombotic, anti-inflammation, antioxidant, antiischemia, antiarrhythmia, antihyperplasia, antiatherosclerosis, and lipid-lowering effect. Clearly, Tan ⅡA appears to be a promising natural cardioprotective agent. Further research is warranted to translate these beneficial effects into clinical practice and definitely address the mechanisms of its multitarget actions.

References

[1] Xu H, Chen KJ. Integrating traditional medicine with biomedicine towards a patient-centered healthcare system. Chinese Journal of Integrative Medicine, 2011, 17 (2): 83-84.

[2] Balasubramani SP, Venkatasubramanian P, Kukkupuni SK, et al. Plant-based Rasayana drugs from Ayurveda. Chinese Journal of Integrative Medicine, 2011, 17 (2): 88-94.

[3] Cheng JT, Chan P, Liu IM, et al. Antihypertension induced by tanshinone ⅡA isolated from the roots of salvia miltiorrhiza, Evidence-based Complementary and Alternative Medicine, 2011, (2011): 392627.

[4] Wu GB, Zhou EX, Qing DX. Tanshinone ⅡA elicited

vasodilation in rat coronary arteriole: roles of nitric oxide and potassium channels. European Journal of Pharmacology, 2009, 617 (1-3): 102-107.

[5] Kim DD, Sánchez FA, Durán RG, et al, Endothelial nitric oxide synthase is a molecular vascular target for the Chinese herb Danshen in hypertension. American Journal of Physiology, 2007, 292 (5): H2131-H2137.

[6] Li YS, Wang ZH, Wang J. Effect of tanshinone ⅡA on angiotensin receptor in hypertrophic myocardium of rats with pressure over-loading. Chinese Journal of Integrated Traditional and Western Medicine, 2008, 28 (7): 632-636.

[7] Li YS, Yan L, Yong YQ. Effect of Tanshinone ⅡA on the transforming growth factor beta1/Smads signal pathway in rats with hypertensive myocardial hypertrophy. Chinese Journal of Integrated Traditional and Western Medicine, 2010, 30 (5): 499.

[8] Yang L, Zou XJ, Gao X et al, Sodium tanshinone ⅡA sulfonate attenuates angiotensin Ⅱ-induced collagen type Ⅰ expression in cardiac fibroblasts in vitro. Experimental and Molecular Medicine, 2009, 41 (7): 508-516.

[9] Fang J, Xu SW, Wang P, et al. Tanshinone Ⅱ-A attenuates cardiac fibrosis and modulates collagen metabolism in rats with renovascular hypertension. Phytomedicine, 2010, 18 (1): 58-64.

[10] Feng J, Zheng Z. Effect of sodium tanshinone ⅡA sulfonate on cardiac myocyte hypertrophy and its underlying mechanism. Chinese Journal of Integrative Medicine, 2008, 14 (3): 197-201.

[11] Zhou D, Liang Q, He X, et al. Changes of c-fos and c-jun mRNA expression in angiotensin Ⅱ-induced cardiomyocyte hypertrophy and effects of sodium tanshinone ⅡA sulfonate. Journal of Huazhong University of Science and Technology, 2008, 28 (5): 531-534.

[12] Takanashi K, Ouyang X, Komatsu K, et al. Sodium Tanshinone ⅡA Sulfonate derived from Danshen (Salvia Miltiorrhiaza) attenuates hypertrophy induced by angiotension Ⅱ in cultured neonatal rat cardiac cells. Biochemical Pharmacology, 2002, 64 (4): 745-749.

[13] Tu EY, Zhou YG, Wang ZH, et al. Effects of tanshinone ⅡA on the myocardial hypertrophy signal transduction system protein kinase B in rats. Chinese Journal of Integrative Medicine, 2009, 15 (5): 365-370.

[14] Li SS, Feng J, Zheng Z, et al. Effect of sodium tanshinone ⅡA sulfonate on phosphorylation of extracellular signal-regulated kinase 1/2 in Angiotensin Ⅱ-induced hypertrophy of myocardial cells. Chinese Journal of Integrative Medicine, 2008, 14 (2): 123-127.

[15] Yang L, Zou X, Liang Q, et al. Sodium tanshinone ⅡA sulfonate depresses angiotensin Ⅱ-induced cardiomyocyte hypertrophy through MEK/ERK pathway. Experimental and Molecular Medicine, 2007, 39 (1): 65-73.

[16] Chen HS, Chen YC, Zeng Z. Effect of Tanshinone ⅡA on vascular smooth muscle cell proliferation in post-injury artery: status and trend, West China Medical Journal, 2003, 18 (4): 602.

[17] Li X, Du JR, Yu Y, et al. Tanshinone ⅡA inhibits smooth muscle proliferation and intimal hyperplasia in the rat carotid balloon-injured model through inhibition of MAPK signaling pathway、Journal of Ethnopharmacology, 2010, 129 (2): 273-279.

[18] Li X, Du JR, Bai B, et al. Inhibitory effects and mechanism of Tanshinone ⅡA on proliferation of rat aortic smooth muscle cells. China Journal of Chinese Materia Medica, 2008, 33 (17): 2146-2150.

[19] Du JR. Effect of Tanshinone ⅡA on proliferation of cultured human smooth muscle cells. West China Journal of Pharmaceutical Sciences, 1999, 14 (1): 1-3.

[20] Zhang HH, Chen YC, Liang L, et al. Tanshinone ⅡA inhibits in vitro cellular proliferation and migration of vascular smooth muscle cell of rabbit. Journal of Sichuan University, 2008, 39 (2): 188-192.

[21] Wang H, Gao X, Zhang B. Tanshinone: an inhibitor of proliferation of vascular smooth muscle cells. Journal of Ethnopharmacology, 2005, 99 (1): 93-98.

[22] Pan YJ, Li XY, Yang GT-Effect of tanshinone ⅡA on the calcineurin activity in proliferating vascular smooth muscle cells of rats. Chinese Journal of Integrated Traditional and Western Medicine, 2009, 29 (2): 133-135.

[23] Jin UH, Suh SJ, Hyen WC, et al. Tanshinone ⅡA from Salvia miltiorrhiza BUNGE inhibits human aortic smooth muscle cell migration and MMP-9 activity through AKT signaling pathway. Journal of Cellular Biochemistry, 2008, 104 (1): 15-26.

[24] Li YS, Liang QS, Wang J. Effect of tanshinone ⅡA on angiotensin Ⅱ induced nitric oxide production and endothelial nitric oxide synthase gene expression in cultured porcine aortic endothelial cells. Chinese

Journal of Integrated Traditional and Western Medicine, 2007, 27 (7): 637-639.

[25] Huang KJ, Wang H, Xie WZ, et al. Investigation of the effect of tanshinone ⅡA on nitric oxide production in human vascular endothelial cells by fluorescence imaging. Spectrochimica Acta Part A, 2007, 68 (5): 1180-1186.

[26] Tang C, Wu AH, Xue HL, et al. Tanshinone ⅡA inhibits endothelin-1 production in TNF-α-induced brain microvascular endothelial cells through suppression of endothelin-converting enzyme-1 synthesis. Acta Pharmacologica Sinica, 2007, 28 (8): 1116-1122.

[27] Chen WY, Tang FT, Chen SR, et al. Phylactic effect of Tanshinone ⅡA on atherogenesis. China Pharmacy, 2008, 19 (12): 884-887.

[28] Tang FT, Cao Y, Wang TQ, et al. Tanshinone ⅡA attenuates atherosclerosis in ApoE-/- mice through downregulation of scavenger receptor expression. European Journal of Pharmacology, 2011, 650 (1): 275-284.

[29] Fang ZY, Lin R, Yuan BX, et al. Tanshinone ⅡA downregulates the CD40 expression and decreases MMP-2 activity on atherosclerosis induced by high fatty diet in rabbit. Journal of Ethnopharmacology, 2008, 115 (2): 217-222.

[30] Tang F, Wu X, Wang T, et al. Tanshinone ⅡA attenuates atherosclerotic calcification in rat model by inhibition of oxidative stress. Vascular Pharmacology, 2007, 46(6): 427-438.

[31] Lin R, Wang WR, Liu JT, et al. Protective effect of tanshinone ⅡA on human umbilical vein endothelial cell injured by hydrogen peroxide and its mechanism. Journal of Ethnopharmacology, 2006, 108 (2): 217-222.

[32] Wang WR, Lin R, Peng N, et al. Protective effect of Tanshinone ⅡA on human vascular endothelial cell injured by hydrogen peroxide. Journal of Chinese Medicinal Materials, 2006, 29 (1): 49-51.

[33] Fang ZY, Lin R, Yuan BX, et al. Tanshinone ⅡA inhibits atherosclerotic plaque formation by down-regulating MMP-2 and MMP-9 expression in rabbits fed a high-fat diet. Life Sciences, 2007, 81 (17-18): 1339-1345.

[34] Jiang KY, Ruan CG, Gu ZL, et al. Effects of tanshinone Ⅱ-A sulfonate on adhesion molecule expression of endothelial cells and platelets in vitro. Acta Pharmacologica Sinica, 1998, 19 (1): 47-50.

[35] Kang YJ, Jin UH, Chang HW, et al. Inhibition of microsomal triglyceride transfer protein expression and atherogenic risk factor apolipoprotein B100 secretion by tanshinone ⅡA in HepG2 cells. Phytotherapy Research, 2008, 22 (12): 1640-1645.

[36] Gong Z, Huang C, Sheng X, et al. The role of Tanshinone ⅡA in the treatment of obesity through peroxisome proliferator-activated receptor γ antagonism. Endocrinology, 2009, 150 (1): 104-113.

[37] Ren ZH, Tong YH, Xu W, et al. Tanshinone ⅡA attenuates inflammatory responses of rats with myocardial infarction by reducing MCP-1 expression. Phytomedicine, 2010, 17 (3-4): 212-218.

[38] Li XH, Tang RY. Relationship between inhibitory action of tanshinone on neutrophil function and its prophylactic effects on mycoardial infarction. Acta Pharmacologica Sinica, 1991, 12 (3): 269-272.

[39] Jang SII, Kim YJ, Jeong SI, et al. Tanshinone ⅡA inhibits LPS-induced NF-κB activation in RAW 264.7 cells: possible involvement of the NIK-IKK, ERK1/2, p38 and JNK pathways-European Journal of Pharmacology, 2006, 542 (1-3): 1-7.

[40] Fan GW, Gao XM, Wang H. et al. The anti-inflammatory activities of Tanshinone ⅡA, an active component of TCM, are mediated by estrogen receptor activation and inhibition of iNOS. Journal of Steroid Biochemistry and Molecular Biology, 2009, 113 (3-5): 275-280.

[41] Li XJ, Zhou M, Li XH, et al. Effects of Tanshinone ⅡA on cytokines and platelets in immune vasculitis and its mechanism. Journal of Experimental Hematology, 2009, 17 (1): 188-192.

[42] Jang SI, Jeong SI, Kim KJ, et al. Tanshinone ⅡA from salvia miltiorrhiza inhibits inducible nitric oxide synthase expression and production of TNF-α, IL-1β and IL-6 in activated RAW 264. 7 Cells, Planta Medica, 2003, 69 (11): 1057-1059.

[43] Li YI, Elmer G, LeBoeuf RC. Tanshinone ⅡA reduces macrophage death induced by hydrogen peroxide by upregulating glutathione peroxidase, Life Sciences, 2008, 83 (15-16): 557-562.

[44] Zhou GY, Zhao BL, Hou JW, et al. Protective effects of sodium tanshinone ⅡA sulphonate against adriamycin-induced lipid peroxidation in mice hearts in vivo and in vitro. Pharmacological Research, 1999, 40 (6): 487-491.

[45] Zhao BL, Jiang W, Zhao Y, et al. Scavenging effects of Salvia miltiorrhiza on free radicals and its protection for myocardial mitochondrial membranes from ischemia-reperfusion injury. Biochemistry and Molecular Biology International, 1996, 38 (6): 1171-1182.

[46] Huang J, Fu, H, Liu J, et al. Tanshinone IIA protects cardiac myocytes against oxidative stresstriggered damage and apoptosis. European Journal of Pharmacology, 2007, 568 (1-3): 213-221.

[47] Zhou G, Jiang W, Zhao Y, et al. Sodium tanshinone IIA sulfonate mediates electron transfer reaction in rat heart mitochondria. Biochemical Pharmacology, 2003, 65 (1): 51-57.

[48] Niu XL, Ichimori K, Yang X, et al. Tanshinone IIA inhibits low density lipoprotein oxidation in vitro. Free Radical Research, 2000, 33 (3): 305-312.

[49] Li XJ, Zhou M, Li XH, et al. Effects of Tanshinone IIa on cytokines and platelets in immune vasculitis and its mechanism. Journal of Experimental Hematology, 2009, 17 (1): 188-192.

[50] Li CZ, Yang SC, Zhao FD, Effect of tanshinone II-A sulfonate on thrombus formation, platelet and coagulation in rats and mice. Acta Pharmacologica Sinica, 1984, 5 (1): 39-42.

[51] Zhang HL, Yang YM, Meng WT. et al. Effects of tanshinone IIA on procoagulant activity of human ECV304 cell line induced by NB4 cells, Journal of Sichuan University, 2006, 37 (1): 55-59.

[52] Jia YH, Sun XG, Chen YY, Effect of Ding Xin Recipe and Tanshinone IIA on expression of platelet membrane adhesive molecule in arrhythmia rat. Journal of Traditional Chinese Medicine, 2002, 43 (2): 140-143.

[53] Xu CQ, Wang XM, Fan JS, et al. Effect of Tanshinone IIA on transmembrane potential and L-type calcium current of single cardiac ventricular myocyte in guinea pig. Chinese Journal of Pathophysiology, 1997, 13 (1): 43-47.

[54] Yu HB, Xu CQ, Shan HL, et al. Effect of Tanshinone IIA on potassium currents in rats ventricular myocytes. Journal of Harbin Medical University, 2002, 36 (2): 112-114.

[55] Shan H, Li X, Pan Z, et al. Tanshinone IIA protects against sudden cardiac death induced by lethal arrhythmias via repression of microRNA-1. British Journal of Pharmacology, 2009, 158 (5): 1227-1235.

[56] Sun DD, Wang HC, Wang XB, et al. Tanshinone IIA: a new activator of human cardiac KCNQ1/KCNE1 (IKs) potassium channels. European Journal of Pharmacology, 2008, 590 (1-3): 317-321.

[57] Huang X, Zang YM, Pharmacological research of Sodium Tanshinone IIA Sulfonate on cardiovascular disease. Foreign Medical Sciences, 1995, 17 (1): 9-12.

[58] Shao RZ, Zeng L, Fu XL, et al. Protective effect of Sodium Tanshinone IIA Sulfonate on myocardium of rat model with hyperthyreosis. Qianwei Journal of Medicine & Pharmacy, 2005, 17 (2): 93-94.

[59] Wan AKS, Leung SWS, Zhu DY, et al. Vascular effects of different lipophilic components of Danshen, a traditional Chinese medicine, in the isolated porcine coronary artery. Journal of Natural Products, 2008, 71 (11): 1825-1828.

[60] Yang Y, Cai F, Lietal-PY, Activation of high conductance Ca²⁺-activated K⁺ channels by sodium tanshinoneII-A sulfonate (DS-201) in porcine coronary artery smooth muscle cells. European Journal of Pharmacology, 2008, 598 (1-3): 9-15.

[61] Sun XG, Jia YH, Zhang LH. The effects of Tanshinone IIA on introcellular free calcium, membrance potential and mitochondria membrance potential of normal and hypoxia myocytes. Chinese Journal of Information on Traditional Chinese Medicine, 2009, 9 (9): 21.

[62] Zhang Y, Wei L, Sun D, et al. Tanshinone IIA pretreatment protects myocardium against ischaemia/reperfusion injury through the phosphatidylinositol 3-kinase/Akt-dependent pathway in diabetic rats, Diabetes. Obesity and Metabolism, 2010, 12 (4): 316-322.

[63] Wu TW, Zeng LH, Fung KP, et al. Effect of sodium tanshinone IIA sulfonate in the rabbit myocardium and on human cardiomyocytes and vascular endothelial cells. Biochemical Pharmacology, 1993, 46 (12): 2327-2332.

[64] Xu W, Yang J, Wu LM. Cardioprotective effects of tanshinone IIA on myocardial ischemia injury in rats, -Pharmazie, 2009, 64 (5): 332-336.

[65] Jiang WD, Yu YZ, Liu WW, Effects of sodium tanshinone II-A sulfonate and propranolol on coronary collaterals in acutely infarcted dogs. Acta Pharmacologica Sinica, 1981, 2 (1): 29-33.

[66] Chen KJ, Shi DZ, Xu H, et al. XS0601 reduces the incidence of restenosis: a prospective study of 335 patients undergoing percutaneous coronary

intervention in China. Chinese Medical Journal, 2006, 119 (1): 6-13.

[67] Xu H, Chen KJ. Integrative medicine: the experience from China. Journal of Alternative and Complementary Medicine, 2008, 14 (1): 3-7.

Clinical Significance of Inflammation Factors in Acute Coronary Syndrome from Pathogenic Toxin[*]

FENG Yan   ZHANG Jing-chun   XI Rui-xi

The theory of Chinese Medicine (CM) proposed the concept of "toxin", which might include the unbalance of yin-yang caused by pathogenic factors and any internal or external adverse factors. Acute coronary syndrome is a series of clinical syndromes originated from acute myocardial ischemia. Its pathomechanism possibly might be the unstable atherosclerotic plaques erosion and bleed, then thrombus form, causing different degrees of blockage and sharply decrease of nutritional supply for cardiaum. In 1999, Prof. Ross issued the theory known as "atherosclerosis is chronic inflammation"[1]. The CM researchers have already begun studies on the similarity of pathogenic toxin and inflammation of ACS.

1. Pathogenic Toxin and ACS Inflammation Response

The occurrence of ACS is closely associated with the stability of plaques. Inflammation response penetrates the whole progression of the formation and ruptures of unstable plaque[1]. As a pathogenic factor, toxin can be classified as external toxin and internal toxin. External toxin is a kind of pathogenic factor coming from outside and causes some body injuries, while internal toxin is produced on basis of endogenous diseases and formed by accumulation of different kinds of pathogens.

1.1 External Toxin and ACS

The main cause of inflammation is infection. The repeated chronic inflammation caused by some microbions such as Chlamydia pneumonia, cytomegalovirus, and the extra-vascular chronic inflammation including ulitis, prostatitis, bronchitis can increase the production of extra-vascular inflammation factors which are able to aggravate atherosclerosis. While intravascular infection inflammation irritants can directly aggravate atherosclerosis[2]. These chronic infections should be grouped in external toxin, and their role in the progression of ACS and atherosclerosis can provide evidence for external pathogenic toxin theory.

1.2 Internal Toxin and ACS

A recent study showed that inflammatory atherosclerotic plaques were hot and their surface temperature correlated with an increased number of macrophages and decreased fibrous-cap thickness[3]. The phenomenon reflects the pathological changes of internal toxin in some degree. Chronic and latent infections induce the production of various cytokines and expression of

* 原载于 Chinese Journal of Integrative Medicine，2009，15（4）：307-312

adhesion factors[4]. All these inflammation factors and cytokines can be grouped in the internal toxin, providing evidence for the association between pathogenic internal toxin and inflammation response of ACS.

1.3　Interaction of Internal and External Toxin

Infective antigens can injury the function of endothelial cells and active monocytes and macrophages to excrete inflammation factors. In contrast, these inflammation factors can trigger production of active oxidize proteinase, causing the instability, even the rupture of plaques[5].

The resent data demonstrated that the production pro-inflammatory cytokines was not counterbalanced by anti-inflammatory cytokines after the stimulation with lipopolysaccharide (LPS) on circulating monocytes in ACS patients[6]. LPS is a kind of endotoxin produced by bacteria, which should belong to external toxin. LPS enters into vivo, inducing the expression of a serial of inflammation cells, motiving the interaction between various factors and target cells, which forms the pathological phenomenon of external toxin inducing internal toxin[7]. These results coincide with the theory of interaction between internal and external toxin.

2.　Inflammation Factors and ACS

Inflammation cells have effects on the atherosclerotic plaques through the production of various inflammation mediators such as inter-cellular adhesion molecular-1 (ICAM-1), vascular cell adhesion molecules (VCAM-1), tumor necrosis factor (TNF-α), macrophage colony stimulating factor (M-CSF), cluster of differentiation 40 ligand (CD40L), interleukin (IL), matrix metalloproteinases (MMPs), oxidize low-density lipoprotein (ox-LDL), nuclear factor kappa B (NF-κB), etc. Detecting their levels can effectively speculate the stability of plaque. Thus, we can take them as specific markers in the diagnosis, prevention, treatment and prognosis of ACS.

2.1　Inflammation Factors and Diagnosis of ACS

With development of inflammation factors studies, the statue of inflammation factors in the diagnosis and prediction of ACS, compared with the traditional ways, will not be neglected. There have been already many studies demonstrated that for the apparently healthy people, detecting the elevation of their inflammation factors level, such as ox-LDL, IL-6, hs-CRP could predict their likelihood of further coronary heart diseases (CHD) occurrence[8-10]. Depending on single factor or multiple factors together were all proposed. With the completion of human genome project, detecting the individual diversity caused by genetic polymorphism may be the significant way for predicting the risk of ACS. The data both in and abroad have demonstrated that the distribution frequency of special allele carriers is much higher in ACS group than in the control group[11]. However, the power of inflammation factors may be affected by age, gender, race and many other factors, thus, to find out the more symbolic and unaffected markers should be one of the directions in the future. As for the published inflammation factors, repeated evaluations are still needed.

2.2　Inflammation Factors and ACS Prevention

2.2.1　Life Styles.　The expression of P-selectin, VCAM-1, monocyte chemoattractant protein-1 were showed to be largely reduced by exercise training[12]and serum levels of IL-6, IL-18 and CRP decreased evidently after losing weight[13], while mental stress and smoking induced increased levels of inflammatory markers[14,15]. In diet, some scholars found that children with hypercholesterolemia might lead early premature of atherosclerosis[16]. Soy-rich food was advised in nutriological studies[17]. It demonstrated that having low-fat diet, strengthening exercise, keeping peaceful state, stopping smoking can all effective reduce the level of inflammation factors, which may be beneficial to the prevention of ACS.

2.2.2 Medicine. (1) Statins: many studies showed that the statins have favorable anti-inflammatory effect independent of the lipid lowering[18]. However, the decreased inflammation level can not be sustained continuously. Diao JL, et al[19]. found that the CRP and IL-6 levels increased again in patients with consistent statin therapy after statin interruption. (2) Aspirin: as a regular medicine in ACS therapy, it also plays an important role in anti-inflammation development of ACS. Solheim S, et al.[20] found that aspirin could significantly lower levels of hs-CRP and TNF-α than warfarin alone over 4 years' after AMI. (3) Clopidogrel: It is also an regular medicine in ACS therapy, and a strategy of clopidogrel with GP IIb/IIIa blockade resulted in superior inhibition of inflammation and cardiac marker release such as TNF-α and CRP[21], and effect are more evident with the combination of aspirin and clopidogrel[22]. (4) Antibiotics: a prospective study demonstrated that using azithromycin on the patients with MI could reduce the serum levels of CRP, IL-1, IL-6, TNF-α, which suggest its role in reducing the risk of acute coronary events[23]. However, a meta-analysis of randomized controlled trials indicated that current evidence could not demonstrated the overall benefit of antibiotic therapy[24].

2.2.3 Other Therapies. Fukushima S, et al.[25] reported that combined antibody therapy inhibited both P-selectin and ICAM-1 via the retrograde intra-coronary route. And pioglitazone had additive anti-inflammatory effects to simvastatin in non-diabetic subjects with cardiovascular diseases and high hs-CRP level[26]. The strategies above could be promising ways for myocardial protection.

2.3 Inflammation Factors and Prognosis of ACS

2.3.1 Single Factor Prediction. Recent studies have shown that high levels of interkleukin-18, CRP, soluble tumor necrosis factor receptor type 1 (sTNFR-1), and P-selectin appeared to be critical factors of short-term prognosis in patients with ACS, and IL-6 levels during the first 48 hrs of ACS were strongly associated with 30-day major cardiovascular end points (MACE)[27,28].

The use of N-terminal pro-brain natriuretic peptide (NT-proBNP) had some sense in the assessment of patients with ACS[29]. Elevated BNP (> 80 pg/mL) at presentation identified patients with non-ST-elevation ACS[30].

2.3.2 Multiple Factors. From the multivariate analysis we could see the interaction of multiple factors, thus, combining the different factors together to predict the clinical end point of ACS might be a better strategy. It was reported that raised plasma hs-CRP and hypoadiponectinemia or cTnI and hs-CRP together might be related to the progression and increasing risk of ACS[31,32]. Putting TnT, CRP and NT-proBNP provided added information to ACS prognosis at 6 months, with a worse outcome for those with two or three elevated biomarkers[33].

2.4 Discussion and Prospect

Above all, inflammation participates the progression of ACS. Some further studies on ACS pathogenesis should be conducted to improve the diagnosis and prediction in ACS. The new studies about many other inflammation factors such as Monocyte Chemoattractant Protein (MCP), myeloperoxidase, serum amyloid A protein, neopterin, pregnancy-associated plasma protein, chemotatic factor ligand 16 (CXCL16), resistin, visfatin lipoprotein-associated phospholipase A_2, lipopolysaccharide-binding protein are also done to find its value in progression of ACS.

At present, the discoveries of new markers mostly depend on the measurement of some known proteins, proteomics can be a promising medical technology. As the different value of various markers in the diagnosis and prediction of ACS, some scholars thought that biochip may be an effective way[34]. Some other scholars even thought to draw out the protein atlas about the expression of various markers with serum proteomics analysis[35].

3. Inflammation Factors and Intervention of ACS with Chinese Medicine

As the association of the theory of pathogenic toxin in CM and the mechanism of ACS issued in inflammation response, the inflammation factors are also paid much attention to in the studies of CM, which may be helpful to provide some objective differentiation markers and induce us to treat ACS from pathogenic toxin.

3.1 Inflammation Factors and Clinical Studies in CM

3.1.1　Syndrome Differentiation.　Yi ZG, et al[36]. found that the serum levels of IL-18、hs-CRP are much higher in patients with syndromes of blood stasis blockade and turbid phlegm blockade than in patients of other kinds of syndromes. These data suggest inflammation factors might be regarded as objective markers in syndrome differentiation of ACS.

3.1.2　Detoxifying methods.　The progression of ACS has similar characteristics of pathogenic toxin in CM. Therefore, detoxifying methods should be studied as an important means for stabling plaques. Huang YS, et al.[37] found that the reduction of serum levels of CRP, TNF-α, IL-6 and syndromes points were much greater than the control group after clearing heat and detoxifying therapy in ACS patients.

3.1.3　Detoxifying medicine.　Geng LM, et al.[38] found that Jiedu Huoxue Pill（解青活血片）could relieve the syndromes of patients with ACS, decreased the levels of CRP and fibrinogen, reduce the risk of coronary events.

3.2 Inflammation Factors and Experimental Studies.

In the studies of ACS, we can take inflammation factors as objective markers, providing objective evidence of some Chinese Medicine and formulas with the functions of detoxinfying, relieving inflammation response, and steady plaques, in order to study and explore some effective medicines and therapies for ACS and provide some guidance for the clinic.

3.2.1　CM formulas.　Some scholars found that in atherosclerosis rabbits, serum levels of CRP, IL-6 and TNF-α decreased obviously, while HDL-C increased obviously, after the treatment of Yiqi Huoxue Jiedu decoction（益气活血解毒汤）[39]. Wu H, et al. reported that high dose huanglianjiedu decoction（黄连解毒汤）could inhibit the progression of atherosclerosis through the resistance of the activation of CRP, TNF-α[40].

3.2.2　Extracts of Chinese Medicine.　There was a report showing that Polydatin (PD, an extract from giant knot weed rhizome for detoxicating) could reduce serum levels of NF-κB, MMP-9 and hs-CRP in ApoE (-/-) mice, and could also reduce the level of in ApoE (-/-) mice in their further study[41,42].

4. Discussion

4.1 Theoretical innovation

ACS has always been the hot spot in cardiovascular studies for its high risk and death rate. CM also pays much attention on it. The proposition of "inflammation response" theory changes the traditional acknowledgement about ACS, and provides new thinking ways and research methods for the related studies, which can set more opportunities for the theoretical innovation in CM. Building our exploration into the pathomechanism of ACS in CM from pathogenic toxin theory, we break through the limitations of single activating blood circulation therapy and develop the new clinical thinking in ACS treatment.

4.2 Improvement on Clinical Diagnosis and Treatment

As the close association between ACS and inflammation factors, detecting the changes of inflammation factors in circulating serum can assist to anticipate morbidity risk, clinical prognosis, and efficacy evaluation and provide a simple and effective way for the diagnosis, treatment, prognosis of ACS in earlier period.

With the development of related studies on

inflammation factors and the coming out of some new markers in succession, people will have much further knowledge on the inflammation response of ACS. Making use of the research achievements about inflammation factors in the systematic intervention of ACS may reduce the incidence rate of cardiovascular events.

Besides, ACS is a complicated pathological progression, associating with the interaction of many factors. On the advantages of multitarget and multilink, CM will play an even significant role in the studies about the systematic intervention on ACS. CM can also make use of the related inflammation factors in clinical practice for the objective observation and evaluation of efficacy.

However, we should also realize that for the disturbance of some factors, in clinical practice, the detection of inflammation factors, clinical syndromes and other related tests should consult with one another. Meanwhile, the exploration of combination of inflammation factors to improve the accuracy for the diagnosis and prognosis of ACS in early stage still needs many further studies.

4.3　Overall Comment

Above all, clinical studies have proved that using integrated method with both Western and Chinese medicine can reduce the fatality of ACS and improve the quality of life, which demonstrated the efficacy advantages of systematic intervention with CM. However, its efficacy in the long term still needs further evaluation. How to use modern medical achievement effectively, choose the rational inflammation factors, and get the approval of the academic circles will be our crucial problems in the future studies.

Integrating the advantages of macroscopic regulating with CM and microscopic regulating with western medicine effectively will strengthen the prevention and treatment of ACS and theoretical innovation of pathogenic toxin theory in CM, which may do some promotion for the academic development of CM.

References

[1] Ross R. Atherosclerosis an inflammatory disisase. N Engl J Med, 1999, 340 (2): 115-126.

[2] Yang SL, He ZY. The significance of inflammation in acute coronary syndrome. Chin J Critl Care Med, 2004, 24 (2): 130-132.

[3] Madjid M, Willerson JT, Casscells SW. Intracoronary thermography for detection of high-risk vulnerable plaques. J Am Coll Cardiol, 2006, 47 (8 Suppl): C80-5.

[4] Nin XX, Sun SR. Infection, inflammation and atherosclerosis. Foreign Med · Geriat Sci, 2000, 21 (4): 173-175.

[5] Go YM, Halvey PJ, Hansen JM, et al. Reactive aldehyde modification of thioredoxin-1 activates early steps of inflammation and cell adhesion. Am J Pathol, 2007, 171 (5): 1670-1681.

[6] Van Haelst PL, Tervaert JW, Bijzet J, et al. Circulating monocytes in patients with acute coronary syndromes lack sufficient interleukin-10 production after lipopolysaccharide stimulation. Clin Exp Immunol, 2004, 138 (2): 364-368.

[7] Xie W, Shao N, Ma X, et al. Bacterial endotoxin lipopolysaccharide induces up-regulation of glyceraldehyde-3-phosphate dehydrogenase in rat liver and lungs. Life Sci, 2006, 79 (19): 1820-1827.

[8] Meisinger C, Baumert J, Khuseyinova N, et al. Plasma oxidized low-density lipoprotein, a strong predictor for acute coronary heart disease events in apparently healthy, middle-aged men from thegeneral population. Circulation, 2005, 112 (5): 651-657.

[9] Ridker PM, Rifai N, Stampfer JM, et al. Plasma concentration of interleukin-6 and the risk of future myocardial infarction among apparently healthy men. Circulation, 2000, 101 (15): 1767-1772.

[10] Bansal S, Ridker PM. Comparison of characteristics of future myocardial infarctions in women with baseline high versus baseline low levels of high-sensitivity C-reactive protein. Am J Cardiol, 2007, 99 (11): 1500-1503.

[11] Horne BD, Camp NJ, Carlquist JF, et al. Multiple-polymorphism associations of 7 matrix metalloproteinase and tissue inhibitor metalloproteinase genes with myocardial infarction and angiographic coronary artery disease. Am Heart, J 2007, 154 (4): 718-724.

[12] Yang AL, Jen CJ, Chen HI. Effects of high-cholesterol diet and parallel exercise training on

第七章

the vascular function of rabbit aortas: a time course study. J Appl Physiol, 2003, 95 (3): 1194 -1200.

[13] Esposito K, Pontillo A, Di Palo C, et al. Effect of weight loss and lifestyle changes on vascular inflammatory markers in obese women: a randomized trial. JAMA, 2003, 289 (14): 1799-1804.

[14] Kop WJ, Weissman NJ, Zhu J, et al. Effects of acute mental stress and exercise on inflammatory markers in patients with coronary artery disease and healthy controls. Am J Cardiol, 2008, 101 (6): 767-773.

[15] Gochman E, Reznick AZ, Avizohar O, et al. Exhaustive exercise modifies oxidative stress in smoking subjects. Am J Med Sci, 2007, 333 (6): 346-353.

[16] Martino F, Pignatelli P, Martino E, et al. Early increase of oxidative stress and soluble CD40L in children with hypercholesterolemia.J Am Coll Cardiol, 2007, 49 (19): 1974-1981.

[17] Fuchs D, Vafeiadou K, Hall WL, et al. Proteomic biomarkers of peripheral blood mononuclear cells obtained from postmenopausal women undergoing an intervention with soy isoflavones. Am J Clin Nutr, 2007, 86 (5): 1369-1375.

[18] Kodama Y, Kitta Y, Nakamura T, et al. Atorvastatin increases plasma soluble Fms-like tyrosine kinase-1 and decreases vascular endothelial growth factor and placental growth factor in association with improvement of ventricular function in acute myocardial infarction. J Am Coll Cardiol, 2006, 48 (1): 43-50.

[19] Diao JL, Pang G Z, Tong QG, et al. Effects of suspending statins on the inflammation factors of acute coronary syndrome. J Clin Inter Med, 2007, 24 (10): 700-702.

[20] Solheim S, Arnesen H, Eikvar L, et al. Influence of aspirin on inflammatory markers in patients after acute myocardial infarction. Am J Cardiol, 2003, 92 (7): 843-845.

[21] Gurbel PA, Bliden KP, Tantry US. Effect of clopidogrel with and without eptifibatide on tumor necrosis factor-alpha and C-reactive protein release after elective stenting: results from the CLEAR PLATELETS 1b study. J Am Coll Cardiol, 2006, 48 (11): 2186-2891.

[22] Chen YG, Xu F, Zhang Y, et al. Effect of aspirin plus clopidogrel on inflammatory markers in patients with non-ST-segment elevation acute coronary syndrome. Chin Med J, 2006, 119 (1): 32-36.

[23] Jia FP, Lei H. Inflammation, immune response and acute coronary syndrome. Foreign Med Sci, 2004, 31 (1): 13-15.

[24] Richard Andraws, Jeffrey SB, David LB, Effects of antibiotic therapy on outcomes of patients with coronary artery disease. JAMA, 2005, 293 (21): 2641-2647.

[25] Fukushima S, Coppen SR, Varela-Carver A, et al. A novel strategy for myocardial protection by combined antibody therapy inhibiting both P-selectin and intercellular adhesion molecule-1 via retrograde intracoronary route. Circulation, 2006, 114 (1 Suppl): 251-256.

[26] Hanefeld M, Marx N, Pfützner A, et al. Anti-inflammatory effects of pioglitazone and/or simvastatin in high cardiovascular risk patients with elevated high sensitivity C-reactive protein: the PIOSTAT Study. J Am Coll Cardiol, 2007, 49 (3): 290-297.

[27] Haim M, Benderly M, Tanne Detc, et al. C-reactive protein, bezafibrate, and recurrent coronary events in patients with chronic coronary heart disease. Am Heart J, 2007, 154 (6): 1095-1101.

[28] Smit JJ, Ottervanger JP, Slingerland RJ, et al. Comparison of usefulness of C-reactive protein versus white blood cell count to predict outcome after primary percutaneous coronary intervention for ST elevation myocardial infarction. Am J Cardiol, 2008, 101 (4): 446-451.

[29] Morrow DA, Braunwald E. Future of biomarkers in acute coronary syndromes: moving toward a multimarker strategy. Circulation, 2003, 108 (3): 275-281.

[30] Morrow DA, deLemos JA, Sabatine MS, et al. Evaluation of B-type natriuretic peptide for risk assessment in unstable angina /non-ST-elevation myocardial infarction: B-type natriuretic peptide and prognosis in TACTICS-TIMI18. J Am Coll Cardiol, 2003, 41 (8): 1264-1272.

[31] Otake H, Shite J, Shinke T, et al. Relation between plasma adiponectin, high-sensitivity C-reactive protein, and coronary plaque components in patients with acute coronary syndrome. Am J Cardiol, 2008, 101 (1): 1-7.

[32] Foussas SG, Zairis MN, Makrygiannis SS, et al. The significance of circulating levels of both cardiac troponin I and high-sensitivity C reactive protein for the prediction of intravenous thrombolysis outcome

in patients with ST-segment elevation myocardial infarction. Heart, 2007 Aug, 93 (8): 952-956.

[33] Tello-Montoliu A, Marín F, Roldán V, et al. A multimarker risk stratification approach to non-ST elevation acute coronary syndrome: implications of troponin T, CRP, NT pro-BNP and fibrin D-dimer levels. J Intern Med, 2007, 262 (6): 651-658.

[34] Di Serio F, Amodiog, Ruggieri E, De Sario R, Varraso L, Antonellig et al. Proteomic approach to the diagnosis of acute coronary syndrome: preliminary results. Clin Chim Acta, 2005, 357 (2): 226-235.

[35] Mateos-Cáceres PJ, García-Méndez A, López Farré A, et al. Proteomic analysis of plasma from patients during an acute coronary syndrome. J Am Coll Cardiol, 2004, 19; 44 (8): 1578-1583.

[36] Yi ZG, Wang Q, Zhang SQ. Associated studies between Chinese syndromes of acute coronary syndrome and IL-18, hs-CRP. Jiangsu J Tradit Chin Med, 2007, 39 (12): 22-23.

[37] Huang YS, Mo HH, Hong YD, et al. Heat-clearing and toxicity-removing therapy for the treatment of acute coronary syndrome: an observation of 55 cases. J Guangzhou University Tradit Chin Med, 2006, 23 (1): 13-16.

[38] Geng LM, Chen FQ. Influence of Jieduhuoxue Pills on prognosis and levels of CRP and Fig in patients with acute coronary syndrome. J Beijing Uni Tradi Chin Med (Clinical Med), 2007, 14 (3): 14-16.

[39] Ge L, Chen XY, Hu YB. Effects of Yiqihuoxuejiedu Decoction on C-reactive protein, interleukin-6, tumor necrosis factor and serum lipid in experimental rabbits with atherosclerosis. Chin J Tradit West Crit Car, 2007, 14 (5): 306-308.

[40] Wu H, Liu YD, Wu W, et al. Effects of clearing heat and detoxifying method on Chlamydia pneumonia infection caused atherosclerosis in rabbits. Jguangzhou Uni Tradit Chin Med, 2006, 23 (2): 151-155.

[41] Zhang JC, Chen KJ , ZhenggJ, et al. Regulatory effect of Chinese herbal compound fur detoxifying and activating circulation expression of NF-κB and MMP-9 in aorta of apolipoprotein E gene knocked-out mice. Chin J Integr Med, 2007, 21 (1): 40-44.

[42] Zhang JC, Chen KJ, Liu JG, et al. Effect of assorted use of Chinese drugs for detoxifying and activating blood circulation on serum high sensitive C-reactive protein in apolipoprotein E gene knock-out mice. Chin J Integr Tradit West Med, 2008, 28 (4): 330-333.

第七章